The Pharmacologic Basis of Anesthesiology

Basic Science and Practical Applications

The Pharmacologic Basis of Anesthesiology

Basic Science and Practical Applications

Edited by

T. Andrew Bowdle, M.D., Ph.D.
Associate Professor
Departments of Anesthesiology
 and Pharmaceutics (Adjunct)
University of Washington
Seattle, Washington

Akira Horita, Ph.D.
Professor
Departments of Pharmacology,
 Psychiatry and Behavioral Sciences
University of Washington
Seattle, Washington

Evan D. Kharasch, M.D., Ph.D.
Associate Professor
Departments of Anesthesiology
 and Medicinal Chemistry (Adjunct)
University of Washington
Seattle, Washington

 Churchill Livingstone
New York, Edinburgh, London, Madrid, Melbourne, Milan, Tokyo

Library of Congress Cataloging-in-Publication Data

The Pharmacologic basis of anesthesiology / edited by T. Andrew
    Bowdle, Akira Horita, Evan D. Kharasch.
       p. cm.
    Includes bibliographical references and index.
    ISBN 0-443-08878-0
    1. Anesthetics—Physiological effect. 2. Anesthesia adjuvants-
- Physiological effect. 3. Anesthetics—Pharmacokinetics.
 4. Anesthesia adjuvants—Pharmacokinetics. 5. Clinical
pharmacology. I. Bowdle, T. Andrew, date.   II. Horita, Akira.
III. Kharasch, Evan D.
[DNLM: 1. Anesthetics—pharmacology. Anesthetics, Local-
- pharmacology. 3. Anesthesia Adjuvants—pharmacology.
 4. Benzodiazepines—pharmacology. 5. Narcotics—pharmacology. QV
81 P5356 1994]
RD85.5.P48 1994
617.9′6—dc20
DNLM/DLC
for Library of Congress   94-20169
                                                  CIP

© Churchill Livingstone Inc. 1994

Distributed in the United Kingdom by Churchill Livingstone, Robert Stevenson House, 1–3 Baxter's Place, Leith Walk, Edinburgh EH1 3AF, and by associated companies, branches, and representatives throughout the world.

Accurate indications, adverse reactions, and dosage schedules for drugs are provided in this book, but it is possible that they may change. The reader is urged to review the package information data of the manufacturers of the medications mentioned.

The Publishers have made every effort to trace the copyright holders for borrowed material. If they have inadvertently overlooked any, they will be pleased to make the necessary arrangements at the first opportunity.

Copy Editor: *Elizabeth Bowman-Schulman*
Production Supervisor: *Patricia McFadden*
Cover Design: *Jeanette Jacobs*

Printed in the United States of America

First published in 1994   7 6 5 4 3 2 1

Contributors

Edmund G. Anderson, Ph.D.

Professor and Head, Department of Pharmacology, University of Illinois College of Medicine at Chicago, Chicago, Illinois

Peter L. Bailey, M.D.

Associate Professor and Director, Division of Cardiothoracic Anesthesia, Department of Anesthesiology, University of Utah School of Medicine, Salt Lake City, Utah

Dan E. Berkowitz, M.D.

Cardiac Anesthesia Fellow, Department of Anesthesiology, Duke University School of Medicine, Durham, North Carolina

David R. Bevan, M.D.

Professor and Head, Department of Anaesthesia, University of British Columbia Faculty of Medicine; Head, Department of Anaesthesia, Vancouver Hospital, Vancouver, British Columbia, Canada

J.G. Bovill, M.D., Ph.D.

Professor, Department of Anaesthesiology, University of Leiden Faculty of Medicine, and University Hospital Leiden, Leiden, The Netherlands

T. Andrew Bowdle, M.D., Ph.D.

Associate Professor, Departments of Anesthesiology and Pharmaceutics (Adjunct), University of Washington, Seattle, Washington

Peter M. Brooks, M.D.

Professor and Head, Department of Medicine, University of New South Wales; Consultant Rheumatologist, St. Vincent's Hospital, Darlinghurst, Sydney, Australia

Burnell R. Brown, Jr., M.D., Ph.D.

Professor and Head, Department of Anesthesiology, and Professor, Department of Pharmacology, University of Arizona College of Medicine, Tucson, Arizona

Anton G.L. Burm, Ph.D.

Associate Professor, Department of Anaesthesiology, University of Leiden Faculty of Medicine; Director, Anaesthesia Research Laboratory, Department of Anaesthesiology, University Hospital Leiden, Leiden, The Netherlands

Sharon E. Corey, Ph.D.

Assistant Professor, Department of Pharmacology and Physiology, University of Pittsburgh School of Dental Medicine, and Pharmacodynamic Research Center, Pittsburgh, Pennsylvania

Mark Dershwitz, M.D., Ph.D.

Assistant Professor, Department of Anaesthesia, Harvard Medical School; Assistant Anesthetist, Department of Anesthesia, Massachusetts General Hospital, Boston, Massachusetts

James P. Dilger, Ph.D.

Associate Professor, Departments of Anesthesiology and Physiology, State University of New York at Stony Brook Health Sciences Center School of Medicine, Stony Brook, New York

Leonard L. Firestone, M.D.

Associate Professor, Department of Anesthesiology and Critical Care Medicine, University of Pittsburgh School of Medicine; Chief of Cardiac Anesthesia, Department of Anesthesiology, Presbyterian University Hospital, Pittsburgh, Pennsylvania

Robert J. Fragen, M.D.

Professor of Clinical Anesthesia, Department of Anesthesia, Northwestern University Medical School; Attending Anesthesiologist, Department of Anesthesiology, Northwestern Memorial Hospital, Chicago, Illinois

Noor Gajraj, M.B., B.S.

Senior Registrar, Queens Medical Center, Nottingham, England

Kelvin W. Gee, Ph.D.

Associate Professor, Department of Pharmacology, University of California, Irvine, College of Medicine, Irvine, California

Tim G. Hales, Ph.D.

Assistant Professor, Department of Anesthesiology, University of California, Los Angeles, UCLA School of Medicine, Los Angeles, California

Yukio Hayashi, M.D.

Department of Anesthesiology, National Cardiovascular Center, Osaka, Japan

Thomas K. Henthorn, M.D.

Associate Professor and Associate Chairman for Research, Department of Anesthesia, Northwestern University Medical School, Chicago, Illinois

R. Joseph Isner, M.D.

Clinical Lecturer, Department of Anesthesiology, University of Arizona College of Medicine; Staff Anesthesiologist, Tucson Medical Center, and Old Pueblo Anesthesiology, Tucson, Arizona

Evan D. Kharasch, M.D., Ph.D.

Associate Professor, Departments of Anesthesiology and Medicinal Chemistry (Adjunct), University of Washington, Seattle, Washington

Aaron F. Kopman, M.D.

Professor of Clinical Anesthesia, New York Medical College, Valhalla, New York; Vice-Chairman, Department of Anesthesiology, St. Vincent's Hospital, New York, New York

Patricia D. Kroboth, Ph.D.

Associate Professor and Chairman, Department of Pharmacy and Therapeutics, University of Pittsburgh School of Pharmacy, and Pharmacodynamic Research Center, Pittsburgh, Pennsylvania

Jerrold Lerman, M.D.

Associate Professor, Department of Anaesthesia, University of Toronto Faculty of Medicine; Anaesthetist-in-Chief, The Hospital for Sick Children, Toronto, Ontario, Canada

Cynthia A. Lien, M.D.

Assistant Professor, Department of Anesthesiology, Cornell University Medical College; Associate Attending Anesthesiologist, Department of Anesthesiology, The New York Hospital, New York, New York

Martin J. London, M.D.

Associate Professor, Department of Anesthesiology, University of Colorado School of Medicine; Chief, Department of Anesthesiology, Veterans Affairs Medical Center, Denver, Colorado

Mervyn Maze, M.D., Ch.B., M.R.C.P. (UK)

Associate Professor, Department of Anesthesia, Stanford University School of Medicine, Stanford, California; Staff Physician, Anesthesiology Service, Veterans Affairs Medical Center, Palo Alto, California

Linda D. McCauley

Department of Pharmacology, University of California, Irvine, College of Medicine, Irvine, California

Thomas F. Murray, Ph.D.

Professor, Department of Pharmacology, Oregon State University College of Pharmacy, Corvallis, Oregon

Toshio Narahashi, Ph.D.

John Evans Professor of Pharmacology and Alfred Newton Richards Professor and Chairman, Department of Pharmacology, Northwestern University Medical School, Chicago, Illinois

Wendel L. Nelson, Ph.D.

Professor and Chairman, Department of Medicinal Chemistry, University of Washington School of Pharmacy, Seattle, Washington

Richard W. Olsen, Ph.D.

Professor, Department of Molecular and Medical Pharmacology, University of California, Los Angeles, UCLA School of Medicine, Los Angeles, California

Gavril W. Pasternak, M.D., Ph.D.

Professor, Departments of Neurology and Pharmacology, Cornell University Medical College; Member, Department of Neurology and The Cotzias Laboratory of Neuro-Oncology, Memorial Sloan-Kettering Cancer Center, New York, New York

Joseph J. Quinlan, M.D.

Assistant Professor, Department of Anesthesiology and Critical Care Medicine, University of Pittsburgh School of Medicine; Staff Anesthesiologist, University of Pittsburgh Medical Center, Pittsburgh, Pennsylvania

Raymond M. Quock, Ph.D.

Professor of Pharmacology, Department of Biomedical Sciences, University of Illinois College of Medicine at Rockford, Rockford, Illinois

Per H. Rosenberg, M.D., Ph.D.

Associate Professor, Department of Anesthesiology, University of Helsinki, and Helsinki University Central Hospital, Helsinki, Finland

Alan N. Sandler, M.B., Ch.B.

Associate Professor, Department of Anaesthesia, University of Toronto Faculty of Medicine; Anaesthetist-in-Chief, The Toronto Hospital, Toronto, Ontario, Canada

John J. Savarese, M.D.

The Joseph F. Artusio, Jr. Professor and Chairman, Department of Anesthesiology, Cornell University Medical College; Anesthesiologist-in-Chief, Department of Anesthesiology, The New York Hospital, New York, New York

Debra A. Schwinn, M.D.

Associate Professor, Department of Anesthesiology, Assistant Professor, Department of Pharmacology, and Director, Molecular Pharmacology Laboratory, Duke University School of Medicine, Durham, North Carolina

Colin A. Shanks, M.D., Ch.B.

Professor, Department of Anesthesiology, Northwestern University Medical School, Chicago, Illinois

Eugene M. Silinsky, Ph.D.

Professor, Department of Pharmacology, Northwestern University Medical School, Chicago, Illinois

Randall B. Smith, Ph.D.
Department of Pharmacy and Therapeutics, University of Pittsburgh School of
Medicine, Pittsburgh, Pennsylvania

James B. Streisand, M.D.
Associate Professor, Department of Anesthesiology, University of Utah School of
Medicine,and University Hospital, Salt Lake City, Utah

Jack W. van Kleef, M.D., Ph.D.
Professor, Department of Anaesthesiology, University of Leiden Faculty of Medicine;
Chairman, Department of Anaesthesiology, University Hospital Leiden, Leiden,
The Netherlands

Paul F. White, M.D., Ph.D.
Professor and McDermott Chair in Anesthesiology, Department of Anesthesiology and
Pain Management, University of Texas Southwestern Medical Center at Southwestern
Medical School, Dallas, Texas; Consultant in Ambulatory Anesthesia and Surgery,
Departments of Anesthesiology and Surgery, Ohio State University College of Medicine,
Columbus, Ohio

Henry I. Yamamura, Ph.D.
Professor, Departments of Pharmacology, Biochemistry, Psychiatry, and Program in
Neuroscience, University of Arizona College of Medicine, Tucson, Arizona

Jie Zhang, Ph.D.
Research Assistant Professor, Department of Anesthesiology, University of Utah School
of Medicine, Salt Lake City, Utah

Preface

One of the editors (TAB) has occasionally enjoyed telling anesthesiology residents that when he began his residency, there was no comprehensive American textbook of anesthesiology (Miller's *Anesthesia* was first published by Churchill Livingstone in 1981). The usual reaction to this story is disbelief. Nevertheless, in the early 1980s there were few books of any kind about anesthesiology. This has changed dramatically in recent years, and books on all subjects relating to the specialty are abundant. Why then would we go to the trouble to produce yet another book? The answer to this question is simple. As clinical anesthesiologists and academic pharmacologists, we could not find a reference book that adequately answered our own questions about the basic science, pharmacokinetics, and clinical pharmacology of anesthetic drugs. We decided to create this book mainly because we wanted to read it!

The Pharmacologic Basis of Anesthesiology focuses on the *unique set of drugs that defines the specialty of anesthesiology.* For each major class of drugs, the reader will find three or more chapters: a chapter describing basic pharmacology at the cellular or molecular level, a chapter describing pharmacokinetics, and a chapter on clinical pharmacology and applications.

During the past decade the technology of molecular biology has produced enormous advances in the understanding of neuropharmacology. Drug receptors that were once abstract concepts have been transformed into specific amino acid sequences. There have also been substantial advances in understanding the pharmacokinetics of anesthetic drugs. These advances, however, have been difficult for most anesthesiologists to assimilate because the relevant information has not been readily accessible. To make information on these advances more available to anesthesiologists, we recruited experts in these fields to write the chapters on basic pharmacology and pharmacokinetics.

Having laid a foundation in basic science and pharmacokinetics, we than joined basic and applied science in chapters that describe the clinical pharmacology and applications of anesthetic drugs as they are used in anesthetic practice. The authors for these chapters were selected based on their expertise as both clinicians and pharmacologists.

Finally, we have highlighted certain promising new areas of research in anesthetic pharmacology under the heading of Emerging Concepts, a section of the book that we believe has potential for enormous growth in the future.

Having said what this book is about, we must also say what this book is not about. The book is not intended to be a handy reference to every drug that an anesthesiologist might ever use. There are already numerous general pharmacology texts. We have excluded most drugs that act primarily in the cardiovascular system. While cardiovascular drugs are certainly very important in anesthetic practice, they are widely used in other medical specialties as well and have been extensively described elsewhere. We have made an exception for the β adrenoceptor blocking drugs because β blockers have been used "in exchange" for anesthetic agents; in such anesthetic regimens, β blocking drugs are given to control autonomic responses, allowing the dose of anesthetic agents to be reduced.

Obviously, the quality of a multi-authored text depends heavily upon the expertise and dedication of the individual authors. We feel fortunate to have been accompanied by an outstanding group of authors from around the world. We extend our sincere thanks to each of them.

We have learned an enormous amount of interesting pharmacology in the process of creating and editing this book. We hope that you will enjoy reading it. We and the authors have endeavored to make the book as accurate as possible, but there is always room for improvement. We would like to receive your comments, corrections, and suggestions. Please send them to us at the Department of Anesthesiology, RN-10, University of Washington, Seattle, WA 98195, USA.

T. Andrew Bowdle, M.D., Ph.D.
Akira Horita, Ph.D.
Evan D. Kharasch, M.D., Ph.D.

Contents

Chapter 1

Fundamentals of Cellular Neuropharmacology

Edmund G. Anderson

The objective of anesthesia is to block pain perception and response while obtaining effective muscle relaxation and a minimal disturbance of homeostasis. Single pharmacologic agents cannot achieve this without unwanted side effects. The skilled use of multiple agents can approach this objective. However, the proper choice and management of multiple agents demand a clear grasp of the mechanisms determining the interactions of each agent with various biologic systems and the kinetics governing the access to those systems.

The major target for anesthetic agents and their adjuvants is the central nervous system and its peripheral pathways. To understand how agents used in anesthesia affect neural function, the reader will find it helpful to review cellular neurobiology and the multiplicity of sites susceptible to pharmacologic alteration. This overview will focus on how neuronal architecture uses electrical and secretory processes to transmit, and sophisticated voltage and chemical detectors to integrate, complex information. Emphasis will be placed on the chemical and physical sites that offer opportunity for selective drug actions.

Recent advances in neurobiology forecast vastly increased possibilities for pharmacologic control of brain function. At the same time, the exploding knowledge base for molecular and cellular neuro-biology amplifies the information needed for optimal use of both existing and forthcoming drugs. Fortunately, this knowledge explosion is now settling toward some cohesive descriptions of receptor and channel function that clarify our understanding of drug actions. Thus, a modest investment of effort toward understanding current concepts of receptor action can pay useful dividends in seeing relationships between drug treatments and clinical events.

The majority of known drug actions in the central nervous system are mediated through effects on membrane proteins that serve as channels, transport molecules, or cell surface receptors. A smaller number of drugs act on cytoplasmic enzyme systems and second messenger transducers. The protein elements of all of these systems are rapidly being characterized, and small structural differences between proteins within a subgroup are being resolved as isoforms of enzymes and subtypes of second messenger transducers or receptors. In addition, new allosteric binding sites for endogenous modulators are being identified. These discoveries have detected new sites for pharmacologic attack, and more selective drugs are being developed. An organized overview of how receptor subunits and allosteric binding sites work together to produce membrane responses will pro-

1

vide a framework for anticipating and interpreting drug actions in therapeutic situations.

MEMBRANE PROPERTIES

Neurobiology rests on our understanding of how neurons generate electrical signals that allow fast communication. Fundamental to this understanding is how the ionic gradients that exist at rest are generated and how they become the basic engines driving electrical activity.

Membrane Composition

Neurons, like all cells, are surrounded by a membrane composed of a phospholipid bilayer with a hydrophobic inner core. The lipid chains composing this inner core have fatty acyl side chains that can undergo reorganization to alter the membrane matrix and the mobility of proteins within the membrane. Narrow temperature changes or lipid-soluble pharmacologic agents can alter the membrane matrix, changing the conformation of the included proteins. Anesthetic agents penetrate this lipid environment and may alter membrane permeability by altering hydrophobic protein segments of ion channels and transport molecules to change their function. Some theories suggest that these effects account for the actions of general anesthetics (see Ch. 23).

Resting Potential

The phospholipid bilayer of the cell membrane serves as an effective electrical insulator by virtue of its impermeability to charged ions. However, a variety of proteins bound to the phospholipid membrane serve as transport molecules or ion channels, conferring permeability on the membrane. These membrane proteins have chains of lipophilic amino acids immersed in the lipid bilayer and polar ends protruding from either or both surfaces. This arrangement allows these proteins to function as transporters or channels for selective permeation of polar ions. Because these proteins select which ions cross the membrane, ionic concentration gradients develop. A key transport molecule is the Na^+/K^+ pump. This pump, driven by adenosine triphosphate hydrolysis, imports two K^+ ions for every three Na^+ ions extruded. This results in an intraneuronal ion concentration high in K^+ and deficient in Na^+. Because of the inequality in cation exchange, this pump contributes to the inward negativity.

However, the key element involved in generating the resting potential is a K^+ channel. This voltage-sensitive channel is widely distributed in membranes and is open at the resting potential. This allows K^+ ions to flow out of the neuron (down their concentration gradient), leaving behind organic anions that cannot leave the cell (impermeant) and a negative charge inside the cell. In contrast, Na^+ channels are mostly closed in a polarized membrane so that minimal Na^+ entry occurs. Thus, K^+ ion gradients are the major determinant of the resting potential. Intracellular anion composition is dominated by large organic molecules that are membrane impermeable. Though Cl^- ions can pass across the membrane, they are repelled by the negativity of the impermeant organic anions located in the cytoplasm, resulting in low intracellular Cl^- concentrations. The Cl^- ions distribute as the sum of their tendency to move inward, down their concentration gradient, and outward as a result of repulsion of their negative charge by intracellular negativity. The Na^+ ions exhibit a small inward leak conductance. The resting potential becomes the electrical potential that establishes an equilibrium between the various ionic conductances and their concentration gradients. It varies between -40 and -90 mV in different cell types. This equilibrium can be disturbed by selective changes in membrane permeability to produce depolarizing or hyperpolarizing responses. Thus, the resting membrane charge and the ionic concentration gradients serve as the driving forces of most neuronal electrical activity. Electrogenic ion pumps also contribute to this activity.[1]

CELLULAR COMPOSITION

Neurons and glia are the basic building blocks of the nervous system. Glia outnumber neurons by about nine to one. However, in comparison with neurons, their function is poorly understood. They are known to provide structure, transport nutrients, and perform cleanup duties by scavenging stray ions and transmitters. They also contact capillaries, where they seal cellular interstices, and contribute to the blood-brain barrier. Active roles in modulating information transfer have been postulated but not established. Glia are affected by pharmacologic agents, and in the future, such actions may become therapeutically important.

Neurons have a plethora of sites that can be selectively affected by pharmacologic agents. Each site offers specific opportunities for therapeutic control. The identification of increasing numbers of cellular and molecular sites at which drugs can alter neuronal function is rapidly increasing our ability to control the brain pharmacologically. At the same time, this information explosion increases the difficulty of mastering the subject of neuropharmacology. Maintaining competency in this field requires a structured approach to organizing this information. A useful strategy is to categorize this information according to the compartments defined by neuron architecture.

NEURON ARCHITECTURE

The highly varied morphology of neurons, reflecting their different roles, can obscure their commonalities in structure. The basic subsystems of the neuron are the dendrites, soma, axon, terminals, and their subsynaptic specializations. Each subsystem serves special functions. Not every neuron contains all of these structures, but when a specific substructure is absent (e.g., the lack of dendrites on most ganglion cells), other structures assume their function (e.g., the soma or an axonal branch becomes the primary target for afferent input).

Dendritic Tree

The tree-like sprouting of dendrites from the cell body vastly expands the surface area available for synaptic contact. In addition, some dendrites also extrude spines that further increase surface area and compartmentalize accumulations of cytoplasmic messengers. The conic shape of the dendrites directs synaptic currents down a path of least resistance toward the soma. This geometry allows currents generated by remote synapses, hundreds of

micrometers from the soma, to influence the soma significantly.

Dendritic membranes are complex. They contain highly specialized subsynaptic areas, some with localized receptors for transmitters. These different receptor systems will be discussed later under postsynaptic specializations. Besides receptor-coupled ion channels, dendritic membranes contain many voltage-sensitive ion channels that increase the dendrites' integrative function. Dendrites are deficient in voltage-sensitive Na^+ channels, and therefore, unlike axons, do not conduct action potentials. However, cells with large dendritic trees (e.g., cortical pyramidal cells and cerebellar Purkinje cells) have specialized patches of membrane at major dendritic branch points that contain voltage-sensitive Ca^{++} channels that are opened when depolarizing currents reach adequate intensities. This generates Ca^{++}-dependent action potentials. These action potentials are confined to the locus containing the Ca^{++} channels, and they serve to boost the current signal on its way to the soma. At the same time, these channels can perform an integrative function by activating only when postsynaptic currents from two dendritic branches arrive simultaneously, boosting generalized afferent stimuli, but not stimuli arriving at only one branch.

Additional integration occurs through the pattern of synaptic distribution to the dendritic arbor. Synapses located on remote dendrites weakly affect somatic currents; those on the proximal dendrites have stronger effects. Inhibitory inputs seem to favor locations at dendritic branch points or on the soma where they have a strategic advantage for shunting currents away from the soma and the axon hillock.

Dendrites are not purely receptive. Some exhibit presynaptic specializations that contain synaptic vesicles. These dendrites can release the transmitter onto adjacent neurons through dendrodendritic synapses and, thus, serve an efferent function.[2]

Cell Soma

The cell body plays a key role in the two major functions of neurons: (1) the reception, modulation, and forwarding of fast electrical signals, and

(2) the synthesis and packaging of proteins involved in secretory processes.

Electrical Functions

The size of the soma offers a low internal resistance pathway for transferring synaptic current from the dendrites to the axon hillock with minimal loss. However, the soma also receives a high density of inhibitory synapses positioned to shunt depolarizing currents away from the axon hillock. Thus, the soma becomes a battleground for competing currents. The axon hillock has a low threshold and, hence, serves as the final arbiter for the opposing currents flowing through the soma. When the sum of these competing currents reaches this lowered threshold a self-generating action potential is initiated. These action potentials progress down the axon, but they also move in a retrograde direction, invading the soma and proximal dendrites. The somatic action potential may involve activation of Na^+ channels, giving rise to a Na^+ spike. However, some neurons, like hippocampal pyramidal cells, exhibit a prominent Ca^{++} spike. This is determined by the nature of the voltage-dependent channels present in different neuronal cell bodies.

During the passage of anterograde synaptic currents and retrograde action potentials through the soma, numerous voltage-sensitive Ca^{++} and K^+ channels are activated. These channels modulate succeeding events. At least four types of voltage-dependent Ca^{++} channels have been identified in neurons. The best characterized are the L, N, and T channels. The L channels have the largest conductances (25 pS; pS = 10^{-12} Siemen, where the Siemen represents a unit of electrical conductance) and are blocked by the dihydropyridine calcium antagonists. The N channels have more moderate conductances (12 to 20 pS) and are blocked by ω-conotoxin. The T channels have the smallest conductance (8 pS) and a more transient activation. They are blocked by flunarizine. More recently, the P channel was characterized and shown to be blocked by funnel-web spider toxin. The activation of these channels allows significant Ca^{++} entry, which can activate calcium-dependent ion channels, enzymes, and secretory processes. The linkages of these Ca^{++} channels with intracellular events are still under investigation, but it is believed that specific channels may supply different

intracellular pools. Hence, different channels may affect specific intracellular pathways.[3–5]

Because a rise in cytoplasmic Ca^{++} affects so many signaling and secretory events, it is critical that cytoplasmic Ca^{++} levels be intensively regulated. This is accomplished by a membrane pump that extrudes Ca^{++} by exchanging it for Na^+ or sequestering it in mitochondria and endoplasmic reticulum.

Molecular biology and patch-clamp techniques are rapidly adding new K^+ channels to the recognized list. Three groups of K^+ channels contribute importantly to somatic events. These are the Ca^{++} activated K^+ channels, the voltage-dependent K^+ channels, and the receptor operated K^+ channels. The Ca^{++}-activated K^+ channels primarily contribute to after hyperpolarizations of varying durations. Increasing neuron activity increases Ca^{++} entry, which activates these channels causing hyperpolarization and terminating a burst of action potentials. The voltage-dependent K^+ channels are a group of inward rectifiers that contribute to repolarization of the action potential and may add to the resting K^+ conductance. These channels modulate the action potential frequency within a burst. The receptor operated K^+ channels are believed to be G protein coupled channels that are affected by endogenous substances. Two examples are the M and S currents (affected by muscarine and serotonin, respectively) that are active at the resting potential but are closed by acetylcholine or serotonin. This decreases membrane conductance and increases the cell's excitability.[6]

The previous classification is oversimplified, and many channels have characteristics of more than one class. For example, many of the Ca^{++}-activated channels are voltage sensitive, and some of the voltage-dependent channels are receptor modulated (e.g., the monoamines can modulate the inward rectifier channel). Perhaps these channels are best viewed as subject to modulation by multiple events, and they offer many specific pharmacologic sites for regulation of soma excitability.

Secretory Functions

The soma contains the organelles that synthesize the macromolecules required for maintenance of neuronal function and integrity. The organelles include the nucleus (containing the genetic information), the ribosomes, endoplasmic reticulum and Nissl substance (required for protein synthesis), and the Golgi apparatus (required for protein packaging). In addition, the soma contains abundant mitochondria for energy production.

Neurons encounter sudden demands for protracted periods of intense transmitter release at remote terminals or dendrites. Transport of newly synthesized transmitter from the soma requires many hours. Thus, a timely response to demands for prolonged transmitter release would require enormous local stores of transmitter or rapid local synthesis. The latter alternative is employed, using two strategies to meet sudden demands. One is to package and transport down the axon the enzymes that are able to synthesize the needed transmitter from locally available substrates. This strategy is used with transmitters (e.g., the monoamines) that require ubiquitous precursors, such as simple amino acids or choline. For the peptide transmitters that require a complex synthesis, a different strategy is used. A complex propeptide is synthesized and transported to the local site. There it is clipped by an appropriate enzyme to make the product(s) that are to be released.

Axon Hillock and Axon

Like the soma, the axon plays an important role in rapidly forwarding electrical signals and transporting protein products to the nerve terminal. However, the axon is much more constrained in its communication processes than is the soma. It is essentially an elongated conduit for electrical activity and protein and organelle transport. The electrical events are executed in seconds; axonal transport requires hours to days.

Action Potential

The synaptic currents generated in the dendrites and soma are graded in nature, and information is encoded in their intensity and temporal-spatial distribution. This information is assembled from the amount of transmitter released by the presynaptic neurons, the number of postsynaptic receptors available, the architectural distribution of the synapses on the cell, the internal resistance of the current pathway, and the leakiness of the membranes confining the current path. The totality of these graded events is summed at the axon hillock, and

when the current intensity activates sufficient voltage-sensitive Na^+ channels, a self-regenerating action potential is evoked. (Because of its lower threshold for excitability, the axon hillock is the first segment to generate an action potential.) In contrast with the preceding events, the action potential is an all-or-nothing event, and information now becomes encoded in action potential frequency rather than in a graded current distribution.

The self-regenerating nature of the action potential confers on the axon the ability to communicate rapidly over long distances without a decrement in signal strength. This ability resides in the simpler ion channel composition of the axon. There is a high density of voltage-sensitive Na^+ channels and a lesser diversity of K^+ channels in the axonal membrane. When the somatic currents depolarize the axon hillock to threshold, voltage-sensitive Na^+ channels are opened, allowing extracellular Na^+ ions to flow inward (down their electrochemical gradient), depolarizing the membrane. This depolarizing wave is recorded as the ascending limb of the action potential. As the membrane depolarizes, the voltage-sensitive Na^+ channels are inactivated. The repolarization process involves two mechanisms. One relies on an increase in the conductance of the K^+ channels that maintain the resting potential. After a slight delay, the second involves the opening of a group of voltage-sensitive K^+ channels known as delayed rectifiers. These channels increase the outflow of K^+ (down its concentration gradient), rapidly repolarizing the membrane. The delayed rectifier channels inactivate on membrane repolarization. This rapid repolarization is recorded as the descending limb of the action potential.

The current generated by the inward flux of Na^+ ions proceeds along the axon by two processes: (1) a fast electrotonic spread, determined by the ohmic properties of the axon and (2) a slower activation of Na^+ channels by the depolarizing electrotonic current. Electrotonic current spread declines with distance as a result of the internal resistance of the axon and the leakiness of the membrane. However, the activation of neighboring Na^+ channels regenerates the depolarizing wave allowing the all-or-nothing movement of the action potential down the axon. The distance of the electrotonic current spread in unmyelinated axons (e.g., C fibers) is small because their high internal resistance and permeable membrane minimizes current spread. Thus, a generalized distribution of Na^+ channels along the axon is required, with sequential activation of adjacent channels to allow for long-distance conduction of the action potential. This consumes time, resulting in slow conduction velocities (less than 1.4 m/sec). Larger fibers are coated with myelin that is interrupted every 1 to 2 mm by nodes of bare axon. The myelin insulation and the lower resistance of the larger axons facilitate fast electrotonic current spread so that the membrane at the next node is adequately depolarized to activate the Na^+ channels. Thus, action potential regeneration jumps from node to node, resulting in conduction velocities that can exceed 100 m/sec.

When the Na^+ channels are inactivated by depolarization, they become refractory and are not reactivated until the membrane is repolarized. This refractory period favors a unidirectional movement of the action potential away from refractory membrane. When the initial action potential is generated in the axon hillock, the exception is that a nonrefractory membrane lies in both directions. Therefore, the action potential proceeds in an anterograde direction down the axon and a retrograde direction to invade the soma.

The highly specialized conductive function of axons depends on the voltage-sensitive Na^+ channel. Thus, the primary site for pharmacologic disruption of the conduction process is the Na^+ channel. The most selective pharmacologic agent for this channel is the puffer fish toxin, tetrodotoxin. This channel is also the target of the local anesthetic drugs (see Ch. 7).

Axonal Transport

The other major role of the axon is to transport proteins and membranous organelles assembled in the soma to the nerve terminal. The fast transport system involves the microtubular system, which serves as a track for small vesicles and particles to move at rates as high as 200 to 400 mm/day. Mitochondrial proteins and enzymes are transported at somewhat slower rates. The slowest transport system proceeds at a rate of 1 mm/day or less. These systems provide the protein machinery that maintains the channels, pumps, and receptors in the nerve membrane and the organelles needed for transmitter synthesis, storage, and release as well as energy functions.

Drugs, such as colchicine and some antineoplastic agents, disrupt the microtubule system, resulting in transport failure. This results in accumulation in the soma of the organelles responsible for transmitter synthesis and storage. Consequently, neurotransmitter levels in the nerve terminal are depleted, and excess transmitter appears in the soma.

Nerve Terminal

As the axon approaches the nerve terminal, the membrane undergoes a number of specialized changes. It loses myelination, adds ion channel diversity, and transmitter receptor systems appear in the membrane. The cytoplasm now contains numerous organelles that synthesize and store transmitters. The primary function of the terminal is to translate the electrical currents generated by the arriving action potentials into a graduated release of neurotransmitter. The cascade of electro-chemical events involved in this translation is subject to extensive physiologic and pharmacologic modulation.

Electrochemical Transduction

The nerve terminal contains an abundance of voltage-sensitive Ca^{++} channels. On the arrival of the depolarizing currents of the action potential, these Ca^{++} channels are opened. The influx of Ca^{++} flowing down its electrochemical gradient elevates cytoplasmic Ca^{++} levels and activates protein kinases to cause fusion of synaptic vesicles with the neuronal membrane. This elicits exocytosis of the vesicles localized near the synaptic juncture of the membrane. The number of quanta (i.e., vesicles) of transmitter released corresponds to the amount of Ca^{++} entering the terminal. These depolarizing Na^+ and Ca^{++} currents then activate voltage-sensitive K^+ channels, which repolarize the membrane. The cytosolic Ca^{++} is rapidly lowered by pumping it into mitochondria or out across the plasma membrane. N, P, and L type Ca^{++} channels appear to be involved in the Ca^{++} influx. Synaptic transmission is blocked in Ca^{++} free or high Mg^{++} media. In some cells, transmission is blocked by the N channel blocker ω-conotoxin and, in others, by the spider toxin. However, the dihydropyridine Ca^{++} antagonists, which block L channels, have limited effects on transmitter release. Thus, the Ca^{++} pool supplied by the L channels does not appear to be required for synaptic transmission.

A critical event regulating Ca^{++} entry is the magnitude of the terminal depolarization induced by the arriving action potentials. This depolarization controls the permeability of the voltage-sensitive Ca^{++} channels and, hence, the cytoplasmic Ca^{++} levels. Consequently, this event is extensively modulated.

Presynaptic Inhibition and Facilitation

The nerve terminal contains a variety of receptors responding to neurotransmitters. These include transmitters released by the neuron itself, secretions from more remote neurons with undirected synapses, and/or neurons making axoaxonal synapses. The presynaptic receptors that respond to transmitter released by their own terminals are known as autoreceptors and exert a negative feedback on transmitter release from that terminal. This prevents excessive build-up of transmitter in the synapse during intense activity. The receptors that respond to transmitter secreted by undirected synapses, sometimes called heteroreceptors, may have negative or positive feedback on the terminal release mechanisms. Both the auto- and heteroreceptors modulate the accumulation of neurotransmitter in the subsynaptic area. These receptors can rapidly compensate for the acute effects of drugs like the monoamine oxidase inhibitors and tricyclic antidepressants, which act on the nerve terminal to increase the synaptic accumulation of neurotransmitter. However, with time, the effectiveness of these receptors is altered, either through down regulation or altered G protein coupling, to remove this compensatory response. This is believed to account for the delayed onset of the antidepressant effect of these drugs.

Axoaxonal synapses are tightly coupled to the presynaptic terminal and allow selective modulation of specific afferents without affecting the excitability of the postsynaptic cell. A prime example of this type of synapse is the γ-aminobutyric acid (GABA) synapse, which is directed toward primary afferents in the spinal cord. At this synapse, the released GABA increases the Cl^- permeability at the terminal. This shunts the action potential current invading the terminal, reducing the opening of voltage sensitive Ca^{++} channels, and diminishes the amount of transmitter released from afferent nerve terminals. A blockade of this site by convulsant drugs like picrotoxin or bicuculline results in clonic seizure activity. In contrast, the benzodiazepine drugs increase the affinity of GABA for these receptors, contributing to their muscle relaxant properties (see Ch. 10).

Synthesis and Storage of Transmitter

The nerve terminal contains mechanisms for the local synthesis, storage, and release of transmitter. The mechanistic details of these processes vary with the transmitter(s) involved. However, the common schemes involve either enzymatic synthesis from a locally available precursor or a precursor transported down the axon. The rate of synthesis is controlled by enzyme and/or substrate availability. For example, catecholamine synthesis is controlled at the first, rate limiting, step in a multienzyme cascade. A negative feedback of the transmitter product on this step reduces the availability of the transmitter. Acetylcholine synthesis is regulated by the availability of the substrate (i.e., choline). These processes offer many opportunities for drugs to reduce the availability of the transmitter to be released. However, to date, drugs inhibiting such synthesis have primarily found experimental rather than therapeutic applications.

Synthesized transmitter is then stored in synaptic vesicles through an active uptake system. This store provides a reservoir to be drawn on during protracted synaptic activity and also protects the transmitter from degradation by intracellular enzymes. The vesicles are another site for drug attack. Drugs such as reserpine reduce synaptic transmission by disrupting the vesicular storage of many monoamine transmitters.

Neurotransmitters, Modulators, and Hormones

The distinction between transmitters and other neuromessengers is somewhat blurred. Transmitters deliver chemical messages from presynaptic to postsynaptic neurons by crossing a narrow synaptic gap. Neurohormones are secreted by neurons and carried by the circulation to their receptor site. The term *neuromodulator* is sometimes used to describe substances that arise from nearby sites to influence synaptic transmission. The lack of a precise application of these terms stems from the lack of complete knowledge of synaptic structures and the multiple roles fulfilled by substances. In addition to the classic tightly coupled directed synapses using classic transmitters, nondirected synapses exist in which the nerve terminals make no clear postsynaptic contacts. For example, there is evidence that some axonal projections of the serotonin system make no synaptic connections and function more as neurosecretory systems; other projections show typical synaptic connectivity.[7] However, serotonin is generally referred to as a neurotransmitter. Similarly, dopamine functions as a transmitter in the caudate but, more frequently, as a hormone in the hypothalamic pituitary tract. Thus, a messenger may serve as a transmitter, a modulator, or a hormone, depending on the system involved.

The number of transmitter candidates is expanding with our growing knowledge of neuronal composition and function. Table 1-1 contains a partial list of transmitter candidates that will continue to expand with time. Furthermore, the number of receptor subtypes associated with each transmitter is increasing even more rapidly. However, the characteristics of the groupings in this table are worth some careful thought because they reveal much about the organizational framework of the brain.

The basic chemical messengers of the brain are the excitatory amino acids, glutamate and aspartate. They function as the principal transmitters for fast synaptic excitation throughout the central nervous system. Thus, they provide the primary excitatory drive that is modified by other transmitter systems. These are the transmitters used by most projection neurons. Animal experiments with the agonists and antagonists for the excitatory amino acid receptors listed in Table 1-1 indicate that the excitatory amino acids play major roles in learning, memory, and seizure activity. There is strong evidence that excessive activity in the excitatory amino acids systems can cause neurotoxicity and may account for significant portions of the pathologic changes induced by brain ischemia and/or anoxia. Drugs blocking the NMDA (N-methyl-

D-aspartate) receptor (a subtype of the glutamate receptor), like phencyclidine and ketamine, can produce temporary learning deficits, exhibit anticonvulsant activity, and anesthesia (see Ch. 16).

The inhibitory amino acids, GABA and glycine, are the principal transmitters for fast synaptic inhibition. They are largely found in intrinsic neurons that are integral parts of local feedback and feedforward circuits requiring rapid execution. Thus, they are complementary to the excitatory amino acids in their generalized distribution and are widely involved in inhibition throughout the central nervous system. Drugs that block these amino acids produce generalized seizure activity. The GABA antagonist, picrotoxin, elicits clonic seizures, and the glycine antagonist strychnine, produces tonic seizures. The tonic seizures produced by strychnine reflect the role that glycine plays in mediating reciprocal inhibition between opposing muscle groups.

The biogenic amine systems are usually characterized by centralized collections of cell bodies (e.g., locus ceruleus for norepinephrinergic neurons and the raphe nuclei for serotoninergic neurons). These neurons project long thin unmyelinated axons, exhibiting multiple varicosities, like beads on a string. These axons conduct impulses very slowly (0.5 m/sec) and visit multiple nuclei along their paths. The strings of varicosities contain synaptic vesicles. These centralized slowly conducting systems are designed to disseminate their messages widely across a fairly slow time scale. Thus, they are not suited for command neurons but rather for global messages regulating sleep and wakefulness, appetite, emotional state, and cognition. However, despite this diffuseness, the local response can be highly specific. It is determined by the receptor subtype(s) present at that site and may be excitatory or inhibitory in effect. This property of the acetylcholine systems resembles the diffuseness of the other biogenic amine systems, except that the cell bodies are not localized but are widely scattered throughout the brain (e.g., nucleus basalis, striatum, medial septal nucleus, and brain stem).[8]

The peptide transmitters usually appear as cotransmitters, frequently with biogenic amines.[9] Individual neurons have been reported to contain as

Table 1-1 Neurotransmitters and Their Attendant Receptors

Transmitters	Receptor Subtypes
Excitatory amino acids	
Glutamate	Kainate, AMPA (quisqualate),
Aspartate	NMDA, metabotropic, and L-AP$_4$
Inhibitory amino acids	
Glycine	Strychnine sensitive glycine
γ-Aminobutyric acid	GABA$_A$ and GABA$_B$
Biogenic amines	
Catecholamines	
Norepinephrine and epinephrine	α_{1A}, α_{1B}, α_{2A}, α_{2B}, β_1, β_2, and β_3
Dopamine	D$_1$, D$_2$, D$_3$, and D$_4$
Serotonin	5-HT$_{1A}$, 5-HT$_{1B}$, 5-HT$_D$, and 5-HT$_{1C}$, 5-HT$_2$, 5-HT$_3$, and 5-HT$_4$
Histamine	H$_1$, H$_2$, and H$_3$
Acetylcholine	Nicotinic (neuronal)
	Muscarinic (M$_1$, M$_2$, and M$_3$)
Nucleotides	
ATP, ADP, and AMP	P$_{2X}$ and P$_Y$
Adenosine	A$_1$ and A$_2$
Peptides (partial list)	
Substance P (tachykinins)	NK$_1$, NK$_2$, and NK$_3$
Bradykinin	B$_1$, B$_2$, and B$_3$
Calcitonin gene related peptide	CGRP$_1$ and CGRP$_2$
Somatostatin	SS$_A$ and SS$_B$
Cholecystokinin	CCK$_A$ and CCK$_B$
Angiotensin II	AT$_1$ and AT$_2$
Vasopressin	V$_{1A}$, V$_{1B}$, and V$_2$ and OT (oxytocin)
Neurotensin	Neurotensin receptor
Neuropeptide Y	NPY receptor
Opioid peptides	
Met-enkephalin	
Leu-enkephalin	
β-Endorphin	μ, δ, κ
Dynorphin A	
Unidentified transmitters with identified receptors	
Benzodiazepine system	BZ$_I$ and BZ$_{II}$ (neuronal receptors)
	BZ ("peripheral" or non-neuronal receptor)
Cannabinoid system	Cannabinoid receptor

many as four peptides, and a given biogenic amine has been found paired with four different peptides at four different projection sites. The interactions of the peptides with their cotransmitters is only partially understood. Demonstrated effects include the differential release of the peptide and the amine and varied but reinforcing postsynaptic effects.

Transmitter Inactivation

There are three basic mechanisms for the termination of transmitter action. These are (1) rapid enzymatic metabolism, (2) rapid reuptake, and (3) diffusion from the sites of release and action. Transmitters involved in fast information transfer (e.g., amino acids and some biogenic amine synapses) require rapid termination of action to allow for the next message. This is accomplished by rapid enzymatic metabolism or reuptake. Slower systems (some biogenic amines and peptide systems) that produce tonic shifts in excitability are adequately controlled by slow transmitter diffusion.

Enzymatic degradation is very important in acetylcholine systems in which acetylcholine esterase, localized at the postsynaptic site, determines the duration of transmitter action. Consequently, choline esterase inhibitors can markedly increase the activity at cholinergic synapses. The primary degradative enzyme for the monoamine systems are the monoamine oxidases. However, these enzymes are located within neuron terminals rather than postsynaptically. Consequently, inhibitors of monoamine oxidase affect the amount of transmitter in the presynaptic pool. The ultimate effect of these inhibitors on released transmitter, however, is modulated by negative feedback systems that reduce the synthesis or release of the transmitter through autoreceptor activation.

Reuptake systems are important in terminating the actions of amino acids and biogenic amines. These systems play a dual role. They assist in terminating transmitter's action, and they recycle transmitter for use by the nerve terminal. High affinity uptake systems in both neurons and glia rapidly reduce amino acid accumulation, and specific neuronal uptake systems regulate synaptic levels of biogenic amine transmitters. These uptake pumps are highly selective, and it is possible to develop pharmacologic agents that selectively block specific uptake systems. Drugs that block amino acid reuptake systems have been useful research tools, confirming the physiologic importance of the reuptake systems. However, only drugs acting on biogenic amine uptake systems have found significant therapeutic application. The tricyclic antidepressant drugs show varying degrees of selective blockade of serotonin and/or norepinephrine uptake and are widely used in the treatment of the affective disorders. More recently, selective reuptake inhibitors for the serotonin system have proved to be clinically effective in depression and in obsessive-compulsive disorders. Cocaine is highly selective in the blockade of dopamine up-

take, and many of its behavioral effects are attributed to this action.

Diffusion probably plays some role in the termination of the action of all transmitters. This role is likely to be dominant in the nondirected synapses in which diffusion must play a role in the onset and offset of the transmitter's action.

Postsynaptic Specialization

The membranes adjacent to the nerve terminal may, or may not, show clear structural specializations. In those in which a classic directed synapse is formed, the junctional membranes show specialized changes, such as presynaptic localization of vesicles and a thickening of the pre- and postsynaptic membranes with a narrow gap between the synapsing neurons. At nondirected synapses, no synaptic specializations are observed, and the nerve terminal, or bouton, appears loosely associated with nearby neurons. However, neurons postsynaptic to directed and nondirected synapses contain receptor systems that respond to neural messengers.

Receptors

Pharmacologic and molecular biologic studies have led to the isolation and cloning of many cell surface receptors. This has exploded our knowledge of receptor function and expanded the number of characterized receptors (Table 1-1). In addition, our understanding of the coupling mechanisms between receptors and cell responses has markedly advanced. Because cell surface receptors are the primary mechanism by which drugs exert selective actions in the brain, it is worth some effort to understand current concepts of receptor structure and function.

Molecular biologic techniques provide the primary structures for an increasing number of cell surface receptor molecules. Certain patterns in these structures have led to the recognition of at least five superfamilies of receptor proteins. Neurotransmitters act primarily on receptors in two of these families: the ligand-gated ion channel and the G protein coupled receptors. Receptors in the first family incorporate an ion channel in their secondary structure, and activation of that receptor directly increases ion channel permeability. Receptors coupled to a G protein usually affect membrane permeability or intracellular chemistry through a second messenger system. The channels that are ultimately affected include those classified as voltage-sensitive channels.

A given transmitter may operate receptors in both family groups. For example, acetylcholine acts on nicotinic receptors, which are incorporated in the Na^+/K^+ ion channel structure, to depolarize the membrane rapidly. Acetylcholine also acts on muscarinic receptors, which are coupled to G proteins that may be directly, or indirectly, coupled to an ion channel, and can increase or decrease ion conductances.[10] Similarly, GABA activates $GABA_A$ receptors, which are incorporated in some chloride ion channels, to increase Cl^- permeability. GABA also activates $GABA_B$ receptors, which are coupled to a G protein that inhibits adenylyl cyclase. The consequent reduction in cyclic adenosine monophosphate (cAMP) increases the permeability of a K^+ channel to hyperpolarize the membrane.[11] Thus, the receptor subtypes listed in Table 1-1 afford a range of membrane effects to any given transmitter.

Sometimes, receptor subtypes are anatomically localized, allowing distinct effects of a given transmitter at different sites. For example, the localization of nicotinic receptors at the neuromuscular junction allows acetylcholine to have a strong localized excitatory action by increasing membrane depolarization at the muscle end plate. The localization of M_2 muscarinic receptors in the cardiac atrium allows acetylcholine to hyperpolarize the atrium selectivity and slow the heart rate.

Ligand Gated Ion Channel Superfamily

This group of receptors contain a transmitter binding site as part of the ion channel structure. Known members of the fast ligand gated ion channel family consist of the acetylcholine nicotinic receptor; the excitatory amino acid receptor subtypes, known as the NMDA, kainate, and AMPS (α-amino-3-hydroxy-5-methyl-4-isoxazolepropionic acid) receptors; the inhibitory amino acid receptors, e.g., glycine and $GABA_A$ receptors; and the $5HT_3$ receptor. Structurally, these receptors consist of a recognition site that binds the transmitter

and a channel formed from several protein subunits (Fig. 1-1). This structure subserves rapid synaptic transmission with fast kinetics for opening and closing channels. Recent research has shown that many of these receptors possess numerous allosteric binding sites that allow elaborate modulation of channel function by endogenous ligands other than the transmitter for which the receptor is named (Fig. 1-1). These modulatory sites offer many opportunities for drugs to modify receptor-induced permeability changes.

The pharmacologic complexity of these receptors is best illustrated by considering the components involved in operating a well defined ligand gated ion channel. Such a description may seem like burdensome detail; however, these details demonstrate a pattern repeated in other receptors. Thus, they illustrate generalized concepts about pharmacologic control of receptor function and suggest where future drugs will be aimed to produce more selective effects.

The $GABA_A$ receptor exemplifies the complexity of the ligand gated family of receptors.[12] Like many ligand-gated ion channels, it has a pentameric structure (i.e., the channel and the receptor binding site are formed from five protein subunits). Functional $GABA_A$ receptors can be assembled from an assortment of a growing number of (currently, 16) different $GABA_A$ subunits. These subunits have been classified on the basis of their amino acid homologies as belonging to at least four major groups designated as α, β, γ, or ∂ subunits. The pentameric structure of a $GABA_A$ receptor is usually composed of at least two β subunits and any three additional subunits. (Cooperativity usually exists between the subunits in binding GABA, that is, most receptors require two molecules of GABA to open the channel.) If the $GABA_A$ receptor also contains an α subunit, it will also bind benzodiazepines. If, in addition, it contains a γ subunit, the benzodiazepine binding will increase the affinity of GABA for its binding site, increasing the Cl^- ion channel's permeability and the intensity of inhibition. Thus, the $GABA_A$ receptor may or may not be modulated by the benzodiazepine drugs, depending on whether it contains both α and γ subunits in its composition (see Ch. 10).[13]

Each type of $GABA_A$ receptor subunit includes

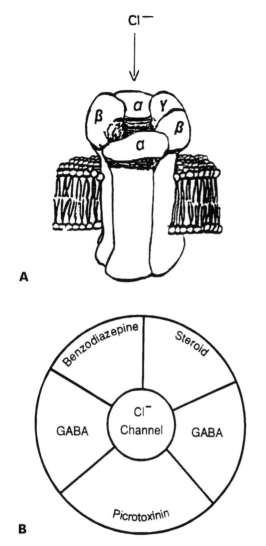

Fig. 1-1 Schematic representations of the GABA receptor. **(A)** This shows how an assembly of five GABA receptor subunits (in this case two α, two β, and one γ subunits) might span the lipid bilayer of the cell membrane and form a Cl⁻ channel. The receptor binding sites are believed to exist on the external (upper) surface of the receptor. Subtype variations in the chemosensitivity of the receptor are thought to be the result of variations in the structure of the subunits making up the pentameric assembly. **(B)** This shows how the pharmacologic binding sites might be distributed around the Cl⁻ channel. Experiments using interactions between these agents suggest that many of these binding sites are in close proximity to the γ-aminobutyric acid binding site, allowing mutual interactions.

several subtypes that exhibit minor structural variations in amino acid composition. Multiple subunits, each with a number of identified subtypes, theoretically allow the assembly of hundreds of unique subunit combinations that can be classified as $GABA_A$ receptors. Some of these variants have altered pharmacologic characteristics. It is not known what combinations of subunits occur naturally. However, there is evidence that $GABA_A$ receptors containing α_1 subunits are associated with benzodiazepine I receptors, which are believed to be responsible for the antianxiety activity. Those receptors containing α_2 subunits exhibit benzodiazepine II receptor activity, which is believed to be responsible for the sedative activity. Ethanol, like the benzodiazepines, also enhances the action of GABA. However, this action requires the presence of a γ_{2s} subunit. In addition, the $GABA_A$ receptors containing β_1 subunits can be phosphorylated on the intracellular projection of those subunits by the AMP-dependent enzyme, protein kinase A. This phosphorylation desensitizes the receptor to GABA. Thus, other transmitters or drugs that activate adenylyl cyclase can modulate $GABA_A$ receptors containing β_1 subunits. Much remains to be learned about the actual number and functional significance of the $GABA_A$ receptor subtypes occurring at different brain sites. However, current findings suggest that the compositions of $GABA_A$ receptors at some sites differ from those at other sites (e.g., cerebellum versus hippocampus) and that pharmacologic agents can be developed that have site specific selectivity.[13,14]

The following briefly summarizes the range of pharmacologic sites on the $GABA_A$ receptor. At the GABA recognition site, muscimol acts as an agonist, and the convulsant drug, bicuculline, acts as a competitive antagonist. The convulsant drug, picrotoxin, acts as a noncompetitive antagonist by binding a site to cause a steric block of the Cl⁻ channel. The actions of these compounds appear to be little influenced by the subunit composition of the receptor. GABA action on the receptor is augmented by benzodiazepines, barbiturates, neurosteroids, volatile anesthetics, and ethanol. As detailed earlier, the actions of the benzodiazepines and ethanol are dependent on the subunit composition of the receptor. Such dependence has not yet been established for the barbiturates, steroids, or volatile anesthetics. Figure 1-1 diagrams an array of receptor binding sites around that Cl^- channel. The exact geometric relationships between these sites is under investigation. The picrotoxin site is believed to be deep within the channel because binding at this site blocks Cl^- permeation. The other sites are believed to be close to the GABA binding sites because their occupation changes the conformation of the GABA sites enough to increase their affinity for GABA.

The benzodiazepine binding site has a complex subpharmacology involving allosteric sites. The benzodiazepine site is blocked by flumazenil, which has no intrinsic antianxiety action. This compound is therapeutically useful in reversing the depressant effects of the benzodiazepines. In contrast, several β carboline derivatives bind at this site but have the opposite effects of the benzodiazepines (i.e., they are anxiety producing and proconvulsant). Thus, they are called inverse agonists. The actions of the inverse agonist are also antagonized by flumazenil. This indicates a close steric relationship between the agonist and inverse agonist sites because both sites are blocked by the same antagonist. The endogenous ligands that act physiologically at the benzodiazepine sites remain to be identified. However, there is growing evidence that some benzodiazepines and β carbolines occur naturally in the brain. The mechanisms for synthesis of these substances remain unknown. However, patients who have died of fulminant hepatic failure exhibit elevated brain levels of diazepam and desmethyldiazepam, and flumazenil can decrease the manifestations of hepatic encephalopathy.[15]

Current observations indicate that extensive variations in $GABA_A$ receptor subtypes exist and that these variants differ in their anatomic distribution and function. Furthermore, these variant receptors may differ in their responsiveness to endogenous substances because they have unique spectra of pharmacologic responsiveness. The $GABA_A$ receptor is not atypical. The ligand gated receptor operated by glutamate, known as the NMDA receptor, exhibits an even more complex array of endogenous regulators, and an extensive pharmacology of this receptor is developing. As the structural characteristics of each of these receptor systems become

better known, it is reasonable to expect that new drugs allow more subtle pharmacologic control of each receptor will become available.

G Protein Coupled Receptors and Their Second Messenger Systems

This group includes the largest number of cell surface receptors by far. More than 100 receptors have been shown to be linked to G proteins, including most of the receptors listed in Table 1-1 (other than the seven listed previously as ligand gated ion channels). These receptors are linked to their second messenger systems by a guanine nucleotide binding protein known as a G protein. This transduction element links the transmembrane receptor to an intracellular messenger system. Each receptor molecule catalyzes the activation of several G protein molecules, thus amplifying the receptor signal. In exchange for this amplification, these receptors accept an increased time constant for response compared with that of ligand gated ion channels. Different G proteins link these receptors to various enzyme cascades, which usually end by phosphorylating a protein to alter its activity. This further amplifies the receptor signal and increases the time delay.

A modulation of the G protein receptors by the binding of endogenous substances to allosteric sites on the receptor protein has not been demonstrated as it has for the ligand gated channels. Rather, these receptor systems appear modulated at various sites along their second messenger pathways. Some of this modulation occurs through cross talk between other second messenger systems. The following examples of the second messenger cascades offer an overview of these receptor systems.[16,17]

The adrenergic β and muscarinic (M_2) receptors in the atrium illustrate two opposing actions on the second messenger system known as the cAMP system (Fig. 1-2A, left). Stimulation of the β receptor activates a stimulatory G protein, which turns on the enzyme adenylyl cyclase. This enzyme converts adenosine triphosphate (ATP) to cAMP, which then activates protein kinase A. In turn, this phosphorylates the target protein, believed to be a Ca^{++} channel. This increases the conductance of this channel and increases cardiac muscle contractility.

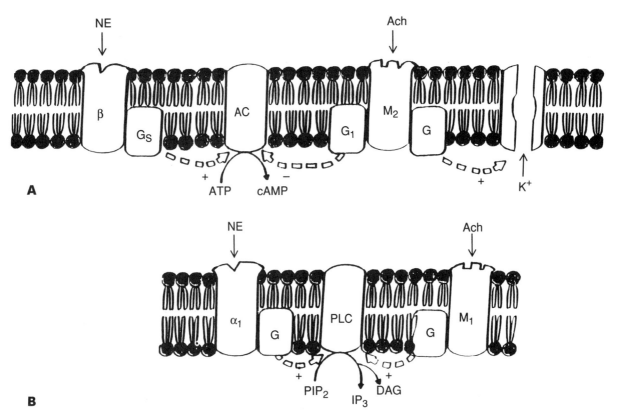

Fig. 1-2 **(A)** This shows how β and muscarinic receptors in cardiac atrial muscle are coupled to two different G proteins. When these receptors are activated, they associate with G proteins that bind guanosine triphosphate and split into subunits that diffuse to act on an effector protein. In this case, the G proteins oppose each others actions on adenylyl cyclase. In addition, the muscarinic receptors are also coupled to a G protein that directly acts on the protein of the K^+ channels of the inward rectifier. This increases their conductance, hyperpolarizes the membrane, and slows the heart rate. **(B)** This shows how α_1 and muscarinic receptors can be coupled to the phosphoinositol second messenger system, possibly through the same G proteins. This allows both acetylcholine and norepinephrine to elevate cytosolic Ca^{++} and induce smooth muscle contraction or initiate secretory activity. The muscarinic receptors are M_1 and M_2 with α and β adrenoceptors. *Abbreviations:* AC, adenylyl cyclase; Ach, acetylcholine; DAG, 1,2-diacylglycerol; G, G proteins (G_i, inhibitory; G_s, stimulatory); IP_3, inositol 1,4,5-trisphosphate; NE, norepinepherine; PIP_2, phosphatidylinositol 4,5-diphosphate; PLC, phospholipase C.

In addition, the kinetics of the pacemaker potential are altered to accelerate the heart rate.

By contrast, the atrial muscarinic receptors are coupled to an inhibitory G protein, which inhibits the enzyme forming cAMP (Fig. 1-2A, middle). This diminishes the activity of protein kinase A and decreases Ca^{++} channel phosphorylation, opposing the actions of the β receptor. In addition, the M_2 receptor also activates a G protein that can act directly on the K^+ channel (Fig. 1-2A, right),

known as the inward rectifier, and increases K^+ conductance. This hyperpolarizes the membrane and slows the heart rate. In this system, two receptors modulate the same second messenger system in opposite directions through opposing G proteins.[18]

Another major second messenger system is the phosphatidylinositol system. The α_1 adrenergic and M_1 muscarinic receptors are coupled to their target proteins through this cascade (Fig. 1-2B). A

G protein, sometimes called G_0, links these receptors to activation of phospholipase C. This enzyme splits phosphatidylinositol 4,5-diphosphate into two different messengers, i.e., inositol trisphosphate and diacylglycerol. The inositol trisphosphate acts on the endoplasmic reticulum (probably through phosphorylation) to release sequestered Ca^{++}. The resulting elevation of cytoplasmic Ca^{++} concentrations can activate a number of enzymes, initiate contraction in smooth muscle cells, and increase secretion. The released diacylglycerol activates cytoplasmic protein kinase C which, in the presence of elevated Ca^{++} levels, is translocated into the membrane where it can phosphorylate receptors or ion channels. Thus, this two pronged second messenger pathway can elevate cytoplasmic Ca^{++} levels, increasing muscle contraction or secretory activity, and phosphorylate receptors and channels to alter their responsiveness. Note that the same transmitter (e.g., acetylcholine) can be linked to pharmacologically similar receptors (muscarinic M_1 and M_2 receptors) that are coupled to different G proteins, affecting different second messenger cascades (phosphatidylinositol and cAMP systems, respectively) with different end organ responses.

It should be recognized that the cAMP and phosphatidylinositol cascades described earlier are not the only second messenger cascades. The arachidonic acid cascade (with its prostaglandin and leukotriene pathways) also exists in the brain, but its role in the central nervous system is not yet well established. The nitric oxide (NO) pathway also exists in neuronal tissue (see Ch.32). In smooth muscle tissue, NO acts like a second messenger by activating the cyclic guanine monophosphate system. In the brain, NO is produced in response to the activation of NMDA receptors by glutamate and is believed by some workers to be released from postsynaptic cells to function as a retrograde transmitter from the postsynaptic cell to inform the presynaptic neuron of the state of excitability. Thus, the NO system has elements of both a transmitter and a second messenger system.

Second Messenger Pharmacology

Because of the role that second messengers play in receptor function, these systems would seem to be a logical pharmacologic target. However, drugs acting beyond the receptor often lack selectivity because they affect generalized systems. Some recent findings suggest that significant specificity might be obtainable through actions on second messenger pathways. An increasing number of G protein variants are being cloned, and greater selectivity of these proteins for specific receptors and second messengers may exist than was at first thought. Multiple forms of adenylyl cyclase and of the phosphodiesterases have been identified, along with multiple isoforms of protein kinase C and phospholipase C. Each of these variants offer potential sites for specific drug action.

There are, to date, few examples of useful drugs that act on second messenger systems, but more are expected to be developed. Lithium chloride may be an example. The concentrations of Li^+ used in bipolar affective disorders are adequate to inhibit the hydrolysis of phosphatidylinositol. This would decrease the availability of inositol trisphosphate and diacylglycerol, which are important second messengers for adrenergic α_1 and some serotonin (5-HT$_{1C}$ and 5-HT$_2$) receptors.[19] Milrinone and amrinone are drugs that selectively inhibit phosphodiesterase type III (an enzyme that metabolizes cAMP but is inhibited by cyclic guanosine monophosphate). These compounds show a selective positive inotropic effect on the heart without increasing the heart rate. They differ from the nonselective phosphodiesterase inhibitors, theophylline and caffeine, which show mixed chronotropic and inotropic effects. Rolipram, which selectively inhibits phosphodiesterase type IV (the enzyme that selectively metabolizes cAMP), shows antidepressant activity in animal studies and is devoid of cardiotonic effects. Though the therapeutic status of some of these drugs remains uncertain, these findings indicate that new therapeutic agents will likely arise from drugs affecting specific elements in second messenger pathways.[20]

Receptor Response and Drug Therapy

The preceding discussion suggests that most drug actions involve interactions with specific cell surface receptors. It is, therefore, tempting to assume that the acute reaction of a drug with an in vitro receptor system is predictive of the pharmacologic response in patients. Unfortunately, a patient's response to chronic drug therapy frequently differs from the acute receptor response found in the laboratory. The differences are sometimes explained by the kinetics of absorption, distribution, and metabolism. With drugs affecting the central nervous system, a patient's response can also be profoundly affected by the dynamic response of the brain to pharmacologic manipulation. Thus, it is important to be mindful of some factors that govern the long term drug response.

Desensitization

Two distinct processes have been demonstrated to reduce response when a system is chronically exposed to a transmitter or a drug-receptor ligand. One type of desensitization occurs when, after prolonged exposure to the ligand, the receptor still binds the ligand, but no cellular response can be detected. This phenomenon has been carefully studied with the β receptor-induced stimulation of adenylyl cyclase. Normally, exposure to epinephrine elevates cAMP. However, prolonged exposure (minutes to hours) to epinephrine results in a diminished response, even though added epinephrine still binds the receptors. This desensitization of the β receptor has been shown to result from phosphorylation of the receptor protein, probably secondary to the excess cAMP generated by the prolonged exposure to epinephrine. This type of desensitization readily reverses on drug withdrawal.[17]

Another type of desensitization occurs when prolonged exposure to a ligand increases an ongoing process of receptor endocytosis. This process removes ligand bound receptors from surface membrane by encapsulating them in vesicles and has been most closely studied with peptide growth factors and β receptors in tissue culture. The bound receptor that is endocytosed into vesicles may be recycled to the surface membrane or transported to lysosomes where it is irreversibly degraded. The recycling of endocytosed receptors results in a temporary down regulation of surface receptor number, which can be reversed in a few hours. However, when the receptor is degraded by the lysosomes, a long term down regulation occurs, which is only reversed by synthesis of new receptor proteins. This may require a period of weeks. For example, when cultured tissues are chronically exposed to a ligand, receptor endocytosis increases. Most of the endocytosed receptors are recycled to the membrane. However, a fraction (about 10 percent with some peptide receptors) are degraded by lysosomes. Thus, if exposure to the ligand is protracted, lysosomes degrade an accumulating number of the endocytosed receptors, causing significant long term down regulation.[17]

Supersensitivity

The deprivation of cell systems from a normal exposure to hormones or transmitters can result in up regulation of receptor numbers and the development of supersensitivity. This is well established at the neuromuscular junction at which denervation results in receptor spread over the muscle fiber and the development of supersensitivity to agonists for the nicotinic receptors. This process is often postulated to explain phenomena observed following brain injury or drug therapy, but little substantive data exist.

The exact role of receptor up or down regulation in the development of drug tolerance and side effects remains to be defined. Changes in drug response over time are frequently attributed to receptor up or down regulation, but supporting data are scarce. The well known tendency of opioid analgesics to produce tolerance is not related to any demonstrable down regulation of opioid receptors. The ability of tricyclic antidepressant drugs to block the reuptake of norepinephrine and/or serotonin does not correlate with therapeutic response. However, a delayed down regulation of brain α_2 and β receptors does correlate with the delayed onset of therapeutic response. The slow development of dyskinetic movements after protracted treatment with antipsychotic drugs (i.e., tardive dyskinesias) is attributed to up regulation of dopamine receptors as a result of chronic receptor blockade by these agents. Though these kinds of explanations are plausible, it is difficult to do decisive experiments in human tissues to provide these inferences.

REFERENCES

1. Hille B: Ionic Channels of Excitable Membranes. Sinauer Associates, Inc., Sunderland, MA 1992

2. Kandel ER, Schwartz JH: Principles of Neuroscience. Elsevier, New York, 1982

3. Hess P: Calcium channels in vertebrate cells. Annu Rev Neurosci 13:337, 1990

4. Tsien RW, Ellinor PT, Horne WA: Molecular diversity of voltage dependent Ca^{2+} channels. Trends Pharmacol Sci 12:349, 1991

5. Llinas R, Sugimori M, Hillman DE, Chersky B: Distribution and functional significance of the P-type voltage-dependent Ca^{2+} channels in the mammalian central nervous system. Trends Neurosci 15:351, 1992

6. Brown AM, Birnbaumer L: Ion channels and their regulation by G protein subunits. Annu Rev Physiol 52:147, 1991

7. Törk I: Anatomy of the serotonergic system: neuropharmacology of serotonin. Ann N Y Acad Sci 600:9, 1990

8. Nicoll RA, Malenka RC, Kauer JA: Functional comparison of neurotransmitter receptor subtypes in mammalian central nervous system. Physiol Rev 70:513, 1990

9. Kupfermann I: Functional studies of cotransmission. Physiol Rev 71:683, 1991

10. Aquilonius S-M, Gillberg P-G (eds): Cholinergic neurotransmission: functional and clinical aspects. In: Progress in Brain Research. Vol. 84. Elsevier, New York, 1990

11. Bowery N: $GABA_B$ receptors and their significance in mammalian pharmacology. Trends Pharmacol Sci 10:401, 1989

12. Olsen RW, Tobin AJ: Molecular biology of $GABA_A$ receptors. FASEB J 4:1469, 1990

13. Sieghart W: $GABA_A$ receptors: ligand-gated Cl^- ion channels modulated by multiple drug-binding sites. Trends Pharmacol Sci 13:446, 1992

14. Lüddens H, Wisden W: Function and pharmacology of multiple $GABA_A$ receptor subunits. Trends Pharmacol Sci 12:49, 1991

15. Basile AS, Jones EA, Skolnick P: The pathogenesis and treatment of hepatic encephalopathy: evidence for involvement of benzodiazepine receptor ligands. Pharmacol Rev 43:27, 1991

16. Freissmuth M, Casey PJ, Gillman AG: G proteins control diverse pathways of transmembrane signaling. FASEB J 3:2125, 1989

17. Kobilka B: Adrenergic receptors as models for G protein-coupled receptors. Annu Rev Neurosci 15:87, 1992

18. Brown AM: A cellular logic for G protein-coupled ion channel pathways. FASEB J 5:2175, 1991

19. Nahorski SR, Ragan CI, Chaliss RAJ: Lithium and the phosphoinositide cycle: example of uncompetitive inhibition and its consequences. Trends Pharmacol Sci 12:297, 1991

20. Beavo JA, Reifsnyder DH: Primary sequence of cyclic nucleotide phosphodiesterase isozymes and the design of selective inhibitors. Trends Pharmacol Sci 11:150, 1990

Chapter 2

Basic Pharmacology of Opioids

Gavril W. Pasternak

The sensation of pain is highly subjective, unique, and dependent on both the nociceptive stimulus and the situation in which it occurs. This is well illustrated by a study comparing the morphine requirements of soldiers wounded in World War II with civilians undergoing elective surgery in the United States. Of the civilians, 80 percent asked for painkillers compared with only 25 percent of the soldiers, despite the more extensive wounds on the battle field. The stress and emotional situation resulting from combat and being wounded dramatically lessened the suffering or the perception of pain.[1] Beecher[1] concluded that situational factors, such as the stress of combat, modify the perception of pain, establishing the lack of a clear correlation between the intensity of nociceptive input and pain. Recently identified pain modulatory systems within the brain may explain these observations. Activation of these systems by electrically stimulating selected brain regions, such as the periaqueductal gray, produces a profound analgesia,[2,3] which is readily reversed by the specific opioid antagonist naloxone.[4] We now know that this system comprises a family of opioid peptides and their receptors and that classic analgesics, such as morphine, act by turning on this sytem.[5]

OPIOID PEPTIDES

The endogenous opioids comprise three major families: the enkephalins, the dynorphins, and β-endorphin (Table 2-1).[6] They can be distinguished by differences in their primary structures, regional localizations, receptor affinities, and behavioral effects. At the same time, they share many features. All have a common N-terminus sequence (Tyr-Gly-Gly-Phe), with the fifth amino acid being either Met or Leu. Despite their similar initial amino acid sequence, the three families of opioid peptides derive from distinct genes.

Although pro-opiomelanocortin, the precursor of β-endorphin, and proenkephalin are distinct proteins, they have some similarities. Both gene products have a molecular weight of approximately 30,000 Daltons, and both are processed to deliver several biologically active peptides. The C-terminal portion of the molecules have the highest concentration of peptides, which are bracketed by double basic residues. The oligonucleotide duplications in the messenger RNA sequences for both precursors suggest that both evolved by gene duplication.[7–13] Pro-opiomelanotropin generates a number of active peptides following processing

Table 2-1 Selected Opioid Peptides

Peptide	Amino Acid Sequence
Natural	
[Leu^5]enkephalin	**Tyr-Gly-Gly-Phe-Leu**
[Met^5]enkephalin	**Tyr-Gly-Gly-Phe-Met**
Dynorphin A	**Tyr-Gly-Gly-Phe-Leu**-Arg-Arg-Ile-Arg-Pro-Lys-Leu-Lys-Trp-Asp-Asn-Gln
Dynorphin B	**Tyr-Gly-Gly-Phe-Leu**-Arg-Arg-Gln-Phe-Lys-Val-Val-Thr
α-Neoendorphin	**Tyr-Gly-Gly-Phe-Leu**-Arg-Lys-Tyr-Pro-Lys
β-Neoendorphin	**Tyr-Gly-Gly-Phe-Leu**-Arg-Lys-Tyr-Pro
β$_h$-Endorphin	**Tyr-Gly-Gly-Phe-Met**-Thr-Ser-Glu-Lys-Ser-Gln-Thr-Pro-Leu-Val-Thr-Leu-Phe-Lys-Asn-Ala-Ile-Ile-Lys-Asn-Ala-Tyr-Lys-Lys-Gly-Glu
Dermorphin	Tyr-D-Ala-Phe-Gly-Tyr-Pro-Ser-NH$_2$
Synthetic	
DAMGO	[D-Ala^2,MePhe^4,Gly(ol)^5]enkephalin
DPDPE	[D-Pen^2,D-Pen^5]enkephalin
DSLET	[D-Ser^2,Leu^5]enkephalin-Thr^6
DADL	[D-Ala^2,D-Leu^5]enkephalin
CTOP	D-Phe-Cys-Tyr-D-Trp-Orn-Thr-Pen-Thr-NH$_2$
FK-33824	[D-Ala^2,N-MePhe^4,Met(O)^5-ol]enkephalin
[D-Ala^2]deltorphin I	Tyr-D-Ala-Phe-Asp-Val-Val-Gly-NH$_2$
[D-Ala^2]deltorphin II	Tyr-D-Ala-Phe-Glu-Val-Val-Gly-NH$_2$
Morphiceptin	Tyr-Pro-Phe-Pro-NH$_2$
PL-017	Tyr-Pro-MePhe-D-Pro-NH$_2$
DALCE	[D-Ala^2,Leu^5,Cys^6]enkephalin

within the cells, including adrenocorticotropic hormone (ACTH) and α-melanocyte-stimulating hormone.[11–14] The pituitary is the primary source of β-endorphin, where it is secreted along with adrenocorticotropic hormone. In addition to β-endorphin, additional opioid peptides have been identified, including α- and γ-endorphin, but their physiologic importance remains unclear. They may represent distinct opioid ligands or simply metabolic side products.

Proenkephalin[8–10] consists of four copies of [met^5]enkephalin and one copy each of [Leu^5]-enkephalin, [Met^5]enkephalin-Arg^6-Phe^7, and [Met^5]enkephalin-Arg^6-Gly^7-Leu^8. All enkephalin-containing peptides are bracketed by double-basic residues. The latter two peptides remain controversial.[15] They have been localized within the brain, but it is unclear whether they reflect distinct transmitters or whether they are further processed to enkephalins. The highest concentrations of proenkephalin are found in the adrenal medulla, where they are coreleased with epinephrine. Like β-endorphin, the enkephalins may have hormonal actions, although these remain obscure.

The dynorphin family derives from yet another precursor, the prodynorphin gene, also known as proenkephalin B. Prodynorphin codes for a 256-amino acid protein, which contains α-neoendorphin, dynorphin A(1-17), and dynorphin B, also known as rimorphin.[16] As in the other precursors, the opioid peptide sequences in prodynorphin are bracketed by double-basic amino acid residues, which are located in the C-terminal half of the precursor. The processing of prodynorphin is complex, with differential processing in different brain regions. The peptides arising from prodynorphin include leumorphin, which corresponds to the C-terminal 29 amino acid residues of prodynorphin with dynorphin B as its first 13 residues, and dynorphin 1-8, which is obtained by cleaving a single basic residue within dynorphin A(1-17).

The pituitary contains the highest concentration of β-endorphin, primarily in the anterior and intermediate lobes.[6] β-Endorphin is also found in the small intestine and placenta; enkephalins are localized in the adrenal medulla, gastrointestinal tract, the carotid body, sympathetic ganglia, parasympathetic preganglionic neurons, and retina. Both β-endorphin and the enkephalins can be measured easily in plasma, raising questions about potential hormonal actions. Although high dynorphin A(1-17) concentrations are present in the pituitary, the immunoreactivity is localized to the posterior lobe, distinguishing it from β-endorphin. Dynorphin was also found in the gastrointestinal tract.

Within the brain, the regional distributions of enkephalin and β-endorphin are different. In general, the enkephalins are widely distributed within the brain; the major sites of β-endorphin are the arcuate nucleus and its projections to the midbrain and brain stem areas. Enkephalin and dynorphin represent separate systems, although some parallel regional distributions exist. For example, high dynorphin levels are present in the supraoptic and paraventricular nuclei of the hypothalamus with only moderate levels in the striatum, an area containing high enkephalin levels. The distributions of dynorphin A(1-17) and α-neoendorphin are similar, with strong evidence for colocalization of both peptides.

The lability of the natural opioid peptides, particularly the enkephalins,[17,18] led to intense efforts to design metabolically stable derivatives. Substituting a D-amino acid, such as D-Ala[2], for the Gly[2] blocks proteolytic enzymes. Amidation of the terminal carboxy group also enhances stability. As additional compounds were designed, many were observed to act preferentially on specific receptor subtypes, and efforts were redirected toward the design of highly selective agents. At the present time, there are numerous highly selective enkephalin derivatives. Although they have not yet made an impact clinically, they have provided valuable experimental tools in studies of the opioid systems.

OPIOIDS

Opioids mimic the actions of the peptides described earlier. Clinically, morphine is the most widely used analgesic and is the "gold standard" against which all opioids are compared. The actions of opioids are unique in that they work selectively on pain and do not change sensory thresholds, as the local anesthetics do. Many patients receiving opioids report that the pain remains, but that it does not "hurt." The synthesis of thousands of opioids led to detailed structure-activity relationships for maintaining analgesic activity, which in turn, led to the development of a number of structurally diverse analgesics.[19–22] Recently, the role of multiple opioid receptors has become more important, and analgesics working through mechanisms distinct from morphine were developed. These agents enhanced our understanding at the molecular and cellular level and within an integrated nervous system and yielded important clinical tools.

Analgesics

Morphine and codeine are the two predominant analgesics found in raw opium (Fig. 2-1). Clinically, codeine is far weaker than morphine. Presumably, the demethylation of codeine at position 3 to yield morphine is responsible for its pharmacologic activity. Heroin (3,6-diacetylmorphine) is indistinguishable from morphine pharmacologically and

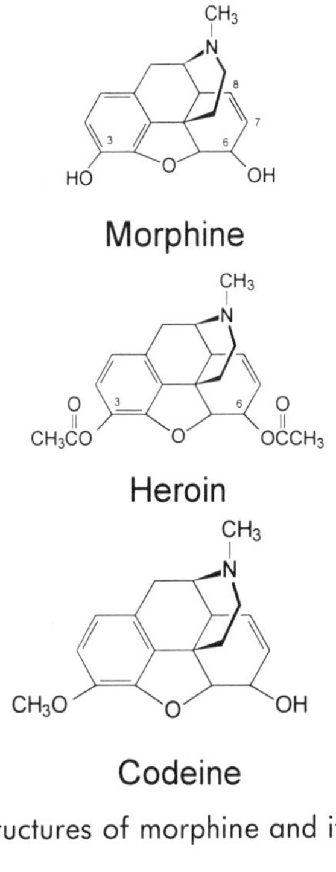

Fig. 2-1 Structures of morphine and its analogs.

offers no clinical advantages.[23] Esterases in the blood rapidly remove the 3-acetyl group, yielding the 6-acetylmorphine, which is active. 6-Acetylmorphine can be further deacetylated to give morphine.

The structure-activity relationships of morphine have been reviewed.[19–22] Reduction of the 7,8 double bond to produce dihydromorphine increases potency, as does the conversion of the 6-hydroxy group to a ketone moiety, yielding dihydromorphone and morphinone. Thebaine is a valuable starting material found in raw opium. Semisynthetic thebaine derivatives include oxymorphone, oxycodone, and the 6,14-endoethano and 6,14-endoetheno drugs,[22] which include etorphine and buprenorphine.

The structure of morphine can be simplified without sacrificing analgesic potency (Fig. 2-2). Levorphanol, a morphinan, lacks the dihydrofuran ring; benzomorphans, like pentazocine, are simpler still, lacking the entire C ring. Benzomorphans are potent analgesics, but their actions extend to a number of different opioid receptor subtypes. Pentazocine, for example, is a mixed κ_1 agonist-μ antagonist (see Ch. 5). In patients tolerant to morphine, pentazocine can acutely precipitate withdrawal. Both ketocyclazocine and N-allylnor-

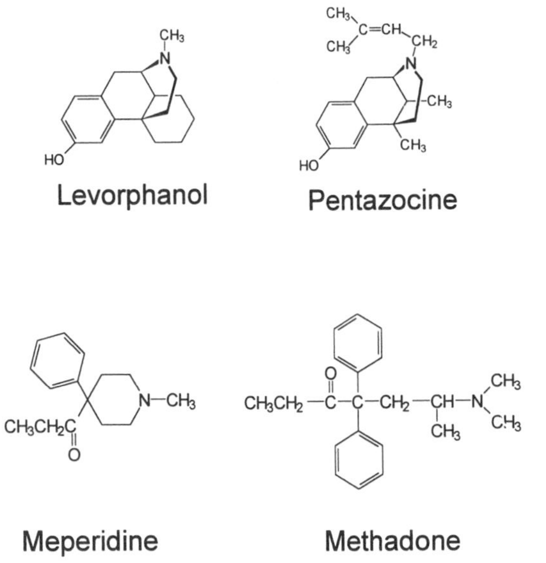

Fig. 2-2 Structures of opioids.

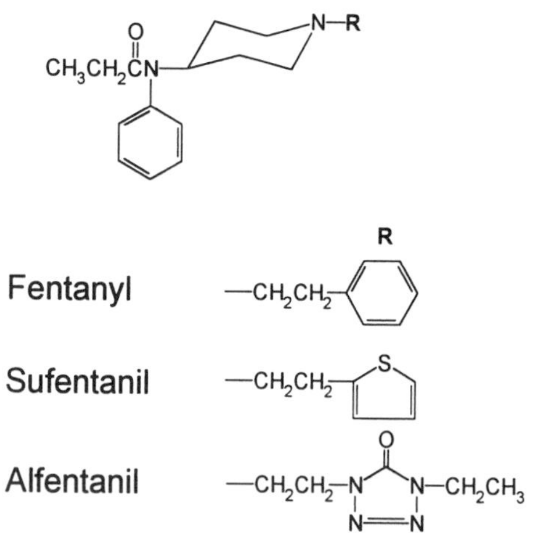

Fig. 2-3 Structures of fentanyl derivatives.

metazocine (SKF 10,047) also belong to this group. Although neither is used clinically, both are important in our understanding and classification of opioid receptor actions.

The phenylpiperidines represent the next simplification in opioid structure and contain the oldest totally synthetic clinical opioid, meperidine and, more recently, fentanyl and its analogs (Fig. 2-3). Meperidine is one of the most widely used opioids in the United States. However, serious problems, such as seizures, may arise from the use of meperidine in patients with impaired renal function as a result of the accumulation of normeperidine, a metabolite that is cleared by the kidneys.[24] The diphenylpropylamines are the second major group of synthetic opioids and include methadone and propoxyphene.

Antagonists

Nalorphine, the N-allyl derivative of morphine, was the first opioid with demonstrable antagonist activity. However, the pharmacology of nalorphine is complex.[25] It is a mixed agonist-antagonist with activity at a wide range of different opioid receptors. Although it potently reverses morphine analgesia and respiratory depression and precipitates withdrawal in morphine-dependent animals, nalorphine is a potent analgesic when given alone.[26,27] The development of naloxone and naltrexone (by substituting the N-methyl group of oxymorphone with an allyl or a methylcyclopropyl group) produced extremely potent pure antagonists, which are valuable experimentally and clinically (see Ch. 5).

MORPHINE AND μ RECEPTORS

Opioid receptors were first hypothesized in 1954,[28–31] based on the receptor concept,[32] almost 20 years before their demonstration in 1973.[33–35] The first proposal of multiple opioid receptor subtypes, "receptor dualism,"[36] was based on studies of interactions of morphine and nalorphine.[26,27] Subsequently, Martin et al.[37] proposed three opioid receptor subtypes. These receptors were confirmed biochemically. Indeed, the receptor sites first described in 1973 correspond to μ receptors because the radioligands were structurally related to morphine. The affinity of a series of opioids for these sites was correlated with their pharmacologic actions.

Two subtypes of μ receptors, μ_1 and μ_2 (Table 2-2), were proposed based on detailed binding and pharmacologic studies,[38–40] and the classification was confirmed by sophisticated computer modeling programs.[41–46] Although the two μ subtypes share many characteristics, such as their high affinity for morphine, they do have differences, including distinct binding profiles for a number of opioids and opioid peptides (Table 2-3).[47] Their regional distributions are similar, but differences were noted.[48,49] Most impressive was the description of CXBK mice, which have a selective deficit in μ_1 opioid receptors.[50] Functionally, several highly selective antagonists are invaluable in defining the pharmacology of the two sites (Table 2-4). β-Funaltrexamine irreversibly inactivates both μ_1 and μ_2 subtypes,[51,52] whereas naloxazone and naloxonazine can selectively antagonize μ_1 receptors.[53–56] These antagonists were used in binding studies and in vivo to define these sites, as described subsequently. The CXBK mouse was used to confirm the distinct roles of the two subtypes in morphine mediated analgesia,[49,50,57] and these reports indicate that the expression of μ_1 and μ_2 receptors is under independent genetic control.

The molecular biology of opioid receptors[58–65] has just begun with the recent cloning of a μ receptor. A member of the G protein superfamily, the receptor has high homology with δ and κ_1 recep-

Table 2-2 Tentative Receptor Classification

Receptor	Agonists	Actions
μ	Morphine	
$\quad\mu_1$		Supraspinal analgesia
$\quad\mu_2$		Spinal analgesia
		Respiratory depression
		Inhibition of gastrointestinal transit
		Guinea pig ileum bioassay
κ		
$\quad\kappa_1$	Dynorphin A	
	U-50,488	Spinal analgesia
	U-69,593	Diuresis
	Spiradoline	
$\quad\kappa_2$		Pharmacology unknown
$\quad\kappa_3$	NalBzoH	Supraspinal analgesia
	Nalorphine	
δ	Enkephalins	Analgesia (spinal systems are more sensitive than supraspinal ones)
		Mouse vas deferens bioassay

Abbreviations: NalBzoH, naloxone benzoylhydrazone; U-50,488, {trans-3,4-dichloro-N-methyl-N-[2-(1-pyrrolindinyl)cyclohexyl]-benzeneacetamide}; U-69,593, [5R-(5,7,8)-(+)-N-methyl-N-[7-(1-pyrrolidinyl)-1-oxaspiro-[4,5]dec-8-yl]benzeneacetamide.

Table 2-3 K_i Values of a Series of Opioids and Opioid Peptides for κ, μ, and δ Receptors

Opioids	K_i (nM)[a]					
	κ_1	κ_2	κ_3	μ_1	μ_2	δ
μ						
Morphine	49 ± 32		32.8 ± 2.2	0.5 ± 0.38	2.5 ± 0.6	278 ± 49
Codeine			>350	>500	>500	
DAMGO	>350		8.2 ± 1.9	0.5 ± 0.68	2.1 ± 0.8	>500
PL-017	>350		88.8 ± 27.8	5.4 ± 1.6	16.5 ± 1.8	>100
(−)Naloxone	5.3 ± 1.1		8.4 ± 0.9	1.3 ± 0.5	3.7 ± 0.7	106 ± 23
(+)Naloxone			>350	>500	>500	>500
Trimu-5	>1,000		314 ± 67	2.9 ±0.9	14 ± 4.9	>500
κ						
(−)Ethylketocyclazocine	0.21 ± 0.03	44 ± 5	1.4 ± 0.5	0.17 ± 0.06	0.24 ± 0.2	4.7 ± 0.5
(+)Ethylketocyclazocine	>350		>350			
Ketocyclazocine	1.8 ± 0.5		4.5 ± 0.8			
U-50,488	6.1 ± 1.3	484 ± 110	>350	370 ± 76	>500	>500
Nalorphine	3.0 ± 1.6		5.4 ± 2.1	0.8 ± 0.6	1.4 ± 0.2	32 ± 16
Tifluadom	0.87 ± 0.24	39 ± 26	6.5 ± 1.2			
Mr2034	1.6 ± 0.14		2.3 ± 0.18			
Mr2266			1.0 ± 0.15			
(−)SKF 10,047	2.9 ± 0.77		6.9 ± 0.97			
(+)SKF 10,047	>350		>350			
WIN44,441	0.32 ± 0.12		0.2 ± 0.06			
(−)Levallorphan	0.95 ± 0.12		2.2 ± 0.56	0.25 ± 0.17	1.0 ± 0.2	5.4 ± 0.8
(+)Levallorphan			>350	>500	>500	>500
Levorphanol	8.1 ± 0.93		5.6 ± 1.2			
NalBzoH	0.60 ± 0.32		0.9 ± 0.19	0.3 ± 0.1	0.8 ± 0.2	
Cyclazocine	0.99 ± 0.16	65 ± 20	1.5 ± 0.59			
Pentazocine	11.8 ± 3.8		79.5 ± 16.8			
Nalbuphine	3.28 ± 1.2		5.8 ± 1.1			
nor-BNI	3.5 ± 0.96		103 ± 8.5	27.5 ± 8.9	115 ± 15	23.5 ± 5.8
δ						
DPDPE	>350	>10,000	>350	82 ± 19	457 ± 149	2.9 ± 0.7
DADL	>350		85.9 ± 17.3	0.9 ± 0.83	7.2 ± 3.1	1.9 ± 0.2
Metkephamid	187 ± 53		4.3 ± 0.51	0.3 ± 0.05	0.9 ± 0.2	2.3 ± 0.2
DSLET			259 ± 121	1.4 ± 0.8	14 ± 6.5	2.3 ± 0.8
Endogenous opioid peptides						
β-Endorphin	80 ± 20		10.7 ± 3.9	0.98 ± 0.14	3.1 ± 0.7	2.6 ± 0.5
α-Neoendorphin			67. ± 39	5.6 ± 1.5	19 ± 7	4.2 ± 1.4
Dynorphin A(1-17)	0.19 ± 0.08	1.7 ± 1.2	14.2 ± 7.9	0.69 ± 0.16	2.2 ± 0.38	8.7 ± 1.5
Dynorphin A(1-8)	4.3 ± 1.7		115. ± 45	11 ± 3.5	53. ± 10.	4.1 ± 1.1
Dynorphin B			63. ± 17	6.0 ± 1.6	17. ± 4.4	6.8 ± 1.3

Abbreviations: DADL, [D-Ala^2,D-Leu^5]enkephalin; DAMGO, [D-Ala^2,MePhe^4,Gly(ol)^5]enkephalin; DPDPE, [D-Pen^2,D-Pen^5]enkephalin; DSLET, [D-Ser^2,Leu^5]enkephalin-Thr^6; Mr2034, (−)-2-(3-furyl)-2^1-hydroxy-5,9-diethyl-6,7-benzomorphan; Mr2266, (−)-2-(3-furylmethyl-2'-hydroxy-5,9-diethyl-6,7-benzomorphan; NalBzoH, naloxone benzoylhydrazone; nor-BNI, nor-binaltorphimine; PL-017, see Table 2-1; SKF 10,047, N-allylnormetazocine; Trimu-5, Tyr-D-Ala-Gyl-NH(Ch$_2$)$_2$-CH(CH$_3$)$_2$; U-50,488, {trans-3,4-dichloro-N-methyl-N-[2-(1-pyrrolidinyl)cyclohexyl]-benzeneacetamide}; WIN 44,441, (2α,6α,11S)-(−)-1-cyclopentyl-5-(1,2,3,4,5,6-hexahydro-8-hydroxy-3,6; 11-trimethyl-2,6-methano-3-benzacin-11-yl)-3-pentanone.

[a] K_i values are an estimate of affinity and represent the concentration of compound needed to occupy 50 percent of receptor sites. The higher the affinity of a drug is, the lower its K_i value.

(Data from Clark et al.,[47] Zukin et al.,[102] and Clark et al.[105])

Table 2-4 Sensitivity of Opioid Analgesia to Antagonists

Antagonists	μ_1	μ_2	δ_1	δ_2	κ_1	κ_3
Selective						
Naloxonazine	Yes	No	No	No	No	No
CTOP	Yes	Yes	No	No	No	No
β-FNA	Yes	Yes	No	No	No	No
Naltrindole	No	No	Yes	Yes	No	No
ICI 174,864	No	No	Yes	Yes	No	No
DALCE	No	No	Yes	No	No	No
Naltrinodole 5′isothiocya-						
nate	No	No	No	Yes	No	No
nor-BNI	No	No	No	No	Yes	No
General						
Naloxone	Yes	Yes	Yes[a]	Yes[a]	Yes[a]	Yes[a]
Naltrexone	Yes	Yes	Yes[a]	Yes[a]	Yes[a]	Yes[a]
Diprenorphine	Yes	Yes	Yes	Yes	Yes	Yes

Abbreviations: CTOP, D-Phe-Cys-Tyr-D-Trp-Orn-Thr-Pen-Thr-NH$_2$; DALCE, [D-Ala^2,Leu^5,Cys^6]enkephalin; β-FNA, β-funaltrexamine; ICI 174,864, N,N diallyl-Tyr-Aib-Aib-Phe-Leu-OH; nor-BNI, nor-binaltorphimine.

[a] Higher antagonist doses needed.

tors (Fig. 2-4). Both transient and stable expression of this receptor yields a receptor with high affinity for morphine and traditional μ drugs, but it is still uncertain whether the clone encodes the μ_1 or the μ_2 receptor. However, it is involved with morphine analgesia. In antisense studies, a short antisense oligodeoxynucleotide directed against the untranslated 5′ region of the clone was microinjected into the periaqueductal gray of rats three times over 5 days; after this, morphine analgesia was exam-

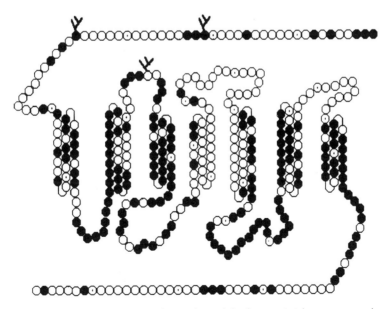

Fig. 2-4 Model of opioid receptor. Hypothetical model of an opioid κ_3 receptor based on hydrophobic analysis. The cloned opioid receptor subtypes differ in regions presumed to be involved with binding, but they share extensive regions of great homology, as indicated by the shaded amino acids.

ined.[170] The antisense treatment blocked morphine analgesia compared with that in control animals. This field is moving rapidly, and many of these issues will soon be resolved.

Localization of Morphine Analgesia

Morphine analgesia is complex. Numerous studies clearly demonstrate the ability of spinal, supraspinal, and peripheral systems to modulate pain when activated by morphine. However, all of these systems do not appear to be equally important. Following systemic administration, supraspinal analgesic systems predominate. The evidence comes from many sources. Morphine is more potent intracerebroventricularly than it is spinally.[66–68] Second, spinal transsections markedly reduce morphine's antinociceptive activity in the tailflick assay, implying the presence of important descending opioid inputs on this spinally mediated reflex.[69–72] Antagonist studies also implicate supraspinal mechanisms. The μ_1 selective antagonists naloxonazine and naloxazone block systemic and supraspinal morphine analgesia without interfering with spinal analgesia.[66,73–76] These results indicate that systemic morphine works supraspinally through μ_1 receptors.

Studies with CXBK mice further confirm the importance of supraspinal mechanisms. CXBK mice have a selective deficit of μ_1 receptors,[50,77] which corresponds to their insensitivity to supraspinal morphine. At the same time, they respond normally to spinal morphine.[77,79] The marked insensitivity of these mice to systemic morphine confirms the importance of supraspinal systems. If spinal systems were playing a significant role, the CXBK mice should respond at standard morphine doses because the sensitivity to spinal morphine is normal. Although the morphine acts supraspinally, it is unclear whether it works by activating the well described morphine-sensitive descending pathways from the brain stem to the dorsal horn of the spinal cord[69–72,80] or whether there are more rostral mechanisms involved.

Within the brain stem, the periaqueductal gray, nucleus raphe magnus, locus ceruleus, and nucleus reticularis gigantocellularis have been implicated in morphine analgesia.[73,81–83] Microinjection studies in conjunction with selective antagonists implicate μ_1 receptors in these regions (Table 2-2).[73] In contrast, μ_2 receptors mediate analgesia at the level of the spinal cord.[67,68] This distinction in the receptors that mediate spinal and systemic/supraspinal morphine analgesia probably will become more important with the increasing clinical use of epidural and intrathecal opioids.

Peripheral mechanisms also contribute to morphine analgesia. Morphine has local analgesic actions in animal studies.[84–85] Clinically, intra-articular morphine is an effective analgesia following arthroscopic knee surgery despite lack of significant systemic absorption.[86]

Synergy

Concomitant injection of morphine both intracerebroventricularly and intrathecally in the rat enhances the analgesic potency of morphine by almost 10-fold.[87] When the role of μ receptor subtypes in spinal/supraspinal synergy was explored,[57] brain stem μ_2 receptors were found to mediate this synergistic action. This contrasts with the analgesia produced by morphine given only supraspinally, which is mediated through brain stem μ_1 receptors. Although the μ_1-selective antagonist naloxonazine blocks the analgesia of supraspinal morphine alone, it does not affect the synergistic system. Furthermore, CXBK mice have a normal spinal/supraspinal synergy despite their deficit of μ_1 receptors.[76,77]

Synergy is not limited to interactions between the spinal cord and brain stem. Microinjection studies now have demonstrated synergy between intrinsic brain stem nuclei, including the periaqueductal gray, nucleus raphe magnus, and locus ceruleus.[88] Unlike spinal/supraspinal synergy, this intrinsic brain stem synergy is mediated through μ_1/μ_1 interactions. Although many questions remain regarding the role of the synergistic interactions among different regions within the central nervous system, their presence emphasizes the importance of examining analgesics in vivo and the problems associated with predicting the analgesic potential of a drug from either binding or bioassay studies.

Spinal/supraspinal synergy may play a role in the dramatic analgesia that occurs with epidural opioids in humans. Epidural injections give high morphine levels at the spinal level at the same time that morphine blood levels approach those following intramuscular administration.[89] Although speculative, the blood levels may be adequate to activate supraspinal systems in addition to the spinal ones (see Ch. 6).

Morphine-6β-Glucuronide

Recent studies reveal some interesting properties of morphine metabolites. Morphine is glucuronidated at both the 3 position and 6 position, with the 3-glucuronide predominating.[90] Although early studies suggested that the 6β-glucuronide analog is active, these were overlooked for many years.[91] Recent studies confirm the activity of morphine-6β-glucuronide.[92,93] Systemically, morphine-6β-glucuronide is approximately twice as potent as morphine. However, when it is administered intracerebroventricularly or intrathecally, morphine-6β-glucuronide is more than 100-fold more active than morphine. The difference in potency between systemic and direct central nervous system administration reflects the greater difficulty morphine-6β-glucuronide has in traversing the blood-brain barrier compared with morphine. These observations are important clinically. Although morphine-6β-glucuronide does not accumulate to appreciable levels with single doses, the blood levels of morphine-6β-glucuronide with chronic oral dosing exceed those of morphine. In view of the greater potency of morphine-6β-glucuronide, these observations imply that morphine-6β-glucuronide is responsible for most of the analgesic activity with chronic oral dosing. The importance of morphine-6β-glucuronide may also help explain the greater sensitivity of patients with renal failure to morphine. Morphine-6β-glucuronide is cleared by the kidneys, and even modest levels of renal insufficiency produce marked increases in the levels of this metabolite.

Side Effects

Side effects can markedly influence the use of opioids. It is important to distinguish between side effects mediated through opioid receptor mechanisms and those resulting from the toxicity of the drugs. Many actions, including respiratory depression and constipation, are receptor mediated and can be antagonized by agents such as naloxone. The ability of a specific drug to elicit these actions

is highly dependent on its receptor profile and, in many cases, can be predicted.

Respiratory Depression

Respiratory depression is rarely a problem in ambulatory patients in the absence of pre-existing respiratory compromise. However, in the surgical setting, it can be clinically significant. Respiratory depression is elicited through μ_2 receptors within the brain stem.[94,95] Thus, drugs with poor affinity for μ_2 receptors or only partial agonist activity at these sites, such as butorphanol or nalbuphine, produce less respiratory depression (see Ch. 5).

Inhibition of Gastrointestinal Transit

Constipation is a common problem with opioid use. Constipation results from a number of factors, but the most important is the decrease in gastrointestinal transit, which is mediated both centrally and peripherally.[96] These actions involve μ_2 receptors in the brain and periphery. Thus, agents with respiratory depressant actions typically also have constipating actions.

Other Actions

Morphine also produces a variety of other effects. The euphoria associated with morphine presumably involves μ receptors. Although some information suggests that reinforcing behavior in rats is mediated through μ_1 receptors,[97] the subtypes involved with euphoria in humans are not established. Sedation also can be a problem, particularly with higher morphine doses. Like most of other opioid actions, it is readily reversed by antagonists such as naloxone. Although nausea and vomiting are commonly seen, it is still unclear whether they involve specific opioid receptor mechanisms and whether they are reversible by naloxone. However, the ability to eliminate nausea and/or vomiting by switching patients from one μ opioid to another suggests that this side effect may not be mediated through traditional μ receptors.

κ RECEPTORS

Studies exploring combinations of nalorphine and morphine led Martin[36] to propose the theory of receptor dualism, which hypothesized the existence of M (morphine) and N (nalorphine) opioid receptors. This classification was later expanded to three types of opioid receptors: μ (morphine), κ (ketocyclazocine), and σ (SKF 10,047).[37] Although the σ site no longer is considered an opioid receptor, the κ receptor family has become increasingly important, as have the dynorphins, their endogenous ligands.[98]

The identification of κ binding sites initially was difficult. Detailed characterizations of κ receptors had to await the development of highly selective ligands[99,100] and the discovery of high levels of κ receptors in guinea pig brain.[101] Binding studies have now identified three major categories of κ receptors.[102–105] The κ_1 receptors have a high affinity for {trans-3,4-dichloro-N-methyl-N-[2-(1-pyrrolindinyl)cyclohexyl]-benzeneacetamide} (U-50,488) and related compounds; the other two subtypes do not. The κ_2 and κ_3 receptors can be readily differentiated by their binding profiles. The κ_1 receptors have been cloned from the mouse and rat.[60,64] Like the cloned μ receptor, the κ_1 receptor is a traditional G protein receptor with the standard seven transmembrane regions. It will be interesting to compare its structure with the other κ subtypes when they are cloned.

κ_1 Receptors

As noted earlier, a number of technical difficulties interfered with the biochemical demonstration of κ receptors, despite extensive pharmacologic findings implicating their existence. The κ_1 receptors are functionally defined by their sensitivity toward U-50,488 and U-69,593, two extraordinarily selective drugs. Kosterlitz et al.[101] first demonstrated κ_1 receptors in the guinea pig cerebellum, a region devoid of other receptor subtypes. Although there is evidence for two subtypes, κ_{1a} and κ_{1b}, using binding approaches,[105] their pharmacology remains unclear.

The pharmacology of κ_1 receptors was widely investigated using the agonists U-50,488 and U-69,593 and the highly selective antagonist norbinaltorphimine.[106–110] The κ_1 receptors mediate substantial analgesia, which is pharmacologically distinct from the other receptor subtypes. In animal studies, κ_1 receptors are localized at the spinal cord and readily reversed by the κ_1 antagonist norbinaltorphimine but not by antagonists selective for μ or δ receptors.[110] Finally, there is no cross tolerance between κ_1 and μ or δ analgesia.

κ_2 Receptors

Zukin et al.[103] first reported the presence of a U-50,488-insensitive κ_2 receptor in rat brain using ^{3}H-ethylketocyclazocine with μ, δ, and κ_1 blockers. These results were confirmed, and the presence of these receptors is established. Unfortunately, the pharmacology of these receptors remains known.

κ_3 Receptors

Another U-50,488-insensitive binding site (κ_3) was reported using the novel opioid derivative, naloxone benzoylhydrazone.[103,105,111,112] Soon afterward, a sophisticated computerized analysis of binding surfaces also revealed a similar site.[104] The receptor density of κ_3 in the brain is high, typically twice that of either μ or δ receptors, making κ_3 receptors the predominant opioid receptor.[105] Although its regional distribution is similar to that of μ receptors, some differences are apparent. Autoradiographic studies reveal low levels of κ_3 binding sites in the periaqueductal gray, a region containing high level of μ receptors. Binding studies also indicate that the selectivity of many agents is not as great as previously thought. This was particularly evident among many μ ligands, including [D-Ala^2, MePhe^4,Gly(ol)^5]enkephalin (Table 2-3).

κ_3 analgesia is distinct. Localized supraspinally, it is insensitive to the selective μ, δ, and κ_1 antagonists.[111–113] Furthermore, κ_3 analgesia shows no cross tolerance with μ or κ_1 drugs. Nalorphine has played a central role in the concept of opioid receptor multiplicity.[26,27,36] Martin[36] based his concept of receptor dualism on distinct morphine and nalorphine receptors. Evidence now indicates that κ_3 receptors represent these nalorphine receptors (see Ch. 5).[25]

δ RECEPTORS

The δ receptors were discovered soon after the enkephalins.[114] Initially classified by bioassays, δ binding sites have been well characterized (Table 2-3),[114–121] and their unique regional localization has been defined.[47,121–124] Enkephalins are labile and have short half-lives in tissues. The development of stabilized analogs[120] greatly facilitated these studies. The selectivity of these synthetic peptides can vary markedly. Some analogs are highly selective for μ receptors, whereas others are specific for δ receptors. Several novel and highly selective δ antagonists have also proved to be valuable.[125–127]

The δ receptors produce analgesia through an independent and distinct mechanism.[122–131] Although relatively weak analgesics supraspinally, δ drugs are potent spinally. Evidence now suggests two subtypes of δ receptors, based on the agonists [D-Pen^2, D-Pen^5] enkephalin (DPDPE, δ_1) and deltorphin II (δ_2)[132–134] with some support for a spinal δ_1 system and supraspinal δ_2 mechanism. The δ analgesia is easily reversed by selective δ antagonists but not by μ or κ_1 antagonists.

TOLERANCE

Repeated opioid use invariably leads to tolerance. However, tolerance is dependent on the receptors being occupied. This is best seen by the lack of cross tolerance between highly selective μ, δ, and κ drugs. Furthermore, tolerance develops at different rates for various actions.[135] Although changes in receptor levels and alterations in second messenger systems have been reported in models of tolerance,[136–145] mounting evidence suggests that tolerance involves the up regulation of antagonistic systems. Cholecystokinin antagonists[146–149] and antidepressants[150–152] enhance morphine analgesia in tolerance animals. However, similar effects are observed in naive animals, implying that they are not directed specifically against the mechanisms of tolerance.

Recently, it was observed that the N-methyl-D-aspartate (NMDA) antagonist dizocilpine (also known as MK-801) blocks morphine tolerance[144] and dependence.[153] Many glutamate actions mediated through NMDA receptors (see Ch. 16) involve the subsequent synthesis and release of nitric oxide (see Ch. 32).[154–157] An inhibitor of nitric oxide synthase, N^G-nitro-L-arginine, prevented morphine tolerance for more than 4 weeks (Fig. 2-5) and even reversed established tolerance.[158,159] N^G-nitro-L-arginine also attenuates dependence.[159,160] Subsequent studies reveal that N^G-nitro-L-arginine

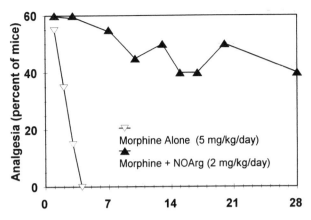

Fig. 2-5 Blockade of morphine tolerance by N^G-nitro-L-arginine. Groups of mice received daily injections of either morphine alone ($\triangle$) or morphine with N^G-nitro-L-arginine. Analgesia was assessed quantally in the tailflick assay. (Data from Kolesnikov et al.[159])

blocks tolerance to morphine and the δ agonist DPDPE but not to κ_1 or κ_3 analgesics.[159] This reinforces the differences in tolerance mechanisms.

GENETIC ISSUES IN OPIOID SENSITIVITY

Clinically, the sensitivity of patients to opioids can vary significantly. Similarly, strains of mice demonstrate marked differences in their sensitivity to opioids (Table 2-5).[161–165] Sensitivity toward one

Table 2-5 Analgesic Sensitivity of Various Strains of Mice^a

Strain	μ	κ_1	κ_3
CD-1	76%	70%	54%
Swiss-Webster	40%	30%	29%
BALB/c	90%	10%	14%
C57/bg^J	62%	0%	0%
C57/+	40%	0%	0%
HS	62%	20%	0%
CXBK	0%	0%	0%

^{a} Mice received fixed subcutaneous doses of morphine (μ; 5 mg/kg), naloxone benzoylhydrazone (κ_3; 50 mg/kg), or U-50,488 (κ_1; 5 mg/kg), and analgesia was assessed quantally in the tailflick assay as the percentage of mice with a doubling or greater of baseline latencies.

(Data from Pick et al.[161])

class of opioid, however, does not predict the sensitivity to another. Sensitivity towards μ, κ_1, and κ_3 opioids appears to be under independent control.[161] The importance of antagonistic systems is growing. Recent evidence now suggests a significant role for σ_1 receptors in the modulation of opioid sensitivity.[166,167] The σ_1 drugs, such as (+)pentazocine, reduce the analgesic response of opioids; σ_1 antagonists reverse this effect (see Ch. 5). Some studies suggest that the sensitivity of strains may reflect the levels of tonic activity of this σ_1 system. Although BALB/c and CD-1 mice have similar sensitivities toward morphine, the BALB/c strain is far less sensitive toward the κ_1 analgesic U-50,488. Blockade of σ_1 actions equalizes the sensitivity of the two strains to U-50, 488.

FUTURE DIRECTIONS

Despite the major advances in our understanding of opioid actions, many questions remain. The recent cloning of several opioid receptors has opened new areas of investigation. The importance of synergy and regional interactions must be explored both in animal models and humans. The identification of novel receptor subtypes helps to explain the pharmacology of drugs that have been used clinically for years. Although levorphanol is a potent μ analgesic, higher doses act through κ_3 receptors.[168] Pentazocine works predominantly through κ_1 receptors; nalbuphine works through a complex combination of κ_3 and κ_1 receptors.[169] At the same time, nalbuphine is an antagonist at μ receptors, capable of blocking the actions of morphine. It is clear that many of our assumptions regarding opioid analgesics have been overly simplistic. Although we have uncovered many secrets about the opioids, many more remain.

REFERENCES

1. Beecher HK: Pain in men wounded in battle. Ann Surg 123:9, 1946
2. Reynolds DV: Surgery in the rat during electrical analgesia induced by focal brain stimulation. Science 164:444, 1969
3. Mayer DJ, Liebeskind JC: Pain reduction by focal electrical stimulation of the brain, an anatomical approach. Brain Res 68:73, 1974
4. Blumberg H, Dayton HB, George M, Rapaport DN: N-allylnoroxymorphone: a potent narcotic antagonist. Fed Proc 20:311, 1961
5. Pasternak GW: Pharmacological mechanisms of opioid analgesics. Clin Neuropharmacol 16:1, 1993
6. Evans CJ, Hammond DL, Frederickson RCA: The opioid peptides. p. 23. In Pasternak GW (ed): The Opiate Receptors. Humana Press, Clifton Park, NJ, 1988
7. Kilpatrick DL, Jones BN, Lewis RV et al: Adrenal opioid proteins of 8,600 and 12,600 Daltons: intermediates in pro-enkephalin processing. Proc Natl Acad Sci U S A 79:307, 1982
8. Gubler U, Seeburg P, Hoffman BJ et al: Molecular cloning establishes pro-enkephalin is a precursor of enkephalin-containing peptides. Nature 295:296, 1982
9. Gubler U, Kilpatrick DL, Seeburg PN et al: Detection and partial characterization of proenkephalin mRNA. Proc Natl Acad Sci U S A 78:5484, 1981
10. Noda M, Furutani Y, Takahashi H et al: Cloning and sequence analysis of cDNA for bovine adrenal proenkephalin. Nature 295:202, 1982
11. Li CH: Lipotropin, a new active peptide from pituitary glands. Nature 201:924, 1964
12. Li CH, Chung D: Isolation and structure of an untriakontapeptide with opiate activity from camel pituitary glands. Proc Natl Acad Sci U S A 3:1145, 1976
13. Nakanishi S, Ione A, Kita T et al: Nucleotide sequence of cloned cDNA for bovine corticotropin-β-lipotropin precursor. Nature 278:423, 1979
14. Bradbury AF, Smyth DG, Snell CR: Lipotropin: precursor to two biologically active peptides. Biochem Biophys Res Commun 69:90, 1976
15. Rossier J, Audigeier Y, Ling N et al: Met-enkephalin-Arg-Phe, present in high amounts in brain of rat, cattle and man, is an opioid agonist. Nature 288:88, 1980
16. Kilpatric DL, Wahlstrom A, Lahm HW et al: Rimorphin, a unique, naturally occurring (Leu)enkephalin-containing peptide found in association with dynorphin and alpha-neo-endorphin. Proc Natl Acad Sci U S A 79:6480, 1982
17. Roemer D, Buescher HH, Pless RC et al: A synthetic enkephalin analogue with prolonged parenteral and oral analgesic activity. Nature 268:47, 1977
18. Pert CB, Bowie DL, Fong BTW et al: Synthetic analogues of Metenkephalin which resist enzymatic destruction. p. 79. In Kosterlitz HW (ed): Opiates and Endogenous Opioid Peptides. North-Holland, Amsterdam, 1976

19. Hahn EF, Pasternak GW: Stereochemistry of opiates and their receptors. p. 441. In Smith D (ed): Handbook of Stereoisomers. CRC Press, Boca Raton, 1984

20. Casey AF: The structure of narcotic analgesic drugs. p. 1. In Clouet D (ed): Narcotic Drugs: Biochemical Pharmacology. Plenum, New York, 1971

21. Harris LS: Structure activity relationships. p. 89. Clouet D (ed): Narcotic Drugs: Biochemical Pharmacology. Plenum, New York, 1971

22. Lewis JW, Bentley KW, Cowan A: Narcotic analgesics and antagonists. Annu Rev Pharmacol 11:241, 1971

23. Kaiko RF, Wallenstein SL, Rogers AG: Analgesic and mood effects of heroin and morphine in cancer patients with post-operative pain. N Engl J Med 304:1501, 1981

24. Szeto HH, Inturrisi CE, Houde RW et al: Accumulation of normeperidine, an active metabolite of meperidine, in patients with renal failure or cancer. Ann Intern Med 86:738, 1977

25. Paul D, Pick CG, Tive LA, Pasternak GW: Pharmacological characterization of nalorphine, a κ_3 analgesic. J Pharmacol Exp Ther 257:1, 1991

26. Houde RW, Wallenstein SL: Clinical studies of morphine-nalorphine combinations. Fed Proc 15:440, 1956

27. Lasagna L, Beecher HK: Analgesic effectiveness of nalorphine and nalorphine-morphine combinations in man. J Pharmacol Exp Ther 112:356, 1954

28. Beckett AH, Casy AF: Synthetic analgesics: stereochemical considerations. J Pharm Pharmacol 6:986, 1954

29. Beckett AH, Casy AF, Harper NJ: Analgesics and their antagonists: some steric and chemical considerations. The influence of the basic group on biological response. J Pharm Pharmacol 8:874, 1956

30. Portoghese PS: A new concept on the mode of interaction of narcotic analgesics with receptors. J Med Chem 8:609, 1965

31. Portoghese PS: Stereochemical factors and receptor interactions associated with narcotic analgesics. J Pharm Sci 55:865, 1966

32. Langley JN: On the contraction of muscle, chiefly in relation to the presence of "receptive" substances. Part IV. The effect of curare and of some other substances on the nicotine response of the sartorius and gastrocnemius muscles of the frog. J Physiol (Lond) 39:235, 1909

33. Pert CB, Snyder SH: Opiate receptor: demonstrated in nervous tissue. Science 179:1011, 1973

34. Terenius L: Characteristics of the "receptor" for narcotic analgesics in synaptic plasma membranes fractions from rab brain. Acta Pharmacol Toxicol 33:377, 1973

35. Simon EJ, Hiller JM, Edelman I: Stereospecific binding of the potent narcotic analgesic ^{3}H-etorphine to rat brain homogenates. Proc Natl Acad Sci U S A 70:1947, 1973

36. Martin WR: Opioid antagonists. Pharmacol Rev 19:463, 1967

37. Martin WR, Eades CG, Thompson JA et al: The effects of morphine and nalorphine-like drugs in the nondependent and morphine-dependent chronic spinal dog. J Pharmacol Exp Ther 197:517, 1976

38. Wolozin BL, Pasternak GW: Classification of multiple morphine and enkephalin binding sites in the central nervous system. Proc Natl Acad Sci U S A 78:6181, 1981

39. Pasternak GW, Wood PL: Multiple μ receptors. Life Sci 38:1889, 1986

40. Pasternak GW, Snyder SH: Identification of noval high affinity opiate receptor binding in rat brain. Nature 253:563, 1975

41. Toll L, Keys C, Polgar W, Loew G: The use of computer modeling in describing multiple opiate receptors. Neuropeptides 5:205, 1984

42. Lutz RA, Cruciani RA, Costa T et al: A very high affinity opioid binding site in rat brain: demonstration by computer modeling. Biochem Biophys Res Commun 122:265, 1984

43. Lutz RA, Cruciani RA, Munson PJ et al: μ_1: a very high affinity subtype of enkephalin binding site in rat brain. Life Sci 36:2233, 1985

44. Fischel SV, Medzihradsy F: Scatchard analysis of opiate receptor binding. Mol Pharmacol 20:269, 1981

45. Rothman RB, Bowen WD, Herkenham M et al: A quanitative study of [^{3}H]D-Ala^2-D-Leu^5-Enkephalin binding to rat brain membranes: evidence that oxymorphone is a noncompetitive inhibitor of the lower affinity δ-binding site. Mol Pharmacol 27:399, 1985

46. Rothman RB, Jacobson AE, Rice KC, Herkenham M: Autoradiographic evidence for two classes of μ opioid binding sites in rat brain using [^{125}I]FK33824. Peptides 8:1015, 1987

47. Clark JA, Houghton R, Pasternak GW: Opiate binding in calf thalamic membranes: a selective μ_1 binding assay. Mol Pharmacol 34:308, 1988

48. Goodman RR, Pasternak GW: Visualization of μ_1 opiate receptors in rat brain using a computerized autoradiographic technique. Proc Natl Acad Sci U S A 82:6667, 1985

49. Moskowitz AS, Goodman RR: Autoradiographic distribution of μ_1 and μ_2 opioid binding in the mouse central nervous system. Brain Res 360:117, 1985

50. Moskowitz AS, Goodman RR: Autoradiographic analysis of μ_1 and μ_2 and δ opioid binding in the central nervous system of C57BL6BY and CXBK (opioid receptor-deficient) mice. Brain Res 360:108, 1985

51. Portoghese PS, Larson DL, Sayer LM et al: A novel opioid receptor site directed alkylating agent with irreversible narcotic antagonistic and reversible agonistic activities. J Med Chem 23:233, 1980

52. Recht LD, Pasternak GW: Effects of β-funaltrexamine on radiolabeled opioid binding. Eur J Pharmacol 230:341, 1987

53. Pasternak GW, Hahn EF: Long acting opiate agonists and antagonists: 14-hydroxydiphydromorphinone hydrazone. J Med Chem 23:674, 1980

54. Ling GSF, Simantov R, Clark JS, Pasternak GW: Naloxonazine actions in vivo, Eur J Pharmacol 129:33, 1986

55. Hahn EF, Carroll-Buatti M, Pasternak GW: Irreversible opiate agonists and antagonists: the 14-hydroxydihydromorphinonazines. J Neurosci 2:572, 1982

56. Pick CG, Paul D, Pasternak GW: Comparison of naloxonazine and β-naloxonazine antagonism of μ_1 and μ_2 opioid actions. Life Sci 48:2005, 1991

57. Pick CG, Nejat RJ, Pasternak GW: Independent expression of two pharmacologically distinct supraspinal μ analgesic systems in genetically different mouse strains. J Pharmacol Exp Ther 265:166, 1993

58. Chen Y, Mestek A, Liu J et al: Molecular cloning and functional expression of a μ-opioid receptor from rat brain. Mol Pharmacol 44:8, 1993

59. Wang JB, Mei Y, Eppler CM et al: μ opiate receptor: cDNA cloning and expression. Proc Natl Acad Sci U S A 90:10230, 1993

60. Thompson RC, Mansour A, Akil H, Watson SJ: Cloning and pharmacological characterization of a rat μ opioid receptor. Neuron 11:1, 1993

61. Fukada K, Kato S, Mori K et al: Primary structures and expression from cDNA's of rat opioid receptor δ and μ subtypes. FEBS Lett 327:311, 1993

62. Evans CJ, Keith DE, Jr, Morrison H et al: Cloning of a δ opioid receptor by functional expression. Science 258:1952, 1992

63. Kieffer BL, Befort K, Gaveriaux-Ruff C, Hirth CG: The δ opioid receptor: isolation of cDNA by expression cloning and pharmacological characterization. Proc Natl Acad Sci U S A 89:12048, 1992

64. Yasuda K, Raynor K, Kong H et al: Cloning and functional comparison of κ and δ opioid receptors from mouse brain. Proc Natl Acad Sci U S A 90:6736, 1993

65. Meng F, Xie GX, Thompson RC et al: Cloning and pharmacological characterization of a rat κ opioid receptor. Proc Natl Acad Sci U S A 90:9954, 1993

66. Ling GSF, Pasternak GW: Spinal and supraspinal opioid analgesia in the mouse: the role of subpopulations of opioid binding sites. Brain Res 271:152, 1983

67. Heyman JS, Williams CL, Burks TF et al: Dissociation of opioid antinociception and central gastrointestinal propulsion in the mouse: studies with naloxonazine, J Pharmacol Exp Ther 245:238, 1988

68. Paul D, Pasternak GW: Differential blockade by naloxonazine of two μ opiate actions: analgesia and inhibition of gastrointestinal transit. Eur J Pharmacol 149:403, 1988

69. Fields HL, Basbaum AI: Brainstem control of spinal pain-transmission neurons. Annu Rev Physiol 40:217, 1978

70. Basbaum AI, Fields HL: Endogenous pain control systems: brainstem spinal pathways and endorphin circuitry. Annu Rev Neurosci 7:309, 1984

71. Fields HL, Heinricher MM, Mason P: Neurotransmitters in nociceptive modulatory circuits. Annu Rev Neurosci 14:219, 1991

72. Yaksh TL, Hammond DL, Tyce GM: Functional aspects of bulbospinal monoaminergic projections in modulating processing of somatosensory information. Fed Proc 40:2786, 1981

73. Bodnar RJ, Williams CL, Lee SJ, Pasternak GW: Role of μ_1-opiate receptors in supraspinal opiate analgesia: a microinjection study. Brain Res 447:25, 1988

74. Pasternak GW, Childers SR, Snyder SH: Opiate analgesia: evidence for mediation by a subpopulation of opiate receptors. Science 208:514, 1980

75. Pasternak GW, Childers SR, Snyder SH: Naloxazone, a long-acting opiate antagonist: effects in intact animals and on opiate receptor binding in vitro. J Pharmacol Exp Ther 214:455, 1980

76. Paul D, Bodnar RJ, Gistrak MA, Pasternak GW: Different μ receptor subtypes mediate spinal and supraspinal analgesia in mice. Eur J Pharmacol 168:307, 1989

77. Vaught JL, Mathiasen JHR, Raffa RB: Examination of the involvement of supraspinal and spinal μ and δ opioid receptors in analgesia using the μ receptor deficient CXBK mouse. J Pharmacol Exp Ther 245:13, 1988

78. Baron A, Shuster L, Elefterhiou BE, Bailey DW: Opiate receptors in mice: genetic differences. Life Sci 17:633, 1975

79. Reith MEA, Sershen H, Vadasz C, Lajtha A: Strain differences in opiate receptors in mouse brain. Eur J Pharmacol 74:377, 1981

80. Besson JM, Chaouch A: Peripheral and spinal mechanisms of nociception. Physiol Rev 67:67, 1987

81. Pert A, Yaksh TL: Sites of morphine induced analgesia in the primate brain. Brain Res 80:135, 1974

82. Lewis VA, Gebhardt GF: Evaluation of the peri-aqueductal gray (PAG) as a morphine-specific locus of action and examination of morphine-induced and stimulation produced analgesia at coincident PAG loci. Brain Res 124:283, 1977

83. Jacquet Y, Lajtha A: Morphine action at central nervous system sites in rat: analgesia or hyperalgesia depending upon site and dose. Science 182:490, 1973

84. Cox BM: Peripheral actions mediated by opioid receptors. p. 357. In Pasternak GW (ed): The Opiate Receptors. Humana Press, Livingston, NJ, 1988

85. Stein C, Millan MJ, Shippenberg TS et al: Peripheral opioid receptors mediating antinociception in inflamation: evidence for involvement of μ, δ and κ receptors. J Pharmacol Exp Ther 248:1269, 1989

86. Stein C, Comisel K, Haimeri E et al: Analgesic effect of intraarticular morphine after arthroscopic knee surgery. N Engl J Med 325:1123, 1991

87. Yeung JC, Rudy TA: Multiplicative interaction between narcotic agonisms expressed at spinal and supraspinal sites of antinocieptive action as revealed by concurrent intrathecal and intracerebroventricular injections of morphine. J Pharmacol Exp Ther 215:633, 1980

88. Bodnar RJ, Paul D, Pasternak GW: Synergistic interactions between the periaqueductal gray and the locus coeruleus. Brain Res 558:224, 1991

89. Foley KM: Pharmacologic approaches to cancer pain management. Adv Pain Res Ther 9:629, 1985

90. Jaffe JH, Marin WR: Opioid analgesics and antagonists. p. 485. In Gilman AG, Rall TW, Nies AS, Taylor P (eds): The Pharmacological Basis of Therapeutics. Pergamon Press, New York, 1990

91. Shimomura K, Kamata O, Ueki S et al: Analgesic effect of morphine glucuronides. Tohoku J Exp Med 105:45, 1971

92. Pasternak GW, Bodnar RJ, Clark JA, Inturrisi CE: Morphine-6β-glucuronide, a potent μ agonist. Life Sci 41:2845, 1987

93. Paul D, Standifer KM, Inturrisi CE, Pasternak GW: Pharmacological characterization of morphine-6β-glucuronide, a very potent morphine metabolite. J Pharmacol Exp Ther 251:477, 1989

94. Ling GSF, Spiegel K, Nishimura S, Pasternak GW: Dissociation of morphine's analgesic and respiratory depressant actions. Eur J Pharmacol 86:487, 1983

95. Ling GSF, Spiegel K, Lockhart SH, Pasternak GW: Separation of opioid analgesia from respiratory depression: evidence for different receptor mechanisms, J Pharmacol Exp Ther 232:149, 1985

96. Gintzler AR, Pasternak GW: Multiple μ receptors: evidence for μ_2 sites in the guinea pig ileum. Neurosci Lett 39:51, 1983

97. Negus SS, Henriksen SJ, Mattox A et al: Effect of antagonist selective for μ, δ and κ opioid receptors on the reinforcing effects of heroin in rats. J Pharmacol Exp Ther 265:1245, 1993

98. Chavkin C, James IF, Goldstein A: Dynorphin is a specific endogenous ligand of the κ opiate receptors. Science 215:413, 1982

99. Von Voightlander PF, Lahti RA, Ludens JH: U50,488: a selective and structurally novel non-μ (κ) opioid agonist, J Pharmacol Exp Ther 224:7, 1983

100. Clark JA, Pasternak GW: U50,488, a κ-selective agent with poor affinity for μ_1 opiate binding sites. Neuropharmacology 27:331, 1988

101. Kosterlitz HW, Paterson SJ, Robson LE: Characterization of the κ-subtype of the opiate receptor in the guinea pig brain. Br J Pharmacol 73:939, 1981

102. Zukin Rs, Eghbali M, Olive D et al: Characterization and visualization of rat and guinea pig brain κ opioid receptors: evidence for κ_1 and κ_2 opioid receptors. Proc Natl Acad Sci U S A 85:4061, 1988

103. Price M, Gistrak MA, Itzhak Y et al: Receptor binding of ^{3}H-naloxone benzoylhydrazone: a reversible κ and slowly dissociable μ opiate. Mol Pharmacol 35:67, 1989

104. Rothman RR, France CP, Bykov V et al: Pharmacological activities of optically pure enantiomers of the κ opioid agonist U50,488 and its cis diastereomer: evidence for three κ receptor subtypes. Eur J Pharmacol 167:345, 1989

105. Clark JA, Liu L, Price M et al: κ Opiate receptor multiplicity: evidence for two U50,488-sensitive κ_1 subtypes and a novel κ_3 subtype. J Pharmacol Exp Ther 251:461, 1989

106. Piercey MF, Varner K, Schroeder LA: Analgesic activity of intraspinally administered dynorphin and ethylketocyclazocine. Eur J Pharmacol 80:283, 1982

107. Han JS, Xie GX, Goldstein A: Analgesia induced by intrathecal injection of dynorphin B in the rat. Life Sci 34:1573, 1984

108. Jhamandas K, Sutak M, Lemaire S: Comparative

spinal analgesia action of dynorphin (1-8), dynorphin (1-13) and a κ-receptor agonist U-50,488H. Can J Physiol Pharmacol 64:263, 1986

109. Piercey MF, Lahti RA, Schroeder LA et al: U-50,488H, a pure κ receptor agonist with spinal analgesic loci in the mouse. Life Sci 31:1197, 1982

110. Takemori AE, Ho BY, Naeseth JS, Portoghese PS: Nor-binaltorphimine, a highly selective κ-opioid antagonist in analgesic and receptor binding assays. J Pharmacol Exp Ther 246:255, 1989

111. Gistrak MA, Paul D, Hahn EF, Pasternak GW: Pharmacological actions of a novel mixed opiate agonist/antagonist: naloxone benzoylhydrazone. J Pharmacol Exp Ther 251:469, 1989

112. Paul D, Levison JA, Howard DH et al: Naloxone benzoylhydrazone (NalBzoH) analgesia. J Pharmacol Exp Ther 255:769, 1990

113. Millan MJ, Czlonkowski A, Lipkowski A, Herz A: κ-opioid receptor-mediated antinociception in the rat. II. Supraspinal in addition to spinal sites of action. J Pharmacol Exp Ther 251:342, 1989

114. Lord JAH, Waterfield AA, Hughes J, Kosterlitz HW: Endogenous opioid peptides: multiple agonists and receptors. Nature 267:495, 1977

115. Chang KJ, Cuatrecasas P: Multiple opiate receptors: enkephalins and morphine bind to receptors of different specificity. J Biol Chem 254:2610, 1979

116. Terenius L: Opioid peptides and opiates differ in receptor selectivity. Psychoneuroendocrinology 2:53, 1977

117. Law PY, Loh HH: ^{3}H-Leu-enkephalin specific binding to synaptic membranes. Comparisons with ^{3}H-dihydromorphine and ^{3}H-naloxone. Res Commun Chem Pathol Pharmacol 21:409, 1978

118. Simantov R, Childers SR, Snyder SH: The opiate receptor binding interactions of ^{3}H-methionine enkephalin, an opiate peptide. Eur J Pharmacol 47:319, 1978

119. Chang KJ, Hazum E, Cuatrecasas P: Possible role of distinct morphine and enkephalin receptors in mediating actions of benzomorphan drugs (putative κ and σ agonists). Proc Natl Acad Sci U S A 77:4469, 1980

120. Pert CB, Pert A, Chang JK, Snyder SH: [D-Ala^2]-Met-enkephalinamide: a potent, long-lasting synthetic pentapeptide analgesic. Science 194:330, 1976

121. Chang KJ, Cooper BR, Hazum E, Cuatrecasas P: Multiple opiate receptors: different regional distribution in the brain and differential binding of opiates and opioid peptides. Mol Pharmacol 16:91, 1979

122. Goodman RR, Snyder SH, Kuhar MJ, Young WS: Differentiation of δ and μ opiate receptor localizations by light microscopic autoradiography. Proc Natl Acad Sci U S A 77:6239, 1980

123. Duka T, Schubert P, Wuster M et al: A selective distribution pattern of different opiate receptors in certain areas of rat brain as revealed by in vitro autoradiography. Neurosci Lett 21:119, 1981

124. Quirion R, Zajac JM, Morgat JL, Rocques BP: Autoradiographic distribution of μ- and δ-opiate receptors in rat brain using highly selective ligands. Life Sci 33:227, 1983

125. Portoghese PS, Sultana M, Nagase H, Takemori AE: Application of the message-address concept in the design of highly potent and selective non-peptide δ opioid receptor antagonists. J Med Chem 31:281, 1988

126. Portoghese PS, Sultana M, Takamori AE: Naltrindole, a highly selective and potent non-peptide δ opioid receptor antagonist. Eur J Pharmacol 146:185, 1988

127. Romer D, Buscher HH, Hill RC et al: A synthetic enkephalin analog with prolonged parenteral and oral analgesic activity. Nature 268:547, 1977

128. Porreca F, Heyman JS, Mosberg HI et al: Role of μ and δ receptors in the supraspinal and spinal analgesic effects of [D-Pen^2,D-Pen^5]enkephalin in the mouse. J Pharmacol Exp Ther 241:393, 1987

129. Porreca F, Mosberg HI, Hurst R et al: Roles of μ, δ and κ opioid receptors in spinal and supraspinal mediation of gastrointestinal transit effects and hot-plate analgesia in the mouse. J Pharmacol Exp Ther 230:341, 1984

130. Schmauss C, Yaksh TL: In vivo studies on spinal opiate receptor systems mediating antinociceptin. II. Pharmacological profile suggesting a differential association of μ, δ and κ receptors with visceral chemical and cutaneous thermal stimuli in the rat. J Pharmacol Exp Ther 228:1, 1984

131. Tung AS, Yaksh TL: In vivo evidence of multiple opiate receptors mediating analgesia in the rat spinal cord. Brain Res 247:75, 1982

132. Mattia A, Farmer SC, Takemori AE et al: Spinal opioid δ antinociception in the mouse: mediation by a 5′-NTII-sensitive δ receptor subtype. J Pharmacol Exp Ther 260:518, 1992

133. Mattia A, Vanderah T, Mosberg HI, Porreca F: Lack of antinociceptive cross-tolerance between [D-Pen^2,D-Pen^5]enkephalin and [D-Ala^2]deltorphin II in mice: evidence for δ receptor subtypes. J Pharmacol Exp Ther 258:583, 1991

134. Jiang Q, Takemori AE, Sultana PS et al: Differential

antagonism of opioid δ antinociception by [D-Ala^2, Leu^5,Cys^6]enkephalin and naltrindole-5'-isothiocyanate: evidence for subtypes. J Pharmacol Exp Ther 257:1069, 1991

135. Ling GSF, Paul D, Simantov R, Pasternak GW: Differential development of acute tolerance to analgesia, respiratory depression, gastrointestinal transit and hormone release in a morphine infusion model. Life Sci 45:1627, 1989

136. Blanchard SG, Chang KJ: Regulation of opioid receptors. p. 425. In Pasternak GW (ed): The Opiate Receptors. Humana Press, Clifton, NJ, 1988

137. Law PY, Hom DS, Loh HH: Opiate regulation of adenosine 3'5'-cyclic monophosphate level in neuroblastoma × glioma NG108-15 hybrid cells. Mol Pharmacol 23:26, 1983

138. Lahti RA, Collins RJ: Chronic naloxone results in prolonged increases in opiate binding sites in brain. Eur J Pharmacol 51:85, 1978

139. Danks JA, Tortella FC, Long JB et al: Chronic administration of morphine and naltrexone up-regulate [^{3}H][D-Ala^2,D-Leu^5]enkephalin binding sites by different mechanisms. Neuropharmacology 27:965, 1988

140. Law PY, Hom DS, Loh HH: Opiate receptor down-regulation and desensitization in neuroblastoma × glioma NG108-15 hybrid cells are two separate cellular adaption processes. Mol Pharmacol 25:413, 1983

141. Sharma SK, Klee WA, Nirenberg M: Dual regulation of adenylate cyclase accounts for narcotic dependence and tolerance. Proc Natl Acad Sci U S A 72:3092, 1975

142. Puttfarcken P, Werling LL, Cox BM: Effects of chronic morphine exposure on opioid inhibition of adenylyl cyclase in 7315c cell membranes: a useful model for the study of tolerance at μ opioid receptors. Mol Pharmacol 33:520, 1988

143. Smith AP, Law PY, Loh HH: Role of opioid receptors in narcotic tolerance/dependence. p. 441. In Pasternak GW (ed): The Opiate Receptors. Humana Press, Clifton, NJ, 1988

144. Trujillo KA, Akil H: Inhibition of morphine tolerance and dependence by the NMDA receptor antagonist MK-801. Science 251:85, 1991

145. Kennedy C, Henderson G: μ-Opioid receptor inhibition of calcium current: development of homologous tolerance in single SH-SY5Y cells after chronic exposure to morphine in vitro. Mol Pharmacol 40:1000, 1991

146. Dourish CT, Hawley D, Iversen SD: Enhancement of morphine analgesia and prevention of morphine

tolerance in the rat by the CCK antagonist, L-364,718. Eur J Pharmacol 147:469, 1988

147. Faris PL, Komisaruk BR, Watkins LR, Mayer DL: Evidence for the neuropeptide cholecystokinin as an antagonist of opiate analgesia. Science 219:310, 1983

148. Panerai AE, Rovati LC, Cocco E et al: Dissociation of tolerance and dependence to morphine: a possible role for cholecystokinin. Brain Res 410:52, 1987

149. Watkins LR, Kinscheck IB, Mayer DJ: Potentiation of opiate analgesia and apparent reversal of morphine tolerance by proglumide, a cholecystokinin antagonist. Science 224:395, 1984

150. Pick CG, Paul D, Eison MS, Pasternak GW: Potentiation of opioid analgesia by the antidepressant nefazodone. Eur J Pharmacol 211:375, 1992

151. Spiegel K, Kourides IA, Pasternak GW: Analgesic activity of tricyclic antidepressants. Ann Neurol 13:462, 1983

152. Botney M, Fields HL: Amitriptyline potentiates morphine analgesia by action on the central nervous system. Ann Neurol 13:160, 1983

153. Higgins GA, Nguyen P, Sellers EM: The NMDA antagonist dizocilpine (MK801) attenuates motivational as well as somatic aspects of naloxone precipitated opioid withdrawal. Life Sci 50:PL167, 1992

154. Garthwaite J, Charles SL, Chess-Williams R: Endothelium-derived relaxing factor release on activation of NMDA receptors suggests role as intercellular messenger in the brain. Nature 336:385, 1988

155. Dawson VL, Dawson TM, London ED et al: Nitric oxide mediates glutamate neurotoxicity in primary cortical cultures. Proc Natl Acad Sci U S A 88:6368, 1991

156. Bredt DS, Snyder SH: Nitric oxide, a novel neuronal messenger. Neuron 8:3, 1992

157. Lancaster JR, Jr: Nitric oxide in cells. Am Scientist 80:248, 1992

158. Kolesnikov YA, Pick CG, Pasternak GW: N^G-Nitro-L-arginine prevents morphine tolerance. Eur J Pharmacol 221:399, 1992

159. Kolesnikov YA, Pick CG, Pasternak GW: Blockade of tolerance to morphine but not κ opioids by a nitric oxide synthase inhibitor. Proc Natl Acad Sci U S A 90:5162, 1993

160. Kimes AS, Vaupel DB, Bruckner M, London ED: Nitroarginine, a nitric oxide synthase inhibitor attenuates morphine withdrawal. Soc Neurosci 17:214.12, 1991

161. Pick CG, Cheng J, Paul D, Pasternak GW: Genetic

influences in opioid analgesic sensitivity in mice. Brain Res 566:295, 1991

162. Baran A, Shuster L, Elfterhiou BE, Bailey DW: Opiate receptors in mice: genetic differences. Life Sci 17:633, 1975

163. Mathiasen JR, Raffa RB, Vaught JL: C57BL/6J-bgj (beige) mice: differential sensitivity in the tailflick test to centrally administered μ and δ opioid receptor agonists. Life Sci 40:1989, 1987

164. Peets JM, Pomerantz B: CXBK mice deficient in opiate receptors show poor electropuncture analgesia. Nature 273:675, 1978

165. Shuster L, Webster GW, Yu G, Elefterhiou BE: Genetic analysis of the response to morphine in mice: analgesia and running. Psychopharmacologica 42:259, 1975

166. Chien CC, Pasternak GW: Functional antagonism of morphine analgesia by (+)pentazocine: evidence for an anti-opioid σ_1 system. Eur J Pharmacol 250:R7, 1993

167. Chien CC, Pasternak GW: Anti-opioid analgesic actions of a σ_1 system. (Submitted)

168. Tive L, Ginsberg K, Pick CG, Pasternak GW: κ_3 receptors and levorphanol analgesia. Neuropharmacology 9:851, 1992

169. Pick CG, Paul D, Pasternak GW: Nalbuphine, a mixed κ_1 and κ_3 analgesic in mice. J Pharmacol Exp Ther 262:1044, 1992

170. Rossi G, Pan Y-X, Cheng J, Pasternak GW: Blockaded morphine analgesia by an antisense oligodeoxynucleotide against the mu receptor. Life Sci (in press)

Chapter 3

Pharmacokinetics of Opioids

J. G. Bovill

Pharmacokinetics is the study of the disposition of a drug in the body, its concentrations in blood and tissues, and how these change with time. It is also the study of those factors, such as absorption, distribution, biotransformation, and elimination, that determine the disposition of the drug. The pharmacologic effects of the opioids are produced by an interaction with one or more of the opioid receptors. For opioids to gain access from the blood to the receptors (situated in the neuronal membranes), they must pass through the capillary endothelial cells into the brain interstitial fluid and, hence, by diffusion to the receptors. The endothelial cells of the brain's microvessels, which form the so-called blood-brain barrier, are characterized by continuous tight endothelial junctions and are much less permeable than are capillaries in other organs. They form an effective barrier, restricting the passage of polar compounds by diffusion. Small polar essential nutrients, such as glucose and amino acids, are transferred by active transport mechanisms and many small polypeptides, such as insulin, by receptor mediated endocytosis.[1] Polar compounds are those containing chemical bonds in which the shared electrons are unevenly distributed between adjacent atoms. The water molecule is a common polar compound. Polar compounds are only soluble in polar solvents; conversely, un-ionized, nonpolar molecules are poorly soluble in water. Despite the barrier formed by the brain's endothelial cells to the entry of polar drugs, the capillary circulation is the major route by which drugs pass from the blood to the brain. How readily individual drugs can cross this barrier is determined by their physical properties, in particular the molecular size, ionization, lipid solubility, and protein binding (Table 3-1).

PHYSICOCHEMICAL PROPERTIES

The opioid analgesics have similar molecular weights, which range from 253 (meperidine) to 416 (alfentanil). The molecular weight correlates highly with the molecular size.[2] Lipid soluble molecules with molecular weights less than about 600 can easily diffuse across the phospholipid and protein layers of cell membranes, including specialized membranes such as the blood-brain barrier and the placental barrier. Poorly lipid soluble drugs, such as morphine, have difficulty in crossing cell membranes, despite a low molecular weight.

Ionization

The degree of ionization of a drug depends on its dissociation constant (pK_a) and the pH of the blood. For basic drugs, the relationship between

Table 3-1 Physicochemical Properties of Opioid Agonists

	Methadone	Morphine	Pethidine	Fentanyl	Alfentanil	Sufentanil
Molecular weight	321	285	253	336	416	387
pK_a	9.3	7.9	8.5	8.4	6.5	8.0
Percent free base (pH 7.4)	1.4	23	7	8.5	89.0	19.7
λ_{ow}	116	1.4	39	816	128	1,757
Protein binding (%)	89	35	70	84	92	93
Bound to AAG (%)	60	<20	60	44	92	83

Abbreviations: AAG, α_1-acid glycoprotein; λ_{ow}, apparent octanol-water partition coefficient at pH 7.4.

the nonionized fraction (F_n) and pH is given by the following equation.

$$F_n = \frac{10^{pH-pK_a}}{1 + 10^{pH-pK_a}}$$

The pK_a of alfentanil is 6.5 so that only 11 percent of its molecules are ionized at pH 7.4 compared with 80 to 92 percent for fentanyl and sufentanil. Morphine is an amphoteric molecule, i.e., it has both basic and acidic properties, with pK_a values of 7.87 and 9.85, respectively. At physiologic pH, however, it acts as an acceptor of protons and can therefore be considered a basic drug. The fourth piperidine ring in the morphine molecule includes a tertiary amine nitrogen, and at pH 7.4, the tertiary amine nitrogen is highly ionized. Approximately 76 percent of the drug is in the ionized form, making the molecule water soluble. In general, it is only nonionized (i.e., free base) molecules that can cross biologic membranes.

The partitioning of a drug between two fluids separated by a biologic membrane is determined by the pK_a of the drug and the pH of the respective fluids. This can be illustrated by looking at the role of the pK_a in determing the absorption of a drug from the gastrointestinal tract. Except for very weak bases (pK_a less than 3), basic drugs are not absorbed from the stomach. As can be seen from Figure 3-1, all opioids will be fully ionized in the acid environment of the stomach (pH 2 to 4). This can be illustrated for fentanyl (pK_a 8.4). In the plasma with a pH 7.4, fentanyl is 91 percent ionized and 9 percent nonionized, whereas any fen-

tanyl in the stomach will be fully ionized. There will be a concentration gradient across the gastric mucosa for nonionized molecules in the plasma that will readily enter the stomach and become ionized and, so, cannot be reabsorbed (ion trapping). If we assume a constant plasma fentanyl concentration of 5 ng/ml, then the concentration of nonionized fentanyl in the plasma not bound to plasma protein (unbound fraction 0.15) will be $5 \times 0.15 \times 0.09 = 0.0675$ ng/ml. At equilibrium, this will also be the concentration of nonionized fentanyl in the gastric juice. However, if the pH of the gastric juice is 2, then the nonionized fraction will only be 3.7×10^{-7} so that the maximum possible concentration of fentanyl (ionized plus nonionized) will be $0.0675/(3.7 \times 10^{-7}) = 182,432$ ng/ml. In practice, this concentration will never be reached because the build-up of fentanyl will be limited by the blood flow to the gastric mucosa. Peak concentrations of fentanyl in gastric juice occurred within about 15 to 30 minutes of intravenous bolus administration and were about 5 to 10 times higher than in the plasma.[3]

The small intestine, where the pH varies between 5 and 8, offers a more favorable opportunity for absorption because of the higher proportion of nonionized molecules and also because of its enormous surface area. These differences in pH within the gastrointestinal tract result in an enterohepatic circulation loop for opioids and other basic drugs. When opioids sequestered in the gastric juice reach the alkaline duodenum and ileum, they can be absorbed into the portal blood stream. It has been suggested that enterohepatic circulation may

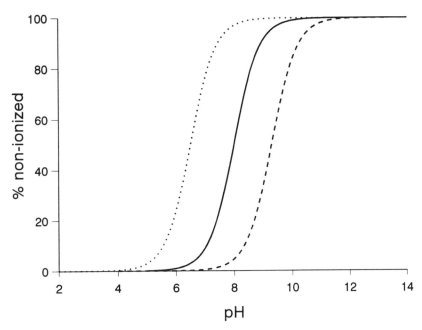

Fig. 3-1 Graphic representation of the change in the nonionized fraction with pH for drugs with different values of pK_a, corresponding to alfentanil (pK_a 6.5; dotted line), sufentanil (pK_a 8.0; solid line), and methadone (pK_a 9.3; dashed line).

be the explanation for observed secondary peaks in the plasma concentration of fentanyl and that this may contribute to the delayed postoperative respiratory depression when opioids are used intraoperatively.[3] However, even if most of the fentanyl that is sequestered in the gastric juice were reabsorbed from the duodenum, because of the large first pass hepatic metabolism, little would reach the systemic circulation. Because of its lower pK_a, conditions for ion trapping and subsequent reabsorption might be more favorable for alfentanil. Furthermore, alfentanil has a lower hepatic extraction than fentanyl so that a higher proportion of the reabsorbed drug might be expected to reach the systemic circulation. However, in rats given fentanyl or alfentanil by infusion to steady state, the differences between fentanyl and alfentanil were minimal; 1.8 ± 0.33 percent of the administered dose of fentanyl and 2.6 ± 0.83 percent of the dose of alfentanil was found in the gut.[4] Simulations by Björkman et al.[4] based on extrapolations of these data from rats to humans suggested that very low amounts of either opioid would be found in the stomachs of humans. Therefore enterohepatic circulation as a cause of delayed respiratory depression is unlikely.

A more likely explanation for the observed secondary peaks in the plasma concentration of fentanyl is the release of fentanyl from body stores, especially muscle, as a result of increased patient activity during the postoperative period. Because of its large mass, muscle can store up to 55 percent of the fentanyl present in the body. The extensive accumulation and slow washout of fentanyl from the muscle compartment provides a depot of drug that can be mobilized if muscle perfusion increases, e.g., during recovery from anesthesia. The muscle-blood partition coefficient for alfentanil is eight times lower than that for fentanyl, and the muscle depot of alfentanil disappears much faster. Therefore, the risk of postoperative respiratory depression should be lower for alfentanil than for fentanyl.[4] Ion trapping can also occur in other body compartments that have a pH lower than that of the blood, e.g., the cerebrospinal fluid, milk, and fetus. Neonates have a lower blood pH than older children (7.30 to 7.35), and hypoxia will result in even lower values (7.2 to 7.25)

Enterohepatic circulation may also occur for drugs that are excreted into the bile either as the parent drug or as metabolites. Hydrolysis of metabolites, particularly conjugates, may subsequently occur in the gut as the result of the action of bacterial enzymes derived from gut flora, and the unconjugated (active) drug may be reabsorbed. There is substantial biliary excretion of morphine, morphine-3-glucuronide (M3G), and morphine-6-glucuronide (M6G); enterohepatic circulation may play a substantial role in the analgesic effects of morphine.[5,6] Enterohepatic circulation may be responsible for the secondary peaks in plasma morphine concentrations observed several hours after oral and intravenous administration of morphine.[6–8]

Lipid Solubility

The lipid solubility of a drug plays a major role in determining the rate at which it can penetrate the central nervous system. It is determined by several factors, including chemical structure. The poor lipid solubility of morphine is related to the presence of two hydroxyl (-OH) groups that confer polar characteristics to the molecule. Polar molecules have poor lipid solubility. The substitution of the hydroxyl groups with acetyl ($CH_3 \cdot CO \cdot O$-) groups produces diamorphine (heroin), a nonpolar, lipid soluble drug (Fig. 3-2). The degree of ionization of a drug is also an important determinant of its lipid solubility. Nonionized molecules are in general 1,000 to 10,000 times more lipid soluble than are the ionized forms and can thus rapidly diffuse across lipid cell membranes. In the laboratory, lipid solubility is estimated by measuring the partitioning of a drug between an organic solvent and an aqueous buffer phase. Unfortunately, there is no organic solvent that fully resembles cell membranes, but good correlations are found between the rates of passage across biologic membranes and partitioning into nonpolar solvents such as n-octanol or n-heptane. The measurements are made first at a pH at which the drug will be fully ionized, e.g., pH 2 for opioids and then at a pH at which the drug will be fully nonionized (pH 10). At any intermediate pH, when the drug will be partially ionized, its lipid solubility can be calculated as the par-

MORPHINE

HEROIN

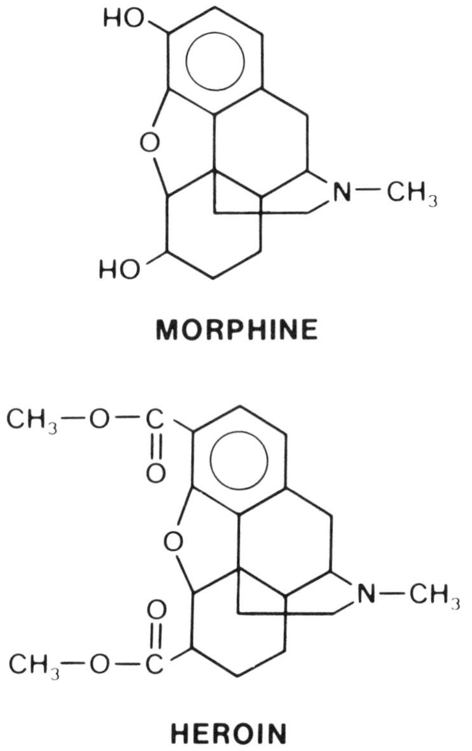

Fig. 3-2 Structure of morphine and heroin.

tition coefficient at that pH, according to the formula.[9]

$$\lambda = \frac{1}{1 + 10^{pH - pK_a}} \cdot \lambda_i + \frac{1}{1 + 10^{pK_a - pH}} \cdot \lambda_{ni}$$

where λ is the partition coefficient at the chosen pH and λ_i and λ_{ni} are the partition coefficients of the fully ionized and fully nonionized drug.

For opioids, the alcohol, n-octanol, is commonly used for the lipid phase so that lipid solubility is frequently represented as the partition coefficient between octanol and water (λ_{ow}). Occasionally, the alcohol, n-heptane, is used for the lipid phase. The value of the partition coefficient when using n-heptane is not the same as with n-octanol, and both will be different from the fat-blood partition coefficient. The fat-plasma partition coefficient for fentanyl is 31 : 1, the λ_{ow} is 955, and the heptane-water partition coefficient is 19.4.[10] The absolute values of the partition coefficients have no direct physiologic meaning; it is the rank order of a series of compounds that is important. In general, when substances are ranked according to their partition coefficient in one solvent, there is approximate correspondence with the rank order in a different solvent.

The octanol-water partition coefficient for alfentanil measured in the laboratory is 128, lower than that of fentanyl or sufentanil. Despite this, alfentanil acts much more rapidly than do these drugs. The half-time for plasma-brain equilibration, estimated using the electroencephalogram (EEG) spectral edge as an effect parameter, is 1.1 minutes for alfentanil and 6.4 minutes for fentanyl.[11] The equilibration half-time for sufentanil is similar to that of fentanyl.[12] The moderate lipid solubility of alfentanil may contribute to its rapid action because fewer molecules will be bound to nonspecific lipid sites in the brain and more will be available in interact with the receptor.

Protein Binding

The degree of protein binding is expressed as the percentage of the drug that is bound to protein in the plasma. An alternative term is the *free fraction*, which is defined as the ratio of the concentration of free (unbound) drug to the concentration of total (sum of free and protein bound) drug in the plasma. Most drug assays measure total drug concentration, i.e., protein bound plus free (unbound) drug. The rate of diffusion of a drug from the blood to the site of action, and thus its effect, is proportional, not to the total concentration, but to the concentration of free drug. The protein binding of the opioids varies from 35 percent for morphine to 93 percent for sufentanil. Morphine binds mainly to albumin, and binding plots show that more than one type of binding site is involved.[13] It is possible that cooperation between binding sites exists because drug binding increases nonproportionally with increasing blood concentrations. As a result of competition for the binding sites, the protein binding of morphine decreases in the presence of methadone or codeine.

Like most basic drugs, fentanyl and its analogs are bound to the acute phase protein α_1 acid glycoprotein (AAG). Binding of fentanyl to AAG (44 percent) is less than that of sufentanil (83 percent)

and alfentanil (92 percent).[9] The contribution of AAG binding as a percentage of total protein binding is less than 20 percent for morphine, about 40 percent for methadone, and 60 percent for meperidine. The concentration of AAG is altered in a variety of disease states. It is elevated following trauma and surgery and in patients with chronic inflammatory diseases or malignancy. It is decreased in neonates, during pregnancy, and in women taking oral contraceptives. The amount of alfentanil required during surgery was significantly higher in patients with Crohn's disease than in other patients undergoing similar surgery.[14] Following surgery, the increase in AAG concentrations may persist for 48 hours or more. In patients with burns, the AAG concentration may be increased by up to 300 percent,[15] and the protein binding of alfentanil was significantly increased (94.2 percent) compared with that in a control group (90.7 percent).[16] The volume of distribution and total clearance of alfentanil was significantly reduced in the burned patients, although the unbound clearance and the elimination half-life were not decreased.

Plasma Disposition

After a bolus intravenous injection or a short intravenous infusion, the plasma concentration of the drug will decrease nonlinearly with time. For most drugs, including opioids, a bi- or triexponential function of the form

$$C(t) = \sum_{i=1}^{2\,or\,3} A_i e^{-\lambda_i t}$$

can be fitted to the concentration time decay curve. This is the basis for the two or three compartment model widely used in pharmacokinetics in which one or two distribution phases are followed by an elimination phase. In the postdistribution phase, the amount of drug remaining in the body can be estimated as the product of plasma concentration and the steady state volume of distribution (V_{ss}). A useful relationship between V_{ss}, clearance (CL), and elimination half-life ($t_{1/2\beta}$) is given by the equation

$$t_{1/2} = \frac{0.693 \cdot V_{ss}}{CL}$$

V_{ss} is directly proportional to the free fraction in the plasma (f_p) and indirectly proportional to the free fraction of the drug in the tissues (f_t), according to the equation[17]

$$V_{ss} = V_p + V_t\left[\frac{f_p}{f_t}\right]$$

where V_p and V_t are the respective plasma and tissues volumes. In general, the greater the degree of protein binding, the less drug will be available to leave the plasma space and, hence, the smaller the volume of distribution. Drugs that are highly bound to plasma proteins but less bound to tissue (f_p/f_t less than 1) have volumes of distributions that are greater than plasma volume but less than the volume of total body water. Conversely, for drugs that are more extensively tissue bound than plasma bound (f_p/f_t more than 1) V_{ss} will be greater than the volume of total body water. For alfentanil, which has high plasma protein binding (91 percent) and moderate lipid solubility (and therefore low tissue binding), V_{ss} is about 30 L. By contrast, for fentanyl, which is less plasma protein bound (85 percent), and highly lipophilic, V_{ss} is on the order of 300 to 400 L. The high lipid solubility of sufentanil might hypothetically be reflected in a volume of distribution larger than that of fentanyl. That this is not the case is due to the higher percentage of sufentanil bound to plasma proteins. This restricts sufentanil to the plasma compartment to a greater extent than fentanyl. Only 8 percent of sufentanil in plasma is distributed in plasma water, and thus is freely mobile throughout the extracellular fluid, compared with 17 percent for fentanyl. Because both drugs have similar clearance values, the lower volume of distribution of sufentanil results in a shorter terminal half-life than that of fentanyl.[19] Obese patients (94.1 ± 14 kg) had an increased volume of distribution of sufentanil (9.1 ± 2.8 L/kg) compared with a control group weighing 70.1 ± 13 kg (5.1 ± 1.7 L/kg) and a prolonged elimination half-life (208 ± 82 versus 135 ± 42 minutes).[19] The altered pharmacokinetics in the obese group was explained by the high lipid solubility of sufentanil.

Changes in pH can alter the disposition of opioids. The Henderson-Hasselbalch equation predicts, for bases, that alkalosis, e.g., as a result of hyperventilation, will increase the nonionized fraction in the plasma. Alkalosis thus increases lipid solubility and may result in an increased volume of distribution. In dogs, hypocarbia decreased the plasma clearance of morphine and fentanyl while increasing their concentration in the brain.[20,21] In humans, hyperventilation caused a decrease in the plasma clearance of fentanyl and prolonged respiratory depression.[22] The volume of distribution of sufentanil was increased in neurosurgical patients hyperventilated to an end tidal CO_2 between 22 and 28 mmHg.[23] Hyperventilation did not influence plasma clearance, but as a result of the increase in the volume of distribution, the elimination half-life increased by 62 percent. Hypocarbia appears to intensify the EEG response to sufentanil in humans.[24] Because the protein binding and lipid solubility of alfentanil are relatively insensitive to pH changes, hyperventilation is unlikely to alter significantly its pharmacokinetics. Changes in blood pH may also alter pharmacodynamic effects. Respiratory alkalosis increased the brain uptake of morphine and enhanced its analgesic effect.[25]

Inherent in the compartmental approach to pharmacokinetics is the concept of half-life. A half-life is defined as the time required for the amount of drug in the body to decrease by 50 percent. This concept is most useful for a drug that can be represented by a one-compartment model, with plasma concentrations declining monoexponentially (for a review of one-compartment kinetics, see Norman[26]). For drugs with multicompartment characteristics, two or more half-lives may be calculated (one for each phase of the multiexponential model), and thus, the concept of half-life is of doubtful clinical usefulness in determining dosage regimens because of the time varying contribution of distribution between compartments.[27] Following multiple or continuous dosing, half-lives provide virtually no insight about the rate of decline in plasma concentration.[28] The route of administration can also affect the terminal half-life. The plasma terminal half-life of fentanyl administered by a transdermal patch was approximately 17 hours after removal of the patch, two to three times that reported after intravenous fentanyl.[29] This was caused by the continued absorption from the depot in the skin; thus, the terminal half-life reflected both the processes of absorption and elimination. The terminal half-life of sufentanil in the plasma is also much longer after epidural injection than after intravenous administration of the same dose.[30,31] For lipophilic drugs, the primary determinant of tissue distribution is tissue blood flow. For alfentanil, a moderately lipophilic opioid, the tissue distribution as measured by intercompartmental clearance is significantly correlated with cardiac output.[32] Cardiac output is likely to be an important factor in determining the response to rapid intravenous administration of alfentanil and other lipid soluble opioids.

To overcome the limited clinical useful of the elimination half-life for drugs with multicompartment kinetics, Hughes et al.[33] devised the concept of "context sensitive half-time," the time required for the drug concentration in the central compartment to decrease by 50 percent following discontinuation of a continuous infusion. The rate of decline in the plasma concentration after stopping an intravenous infusion is not the same as after a bolus injection of the same drug. After a bolus in-

jection, the peripheral compartments are initially empty so that drug can rapidly distribute into them from the central compartment. During an infusion, these peripheral compartments gradually fill up. Therefore, when the infusion is stopped, the contribution made by distribution to the fall in plasma concentration will be correspondingly less. These differences are a function of the duration of the infusion (Fig. 3-3) and reflect the influence of the distribution process on drug disposition. For drugs that have a large peripheral compartment with a slow compartmental clearance, the drug will continue to accumulate in this compartment after stopping even a very long infusion for as long as the concentration in the peripheral compartment is lower than that in the plasma. To use engineering terminology, the peripheral compartment acts as a sink. When the plasma concentration falls below that in the peripheral compartment, the latter will then act as a source, releasing the drug slowly back into the plasma, maintaining the plasma concentration, and thus, prolonging the terminal half-life. Even if an infusion were continued indefinitely, we would still observe a distribution phase in

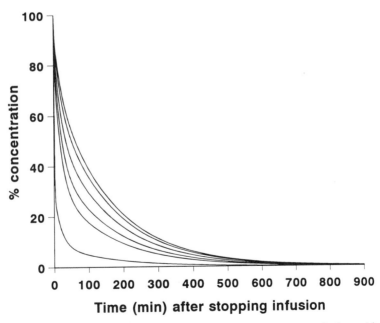

Fig. 3-3 Plasma alfentanil decay curves after cessation of intravenous infusion with constant plasma concentrations (normalized to 100%), for infusions lasting 1 minute (lowest curve) and 15, 30, 60, 120, or 480 minutes (upper curve).

the plasma disposition because the intercompartmental transfer rate constant that determines the rate at which drug can re-enter the central compartment (k_{31} for a 3 compartment model) is always less than the rate constant for drug elimination from the central compartment (k_{10}). Context-sensitive half-times, plotted as a function of infusion duration, are shown in Fig. 3-4 for three opioids. This figure demonstrates the marked differences between this parameter and the elimination half-life. The context-sensitive half-time for alfentanil was significantly longer than that of sufentanil, although the latter has a much longer elimination half-life. Furthermore, fentanyl appeared much less suitable than either alfentanil or sufentanil for long term infusions. These differences arise from the complex effects of the rate constants governing transfer of these drugs between the different compartments.

Shafer and Varvel[27] used computer simulations to predict the rates of decrease in the effect site, and thus the pharmacologic effect, after infusions of alfentanil, sufentanil, and fentanyl. They demonstrated that simply comparing pharmacokinetic parameters, such as half-lives, of different drugs will not reliably predict the rate of change in effect after either a bolus or an infusion. Their analysis suggests that alfentanil by infusion is best used for operations lasting longer than 6 to 8 hours when a rapid decrease in the effect site concentration is desired after stopping the infusion. Alfentanil may also be the most appropriate opioid to provide a transient peak effect after a single bolus. Despite a longer distribution and elimination half-life, sufentanil may be the opioid of choice for intravenous infusion for operations shorter than 6 to 8 hours, with recovery expected to be more rapid than after an infusion of alfentanil. There is good agreement between the context sensitive half-time versus the duration of infusion predicted by Hughes et al.[33] and the recovery curves describing the time required for decreases of 50 percent in the effect site concentrations of fentanyl, alfentanil, and sufentanil described by Shafer and Varvel[27] (Fig. 3-5). Nonetheless these hypotheses still need to be tested in the clinical situation.

In the single compartment model, both the half-life and the clearance serve as meaningful measures of drug elimination, but in a multicompartment system, the half-life does not necessarily

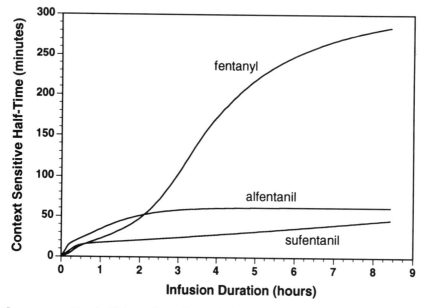

Fig. 3-4 Context sensitive half-times for sufentanil, fentanyl, and alfentanil. Context sensitive half-time is the time required for the central compartment drug concentration to decrease by 50 percent following infusions of varying durations. (Modified from Hughes et al.,[33] with permission.)

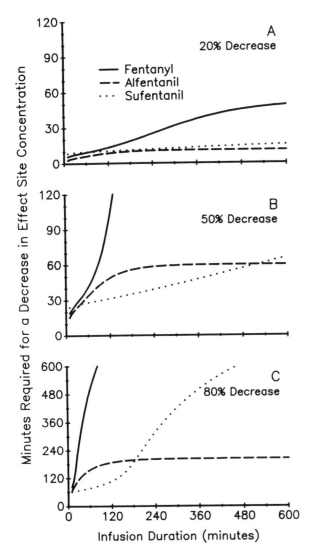

Fig. 3-5 Overlay of the fentanyl, alfentanil, and sufentanil, recovery curves describing the time required for decreases of (A) 20, (B) 50, and (C) 80 percent from the maintained intraoperative effect site concentration after termination of the infusion. (From Shafer and Varvel,[27] with permission.)

reflect the metabolic removal of a drug. On the other hand, clearance, defined as the rate of drug elimination per unit concentration, is a direct measure of this activity and has the advantage that it is independent of any assumptions concerning the pharmacokinetic model. A term related to clearance is *extraction ratio*, which is the fraction of blood

extracted from each unit volume of perfusing blood (maximum value of the extraction ratio = 1). The product of the extraction ratio and organ blood flow equals organ clearance. Hepatic clearance is a function of hepatic blood flow and the ability of the liver to extract the drug as it perfuses hepatic capillaries. To overcome the modifying effect of flow on the removal of drug, the term *intrinsic clearance* (CL_{int}) is used. This term indicates the maximum ability of the liver to remove drug in the absence of flow limitations.[34] Rowland et al.[35] used the more descriptive term metabolizing capacity.

For drugs with a high extraction ratio (approaching unity), the hepatic clearance will be virtually independent of protein binding because almost all drug passing through the liver is extracted. This implies that the drug must be "stripped" from the plasma proteins during its passage through the liver, and therefore, hepatic clearance is not restricted by binding to proteins. Restrictive clearance, i.e., clearance that is restricted by the degree of protein binding, occurs when the hepatic extraction ratio is less than the free fraction in the plasma. Under conditions of restrictive clearance, $CL = f_b \cdot CL_{int}$ where f_b is the free fraction in the blood.

The hepatic extraction of fentanyl and sufentanil is high, and intrinsic hepatic clearance is greater than the hepatic blood flow. The clearance of these drugs will, therefore, be dependent mainly on hepatic blood flow. Anesthesia and surgery decrease hepatic blood flow and drug clearance.[37–39] Conversely, because the liver has such a large reserve capacity of metabolizing enzymes, the elimination of these drugs is unlikely to be significantly altered in patients with hepatic disease until hepatic function becomes severely compromised. In contrast with fentanyl and sufentanil, alfentanil has an intermediate hepatic extraction of 0.3 to 0.5, and alfentanil clearance could be influenced by alterations of plasma protein binding, hepatic blood flow, or hepatic enzyme activity.[40]

Epidural and Intrathecal Opioids

Drugs injected into the epidural or intrathecal space also undergo processes of absorption, distribution, and elimination, although these processes are often more complex than after administration by other routes. After epidural injection, an opioid may undergo transfer into the blood stream or into the cerebrospinal (CSF), or it may be bound to epidural fat, which will act as a reservoir for epidural opioids, the extent depending on their lipophilicity. Transfer into the CSF may take place by direct penetration through the dura and also by diffusion along the perineural cuffs of the dura. Opioids in the CSF will undergo distribution within the CSF space as a result of passive diffusion and CSF bulk flow. Ultimately, all spinally administered opioids will be eliminated by systemic absorption into blood vessels in the spinal canal. In the case of a drug given as an intravenous bolus, there is a fairly rapid and uniform distribution in the blood so that the distribution and elimination phases can be clearly described. In the case of epidural or intrathecal administration, the distribution is neither rapid nor uniform. In particular, absorption from the epidural space into the blood will continue for a relatively long time, overlapping the time when calculations of the elimination half-life and other pharmacokinetic parameters typically are being made.[41] Despite these difficulties, in recent years we have obtained considerable insights into the pharmacokinetics of many spinally administered opioids in humans.

Lipid solubility is important in determining the ability of opioids and other analgesic drugs to move from the epidural space across the spinal meninges to reach their sites of action in the dorsal horn of the spinal cord. The arachnoid mater, which is the principal permeability barrier for drugs diffusing across the meninges,[42] has a structure in many ways resembling that of the endothelial layer of the cerebral capillaries forming the blood-brain barrier. It consists of multiple tiers of overlapping cells connected to one another by tight and occluding junctions.[2] This cellular barrier can be considered to consist of a hydrophilic region (extracellular and intracellular water) and a lipophilic region (cell membrane lipids). Bernards and Hill[2] demonstrated that the permeability of a drug through the meninges was not related to molecular size but was correlated with lipid solubility, though in a nonlinear fashion (Fig. 3-6). There was a biphasic relationship between the octanol-buffer partition coefficient and a drug's permeability coefficient. Drugs

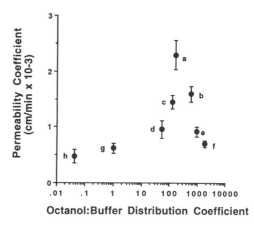

Fig. 3-6 Plot of octanol-buffer (pH, 7.4) distribution coefficient versus experimentally determined permeability coefficient for monkey spinal meninges. The individual data points are: a = alfentanil; b = bupivacaine; c = lidocaine; d = haloperidol; e = fentanyl; f = sufentanil; g = morphine; and h = tetracycline. (From Bernards and Hill,[2] with permission.)

that were either very hydrophobic or hydrophilic were significantly less permeable than were those with intermediate lipid solubilities. Maximum meningeal permeability was associated with λ_{ow} values between 129 (alfentanil) and 560 (bupivacaine). The authors concluded that the aqueous-lipid interface is the rate limiting step in the diffusion of drugs through the meninges. Very hydrophilic molecules will be excluded entirely from the lipid barrier, whereas very highly lipophilic molecules, although they easily enter the lipid region, will have great difficulty in entering the aqueous phase of the CSF.

Morphine appears rapidly in the plasma after epidural or intrathecal injection, with peak plasma concentrations being attained within 5 to 10 minutes.[43–46] The systemic absorption of morphine does not appear to be significantly affected by the volume in which it is administered, but the addition of epinephrine to solutions for intrathecal use significantly reduces systemic absorption.[47] The peak morphine concentration in the plasma after 3 mg of morphine in 1 ml of solution (33.3 ± 7.4 ng/ml; mean ± standard error of the mean) was similar to that when the same dose was given in a volume of

10 ml (39.5 ± 2.9 ng/ml).[45] When morphine 0.3 mg was injected intrathecally, plasma concentrations were low (4.5 ± 1.1 ng/ml).[46] By contrast, the maximum concentration of morphine in the CSF was 6,410 ng/ml.[46] The minimum analgesic concentration of morphine in plasma is about 20 to 40 ng/ml,[48,49] thus morphine absorbed into the plasma after intrathecal administration is unlikely to contribute significantly to the analgesic effect. In the studies from Sjöström et al.,[45,46] referred to earlier, blood samples were obtained from the superior vena cava. Blood from the epidural venous plexus is drained to the superior vena cava through the azygos vein, and it is probable that the concentrations would have been lower in peripheral venous or arterial blood.

After epidural administration, morphine passes relatively slowly into the CSF with an absorption half-life of 22 minutes. Maximum CSF concentrations were only attained 60 to 90 minutes after injection of morphine (Fig. 3-7). CSF concentrations also fell slowly with a terminal half-life of 370 minutes (Fig. 3-8). This slow transfer explains the slow onset and prolonged duration of analgesia associated with epidural morphine. Only about 4 percent of an epidural dose of morphine crosses the dura; therefore, the dose of intrathecal morphine required to produce effective analgesia should also be about 4 to 5 percent of the effective epidural dose. This is borne out by clinical experience.

The amount of meperidine that is transferred into the CSF after epidural injection is also about 4 percent, the same as for morphine. However, the major difference between epidural meperidine and morphine is that meperidine rapidly crosses the dura, with an absorption half-life of about 8 minutes, three times shorter than that of morphine.[45] This difference between these two opioids reflects the key role of lipophilicity in dural transfer. Similarly, meperidine concentrations decreased in the CSF four times faster than did those of morphine. The more rapid transfer and faster decline in CSF concentration account for the more rapid onset and shorter duration of analgesia with epidural meperidine compared with morphine. It also supports the view that the analgesic action of these drugs given epidurally is predominantly the result of a spinal action. The rapid clearance of the more

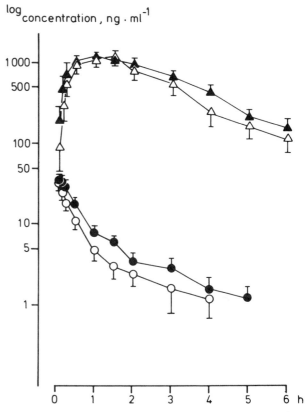

Fig. 3-7 Mean morphine cerebrospinal fluid (*open triangles*, group I; *solid triangles*, group II) and plasma concentrations (*open circles*, group I; *solid circles*, group II) after epidural administration of morphine, 3 mg in 1 ml (group I) or 3 mg in 10 ml (group II). (From Sjöström et al.,[46] with permission.)

lipophilic meperidine from the lumbar CSF means that it is less likely to migrate cephalad within the CSF to cause direct brain stem mediated respiratory depression. However, significant amounts of meperidine have been measured at the C7–T1 level after lumbar epidural injection, and the peak concentration at this level occurred earlier than for morphine.[50] Meperidine concentrations in the cervical CSF decreased more rapidly than did those of morphine so that respiratory depression caused by a rostral spread of meperidine is likely to occur earlier and be of shorter duration than with morphine.

Sufentanil is a highly lipophilic opioid that has been given extensively by the spinal route in hu-

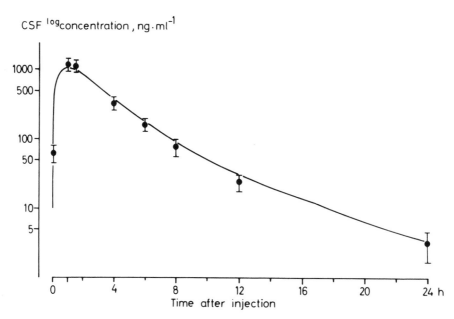

Fig. 3-8 Mean morphine cerebrospinal fluid concentrations after epidural administration of morphine, 3 mg. (From Sjöström et al.,[46] with permission.)

mans. Sufentanil can be detected in the plasma within 2 minutes after epidural injection.[30,31,51] Plasma concentrations of sufentanil were similar within 15 minutes after injection when sufentanil 150 μg was injected either epidurally or intravenously 5 to 10 minutes before skin incision in patients undergoing elective major abdominal surgery.[30,31] In rats, significant binding of sufentanil in the brain was detected after lumbar epidural injection, although the amount bound was three to seven times less than after intravenous sufentanil in all areas of the brain except the medulla oblongata.[52] In the lumbar spinal cord, sufentanil binding was about three times higher after epidural than after intravenous administration, whereas binding to the thoracic and cervical cord was similar with both routes. This suggests that at least part of the analgesic effects produced by epidural sufentanil is the result of a supraspinal action consequent to systemic absorption from the epidural space.

The transfer of sufentanil from the epidural space into the CSF occurs more slowly than into the plasma, peak CSF concentration being attained at about 50 minutes.[31] This may be related to the high lipid solubility of sufentanil.[2] As with other epidu-

ral opioids, there is considerable interpatient variability in dural transfer, possibly reflecting differences in the amount of epidural fat and the proximity of the injection drug to epidural arachnoid granulations through which a large amount of the injected dose could rapidly reach the CSF. This variability highlights the need to individualize the dose of spinal opioids to minimize the risk of respiratory depression. The ratio between the spinal dose of an opioid producing effective analgesia and the dose that causes severe respiratory depression is not much in excess of two.[41] After intravenous injection of sufentanil only minimal amounts reach the CSF; the concentrations were below the detection limit in 7 of 10 patients given a single intravenous bolus of 150 μg of sufentanil.

After intrathecal injection of sufentanil 150 μg, transfer from the CSF into the blood is rapid (C_{max} 0.54 ± 0.21 ng/ml, T_{max} 6.6 ± 0.3 minutes; mean $\pm$ standard deviation), although plasma concentrations of sufentanil during the first hour after injection were significantly less than after the same dose given epidurally.[30] After 1 hour, plasma sufentanil concentrations were higher in the patients given sufentanil intrathecally than in those who received it epidurally. The rapid and sustained uptake of sufentanil from the CSF into the central circulation may be because the CSF is protein free; therefore, all sufentanil will be unbound or free in the CSF. However, it may also be related to the high dose of sufentanil administered by Ionescu et al.[30] In patients given sufentanil 15 μg intrathecally, the maximum concentrations in the plasma was 0.15 ± 0.02 ng/ml (mean ± standard error of the mean [SEM]), which was reached at 39 ± 10 minutes.[53] In that study, the concentration in the CSF was always considerably higher than in the plasma, but it declined more rapidly. The mean residence time of sufentanil in the CSF was 0.9 ± 0.8 hours compared with 6.8 ± 0.6 hours in the plasma.

Epidural Fentanyl

Although epidural fentanyl has become widely used in recent years, especially in obstetrics, information about the pharmacokinetics of this route of administration is limited. In the goat, after epidural administration, morphine and fentanyl are absorbed into the CSF at the same rate, with maximum CSF concentrations being reached at about 12 to 15 minutes.[54] When epidural fentanyl 80 μg was given to patients during the first stage of labor, the mean (± SEM) maximum plasma fentanyl concentrations of 1.01 ± 0.16 ng/ml (range, 0.12 to 1.55 ng/ml) were reached in 5 to 20 minutes.[55] Plasma concentrations were higher and rose faster after epidural administration compared with the same dose of fentanyl given intramuscularly. By contrast, Gourlay et al.[56] reported minimal vascular uptake of fentanyl after giving epidural fentanyl 1 μg/kg through a lumbar epidural catheter to patients with chronic noncancer pain. There was rapid penetration of the fentanyl across the dura mater, with mean maximum lumbar CSF concentrations of 19 ng/ml at 22 minutes. The fentanyl that reached the lumbar CSF underwent cephalad migration, albeit to a small extent. The mean maximum cervical CSF concentrations of fentanyl were only 10 percent of the lumbar CSF concentrations. Maximum concentrations in the cervical CSF occurred between 10 and 45 minutes after epidural injection.

The duration of analgesia with a single shot epidural injection of fentanyl is relatively short (2 to 4 hours), reflecting its lipophilicity. Rostaing et al.[57] investigated the consequences of the combination of clonidine, an α_2 adrenoceptor agonist, with epidural fentanyl. Clonidine enhances opioid-induced analgesia in laboratory animals.[58] Patients recovering from abdominal aortic surgery were given epidural fentanyl 100 μg either alone or in combination with clonidine 150 μg. The onset of analgesia was similar in both groups, around 13 minutes, but the duration was more than doubled in patients receiving clonidine (543 ± 183 versus 250 ± 64 minutes). Peak plasma fentanyl concentrations were comparable in the two groups (0.29 ± 0.15 ng/ml at 16.2 ± 14.8 minutes in the fentanyl only group and 0.27 ± 0.11 ng/ml at 8.3 ± 5.5 minutes in the fentanyl and clonidine group).

To overcome the short duration of epidural fentanyl, it may be given as a continuous epidural infusion. A continuous epidural infusion of fentanyl 100 μg/h given to patients after knee surgery resulted in plasma fentanyl concentrations of 1.7 ng/ml after 18 hours, which was similar to that produced by an intravenous infusion of fentanyl at the same rate.[59] The degree of analgesia and the incidence of side effects were similar with the two routes of administration, and it was concluded that the continuous epidural administration of fentanyl offered no clinical advantages over the intravenous route for the management of postoperative pain. Similar conclusions were reached by others who compared continuous epidural and intravenous infusion of fentanyl in patients after thoracotomy[60] or cesarean section.[61] By contrast, Salomäki et al.[62] found that there was a clinical advantage with continuous epidural fentanyl after thoracotomy because patients in their epidural group required lower fentanyl infusion rates and had lower plasma concentrations than did those receiving intravenous infusions of fentanyl. In these studies, the fentanyl infusion rates were adjusted to obtain maximum patient comfort. In general, epidural infusions of fentanyl of about 1 μg/kg/h provided good analgesia and resulted in plasma fentanyl concentrations of about 1 ng/ml.

Plasma alfentanil concentrations in volunteers were similar after epidural and intramuscular alfentanil 15 μg/kg (15 to 22 ng/ml in the epidural group and 14 to 24 ng/ml in the intramuscular group).[63] Chauvin et al.[64] compared epidural alfentanil, 15 μg/kg and 30 μg/kg, with intramuscular alfentanil, 15 μg/kg, in patients with postoperative pain. Maximum plasma alfentanil concentrations were 54.3 ± 10.8 ng/ml (mean ± SEM), 155 ± 28 ng/ml, and 74.2 ± 18.4 ng/ml, respectively, in the three groups. The times to peak concentrations were similar in each group, about 16 minutes. Both epidural doses provided effective analgesia, although the duration was short, 45 to 80 minutes. None of the patients given intramuscular alfentanil obtained pain relief. In pregnant women undergoing normal vaginal delivery given epidural analgesia with a loading dose of alfentanil 30 μg/kg followed by a continuous epidural infusion of 30 μg/kg/h, maternal plasma concentrations of alfentanil at birth were between 21 and 48 ng/ml.[65] Umbilical venous total alfentanil concentrations were between 4.8 and 16.2 ng/ml. In patients after abdominal hysterectomy, a loading dose of epidural alfentanil 15 μg/kg followed by a constant rate infusion of 18 μg/kg/h for 20 hours resulted in plasma concentrations that varied between 23 and 68 ng/ml.[66]

The studies described suggest that systemic absorption of alfentanil after epidural administration is substantial and will likely make a significant contribution to the analgesia produced. Burm et al.[67] studied the systemic absorption of alfentanil following epidural administration using a stable isotope method in patients undergoing abdominal surgery. Patients received a bolus dose of deuterium labeled alfentanil, 1 mg, injected into the epidural space and, at the same time, an intravenous infusion of unlabeled alfentanil was given at 1 mg/h for 1 hour. Blood samples were collected for 12 hours, and plasma concentrations of labeled and unlabeled alfentanil were determined with a combination of gas chromatography and mass fragmentography. From these data, the absorption profile of alfentanil was determined using constrained point area deconvolution. All of the epidurally administered alfentanil was recovered in the plasma. Alfentanil was slowly absorbed from the epidural space into the systemic circulation, with an absorption half-life of 92 ± 29 minutes (mean ± standard deviation [SD]).

Metabolism and Excretion

There are two main mechanisms whereby drugs are removed from the body, metabolism and excretion. For the opioids, as for most drugs, the liver is the main organ responsible for metabolism. Excretion of the metabolic products and, to a lesser extent, the parent drug occurs primarily through the kidney; other routes of excretion are the biliary system and the intestines. In general, only water soluble polar substances can be excreted by these routes, and a characteristic of metabolic transformation is that the products are more polar than the parent drug. The reactions involved in drug metabolism are classified into two groups. Phase I reactions are oxidative or reductive reactions that alter and create new functional groups and hydrolytic reactions that metabolize esters and amides. Phase II reactions are conjugation reactions in which the drug, or more often its metabolite, is coupled to an endogenous substrate, such as glucuronic acid or sulfuric acid. For the phenylpiperidine opioids, i.e., meperidine and the fentanyl analogs, biotransformation occurs primarily by hepatic phase I metabolism, catalyzed by cytochrome P-450 isoenzymes. The major metabolic pathways are N-dealkylation and O-demethylation, both in animals[68,69] and humans.[70,71] The cytochrome P-450 enzymes are membrane proteins associated with the endoplasmic reticulum. They are a heterogeneous class of enzymes, but each enzyme contains one molecule of heme, which functions in the reduction of oxygen and the subsequent oxidation process.

Some drugs and xenobiotics inhibit drug metabolism by forming metabolic intermediate complexes with cytochrome P-450. The H_2 receptor antagonist cimetidine inhibits the P-450 mediated metabolism of a variety of drugs, including morphine[72] and fentanyl.[73] Borel et al.[74] studied dogs pretreated with cimetidine, 10 mg/kg intramuscularly, the night before and 5 mg/kg intramuscularly 90 minutes before receiving fentanyl, 100 μg/kg intravenously. The dogs served as their own controls in a double crossover protocol with a minimum of 3 weeks between studies. Cimetidine significantly increased the elimination half-life of fentanyl from 155 to 340 minutes. In addition to inhibiting cytochrome P-450 mediated oxidation, cimetidine also causes a considerable reduction in hepatic blood flow, interfering further with drug metabolism.[75] Cimetidine inhibits metabolism by binding to the heme of cytochrome P-450 through its imidazole and cyano groups.[76] Ranitidine, another H₂ receptor antagonist, does not contain an imidazole ring and impairs drug metabolism much less than does cimetidine. Both drugs, however, reduce hepatic blood flow by similar amounts. The antibiotic erythromycin is also an inhibitor of hepatic metabolic processes. The elimination of alfentanil is significantly slowed in patients treated with erythromycin,[77] and this can delay recovery and result in prolonged postoperative respiratory depression.[78]

The P-450 monoxygenases are a complex family of hepatic enzymes that are responsible for metabolizing a wide range of substances, including many drugs. The classification of these enzymes has often been confusing; this chapter adheres to the recent classification described by Nebert et al.[79] About 5 to 10 percent of whites have a genetic deficiency of the P-450 2D6 enzyme and are poor metabolizers of the antihypertensive drug debrisoquin. The abnormal phenotype is inherited as an autosomal recessive trait. There is considerable ethnic variation in the incidence of the phenotype, even among whites. The incidence is about 3 percent in Sweden, 12 to 15 percent in West Africa, and only 1.5 percent in Egypt; it also thought to be very low in Japan.[80,81] The cytochrome P-450 2D6 enzyme is involved in the formation of morphine from codeine.[82,83] Metabolically formed morphine is thought to be responsible for most of the analgesic effect of codeine, and in subjects who are poor metabolizers of debrisoquin, codeine is without analgesic effect.[84]

It had been suggested that the metabolism of alfentanil, and possibly also that of fentanyl, might be subject to polymorphic oxidation by P-450 2D6 enzyme.[85] However, it is now known that this is not the case, both from in vitro studies using human hepatic[86] and rat microsomes[68] and from evidence in subjects, who, although poor metabolizers of debrisoquin, had normal metabolic patterns for al-

fentanil.[32,71] A recent study has clearly demonstrated that the liver enzyme responsible for oxidative metabolism of alfentanil is P-450 3A4.[87] The main metabolic pathway for alfentanil is oxidation (N-dealkylation) with the formation of noralfentanil.[68,88] Fentanyl, sufentanil, and meperidine also undergo oxidation to norfentanyl, norsufentanil, and normeperidine. Normeperidine is toxic, producing tremor, hyperactive reflexes, and convulsions. Neither fentanyl or alfentanil have metabolites that are pharmacologically active. However, one of the metabolites of sufentanil, desmethyl sufentanil, is pharmacologically active with a potency about one-tenth that of the parent drug. This metabolite is thus approximately equipotent with fentanyl.[89] However, desmethyl sufentanil is a relatively minor metabolite of sufentanil, and its contribution to the overall pharmacologic effect is likely to be negligible. After sufentanil, 3 μg/kg, desmethyl sufentanil cannot be detected in the plasma; in the urine, it amounts to not more than 0.3 percent of the administered dose.[90] Among other important drugs metabolized by cytochrome P-450 3A4 are midazolam, lidocaine, and several antibiotics, including erythromycin. It is possible that the interactions between alfentanil and erythromycin described earlier are related to this common metabolic pathway. Markedly raised plasma concentrations of midazolam, associated with unconsciousness, occurred in an 8-year-old boy given oral midazolam 0.5 mg/kg as premedication, followed by an intravenous infusion of erythromycin.[91] It was assumed that this was the result of an altered hepatic clearance of midazolam caused by the erythromycin.

Remifentanil (GI87084B), a new opioid undergoing clinical trials at the time of writing this chapter, has a novel metabolism for an opioid. Remifentanil is a phenylpiperidine that contains an ester linkage that allows it to be broken down by blood and tissue esterases. It undergoes extremely rapid metabolism, with a clearance of 2 to 7 L/min and an elimination half-life of only 5 to 12 minutes.[92,93] Remifentanil also has a fast onset of action with a plasma-brain equilibration half-life of 1.3 minutes,[92] similar to that of alfentanil. This novel new opioid could have promising clinical potential, particularly when a rapid onset and offset of opioid effect is desirable.

Morphine Conjugation

In contrast with the phenylpiperidine opioids, the major metabolic route for morphine biotransformation is by phase II conjugation. In adults, more than 70 percent of morphine undergoes glucuronide conjugation to M3G, the major metabolite, and M6G. Five to 10 percent is sulfate conjugation. About 1 to 2 percent is excreted by the kidneys as unconjugated drug.[94,95] In dogs, there is evidence that the enzyme system responsible for glucuronidation of morphine is saturable; therefore, the systemic availability of oral morphine increases with increasing doses.[96] However, there is no evidence of enzyme saturability in humans, and the systemic availability of morphine in humans appears to be independent of the dose or duration of treatment.[5,97] Two different sites have been suggested for morphine metabolism, the liver and kidney. Although classically the liver has been considered the primary metabolizing organ, normal morphine metabolism has been described in patients with hepatic disease,[98] although others have reported a decreased clearance of morphine in patients with cirrhosis.[99] The importance of hepatic metabolism has been emphasized by studies of patients undergoing liver transplantation. Bodenham et al.[100] studied the pharmacokinetics of morphine and its metabolites in seven adult patients undergoing orthotopic hepatic transplantation. Patients were given morphine, 10 mg intravenously, at the beginning of the anhepatic phase. Plasma concentrations decreased rapidly as a result of distribution. Small, but measurable, concentrations of M3G and M6G were found in the plasma and urine during this phase. Morphine's metabolism increased markedly when the new donor liver was reperfused; plasma M3G concentrations increased from less than 7 ng/ml during the anhepatic phase to a maximum of 236 ng/ml within 30 to 50 minutes after reperfusion. The pharmacokinetics and metabolism of morphine in the immediate postoperative period after liver transplantation were similar to those in other postsurgical patients.[101]

Although the liver is the primary organ of conjugation, extrahepatic metabolism of morphine may occur. Conjugation of morphine to glucuronide has been demonstrated in the kidneys and gut wall in animals[102] and in the human fetus.[103] More recently, Mazoit et al.[95] studied morphine pharmacokinetics in six patients in whom catheters were placed in the portal and hepatic veins and the superior mesenteric vein. After a bolus injection of morphine, no concentration gradient was observed between the arterial and mesenteric venous blood, indicating that no gut wall metabolism of morphine was occurring. The total body clearance of morphine exceeded the hepatic clearance by 38 percent, and it was concluded that the extrahepatic clearance probably occurred through the kidney. This may have important therapeutic implications in patients after renal transplantion and can explain the findings of normal clearance of morphine in patients with cirrhosis and liver failure.[98,104]

The lung has been investigated as a potential site of morphine metabolism. The lung in humans is capable of the uptake of morphine and other opioids,[105,106] but there is no evidence for actual pulmonary metabolism of morphine.[107,108] The human brain also contains a uridine diphosphate glucuronyl transferase system, and glucuronidation of morphine and naloxone has been found in microsomal fractions from various parts of the brain known to contain endorphin systems and opioid receptors.[109] The formation rate of M3G was 10 to 25 times lower than in hepatic tissue. Although the formation rate of M6G was only 10 percent that of M3G, the formation of this pharmacologically active metabolite in close proximity to the opioid receptor rich areas, where even minute amounts may produce pharmacologic effects, could be of clinical relevance.

M3G has no analgesic activity but may antagonize the analgesic effects of morphine.[110] M6G is pharmacologically active with a potency about 45 times higher than that of morphine when administered intracerebrally to the mouse.[111] Its affinity for μ_1 and μ_2 receptors in the rat brain was similar to that of morphine,[112] and it was only three times less potent than morphine in displacing naloxone binding from opioid receptors in the bovine brain.[113] Despite its polarity, M6G can cross the blood-brain barrier, and it was found in the CSF within 2 hours of a parenteral dose of morphine.[114]

It was eliminated more slowly than morphine from the CSF, with an average half-life of 10.5 hours.[115] M6G occurs in significant quantities after the administration of morphine, and its concentration in plasma exceeded that of the parent drug by a factor of 9:1 within 30 minutes of the intravenous administration of morphine.[116] When administered intravenously[117] or intrathecally[115] to patients with cancer, M6G produced significant analgesia, and there is evidence that it contributes to the analgesic effect of morphine.[118] In healthy subjects, the pharmacokinetics of morphine and M6G are similar after intravenous administration,[116,119] but the elimination half-life of M6G in patients with cancer was twice that reported in healthy subjects.[117] After oral administration of morphine, the terminal half-life of both glucuronide metabolites are markedly prolonged.[116] After intravenous injection, these were 1.7 ± 0.9 hours (mean ± SD), 3.9 ± 1.5 hours, and 2.6 ± 0.7 hours for morphine, M3G, and M6G, respectively. The corresponding values after oral morphine were 1.3 ± 0.5, 9.5 ± 8.6, and 10.7 ± 9.2 hours (Fig. 3-9) The bioavailability of morphine after oral administration was 20 ± 8.7 percent. M6G is a ventilatory depressant with a potency substantially in excess of morphine. Even allowing for its slower penetration into the brain, it may be that 50 percent or more of the respiratory depression observed by 1 hour following systemic administration of morphine is the result of this metabolite, and this contribution will subsequently increase with time.[120]

Patients with renal insufficiency have relatively normal metabolism and elimination of morphine, but they do have impaired elimination of morphine glucuronides[94,121] with a significant correlation between the M3G half-life and renal function, as estimated by the serum urea level.[94] The elimination half-life of M3G varied between 14.5 and 119 hours (mean, 49.6 hours) in uremic patients compared with 2.4 to 6.7 hours (mean, 4.0 hours) in patients with normal kidney function. Shelley et al.[104] studied two children in end stage hepatic failure, one of whom was also in renal failure and oliguric. Both patients metabolized morphine rapidly, but in the patient with renal failure, there was an accumulation of the metabolites. She continued to be unresponsive to painful stimuli and had pinpoint pupils for 24 hours after a single dose of morphine, 1 mg/kg. She became responsive to stimuli and her pupils enlarged within 1 hour after she developed a large diuresis. Accumulation of M6G is thought to be responsible for the prolonged action of morphine in patients with renal

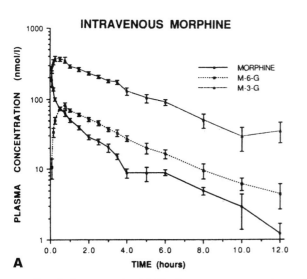
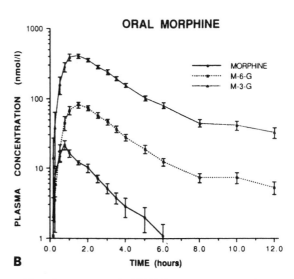

Fig. 3-9 Mean (± SEM) plasma concentrations of morphine (lowest curve), M3G (uppermost curve), M6G after administration of morphine **(A)** 5 mg intravenously or **(B)** 11.7 mg orally. (From Osborne et al.,[116] with permission.)

failure. Osborne et al.[122] described three patients with impaired renal function who experienced prolonged respiratory depression after treatment with morphine. Each patient had high concentrations of M6G in the plasma, whereas there were no measurable amounts of morphine. Hasselström et al.[123] reported on a patient with postoperative renal failure, who was given 165 mg of morphine over 3 days and who required a naloxone infusion for 10 days to counteract the respiratory depression. This patient had high plasma concentrations of morphine metabolites. These decayed with a half-life of 2 to 5 days and were unaffected by peritoneal dialysis. General anesthesia with nitrous oxide and halothane did not influence the disposition of morphine in patients without renal disease but was associated with significant increases in the area under the concentration time curve for M3G and M6G.[124] The peak concentration of M6G, but not M3G, was also greater in anesthetized patients. These changes were attributed to decreases in renal blood flow and the glomerular filtration rate during halothane anesthesia. The influence of general anesthesia on the disposition of morphine and its metabolites might be more pronounced in patients with pre-existing impaired renal function.

PHARMACOKINETICS IN NEONATES AND INFANTS

In premature infants and during the first 2 weeks in normal infants, the activities of the hepatic enzymes responsible for the biotransformation of many drugs is low. Cytochrome P-450 activity in neonates is only 25 to 50 percent of that in adults. Halothane decreases the metabolic capacity of cytochrome P-450 isoenzymes, and its coadministration will further reduce the clearance of opioids in neonates.[125] The pharmacokinetics of meperidine showed great variability in neonates and premature infants.[126] The elimination half-life of meperidine in patients younger than 1 week of age varied from 3.3 to 59.4 hours compared with a mean of 2.3 hours in infants aged 3 to 18 months. The clearance of fentanyl increased during the neonatal period, most of the increase occurring during the first 2 weeks (Fig. 3-10).[127] In the study of Gauntlett et al.,[127] two neonates who underwent

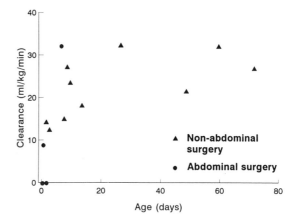

Fig. 3-10 Values of clearance of fentanyl in human neonates and infants plotted against age. Note that two neonates had virtually no clearance. (From Gauntlett et al.,[127] with permission.)

intra-abdominal surgery had no clearance of fentanyl, and plasma fentanyl concentrations remained constant for approximately 10 hours after an initial distribution phase. Koehntop et al.[128] also reported that the terminal half-life of fentanyl was markedly prolonged in the presence of increased abdominal pressure. The clearance of fentanyl is a function of both the ability of the liver to metabolize fentanyl and the blood flow to the liver. Increased abdominal pressure and/or abdominal surgery can significantly decrease blood flow through the portal vein.[129] Because of their reduced clearance, neonates will achieve higher plasma concentrations than will older infants given the same dose. The dose of fentanyl needed in neonatal anesthesia is considerably lower than that for older children or adults.[130] Additional factors that contribute to a lower requirement for opioids in neonates may be an increased permeability of the blood-brain barrier and lower plasma protein binding. There is a significant correlation between the free fraction in the plasma and the brain's extraction of a drug and its pharmacodynamic effect.[131,132] The free fraction of sufentanil is about 2.5 times greater in neonates than in children and adults.[133] This is due to the much lower concentration of AAG in neonates than in children and adults. The AAG concentration is dependent on gestational age; the concentration in premature infants born at 30 to 35 weeks of gestation is only 60 percent of that in full term infants.[134]

In pediatric cardiovascular patients, sufentanil clearance in children aged older than 2 months varied between 13 and 18 ml/min/kg, values not dissimilar from those in young adults.[135] Dixon et al.[136] studied the pharmacokinetics of high dose sufentanil (15 μg/kg given over 1 minute) in children undergoing cardiac surgery for the repair of congenital heart defects. Elimination half-lives and plasma clearance were similar in infants younger than 10 months and those older than 10 months who were not surface cooled. The mean half-life was 54 minutes, considerably shorter than in adults, and the clearance was also higher than the adult value, 23 ml/min/kg. The younger patients, however, had a smaller distribution volume. In children in whom surface cooling was used, the elimination half-life of sufentanil was markedly prolonged (120 ± 36 minutes; mean ± SD).

Important differences exist in the pharmacokinetics of sufentanil between neonates and older children. Greeley and de Bruijn[137] studied sequential sufentanil pharmacokinetics in three patients who underwent surgery for complex cardiac malformations during the first week of life and a second procedure 16 to 25 days later. Sufentanil, 10 μg/kg, was given as a single bolus, combined with pancuronium and oxygen, for each procedure, and arterial blood concentrations were measured by radioimmunoassay for up to 20 hours. The clearance of sufentanil during the first study in the three infants was 1.7, 4.3, and 6.7 ml/min/kg, and this increased dramatically during the second study of 12.9, 18.8, and 19.3 ml/min/kg. There were corresponding decreases in the terminal half-life and a small increase in V_{ss}. The authors attributed these changes to improved hepatic blood flow and improved hepatic metabolism. In a previous study by the same authors, the clearance of sufentanil in children younger than 1 month was 6.7 ml/min/kg, about 40 percent of the value in infants and older children.[135]

There are conflicting reports on the effect of age on alfentanil's pharmacokinetics in children. In a study of 18 children aged 3 months to 14 years, there was a weak but significant correlation between age and alfentanil clearance, but the mean clearance for the whole group (7.9 ml/min/kg) was within the adult range.[138] Meistelman et al.[139] also found the clearance of alfentanil in children to be similar to that in adults, although there was considerable variability in clearance rates (between 2.7 and 8.3 ml/min/kg); a reduced volume of distribution resulted in a significantly shorter elimination half-life of 40 minutes and rapid disappearance of alfentanil from the blood. Roure et al.[140] compared the pharmacokinetics of alfentanil in children aged between 10 months and 6.5 years with those in 10 adults. The apparent V_{ss} did not differ between the two groups. However, the elimination half-life was significantly shorter, and plasma clearance of alfentanil was greater in the children. The increased clearance in these young children might be explained by an increase in hepatic microsomal enzyme activity. There is a marked increase in oxidative metabolic activity after birth, and the metabolic capacity of children aged between 2 months and 3 years often exceeds that in adults.[141] On the other hand, in very young premature infants, alfentanil's clearance is significantly lower than that in children or adults.[142,143] The lower clearance results in a prolonged elimination half-life (five times the adult value). Den Hollander et al.[144] studied alfentanil's pharmacokinetics in children with congenital heart defects, who were given a continuous infusion of alfentanil during surgery with cardiopulmonary bypass. They found pharmacokinetic parameters comparable to those reported by Goresky et al.[138] in children of the same age group undergoing noncardiac surgery.

Morphine is a popular analgesic for pediatric patients, including neonates. Neonates are often considered to be more sensitive to the respiratory depressant effects of morphine.[145] This might be explained, at least partially, by age related differences in the development of opioid receptors, but it is equally likely that impaired clearance, and thus higher morphine concentrations, also contribute.[146] On the other hand, there is evidence that neonates require much higher plasma concentrations of morphine for adequate sedation and analgesia compared older children or adults.[147,148] However, the study by Olkkola et al.[148] showed that, contrary to previous views, neonates were not more susceptible to the respiratory depressant effects of morphine compared with adults. Neonates in that study were judged to have pain when the mean plasma morphine concentration was about sevenfold higher than that in older patients. Neonates being ventilated for respiratory distress syndrome required mean morphine concentrations of 127 ng/ml to produce sedation and analgesia.[147] The requirement for higher morphine concentrations may be partly explained by the absence or markedly reduced production of M6G in neonates. Both morphine and M6G contribute to the analgesic effect of morphine.[39,117,118,149] The elimination half-life, total plasma clearance, and V_{ss} (mean ± SD) were 9.6 ± 3.0 hours, 2.09 ± 1.19 ml/min/kg, and 2.05 ± 1.05 L/kg, respectively, and they were not significantly different between preterm and term neonates. However, in neonates with adverse effects of morphine, the plasma clearance was increased twofold. In neonates, and especially in premature infants, the mechanism for glucuronide conjugation is poorly developed.[103,146] At the same time, renal function (both glomerular filtration and tubular secretion) is also inefficient. Not surprisingly, therefore, the pharmacokinetic profile of morphine in neonates is markedly different from that in older children and adults.

In neonates, the deficiency of glucuronidation is compensated for by an increased ability to form the sulfate conjugate of morphine.[150,151] Preterm infants, even of 24 to 25 weeks of gestation, can metabolize morphine by glucuronidation, albeit at much lower levels than do children.[152] The M3G/morphine ratios in plasma and urine and the M6G/morphine ratio in urine were significantly higher in children than in neonates.[152] For children, the mean (± SD) M3G/M ratio in plasma was 23.6 ± 5.9, and in urine, it was 12.9 ± 5.0. The corresponding ratios in neonates were 5.0 ± 4.3 and 2.3 ± 2.1. In adults, there is a direct correlation between the in vitro glucuronidation of morphine to M3G in human hepatic microsomes and the M3G/morphine ratios in plasma and urine.[153] In a study of preterm infants younger than 5 days of age who were born at 26 to 40 weeks of gestation, the clearance rate of morphine increased as a function of gestational age at a rate of 0.9 ml/min/kg per week of gestation.[154] In 10 infants whose gestational age was younger than 30 weeks, the mean (±

SD) morphine clearance was 3.4 ± 3.3 ml/kg/min compared with a clearance of 15.5 ± 10 ml/min/kg in three term infants. The significantly lower plasma clearance of morphine in neonates compared with that in children also has been reported by Lynn and Slattery[150] (6.3 and 23.8 ml/min/kg) and Choonara et al.[152] (4.7 and 25.7 ml/min/kg). The M3G and M6G that is formed in neonates will be excreted more slowly as a result of reduced renal function.[94,155]

PHARMACOKINETICS IN ELDERLY PATIENTS

Elderly patients are believed to be more sensitive to the depressant effects of opioids, but it is not certain whether this is caused by age related changes in pharmacodynamics or pharmacokinetics, both of which may be altered by concomitant disease, which is often present in elderly patients. There was a 35 percent decrease in morphine clearance and a smaller volume of distribution in older patients.[156] After oral doses of morphine, the plasma concentrations were higher in elderly patients compared with patients in a younger age group; bioavailability was not affected by aging. The clearance of fentanyl was reported to be decreased, and the elimination was half-life prolonged in elderly patients,[157] although in another study the plasma clearance of fentanyl was similar in elderly and young patients.[158] The most likely explanation for a decreased clearance in older patients is a reduction in hepatic blood flow, which decreases with aging.[159] Fentanyl has an extraction ratio close to one; therefore, the clearance of fentanyl depends on hepatic blood flow.[160] Based on the data of Bentley et al.,[157] the time to reach a threshold concentration for respiratory depression of 1 ng/ml[161] after fentanyl 10 μg/kg would take 150 minutes in younger patients and approximately 560 minutes in elderly ones. These differences will be even more pronounced after doses of 50 to 100 μg/kg, which are often used in cardiac surgery.

Lemmens et al.[88] found decreased dose requirements for alfentanil in elderly patients but no difference in pharmacodynamics compared with those in young adults. They concluded that pharmacokinetic differences were responsible for the decreased dose requirement in elderly patients. By contrast, Scott and Stanski[162] found no age related changes in the pharmacokinetics of alfentanil, but reported that brain sensitivity, as determined by electroencephalographic changes, decreased significantly with age. In a subsequent study, Lemmens et al.[163] found no pharmacokinetic differences between older and younger male patients, but there was a significant negative correlation (r = −0.79) between the clearance of plasma alfentanil and age in women. Clearance in the older women was only 60 percent of that in younger women. Sitar et al.[164] found that older patients metabolize alfentanil more slowly than do young adults. Maitre et al.[165] investigated the population pharmacokinetics of alfentanil using data from four previously published studies involving 45 anesthetized patients. They found that age had no influence on alfentanil's clearance up to the age of 40 years, but beyond 40 years, the clearance decreased according to the equation

$$CL = CL_{40} - 0.00258 \, (age - 40)$$

where CL_{40} is the mean population clearance of patients younger than 40 years old (356 ml/min). The terminal half-life, total volume of distribution, and plasma clearance of sufentanil were similar in patients aged 70 to 80 years and those aged 22 to 57 years,[166] although elderly patients had significantly smaller initial volumes of distribution.

The effect of age on the concentration of AAG, the principle binding protein for the phenylpiperidine opioids, has not been well established. Discrimination between between pure age related changes and those caused by factors such as concomitant disease or medication is difficult. Veering et al.[167] have provided evidence that age per se has no effect on the concentration of AAG. They studied plasma AAG and human serum albumin concentrations in 68 healthy subjects, aged 20 to 90 years. None had taken any medication for at least 1 month before the study, and patients with diseases or conditions known or suspected to be associated with alterations in serum proteins were excluded. The authors found that, in healthy subjects, albumin concentrations decreased with increasing age, whereas age did not influence the concentration of AAG.

PREGNANCY AND LACTATION

Fentanyl and its newer analogues cross the placental barrier rapidly. In a maternal fetal sheep preparation, fentanyl was detected in fetal blood as early as 1 minute after intravenous administration to the ewe, and peak fetal concentrations occurred at 5 minutes.[168] Plasma levels were always lower in the fetus. In humans, plasma concentrations of alfentanil and sufentanil are also higher in maternal than in neonatal blood.[169,170] However, because of the lesser protein binding in the neonates caused by lower concentrations of AAG, free (unbound) concentrations were similar in mothers and neonates. There is an overall fall in AAG levels during pregnancy, with about a 30 percent reduction at term.[134] This will result in higher free fractions of opioids and, possibly, increased sensitivity to their effects.

Neonates may potentially be at risk when opioids are administered to lactating mothers. The mean pH of milk (7.2) is lower than that of plasma so that ion trapping of basic drugs will occur in the milk. Wittels et al.[171] studied opioid concentrations in breast milk and neonatal neurobehavior following administration of meperidine or morphine intravenously by patient-controlled analgesia and orally to mothers after elective cesarian section. Significant concentrations of opioids and metabolites were found in specimens of milk obtained from 12 to 96 hours postpartum. In the meperidine group, the metabolite normeperidine was persistently elevated. Neonates in this group had significantly more neurobehavioral depression; those in the morphine group were more alert and better oriented on their 3rd day of life.

CARDIOPULMONARY BYPASS AND OPIOID PHARMACOKINETICS

Hemodilution, hypotension and altered regional blood flow, nonpulsatile flow, and hypothermia can be expected to alter the pharmacokinetics of drugs profoundly, which are given during cardiac anesthesia.[172] In dogs, the elimination half-life of morphine is significantly increased, and the distribution volume and total body clearance are decreased during hypothermia to 30°C.[173] This resulted in significantly higher plasma concentrations of morphine than following similar doses given during normothermia. When patients were given a single large bolus of fentanyl at the start of anesthesia, there were large falls in plasma fentanyl concentrations at the onset of cardiopulmonary bypass, probably as a result of hemodilution. Thereafter, during bypass, fentanyl concentrations remained fairly constant, suggesting that clearance by the liver was markedly reduced.[174,175] Koska et al.[175] found an elimination half-life of fentanyl of 5.2 hours in cardiac patients compared with 3.3 hours in a control group undergoing vascular surgery without cardiopulmonary bypass. Indocyanine green clearance, which is closely related to hepatic plasma flow, was reduced by about 30 percent during and after bypass. Other studies of fentanyl during cardiac surgery have reported even longer elimination half-lives, 7.1 hours[174] and 11 hours.[176] Clearance was decreased (7.6 ml/min/kg), and the volume of distribution (7.9 L/kg) was increased.[176]

The average terminal half-life of alfentanil following infusion for coronary artery surgery was 5.1 hours (range, 1.5 to 10 hours).[177] Hug et al.[178] assessed alfentanil pharmacokinetics before and after bypass. Alfentanil, 125 μg/kg, was injected as a bolus at the induction of anesthesia, and a second 125-μg/kg bolus was given approximately 30 minutes after the end of bypass. The pharmacokinetic parameters prebypass were similar to those in noncardiac surgical patients. After bypass, the terminal half-life was significantly prolonged compared with the prebypass period (195 ± 31 versus 72 ± 6 minutes; mean ± standard error of the mean). This was the result of an increased volume of distribution because alfentanil clearance did not change. The initiation of cardiopulmonary bypass with hemodilution causes profound changes in the concentration of plasma proteins and, thus, of the free concentration of drugs. Alfentanil's total plasma concentrations decreased from 177 ng/ml before bypass to 92 ng/ml after the commencement of bypass and rose to 155 ng/ml at the end of bypass 2

hours later. However, during this period, the unbound concentration of alfentanil remained essentially unchanged because the unbound fraction rose from 0.16 to 0.35 two minutes after the start of bypass and then fell gradually to 0.22.[179] Generally, the unbound fraction of a drug is responsible for the pharmacologic effect.

The pharmacokinetics of alfentanil in infants and children are markedly different before and after cardiopulmonary bypass. The initial volume of distribution before bypass was smaller (68 ± 37 ml/kg in infants and 80 ± 32 ml/kg in children) than after bypass (235 ± 58 ml/kg in infants and 179 ± 99 ml/kg in children).[144] However, the total sampling time before bypass in the clinical situation is too short to allow full characterization of the pharmacokinetics of alfentanil. The same authors compared the pharmacokinetics of alfentanil before and after cardiopulmonary bypass in pigs in which sufficiently long sampling times were possible.[180] As in the children, there were significant differences between the two periods (Fig. 3-11). The V_{ss} (258 ± 70 ml/kg), elimination clearance (CL_e, 10.7 ± 3.0 ml/min/kg), and distribution clearance (CL_d, 6.8 ± 3.3 ml/kg/min) before bypass were smaller than after bypass (V_{ss}, 1107 ± 373 ml/kg; CL_e, 20.0 ± 3.0 ml/min/kg; CL_d, 23.0 ± 6.7 ml/kg/min). The elimination half-life was shorter before than after bypass (36.8 ± 8 versus 68 ± 20 minutes).

The concentration of sufentanil fell by 30 to 55 percent with the start of cardiopulmonary bypass and then remained stable during the period of hypothermia.[181] Plasma concentrations increased during rewarming and were similar in the first post-cardiopulmonary bypass sample to the value immediately prior to cardiopulmonary bypass. Flezzani et al.[182] investigated sufentanil disposition during cardiopulmonary bypass in 10 patients undergoing coronary artery surgery anesthetized with diazepam and enflurane. Ten minutes before the expected start of cardiopulmonary bypass, a computer controlled infusion of sufentanil was set to reach and maintain a plasma sufentanil concentration of 5 ng/ml. Plasma concentrations (mean ± SEM) immediately before cardiopulmonary bypass were 3.8 ± 0.4 ng/ml, fell to 2.5 ± 0.3 ng/ml immediately after the start of cardiopulmonary bypass,

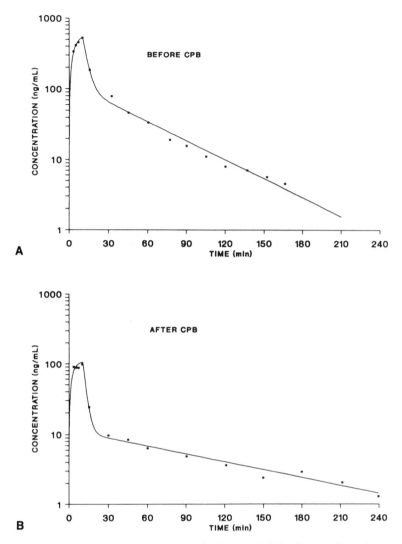

Fig. 3-11 Alfentanil plasma concentrations **(A)** before and **(B)** after cardiopulmonary bypass in a pig. (From den Hollander et al.,[180] with permission.)

and then slowly rose to 4.7 ± 0.4 ng/ml by the end of cardiopulmonary bypass. The accumulation of sufentanil when infused in this manner during cardiopulmonary bypass suggests that pharmacokinetic parameters from healthy normothermic patients are not entirely appropriate for use by computer controlled infusion schemes for cardiac surgery. Fentanyl plasma concentrations in children undergoing cardiac surgery remained essentially unchanged over a 140-minute period during cardiopulmonary bypass with profound hypother-

mia to 18°C to 25°C.[183] These authors also investigated the disposition of fentanyl, 30 μg/kg, given as a bolus over 1 minute in four piglets during normothermia (37°C) and hypothermia (29°C). Each piglet served as its own control. During hypothermia, fentanyl plasma concentrations were considerably higher than during normothermia. Terminal half-lives were similar, but distribution volume and total body clearance were significantly smaller during hypothermia.

Apart from the effects of hypothermia and hemodilution, sequestration of opioids in the extra-corporeal circuit may be a factor in drug disposition during cardiopulmonary bypass. Fentanyl, but not alfentanil, is absorbed into a Shiley bubble oxygenator circuit.[184] Both fentanyl and sufentanil are sequestered onto the Scimed membrane oxygenator circuit.[185,186] At 25°C, the capacity of this membrane for sufentanil uptake was 11 ng/cm², increasing to 24 ng/cm² at 37°C. This is much less than the capacity of the same device for fentanyl, 130 ng/cm².[185] This is an enormous capacity, corresponding to a saturated absorption of 5 to 6 mg of fentanyl for a standard adult oxygenator, approximately the total amount of fentanyl in an adult patient with a steady state fentanyl plasma concentration of 20 ng/ml. The amount of fentanyl that will be absorbed onto such a membrane in actual practice will be considerably less because of coating of the membrane with plasma proteins and platelets that reduce the absorptive capacity. We cannot, of course, extrapolate these findings to oxygenators from different manufacturers because opioid binding will be dependent on the composition and structure of the material used, and this differs among manufacturers. There was a wide variability in fentanyl absorption by different membrane oxygenators.[185] Alfentanil was sequestered by oxygenators to a lesser degree than was fentanyl.

Data from the study of Okutani et al.[181] suggested that relatively large amounts of sufentanil were sequestered during hypothermic cardiopulmonary bypass, although the authors thought that absorption in the bypass circuit was unlikely to have been a major factor. They suggested that significant pulmonary sequestration may have occurred, with subsequent release with rewarming and restoration of ventilation. Substantial quantities of many drugs, including opioids, can be retained in the lungs. The first pass uptake of fentanyl, meperidine, alfentanil, and sufentanil in the lungs exceeds 60 to 90 percent.[105,106,187] Propranolol reduced the uptake of fentanyl by the lungs from 83 percent in patients receiving no propranolol to 53 percent in those receiving 30 to 120 mg per day.[188] One patient who received 120 mg of propranolol per day had a first pass pulmonary uptake of fentanyl of only 23 percent of the in-jected dose. The pharmacodynamic implications of such interactions need to be assessed.

THE INFLUENCE OF LIVER DISEASE

Drug clearance may be modified by three factors that are altered in hepatic disease as follows: (1) reduced hepatic blood flow, (2) diminished activity of metabolizing enzymes, and (3) changes in plasma proteins. For drugs such as fentanyl and sufentanil, with high hepatic extraction ratios and an intrinsic hepatic clearance greater than the hepatic blood flow, clearance will be dependent on hepatic blood flow; factors decreasing hepatic blood flow, such as anesthesia and cardiac failure, will reduce clearance. Conversely, because the liver has such a large reserve capacity of metabolizing enzymes, the elimination of these drugs is unlikely to be significantly altered in patients with hepatic disease until hepatic function becomes severely compromised.

Sufentanil's pharmacokinetics were unaltered in patients with cirrhosis,[189] suggesting that hepatic blood flow was maintained in a normal range in these particular subjects. Fentanyl's plasma clearance was also unchanged in patients with cirrhosis.[190] Anhepatic dogs had a marked prolongation of the elimination half-life of fentanyl.[191] Interestingly, in these dogs, 8 percent of the administered dose of fentanyl was excreted in the urine as fentanyl metabolites, indicating extrahepatic sites of metabolism for fentanyl.

By contrast with fentanyl and sufentanil, alfentanil has an hepatic extraction of only 0.3 to 0.5,[40] and alfentanil's clearance could be influenced by hepatic blood flow, hepatic enzyme capacity, and plasma protein binding. Ferrier et al.[192] reported that, compared with control patients, patients with cirrhosis had lower total plasma clearances (1.6 versus 3.06 ml/min/kg) and a more prolonged elimination half-life (219 versus 97 minutes) but similar volumes of distribution. Reduced clearance of alfentanil and a prolonged elimination have also been reported in patients with mildly abnormal hepatic function tests but without clinically significant hepatic disease;[193] 30 percent of the patients with abnormal hepatic function test results required naloxone postoperatively for respiratory depression compared with 6 percent of the patients with normal ones. Bower et al.[113] compared the effect of different hepatic pathologic conditions on the disposition of alfentanil and found that patients with nonalcoholic liver disease had lesser plasma clearance (115 ml/min) than did those with alcoholic liver disease (159 ml/min) or healthy control subjects (187 ml/min). Free drug clearance was reduced in both hepatic dysfunction groups compared with controls. Alfentanil pharmacokinetics were not significantly disturbed in children with cholestatic disease.[194]

The elimination half-life of morphine in patients with alcohol related cirrhosis of the liver was double that in a group of healthy volunteers (201 versus 111 minutes),[99] as a result of a lower total body clearance without a significant change in the volume of distribution. These results are in contrast with those reported by Patwardhan et al.,[98] who observed similar elimination half-lives in cirrhotic patients and volunteers. All pharmacokinetic parameters were similar between the two groups, despite decreased clearance of indocyanine green, an indicator of hepatic blood flow, in the patients with cirrhosis. The authors concluded that this was evidence of extrahepatic metabolism of morphine in both normal individuals and in patients with cirrhosis. Elimination half-lives of morphine in patients with renal failure are comparable to those of normal patients.[94,195]

INFLUENCE OF RENAL DISEASE

Although the kidneys play a minor role in the elimination of most opioids, renal disease can nonetheless influence their pharmacokinetic profile, secondary to alterations in distribution or clearance, caused mainly by alterations in plasma protein binding. There are limited data concerning the influence of renal disease on fentanyl pharmacokinetics. Accumulation of fentanyl's metabolites might occur in patients with impaired renal function, but this is unlikely to have clinical consequences because they are pharmacologically inactive. Fentanyl has been given to anephric patients without untoward side effects.[196] Fentanyl's clearance was higher in these patients than in surgical patients with normal renal function.

The effect of renal failure on the pharmacokinetics of alfentanil appears to be variable, possibly because of alterations in plasma protein binding. Although chronic renal failure generally causes a decrease in the plasma protein binding of acid drugs (e.g., thiopental), basic drug binding is less predictable. Plasma protein binding in renal failure may be affected by changes in the concentrations of binding proteins, structural changes in the binding proteins, or by the presence of competitive inhibitors of drug binding. Endogenous inhibitors of binding that accumulate in renal failure may be reduced by dialysis; thus, plasma protein binding may vary in relationship to the dialysis schedule. AAG levels were found to be elevated during chronic renal failure in some patients[197] but not in others.[198] The alfentanil free fraction was reported to be increased.[199,200] The clearance of alfentanil was found to be increased[200] or unchanged[194,199,201] by renal failure. The V_{ss} of alfentanil has been reported variously as increased,[194,199] decreased,[201] or unchanged.[200]

The pharmacokinetics of sufentanil were not altered in patients with chronic renal disease undergoing renal transplant surgery.[198,202,203] The pharmacokinetics of morphine were not altered in patients with advanced renal failure,[94,155,195] although V_{ss} was decreased in patients with end-stage renal failure.[155] However, the terminal half-lives of M3G and M6G were significantly prolonged, from about 4 hours in nonuremic patients to between 14 and 119 hours in patients with renal failure.[94] Because glucuronides are water soluble compounds excreted by the kidneys, this finding is not surprising. Impaired elimination of morphine glucuronide was also reported by Wolff et al.[121] Morphine glucuronide was increased during general anesthesia.[124] There is a linear relationship between creatinine clearance and the renal clearances of morphine, M3G, and M6G.[204] M6G is pharmacologically active with a high affinity for opioid receptors. It can cross the blood-brain barrier, and its accumulation is thought to be responsible for the prolonged action of morphine in patients with renal failure.[122] The influence of renal failure on the pharmacokinetics of morphine and metabolites is clinically relevant, especially when repeated doses or infusions are given. The accumulation of the parent drug, and perhaps more importantly the active metabolite M6G, may result in prolonged sedation and respiratory depression.[122,123]

PHARMACOKINETICS OF INDIVIDUAL OPIOIDS

Morphine

Morphine is the most abundant of the natural alkaloids present in opium. Opium contains more than 50 natural alkaloids, which can be divided into two distinct classes: the phenanthrenes and the benzylquinolines. Morphine, along with codeine and thebaine, belongs to the phenanthrene group and constitutes approximately 10 percent of raw opium. It was first isolated from opium in 1806 by Sertürner, a German chemist, who also gave morphine its name, after the Greek god of dreams, Morpheus. Many semisynthetic derivatives are made by simple modifications of the morphine molecule. Codeine (methylmorphine), hydromorphone, oxymorphone, and hydrocodone are obtained by substitution of side chains at the C3, C6, or C17 position of the morphine molecule. Morphine is considered the prototype opioid agonist to which all opioids are compared.

Morphine occurs as colorless crystals or as a white crystalline powder, and it is available either as the sulfate or hydrochloride salt. The structure of morphine is shown in Figure 3-2. Morphine is poorly lipid soluble, with a partition coefficient of 1 : 4 in a buffered solution of octanol and water at pH 7.4.

The pharmacokinetics of morphine have been extensively studied, but data from many of the earlier studies are unreliable because the radioimmunoassay used did not adequately discriminate between morphine and its metabolites. Stanski et al.[205] reported a mean value for the elimination half-life of 4.5 hours, whereas more recent studies, using an improved assay technique, have found that the elimination half-life is on the order of 2 hours (Table 3-2).

Morphine is metabolized primarily in the liver, principally by conjugation to form water soluble glucuronides. It has a hepatic extraction ratio of 0.65 and a hepatic clearance of 635 ml/min, whereas the systemic clearance is 900 to 2300 ml/min.[95] Extrahepatic clearance accounts for 32 percent of the total body clearance. Significant renal glucuronidation of morphine has been demonstrated in dogs.[208] Morphine is cleared from the body mainly through urinary excretion of the metabolized drug. Less than 10 percent of the morphine cleared by the kidneys is free morphine, and 65 to 70 percent of the dose is excreted as morphine glucuronides. Peak concentrations of M3G and M6G are significantly higher in patients with renal insufficiency. There was a significant correlation between the half-life of M3G and renal function.[195] Compared with morphine, M6G had a smaller volume of distribution, a lower clearance, and a similar half-life.[119] Morphine first pass uptake in the lungs after intravenous bolus administration was insignificant.[105,106]

Morphine disposition is altered during hypothermia (30°C). Compared with normothermic or hyperthermic (40°C) dogs, the elimination half-life in hypothermic dogs was prolonged from 80 to 180 minutes; the volume of distribution decreased from 8.5 to 5.7 L/kg and clearance decreased from 84 to 25 ml/kg/min.[173] A significant and sustained decrease in mean arterial blood pressure was observed in the hypothermic dogs during the experiment. Whether the decreased clearance of morphine was secondary to the hemodynamic changes or to a change in hepatic metabolic activity remains unclear. Morphine clearance was not influenced by halothane[208] or balanced anesthesia.[195]

Meperidine

Meperidine (pethidine) was the first totally synthetic opioid. It is well absorbed from the gastrointestinal tract, but the bioavailability is low (47 to 73 percent) because of presystemic (first pass) metabolism.[209] Peak plasma concentrations after oral administration occur after about 1 hour. Absorption after intramuscular injection is complete with maximum concentrations within 5 to 15 min; thereafter, plasma concentrations are essentially the same as after intravenous administration of the same

Table 3-2 Pharmacokinetic Parameters for Morphine[a]

Authors	Patients	$t_{1/2}$ (min)	CL (ml/min)	V_{ss} (L)
Murphy and Hug[206]	Adult surgical patients	104 ± 15.8	1,269 ± 330	192 ± 66
Säwe et al.[8]	Patients with cancer	204 ± 114	551 ± 210	147 ± 84
Stanski et al.[205]	Volunteers	174 ± 30	1,030 ± 63	224 ± 21
Dahlström et al.[48]	Adult surgical patients	228 ± 138	1,435 ± 490	434 ± 245
Sear et al.[195]	Anesthetized adults	153 ± 61	766 ± 212	157 ± 42
	Awake adults	208 ± 74	587 ± 192	161 ± 40
Säwe et al.[94]	Patients with renal failure	144 ± 66	1,477 ± 434	308 ± 119
	Adult surgical patients	102 ± 48	1,260 ± 392	280 ± 161
Wolff et al.[121]	Patients with renal insufficiency	372 ± 150	876 ± 151	439 ± 174
Aitkenhead et al.[207]	Patients with renal failure	191 (61–396)	605 (311–1,197)	106 (35–215)
	Adult controls	210 (100–442)	720 (482–1,090)	175 (104–275)
Patwardhan et al.[98]	Patients with liver cirrhosis	132 ± 78	1,022 ± 308	161 ± 91
	Healthy adult controls	180 ± 90	1,134 ± 392	203 ± 168
Mazoit et al.[99]	Patients with liver cirrhosis	201 ± 39	1,470 ± 525	314 ± 62
	Healthy adult controls	111 ± 32	2,345 ± 540	295 ± 65
Chay et al.[147]	Neonates	575 ± 172	2.1 ± 1.2[b]	2.1 ± 1.0[c]
Lynn and Slattery[150]	Neonates	409 ± 98	6.3 ± 2.2[b]	3.4 ± 1.0[c]
Bhat et al.[154]	Preterm neonates			
	Gestational age, 28 weeks	600 ± 22	3.4 ± 3.3[b]	1.8 ± 0.84[c]
	Gestational age, 33 weeks	444 ± 102	9.6 ± 4.0[b]	5.2 ± 1.6[c]
	Gestational age, 40 weeks	402 ± 276	15.5 ± 10.0[b]	2.9 ± 2.1[c]
Choonara et al.[152]	Neonates (2–12 days)		4.7 ± 2.8[b]	
	Children (1–16 yr)		26 ± 4.7[b]	

Abbreviations: CL, clearance; $t_{1/2}$, half-life; V, volume of distribution.

[a] Values are mean ± standard deviation.

[b] ml/min/kg.

[c] L/kg.

dose. Meperidine is moderately lipid soluble, and plasma proteins binding is about 70 percent, with binding to albumin, lipoprotein, and AAG.[210] The volume of distribution is large, reflecting the extensive binding to tissues (Table 3-3). The clearance of meperidine is about 600 to 800 ml/min, reflecting a high hepatic extraction ratio. The terminal elimination half-life is between 3 and 5 hours. Meperidine is metabolized mainly by the liver, and only about 7 percent of a dose is excreted unchanged in the urine. This amount is, however, markedly influenced by urinary pH. Acidification of the urine reduced the excretion of unchanged meperidine to less than 1 percent, whereas with urinary alkalinization, this was increased to 20 to 25 percent.[209]

There are two hepatic metabolic routes, hydrolysis to meperidinic acid and N-demethylation to normeperidine. Meperidinic acid is pharmacologically inactive, but normeperidine, the predominant metabolite, is active and potentially toxic. Normeperidine causes central nervous system excitability, including tremors, myoclonus, and grand mal convulsions. These toxic effects are not reversed by naloxone.[220,221] Because normeperidine is excreted

Table 3-3 Pharmacokinetic Parameters for Meperidine[a]

Authors	Patients	$t_{1/2}$ (min)	CL (ml/min)	V_{ss} (L)
Verbeeck et al.[209]	Adult volunteers	408 ± 47	574 ± 86	270 ± 20
Stambaugh et al.[211]	Adult volunteers	236 ± 20	710 ± 110	198 ± 94
Mather et al.[212]	Adult surgical patients	186 ± 84	830 ± 410	203 ± 99
	Adult volunteers	222 ± 96	1,020 ± 400	305 ± 120
Herman et al.[213]	Elderly volunteers (60–79 yr)	419 ± 112	615 ± 157	326 ± 64
Bloedow et al.[214]	Burns patients			
	Acute	246 ± 72	420 ± 120	140 ± 44
	Convalescent	180 ± 102	600 ± 220	130 ± 45
	Control	222 ± 96	1,020 ± 400	276 ± 100
Kirkwood et al.[215]	Acute trauma patients		684 ± 206	
Kuhnert et al.[216]	Full term pregnant women	152	1,010 ± 381	217 ± 90
	Control nonpregnant women	177	964 ± 300	233 ± 64
Husemeyer et al.[217]	Full term pregnant women	157	1,190 ± 421	231 ± 61
Chan et al.[218]	Patients with renal disease			
	Severe renal dysfunction	1,242 ± 764	100 ± 33	
	Moderate renal dysfunction	870 ± 470	121 ± 102	
	Mild renal dysfunction	636 ± 148	124 ± 76	
	Healthy volunteers	474 ± 171	343 ± 198	
Klotz et al.[219]	Patients with liver cirrhosis	422 ± 55	664 ± 293	406 ± 177
	Adult volunteers	193 ± 48	1,316 ± 383	330 ± 99
Pokela et al.[126]	Neonates and infants			
	< 1 week old	642 (294–1,008)	7.2 (5.3–13.8)[b]	5.6 (3.7–9.2)[c]
	> 3 weeks old	492 (342–1,900)	9.7 (4.1–20.5)[b]	8.0 (4.9–11.0)[c]

Abbreviations: CL, clearance; $t_{1/2}$, half-life; V, volume of distribution.
[a] Values are mean ± standard deviation.
[b] ml/min.
[c] L/kg.

in the urine, the risk of toxic side effects with prolonged or high doses of meperidine will be greater in patients with renal dysfunction. The elimination half-life of normeperidine is on the order of 15 to 20 hours in patients with normal renal function, but it may be as long as 30 to 40 hours in those in renal failure.[222] Both meperidine and normeperidine readily cross the placenta and can accumulate in the fetus. Because both compounds are weak bases (the pK_a of meperidine is 8.5 and that of normeperidine is higher), ion trapping in the fetal plasma occurs. The elimination of meperidine in neonates is slower than in adults and children, with half-lives prolonged up to 24 hours, and neonates whose mothers have received meperidine during labor may take 3 to 6 days to eliminate the drug completely. The pharmacokinetic disposition and elimination of meperidine appeared to be little altered by pregnancy.[223] However, a recent study in which blood samples were collected for 48 hours after a single 50-mg intravenous bolus of meperidine to term pregnant women reported a terminal half-life of 13.3 hours.[224] This is considerably longer than previously reported half-lives based on data collected over less than 8 hours. Unfortunately, no control nonpregnant patients were studied, and it is difficult to know whether these authors found a truly prolonged elimination half-life or whether this was just a consequence of a long sampling period. Generally, in pharmacokinetic studies, the terminal half-life is correlated with the duration of sampling.

Although renal excretion plays only a minor role in the elimination of meperidine, nonetheless renal disease may result in significant pharmacokinetic changes. Chan et al.[218] administered meperidine, 150 μg/kg, intravenously to healthy volunteers and patients with varying degrees of renal disease, the latter subdivided into those with severe, moderate, or mild dysfunction. The plasma concentrations of meperidine in the patients were considerably higher than in the volunteers, and the elimination half-lives were significantly longer; 7.9, 20.2, 16.6, and 14.3 hours, respectively, for healthy volunteers and patients with severe, moderate, or mild renal dysfunction. The mean plasma clearance of meperidine was 342 ml/min in the healthy volunteers and varied between 100 and 124 ml/min in the patients. The volume of distribution was increased in patients with renal dysfunction as a result of reduced plasma protein binding. The bound fraction was 58 percent in volunteers and 32 to 42 percent in renal patients.

The V_{ss} of meperidine was reduced by about one-half in burn injuries, and the plasma clearance was lower.[214] Meperidine's clearance was not altered in patients after acute trauma if renal and hepatic function were normal.[215]

Methadone

Methadone is a synthetic opioid with a chemical structure that does not resemble that of other opioids, when viewed in two dimensions (Fig. 3-12). However, in three dimensions, the molecule

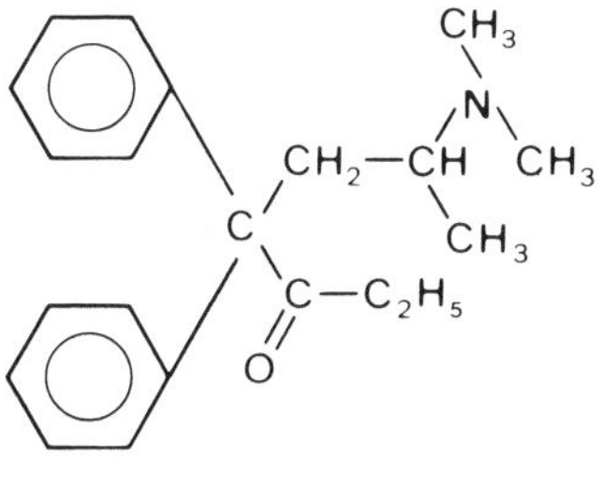

METHADONE

Fig. 3-12 Structure of methadone.

has an opioid-like pseudopiperidine configuration. Methadone is commercially available as a racemic mixture, but almost all of its pharmacologic activity resides in the L-isomer, which is about 50 times more potent than is the D-isomer. Methadone is rapidly absorbed from the gastrointestinal tract, and the bioavailability is high, about 80 percent, but can vary among individuals from 40 to 99 percent.[225] The high bioavailability after oral administration coupled with a long duration of analgesia makes methadone particularly useful in the management of severe cancer-induced pain. Measurable plasma concentrations occur within 30 minutes after oral administration with peak concentrations at about 3 hours (range, 1 to 5 hours). About 85 percent of methadone in the plasma is protein bound; AAG is the main determinant of the free fraction.[226] A lower free fraction of methadone, caused by elevated concentrations of AAG, has been shown in patients with cancer[227] and in patients with rheumatoid arthritis[226] compared with healthy volunteers. Methadone is a lipophilic drug, and it is highly bound to tissues, resulting in a large volume of distribution[217,220] (Table 3-4).[225,228] Total body clearance is low, 100 to 178 ml/min,[225,228,231] and this, together with the large volume of distribution, results in a long elimination half-life, which in postoperative patients averaged 35 hours (range, 9 to 87 hours) and correlated with age.[228] Caution should be exercised with repeated doses, especially in elderly patients, to avoid accumulation. Higher clearance values have been reported in patients with severe burns.[229] However, in that study, blood samples were only obtained for 24 hours, too short a sampling period for a drug with such a long half-life.

Methadone undergoes hepatic biotransformation to diphenylpyrrolidine, which undergoes further demethylation to form pyrroline. This is the major metabolic pathway, but reduction to form the pharmacologically active metabolites methadole and normethadole also occurs. Renal and fecal excretion is also important, the latter accounting for the excretion of 10 to 45 percent of an orally administered dose of methadone. In patients with renal disease who are receiving prolonged oral methadone treatment, plasma concentrations were within the expected range for the adminis-

Table 3-4 Pharmacokinetic Parameters for Methadone[a]

	Patients	$t_{1/2}$ (min)	CL (ml/min)	V_{ss} (L)
Gourlay et al.[228]	Adult surgical patients	35 ± 22 h	178 ± 100	410 ± 156
Denson et al.[229]	Burned patients[b]	2.6 ± 0.15 h	53 ± 19	180 ± 68
Nilsson[230]	Patients with chronic pain	30 ± 7.7 h	96 ± 30	250 ± 49

Abbreviations: CL, clearance; $t_{1/2}$, half-life; V, volume of distribution.
[a] Values are mean ± standard deviation.
[b] Sampling only for 24 hours.

tered dose.[232] Less than 1 percent of the daily dose was removed by peritoneal dialysis or hemodialysis. The elimination half-life of methadone was longer in patients with severe liver disease compared with mild or moderate liver disease, but dose adjusted plasma concentrations were not significantly different.[233] Although few studies have focused on the clinical implications of renal or hepatic disease for the use of methadone, clinical experience suggests that patients with renal or hepatic dysfunction and elderly patients tend to have an exaggerated response to the drug, and caution with dosing is advised.[225]

Fentanyl

Fentanyl is a synthetic phenylpiperidine belonging to the 4-anilopiperidine series. Fentanyl occurs as a white powder and is readily soluble in water. It is commercially available as the citrate salt in an aqueous preservative free solution containing 50 μg/ml of fentanyl base. It is a basic amine with a pK_a of 8.43; at physiologic pH, only 8.4 percent of the drug is in its un-ionized form. On a milligram basis, fentanyl is considerably more potent than is morphine; estimates of potency ratios have ranged from 60 to 270, depending on species. Fentanyl is 60 to 80 times more potent than morphine in humans. At the opioid receptor, however, the intrinsic affinities of fentanyl and morphine differ only by a factor of two to three.[234] The differences between the receptor affinities and clinical potency ratios arise from differing physicochemical and pharmacokinetic properties of these drugs, and in particular, the differences in lipid solubility.

Fentanyl is highly lipid soluble with an octanol-water partition coefficient of 816.[9] At pH 7.4, fentanyl is 80 to 85 percent bound to plasma proteins. The acute phase protein, AAG, accounts for about 44 percent of the protein binding of fentanyl. Within the concentration ranges encountered clinically, protein binding of fentanyl is independent of drug concentration. Fentanyl is rapidly transferred across the blood-brain barrier, resulting in a rapid onset of action after intravenous injection. The relative potential for entering the central nervous system is 156 times greater for fentanyl than for morphine. However, the large quantities of fentanyl taken up by adipose tissues act as a reservoir that releases fentanyl back into the circulation as plasma concentrations fall. This re-entry serves to maintain the plasma concentration and is one factor in the relatively long plasma elimination half-life of fentanyl, 3.1 to 3.7 hours in volunteers.[160,161] The properties that enable fentanyl to cross the blood-brain barrier also ensure rapid penetration across the placental barrier.[168,235] Fentanyl is rapidly and extensively metabolized by the liver to inactive metabolites.

The disposition of fentanyl in the plasma has been extensively studied in animals and humans, both in healthy volunteers and in patients undergoing surgery (Table 3-5). After a bolus intravenous injection, plasma fentanyl concentrations decrease rapidly as a result of distribution from the plasma to tissues. In volunteers, 98.6 percent of a 10-μg/kg intravenous dose is eliminated from plasma in 60 minutes.[161] This rapid distribution of fentanyl explains why, after moderate (up to 10 μg/kg) doses, fentanyl has a short duration of action. The mechanism is analogous to the rapid

Table 3-5 Pharmacokinetic Parameters for Fentanyl[a]

Authors	Patients	$t_{1/2}$ (min)	CL (ml/min)	V_{ss} (L)
Bower and Hull[160]	Adult volunteers	184 ± 70	1,530 ± 246	335 ± 143
McClain and Hug[161]	Adult volunteers	219 ± 22	956 ± 145	257 ± 42
Scott and Stanski[162]	Adult surgical patients	475 ± 193	574 ± 214	339 ± 139
Koska et al.[175]	Adult surgical patients	198 ± 66	830 ± 263	227 ± 104
Bentley et al.[157]	Adult, young	265 ± 49.2	991 ± 248	381 ± 123
	Adult, elderly	945 ± 128	275 ± 114	328 ± 54
Singleton et al.[158]	Adult, young[b]	133 ± 47	973 ± 210	159 ± 57.4
	Adult, elderly[b]	103 ± 52	917 ± 287	95 ± 31
Hudson et al.[236]	Aortic surgery patients	522 ± 150	769 ± 141	424 ± 149

Abbreviations: CL, clearance; $t_{1/2}$, half-life; V, volume of distribution.
[a] Values are mean ± standard deviation.
[b] Only sampled for 4 hours.

recovery from thiopental as a result of redistribution. However, attempts to increase the intensity of effect by giving a larger initial dose converts fentanyl from a short acting to a long acting drug. A 10-fold increment in dose produces an 8-fold increase in the time that plasma levels remain above the threshold for respiratory depression. With the larger dose, the distribution phase is completed before the fentanyl concentration declines to threshold levels; therefore, the duration of action now becomes dependent on the decrease in concentration during the much slower elimination phase.

Fentanyl undergoes significant first pass uptake in the lungs (70 to 85 percent of the injected dose).[105,106,187] Pulmonary accumulation of fentanyl is temporary, and fentanyl is released bimodally, with a fast release half-time of 0.2 minutes and a slower release half-time of 5.8 minutes.[187] First pass pulmonary uptake of fentanyl is lower in patients taking propranolol, indicating that there is competition between the drugs for uptake in the lung.[188]

There is a large variability in the reported pharmacokinetic parameters for fentanyl. Estimates of the elimination half-life range from 100 to 347 minutes; the volume of distribution, from 55 to 257 L; and the total body clearance, from 194 to 1,530 ml/min. This probably reflects differences in methodology, analytic techniques, and subjects studied. Some investigators have studied groups of healthy young volunteers, whereas others have studied patients undergoing a variety of surgical procedures under general anesthesia. Anesthesia and surgery influence hepatic blood flow and drug metabolism. Hepatic clearance of fentanyl is blood flow dependent and is thus sensitive to a reduction in hepatic perfusion. Halothane and enflurane inhibited fentanyl's biotransformation in rat hepatic tissue homogenates, and halothane altered fentanyl disposition in humans.[237]

The nature of the surgery may also influence fentanyl's disposition. Major surgery may be associated with blood loss and changes in the volume of distribution. Patients undergoing abdominal aortic surgery anesthetized with fentanyl, 100 μg/kg, had an elimination half-life of fentanyl of 8.7 hours, about double that of normal volunteers.[236] This was due to a lower clearance and a greater volume of distribution.

Few studies have investigated the effects of other drugs on fentanyl's pharmacokinetics. Patients anesthetized with halothane or enflurane had a reduced fentanyl clearance compared with a control group receiving only intravenous anesthesia.[237] In sheep, general anesthesia with 1.5 percent halothane caused a 71 percent decrease in hepatic blood flow from the awake control value.[238] Decreases in hepatic blood flow of 30 to 40 percent occur during halothane or isoflurane anesthesia in humans.[239] Hepatic arterial blood flow, of prime importance for hepatic clearance of drugs, is more compromised than portal blood flow during halothane anesthesia.[238]

Alfentanil

Alfentanil is a phenylpiperidine analog of fentanyl. Alfentanil hydrochloride is an almost white powder and is supplied as an aqueous solution containing 500 μg/ml of alfentanil base. Alfentanil is between 5 and 10 times less potent than is fentanyl when single intravenous boluses are compared. It acts rapidly, the peak effect being reached approximately five times faster than fentanyl. When given by bolus injection, its effects are of short duration, making it a versatile opioid for use in anesthesia.

The physiochemical properties of alfentanil are summarized in Table 3-1. Alfentanil is 92 percent bound to plasma proteins, principally AAG.[9] The pK$_a$ is 6.5 so that 89 percent of the molecules are unionized at pH 7.4 compared with 9 percent for fentanyl and 20 percent for sufentanil. The half-time for plasma-brain equilibration is 1.1 minute for alfentanil compared with 5.8 minutes for sufentanil and 6.4 minutes for fentanyl.

Pharmacokinetic data from human studies with alfentanil are given in Table 3-6. The volume of distribution of the central compartment (V$_c$), 0.13 to 0.88 L/kg, is much smaller than that of fentanyl, and the volume of distribution at steady state (V$_{ss}$) is 6 to 12 times smaller than that of fentanyl.[160] Total body clearance is also approximately 6 times lower than that of fentanyl. Although alfentanil is moderately lipophilic, alfentanil's pharmacokinetics are not altered by obesity.[246] The apparent volume of distribution of alfentanil in the brain is about 20 times less than that of fentanyl,[203] and thus the brain compartment will fill more rapidly with alfentanil than with fentanyl. Using simulated brain concentration curves for humans, based on tissue/blood partition data measured in rats, Björkman et al.[4] found that the maximum fentanyl concentrations after a single intravenous bolus were reached after 10 minutes compared with only 1 minute in the case of alfentanil.

After intravenous administration, alfentanil undergoes minimal to moderate pulmonary first pass uptake,[106,187] but pulmonary retention is only temporary. The release half-time is less than 1 minute. Alfentanil's metabolism in the lung is probably insignificant. Alfentanil is primarily eliminated from the body by renal excretion of the metabolized drug (90 percent of the dose) and only to a very minor extent (0.2 to 0.5 percent) as unmetabolized drug.[70,71] Alfentanil is mainly excreted as noralfentanil (31 to 48 percent).

Sufentanil

Sufentanil is a phenylpiperidine fentanyl analog, 8 to 10 times more potent than fentanyl. It is supplied as the aqueous solution of the citrate salt containing 50 μg/ml of sufentanil base; in a limited number of countries, it is also available in a concentration of 5 μg/ml. Sufentanil is a basic amine, with a pK$_a$ of 8.01. At physiologic pH, 20 percent of the drug in solution is in the un-ionized form. It is extremely lipid soluble with an octanol-water partition coefficient of 1,757.[9] The physiochemical properties of sufentanil are summarized in Table 3-1.

After intravenous administration, plasma sufentanil concentrations rapidly decrease so that, within 30 minutes, 98 percent of the injected dose will have left the plasma.[18] After intravenous administration, sufentanil undergoes significant first pass uptake in the lungs.[106] Of the injected dose, 65 percent remains in the lungs after the first pass, to be released within minutes after injection. The pharmacokinetic parameters of sufentanil are given in Table 3-7. Sufentanil is highly bound (93 percent) to plasma proteins, mainly AAG, which accounts for 83 percent of the total binding.[9] The metabolic pathways of sufentanil are similar to those of fentanyl. In rats and dogs, sufentanil is rapidly metabolized by dealkylation and aromatic hydroxylation.[69] The metabolism in humans has not been studied.

In patients undergoing elective abdominal aortic aneurysm repair, the elimination half-life of sufentanil was markedly prolonged, to 12 ± 5.8 hours.[247] The clearance was similar to values reported for patients undergoing general surgery, but the volume of distribution was larger, accounting for the

Table 3-6   Pharmacokinetic Parameters for Alfentanil[a]

Authors	Patients	$t_{1/2}$ (min)	CL (ml/min)	V_{ss} (L)
Bovill et al.[240]	Adult surgical patients	94 ± 18	457 ± 328	62 ± 45
Bower and Hull[160]	Adult volunteers	98 ± 25	238 ± 87	27 ± 7
Scott and Stanski[162]	Adult surgical patients	118 ± 32	195 ± 111	22 ± 8
Hudson et al.[241]	Aortic surgery patients	222 ± 156	448 ± 133	44 ± 23
Persson et al.[242]	Adult surgical patients	112 ± 28	249 ± 106	31 ± 8
Gepts et al.[65]	Pregnant patients	102 ± 67	416 ± 55	35 ± 11
	Nonpregnant surgical patients	104 ± 50	379 ± 133	32 ± 10
Bower and Sear[200]	Renal transplant patients	142 ± 50	342 ± 160	41 ± 18
	Adult surgical patients	120 ± 28	212 ± 56	28 ± 5
van Peer et al.[201]	Patients with renal failure	58 ± 16	371 ± 175	21 ± 12
Chauvin et al.[199]	Patients with renal failure	107 ± 44	189 ± 98	25 ± 5
	Adult surgical patients	90 ± 18	183 ± 94	17 ± 6
Shafer et al.[243]	Patients with hepatic dysfunction	176 ± 119	161 ± 91	33 ± 15
	Adult surgical patients	104 ± 72	294 ± 140	33 ± 18
Lemmens et al.[163]	Male surgical patients	132 ± 82	283 ± 66	35 ± 11
	Female surgical patients	133 ± 55	315 ± 111	39 ± 14
Kent et al.[244]	Elderly surgical patients	117 ± 24	126 ± 40	17 ± 4
Goresky et al.[138]	Children 3 mo–14 yr	76 ± 27	7.9 ± 0.12[b]	0.42 ± 0.12[c]
Meistelman et al.[139]	Children 4–8 yr	40 ± 9	4.7 ± 0.6[b]	0.16 ± 0.1[c]
	Adults	97 ± 22	4.2 ± 1.7[b]	0.5 ± 0.16[c]
Roure et al.[140]	Children 10 mo–6.5 yr	63 ± 24	11.1 ± 3.9[b]	0.8 ± 0.3[c]
	Adults	95 ± 20	5.9 ± 1.6[b]	1.0 ± 0.7[c]
den Hollander et al.[245]	Cardiac surgical infants	69 ± 25	8.2 ± 2.2[b]	0.5 ± 0.12[c]
	Cardiac surgical children	62 ± 59	6.3 ± 0.8[b]	0.3 ± 0.08[c]

Abbreviations: CL, clearance; $t_{1/2}$, half-life; V, volume of distribution.

[a] Values are mean ± standard deviation.

[b] ml/min/kg.

[c] L/kg.

slower elimination. Several factors could explain the altered pharmacokinetics of sufentanil in these patients. The investigators sampled blood for up to 24 hours, possibly resulting in a more accurate estimation of the terminal phase of elimination and, thus, more accurate pharmacokinetic parameters. This is unlikely, however, to be the whole story. The increased V_{ss} may have been related to fluid shifts and hemodilution.

PHARMACOKINETICS OF OPIOID AGONIST-ANTAGONISTS

Pentazocine

Pentazocine, a benzomorphan compound, was the first clinically successful member of the so-called agonist-antagonist group of opioids. Its analgesic potency is approximately one-third that of morphine. Pentazocine is a racemic mixture, and anal-

Table 3-7 Pharmacokinetic Parameters for Sufentanil[a]

Authors	Patients	$t_{1/2}$ (min)	CL (ml/min)	V_{ss} (L)
Bovill et al.[18]	Adult surgical patients	164 ± 22	890 ± 223	118 ± 32
Hudson et al.[247]	Aortic surgery patients	726 ± 348	1,116 ± 238	647 ± 344
Sear[198]	Renal transplant patients	201 ± 151	1,090 ± 446	206 ± 163
	Adult surgical patients	185 ± 90	1,196 ± 420	196 ± 64
Fyman et al.[202]	Renal transplant patients[b]	176 ± 275	776 ± 249	57 ± 10.8
Davis et al.[203]	Adolescent renal transplant patients[b]	76 ± 33	12.8 ± 12.0[c]	1.28 ± 0.62[d]
	Adolescent surgical patients[b]	90 ± 16	16.4 ± 6.1[c]	1.65 ± 0.6[d]
Chauvin et al.[189]	Patients with cirrhosis	246 ± 36	762 ± 311	280 ± 107
	Adult surgical patients	210 ± 54	740 ± 161	221 ± 57
Matteo et al.[166]	Elderly neurosurgical patients	113 ± 89	1,125 ± 522	137 ± 64
	Young neurosurgical patients	137 ± 68	1,226 ± 469	217 ± 74
Schwartz et al.[23]	Neurosurgical patients, hypocapnic	232 ± 60	1,170 ± 435	380 ± 131
	Neurosurgical patients, hormocapnic	143 ± 51	1,253 ± 203	255 ± 79
Schwartz et al.[19]	Obese surgical patients	208 ± 82	1,990 ± 860	547 ± 178
	Adult surgical patients	135 ± 42	1,780 ± 520	346 ± 144
Greeley et al.[135]	Pediatric patients			
	0 mo–1 mo	737 ± 346	6.7 ± 6.1[c]	4.2 ± 1.01[d]
	1 mo–23 mo	214 ± 41	18.1 ± 2.8[c]	3.1 ± 0.95[d]
	3–12 yr	140 ± 30	16.9 ± 3.2[c]	2.7 ± 0.50[d]
	13–18 yr	209 ± 23	13.1 ± 3.6[c]	2.8 ± 0.53[d]

Abbreviations: CL, clearance; $t_{1/2}$, half-life; V, volume of distribution.
[a] Values are mean ± standard deviation.
[b] Limited sampling time.
[c] ml/min/kg.
[d] L/kg.

gesia resides exclusively in the L-isomer.[248] Pentazocine is available for oral and parenteral administration. After oral administration, peak concentrations in the blood are reached within 1 to 3 hours and within 15 to 45 minutes after intramuscular administration. The oral bioavailability is about 20 percent, indicating a large hepatic first pass effect. Clearance has ranged from 768 to 1,500 ml/min in various studies (Table 3-8). The renal clearance of pentazocine was low (45 ml/min) in normal subjects.[250] In patients with cirrhosis of the liver, clearance values were about one-half that in normal subjects, and oral availability increased to about 70 percent.[250,251] Clearance of pentazocine in elderly subjects (age 60 to 90 years) was 11.7 ± 3.6 ml/min/kg compared with 22.1 ± 4.1 ml/min/kg in a younger group aged 22 to 48 years.[258] The elimina-

tion half-life in the elderly subjects was 4.1 ± 1.2 hours and it was 2.5 ± 0.7 hours in the younger subjects. Pentazocine is 60 percent bound to plasma proteins.[259]

Butorphanol

Butorphanol is a fully synthetic morphinan derivative available as the tartrate salt. One milligram of the salt is equivalent to 0.68 mg of butorphanol base. Butorphanol is 3.5 to 5 times more potent than is morphine. Butorphanol is about 80 percent bound to plasma proteins. Metabolism is by N-dealkylation, hydroxylation, and conjugation, and considerable quantities of the conjugated drug are present in the blood 5 minutes after intravenous injection in humans.[252] Studies in which blood samples were obtained for 8 hours reported an elimi-

Table 3-8 Pharmacokinetic Parameters for Mixed Agonist-Antagonist Opioids[a]

	Patients	$t_{1/2}$ (min)	CL (ml/min)	V_{ss} (L)
Pentazocine				
Ehrnebro et al.[249]	Adult volunteers	203 ± 72	$1,380 \pm 320$	396 ± 136
Neal et al.[250]	Adult volunteers	230 ± 28	$1,246 \pm 236$	342 ± 188
	Patients with liver cirrhosis	396 ± 115	675 ± 296	306 ± 77
Pond et al.[251]	Adult volunteers	342 ± 84	768 ± 130	
	Patients with liver cirrhosis	720 ± 180	398 ± 121	
Butorphanol				
Pittman et al.[252]	Adult volunteers	159 ± 23		
Gaver et al.[253]	Adult volunteers	180 ± 240	$4,065$	
Bullingham et al.[248]		162	$2,700$	350
Nalbupine				
Aitkenhead et al.[254]	Adult volunteers	$222\ (110–459)$	$1,500\ (820–2,290)$	$315\ (162–498)$
Lo et al.[255]	Adult volunteers	138 ± 72	$1,642 \pm 380$	
Sear et al.[256]	Adult surgical patients	136 ± 55	$1,095 \pm 277$	160 ± 40
Buprenorphine				
Bullingham et al.[257]		184 ± 117	$1,275 \pm 281$	188 ± 111

Abbreviations: CL, clearance; $t_{1/2}$, half-life; V, volume of distribution.

[a] Values are mean ± standard deviation.

nation half-life of about 160 minutes, and a plasma clearance of 2,700 to 4,000 ml/min,[248,253] much greater than normal hepatic blood flow. Ramsey et al.[260] studied butorphanol kinetics in healthy male subjects following an intravenous bolus of 2 mg and collected blood samples for 24 hours. The blood clearance was 21 ml/min/kg. Blood clearance did not differ statistically between subjects aged 23 to 34 years and those aged 65 to 79 years. However, there were positive correlations between age and both elimination half-life and V_{ss}.

Nalbuphine

Nalbuphine hydrochloride is the N-cyclobutylmethyl analog of oxymorphone. It is approximately equipotent with morphine. Nalbuphine binding to plasma protein is 25 to 40 percent.[256] The reported elimination half-life of nalbuphine in healthy adult volunteers varied between 1.9 and 3.7 hours.[254,255,261] Total body clearance is about 1,500 ml/min. In patients undergoing general anesthesia, Sear et al.[256] found an elimination half-life of 136 minutes and a total body clearance of 1,095 ml/min, the shorter half-life in comparison with awake subjects being the result of a lower volume of distribution. In patients undergoing cardiac sur-

gery, the elimination half-life was 3 to 3.5 hours.[262] In children younger than 9 years of age, the elimination half-life (0.9 hours) was significantly shorter than in young adults (1.9 hours) or elderly patients (2 to 3 hours).[261] The bioavailability of oral nalbuphine was 12 to 17 percent in young adults[255,261] but increased to 46 percent in patients aged older than 65 years.[261] The elimination half-life following oral administration was considerably longer than after intravenous administration (2.3 versus 6.9 to 7.7 hours).[255] The low bioavailability and the prolonged half-life of nalbuphine after oral administration are likely the result of extensive first pass metabolism and enterohepatic circulation.[255] In mothers given nalbuphine intramuscularly in the postpartum period, only about 0.01 percent of the dose was recovered in breast milk during a 24-hour period.[263]

Buprenorphine

Buprenorphine is a semisynthetic derivative of thebaine, an opium alkaloid. Buprenorphine is lipophilic and extensively bound to plasma proteins, with a bound fraction of 95 to 98 percent.[264] Its pK_a is 9.24. It is metabolized in humans by N-dealkylation and conjugation. There are no data on oral bioavailability in humans, but in the dog it is only 3 to 6 percent.[265] In humans, the hepatic extraction ratio is 0.85 so that oral systemic availability would be expected to be about 15 percent or less.[257,266] When given sublingually, the average bioavailability is about 55 percent, but absorption is slow and the time to achieve peak plasma concentrations is variable, with a range of 90 to 360 minutes.[266] The use of the sublingual route for initiating therapy with buprenorphine will result in an appreciable delay in the onset of analgesia. However, when used for maintenance after parenteral loading, postoperative analgesia is smooth and uniform.[267] When buprenorphine is given intramuscularly, absorption is rapid, and peak plasma levels can occur within 5 minutes. Beyond this time, plasma levels differ little from those seen after intravenous administration of the same dose.[257] The elimination half-life of buprenorphine after intravenous administration is about 5 hours.[266] Plasma clearance, calculated from the data reported by Bullingham et al.[266] is 1,400 ml/min, consistent with a high hepatic extraction ratio. The clearance of buprenorphine will therefore be dependent on hepatic blood flow, and plasma clearance in patients under general anesthesia with halothane was about 70 percent that in awake subjects. This is consistent with a 30 percent reduction in hepatic blood flow during halothane anesthesia.[268] It should be noted that, because of the extremely slow dissociation of buprenorphine from the opioid receptor, the pharmacologic effect may persist without a direct relationship to the plasma concentration (see Ch. 5).[269]

REFERENCES

1. Pardridge WM, Oldendorf WH: Transport of metabolic substrates through the blood brain barrier. J Neurochem 28:5, 1977
2. Bernards CM, Hill HF: Physical and chemical properties of drug molecules governing their diffusion through the meninges. Anesthesiology 77:750, 1992
3. Stoeckel H, Hengstman JH, Schüttler J: Pharmacokinetics of fentanyl as a possible explanation of recurrence of respiratory depression. Br J Anaesth 51:741, 1979
4. Björkman S, Stanski DR, Verotta D, Harashima H: Comparative tissue concentration profiles of fentanyl and alfentanil in humans predicted from tissue/blood partition data obtained in rats. Anesth Analg 72:865, 1990
5. Hanks GW, Wand PJ: Enterohepatic circulation of opioid drugs. Is it clinically relevant in the treatment of cancer patients. Clin Pharmacokinet 17:65, 1989
6. Hanks GW, Hoskin PJ, Aherne GW et al: Enterohepatic circulation of morphine. Lancet 1:469, 1988
7. Leslie ST, Rhodes A, Black FM: Controlled release morphine sulphate tablets—a study in normal volunteers. Br J Clin Pharmacol 9:631, 1980
8. Säwe J, Dahlstrom B, Paalzow L, Rane A: Morphine kinetics in cancer patients. Clin Pharmacol Ther 30:629, 1981
9. Meuldermans WEG, Hurkmans RMA, Heykants JJP: Plasma protein binding and distribution of fentanyl, sufentanil, alfentanil and lofentanil in blood. Arch Int Pharmacodyn Ther 257:4, 1982
10. Hug CC Jr, Murphy MR: Tissue distribution of fentanyl and termination of its effect in rats. Anesthesiology 55:369, 1981
11. Scott JC, Ponganis KV, Stanski DR: EEG quantitation of narcotic effect: the comparative pharmacodynamics of fentanyl and alfentanil. Anesthesiology 62:234, 1985
12. Scott JC, Cooke JE, Stanski DR: Electroencephalographic quantitation of opioid effects: comparative pharmacodynamics of fentanyl and sufentanil. Anesthesiology 74:34, 1991
13. Judis J: Binding of codeine, morphine, and methadone to human serum proteins. J Pharm Sci 6:802, 1977
14. Gesink-van der Veer BJ, Burm AGL, Hennis PJ, Bovill JG: Alfentanil requirement in Crohn's disease: increased alfentanil dose requirement in patients with Crohn's disease. Anaesthesia 44:209, 1989
15. Bloedow DC, Hansbrough JF, Hardin T, Simons M: Postburn serum drug binding and serum protein concentrations. J Clin Pharmacol 26:147, 1986
16. Macfie AG, Magides AD, Reilly CS: Disposition of alfentanil in burns patients. Br J Anaesth 69:447, 1992
17. Gibaldi M, McNamara PJ: Apparent volumes of distribution and drug binding to plasma proteins and tissues. Eur J Clin Pharmacol 13:373, 1978
18. Bovill JG, Sebel PS, Blackburn CL et al: The pharmacokinetics of sufentanil in surgical patients. Anesthesiology 61:502, 1984
19. Schwartz AE, Matteo RS, Ornstein E et al: Pharma-

cokinetics of sufentanil in obese patients. Anesth Analg 73:790, 1991

20. Nishitateno K, Ngai SH, Finck AD, Berkowitz BA: Pharmacokinetics of morphine: concentrations in the serum and brain of the dog during hyperventilation. Anesthesiology 50:520, 1979

21. Ainslie SG, Eisele JH, Corkill G: Fentanyl concentrations in brain and serum during respiratory acid-base changes in the dog. Anesthesiology 51:293, 1979

22. Cartwright P, Prys-Roberts C, Gill K et al: Ventilatory depression related to plasma fentanyl concentrations during and after anesthesia in humans. Anesth Analg 62:966, 1983

23. Schwartz AE, Matteo RS, Ornstein E et al: Pharmacokinetics of sufentanil in neurosurgical patients undergoing hyperventilation. Br J Anaesth 63:385, 1989

24. Matteo RS, Ornstein E, Schwartz AE et al: Effects of hypocarbia on the pharmacodynamics of sufentanil in humans. Anesth Analg 75:186, 1992

25. Schulman DS, Kaufman JJ, Eisenstein MM, Rapoport SI: Blood pH and brain uptake of 14C-morphine. Anesthesiology 61:540, 1984

26. Norman J: One-compartment kinetics. Br J Anaesth 69:387, 1992

27. Shafer SL, Varvel JR: Pharmacokinetics, pharmacodynamics, and rational opioid selection. Anesthesiology 74:53, 1991

28. Shafer SL, Stanski DR: Improving the clinical utility of anesthetic drug pharmacokinetics. Anesthesiology 76:327, 1992

29. Varvel JR, Shafer SL, Hwang SS et al: Absorption characteristics of transdermally administered fentanyl. Anesthesiology 70:928, 1989

30. Ionescu TI, Taverne RH, Houweling PL et al: Pharmacokinetic study of extradural and intrathecal sufentanil anaesthesia for major surgery. Br J Anaesth 66:458, 1991

31. Taverne RHT, Ionescu TI, Nuyten STM: Comparative absorption and distribution pharmacokinetics of intravenous and epidural sufentanil for major abdominal surgery. Clin Pharmacokinet 23:231, 1992

32. Henthorn TK, Krejcie TC, Avram MJ: The relationship between alfentanil distribution kinetics and cardiac output. Clin Pharmacol Ther 52:190, 1992

33. Hughes MA, Glass PS, Jacobs JR: Context-sensitive half-time in multicompartment pharmacokinetic models for intravenous anesthetic drugs. Anesthesiology 76:334, 1992

34. Wilkinson GR, Shand DG: A physiological approach to hepatic drug clearance. Clin Pharmacol Ther 18:377, 1975

35. Rowland M, Benet LZ, Graham GG: Clearance concepts in pharmacokinetics. J Pharmacokinet Biopharm 1:123, 1973

36. Gibaldi M, Levy G, McNamara PJ: Effect of plasma protein and tissue binding on the biologic half-life of drugs. Clin Pharmacol Ther 24:1, 1978

37. Runciman WB, Mather LE: Effects of anaesthesia on drug disposition. p. 86. In Feldman SA, Scurr CF, Paton W (eds): Drugs in Anaesthesia: Mechanisms of Action. Edward Arnold, London, 1987

38. Juhl B, Einer-Jensen N: Hepatic blood flow and cardiac output during halothane anaesthesia: an animal study. Acta Anaesthesiol Scand 18:114, 1974

39. Sullivan AF, McQuay HJ, Bailey D, Dickenson AH: The spinal antinociceptive actions of morphine metabolites morphine-6-glucuronide and normorphine in the rat. Brain Res 482:219, 1989

40. Chauvin M, Bonnett F, Montembault C et al: The influence of hepatic plasma flow on alfentanil plasma concentration plateaus achieved with an infusion model in humans: measurement of alfentanil hepatic extraction coefficient. Anesth Analg 65:999, 1986

41. Cousins MJ: Comparative pharmacokinetics of spinal opioids in humans: a step toward determination of relative safety. Anesthesiology 67:875, 1987

42. Bernards CM, Hill HF: Morphine and alfentanil permeability through the spinal dura, arachnoid, and pia mater of dogs and monkeys. Anesthesiology 73:1214, 1990

43. Nordberg G, Hedner T, Mellstrand T, Dahlström B: Pharmacokinetic aspects of intrathecal morphine analgesia. Anesthesiology 60:448, 1984

44. Nordberg G, Hedner T, Mellstrand T, Borg L: Pharmacokinetics of epidural morphine in man. Eur J Clin Pharmacol 26:233, 1984

45. Sjöström S, Tamsen A, Persson MP, Hartvig P: Pharmacokinetics of intrathecal morphine and meperidine in humans. Anesthesiology 67:889, 1987

46. Sjöström S, Hartvig P, Persson MP, Tamsen A: Pharmacokinetics of epidural morphine and meperidine in humans. Anesthesiology 67:877, 1987

47. Zakowski MI, Ramanathan S, Sharnick S, Turndorf H: Uptake and distribution of bupivacaine and morphine after intrathecal administration in parturients: effects of epinephrine. Anesth Analg 74:664, 1992

48. Dahlström B, Tamsen A, Paalzow L, Hartvig P: Patient-controlled analgesic therapy, part IV: pharma-

cokinetics and analgesic plasma concentrations of morphine. Clin Pharmacokinet 7:266, 1982

49. Graves DA, Arrigo JM, Foster TS et al: Relationship between plasma morphine concentrations and pharmacologic effects in postoperative patients using patient-controlled analgesia. Clin Pharm 4:41, 1985

50. Gourlay GK, Cherry DA, Plummer JL et al: The influence of drug polarity on the absorption of opioid drugs into CSF and subsequent cephalad migration following lumbar epidural administration: application to morphine and pethidine. Pain 31:297, 1987

51. Koren G, Sandler AN, Klein J et al: Relationship between the pharmacokinetics and the analgesic and respiratory pharmacodynamics of epidural sufentanil. Clin Pharmacol Ther 46:458, 1989

52. Colpaert FC, Leysen JE, Michiels M, van den Hoogen RH: Epidural and intravenous sufentanil in the rat: analgesia, opiate receptor binding, and drug concentrations in plasma and brain. Anesthesiology 65:41, 1986

53. Hansdottir V, Hedner T, Woestenborghs R, Nordberg G: The CSF and plasma pharmacokinetics of sufentanil after intrathecal administration. Anesthesiology 74:264, 1991

54. Andersen HB, Christensen B, Findlay JW, Jansen JA: Pharmacokinetics of intravenous, intrathecal and epidural morphine and fentanyl in the goat. Acta Anaesthesiol Scand 30:393, 1986

55. Justins DM, Knott C, Luthman J, Reynolds F: Epidural versus intramuscular fentanyl. Analgesia and pharmacokinetics in labour. Anaesthesia 38:937, 1983

56. Gourlay GK, Murphy TM, Plummer JL et al: Pharmacokinetics of fentanyl in lumbar and cervical CSF following lumbar epidural and intravenous administration. Pain 38:253, 1989

57. Rostaing S, Bonnet F, Levron JC et al: Effect of epidural clonidine on analgesia and pharmacokinetics of epidural fentanyl in postoperative patients. Anesthesiology 75:420, 1991

58. Ossipov MH, Suarez LJ, Spaulding T: Antinociceptive interactions between alpha 2-adrenergic and opiate agonists at the spinal level in rodents. Anesth Analg 68:194, 1989

59. Loper KA, Ready B, Downey M et al: Epidural and intravenous fentanyl infusions are clinically equivalent after knee surgery. Anesth Analg 70:72, 1990

60. Sandler AN, Stringer D, Panos L et al: A randomized, double-blind comparison of lumbar epidural and intravenous fentanyl infusions for postthora-

cotomy pain relief. Analgesic, pharmacokinetic, and respiratory effects. Anesthesiology 77:626, 1992

61. Ellis DJ, Millar WL, Reisner LS: A randomized double-blind comparison of epidural versus intravenous fentanyl infusion for analgesia after caesarean section. Anesthesiology 72:981, 1990

62. Salomäki TE, Laitinen JO, Nuutinen LS: A randomized double-blind comparison of epidural versus intravenous fentanyl infusion for analgesia after thoracotomy. Anesthesiology 75:790, 1991

63. Penon C, Negre I, Ecoffey C et al: Analgesia and ventilatory response to carbon dioxide after intramuscular and epidural alfentanil. Anesth Analg 67:313, 1988

64. Chauvin M, Salbaing J, Perrin D et al: Clinical assessment and plasma pharmacokinetics associated with intramuscular or extradural alfentanil. Br J Anaesth 57:886, 1985

65. Gepts E, Heytens L, Camu F: Pharmacokinetics and placental transfer of intravenous and epidural alfentanil in parturient women. Anesth Analg 65:1155, 1986

66. Camu F, Debucquoy F: Alfentanil infusion for postoperative pain: a comparison of epidural and intravenous routes. Anesthesiology 75:171, 1991

67. Burm AGL, Haak-van der Lely F, van Kleef JW et al: Pharmacokinetics of alfentanil following epidural administration. Reg Anesth 1993:70(Suppl 1):76, 1993 (abstracts)

68. Lavrijsen K, van Houdt J, Meuldermans W, Knaeps F: Metabolism of alfentanil by isolated hepatocytes of rat and dog. Xenobiotica 18:183, 1988

69. Meuldermans W, Hendrickx J, Lauwers W et al: Excretion and biotransformation of alfentanil and sufentanil in rats and dogs. Drug Metab Dispos 15:905, 1987

70. Bovill JG, Odoom JA, Heykants J: Biotransformation of alftentanil in man. Anesthesiology 69:A467, 1988

71. Meuldermans W, van Peer A, Hendrickx J et al: Alfentanil pharmacokinetics and metabolism in humans. Anesthesiology 69:527, 1988

72. Sadman AJ: Cimetidine—drug interactions. Am J Med 76:109, 1984

73. Lauven PM, Stoeckel H, Schüttler J, Schwilden H: Prevention of fentanyl rebound by administration of cimetidine. Anaesthetist 30:467, 1981

74. Borel JD, Bentley JB, Nenad RE: Cimetidine alteration of fentanyl pharmacokinetics in the dog. p. 149. In Proceedings of the 56th Annual Meeting, International Anesthetic Research Society, 1982

75. Feely J, Wilkinson GR, Wood AJJ: Reduction of

liver blood flow and propranolol metabolism by cimetidine. N Engl J Med 304:692, 1981

76. Rendic S, Kajfez F, Ruf HH: Characterization of
cimetidine, ranitidine, and related structures' interaction with cytochrome P-450. Drug Metab Dispos
11:137, 1983

77. Bartkowski RR, Goldber ME, Larijani GE: Inhibition of alfentanil metabolism by erythromycin. Clin
Pharmacol Ther 46:99, 1989

78. Bartkowski RR, McDonnell TE: Prolonged alfentanil effect following erythromycin administration.
Anesthesiology 73:566, 1990

79. Nebert DW, Nelson DR, Coon MJ et al: The P450
superfamily: update on new sequences, gene mapping and recommended nomenclature. DNA Cell
Biol 10:1, 1991

80. Kalow W: Ethnic differences in drug metabolism.
Clin Pharmacokinet 7:373, 1982

81. Nakamura K, Goto F, Ray WA et al: Interethnic
differences in genetic polymorphism of hydroxylation between Japanese and Caucasians. Clin Pharmacol Ther 38:402, 1985

82. Mortimer Ö, Persson K, Ladona MG et al: Polymorphic formation of morphine from codeine in poor
and extensive metabolizers of dextromethorphan:
relationship to the presence of immunoidentified
cytochrome P-450IID1. Clin Pharmacol Ther 47:27,
1990

83. Dayer P, Desmeules HW, Leemann T, Striberni R:
Bioactivation of the narcotic drug codeine in human
liver is mediated by the polymorphic onooxygenase
catalyzing debrisoquine 4-hydroxylation (cytochrome P-450 dbl/bufl). Biochem Biophys Res
Commun 152:411, 1988

84. Desmeules HW, Dayer P, Gascon M-P, Magistris M:
Impact of genetic and environmental factors on codeine analgesia. Clin Pharmacol Ther 45:122, 1989

85. Henthorn TK, Spina E, Dumont E, von Bahr C: In
vitro inhibition of a polymorphic human liver P-450
isoenzyme by narcotic analgesics. Anesthesiology
70:339, 1989

86. Lavrijsen KLM, van Houdt JMG, van Dyck DMJ et
al: Is the metabolism of alfentanil subject to debrisoquine polymorphism? A study using human liver
microsomes. Anesthesiology 69:535, 1988

87. Yun C-H, Wood M, Wood AJJ, Guengerich FP:
Identification of the pharmacogenetic determinants
of alfentanil metabolism: cytochrome P-450 3A4.
Anesthesiology 77:467, 1992

88. Lemmens HJM, Bovill JG, Hennis PJ, Burm AGL:
Age has no effect on the pharmacodynamics of alfentanil. Anesth Analg 67:956, 1988

89. Weldon ST, Perry DF, Cork RC, Gandolfi AJ: Detection of picogram levels of sufentanil by capillary
gas chromatography. Anesthesiology 65:684, 1985

90. Heykants J, Woestenborghs R, Timmerman P: Reliability of sufentanil plasma level assays in patients.
Anesthesiology 65:112, 1986

91. Hiller A, Olkkola KT, Isohanni P, Saarnivaara L:
Unconsciousness associated with midazolam and
erythromycin. Br J Anaesth 65:826, 1990

92. Egan TD, Lemmens HJM, Fiset P et al: The pharmacokinetics and pharmacodynamics of G187084B.
Anesthesiology 77:A369, 1992

93. Westmorland C, Sebel PS, Hug CC Jr et al: Pharmacokinetics and histamine release following
G187084B, a new ultra-short acting opioid. Anesthesiology 77:A395, 1992

94. Säwe J, Odar-Cederlöf I: Kinetics of morphine in
patients with renal failure. Eur J Clin Pharmacol
32:377, 1987

95. Mazoit JX, Sandouk P, Scherrmann J-M, Roche A:
Extrahepatic metabolism of morphine occurs in humans. Clin Pharmacol Ther 48:613, 1990

96. Garrett ER, Jackson AJ: Pharmacokinetics of morphine and its surrogates III: morphine and mor-
phine-3-monoglucuronide pharmacokinetics in the
dog as a function of dose. J Pharm Sci 68:753, 1979

97. Säwe J, Rane A, Svensson A-O: Morphine metabolism in cancer patients on increasing doses—no evidence of autoinduction or dose dependence. Br J
Clin Pharmacol 16:85, 1983

98. Patwardhan RV, Johnson RF, Hoyumpa A et al:
Normal metabolism of morphine in cirrhosis. Gastroenterology 81:1006, 1981

99. Mazoit JX, Sandouk P, Zetlaoui P, Scherrmann JM:
Pharmacokinetics of unchanged morphine in normal and cirrhotic subjects. Anesth Analg 66:293,
1987

100. Bodenham A, Guinn K, Park GR: Extrahepatic
morphine metabolism in man during the anhepatic
phase of orthotopic liver transplantation. Br J
Anaesth 63:308, 1989

101. Shelly MP, Quinn KG, Park GR: Pharmacokinetics
of morphine in patients following orthotopic liver
transplantation. Br J Anaesth 63:375, 1989

102. Iwamato K, Klassen CD: First-pass effect of morphine in rats. J Pharmacol Exp Ther 200:236, 1977

103. Pacifici GM, Rane A: Renal glucuronidation of morphine in the human fetus. Acta Pharmacol Toxicol
50:155, 1982

104. Shelly MP, Cory EP, Park GR: Pharmacokinetics of
morphine in two children before and after liver
transplantation. Br J Anaesth 58:1218, 1986

105. Roerig DL, Kotrly KJ, Vucins EJ et al: First pass uptake of fentanyl, meperidine, and morphine in the human lung. Anesthesiology 67:466, 1987

106. Boer F, Bovill JG, Burm AGL, Mooren RAG: Uptake of sufentanil, alfentanil and morphine in the lungs of patients about to undergo coronary artery surgery. Br J Anaesth 68:370, 1992

107. Persson MP, Wiklund L, Hartvig P, Paalzow L: Potential pulmonary uptake and clearance of morphine in postoperative patients. Eur J Clin Pharmacol 30:567, 1986

108. Ratcliffe FM: Absence of morphine glucuronidation in the human lung. Eur J Clin Pharmacol 37:537, 1989

109. Wahlström A, Winblad B, Bixo M, Rane A: Human brain metabolism of morphine and naloxone. Pain 35:121, 1988

110. Smith MT, Watt JA, Cramond T: Morphine-3-glucuronide—a potent antagonist of morphine analgesia. Life Sci 47:579, 1990

111. Yoshimura H, Natsuki R, Ida S, Oguri K: Chemical reactivity of morphine-6-conjugates and their binding to rat brain. Chem Pharm Bull (Tokyo) 24:901, 1976

112. Abbott FV, Palmour RM: Morphine-6-glucuronide: analgesic effects and receptor binding profile in rats. Life Sci 43:1685, 1988

113. Bower S, Sear JW, Roy RC, Carter RF: Effects of different hepatic pathologies on disposition of alfentanil in anaesthetized patients. Br J Anaesth 68:462, 1992

114. Hand CW, Blunnie WP, Claffey LP et al: Potential analgesic contribution from morphine 6 glucuronide in CSF. Lancet 2:1207, 1987

115. Hanna MH, Peat SJ, Woodham M et al: Analgesic efficacy and CSF pharmacokinetics of intrathecal morphine-6-glucuronide: comparison with morphine. Br J Anaesth 64:547, 1990

116. Osborne R, Joel S, Trew P, Slevin M: Morphine and metabolite behavior after different routes of morphine administration: demonstration of the importance of the active metabolite morphine-6-glucuronide. Clin Pharmacol Ther 47:12, 1990

117. Osborne R, Thompson P, Joel S et al: The analgesic activity of morphine-6-glucuronide. Br J Clin Pharmacol 34:130, 1992

118. Portenoy RK, Thaler HT, Inturrisi CE et al: The metabolite morphine-6-glucuronide contributes to the analgesia produced by morphine infusion in patients with pain and normal renal function. Clin Pharmacol Ther 51:422, 1992

119. Hanna MH, Peat SJ, Knibb AA, Fung C: Disposition of morphine-6-glucuronide and morphine in healthy volunteers. Br J Anaesth 66:103, 1991

120. Pelligrino DA, Riegler FX, Albrecht RF: Ventilatory effects of fourth cerebroventricular infusions of morphine-6- or morphine-3-glucuronide in the awake dog. Anesthesiology 71:936, 1989

121. Wolff J, Bigler D, Christensen BC et al: Influence of renal function on the elimination of morphine and morphine glucuronides. Eur J Clin Pharmacol 34:353, 1988

122. Osborne RJ, Joel SP, Slevin ML: Morphine intoxication in renal failure: the role of morphine-6-glucuronide. BMJ 292:1548, 1986

123. Hasselström J, Berg V, Löfgren A, Säwe J: Long lasting respiratory depression induced by morphine-6-glucuronide. Br J Clin Pharmacol 27:515, 1989

124. Sear JW, Hand CW, Moore RA, McQuay HJ: Studies on morphine disposition: influence of general anaesthesia on plasma concentrations of morphine and its metabolites. Br J Anaesth 62:22, 1989

125. Krieter PA, van Dijke RA: Cytochrome P-450 and halothane metabolism. Decrease in rat liver microsomal P-450 in vitro. Chem Biol Interact 44:219, 1983

126. Pokela M-L, Olkkola KT, Koivisto M, Ryhänen P: Pharmacokinetics and pharmacodynamics of meperidine in neonates and infants. Clin Pharmacol Ther 52:342, 1992

127. Gauntlett IS, Fisher DM, Hertzra RE et al: Pharmacokinetics of fentanyl in neonatal humans and lambs: effects of age. Anesthesiology 69:683, 1988

128. Koehntop DE, Rodman JH, Brundage DM et al: Pharmacokinetics of fentanyl in neonates. Anesth Analg 65:227, 1986

129. Masey SA, Koehler RC, Buck JR et al: Effect of abdominal distension on central and regional hemodynamics in neonatal lambs. Pediatr Res 19:1244, 1985

130. Yaster M: The dose response of fentanyl in neonatal anesthesia. Anesthesiology 66:433, 1987

131. Robinson PJ, Rapoport SI: Kinetics of protein binding determine rates of uptake of drugs by brain. Am J Physiol 251:R1212, 1986

132. Lemmens HJ, Burm AG, Bovill JG et al: Pharmacodynamics of alfentanil. The role of plasma protein binding. Anesthesiology 76:65, 1992

133. Meistelman C, Benhamou D, Barre J et al: Effects of age on plasma protein binding of sufentanil. Anesthesiology 72:470, 1990

134. Notarianni LJ: Plasma protein binding of drugs in

pregnancy and in neonates. Clin Pharmacokinet 18:20, 1990

135. Greeley WJ, de Bruijn NP, Davis DP: Sufentanil pharmacokinetics in pediatric cardiovascular patients. Anesth Analg 66:1067, 1987

136. Dixon R, Howes J, Gentile J et al: Nalmefene: intravenous safety and kinetics of a new opioid antagonist. Clin Pharmacol Ther 39:49, 1986

137. Greeley WJ, de Bruijn NP: Changes in sufentanil pharmacokinetics within the neonatal period. Anesth Analg 67:86, 1988

138. Goresky GV, Koren G, Sabourin MA et al: The pharmacokinetics of alfentanil in children. Anesthesiology 67:654, 1987

139. Meistelman C, Saint-Maurice C, LePaul M et al: A comparison of alfentanil pharmacokinetics in children and adults. Anesthesiology 66:13, 1987

140. Roure P, Jean N, Leclerc AC et al: Pharmacokinetics of alfentanil in children undergoing surgery. Br J Anaesth 59:1437, 1987

141. Morselli PL, Franco-Morselli R, Bossi L: Clinical pharmacokinetics in newborns and children. Age-related differences and their therapeutic implications. Clin Pharmacokinet 5:485, 1980

142. Davis PJ, Killian A, Stiller RL et al: Pharmacokinetics of alfentanil in newborn premature infants and older children. Dev Pharmacol Ther 13:21, 1989

143. Killian A, Davis PJ, Stiller RL et al: Influence of gestational age on pharmacokinetics of alfentanil in neonates. Dev Pharmacol Ther 15:82, 1990

144. den Hollander JM, Hennis PJ, Burm AG et al: Pharmacokinetics of alfentanil before and after cardiopulmonary bypass in pediatric patients undergoing cardiac surgery: part I. J Cardiothorac Vasc Anesth 6:308, 1992

145. Yaster M, Deshpande JK: Management of pediatric pain with opioid analgesics. J Pediatr 113:421, 1988

146. Besunder JB, Reed MD, Blumer JL: Principles of drug biodisposition in the neonate. A critical evaluation of the pharmacokinetic-pharmacodynamic interface (part I). Clin Pharmacokinet 14:189, 1988

147. Chay PC, Duffy BJ, Walker JS: Pharmacokinetic-pharmacodynamic relationships of morphine in neonates. Clin Pharmacol Ther 51:334, 1992

148. Olkkola KT, Maunuksela EL, Korpela R, Rosenberg PH: Kinetics and dynamics of postoperative intravenous morphine in children. Clin Pharmacol Ther 44:128, 1988

149. Pasternak GW, Bodnar RJ, Clark JA, Inturrisi CE: Morphine-6-glucuronide, a potent mu agonist. Life Sci 41:2845, 1987

150. Lynn AM, Slattery JT: Morphine pharmacokinetics in early infancy. Anesthesiology 66:136, 1987

151. Choonara I, Ekbom Y, Lindström B, Rane A: Morphine sulphation in children. Br J Clin Pharmacol 30:897, 1990

152. Choonara IA, McKay P, Hain R, Rane A: Morphine metabolism in children. Br J Clin Pharmacol 28:599, 1989

153. Säwe J, Kager L, Svensson JO, Rane A: Oral morphine in cancer patients: in vivo kinetics and in vitro hepatic glucuronidation. Br J Clin Pharmacol 19:495, 1985

154. Bhat R, Chari G, Gulati A et al: Pharmacokinetics of a single dose of morphine in preterm infants during the first week of life. J Pediatr 117:477, 1990

155. Chauvin M, Sandouk P, Scherrmann JM et al: Morphine pharmacokinetics in renal failure. Anesthesiology 66:327, 1987

156. Baillie SP, Bateman DN, Coates PE, Woodhouse KW: Age and the pharmacokinetics of morphine. Age Ageing 18:258, 1989

157. Bentley JB, Borel JD, Nenad RE, Gillespie TJ: Age and fentanyl pharmacokinetics. Anesth Analg 61:968, 1982

158. Singleton MA, Rosen JI, Fisher DM: Pharmacokinetics of fentanyl in the elderly. Br J Anaesth 60:619, 1988

159. Greenblatt DJ, Sellers EM, Shader RI: Drug disposition in old age. N Engl J Med 306:1081, 1982

160. Bower S, Hull CJ: Comparative pharmacokinetics of fentanyl and alfentanil. Br J Anaesth 54:871, 1982

161. McClain DA, Hug CC Jr: Intravenous fentanyl kinetics. Clin Pharmacol Ther 28:106, 1980

162. Scott JC, Stanski DR: Decreased fentanyl and alfentanil dose requirements with age. A simultaneous pharmacokinetic and pharmacodynamic evaluation. J Pharmacol Exp Ther 240:159, 1987

163. Lemmens HJM, Burm AGL, Hennis PJ et al: Influence of age on the pharmacokinetics of alfentanil. Gender dependence. Clin Pharmacokinet 19:416, 1990

164. Sitar DS, Duke PC, Benthuysen JL et al: Aging and alfentanil disposition in healthy volunteers and surgical patients. Can J Anaesth 36:149, 1989

165. Maitre PO, Vozeh S, Heykants J et al: Population pharmacokinetics of alfentanil: the average dose-plasma concentration relationship and interindividual variability in patients. Anesthesiology 66:3, 1987

166. Matteo RS, Schwartz AE, Ornstein E et al: Pharmacokinetics of sufentanil in the elderly surgical patient. Can J Anaesth 37:852, 1990

167. Veering BT, Burm AGL, Souverign JHM et al: The effect of age on serum concentrations of albumin and α1-acid glycoprotein. Br J Clin Pharmacol 29:201, 1990

168. Craft JB, Coaldrake LA, Bolan JC et al: Placental passage and uterine effects of fentanyl. Anesth Analg 62:894, 1983

169. Meuldermans W, Woestenborghs R, Noorduin H et al: Protein binding of the analgesics alfentanil and sufentanil in maternal and neonatal plasma. Eur J Clin Pharmacol 30:217, 1986

170. Gepts E, Heytens L, Camu F: Pharmacokinetics and placental transfer of intravenous and epidural alfentanil in parturient women. Anesth Analg 65:1155, 1986

171. Wittels B, Scott DT, Sinatra RS: Exogenous opioids in human breast milk and acute neonatal neurobehavior: a preliminary study. Anesthesiology 73:864, 1990

172. Buylaert WA, Herregods LL, Mortier EP, Bogaert MG: Cardiopulmonary bypass and the pharmacokinetics of drugs. An update. Clin Pharmacokinet 17:10, 1989

173. Bansinath M, Turndorf H, Puig MM: Influence of hypo- and hyperthermia on disposition of morphine. J Clin Pharmacol 28:860, 1988

174. Bovill JG, Sebel PS: Pharmacokinetics of high-dose fentanyl. Br J Anaesth 52:795, 1980

175. Koska AJ, Romagnoli A, Kramer WG: Effect of cardiopulmonary bypass on fentanyl disposition and elimination. Clin Pharmacol Ther 29:100, 1981

176. Hug CC Jr, Moldenhauer CC: Pharmacokinetics and dynamics of fentanyl infusions in cardiac surgical patients, abstracted. Anesthesiology 57:A45, 1982

177. Robbins GR, Wynands JE, Whalley DG et al: Pharmacokinetics of alfentanil and clinical responses during cardiac surgery. Can J Anaesth 37:52, 1990

178. Hug CC, de Lange S, Burm AGL: Alfentanil pharmacokinetics in patients before and after cardiopulmonary bypass (CPB). Anesth Analg 62:245, 1983

179. Kumar K, Crankshaw DP, Morgan DJ, Beemer GH: The effect of cardiopulmonary bypass on plasma protein binding of alfentanil. Eur J Clin Pharmacol 35:47, 1988

180. den Hollander JM, Burm AG, Vletter AA, Bovill JG: Pharmacokinetics of alfentanil before and after cardiopulmonary bypass in pigs: part II. J Cardiothorac Vasc Anesth 6:313, 1992

181. Okutani R, Philbin DM, Rosow CE et al: Effect of hypothermic hemodilutional cardiopulmonary bypass on plasma sufentanil and catecholamine concentrations in humans. Anesth Analg 67:667, 1988

182. Flezzani P, Alvis MJ, Jacobs JR et al: Sufentanil disposition during cardiopulmonary bypass. Can J Anaesth 34:566, 1987

183. Koren G, Barker C, Goresky G et al: The influence of hypothermia on the disposition of fentanyl—human and animal studies. Eur J Clin Pharmacol 32:373, 1987

184. Skacel M, Knott C, Reynolds F, Aps C: Extracorporeal circuit sequestration of fentanyl and alfentanil. Br J Anaesth 58:947, 1986

185. Rosen D, Rosen K, Davidson B, Broadman L: Fentanyl uptake by the Scimed membrane oxygenator. J Cardiothorac Anesth 5:619, 1988

186. Hynynen M: Binding of fentanyl and alfentanil to the extracorporeal circuit. Acta Anaesthesiol Scand 31:706, 1987

187. Taeger K, Weninger E, Schmelzer F et al: Pulmonary kinetics of fentanyl and alfentanil in surgical patients. Br J Anaesth 61:425, 1988

188. Roerig DL, Kotrly KJ, Ahlf SB et al: Effect of propranolol on the first pass uptake of fentanyl in the human lung. Anesthesiology 71:62, 1989

189. Chauvin M, Ferrier C, Haberer JP et al: Sufentanil pharmacokinetics in patients with cirrhosis. Anesth Analg 68:1, 1989

190. Haberer JP, Schoeffler P, Couderc E, Duvaldestin P: Fentanyl pharmacokinetics in anaesthetized patients with cirrhosis. Br J Anaesth 54:1267, 1982

191. Hug CC Jr, Murphy MR, Sampson JF: Biotransformation of morphine and fentanyl in anhepatic dogs. Anesthesiology 55:A261, 1981

192. Ferrier C, Marty J, Bouffard Y et al: Alfentanil pharmacokinetics in patients with cirrhosis. Anesthesiology 62:480, 1985

193. Shafer A, Sung ML, White PF: Pharmacokinetics and pharmacodynamics of alfentanil infusions during general anesthesia. Anesth Analg 65:1021, 1986

194. Davis PJ, Stiller RL, Cook DR et al: Effects of cholestatic hepatic disease and chronic renal failure on alfentanil pharmacokinetics in children. Anesth Analg 68:579, 1989

195. Sear JW, Hand CW, Moore RA, McQuay HJ: Studies on morphine disposition: influence of renal failure on the kinetics of morphine and its metabolites. Br J Anaesth 62:28, 1989

196. Corall IM, Moore AR, Strunin L: Plasma concentrations of fentanyl in normal surgical patients and

those with severe renal and hepatic disease. Br J Anaesth 52:101P, 1980

197. Henriksen HJO, Petersen MU, Pedersen I-B: Serum alpha 1-acid glycoprotein (orosomucoid) in uraemic patients on hemodialysis. Nephron 31:24, 1982

198. Sear JW: Sufentanil disposition in patients undergoing renal transplantation: influence of choice of kinetic model. Br J Anaesth 63:60, 1989

199. Chauvin M, Lebrault C, Levron JC, Duvaldestin P: Pharmacokinetics of alfentanil in chronic renal failure. Anesth Analg 66:53, 1987

200. Bower S, Sear JW: Disposition of alfentanil in patients receiving a renal transplant. J Pharm Pharmacol 41:654, 1989

201. van Peer A, Vercauteren M, Noorduin H et al: Alfentanil kinetics in renal insufficiency. Eur J Clin Pharmacol 30:245, 1986

202. Fyman PN, Reynolds JR, Moser F et al: Pharmacokinetics of sufentanil in patients undergoing renal transplantation. Can J Anaesth 35:312, 1988

203. Davis PJ, Stiller RL, Cook DR et al: Pharmacokinetics of sufentanil in adolescent patients with chronic renal failure. Anesth Analg 67:268, 1988

204. Milne RW, Nation RL, Somogyi AA et al: The influence of renal function on the renal clearance of morphine and its glucuronide metabolites in intensive-care patients. Br J Clin Pharmacol 34:53, 1992

205. Stanski DR, Greenblatt DJ, Lowenstein E: Kinetics of intravenous and intramuscular morphine. Clin Pharmacol Ther 24:52, 1978

206. Murphy MR, Hug CC Jr: Pharmacokinetics of intravenous morphine in patients anesthetized with flurane-nitrous oxide. Anesthesiology 54:187, 1981

207. Aitkenhead AR, Vater M, Achola K et al: Pharmacokinetics of single-dose i.v. morphine in normal volunteers and patients with end-stage renal failure. Br J Anaesth 56:813, 1984

208. Merrell WJ, Gordon L, Wood AJ et al: The effect of halothane on morphine disposition: relative contributions of the liver and kidney to morphine glucuronidation in the dog. Anesthesiology 72:308, 1990

209. Verbeeck RK, Branch RA, Wilkinson GR: Meperidine disposition in man: influences of urinary pH and route of administration. Clin Pharmacol Ther 30:619, 1981

210. Nation RL: Meperidine binding in maternal and fetal plasma. Clin Pharmacol Ther 29:472, 1981

211. Stambaugh JE, Wainer IW, Sanstead JK, Hemphill DM: The clinical pharmacology of meperidine—comparison of routes of administration. J Clin Pharmacol 16:245, 1976

212. Mather LE, Tucker GT, Pflug AE et al: Meperidine kinetics in man. Intravenous injection in surgical patients and volunteers. Clin Pharmacol Ther 17:21, 1975

213. Herman RJ, McAllister CB, Branch RA, Wilkinson GR: Effects of age on meperidine disposition. Clin Pharmacol Ther 37:19, 1985

214. Bloedow DC, Goodfellow LA, Marvin J, Heimbach D: Meperidine disposition in burn patients. Res Commun Chem Pathol Pharmacol 54:87, 1986

215. Kirkwood CF, Edwards DJ, Lalka D et al: The pharmacokinetics of meperidine in acute trauma patients. J Trauma 26:1090, 1986

216. Kuhnert BR, Kuhnert PM, Prochaska AL, Sokol RJ: Meperidine disposition in mother, neonate and non-pregnant females. Clin Pharmacol Ther 27:486, 1980

217. Husemeyer RP, Cummings AJ, Romankiewicz JR, Davenport HT: A study of pethidine kinetics and analgesia in women in labour following intravenous, intramuscular and epidural administration. Br J Clin Pharmacol 13:171, 1982

218. Chan K, Tse J, Jennings F, Orme ML: Pharmacokinetics of low-dose intravenous pethidine in patients with renal dysfunction. J Clin Pharmacol 27:516, 1987

219. Klotz U, McHorse TS, Wilkinson GR, Schenker S: The effect of cirrhosis on the disposition and elimination of meperidine in man. Clin Pharmacol Ther 16:667, 1974

220. Kaiko RR, Foley KM, Grabinski PY et al: Central nervous system excitatory effects of meperidine in cancer patients. Ann Neurol 13:180, 1983

221. Armstrong PJ, Bersten A: Normeperidine toxicity. Anesth Analg 65:536, 1986

222. Szeto HH, Inturrisi CE, Houde R et al: Accumulation of normeperidine, an active metabolite of meperidine, in patients with renal failure or cancer. Ann Intern Med 86:738, 1977

223. Cummings AJ: A survey of pharmacokinetic data from pregnant women. Clin Pharmacokinet 8:344, 1983

224. Todd EL, Stafford DT, Bucovaz ET, Morrison JC: Pharmacokinetics of meperidine in pregnancy. Int J Gynaecol Obstet 29:143, 1989

225. Säwe J: High-dose morphine and methadone in cancer patients. Clinical pharmacokinetic considerations of oral treatment. Clin Pharmacokinet 11:87, 1986

226. Romach MK, Piafky KM, Abel JG et al: Methadone

binding to orosomucoid (α1-acid glycoprotein). Determinant of free fraction in the plasma. Clin Pharmacol Ther 29:211, 1981

227. Abramson F: Methadone plasma protein binding: alterations in cancer and displacement from α1-acid glycoprotein. Clin Pharmacol Ther 32:652, 1982

228. Gourlay GK, Wilson PR, Glynn CJ: Pharmacodynamics and pharmacokinetics of methadone during the postoperative period. Anesthesiology 57:458, 1982

229. Denson DD, Concilus RR, Warden G, Raj PP: Pharmacokinetics of continuous intravenous infusion of methadone in the early post-burn period. J Clin Pharmacol 30:70, 1990

230. Nilsson MJ: Clinical Pharmacokinetics of Methadone, thesis. Uppsala University, Uppsala, Sweden, 1982

231. Bullingham RES, McQuay HJ, Porter EJB et al: Acute i.v. methadone kinetics in man. Relationship to chronic studies. Br J Anaesth 54:1271, 1982

232. Kreek MJ, Gutjahr CL, Schecter AJ, Hecht M: Methadone use in patients with chronic renal disease. Drug Alcohol Depend 5:197, 1980

233. Novic DM, Kreek MJ, Fanizza AH et al: Methadone disposition in patients with chronic liver disease. Clin Pharmacol Ther 30:353, 1981

234. Leysen JE, Gommeren W, Niemegeers CJE: [3H] Sufentanil, a superior ligand for μ-opiate receptors. Binding properties and regional distribution in rat brain and spinal cord. Eur J Pharmacol 87:209, 1983

235. Eisele JH, Wright R, Rogge P: Newborn and maternal fentanyl levels at caesarean section. Anesth Analg 61:179, 1982

236. Hudson RJ, Thomson IR, Cannon JE et al: Pharmacokinetics of fentanyl in patients undergoing abdominal aortic surgery. Anesthesiology 64:334, 1986

237. Lehmann KA, Weski C, Hunger L et al: Biotransformation von Fentanyl II. Akute Arzneimittelinteraktionen—Untersuchungen bei Ratte und Mensch. Anaesthetist 31:221, 1982

238. Runciman WB, Mather LE, Ilsley AH et al: A sheep preparation for studying interactions between blood flow and drug disposition. III: Effects of general and spinal anaesthesia on regional blood flow and oxygen tensions. Br J Anaesth 56:1247, 1984

239. Gelman S, Dillard E, Bradley EL: Hepatic circulation during surgical stress and anesthesia with halothane, isoflurane or fentanyl. Anesth Analg 66:936, 1987

240. Bovill JG, Sebel PS, Blackburn CL, Heykants J: The pharmacokinetics of alfentanil (R39209): a new opioid analgesic. Anesthesiology 57:439, 1982

241. Hudson RJ, Thompson IR, Burgess PM, Rosenbloom IR: Alfentanil pharmacokinetics in patients undergoing abdominal aortic surgery. Can J Anaesth 38:61, 1991

242. Persson MP, Nilsson A, Hartvig P: Pharmacokinetics of alfentanil in total i.v. anaesthesia. Br J Anaesth 60:755, 1988

243. Shafer A, Sung M-L, White PF: Pharmacokinetics and pharmacodynamics of alfentanil infusions during general anesthesia. Anesth Analg 65:1021, 1986

244. Kent AP, Dodson ME, Bower S: The pharmacokinetics and clinical effects of a low dose of alfentanil in elderly patients. Acta Anaesthesiol Belg 39:25, 1988

245. den Hollander JM, Hennis PJ, Burm AGL, Bovill JG: Alfentanil in infants and children with congenital heart defects. J Cardiothorac Anesth 2:12, 1988

246. Bentley JB, Finley JH, Humphrey LR et al: Obesity and alfentanil pharmacokinetics. Anesth Analg 62:245, 1983

247. Hudson RJ, Bergstrom RG, Thomson IR et al: Pharmacokinetics of sufentanil in patients undergoing abdominal aortic surgery. Anesthesiology 70:426, 1989

248. Bullingham RES, McQuay HJ, Moore RA: Clinical pharmacokinetics of narcotic agonist-antagonist drugs. Clin Pharmacokinet 8:332, 1983

249. Ehrnebro M, Boreus LO, Lonroth U: Bioavailability and first-pass metabolism of oral pentazocine in man. Clin Pharmacol Ther 22:888, 1977

250. Neal EA, Meffin PJ, Gregory PB, Blascke TF: Enhanced bioavailability and decreased clearance of analgesics in patients with cirrhosis. Gastroenterology 77:96, 1979

251. Pond SM, Tong T, Benowitz NL, Jacob P: Enhanced bioavailability of pethidine and pentazocine in patients with cirrhosis of the liver. Aust N Z J Med 10:515, 1980

252. Pittman KA, Smyth RD, Mayol RF: Serum levels of butorphanol by radioimmunoassay. J Pharm Sci 69:160, 1980

253. Gaver RC, Vasiljev M, Wong H et al: Disposition of parenteral butorphanol in man. Drug Metab Dispos 8:230, 1980

254. Aitkenhead AR, Lin ES, Achola KJ: The pharmacokinetics of oral and intravenous nalbuphine in healthy volunteers. Br J Clin Pharmacol 25:264, 1988

255. Lo MW, Schary WL, Whitney CC Jr: The disposition and bioavailability of intravenous and oral nalbuphine in healthy volunteers. J Clin Pharmacol 27:866, 1987

256. Sear JW, Keegan M, Kay B: Disposition of nalbupine in patients undergoing general anaesthesia. Br J Anaesth 59:572, 1987

257. Bullingham RES, McQuay HJ, Moore A, Bennett MRD: Buprenorphine kinetics. Clin Pharmacol Ther 28:667, 1980

258. Ritschel WA, Hoffmann KA, Willig JL et al: The effect of age on the pharmacokinetics of pentazocine. Methods Find Exp Clin Pharmacol 8:497, 1986

259. Ehrnebro M, Agurell S, Boreus LO et al: Pentazocine binding to blood cells and plasma proteins. Clin Pharmacol Ther 16:424, 1974

260. Ramsey R, Higbee M, Maesner J, Wood J: Influence of age on the pharmacokinetics of butorphanol. Acute Care, suppl. 1:8, 1988

261. Jaillon P, Gardin ME, Lecocq B et al: Pharmacokinetics of nalbuphine in infants, young healthy volunteers, and elderly patients. Clin Pharmacol Ther 46:226, 1989

262. Lake CL, DiFazio CA, Duckworth EN et al: High-performance liquid chromatographic analysis of plasma levels of nalbuphine in cardiac surgical patients. J Chromatogr 233:410, 1982

263. Wischnik A, Wetzelsberger N, Lucker PW: [Elimination of nalbuphine in human milk] Elimination von Nalbuphin in die Muttermilch. Arzneimittelforschung 38:1496, 1988

264. Garrett ER, Chandran VR: Pharmacokinetics of morphine and its surrogates. VI: Bioanalysis, solvolysis kinetics, solubility, pK_a values, and protein binding of buprenorphine. J Pharm Sci 74:515, 1985

265. Garrett ER, Chandran VR: Pharmacokinetics of morphine and its surrogates. X: Analyses and pharmacokinetics of buprenorphine in dogs. Biopharm Drug Dispos 11:311, 1990

266. Bullingham RES, McQuay HJ, Porter EJB et al: Sublingual buprenorphine used postoperatively: ten hour plasma drug concentration analysis. Br J Clin Pharmacol 13:665, 1982

267. Bullingham RES, McQuay HJ, Dwyer D et al: Sublingual buprenorphine used postoperatively: clinical observations and preliminary pharmacokinetic analysis. Br J Clin Pharmacol 12:117, 1981

268. Reilly CS, Wood AJJ, Koshakji RP, Wood M: The effect of halothane on drug disposition: contribution of changes in intrinsic drug metabolizing capacity and hepatic blood flow. Anesthesiology 63:70, 1985

269. Boas RA, Villiger JW: Clinical actions of fentanyl and buprenorphine. The significance of receptor binding. Br J Anaesth 57:192, 1985

Chapter 4

Clinical Pharmacology and Applications of Opioid Agonists

Peter L. Bailey

Opioids have been used to treat pain for hundreds of years. Today, many opioid agonists are employed clinically in a host of settings. They are the "gold standard" of analgesics, but their application in anesthesia involves much more than producing pain relief. They are often administered in high doses as the primary anesthetic agent, supplemented at times by only small doses of other anesthetics. This practice is based primarily on the expectation that hemodynamic function will be minimally disturbed. Many advances in pharmacokinetics, new drug development, and drug delivery technology have occurred. These have contributed significantly to improvements in intravenous anesthesia. Continued progress in the area of intravenous anesthesia is likely to occur. Opioids will continue to play an important role.

THERAPEUTIC DRUG EFFECTS

Therapeutic opioid actions that accompany analgesia in a dose-related fashion include sedation, anxiolysis (especially anxiety elicited by pain or fear of pain), cough suppression, and the relief of dyspnea. High doses of opioid agonists produce sleep, unconsciousness, and anesthesia. The neurophysi-

ologic state produced by high doses of potent opioids is different from that induced by potent inhaled anesthetics. Inhaled anesthetics produce a dose-dependent continuum of electrocephalographic (EEG) changes, eventually resulting in burst suppression and a silent EEG. Opioids, in contrast, produce minimal changes at low doses and high voltage slow (δ) waves with high doses. These EEG effects have been documented to be consistent with general anesthesia.[1,2]

It continues to be debated whether or not opioids are "anesthetics." Though an academic point of pharmacologic interest on the one hand, the responsibility of anesthesiologists to ensure amnesia for their patients makes this issue real on the other. Opioids do not possess strong amnestic properties, and it is argued that amnesia can and should only be achieved with other agents. However, sufentanil can be substituted for halothane in rats, supporting the notion that opioids, such as sufentanil, are anesthetics (Fig. 4-1).[3] Unconsciousness and amnesia have been produced by opioids alone in human volunteers who received no other drugs.[4] In addition, there are no data associating the use of opioids with an increased incidence of intraoperative awareness.

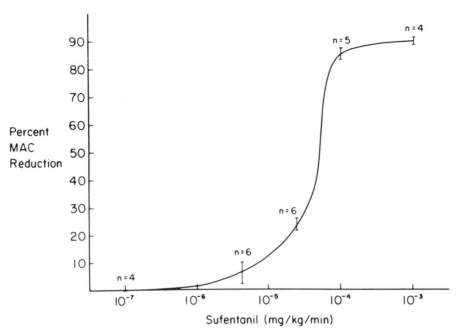

Fig. 4-1 Reduction of halothane minimum alveolar concentration (MAC) in the rat observed with progressively increased sufentanil dosage. (From Hecker et al.,[3] with permission.)

Cardiovascular Effects

The rationale behind the application of opioids in anesthesia is to produce analgesia and stable hemodynamics. Opioids are arguably superior to most other agents in achieving this goal. Central cardiovascular regulatory centers, the sympathetic nervous system, vagal nuclei, and the adrenal medulla are among the key sites that possess opioid receptors and contribute to the ability of opioids to blunt or eliminate significant hemodynamic responses to noxious stimuli.[5] The potent opioids applied in anesthesia produce minimal cardiac depression modest or no decrease in preload and afterload,[6–8] little depression of great vessel and atrial baroreceptors,[9] and no effect on coronary vasomotion.

Because increases in heart rate simultaneously increase myocardial oxygen consumption and decrease myocardial oxygen supply (decreased diastolic filling time), controlling the heart rate is an important goal when caring for patients at risk for myocardial ischemia. Some studies have found a relationship between intraoperative tachycardia and outcome.[10] Opioids (excluding meperidine) are excellent agents in this regard because they tend to lower the heart rate. Central stimulation of the vagal nuclei is most likely the primary mechanism of opioid-induced heart rate slowing. Bilateral vagotomy[11] and vagal pharmacologic blockade with anticholinergic agents[12] prevents this opioid action. However, significant evidence linking the choice of anesthetic agent(s) and the cardiovascular outcome after coronary artery surgery has not been found.[13,14]

Respiratory Effects

The respiratory depressant actions of opioids represent their single greatest disadvantage (see Nontherapeutic Drug Effects). However, some significant therapeutic respiratory effects are obtained by the use of opioids. The lack of adequate pain relief can also cause postoperative respiratory dysfunction.[15]

Opioids are excellent agents for depressing upper airway and tracheal reflexes. This action may be beneficial during anesthesia and in the intensive care setting. Opioids allow patients to tolerate endotracheal tubes without coughing or "bucking," which can lead to hypoxemia, hypercarbia, hemodynamic instability, and other deleterious effects. Impaired gas exchange results from the marked disturbance in ventilatory pattern and the loss of lung volume. Thus, upon emergence from general anesthesia, patients anesthetized with a potent inhalation agent and no opioid will routinely cough and buck prior to regaining consciousness and responsiveness; patients adequately treated with opioids can awaken without such disturbances, even while they are still tracheally intubated.

Opioids can also help quiet the lower respiratory tract and avoid increases in bronchomotor tone. Although some evidence exists to document the airway smooth muscle relaxing properties of opioids such as fentanyl[16] and opioids have long been used in the treatment of acute asthma, adequate documentation of this effect is lacking. Opioids minimally alter pulmonary gas exchange,[17,18] in contrast to the potent inhalation agents. The capacity of the lungs to filter air emboli was significantly greater during fentanyl anesthesia in dogs compared with halothane anesthesia; presumably, intrapulmonary shunting was greater with halothane.[19]

Endocrine Effects

The endocrine response to surgery results in augmented metabolism and increased mobilization of energy stores. This "stress response," although at times appropriate and beneficial, can contribute to perioperative hemodynamic and metabolic instability. The response to an injury includes the release of adrenocorticotropic hormone, growth hormone, prolactin, endorphin, and antidiuretic hormone. The catabolic hormones released include cortisol, catecholamines, glucagon, and thyroxine.[20] Under the assumption that control of the stress response will benefit patients, numerous studies have evaluated the effects of opioids on various hormones. Opioids might be expected to be therapeutic in this regard because opioid receptors exist at multiple sites and levels in the neuraxis and in some endocrine organs (e.g., the adrenal gland), opioid peptides (β-endorphin) are cosynthesized with adenocorticotropic hormone, (ACTH), endogenous opioids are stress hormones themselves, and opioids modulate the secretion of other hormones.

Opioids in high doses can blunt the stress response, as indicated by perioperative blood levels of cortisol, catecholamines, vasopressin, and growth hormone.[21-23] Protein catabolism may also be reduced. Nevertheless, until recently, little data existed to suggest that the benefits of applying high doses of opioids in anesthesia outweighed the disadvantages that include, most notably, the need for extended mechanical ventilatory support. However, recent reports have found significant associations between the extension of intense anesthesia or analgesia with sufentanil into the postoperative period and reductions in morbidity and mortality rates.[24,25] It is hoped that future studies will determine which patient populations are most susceptible to this intervention.

NONTHERAPEUTIC DRUG EFFECTS

Lethargy, dysphoria, euphoria, pruritus, and miosis are some of the most frequent nontherapeutic opioid actions. Nausea and vomiting and respiratory depression are often the greatest concerns and will be discussed later.

Muscle Rigidity

Opioids can cause increases in skeletal muscle tone, which at times may be severe. One or more central neurologic sites, including the nucleus raphe pontis, are responsible for this opioid effect.[26] The occurrence of opioid induced rigidity is dose dependent and patient age related. Fentanyl, 15 μg/kg, produced rigidity 50 percent of the time in healthy, young adult volunteers, which was not related to plasma levels, and abated spontaneously in 10 to 20 minutes with decreasing blood drug levels.[4] Older patients experienced a higher incidence of rigidity after intravenous opioids.[27] The potent and rapidly acting opioids (e.g., sufentanil, fentanyl, and especially, alfentanil) are likely to trigger rigidity as the dose increases above 0.3, 3.0, and 30 μg/kg, respectively, in humans. The concomitant use of nitrous oxide may exacerbate opioid-induced rigidity.

Opioid induced rigidity is characterized by upper extremity flexion, especially at the fingers, wrist, and elbow; significant decreases in abdominothoracic compliance; and unconsciousness. When rigidity is moderate to severe, ventilation by mask, and even via an endotracheal tube, may be difficult or impossible. Although various agents may attenuate or, at times, prevent rigidity, only the administration of intubating doses of neuromuscular blocking agents is reliably effective. Naloxone can antagonize opioid-induced rigidity. Rigidity may also rarely occur postoperatively (see subsequent discussion).

Opioid induced rigidity can increase pulmonary artery, central venous, and intracranial pressures.[28,29] These adverse effects are reversed with the adequate treatment of rigidity. Rigidity and its effects during anesthesia are best approached by being prepared to complete rapidly the induction of anesthesia with muscle relaxation if significant rigidity occurs.

Other Neuroexcitatory Effects

Various neuroexcitatory phenomena can occasionally occur in association with opioid administration. These actions are also dose related and more apparent with the use of high doses of potent opioids. These effects range from nystagmus and nonspecific eye movements to single extremity myoclonus to generalized myoclonic activity that may resemble a grand mal seizure in appearance. Detailed studies with surface electrodes have failed to document any EEG evidence of seizure activity in humans after high doses of either fentanyl, alfentanil, or sufentanil.[1,2,29] In addition, no permanent neurologic deficit has ever been reported in association with opioid induced neuroexcitation. Nevertheless, some concerns remain. Focal increases in cerebral blood flow,[30] and metabolism[31] can occur with opioids in animal models. Fentanyl has produced electrical seizure activity in temporal lobe structures of patients with complex partial seizure disorders, but there was no cortical seizure activity or motor activity.[32]

Until recently, it was generally believed that opioids produced no change or modest reductions in cerebral blood flow and cerebral metabolic oxygen consumption. However, Milde et al.[33] reported that sufentanil caused substantial increases in cerebral blood flow in normocapnic dogs anesthetized with small doses of halothane. For the most part, the increase in cerebral blood flow was not explained by concomitant changes in cerebral oxygen consumption, implying that sufentanil was dilating cerebral vessels directly.

Sperry et al.[34] studied the intracranial pressures in patients with severe head trauma. The patients were paralyzed with vecuronium, and their intracranial pressures were controlled by standard clinical procedures, including hyperventilation, elevation of the head, sedation with midazolam, and osmotic agents. Intracranial pressure was monitored by subarachnoid bolt device. Administration of fentanyl (3.0 μg/kg) or sufentanil (0.6 μg/kg) resulted in a mean increase in intracranial pressure of about 10 mmHg. Mean blood pressure declined by about 10 mmHg. The maximum increase in intracranial pressure occurred about 5 minutes after opioid administration and persisted for about 20 minutes.

The explanation for the apparent increase in cerebral blood flow or intracranial pressure in these studies is unknown. It is interesting that feline cerebrovascular smooth muscle was reported to dilate in response to direct microapplication of μ or δ agonists.[35] Localized electrical seizure activity could be associated with increases in regional cerebral blood flow.[32]

The subject of opioid effects on the cerebral circulation has become very complex and controversial because of unexplained discrepancies between studies.[34] Some recent studies have not found increased cerebral blood flow or increased intracranial pressure following opioid administration.[36] The effects of opioids on the cerebral circulation may be highly variable, depending upon the circumstances. Until this issue is resolved, opioids should be used cautiously in patients with critically reduced intracranial compliance.

The N-demethylated metabolite of meperidine, normeperidine, can cause central nervous system excitation and true convulsions. Because normeperidine has a long half-life and its elimination is predominantly via the kidney, prolonged meperidine administration, especially in patients with impaired renal function, may increase the risk of this problem.[37]

Nontherapeutic Cardiovascular Effects

Understanding the adverse actions of opioids includes an appreciation of the fact that certain effects (e.g., slow heart), although desirable in some patients, may not be so in others. Thus, whereas opioids may be chosen as anesthetic agents to promote hemodynamic stability, their cardiovascular effects may be exaggerated or undesirable.

Hypotension can occur after opioid administration, probably mediated primarily by reductions in sympathetic tone.[38] This is especially true in vasoconstricted, hypovolemic patients, whose hemodynamic stability is dependent on high sympathetic tone. Opioids may also have direct effects on vascular smooth muscle and myocardium,[40] although the contribution of these actions to hypotension in the clinical setting is probably minimal, except in the case of meperidine. Meperidine is a relatively potent direct myocardial depressant. Opioid induced bradycardia may exacerbate hypotension. Morphine and meperidine can release histamine, resulting in vasodilatation and hypotension. Both the dose and rate of morphine infusion, and pretreatment with H_1 and H_2 blockers, affect the severity of the hypotension.[41,42] Fentanyl, alfentanil, and sufentanil do not stimulate histamine release.[43–45] Meperidine is particularly undesirable as an anesthetic agent because of its histamine releasing and myocardial depressant properties.[46]

Hypotension, usually of moderate degree, may occur with fentanyl, sufentanil, or alfentanil. Differences between these three opioids is difficult to assess from the numerous but often conflicting animal and human studies. The dose and rate of drug administration, the volume status of the patient, and a host of other factors, especially concomitant administration of other drugs (see Drug Interactions) are important factors contributing to hypotension. Although sufentanil alone may be a more "complete anesthetic" compared with fentanyl,[47] this may also account for reports of lower blood pressures and decreased myocardial contractility associated with it.[48] High dose alfentanil anesthesia may produce greater hypotension than either fentanyl or sufentanil.[48]

Hypertension may occur during high dose opioid anesthesia, as with other anesthetic techniques. Most often this is the result of an inadequate dose of opioid or improper timing of drug administration (Fig. 4-2), but it can be related to inadequate opioid effect, regardless of dose.[49] Patients with good left ventricular function become hypertensive more frequently.[50] Occasionally, sympathetic activation occurs during induction of anesthesia with fentanyl analog; the mechanism is un-

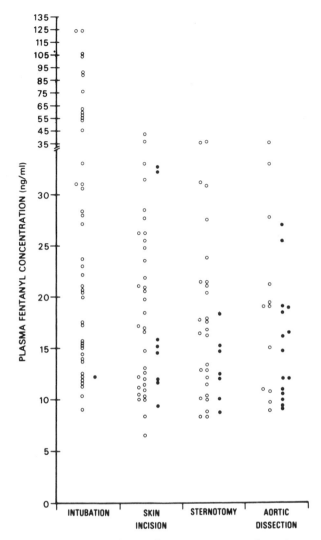

Fig. 4-2 Plasma fentanyl concentration and number of patients with a hypertensive response at each event during coronary artery surgery. ●, hypertensive; ○, normotensive. (From Wynands et al.,[242] with permission.)

known.[51] Sufentanil has caused adrenal gland catecholamine release in cats.[52] Specific cardiogenic reflexes elicited during surgery, aortic root manipulation for example, may stimulate hypertensive episodes during opioid anesthesia (Fig. 4-2).[53] Hypertension may be less likely during sufentanil anesthesia compared with fentanyl.[54] A host of other factors (premedication, the degree of β-adrenergic or calcium channel blockade and, other anesthetic agents) are likely to influence the occurrence of hypertension. Alfentanil was less reliable in controlling hypertensive episodes when used for cardiac anesthesia.[48]

Many opioids decrease heart rate as a result of vagal stimulation; meperidine is a notable exception. Severe bradycardia or even asystole can occur, especially in conjunction with other vagal stimuli (e.g., laryngoscopy or nasal stimulation[55]) or other drugs that lower heart rate.[56] Alfentanil and sufentanil seem to carry somewhat greater risks for this complication. Alfentanil may also carry a greater risk for bradycardia compared with sufentanil and fentanyl when used to induce anesthesia in patients with known coronary artery disease.[48]

Nontherapeutic Respiratory Effects

All μ receptor opioid agonists produce dose-dependent depression of ventilation, primarily through a direct action on the medullary respiratory center.[57,58] The responsiveness of the respiratory center to CO_2 is significantly reduced by opioids. The slope of the ventilatory response to CO_2 is decreased and shifted to the right (Fig. 4-3). The apneic threshold and resting $PaCO_2$ are increased by opioids. Opioids decrease hypoxic ventilatory drive[59,60] and blunt the increase in respiratory drive normally associated with increased loads, such as increased airway resistance.[60] Opioid effects on respiratory rhythm include pauses, delays

Table 4-1 Factors Increasing the Magnitude and/or Duration of Opioid Induced Respiratory Depression

↑ Dose

Intermittent bolus (versus continuous infusion)

↑ Brain penetration and drug delivery
  ↓ Distribution (↓ cardiac output)
  ↑ Un-ionized fraction (respiratory alkalosis)

↓ Reuptake from the brain (intraoperative respiratory alkalosis)

↓ Clearance (↓ hepatic blood flow, e.g., intra-abdominal surgery)

Secondary peaks in plasma opioid levels (reuptake of opioid from muscle, lung, fat, and intestine)

↑ Ionized opioid at receptor site (postoperative respiratory acidosis)

Sleep

↑ Age

Metabolic alkalosis

in expiration, and irregular or periodic breathing. High doses of opioids produce apnea; patients who remain conscious may still respond to verbal commands to breathe.

Many factors can affect the magnitude and duration of respiratory depression after opioid administration (Table 4-1). Even small doses of opioids markedly potentiate the normal right shift of the CO_2 response curve that occurs during natural sleep.[61,62] Interestingly, both sleep and morphine decrease the thoracic (rib cage) component of breathing, although the diaphragm is relatively unaffected. Sleep also impairs the tonic and phasic activity of upper airway muscles that accompanies breathing.[63] This combination of factors can be worrisome when patients have an opioid-based anesthetic and undergo an operation that results in little or no postoperative pain or receive an analgesic regimen that results in an excessive opioid effect. Apparently adequate breathing can become insufficient when these patients fall asleep.

Delayed or recurrent respiratory depression can occasionally occur with most opioids including fentanyl,[64,65] morphine,[66] meperidine,[67] alfentanil,[68] and sufentanil.[69] Proposed explanations for this phenomenon have included lack of stimulation or pain, combined effects with other medications

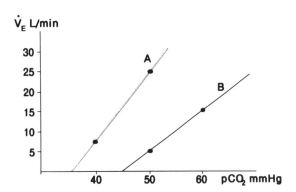

Fig. 4-3 Ventilatory response to progressive increases in CO_2 (*A*) before and (*B*) after an opioid agonist. Note that after opioid administration the apneic threshold is increased (elevated $PaCO_2$ intercept) and the response curve is both shifted to the right and of a lesser slope.

(such as benzodiazepines), release of opioids from muscles or other tissue compartments, hypothermia, hypovolemia, and hypotension. Secondary peaks in plasma fentanyl levels have been noted during the elimination phase,[70] along with parallel changes in CO_2 responsiveness and breathing (Fig. 4-4).[71]

Some authors have suggested that the intraoperative or postoperative use of opioids leads to an increased incidence of postoperative respiratory problems, such as hypoxemia.[72,73] However, the vast majority of studies have not implicated opioids as especially hazardous compared with other anesthetic agents.[74] The recommendation to minimize or avoid opioids in anesthesia should be considered in view of recent studies revealing the significant morbidity and mortality rates that can be associated with inadequate analgesia.[23,24,75] The inadequate treatment of pain is a well documented problem.[75] Every clinician involved in the treatment of pain should be thoroughly familiar with both the respiratory and analgesic pharmacology of opioids to maximize their benefits and minimize adverse effects.

A brief coughing episode occurs almost immediately after central intravenous administration of fentanyl and sufentanil. This clinical curiosity may be induced via a pulmonary chemoreflex.[76] It is especially interesting in light of the fact that opioids also have cough suppressant properties.

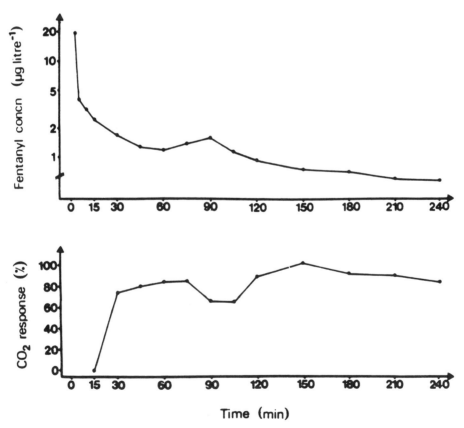

Fig. 4-4 Fentanyl plasma concentrations (upper panel) after a single bolus injection of fentanyl 0.5 mg and the CO_2 ventilatory response slopes as percentages of the control slope (lower panel) in a volunteer with a second, delayed decrease in the response to carbon dioxide. (From Stoeckel et al.,[71] with permission.)

Nontherapeutic Gastrointestinal Effects

Opioids have gastrointestinal actions that may be applied therapeutically (e.g., antidiarrheal agents), but these more often represent undesirable side effects. Chief among these is nausea and/or vomiting. After pain, nausea and vomiting ranks as a principal problem for many surgical patients.[77] The use of opioids in a balanced anesthetic technique contributes to the significant incidence (15 to 60 percent) of nausea and vomiting after surgery. However, many other factors predispose patients to this problem (see Ch. 30).[77] A particular opioid agonist has not proven to be more or less emetogenic. The method of opioid administration is not proven to affect the incidence of nausea and vomiting, but in one study, the use of a continuous alfentanil infusion appeared to exacerbate nausea and vomiting.[78] Reducing opioid requirements by administering nonsteroidal anti-inflammatory drugs when they are appropriate may help reduce the incidence of nausea and vomiting.[79]

Strategies for minimizing nausea and vomiting include combining opioids with agents such as propofol that are associated with a low incidence of nausea and vomiting and the use of prophylactic antiemetic agents. Ondansetron, a relatively new antiemetic that blocks serotonin receptors, may be superior to droperidol or metoclopramide (see Ch. 30).[80]

The neurophysiology and pharmacology of nausea and vomiting is very complex. The vomiting center in the medulla receives input from the cerebral cortex, the gut, the vestibular system, and the chemoreceptor trigger zone. The chemoreceptor trigger zone is located in the floor of the fourth ventricle, outside the blood-brain barrier. The chemoreceptor trigger zone contains many types of receptors, including opioid receptors, that promote vomiting. Experiments in cats have suggested that opioids have an antiemetic effect on the vomiting center that is reversible by naloxone.[81] Intravenous naloxone appeared to reverse the antiemetic effects of opioids on the vomiting center but not the emetic effect of opioids on the chemoreceptor trigger zone, thereby promoting emesis. For exam-

ple, fentanyl did not produce emesis in cats until they were pretreated with intravenous naloxone.[81] This is consistent with the clinical observation that naloxone frequently resulted in vomiting when administered to antagonize morphine.[82]

Opioids increase gastrointestinal secretions, decrease gastrointestinal activity, lower esophageal sphincter tone, and delay gastric emptying. Naloxone, but not metoclopramide, can fully reverse the effect of opioids on gastric emptying. The clinical significance, if any, of the constipating effect of opioids (caused by decreased propulsion and augmented resting tone) administered in the perioperative period is unknown.

Opioid induced increases in biliary duct pressure and sphincter of Oddi tone can produce biliary spasm and colic and also contribute to nausea and vomiting. Opioid induced spasm of the sphincter may prevent radiographic dye from entering the duodenum during intraoperative cholangiography, simulating the presence of a gallstone in the common bile duct. Some anesthesiologists prefer to avoid opioid balanced anesthesia for cholecystectomy because of the possibility of interfering with the cholangiogram. However, this is a relatively uncommon problem[83] and may be resolved by administering glucagon (alternatively, naloxone or nalbuphine), which relaxes the sphincter of Oddi. The obstruction of the common bile duct that persists after glucagon administration is unlikely to be related to opioid effects.

Other Nontherapeutic Opioid Effects

Studies in dogs suggested that fentanyl might have adverse renal effects, including increased renovascular resistance and decreased renal plasma flow, glomerular filtration rate, and urine volume.[84] Alfentanil also impaired renal blood flow in dogs.[85] These effects may have been caused by opioid induced antidiuretic hormone (ADH) release or decreased systemic arterial pressure with blunted renal circulatory autoregulation.[85,86] Morphine may increase ADH release in humans[87] and ADH levels also increase in response to surgery. Morphine, 2 mg/kg, had little effect on renal function in human volunteers if hemodynamic stability was maintained by fluid administration.[88] The lack of reports of renal dysfunction associated with opioid anesthesia, after thousands of high dose opioid anesthetics, supports its safety in this regard. However, two case reports involving a total of three patients documented dihydrocodeine and papaveretum induced renal failure that was reversible by naloxone.[89]

The lower urinary tract can be significantly affected by opioids. Disturbances in micturition include increased detrusor muscle tone (sometimes resulting in urgency) and increased vesical sphincter and ureteral tone (sometimes making urination difficult). Intrathecal administration of opioids also commonly causes urinary retention. The problem is often responsive to naloxone or mixed agonist-antagonist opioids.

Opioids, like most anesthetics, may exacerbate hepatic injury associated with hypoxia in animals.[90] Small degrees of hepatic dysfunction may be associated with most anesthetics, including fentanyl.[91] Nevertheless, there is little evidence implicating opioids as having any significant adverse hepatic effect in humans.

The teratogenecity of opioids in humans is uncertain. Older studies implicated morphine, meperidine, and methadone as teratogenic,[92] but fentanyl, sufentanil, and alfentanil failed to induce abnormalities in rat studies.[93,94] Small doses of fentanyl had little or no effect on uterine blood flow, uterine tone, or maternal/fetal acid base balance in sheep.[95] Nevertheless, opioids cross the placenta easily, especially if they are lipophilic. Fetal plasma fentanyl levels rapidly approximated (but did not reach) maternal plasma levels.[95] Newborns of addicted mothers can exhibit opioid effects and/or withdrawal. Newborns of mothers receiving opioids prior to delivery are at risk for respiratory depression. The milk of lactating mothers receiving parenteral morphine for postoperative analgesia contained low concentrations of morphine that were not likely to harm an infant.[96]

Serious allergic responses to opioids are rare, although anaphylaxis after fentanyl, meperidine, and papaveretum has been reported.[97,98] Wheal and flare responses to opioids vary, are independent of analgesic potency, and are dependent upon histamine release from most cells and direct vascular effects.[99] Pruritus often accompanies opioid administration and is not usually indicative of an allergic response. The underlying mechanism for opioid induced pruritus is poorly understood.

DOSE-EFFECT RELATIONSHIPS

The opioid dose is a very poor predictor of target organ drug concentrations. Recent attempts to relate plasma concentration to drug effects have employed the EEG to quantify drug effect.[100] The relationship of the EEG to other opioid actions is unknown. Although simple potency ratios may adequately describe the differences between opioid agonists with regard to analgesic dose requirements, other actions, such as hypnosis or cardiovascular effects, may not adhere to the same potency ratios as those of analgesia. Analgesia and respiratory depression have traditionally been assumed to be proportional. However it has been shown that sufentanil may produce relatively greater analgesia with less respiratory depression compared with fentanyl.[101] The μ receptor subtypes designated μ_1 and μ_2, are separately responsible for analgesia and respiratory depression in rodents (see Chs. 2 and Ch. 5).[102] Whether the μ receptor subtypes account for the differing effects of opioid agonists in humans is unknown.

Opioid agonists produce a spectrum of effects in a dose dependent fashion. Lower doses produce analgesia, cough suppression, mild to moderate respiratory depression, and sedation. As the dose increases, analgesia and respiratory depression intensify. Eventually, apnea, rigidity, loss of response to commands, unconsciousness, and an anesthetic or near anesthetic state occurs.

A central issue when considering the dose effect relationships of opioids when they are used as a major component or sole agent in an anesthetic is which opioid produces the greatest hemodynamic stability or the best outcome. Although the vast majority of outcome studies conclude that the anesthetic type does not affect outcome,[13,14,103] studies by Benefiel et al.,[104] Anand et al.,[25] and Mangano et al.,[24] suggest that the application of opioid (sufentanil) based anesthetic techniques can reduce complications. Opioid based anesthetic techniques are often chosen in an effort to control the indices of myocardial oxygen supply and demand and reduce the risks of cardiac complications. Whether these techniques are successful will continue to be the subject of clinical studies.

Lowenstein et al.[105] introduced the concept that high doses of opioids (morphine) could be applied as the primary or sole anesthetic agent. In patients with minimal circulatory reserve, morphine, 1.0 mg/kg, actually improved the cardiac index with little change in blood pressure. However, there was a requirement for prolonged postoperative ventilatory support, occasional profound hypotension, and inadequate anesthesia with morphine in healthier patients. Morphine (up to 4.4 mg/kg) provided unsatisfactory hemodynamic control compared with fentanyl and sufentanil.[106] Patients receiving morphine for cardiac surgery experienced much greater changes in key hemodynamic indices, such as blood pressure (hypotension and hypertension), heart rate (tachycardia), and cardiac index (elevations).[106]

Stanley and Webster[6] are most frequently credited with popularizing fentanyl as an anesthetic for cardiac surgery. Many investigations have evaluated this agent, alone and in combination with other anesthetics, in the dose range of 15 to 150 μg/kg, given either as a single bolus, multiple intermittent boluses, or continuous infusion.[50,107–109] The ability of fentanyl to block hemodynamic responses is dose (and plasma level) dependent to a certain extent (Fig. 4-2). Sprigge et al.[109] demonstrated that fentanyl 50 μg/kg followed by an infusion of 0.5 μg/kg/min could maintain an arterial fentanyl level of at least 15 ng/ml. This level (C_p50) was described as analogous to the minimum alveolar concentration of inhalation agents because it prevented increases in blood pressure requiring treatment in 50 percent of patients undergoing coronary artery surgery. However, fentanyl cannot block responses to all noxious stimuli in all subjects.[110] Some authors have suggested that all noxious stimuli could be blocked, given high enough opioid levels, but proof is lacking. Fentanyl plasma levels of at least 30 ng/ml at the time of the most potent noxious stimuli[50] (Fig. 4-2) may be required for an optimal opioid effect.

Sufentanil is more potent than fentanyl and may also produce greater maximal effect. Doses of 10 to 30 μg/kg can provide stable hemodynamic conditions for tracheal intubation,[48] sternotomy,[54] and cardiopulmonary bypass.[54] Many studies have investigated the efficacy of sufentanil and fentanyl, primarily in patients undergoing cardiac surgery. A problem with all these studies is that rigorous protocols must be adhered to, eliminating the ability of clinicians to titrate their drugs in a flexible, adaptive, and arguably, more logical and effective manner.[111]

Some investigators have found sufentanil to be inadequate at times as a sole anesthetic agent in cardiac surgery.[49,110,112,113] Philbin et al.[49] suggested that no relationship exists between the fentanyl or sufentanil dose and the suppression of hemodynamic or hormonal responses during surgery. However, others have suggested that dose related effects do exist.[48,54,114,115] A reinterpretation of the data reported by Philbin et al.[49] has also been made in support of a dose effect relationship.[111] Some authors found sufentanil superior to fentanyl with regard to controlling hypertensive episodes intraoperatively[47,54,106,110] and postoperatively[116] and other anesthetic considerations.[117,118] Sufentanil was at times associated with lower blood pressures, which can be desirable,[118] potentially deleterious,[119] or of no consequence.[48]

Dose effect relationship for alfentanil anesthesia for general surgery have been well defined. Ausems et al.[120] found that the Cp50s for alfentanil, combined with 66% nitrous oxide in oxygen, were 475 ± 28 and 279 ± 20 ng/ml for intubation and skin incision, respectively, in patients undergoing abdominal or breast surgery. Superficial surgery required lower alfentanil levels (270 ± 63 mg/ml) than did lower abdominal surgery (309 ± 44 ng/ml) or upper abdominal surgery (412 ± 135 ng/ml). The skin closure Cp50 was 150 ± 23 ng/ml. Alfentanil appeared to be inadequate as a sole anesthetic for cardiac surgery.[48,121] Several studies have compared alfentanil with fentanyl or sufentanil for cardiac surgery. Alfentanil was associated with higher incidence of hypertensive episodes during sternotomy,[122] the need for very high plasma levels (leading to an expensive technique),[123] and most importantly a greater incidence of hypotension and myocardial ischemia.[48]

McDonnell et al.[124] and Vinik et al.[125] have reported dose effect studies of alfentanil for the induction of anesthesia. McDonnell et al.[124] determined the ED_{50} and ED_{90} for unconsciousness in unpremedicated young adults by using both loss of response to verbal commands and loss of response to a nasopharyngeal airway as end points to identify unconsciousness. The ED_{50} and ED_{90} were 92 and 111 $\mu g/kg$, respectively, for loss of response to a verbal stimulus and 111 and 169 $\mu g/kg$, respectively, for loss of response to a nasopharyngeal airway.

DRUG INTERACTIONS

The clinical effects of opioids can be profoundly altered by the concomitant administration of many other drugs. Most notably, hemodynamic stability can be compromised and respiratory depression exacerbated. Some drug interactions may be used to advantage; for example, modest doses of opioids usually reduce the requirements for other agents used to induce loss of consciousness. Alfentanil, 50 $\mu g/kg$, reduced the required induction dose of propofol from 2 to 3 mg/kg[126] to less than 1 mg/kg.[127] Fentanyl and, to an even greater extent, sufentanil decreased the sleep inducing dose of thiopental (Fig. 4-5).[128] It is not entirely clear whether and when similar type interactions are only additive[129] or synergistic.[130] Although other drug interactions may be employed toward favorable ends (e.g., adding a benzodiazepine to increase amnesia or reduce hypertensive episodes during opioid anesthesia), the purpose of this section will be to concentrate on potentially unfavorable or undesirable drug interactions.

Monoamine Oxidase Inhibitors

At the top of the list of opioid drug interactions should be the issue of meperidine administration during monoamine oxidase inhibitor (MAOI) drug therapy because of potentially fatal consequences. Two recent reviews carefully documented reports that demonstrate the safety of opioids other than meperidine in patients receiving MAOIs.[131,132] Two forms of the MAOI-meperidine interaction exist. One is an "excitatory" form characterized by agitation, rigidity, hyperpyrexia, convulsions, he-

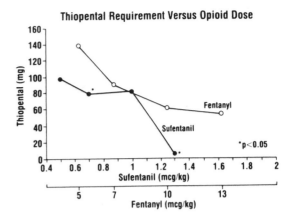

Fig. 4-5 Thiopental requirement for induction of sleep versus opioid dose in surgical patients. Thiopental was administered intravenously in 25-mg increments every 30 seconds until the subject was unconscious. Sufentanil and fentanyl doses were plotted on the same scale, using a potency ratio of 1:8. Thiopental requirements were significantly less ($P < 0.0001$) for sufentanil (0.7 and 1.3 $\mu g/kg$) compared with equipotent doses of fentanyl (5 and 10 $\mu g/kg$, respectively). Only 1 of the 10 patients receiving sufentanil (1.3 $\mu g/kg$) required any thiopental compared with 10 of 10 in the fentanyl 10-$\mu g/kg$ group and 8 of 10 in the fentanyl 13-$\mu g/kg$ group ($P < 0.0001$). (From Bowdle and Ward.,[128] with permission.)

modynamic instability, and coma. It is thought to be related to the blockade of neuronal uptake of serotonin by meperidine. The second type of interaction is "depressive" and manifests as respiratory depression, hypotension, and coma, perhaps as a result of hepatic microsomal enzyme inhibition by the MAOI and resultant meperidine accumulation. Successful therapies for these conditions are unsubstantiated but would likely include common supportive measures.

Respiratory Effects of Drug Interactions

Many central nervous system depressants increase the magnitude of opioid induced respiratory depression. Even small doses of benzodiazepines, barbiturates, and other anesthetic induction agents, such as propofol,[133] can result in significant respiratory depression when combined with opioids. Fentanyl (2.0 $\mu g/kg$ IV) and midazolam (0.05 mg/

kg IV) given separately to human volunteers did not result in apnea, but when combined they produced apnea 50 percent of the time (Fig. 4-6).[134] The administration of even small doses of benzodiazepines in the immediate preinduction phase of anesthesia increased the incidence of inadequate postoperative ventilation after anesthetic induction with alfentanil.[135] Some other centrally acting drugs, such as droperidol, tricyclic antidepressants, and α_2 agonists (such as clonidine), do not significantly potentiate opioid induced ventilatory depression.[136]

Nitrous oxide adds to opioid induced respiratory depression.[137] Sufentanil significantly reduced ventilation while minimally effecting hemodynamics in dogs anesthetized with isoflurane.[138] Even small doses of fentanyl (0.3 μg/kg IV) administered during inhalation anesthesia (enflurane plus nitrous oxide) significantly depressed ventilation in humans by increasing expiratory time and, thus, decreasing minute ventilation.[139] Apnea often occurs in patients breathing spontaneously under general anesthesia with a potent inhalation agent when analgesic doses of opioids are added.

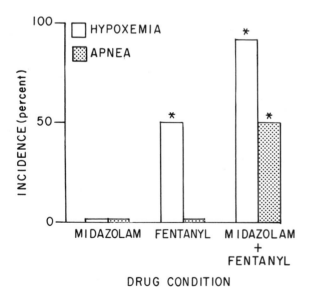

Fig. 4-6 Incidence of hypoxemia and apnea after midazolam (0.05 mg/kg IV), fentanyl (2 μg/kg IV), or both drugs, in young adult volunteers. (From Bailey et al.,[134] with permission.)

Cardiovascular Effects of Drug Interactions

Intravenous sedative hypnotic agents are often administered with opioids, including barbiturates, benzodiazepines, ketamine, etomidate, and propofol. Hypotension frequently results after barbiturate administration, as a result of venodilatation, decreased cardiac filling, myocardial depression, and decreased sympathetic nervous system activity. Attempts to ensure amnesia by combining barbiturates with opioids can significantly compromise hemodynamic stability and result in hypotension and reduced cardiac output despite increased peripheral vascular resistance and heart rate.[140,141] Reducing the dose of thiopental administered in the presence of opioids to 0.5 to 1.0 mg/kg may help to minimize this problem.

Much information exists with regard to benzodiazepine-opioid combinations and hemodynamic effects. Benzodiazepines and opioids are synergistic when administered to induce anesthesia.[142,143] However, hemodynamic stability can be compromised, especially in patients with little cardiovascular reserve. Hypotension can result from combinations of diazepam, midazolam, or lorazepam with virtually all opioids, including morphine,[144] fentanyl[6,27] and sufentanil.[119] Hemodynamic consequences may include decreased heart rate, mean arterial pressure, central venous pressure, and cardiac output. Mechanisms may include decreased sympathetic tone,[39] decreased circulating catecholamines,[144,145] additive negative inotropic effects,[146] depression of baroreceptor function,[147] and higher opioid plasma levels secondary to the pharmacokinetic consequences of decreased cardiac output.[148] In addition, the order of drug administration has been suggested to be important. Lorazepam-sufentanil combinations resulted in hypotension when lorazepam preceded sufentanil,[119,149,150] but not when it followed both anesthetic induction with sufentanil and endotracheal intubation.[151,152]

Propofol can produce significant cardiovascular depression that may not resolve immediately with decreasing blood levels.[153] Although propofol-fentanyl[154] and propofol-sufentanil[155] anesthesia for coronary artery bypass surgery may provide acceptable conditions, mean arterial pressure can decrease, especially during induction, to levels that might jeopardize coronary perfusion.[154] Etomidate and ketamine can be combined with opioids and, generally, result in little cardiovascular instability. Alone, these agents inadequately block responses to noxious stimuli, but in low doses, they can enhance amnesia and preserve the hemodynamic stability sought with high doses of opioids.

Frequently, nitrous oxide or a potent inhaled anesthetic agent is administered in conjunction with opioid anesthesia. Nitrous oxide often, but not always, preserves cardiovascular function.[156] Nitrous oxide combined with morphine or fentanyl in humans has produced concentration dependent decreases in cardiac output and arterial blood pressure.[157,158] Deterioration of cardiac function with nitrous oxide-opioid combinations may be caused by increased afterload (systemic and pulmonary vascular resistance increases),[159,160] increased coronary vascular resistance and impaired coronary blood flow,[161] lower inspired oxygen concentration associated with the use of nitrous oxide,[162] or direct myocardial depression.[163,164] Nevertheless, the use of nitrous oxide in conjunction with fentanyl for cardiac surgery has not been associated with increased myocardial ischemia.[165,166]

Numerous reports have documented the hemodynamic consequences of concomitantly administered opioids and muscle relaxants. Pancuronium can result in increases in heart rate and myocardial ischemia.[150,167–169] Thus some authors recommend avoiding pancuronium in patients with coronary artery disease,[167] but at times, pancuronium may be employed to advantage if increases in heart rate and blood pressure are desirable.[170] Vecuronium-opioid combinations can result in a greater need for vasopressor support than pancuronium opioid combinations.[170,171] Metocurine can produce hypotension,[169,172] but metocurine pancuronium mixtures produce minimal hemodynamic effects.[173] Newer muscle relaxants have been developed with the aim of eliminating cardiovascular effects (see Ch. 21).[174–178] Muscle relaxant selection should be based on multiple factors, including the patient's status and pathologic condition, concomitant medications (e.g., β-adrenergic blockers), anesthetic premedication, and anesthetic agents used. No

drug regimen or drug combination is suitable for all patients. For example, patients with ischemic heart disease are best served by slow heart rates and adequate coronary artery pressure; patients with regurgitant valvular disorders may require faster heart rates and reduced afterload.

Many other drugs, including nonanesthetic agents, alter the hemodynamic actions of opioids. β-Adrenergic blockers, either as premedication[179] or administered intraoperatively,[180] can contribute to hemodynamic stability, especially with regard to heart rate (see Ch. 28). During high dose opioid anesthesia for coronary surgery, β blockade can reduce opioid requirements and the need for other supplements and decrease intraoperative and postoperative myocardial ischemia.[179,181,182] The incidence of arrhythmias may also be reduced.[183] Intraoperative nitroglycerin administration may[184] or may not[185] ameliorate myocardial ischemia during opioid anesthesia.

Clonidine, dexmedetomidine, and other α_2 agonist agents act synergistically with opioids and hold promise as anesthetic adjuncts (see Ch. 27). α_2 Agonists reduced opioid requirements while improving hemodynamic stability in patients undergoing coronary surgery.[186,187] There were also benefits in the postoperative period, including higher cardiac output, earlier extubation, reduced plasma catecholamine levels, and less shivering.[186] Bradycardia and hypotension are side effects that can occur when α_2 agonists are administered alone or in combination with opioids.

CLINICAL APPLICATIONS

Morphine

Morphine is frequently administered intravenously in the perioperative period primarily to control pain, in doses ranging from 0.1 to 0.25 mg/kg. Higher doses (0.25 to 3 mg/kg) are infrequently used. Although some subjective central nervous system effects may be noted within minutes of injection, morphine does not easily penetrate the blood-brain barrier. Thus, peak effects require at least 10 to 30 minutes to develop. Titration of morphine to clinical end points should take this into consideration. Sensations of euphoria, warmth, visceral burning, sedation, or itching may occur. Rarely, dysphoria occurs. Histamine release, especially if large doses of morphine are rapidly administered, may result in hypotension, particularly in hypovolemic patients or those who sit up or ambulate. Intravenous doses of morphine of 0.2 mg/kg produce analgesic and respiratory effects that peak in less than 1 hour and last for up to 4 to 6 hours.[188]

Excessive doses of morphine produce significant lethargy and respiratory depression. Unresponsiveness with or without pinpoint pupils may result. The absence of pinpoint pupils may be the result of sympathetic stimulation caused by unrecognized hypoxemia and/or hypercarbia. Anormal respiratory patterns include rapid, very shallow abdominal breathing, slow Cheyne-Stokes type breathing with relatively normal or large tidal volumes, and intermittent apnea. Respiratory arrest is always a risk with excessive opioid agonist doses.

Fentanyl Analogs

The opioid agonists most frequently employed in operative anesthesia today are fentanyl, alfentanil, and sufentanil. There are major differences in the speed of onset and duration of action of these closely related analogs of fentanyl (see Ch. 3). Scott et al.[189] fitted EEG data to a pharmacodynamic model and reported a half-time for onset of 6.4

minutes for fentanyl and 1.1 minutes for alfentanil (Fig. 4-7).[189] Similar data for sufentanil suggest that the speed of onset of sufentanil and fentanyl are comparable. Bowdle and Ward[128] reported that the peak EEG effects of fentanyl or sufentanil occurred less than 2 minutes after an intravenous bolus, the 2 minutes including 1 minute taken to administer the drug. They also observed that the speed of onset was dose related; larger doses had earlier peak effects.

After a bolus injection, effect site concentrations for sufentanil and, especially, alfentanil decrease more rapidly compared with fentanyl, according to computer simulations (Fig. 4-8).[190] This disparity between fentanyl on the one hand and alfentanil and sufentanil on the other becomes even more significant if drug infusions are administered (Fig. 4-9). For significant (50 and 80 percent in Fig. 4-9) decreases in target organ (effect site) opioid levels to occur after drug infusions of 2 to 4 hours, fentanyl requires more time than either alfentanil or sufentanil. Infusions of sufentanil will require less time than alfentanil to decrease 50 and 80 percent if the infusion duration is less than 8 and 3 hours, respectively (Fig. 4-9).

The rapid blood-brain equilibration for alfentanil (Fig. 4-10)[189-191] predicts that this opioid will be the most suitable choice when a rapid, pro-

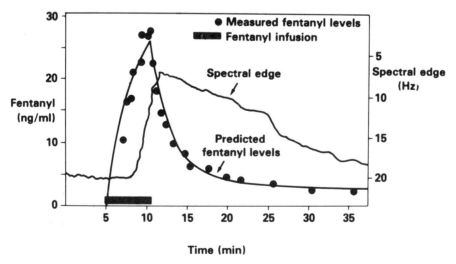

Fig. 4-7 Time course of the EEG spectral edge and serum fentanyl concentrations. Note that the spectral edge axis is inverted. Changes in the spectral edge lag behind the changes in serum concentration. The fentanyl infusion rate = 150 μg/min (solid bar). (From Scott et al.,[189] with permission.)

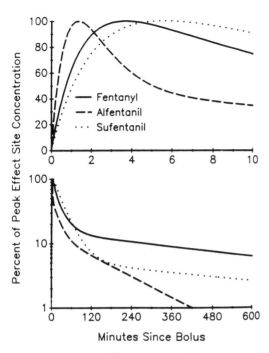

Fig. 4-8 Predicted effect site opioid concentrations over time, as a percentage of the peak effect site concentration, after a bolus. (From Shafer et al.,[190] with permission.)

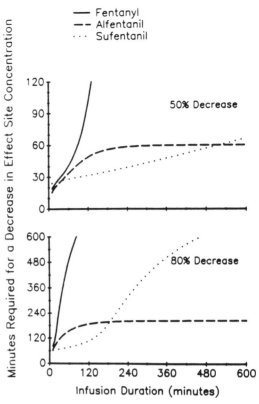

Fig. 4-9 Overlay of fentanyl, alfentanil, and sufentanil recovery curves describing the time required for decreases of 50 percent and 80 percent from the maintained intraoperative effect site concentration after termination of the infusion. (From Shafer et al.,[190] with permission.)

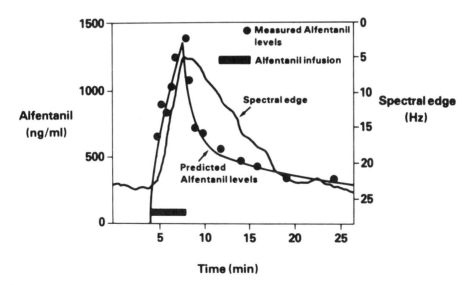

Fig. 4-10 Time course of the EEG spectral edge and serum alfentanil concentrations. Note that the spectral edge axis is inverted. Changes in the spectral edge closely parallel the serum concentrations. The alfentanil infusion rate is 1,500 μg/min (solid bar). (From Scott et al.,[189] with permission.)

found, but brief opioid effect is desired. Because alfentanil gets into the brain most rapidly (most rapid blood-brain equilibration), a relatively larger peak effect site concentration will be achieved.[190] This is a result of the fact that blood levels for all the opioids peak and then diminish rapidly. The peak effect site concentrations for drugs with more rapid blood-brain equilibration will reflect higher plasma drug levels than those with slower blood-brain equilibration times. Thus a greater percent of the drug administered (or the peak plasma drug level) reaches the effect site. This permits the physician to reduce the alfentanil dose, enhancing the patient's recovery from the drug's effects.[190]

Although sufentanil does not reach the brain any faster than does fentanyl, the more rapid decrease in effect site concentrations allows greater amounts of the drug to be administered without prolonging the effects. In addition sufentanil may provide longer lasting analgesia with less respiratory depression than does fentanyl[101,192]

Careful titration of fentanyl, sufentanil, and alfentanil are important, especially if the immediate induction of anesthesia is not anticipated. Because opioid pharmacokinetics[193] and pharmacodynamics are so variable, occasionally, modest doses of alfentanil (5 to 20 μg/kg) or sufentanil (0.1 to 0.4 μg/kg) can render patients apneic and rigid.

Premedication

Routine premedication has decreased as a result of the large increase in same day or outpatient surgery. Nevertheless, many patients receive premedication, often with an opioid. Premedication with opioid agonists can serve multiple purposes. Anxiety may be relieved, particularly in patients experiencing pain preoperatively. Although, benzodiazepines are more potent and specific anxiolytics, the sedation produced by opioids can be effective. Other goals sought with opioid premedication include the relief of pain associated with the insertion of intravascular or regional block needles; the blunting of cardiovascular responses to anesthetic induction, laryngoscopy, and intubation; the reduction of anesthetic requirements; and the provision of postoperative analgesia. Numerous existing reports do not permit uniform conclusions as to the efficacy of opioid agonists as premedicants.[194,195] Some authors contend that premedica-

tion with opioids should be restricted to the relief of pain.

Intramuscular injections of morphine or meperidine have been used most often. Recommended doses for morphine and meperidine range from 0.1 to 0.2 and 0.75 to 1.25 mg/kg IM, respectively. The onset and peak effect require 15 to 45 minutes. Fentanyl can be administered intramuscularly as a premedicant in a dose range of 0.05 to 0.2 mg in adults. The onset of action with fentanyl will be more rapid than with morphine. Depending on the fentanyl dose, the duration of effect (usually 2 to 4 hours) may be longer or shorter than that of meperidine.[196] Fentanyl is less likely to cause cardiovascular side effects than meperidine.[197,198] Innovar, a proprietary combination of fentanyl (50 μg/mL) and droperidol (2.5 mg/ml) has also been used as a premedicant. Good to excellent sedation and cooperation can be achieved with Innovar for procedures only requiring local or regional anesthesia[198–200] but postoperative somnolence was less and patient satisfaction was greater with midazolam compared with Innovar.[201,202] Innovar has been favorably compared with meperidine[198] and morphine.[203] The usual dose of Innovar in adults is 1 to 2 ml IM or IV. Fentanyl and droperidol peak plasma levels occur 10 to 30 minutes after the intramuscular injection.

Reduced enthusiasm for intramuscular injections, combined with the availability of newer routes of drug delivery, has led to other approaches for premedication. Transmucosal routes of drug delivery can be employed for premedication (see Ch. 31). Sublingual, buccal, gingival, nasal, and rectal mucosal sites have all found application. Although these routes are more often employed for postoperative or cancer pain management, transmucosal administration holds promise for premedication in certain patient populations. Fentanyl has been incorporated into a palatable lozenge on a stick that can be applied to the oral mucosa and titrated to effect.[204–206] The onset of its effect is observed in 20 to 40 minutes. This particular mode of delivery is particularly appealing in pediatric surgical patients. Oral transmucosal fentanyl (15 to 20 μg/kg) in children was compared with a swallowed solution of meperidine (1.5 mg/kg), diazepam (0.2 mg/kg), and atropine (0.02 mg/kg). Either treatment produced similar

degrees of sedation and anxiolysis, lower requirements for postoperative analgesics, and no change
in preoperative oxygen saturation, but fentanyl
produced more (37 percent versus 5 percent) vomiting.[206] Optimal methods of controlling the increased nausea and vomiting associated with oral
transmucosal fentanyl remain to be defined; reducing fentanyl doses to 10 to 15 μg/kg, administering
antiemetics, and minimizing early ambulation may
all be important factors.

The delivery of opioids through the nasal mucosa has also been reported.[207] Sufentanil is effective in a dose range of 0.05 to 2 μg/kg.[208-209] The
onset of drug effect is rapid (10 to 20 minutes), and
the bioavailability is high (78 percent).[209] Unfortunately, children often cry upon nasal drug administration, and the risk of chest wall rigidity increases
with higher doses (more than 2.0 μg/kg). Fentanyl
may also be aerosolized or nebulized and inhaled.[210,211] Inhaled morphine was not satisfactory
because of its erratic bioavailability.[212]

Buccal morphine as a perioperative opioid
analgesic delivery method has had its proponents.[213] Others have not found buccal morphine
to be effective in reducing postoperative analgesic
requirements.[214] Problems with this approach include the poor taste, variable dissolution, and
washout of buccal morphine in the saliva. Sublingual buprenorphine, 0.4 mg, was similar to intramuscular morphine (7.5 to 10 mg) as a premedicant in female patients undergoing orthopedic
surgery.[215]

The rectal mucosa is a potential site for drug
delivery. Although morphine is poorly absorbed
via this site,[216] sustained release technology[217] or a
starch Hydrogel preparation[218] can overcome this
problem. Therapeutic blood levels can be achieved
in 1 hour and maintained for hours. Rectal premedication with other opioids, including meperidine,[218] has also been tried. Children may not accept rectal administration without crying and
struggling.

Induction of Anesthesia

The reasons for the use of opioids for the induction and maintenance of anesthesia are listed in
Table 4-2. The primary goal of employing opioids
during anesthetic induction is to blunt the cardiovascular responses (e.g., hypertension and tachy-

Table 4-2 Rationale Behind the Use of Opioids in Anesthesia

Provide preinduction sedation and analgesia

Provide analgesia for additional vascular line placement

Blunt hemodynamic and stress response to laryngoscopy and intubation

Reduce requirements for other anesthetics

Promote perioperative hemodynamic stability

Provide for a smooth emergence

Provide analgesia in the postoperative phase

cardia) to laryngoscopy and tracheal intubation.
Few anesthetic agents are able to blunt these responses as effectively as opioids, without causing
cardiovascular depression. The choice of opioid for
induction depends upon the specific circumstances. Few studies have compared three or more
opioids.[220-222] Nevertheless, certain opioids are
rarely desirable as induction agents. Meperidine
produces significant cardiovascular side effects, including hypotension and tachycardia.[222] Morphine
has a very slow onset and may cause hypotension as
a result of the release of histamine. Generally, fentanyl, sufentanil, or alfentanil are preferred because of rapid onset and relative lack of cardiovascular side effects.

Maintenance of Anesthesia

Three main approaches are used to maintain the
opioid component of balanced anesthesia. The
most simple technique is the administration of a
single large bolus. Fentanyl, sufentanil, or alfentanil administered as a single large bolus during
induction will produce effects that carry over into
the maintenance phase of anesthesia; such induction bolus doses of fentanyl, alfentanil, and sufentanil typically range from 5 to 50, 50 to 150, and 1
to 10 μg/kg, respectively. Although simple and
practical, this approach has several disadvantages,
including a substantial incidence of muscle rigidity,
a risk of hypotension, and drug wastage. Drug
wastage is illustrated in Figure 4-11. Alfentanil levels were maintained in the therapeutic range
longer when 200 μg/kg was administered as an 80-
μg/kg bolus, followed by a 3-μg/kg/min infusion

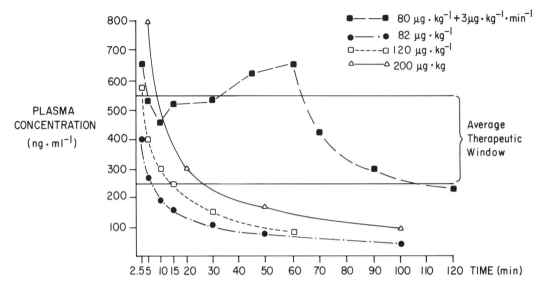

Fig. 4-11 Plasma alfentanil levels after three different bolus injections and a bolus plus continuous infusion for 1 hour.

for 40 minutes than when all 200 μg/kg was given as a single bolus. The administration of a large single bolus produces high blood and effect site drug levels, but rapid distribution results in much of the administered dose being delivered to nontarget organ tissues, representing drug wastage.

A second approach to maintenance is intermittent administration of small bolus doses at regular time intervals (e.g., every 15 to 30 minutes) or titrated to the response to surgical stimuli. Fentanyl (e.g., 25 to 100 μg) and sufentanil (e.g., 5 to 25 μg) are frequently employed in this manner. This approach is nearly as simple as the single large bolus

technique, and it will narrow the range between the peaks and valleys in drug levels. Though clinically this approach is often effective, fluctuations in plasma levels will still be significant.

A third approach to maintenance opioid administration is variable continuous infusion. The potential advantages of this method are listed in Table 4-3. Much work has been directed toward the clinical application of opioid infusions.[190,193,223–229] These efforts include defining population based pharmacokinetic parameters, developing computer software programs and pumps to deliver drugs, and determining therapeutic plasma drug levels for various stimuli. Computer simulations have been used to explore the pharmacokinetic properties of opioid infusions.[190] Drug regimens may be described by a calculated* or clinically esti-

Table 4-3 Potential Advantages of Continuous Infusions Versus Intermittent Boluses of Opioids in Anesthesia

Decreased total dose

Greater hemodynamic stability

Decreased side effects

Decreased need for supplementation

More rapid recovery of consciousness

Less respiratory depression and need for antagonists

Less pain in the immediate postoperative period

Decreased discharge time

---

* Dose calculation targeting alfentanil 300 ng/ml

Loading dose = Desired plasma concentration: volume of distribution
= Css·Vdβ
= 0.3 μg/ml·380 ml/kg
= 114 μg/kg

Infusion rate = Desired plasma concentration·clearance
= Css·Cl$_E$
= 0.3 μg/ml·32 mg/kg/min
= 0.96 μg/kg/min

Table 4-4 Approximate Plasma Opioid Levels (in Nanograms/Milliliter) Required in Balanced Anesthesia With Nitrous Oxide

	Noxious and Surgical Stimulus Level (1–10 Scale)			
	1–2	3–5	6–8	9–10
Alfentanil	50–150	100–300	200–500	400–800
Fentanyl	1–2	3–6	4–10	6–20
Sufentanil	0.1–0.3	0.25–1.5	1.0–3.0	3.0–6.0

mated (1) loading dose that is titrated to effect over several minutes and (2) variable rate continuous infusion to maintain targeted plasma and effect site drug levels (Table 4-4). Additional small boluses that adjust plasma drug levels upward in anticipation of greater stimulation are also employed. Several computerized drug infusion pumps have been used experimentally to deliver opioids.[227]

Intraoperative cardiovascular stability and a smooth, pain free emergence after surgery can usually be achieved when fentanyl, sufentanil, or alfentanil are administered in a balanced technique employing low doses of isoflurane (0.2 to 0.6 percent) with or without nitrous oxide (50 to 70 percent) in oxygen. The addition of nitrous oxide and/or a potent inhalation agent can alter opioid requirements significantly. Without even small concentrations of isoflurane, for example, opioid requirements may increase 50 to 100 percent. It is often advantageous to "balance" the anesthetic technique with nonopioid agents rather than to persist in progressively increasing opioid doses. Table 4-5 depicts suggested loading and maintenance drug doses. Note that drug levels required

for particular degrees of noxious stimuli not only overlap (Table 4-4), but that they also tend to become greater in range as the pain intensity increases. This reflects the larger variability in requirements as surgical stimulus increases.[120]

Rapid emergence is preferred following most general anesthetics. Therefore, a rapid decline in plasma drug levels when an infusion is terminated is advantageous. Sufentanil has an elimination half-life similar to fentanyl, but sufentanil levels decrease more rapidly when infusions are stopped.[190,228,229]

Residual postoperative respiratory depression is the main disadvantage of opioid anesthesia. Opioid antagonists will restore adequate ventilation; however, analgesia may not be preserved. In addition, cardiovascular side effects are commonly associated with the use of antagonists (see Ch. 5).[230] Therefore, it is desirable to administer opioids so that plasma levels at the end of surgery permit adequate spontaneous ventilation; this goal is difficult to achieve at times, for several reasons. Plasma opioid levels that result in analgesia overlap considerably with those that result in respiratory depression, patient sensitivity varies greatly, and the abil-

Table 4-5 Suggested Opioid Loading, Maintenance Infusion, and Additional Bolus Doses for Maintenance of Balanced Anesthesia

	Loading Dose (μg/kg)	Maintenance Dose	Additional Bolus
Alfentanil	50–100	1–3 μg/kg/min	5–10 μg/kg
Sufentanil	0.5–3	0.5–2 μg/kg/h	2.5–10 μg
Fentanyl	4–20	2–10 μg/kg/h	25–100 μg

ity to predict and produce appropriate opioid plasma levels remains largely based on clinical experience. Until computer assisted opioid infusion is adequately refined, much clinical skill and an element of luck will be needed to employ opioids successfully by infusion. Real time measurement of plasma drug concentrations would be a major advance in the clinical application of intravenous anesthetics, analogous to the measurement of anesthetic gases in the breathing circuit. However, the technology for online plasma level analysis does not exist.

The clinician must actively search for the minimum infusion rate that provides adequate conditions to avoid excessive drug administration. Doses for sufentanil infusion should be generally restricted to 1 μg/kg/h or less if adequate spontaneous ventilation at the end of surgery is desired.[231] Alfentanil infusions should be lowered to 0.5 to 1 μg/kg/min in anticipation of the end of surgery; premature termination of an alfentanil infusion will result in a short duration of residual analgesia.

Total intravenous anesthesia (TIVA) is general anesthesia without inhalational anesthetic agents. Because no single intravenous agent produces satisfactory anesthesia, combinations of two or more drugs are required. The development of shorter acting opioids and nonopioid intravenous anesthetic agents, and techniques for administering them, has made TIVA a more practical anesthetic technique.[231] TIVA has particular appeal where the delivery of inhalation agents is impaired, for example, in airway procedures requiring jet ventilation or in conditions in which ventilation-perfusion abnormalities markedly delay the uptake and washout of inhalation agents.

The combination of propofol and alfentanil for TIVA is well documented.[232–236] Propofol and alfentanil provide most, if not all, the desired components of anesthesia even without supplementation with nitrous oxide.[235] Propofol also reduces nausea and vomiting.[238] The addition of even small doses of adjuncts such as a benzodiazepine, can increase recovery time after propofol-alfentanil TIVA.[236] Propofol also had better characteristics for TIVA compared with barbiturates or benzodiazepines.[239,240] Propofol and alfentanil should be administered by continuous infusion, after loading doses. Alfentanil, 25 to 100 μg/kg may be titrated in 25-μg/kg increments, followed by propofol, 0.5 to 1.5 mg/kg, for induction of anesthesia. Maintenance infusions for alfentanil (1 to 2 μg/kg/min) and propofol (60 to 120 μg/kg/min) are best initiated just prior to induction because the effect of the induction boluses rapidly dissipates.

During the maintenance phase of TIVA, the infusions may be adjustmented, and if necessary, small drug boluses may be titrated to patient responsiveness. Alfentanil boluses of 5 to 15 μg/kg will raise blood levels by 50 to 100 ng/ml. Propofol infusion should be terminated 10 to 20 minutes prior to the desired time of emergence, especially if nitrous oxide can be employed. The alfentanil infusion should be kept at a low rate (0.5 to 1.0 μg/kg/min) but not turned off until surgery is finished, especially if substantial postoperative pain is anticipated. Skillfully administered TIVA with alfentanil and propofol results in a rapid and pleasant emergence from anesthesia.

High Dose Opioid Anesthesia

The use of high doses of opioids as sole anesthetics has been attributed to Lowenstein et al.[105] and Stanley and Webster.[6] The merits, usefulness, and validity of "opioid anesthesia" continue to be debated and evaluated.[49,111] Although some authors have argued that opioids should not be expected to produce anesthesia,[241] others believe that "cookbook" approaches underlie failed techniques. Adherence to rigid administration regimens ignores the necessity for producing plasma and effect site opioid levels in accordance with the level of surgical stimulation. Many rigid drug administration schemes result in relatively low blood opioid levels at points of maximal surgical stimulation. Nevertheless, opioids may not block responses to surgical stimuli in all patients, regardless of dose.[49,241]

Bolus doses of fentanyl (injected in less than 1 minute) range from 15 to 75 μg/kg. Loading doses of 20 to 40 μg/kg establish plasma fentanyl concentrations (10 to 20 ng/ml) that are often sufficient to provide stable hemodynamics throughout the induction and intubation sequence. Some clinicians prefer to infuse rapidly a single large bolus of fentanyl (up to 150 μg/kg) to provide for both the induction and maintenance of anesthesia. Others prefer a lower loading dose of fentanyl followed by a maintenance infusion ranging from 0.3 to 1.0 μg/kg/min. Very high fentanyl doses (greater than 100 μg/kg) prolong ventilator dependency and may increase the need for postoperative vasopressors and intravenous fluids.[243]

Induction doses of sufentanil range from 2 to 20 μg/kg administered as a bolus or infused over 2 to 10 minutes. Additional sufentanil may be required in anticipation of provocative stimuli, e.g., before skin incision and sternotomy. Total doses of sufentanil for cardiac surgery usually range from 15 to 30 μg/kg.

High dose alfentanil has been less frequently applied as an anesthetic technique for cardiac surgery and is not generally recommended.[46] Unconsciousness is produced with 100 to 200 μg/kg. Rigidity, bradycardia, and other opioid side effects occur at least as frequently as after sufentanil and fentanyl. Continuous infusions (2 to 12 μg/kg/min) have been employed to maintain adequate plasma alfentanil concentrations (up to 2,000 ng/ml) during cardiac surgery. Hemodynamic control may be more difficult with intermittent bolus techniques using alfentanil.[123]

Postoperative Pain Control

The parenteral administration of opioids continues to be the standard method of surgical pain control. The use of other agents such as mixed agonist-antagonist opioids (see Ch. 5) or nonsteroidal anti-inflammatory drugs (see Ch. 29) and other routes of administration, such as neuraxial opioids (see Ch. 6) do represent significant therapeutic alternatives. Such options may at times provide superior pain relief. Studies by Yeager et al.[244] and Baron et al.[245] suggest the postoperative application of neuraxial opioids and local anesthetics can reduce complications and health care costs. Other emerging, potentially important, concepts include pre-emptive analgesia. Pre-emptive analgesia refers to the observation that analgesics may be more effective when administered in advance of a painful stimulus, rather than after the painful stimulus. Although there is evidence supporting pre-emptive analgesia, its clinical value is uncertain.[245–248] Confirmation of such suggested benefits should pre-cede the routine clinical application of such therapies.[249]

The opioid drug, dose, route, and frequency of administration and side effect management scheme must all be tailored to the individual patient. Two pharmacologic principles underlie the application of opioid analgesia: (1) titration to effect and (2) dosing to maintain effect. Patient-controlled analgesia (PCA) has achieved great popularity for this purpose. The ideal opioid for PCA, one that has a rapid onset of effect, is highly efficacious, has an intermediate duration of action (to enhance control), and produces few side effects, does not exist. Morphine, fentanyl, and meperidine are most widely used.

Fentanyl via PCA may be as effective as lumbar epidural fentanyl administration (and, obviously, more simple) because systemic absorption contributes significantly to epidural fentanyl action.[254] Minimal effective analgesic blood concentrations for fentanyl and morphine are 1 to 2 and 15 to 20 ng/ml, respectively. Once established, effective concentrations remain relatively stable with PCA.[251]

Loading doses prior to initiation of PCA are best titrated to effect at the bedside by physicians or nurses. (Table 4-6). The titration of loading doses must consider the time required for peak opioid effects. Whereas fentanyl will produce significant and peak effects within a few minutes of administration, morphine requires a longer time. Stacking morphine loading doses at intervals of less than 5 minutes may result in overdosage. PCA lockout intervals (minimum time between doses) ranging from 6 to 12 minutes are usually appropriate.

PCA maintenance doses are typically small. Morphine interval doses of 1 mg are often used. Lower doses may be less effective and higher doses may increase side effects. A background continuous opioid infusion during PCA does not appear to improve analgesia or reduce side effects.[252–254] If employed, background infusion rates during PCA are typically 0.5 to 2 mg/h for morphine. Daily PCA morphine requirements vary greatly and, at times, are more than 3 to 4 mg/h.

PCA has been administered via subcutaneous, intramuscular, epidural, and intrathecal routes, in addition to the conventional intravenous route.

Table 4-6 Loading and Initial Interval Dose for PCA Morphine, Meperidine, and Fentanyl[a]

Drug	Loading Dose		Interval Dose	
	Adult	By Weight	Adult	By Weight
Morphine	2–4 mg every 10 min (total, 6–16 mg)	0.05 mg/kg (total, 0.05–0.2 mg/kg)	0.5–2 mg	10–20 μg/kg
Fentanyl	25–50 μg every 5 min (total, 50–300 μg)	0.05–2.0 μg/kg (total, 0.5–4 μg/kg)	10–30 μg	0.25–0.5 μg/kg
Meperidine	12.5–25 mg every 10 min (total, 50–125 mg)	0.5–1.5 mg/kg	5–10 mg	0.1–0.2 mg/kg

[a] Lockout Intervals Generally Range from 6 to 12 Minutes.

PCA devices have been used for the evaluation of patient and analgesic requirements, for predicting correct analgesic dose when converting to oral therapy, and in pain research efforts. The management of acute pain via PCA requires well trained personnel. Efficacy must be assessed at regular intervals and appropriate adjustments made. Alternative therapies should be considered if necessary. Side effect management must be organized and deliberate.

The complications of PCA therapy should theoretically be less frequent than those of traditional opioid administration regimens. However, overdosage with its attendant respiratory depression, and rarely death, can occur. Patient assessment at regular intervals, preferably by a well trained and organized acute pain service, is recommended. Monitoring of respiratory function, though not standardized, is recommended by some. Errors by health care providers and patients and mechanical problems contribute to the risks associated with PCA usage.[255,256]

Conventional intermittent parenteral administration of opioids is still frequently employed. However, it is generally less efficacious compared with PCA. Intermittent intramuscular injections of morphine frequently result in periods of relative underdosage when prescribed on an as needed basis or overdosage if administered at regular intervals. Injection site pain, and more rarely, infection may also accompany intramuscular therapy. Morphine is often recommended as the opioid agonist of choice for intramuscular administration.[66] Meperidine is less desirable because of its potential for toxicity. A metabolite of meperidine, normeperidine, produces central nervous system excitation. Normeperidine can accumulate and cause seizures, especially in the presence of renal dysfunction. Occasionally, even healthy patients will experience significant dysphoria or other signs of central nervous system excitation after receiving meperidine for several days. Opioid agonists can also be taken orally (Table 4-7).

Geriatrics

Elderly patients present their own unique set of problems. The prevalence of pain increases in elderly patients because of medical and surgical conditions. Nevertheless, pain assessment in this age group can be more difficult; myths, such as a purported increase in pain threshold, remain largely unsubstantiated. The variation between patients in many physiologic and pharmacologic parameters may increase with age, rendering the elderly patient at greater risk for drug under- and overdosage. Organ function and physiologic reserve may be reduced with age. Judicious administration of anesthetic drugs and attentive monitoring is required when caring for aged patients if physiologic homeostasis is to be maintained and complications avoided. The simplest distillation of all information available is based on the principle and practice of drug titration, "administer one-half the usual dose and wait twice as long" is a rule of thumb that works well in clinical geriatric anesthesia.

Opioid agonists will generally have greater effects in the elderly patient. Bellville et al.[257] found that 10 mg of morphine produced greater pain re-

Table 4-7 Average Recommended Starting Doses for Opioid Analgesics

Opioid	Oral Dose		Parenteral Dose	
	Adult	By Weight	Adult	By Weight
Morphine	30 mg every 3–4 h	0.3 mg/kg	10 mg every 3–4 h	0.1 mg/kg every 3–4 h
Hydromorphone	6 mg every 3–4 h	0.06 mg/kg every 3–4 h	1.5 mg every 3–4 h	0.015 mg/kg every 3–4 h
Codeine	60 mg every 3–4 h	1 mg/kg every 3–4 h	60 mg every 2–3 h SC for IM only	Not recommended
Hydrocodone	10 mg every 3–4 h	0.2 mg/kg every 3–4 h	Not available	Not available
Meperidine	Not recommended	Not recommended	100 mg every 3–4 h	0.75–1.5 mg/kg every 2–3 h
Methadone	20 mg every 6–8 h	0.2 mg/kg every 6–8 h	10 mg every 6–8 h	0.1 mg/kg every 6–8 h
Oxycodone	10 mg every 3–4 h	0.2 mg/kg every 3–4 h	Not available	Not available

lief in elderly postoperative patients. Older subjects sustained higher tissue concentrations of morphine for approximately 1.5 hours after a 10-mg dose compared with younger individuals.[258] Morphine requirements during PCA were also reduced in older subjects.[259] Older patients had more apnea, periodic breathing, and airway obstruction after morphine compared with young adults.[260] Similar findings exist with regard to meperidine[67] (Fig. 4-12), alfentanil,[261-264] fentanyl,[261,265,266] and perhaps sufentanil.[267] Pharmacokinetic changes sometimes, but not always, explain the decreased opioid requirements. Decreased initial volumes of distribution, intravascular volume, cardiac output, plasma protein binding, or red cell binding can all lead to increased drug delivery to the brain. Pharmacodynamic changes (increased brain sensitivity) may also underlie decreased drug requirements in the elderly.[262]

Obstetrics

The parenteral administration of opioid agonists persists as a method of providing analgesia in obstetrics. Hypotension associated with aortocaval compression may be exacerbated by morphine or meperidine. Effects on the fetus include decreased fetal heart rate variability, neonatal respiratory acidosis, lower Apgar scores, and neurobehavioral deficits in the newborn.[208,209] Neonatal problems may be minimized by avoiding opioid administration beyond the first stage of labor.

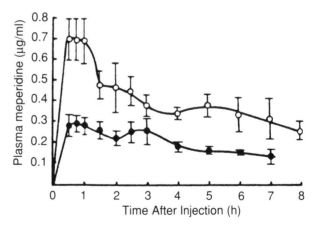

Fig. 4-12 Mean plasma meperidine concentration (± standard error of mean) after an intramuscular injection (1.5 mg/kg) in a group of young (●, 16 to 40 years, n = 7) and old (○, older than 70 years, n = 10) subjects. (From Chan et al.,[67] with permission.)

Morphine, meperidine, and fentanyl are the most frequently used opioid agonists in obstetrics. Morphine (2 to 6 mg IV or 4 to 10 mg IM) is not employed as often as meperidine (25 to 50 mg IV or 50 to 125 mg IM) because of the suggestion that morphine produces more neonatal respiratory depression.[270] Nevertheless, both morphine and meperidine achieve significant levels in the fetus and neonate soon after maternal injection,[271] and drug elimination for both agents is impaired in the neonate.[268,272] Multiple maternal doses of meperidine result in significant fetal accumulation of meperidine and normeperidine.[269] The neonatal elimination half-life of meperidine can be as long as 23 hours.[272] The neonatal effects of maternally administered meperidine can last up to three days.[273] Studies of exogenous opioids in the breast milk of mothers receiving PCA demonstrated that meperidine produced more neonatal neurobehavioral depression than did morphine.[274] Thus adverse neonatal effects can occur after either morphine or meperidine.[268] The shorter duration of action of analgesic doses of fentanyl (1 to 2 μg/kg) may represent an advantage.

Opioids are commonly avoided during general anesthesia for cesarian section until after delivery. However, in cases of severe hypertension, opioid agonists, such as alfentanil have been employed during induction to improve hemodynamic control. The newborn will most likely require resuscitation and administration of naloxone in these circumstances.

Pediatrics

Pediatric patients in general, are probably undermedicated with opioids for pain. The presence or absence of pain in neonates and infants may be difficult to confirm. Nevertheless, noxious or invasive procedures in young children evoke behaviors and neurologic and sympathetic responses that are identical to those in older individuals. Thus, although some have argued that neither anesthesia nor analgesia is necessary for newborns undergoing surgery,[275] others believe that this approach is inhumane.

Reduced opioid clearance in premature infants results in an altered response to opioids.[276] Full term neonates also require reduced initial doses of the opioids, alfentanil[276] and sufentanil[277] for pharmcokinetic reasons. Twenty- to 28-day-old neonates do possess an active cytochrome oxidase system and better hepatic blood flow, resulting in improved opioid clearance.[278] Abdominal surgery, increased intra-abdominal pressure,[279] and an open ductus venosus may reduce drug clearance and prolong drug action. Opioid pharmacokinetics are variable in children and adults.

Whether pediatric patients are more sensitive to opioids continues to be debated. The lethal dose of morphine on a weight basis in rats increased with age.[280] Rat brain morphine levels were also found to be greater in the newborn rat compared with the adults. Perhaps, an immature blood-brain barrier permitted morphine to penetrate the brain more readily. Way et al.[270] studied ventilation in (8) newborns given morphine (0.05 mg/kg IM) or meperidine (0.5 mg/kg IM) and concluded that ventilatory depression was greater with morphine. The number of subjects studied was small, and no statistical test of a difference was offered. Nevertheless, this report promoted the belief that infants were extremely sensitive to opioids, especially morphine. Subsequently, Hertzka et al.[281] demonstrated that infants 3 months of age or older were not more sensitive to the ventilatory depressant effects of fentanyl than were older children and young adults; the infants experienced less apnea than did the older patients. The causes of perioperative apnea and its management in pediatric patients younger than 60 weeks of total gestational age remains somewhat controversial.

Small doses of morphine (0.05 to 0.15 mg/kg IV or IM), fentanyl (1 to 2 μg/kg IV or IM), or meperidine (0.5 to 1.5 mg/kg IV or IM) usually provide safe and effective postoperative analgesia in infants with mild to moderate pain. Infusions of alfentanil or sufentanil, in combination with other intravenous or inhalated agents, can provide anesthesia, as in adults. Intravenous anesthesia for routine pediatric operations has not been well studied. Induction of anesthesia in children is often by inhalation, but conversion to intravenous anesthesia is an option. Alfentanil infusions have been employed for herniorrhaphy in pediatric patients.[282] Alfentanil based anesthesia in children undergoing oral surgery has been reported.[283] Postoperative emesis may be increased by opioids, especially if no prophylaxis is administered. Thus, prophylactic therapy for nausea and vomiting should be provided. Doses of opioids on a weight basis are described in Tables 4-5, 4-6, and 4-7.

High dose opioid anesthesia has had an important role in major pediatric operations.[284] Doses based on weight and effective plasma levels are similar to those for adults for morphine,[285] fentanyl,[286,287] and sufentanil.[288,289] Anand et al.[25] reported data suggesting that the stress response, morbidity, and mortality were reduced in neonates undergoing cardiac surgery when they received high dose sufentanil compared with halothane-morphine anesthesia. Curiously, this report and the accompanying editorial[290] characterized the high dose sufentanil anesthesia group as "deep" and the halothane-morphine anesthesia group as "light," in direct contradistinction to how these two types of anesthetic techniques have always been described in the past. The rationale for this change in terminology was not made clear. Maintenance of postoperative sedation and intense analgesia in *intubated* pediatric patients can be achieved with initial infusions of morphine (0.05 to 0.4 mg/kg/h), fentanyl (1 to 5 μg/kg/h), sufentanil (0.1 to 0.5 μg/kg/h), or alfentanil (0.5 to 1.5 μg/kg/min), followed by appropriate adjustments.

Disease States

Many diseases and surgery itself[290] may alter drug pharmacokinetics. The many reports delineating the pharmacokinetic changes associated with specific disease states are addressed in Chapter 3.

Acid Base Changes

Acid base changes can alter drug action through pharmacokinetic mechanisms. Opioid elimination half-lives are prolonged by hypocapnic hyperventilation in dogs[292] and humans.[293] In addition, a sudden acidosis, as frequently occurs after the termination of artificial ventilation, may result in an augmentation of opioid action.[294] A vicious cycle of acidosis, increased opioid action, further ventilatory depression, and worse acidosis may result. It is common, but usually unwarranted, to produce mild to moderate hypocapnic hyperventilation during controlled mechanical ventilation in-

traoperatively. The intraoperatively maintenance of normocarbia or even mild hypercapnia ($PaCO_2$ 42 to 46 mmHg) may be desirable with regard to avoiding prolonged or exaggerated opioid effects.

Plasma Protein Binding

Changes in plasma protein binding may also alter drug action. The clinical impact of this phenomenon is complex and poorly appreciated. Protein binding not only limits the amount of drug available ("free drug") for receptor interaction but also reduces drug distribution volumes.[295] Many drugs bind to plasma proteins. For example, propranolol, lidocaine, verapamil, meperidine, sufentanil, fentanyl, and alfentanil all bind to varying degrees to α-1 acid glycoprotein.[296] Complicating matters is the fact that a host of pathophysiologic states alter plasma protein concentrations (Table 4-8). Meistelman et al.[277] have demonstrated, for example, that lower concentrations of α-1 acid glycoprotein in neonates and infants leads to significantly higher plasma free fractions of sufentanil (19.5 and 11.5 percent, respectively) compared with those in children and adults (8.1 and 7.8 percent, respectively). Fentanyl, sufentanil, and alfentanil are 84.4, 92.5, and 92.1 percent protein (albumin, α and β globulins, and α-1 acid glycoprotein) bound in humans.[297] Plasma protein dilution increases free opioid levels.

Obesity

Obesity may alter opioid pharmacology. Few studies exist to clarify this issue with regard to opioids, and the results have not been consistent.[298–300] The usual recommendation is to reduce the administered dose based on weight for obese patients, especially with regard to maintenance doses, to account for possible decreased drug clearance and increased volumes of distribution and elimination half-lives.

Renal and Hepatic Pathology

Renal and hepatic pathologic conditions frequently alter drug action by affecting pharmacokinetics (see Ch. 3). Hepatic dysfunction may result in decreased opioid clearance and an increase elimination half-life for some opioids (morphine and alfentanil)[301–303] but not for others (fentanyl and

Table 4-8 Pathophysiologic States Associated With Alterations in Plasma Proteins to Which Drugs Are Bound

Decreased Albumin	Increased AAG	Decreased AAG
Burns	Burns	Neonates
Renal disease	Crohn's disease	Oral contraceptives
Hepatic disease	Renal transplantation	Pregnancy
Inflammatory disease	Infection	
Nephrotic syndrome	Trauma	
Cardiac failure	Chronic pain	
Postoperative period	Myocardial infarction	
Malnutrition	Postoperative period	
Malignancy	Malignancy	
Neonates	Rheumatoid arthritis	
Elderly patients	Ulcerative colitis	
Pregnancy		

Abbreviation: AAG, α-1 acid glycoprotein.

sufentanil).[304,305] Severe hepatic disease results in a host of changes, including abnormalities in plasma protein concentrations and drug binding. For example, excessive morphine effects may result from hypoalbuminemia combined with increased bilirubin, which competes with morphine for albumin binding sites.[306] Some evidence suggests that alcoholic patients may be pharmacodynamically less sensitive to opioids such as alfentanil.[307]

The intrinsic variability associated with human opioid pharmacokinetics and pharmacodynamics mandates careful drug titration. Myriad potential factors affecting drug action render patients somewhat different in their responses. Even apparently insignificant considerations, such as antibiotic therapy with erythromycin, can prolong alfentanil action via hepatic enzyme inhibition.[308] Assimilation of such information into clinical practice is rendered even more complicated by the fact that sufentanil is not similarly affected by the same antibiotic.[309] Such divergence in findings is the case for many issues concerning opioid agonist pharmacology. Only by continually refining our knowledge can we hope to achieve the desired results of opioid, and indeed, all drug therapy.

REFERENCES

1. Smith NT, Dec-Silver H, Sanford TJ et al: EEGs during high-dose fentanyl-, sufentanil-, or morphine-oxygen anesthesia. Anesth Analg 63:386, 1984
2. Sebel PS, Bovill JG, Wauquier A, Rog P: Effects of high dose fentanyl anesthesia on the electroencephalogram. Anesthesiology 55:203, 1981
3. Hecker BR, Lake CL, DiFazio CA et al: The decrease of the minimum alveolar anesthetic concentration produced by sufentanil in rats. Anesth Analg 62:987, 1983
4. Streisand JB, Bailey PL, LeMaire L et al: Fentanyl induced rigidity and unconsciousness in human volunteers. Anesthesiology 78:629, 1983
5. Parratt JR: Opioid receptors in the cardiovascular system. In van Zwielen P, Schönbaum E (eds): Progress in Pharmacology. Vol. 6/2. Gustar Fischer, New York, 1986
6. Stanley TH, Webster LR: Anesthetic requirements and cardiovascular effects of fentanyl-oxygen and fentanyl-diazepam-oxygen anaesthesia in man. Anesth Analg 57:411, 1978
7. Sebel PS, Bovill JG: Cardiovascular effects of sufentanil anesthesia: a study in patients undergoing cardiac surgery. Anesth Analg 61:115, 1982

8. Nauta J, Stanley TH, de Lange S et al: Anaesthetic induction with alfentanil: comparison with thiopental, midazolam, and etomidate. Can J Anaesth 30:53, 1983

9. Ebert TJ, Kotrly KJ, Madsen KE et al: Fentanyl-diazepam anesthesia with or without N_2O does not attenuate cardiopulmonary baroreflex-mediated vasoconstrictor responses to controlled hypovolemia in humans. Anesth Analg 67:548, 1988

10. Slogoff S, Keats AS: Does perioperative myocardial ischemia lead to postoperative myocardial infarction? Anesthesiology 62:107, 1985

11. Reitan JA, Stengert KB, Wymore ML, Martucci RW: Central vagal control of fentanyl induced bradycardia during halothane anesthesia. Anesth Analg 57:31, 1978

12. Liu WS, Bidwai AV, Stanley TH, Isern-Amaral S: Cardiovascular dynamics after large doses of fentanyl and fentanyl plus N_2O in the dog. Anesth Analg 55:168, 1976

13. Slogoff S, Keats AS: Randomized trial of primary anesthetic agents on outcome of coronary artery bypass operations. Anesthesiology 70:179, 1989

14. Tuman KJ, McCarthy RJ, Spiess BD et al: Does choice of anesthetic agent significantly affect outcome after coronary artery surgery? Anesthesiology 70:189, 1989

15. Tyler DC: Respiratory effects of pain in a child after thoracotomy. Anesthesiology 70:873, 1989

16. Toda N, Hatano Y: Contractile responses of canine tracheal muscle during exposure to fentanyl and morphine. Anesthesiology 53:93, 1980

17. Anjou-Lindskog E, Broman L, Broman M et al: Effects of intravenous anesthesia on Va/Q distribution: a study performed during ventilation with air and with 50% oxygen, supine and in the lateral position. Anesthesiology 62:485, 1985

18. Bjertraes LJ: Hypoxia-induced vasoconstriction in isolated perfused lungs exposed to injectable or inhalation anesthetics. Acta Anaesthesiol Scand 21:133, 1977

19. Yahagi N, Furuya H, Sai Y, Amakata Y: Effect of halothane, fentanyl, and ketamine on the threshold for transpulmonary passage of venous air emboli in dogs. Anesth Analg 75:720, 1992

20. Oyama T, Wakayama S: The endocrine responses to general anesthesia. Int Anesthesiol Clin 26:176, 1988

21. Reier CE, George JM, Kilman JW: Cortisol and growth hormone response to surgical stress during morphine anesthesia. Anesth Analg 52:1003, 1973

22. Haxholdt O, Kehlet H, Dyrberg V: Effect of fentanyl on the cortisol and hyperglycaemic response to abdominal surgery. Acta Anaesthsiol Scand 25:434, 1981

23. Anand K: The stress response to surgery and trauma: from physiologic basis to therapeutic implications. Prog Food Nutr Sci 10:67, 1986

24. Mangano DT, Siliciano D, Hollenberg M et al: Postoperative myocardial ischemia: therapeutic trials using intensive analgesia following surgery. Anesthesiology 76:342, 1992

25. Anand KJS, Phil D, Hickey PR: Halothane-morphine compared with high-dose sufentanil for anesthesia and postoperative analgesia in neonatal cardiac surgery. N Engl J Med 326:1, 1992

26. Blasco TA, Lee D, Amalric M et al: The role of the nucleus raphe pontis and the caudate nucleus in alfentanil rigidity in the rat. Brain Res 386:280, 1986

27. Bailey PL, Wilbrink J, Zwanikken P et al: Anesthetic induction with fentanyl. Anesth Analg 64:48, 1985

28. Benthuysen JL, Kien ND, Quam DD: Intracranial pressure during alfentanil-induced rigidity. Anesthesiology 68:438, 1988

29. Benthuysen JL, Smith NT, Sanford TJ et al: Physiology of alfentanil-induced rigidity. Anesthesiology 64:440, 1986

30. Safo Y, Greenberg J, Young M et al: Effects of high dose fentanyl on regional cerebral blood flow. Anesthesiology 59:A306, 1983

31. Tommasino C, Mackawa T, Shapiro HM: Fentanyl-induced seizures activate subcortical brain metabolism. Anesthesiology 60:283, 1984

32. Tempelhoff R, Modica PA, Bernardo KL, Edwards I: Fentanyl-induced electrocorticographic seizures in patients with complex partial epilepsy. J Neurosurg 77:201, 1992

33. Milde L, Milde J, Gallagher W: Effects of sufentanil on cerebral circulation and metabolism in dogs. Anesth Analg 70:13B, 1990

34. Sperry RJ, Bailey PL, Reichman MV et al: Fentanyl and sufentanil increase intracranial pressure in head trauma patients. Anesthesiology 77:416, 1992

35. Wahl M: Effects of enkephalins, morphine and naloxone on pial arteries during perivascular microapplication. J Cereb Blood Flow Metab 5:451, 1985

36. Weinstabl C, Mayer N, Richling B et al: Effect of sufentanil on intracranial pressure in neurosurgical patients. Anesthesia 46:837, 1991

37. Armstrong PJ, Bersten A: Normeperidine toxicity. Anesth Analg 65:536, 1986

38. Flacke JW, David LJ, Flacke WE et al: Effects of fentanyl and diazepam in dogs deprived of autonomic tone. Anesth Analg 64:1053, 1985

39. Lowenstein E, Whiting RB, Bittar DA et al: Local and neurally mediated effects of morphine on skeletal muscle vascular resistance. J Pharmacol Exp Ther 180:359, 1972

40. Rendig SV, Amsterdam EA, Henderson GL, Mason DT: Comparative cardiac contractile actions of six narcotic analgesics: morphine meperidine, pentazocine, fentanyl, methadone and L-α-acetylmethadol (LAAM). J Pharmacol Exp Ther 215:259, 1980

41. Lappas DG, Geha D, Fischer JE et al: Filling pressures of the heart and pulmonary circulation of the patient with coronary-artery disease after large intravenous doses of morphine. Anesthesiology 42:153, 1975

42. Philbin DM, Moss J, Akins CW et al: The use of H1 and H2 histamine antagonists with morphine anesthesia: a double-blind study. Anesthesiology 55:292, 1981

43. Flacke JW, Van Etten AP, Bloor BC et al: Histamine release by four narcotics: a double blind study in humans. Anesth Analg 66:723, 1987

44. Rosow CE, Moss J, Philbin DM, Savarese JJ: Histamine release during morphine and fentanyl anesthesia. Anesthesiology 56:93, 1982

45. Moss J, Rosow CE: Histamine release by narcotics and muscle relaxants in humans. Anesthesiology 59:330, 1983

46. King BD, Elder JD, Dripps RD: The effect of the intravenous administration of meperidine upon the circulation of man and upon the circulatory response to tilt. Surg Gynecol Obstet 94:591, 1952

47. Lake CL, DiFazio CA: Sufentanil versus fentanyl: hemodynamic effects in valvular heart disease. Anesth Analg 66:S99, 1987

48. Miller DR, Wellwood M, Teasdale SJ et al: Effects of anaesthetic induction on myocardial function and metabolism: a comparison of fentanyl, sufentanil and alfentanil. Can J Anaesth 35:219, 1988

49. Philbin DM, Rosow CE, Schneider RC et al: Fentanyl and sufentanil anesthesia revisited: how much is enough? Anesthesiology 73:5, 1990

50. Wynands JE, Wong P, Whalley DG et al: Oxygen-fentanyl anesthesia in patients with poor left ventricular function, hemodynamics and plasma fentanyl concentrations. Anesth Analg 62:476, 1983

51. Thomson IR, Putnins CL, Friesen RM: Hyperdynamic cardiovascular response to anesthetic induction with high dose fentanyl. Anesth Analg 65:91, 1986

52. Gaumann DM, Yaksh TL, Tyce GM, Lucas DL: Opioids preserve the adrenal medullary response evoked by severe hemorrhage: studies on adrenal catecholamines and met-enkephalin secretion in halothane anesthetized cats. Anesthesiology 68:743, 1988

53. James TN, Isobe JH, Urthaler F: Analysis of components in a cardiogenic hypertensive chemoreflex. Circulation 52:179, 1975

54. de Lange S, Stanley TH, Boscoe MJ, Pace NL: Comparison of sufentanil-O_2 and fentanyl-O_2 for coronary artery surgery. Anesthesiology 56:112, 1982

55. Bailey PL: Sinus arrest induced by nasal stimulation during alfentanil-nitrous oxide anesthesia. Br J Anaesth 65:718, 1990

56. Sherman EP, Leobwitz PW, Street WC: Bradycardia following sufentanil-succinylcholine. Anesthesiology 66:106, 1987

57. Ngai SH: Effects of morphine and meperidine on the central respiratory mechanisms in the cat, the action of levallorphan in antagonizing these effects. J Pharmacol Exp Ther 131:91, 1961

58. Hickey RF, Severinghaus JW: Regulation of breathing. p. 1251. In Hornbein J (ed): Drug Effects, Lung Biology in Health and Disease. Vol. 17. Part II. Marcel Dekker, New York 1981

59. Weil JV, McCullough RE, Kline JS, Sodal IE: Diminished ventilatory response to hypoxia and hypercapnia after morphine in normal man. N Engl J Med 292:1103, 1975

60. Kryger MH, Yacoub O, Dosman J et al: Effect of meperidine on occlusion pressure responses to hypercapnia and hypoxia with and without external inspiratory resistance. Am Rev Respir Dis 114:333, 1976

61. Reed DJ, Kellog RH: Changes in respiratory response to CO_2 during natural sleep at sea level and at altitude. J Appl Physiol 13:325, 1958

62. Forrest WH, Bellville JW: The effect of sleep plus morphine on the respiratory response to carbon dioxide. Anesthesiology 25:137, 1964

63. Longobardo GE, Gothe B, Goldman MD, Cherniak NS: Sleep apnea considered as a control system instability. Respir Physiol 50:311, 1982

64. Becker LD, Paulson BA, Miller RD et al: Biphasic respiratory depression after fentanyl-droperidol or fentanyl alone used to supplement nitrous oxide anesthesia. Anesthesiology 44:291, 1976

65. Adams AP, Pybus DA: Delayed respiratory depression after use of fentanyl during anaesthesia BMJ 1:278, 1978

66. Stanski DR, Greenblatt DJ, Lowenstein E: Kinetics

of intravenous and intramuscular morphine. Clin Pharmacol Ther 24:52, 1978

67. Chan K, Kendall MJ, Mitchard M, Will WDE: The effect of aging on plasma pethidine concentration. Br J Clin Pharmacol 2:297, 1975

68. Mahla ME, Maj MC, Maj SEW, Moneta MD: Delayed respiratory depression after alfentanil. Anesthesiology 69:593, 1988

69. Chang J, Fish KJ: Acute respiratory arrest and rigidity after anesthesia with sufentanil: a case report. Anesthesiology 63:710, 1985

70. McClain DA, Hug CC Jr: Intravenous fentanyl kinetics. Clin Pharmacol Ther 28:106, 1980

71. Stoeckel H, Schuttler J, Magnussen H, Hengstmann JH: Plasma fentanyl concentrations and occurrence of respiratory depression in volunteers. Br J Anaesth 54:1087, 1982

72. Severinghaus JW, Kelleher JF: Recent developments in pulse oximetry. Anesthesiology 76:1018, 1992

73. Catley D, Thornton C, Jordan C et al: Pronounced, episodic oxygen desaturation in the postoperative period: its association with ventilatory pattern and analgesic regimen. Anesthesiology 63:20, 1985

74. Bailey PL: The use of opioids in anesthesia is not especially associated with nor predictive of postoperative hypoxemia (letter to the editor). Anesthesiology 77:1235, 1992

75. Marks RM, Sachar EJ: Undertreatment of medical in patients with narcotic analgesics. Ann Intern Med 78:173, 1973

76. Böhrer H, Fleischer F, Werning P: Tussive effect of a fentanyl bolus administered through a central venous catheter. Anaesthesia 45:18, 1990

77. Watcha MF, White PF: Postoperative nausea and vomiting: its etiology, treatment and prevention. Anesthesiology 77:162, 1992

78. Okum GS, Colonna-Romano P, Horrow JC: Vomiting after alfentanil anesthesia: effect of dosing method. Anesth Analg 75:558, 1992

79. Watcha MF, Jones MB, Lagueruela RG et al: Comparison of ketorolac and morphine as adjuvants during pediatric surgery. Anesthesiology 76:368, 1992

80. Alon E, Himmelseher S: Ondansetron in the treatment of postoperative vomiting: a randomized, double-blind comparison with droperidol and metoclopramide. Anesth Analg 75:561, 1992

81. Costello DJ, Borison HL: Naloxone antagonizes narcotic self-blockade of emesis in the cat. J Pharmacol Exp Ther 203:222, 1977

82. Longnecker D, Grazis P, Eggers G: Naloxone antagonism of morphine induced respiratory depression. Anesth Analg 52:477, 1973

83. Jones R, Detmer M, Hill A et al: Incidence of choledochoduodenal sphincter spasm during fentanyl-supplemental anesthesia. Anesth Analg 60:638, 1981

84. Hunter JM, Jones RS, Utting JE: Effect of anaesthesia with nitrous oxide in oxygen and fentanyl on renal function in the artificially ventilated dog. Br J Anaesth 52:343, 1980

85. Kien ND, Reitan JA, White DA et al: Hemodynamic responses to alfentanil in halothane-anesthetized dogs. Anesth Analg 65:765, 1986

86. Bidwai AV, Wen-Shin L, Stanley TH et al: The effects of large doses of fentanyl with nitrous oxide on renal function in the dog. Can J Anaesth 23:296, 1976

87. Deutch S, Bastron RD, Pierce EC, Vandam LD: The effects of anaesthia with thiopentone, nitrous oxide, narcotics, and neuromuscular blocking drugs on renal function in normal man. Br J Anaesth 41:807, 1969

88. Stanley TH, Gray NH, Bidwai AV, Lordon R: The effects of high dose morphine and morphine plus nitrous oxide on urinary output in man. Can J Anaesth 21:379, 1974

89. Hill SA, Quinn K, Shelly MP, Park GR: Reversible renal failure following opioid administration. Anaesthesia 46:938, 1991

90. Shingu K, Eger EI, Brynte H et al: Effect of oxygen concentration, hyperthermia, and choice of vendor on anesthetic-induced hepatic injury in rats. Anesth Analg 62:146, 1983

91. Baden JM, Kundomal YR, Luttropp ME Jr et al: Effects of volatile anesthetics or fentanyl on hepatic function in cirrhotic rats. Anesth Analg 64:1183, 1985

92. Harpel HS, Gautieri RF: Morphine-induced fetal malformations. J Pharm Sci 57:1590, 1968

93. Fujinaga M, Stevenson JB, Mazze RI: Reproductive and teratogenic effects of fentanyl in Sprague-Dawley rats. Teratology 34:51, 1986

94. Fujinaga M, Mazze RI, Jackson EL, Baden JM: Reproductive and teratogenic effects of sufentanil and alfentanil in Sprague-Dawley rats. Anesth Analg 67:166, 1988

95. Craft JB, Coaldrake LA, Bolan JC et al: Placental passage and uterine effects of fentanyl. Anesth Analg 62:894, 1983

96. Feilberg VL, Rosenborg D, Christensen CB, Mogensen JV: Excretion of morphine in human breast mild. Acta Anaesthesiol Scand 33:426, 1989

97. Levy JH, Rockoff MA: Anaphylaxis to meperidine. Anesth Analg 61:301, 1982

98. Harle DG, Baldo BA, Coroneos NJ, Fisher MM: Anaphylaxis following administration of papaveretum. Case report: implication of IgE antibodies that react with morphine and codeine, and identification of an allergenic determinant. Anesthesiology 71:489, 1989

99. Levy JH, Brister NW, Shearin A et al: Wheal and flare responses to opioids in humans. Anesthesiology 70:756, 1989

100. Scott JC, Cooke JE, Stanski DR: Electroencephalographic quantitation of opioid effect: comparative pharmacodynamics of fentanyl and sufentanil. Anesthesiology 74:34, 1991

101. Bailey PL, Streisand JB, East KA et al: Differences in magnitude and duration of opioid-induced respiratory depression and analgesia with fentanyl and sufentanil. Anesth Analg 70:8, 1990

102. Ling GSF, Spiegel K, Lockhart SH, Pasternak GW: Separation of opioid analgesia from respiratory depression: evidence for different receptor mechanisms. J Pharmacol Exp Ther 232:149, 1985

103. Mangano DT: Anesthetics, coronary artery disease, and outcome: unresolved controversies. Anesthesiology 70:175, 1989

104. Benefiel DJ, Roizen MF, Lampe GH et al: Morbidity after aortic surgery with sufentanil vs isoflurane anesthesia. Anesthesiology 65:A516, 1986

105. Lowenstein E, Hallowell P, Levine FH et al: Cardiovascular response to large doses of intravenous morphine in man. N Engl J Med 281:1389, 1969

106. Benthuysen JL, Foltz BD, Smith NT et al: Prebypass hemodynamic stability of sufentanil-O_2, fentanyl-O_2 and morphine-O_2 anesthesia during cardiac surgery: a comparison of cardiovascular profiles. J Cardiothoracic Vasc Anesth 12:749, 1988

107. Bazaral MG, Wagner R, Abi-Nader E, Estafanous FG: Comparison of effects of 15 and 60 μg/kg fentanyl used for induction of anesthesia in patients with coronary artery disease. Anesth Analg 64:312, 1985

108. Murkin JM, Moldenhauer CC, Hug CC Jr: High-dose fentanyl for rapid induction of anaesthesia in patients with coronary artery disease. Can J Anaesth 32:320, 1984

109. Sprigge JS, Wynands JE, Whalley DG et al: Fentanyl infusion anesthesia for aortocoronary bypass surgery: plasma levels and hemodynamic response. Anesth Analg 61:972, 1982

110. Boulton AJ, Wilson N, Turnbull KW, Yip RW: Haemodynamic and plasma vasopressin responses during high-dose fentanyl or sufentanil anaesthesia. Can J Anaesth 33:475, 1986

111. Stanley T, Bailey P: Fentanyl and sufentanil anesthesia revisited: establish an effective plasma concentration and achieve it at the right time (letter). Anesthesiology 74:388, 1991

112. Sonntag H, Stephan H, Lange H et al: Sufentanil does not block sympathetic responses to surgical stimuli in patients having coronary artery revascularization surgery. Anesth Analg 68:584, 1989

113. Moore RA, Yang SS, McNicholas KW et al: Hemodynamic and anesthetic effects of sufentanil as the sole anesthetic for pediatric cardiovascular surgery. Anesthesiology 62:725, 1985

114. Giesecke K, Hamberger B, Jarnberg P et al: High- and low-dose fentanyl anaesthesia: hormonal and metabolic responses during cholecystectomy. Br J Anaesth 61:575, 1988

115. Moffitt EA, Scovil JE, Barker RA et al: Myocardial metabolism and haemodynamic responses during high-dose fentanyl anesthesia for coronary patients. Can J Anaesth 31:611, 1984

116. Howie MB, Smith DF, Reiley TE et al: Postoperative course after sufentanil or fentanyl anesthesia for coronary artery surgery. J Cardiothorac Vasc Anesth 5:485, 1991

117. Sanford TJ, Smith NT, Dec-Silver H, Harrison WK: A comparison of morphine, fentanyl, and sufentanil anesthesia for cardiac surgery: induction, emergence, and extubation. Anesth Analg 65:259, 1986

118. Mathews HML, Furness G, Carson IW et al: Comparison of sufentanil-oxygen and fentanyl-oxygen anaesthesia for coronary artery bypass grafting. Br J Anaesth 60:530, 1988

119. Spiess BD, Sathoff RH, El-Ganzouri ARS, Ivankovich AD: High-dose sufentanil: four cases of sudden hypotension on induction. Anesth Analg 65:703, 1986

120. Ausems ME, Hug CJ, Stanski DR, Burm AG: Plasma concentrations of alfentanil required to supplement nitrous oxide anesthesia for general surgery. Anesthesiology 65:362, 1986

121. Hug CCJ, Hall RI, Angert KC et al: Alfentanil plasma concentration v. effect relationships in cardiac surgical patients. Br J Anaesth 61:435, 1988

122. de Lange S, Stanley TH, Boscoe MJ: Alfentanil-oxygen anaesthesia for coronary artery surgery. Br J Anaesth 53:1291, 1981

123. de Lange S, de Bruijn N: Alfentanil-oxygen anesthesia: plasma concentration and clinical effects during variable rate continuous infusion for coronary artery surgery. Br J Anaesth 55:S183, 1983

124. McDonnell T, Bartowski R, Williams J: ED_{50} for alfentanil for induction of anesthesia in unpremedicated young adults. Anesthesiology 60:136, 1984

125. Vinik H, Bradley E, Kissin I: Midazolam-alfentanil synergism for anesthetic induction in patients. Anesth Analg 69:213, 1989

126. Leslie K, Crankshaw DP: Potency of propofol for loss of consciousness after a single dose. Br J Anaesth 64:734, 1990

127. Richards MJ, Skues MA, Jarvis AP, Prys-Roberts C: Total I.V. anaesthesia with propofol and alfentanil: dose requirements for propofol and the effect of premedication with clonidine. Br J Anaesth 65:157, 1990

128. Bowdle TA, Ward RJ: Induction of anesthesia with small doses of sufentanil or fentanyl: dose versus EEG response, speed of onset and thiopental requirement. Anesthesiology 70:26, 1989

129. Tverskoy M, Fleyshman G, Ezry J et al: Midazolam-morphine sedative interaction in patients. Anesth Analg 68:282, 1989

130. Kissin I, Brown P, Bradley E et al: Diazepam-morphine hypnotic synergism in rats. Anesthesiology 70:689, 1989

131. Stack CG, Rogers P, Linter SPK: Monoamine oxidase inhibitors and anaesthesia. Br J Anaesth 60:222, 1988

132. Wells DG, Bjorksten AR: Monoamine oxidase inhibitors revisited (review article). Can J Anaesth 36:64, 1989

133. Taylor MB, Grounds RM, Mulrooney PD, Morgan M: Ventilatory effects of propofol during induction of anaesthesia. Anaesthesia 41:816, 1986

134. Bailey PL, Pace NL, Ashburn MA et al: Frequent hypoxemia and apnea after sedation with midazolam and fentanyl. Anesthesiology 73:826, 1990

135. Silbert B, Rosow CE, Keegan CR et al: The effect of diazepam on induction of anesthesia with alfentanil. Anesth Analg 65:71, 1986

136. Bailey PL, Sperry RJ, East KA et al: Respiratory effects of clonidine and morphine, alone and in combination. Anesthesiology 73:43, 1991

137. Andrews CJH, Sinclair M, Dye A et al: The additive effect of nitrous oxide on respiratory depression in patients having fentanyl or alfentanil infusion. Br J Anaesth 54:1129, 1982

138. Abdul-Rasool IH, Ward DS: Ventilatory and cardiovascular responses to sufentanil infusion in dogs anesthetized with isoflurane. Anesth Analg 69:300, 1989

139. Drummond GB: Comparison of decreases in ventilation caused by enflurane and fentanyl during anesthesia. Br J Anaesth 55:825, 1983

140. Takkunen O, Meretoja OA: Thiopentone reduces the haemodynamic response to induction of high-dose fentanyl-pancuronium anaesthesia in coronary artery surgical patients. Acta Anaesthesiol Scand 32:222, 1988

141. Pomane C, Paulin M, Lena P et al: Comparison of the hemodynamic effects of a midazolam-fentanyl and thiopental-fentanyl combination for induction of general anesthesia. Anesthesiology 2:75, 1983

142. Vinik HR, Bradley EL, Kissin I: Midazolam-alfentanil synergism for anesthetic induction in patients. Anesth Analg 69:213, 1989

143. Ben-Shlomo I, Abd-El-Khalim H, Ezry J et al: Midazolam acts synergistically with fentanyl for induction of anaesthesia. Br J Anaesth 64:45, 1990

144. Hoar PF, Nelson NT, Mangano DT et al: Adrenergic response to morphine-diazepam anesthesia for myocardial revascularization. Anesth Analg 60:406, 1981

145. Tomichek RC, Rosow CE, Philbin DM et al: Diazepam-fentanyl interaction—hemodynamic and hormonal effects in coronary artery surgery. Anesth Analg 62:881, 1983

146. Reves JG, Kissin I, Fournier SE, Smith LR: Additive negative inotropic effect of a combination of diazepam and fentanyl. Anesth Analg 63:97, 1984

147. Marty J, Gauzit R, Lefevre P et al: Effects of diazepam and midazolam on baroreflex control of heart rate and on sympathetic activity in humans. Anesth Analg 65:113, 1986

148. Thomson IR, Bergstrom RG, Rosenbloom M, Meatherall RC: Premedication and high-dose fentanyl anesthesia for myocardial revascularization: a comparison of lorazepam versus morphine-scopolamine. Anesthesiology 68:194, 1988

149. Butterworth JF, Bean VE, Royster RL: Premedication profoundly influences hemodynamics during rapid sequence induction with sufentanil-succinylcholine for aortocoronary bypass grafting. Anesthesiology 69:A65, 1988

150. Thomson IR, MacAdams CL, Hudson RJ, Rosenbloom M: Drug interactions with sufentanil. Hemodynamic effects of premedication and muscle relaxants. Anesthesiology 76:922, 1992

151. Heikkilä H, Jalonen J, Laaksonen V et al: Lorazepam and high-dose fentanyl anaesthesia: effects on haemodynamics and oxygen transportation in patients undergoing coronary revascularization. Acta Anaesthesiol Scand 28:357, 1984

152. Benson KT, Tomlinson DL, Goto H, Arakawa K:

Cardiovascular effects of lorazepam during sufentanil anesthesia. Anesth Analg 67:996, 1988

153. Coetzee A, Fourie P, Coetzee J et al: Effect of various propofol plasma concentrations on regional myocardial contractility and left ventricular afterload. Anesth Analg 69:473, 1989

154. Lepage J-Y, Pinaud M, Helias J et al: Left ventricular function during propofol and fentanyl anesthesia in patients with coronary artery disease: assessment with a radionuclide approach. Anesth Analg 67:949, 1988

155. Hall RI, Murphy JT, Moffitt EA et al: A comparison of the myocardial metabolic and haemodynamic changes produced by propofol-sufentanil and enflurane-sufentanil anaesthesia for patients having coronary artery bypass graft surgery. Can J Anaesth 38:996, 1991

156. Eisele JH, Smith NT: Cardiovascular effects of 40 percent nitrous oxide in man. Anesth Analg 51:956, 1972

157. Stoelting RK, Gibbs PS, Creasser CW, Peterson C: Hemodynamic and ventilatory response to fentanyl, fentanyl-droperidol, and nitrous oxide in patients with acquired valvular heart disease. Anesthesiology 42:319, 1975

158. McDermott RW, Stanley TH: Cardiovascular effects of low concentrations of nitrous oxide during morphine anesthesia. Anesthesiology 41:89, 1974

159. Lunn JK, Stanley TH, Webster LR et al: High dose fentanyl anesthesia for coronary artery surgery: Plasma fentanyl concentration and influence of nitrous oxide on cardiovascular responses. Anesth Analg 58:390, 1979

160. Wong KC, Martin WE, Hornbein TF et al: The cardiovascular effects of morphine sulfate with oxygen and with nitrous oxide in man. Anesthesiology 38:542, 1973

161. Moffitt EA, Scovil JE, Barker RA et al: Myocardial metabolism and hemodynamics of nitrous oxide in fentanyl or enflurane anesthesia in coronary patients. Anesthesiology 59:A31, 1983

162. Michaels I, Barash PG: Does nitrous oxide or a reduced FiO_2 alter hemodynamic function during high-dose sufentanil anesthesia? Anesth Analg 62:275, 1983

163. Stowe DF, Monroe SM, Marijic J et al: Effects of nitrous oxide on contractile function and metabolism of the isolated heart. Anesthesiology 73:1220, 1990

164. Lawson D, Frazer MJ, Lynch C: Nitrous oxide effects on isolated myocardium: a reexamination in vitro. Anesthesiology 73:930, 1990

165. Cahalan MK, Prakash O, Rulf E et al: Addition of nitrous oxide to fentanyl anesthesia does not induce myocardial ischemia in patients with ischemic heart disease. Anesthesiology 67:925, 1987

166. Mitchell MM, Prakash O, Rulf EN et al: Nitrous oxide does not induce myocardial ischemia in patients with ischemic heart disease and poor ventricular function. Anesthesiology 71:526, 1989

167. Thomson IR, Putnins CI: Adverse effects of pancuronium during high-dose fentanyl anesthesia for coronary artery bypass grafting. Anesthesiology 62:708, 1985

168. Sethna DH, Starr NJ, Estafanous FG: Cardiovascular effects of non-depolarizing neuromuscular blockers in patients with coronary artery disease. Can J Anaesth 33:280, 1986

169. Atlee JL, Laravuso RB: Muscle relaxants and high-dose fentanyl: hemodynamics during coronary bypass surgery. Anesth Analg 63:181, 1984

170. Oikkonen M: Alfentanil combined with vecuronium or pancuronium: haemodynamic implications. Acta Anaesthesiol Scand 36:406, 1992

171. Gravlee GP, Ramsey FM, Roy RC et al: Pancuronium is hemodynamically superior to vecuronium for narcotic/relaxant induction. Anesthesiology 65:A46, 1986

172. Hill AEG, Muller BJ: Optimum relaxant for sufentanil anesthesia. Anesthesiology 61:A393, 1984

173. Lebowitz PW, Ramsey FM, Savarese JJ et al: Combination of pancuronium and metocurine: neuromuscular and hemodynamic advantages over pancuronium alone. Anesth Analg 60:12, 1981

174. Emmott RS, Bracey BJ, Goldhill DR et al: Cardiovascular effects of doxacurium, pancuronium and vecuronium in anaesthetized patients presenting for coronary artery bypass surgery. Br J Anaesth 65:480, 1990

175. Murray DJ, Mehta MP, Choi WW et al: The neuromuscular blocking and cardiovascular effects of doxacurium chloride in patients receiving nitrous oxide narcotic anesthesia. Anesthesiology 69:472, 1988

176. Savarese JJ, Ali HH, Basta SJ et al: The cardiovascular effects of mivacurium chloride (BW B1090U) in patients receiving nitrous oxide-opiate-barbiturate anesthesia. Anesthesiology 70:386, 1989

177. Wierda JMKH, Richardson FJ, Agoston S: Dose-response relation and time course of action of pipecuronium bromide in humans anesthetized with nitrous oxide and isoflurane, halothane, or droperidol and fentanyl. Anesth Analg 68:208, 1989

178. Rupp SM, Fahey MR, Miller RD: Neuromuscular

and cardiovascular effects of atracurium during nitrous oxide-fentanyl and nitrous oxide-isoflurane anaesthesia. Br J Anaesth 55:67S, 1983

179. Stanley TH, de Lange S, Boscoe MJ, de Bruijn N: The influence of chronic preoperative propranolol therapy on cardiovascular dynamics and narcotic requirements during operation in patients with coronary artery disease. Can J Anaesth 29:319, 1982

180. Newsome LR, Roth JV, Hug CC Jr, Nagle D: Esmolol attenuates hemodynamic responses during fentanyl-pancuronium anesthesia for aortocoronary bypass surgery. Anesth Analg 65:451, 1986

181. Sebel PS, Bovill JG, Schellekens APM, Hawker CD: Hormonal responses of high-dose fentanyl anaesthesia: a study in patients undergoing cardiac surgery. Br J Anaesth 53:941, 1981

182. Stoelting RK, Creasser CW, Gibbs PS, Peterson C: Circulatory effects of halothane added to morphine anesthesia in patients with coronary-artery disease. Anesth Analg 53:449, 1974

183. Harrison L, Ralley F, Wynands JE et al: The role of an ultra short-acting adrenergic blocker (esmolol) in patients undergoing coronary artery bypass surgery. Anesthesiology 66:413, 1987

184. Coriat P, Daloz M, Bousseau D et al: Prevention of intraoperative myocardial ischemia during noncardiac surgery with intravenous nitroglycerin. Anesthesiology 61:193, 1984

185. Thomson IR, Mutch AC, Culligan JD: Failure of intravenous nitroglycerin to prevent intraoperative myocardial ischemia during fentanyl-pancuronium anesthesia. Anesthesiology 61:385, 1984

186. Flacke JW, Bloor BC, Flacke WE et al: Reduced narcotic requirement by clonidine with improved hemodynamic and adrenergic stability in patients undergoing coronary bypass surgery. Anesthesiology 67:11, 1987

187. Ghignone M, Quinton L, Duke PC et al: Effects of clonidine on narcotic requirements and hemodynamic response during induction of fentanyl anesthesia and endotracheal intubation. Anesthesiology 64:36, 1986

188. Bailey PL, Clark NJ, Pace NL et al: Failure of nalbuphine to antagonize morphine. Anesth Analg 65:605, 1986

189. Scott JC, Ponganis KV, Stanski DR: EEG quantitation of narcotic effect: the comparative pharmacodynamics of fentanyl and alfentanil. Anesthesioloy 62:234, 1985

190. Shafer SL, Varvel JR: Pharmacokinetics, pharmacodynamics, and rational opioid selection. Anesthesiology 74:53, 1991

191. Ebling WF, Lee EN, Stanski DR: Understanding pharmacokinetics and pharmacodynamics through computer stimulation: I. The comparative clinical profiles of fentanyl and alfentanil. Anesthesiology 72:650, 1990

192. Clark NJ, Meuleman T, Liu W et al: Comparison of sufentanil-N_2O and fentanyl-N_2O in patients without cardiac disease undergoing general surgery. Anesthesiology 66:130, 1987

193. Maitre PO, Vozeh S, Heykants J et al: Population pharmacokinetics of alfentanil: the average dose-plasma concentration relationship and interindividual variability in patients. Anesthesiology 66:3, 1987

194. Conner JT, Herr G, Katz RL et al: Droperidol, fentanyl and morphine for I.V. surgical premedication. Br J Anaesth 50:463, 1978

195. Van de Velde A, Camu F, Claeys M: Midazolam for intramuscular premedication: dose-effect relationships compared to diazepam, fentanyl and fentanyl-droperidol in a placebo controlled study. Acta Anaesthesiol Belg 37:127, 1986

196. Downes JJ, Kemp RA, Lambertsen CJ: The magnitude and duration of respiratory depression due to fentanyl and meperidine in man. J Pharmacol Exp Therap 158:416, 1967

197. Grell FL, Koons DA, Denson JS: Fentanyl in anesthesia: a report of 500 cases. Anesth Analg 49:523, 1970

198. Catton D, Browne R: Premedication with fentanyl and droperidol, or meperidine. Anesth Analg 49:389, 1970

199. Shamash R, Gutman D, Birkham J: Neuroleptanalgesia: a new concept in premedication. J Oral Maxillofac Surg 29:405, 1971

200. Sloan JB: Innovar as a preoperative medication. South Med J 68:1407, 1975

201. Van Wijhe M, De Voogt-Frenkel E, Stijnen T: Midazolam versus fentanyl/droperidol and placebo as intramuscular premedicant. Acta Anaesthesiol Scand 29:409, 1985

202. Wyant GM, Lewis GBH: Observations on Innovar as preoperative medication. Can J Anaesth 16:377, 1969

203. Norris W, Telfer ABM: Thalamonal as a pre-operative sedative. Br J Anaesth 40:517, 1968

204. Stanley TH, Hague BH, Mock DL et al: Oral transmucosal fentanyl citrate (lollipop) premedication in human volunteers. Anesth Analg 69:21, 1989

205. Streisand JB, Stanley TH, Hague B et al: Oral transmucosal fentanyl citrate premedication in children. Anesth Analg 69:28, 1989

206. Nelson P, Streisand JB, Mulder S et al: Comparison of oral transmucosal fentanyl citrate and an oral solution of meperidine, diazepam and atropine for premedication in children. Anesthesiology 70:616, 1989

207. Ralley FE: Intranasal opiates: old route for new drugs. Can J Anaesth 36:491, 1989

208. Henderson JM, Brodsky DA, Fisher DM et al: Pre-induction of anesthesia in pediatric with nasally administered sufentanil. Anesthesiology 68:671, 1988

209. Helmers JHJH, Noorduin H, Van Peer A et al: Comparison of intravenous and intranasal sufentanil absorption and sedation. Can J Anaesth 36:494, 1989

210. Worsley MH, Macleod AD, Brodie MJ et al: Inhaled fentanyl as a method of analgesia. Anaesthesia 45:449, 1990

211. Higgins MJ, Asbury AJ, Brodie MJ: Inhaled nebulised fentanyl for postoperative analgesia. Anaesthesia 46:973, 1991

212. Chrubasik J, Wüst H, Friedrich G, Geller E: Absorption and bioavailability of nebulized morphine. Br J Anaesth 61:228, 1988

213. Bell MDD, Mishra P, Weldon BD et al: Buccal morphine—a new route for analgesia? Lancet 1:71, 1985

214. Manara AR, Bodenham AR, Park GR: Analgesic efficacy of perioperative buccal morphine. Br J Anaesth 64:551, 1990

215. Risbo A: Sublingual buprenorphine for premedication and postoperative pain relief in orthpedic surgery. Acta Anaesthesiol Scand 29:180, 1985

216. Lindahl S, Olsson A-K, Thomson D: Rectal premedication in children. Use of diazepam, morphine and hyoscine. Anaesthesia 36:376, 1981

217. Hanning CD, Vickers AP, Smith G et al: The morphine hydrogel suppository. Br J Anaesth 61:221, 1988

218. Westerling D: Rectally administered morphine: plasma concentrations in children premedicated with morphine in hydrogel and in solution. Acta Anaesthesiol Scand 29:653, 1985

219. Jacobsen J, Flachs H, Dich-Nielsen JO et al: Comparative plasma concentration profiles after I.V., I.M. and rectal administration of pethidine in children. Br J Anaesth 60:623, 1988

220. Choneim MM, Dhanaraj J, Choi WW: Comparison of four opioid analgesics as supplements to nitrous oxide anesthesia. Anesth Analg 63:405, 1984

221. Holmes CM: Supplementation of general anaesthesia with narcotic analgesics. Br J Anaesth 48:907, 1976

222. Flacke JW, Bloor BC, Flacke WE et al: Comparison of morphine, meperidine, fentanyl, and sufentanil in balanced anesthesia: a double-blind study. Anesth Analg 64:897, 1985

223. Stanski DR, Hug CCJ: Alfentanil—a kinetically predictable narcotic analgesic. Anesthesiology 57:435, 1982

224. Maitre PO, Stanski DR: Bayesian Forecasting improves the prediction of intraoperative plasma concentrations of alfentanil. Anesthesiology 69:652, 1988

225. Maitre PO, Shafer SL: A simple pocket calculator approach to predict anesthetic drug concentrations from pharmacokinetic data. Anesthesiology 73:332, 1990

226. Stanski DR: Narcotic pharmacokinetics and dynamics: the basis of infusion applications. Anaesth Intensive Care 15:23, 1987

227. Glass PSA, Jacobs JR, Quill TJ: Intravenous drug delivery systems. p. 23. In Fragen RJ (ed): Drug Infusions in Anesthesiology. Raven Press, New York, 1991

228. Shafer SL, Stanski DR: Improving the clinical utility of anesthetic drug pharmacokinetics. Anesthesiology 76:327, 1992

229. Hughes MA, Glass PSA, Jacobs JR: Context-sensitive half-time in multicompartment pharmacokinetic models for intravenous anesthetic drugs. Anesthesiology 76:334, 1992

230. Bailey PL, Clark NJ, Pace NL et al: Antagonism of postoperative opioid induced respiratory depression: nalbuphine vs. naloxone. Anesth Analg 66:1109, 1987

231. Murkin JM: Multicentre trial—sufentanil anaesthesia for major surgery: the multicentre Canadian clinical trial. Can J Anaesth 36:343, 1989

232. Mallon JS, Edelist G: Editorial: total intravenous anaesthesia. Can J Anaesth 37:279, 1990

233. Steegers PA, Foster PA: Propofol in total intravenous anaesthesia without nitrous oxide. Anaesthesia 43:94, 1988

234. Mayné A, Joucken J, Collard E, Randour P: Intravenous infusion of propofol for induction and maintenance of anaesthesia during endoscopic carbon dioxide laser ENT procedures with high frequency jet ventilation. Anaesthesia 43:97, 1988

235. van Leeuwen L, Zuurmond WWA, Deen L, Helmers HJ: Total intraveous anaesthesia with propofol, alfentanil, and oxygen-air: three different dosage schemes. Can J Anaesth 37:282, 1990

236. Bailie R, Christmas L, Price N et al: Effects of temazepam premedication on cognitive recovery follow-

ing alfentanil-propofol anaesthesia. Br J Anaesth 63:68, 1989

237. Manara AR, Monk CR, Bolsin SN, Prys-Roberts C: Total I.V. anaesthesia with propofol and alfentanil for coronary artery bypass grafting. Br J Anaesth 66:716, 1991

238. Raftery S, Sherry E: Total intravenous anaesthesia with propofol and alfentanil protects against postoperative nausea and vomiting. Can J Anaesth 39:37, 1992

239. Kashtan H, Edelist G, Mallon J, Kapala D: Comparative evaluation of propofol and thiopentone for total intravenous anaesthesia. Can J Anaesth 37:170, 1990

240. Vuyk J, Hennis PJ, Burm AGL et al: Comparison of midazolam and propofol in combination with alfentanil for total intravenous anesthesia. Anesth Analg 71:645, 1990

241. Wong KC: Narcotics are not expected to produce unconsciousness and amnesia (editorial). Anesth Analg 62:625, 1983

242. Wynands JE, Wong P, Townsend GE et al: Narcotic requirements for intravenous anesthesia. Anesth Analg 63:101, 1984

243. Tuman KJ, Keane DM, Silins AI et al: Effects of high dose fentanyl on fluid and vasopressor requirements after cardiac surgery. Anesth Analg 67:S236, 1988

244. Yeager MP, Glass DD, Neff RK, Brinck-Johnsen T: Epidural anesthesia and analgesia in high-risk surgical patients. Anesthesiology 66:729, 1987

245. Baron J-F, Bertrand M, Barre E et al: Combined epidural and general anesthesia versus general anesthesia for abdominal aortic surgery. Anesthesiology 75:611, 1991

246. McQuay HJ: Pre-emptive analgesia, Br J Anaesth 69:1, 1992

247. Dahl JB, Hansen BL, Hjorts ONC et al: Influence of timing on the effect of continuous extradural analgesia with bupivacaine and morphine after major abdominal surgery. Br J Anaesth 69:4, 1992

248. Katz J, Kavanagh BP, Sandler AN et al: Preemptive analgesia: clinical evidence of neuroplasticity contributing to postoperative pain. Anesthesiology 77:439, 1992

249. Pace NL: Adverse outcomes and the multicenter study of general anesthesia: II. Anesthesiology 77:394, 1992

250. Sandler AN, Stringer D, Panos L et al: A randomized, double-blind comparison of lumbar epidural and intravenous fentanyl infusions for postthoracotomy pain relief. Anesthesiology 77:626, 1992

251. Gourlay GK, Kowalski SR, Plummer JL et al: Fentanyl blood concentration-analgesic response relationship in the treatment of postoperative pain. Anesth Analg 67:329, 1988

252. Vickers AP, Derbyshire DR, Burt DR et al: Comparison of the Leicester micropalliator and the Cardiff palliator in the relief of postoperative pain. Br J Anaesth 59:503, 1987

253. Owen H, Szelkely SM, Plummer JL et al: Variables of patient-controlled analgesia: 2. Concurrent infusion. Anaesthesia 44:11, 1989

254. Parker RK, Holtmann B, White PF: Patient-controlled analgesia. Does a concurrent opioid infusion improve pain management after surgery? JAMA 266:1947, 1991

255. White PF: Use of patient-controlled analgesia for management of acute pain. JAMA 259:243, 1988

256. Notcutt WG, Knowles P, Kaldas R: Overdose of opioid from patient-controlled analgesia pumps. Br J Anaesth 69:95, 1992

257. Bellville JW, Forrest WH, Miller E, Brown BW: Influence of age on pain relief from analgesics. A study of postoperative patients. JAMA 217:1835, 1971

258. Owen JA, Sitar DS, Berger L et al: Age-related morphine kinetics. Clin Pharmacol Ther 34:364, 1983

259. Monk TG, Parker RK, White PF: Use of PCA in geriatric patients—effect of aging on the postoperative analgesic requirement. Anesth Analg 70:S272, 1990

260. Arunasalam K, Davenport HT, Painter S, Jones JG: Ventilatory response to morphine in young and old subjects. Anaesthesia 38:529, 1983

261. Lemmens HJM, Bovill JG, Hennis P, Burm GL: Age has no effect on pharmacodynamics of alfentanil. Anesth Analg 67:956, 1988

262. Scott JC, Stanski DR: Decreased fentanyl and alfentanil dose requirements with age. A simultaneous pharmacokinetic and pharmacodynamic evaluation. J Pharmacol Exper Ther 240:159, 1987

263. Lemmens HJM, Bovill JG, Hennis PJ, Burm AGL: Influence of age on the pharmacokinetics of alfentanil. Anesthesiology 69:A629, 1988

264. Helmers H, Van Peer A, Woestenborghs R et al: Alfentanil kinetics in the elderly. Clin Pharmacol Ther 36:239, 1984

265. Singleton MA, Rosen JI, Fisher Dm: Pharmacokinetics of fentanyl in the elderly. Br J Anaesth 60:619, 1988

266. Bentley JB, Borel JD, Nenad REJ, Gillespie TJ: Age and fentanyl pharmacokinetics. Anesth Analg 61:968, 1982

267. Matteo RS, Schwartz AE, Ornstein E et al: Pharmacokinetics of sufentanil in the elderly surgical patient. Can J Anaesth 37:852, 1990

268. Kuhnert BR, Kuhnert PM, Philipson EH et al: Disposition of meperidine and normeperidine following multiple doses during labor. Am J Obstet Gynecol 151:410, 1985

269. Kuhnert BR, Linn PL, Kennard MJ, Kuhnert PM: Effects of low doses of meperidine on neonatal behavior. Anesth Analg 64:335, 1985

270. Way WL, Costley EC, Way EL: Respiratory sensitivity of the newborn to meperidine and morphine. Clin Pharmacol Ther 6:454, 1965

271. Crawford JS, Rudofsky S: The placental transmission of pethidine. Br J Anaesth 37:929, 1965

272. Caldwell J, Wakile LA, Notarianni LJ et al: Maternal and neonatal disposition of pethidine in childbirth—a study using quantitative gas chromatography-mass spectrometry. Life Sci 22:589, 1978

273. Hodgkinson R, Husain FJ: The duration of effect of maternally administered meperidine on neonatal neurobehavior. Anesthesiology 56:51, 1982

274. Wittels B, Scott DT, Sinatra RS: Exogenous opioids in human breast mild and acute neonatal neurobehavior: a preliminary study. Anesthesiology 73:864, 1990

275. Lippmann N, Nelson RJ, Emmanoulides GC et al: Ligation of patent ductus arteriosus in premature infants. Br J Anaesth 48:365, 1976

276. Davis PJ, Killian A, Stiller RL et al: Alfentanil pharmacokinetics in premature infants and older children. Anesthesiology 69:A758, 1988

277. Meistelman C, Benhamou D, Barre J et al: Effects of age on plasma protein binding of sufentanil. Anesthesiology 72:470, 1990

278. Greeley WJ, de Bruijn NP, Davis DP: Pharmacokinetics of sufentanil in pediatric patients. Anesthesiology 65:A422, 1986

279. Koehntop DE, Rodman JH, Brundage DM et al: Pharmacokinetics of fentanyl in neonates. Anesth Analg 65:227, 1986

280. Kupferberg HG, Way EL: Pharmacologic basis for the increased sensitivity of the newborn rat to morphine. J Pharmacol Exp Ther 141:109, 1963

281. Hertzka RE, Gauntlett IS, Fisher DM, Spellman MJ: Fentanyl-induced ventilatory depression: effects of age. Anesthesiology 70:213, 1989

282. Gronert B, Davis PJ, Cook DR: Continuous infusions of alfentanil in infants undergoing inguinal herniorrhaphy. Paediatr Anaesth 2:105, 1992

283. Davis PJ, Chopyk J-C, Nazif M, Cook DR: Continuous alfentanil infusion in pediatric patients undergoing general anesthesia for complete oral restoration. J Clin Anesth 3:125, 1991

284. Robinson S, Gregory GA: Fentanyl-air-oxygen anesthesia for ligation of patent ductus arteriosus in preterm infants. Anesth Analg 60:331, 1981

285. Dahlström B, Bolme P, Feychting H et al: Morphine kinetics in children. Clin Pharmacol Ther 26:354, 1979

286. Koren G, Goresky G, Crean P et al: Pediatric fentanyl dosing based on pharmacokinetics during cardiac surgery. Anesth Analg 63:577, 1984

287. Collins C, Koren G, Crean P et al: Fentanyl pharmacokinetics and hemodynamic effects in preterm infants during ligation of patent ductus arteriosus. Anesth Analg 64:1078, 1985

288. Davis PJ, Cook DR, Stiller RL, Davin-Robinson KA: Pharmacodynamics and pharmacokinetics of high-dose sufentanil in infants and children undergoing cardiac surgery. Anesth Analg 66:203, 1987

289. Greeley WJ, de Bruijn NP, Davis DP: Sufentanil pharmacokinetics in pediatric cardiovascular patients. Anesth Analg 66:1067, 1987

290. Rogers MC: Do the right thing. Pain relief in infants and children (editorial). N Engl J Med 326:55, 1992

291. Hudson RJ, Bergstrom RG, Thomson IR et al: Pharmacokinetics of sufentanil in patients undergoing abdominal aortic surgery. Anesthesiology 70:426, 1989

292. Nishitateno K, Ngai SH, Finck AD, Berkowitz BA: Pharmacokinetics of morphine: concentrations in the serum and brain of the dog during hyperventilation. Anesthesiology 50:520, 1979

293. Cartwright P, Prys-Roberts C, Gill K et al: Ventilatory depression related to plasma fentanyl concentrations during and after anesthesia in humans. Anesth Analg 62:966, 1983

294. Lüllmann H, Martins B-S, Peters T: pH-dependent accumulation of fentanyl, lofentanil, and alfentanil by beating guinea pig atria. Br J Anaesth 57:1012, 1985

295. Wood M: Plasma binding and limitation of drug access to site of action. Anesthesiology 75:721, 1991

296. Wood M: Review article: plasma drug binding: implications for anesthesiologists. Anesth Analg 65:786, 1986

297. Meuldermans WEG, Hurkmans RMA, Heykants JJP: Plasma protein binding and distribution of fentanyl, sufentanil, alfentanil and lofentanil in blood. Arch Int Pharmacodyn Ther 257:4, 1982

298. Bentley JB, Finley JH, Humphrey LR et al: Obesity and alfentanil pharmacokinetics. Anesth Analg 62:251, 1983

299. Schwartz AE, Matteo RS, Ornstein E et al: Pharmacokinetics of sufentanil in obese patients. Anesth Analg 73:790, 1991

300. Bentley JB, Borel JD, Gillespie TJ et al: Fentanyl pharmacokinetics in obese and nonobese patients. Anesthesiology 55:A177, 1981

301. Mazoit J-X, Sandouk P, Zetlaoui P, Scherrmann J-M: Pharmacokinetics of unchanged morphine in normal and cirrhotic subjects. Anesth Analg 66:293, 1987

302. Olsen GD, Bennett WM, Porter GA: Morphine and phenytoin binding to plasma proteins in renal and hepatic failure. Clin Pharmacol Exp Ther 17:677, 1975

303. Ferrier C, Marty J, Bouffaud Y et al: Alfentanil pharmacokinetics in patients with cirrhosis. Anesthesiology 62:480, 1985

304. Haberer JP, Schoeffler P, Coudere E, Duvaldstein P: Fentanyl pharmacokinetics in anaesthetized patients with cirrhosis. Br J Anaesth 54:1267, 1982

305. Chauvin M, Ferrier C, Haberer JP et al: Sufentanil pharmacokinetics in patients with cirrhosis. Anesth Analg 68:1, 1989

306. Hug CC Jr, Aldrete JA, Sampson JF, Murphy MR: Morphine anesthesia in patients with liver failure. Anesthesiology 51:S30, 1979

307. Lemmens HJM, Bovill JG, Hennis PJ et al: Alcohol consumption alters the pharmacodynamics of alfentanil. Anesthesiology 71:669, 1989

308. Bartkowski RR, Larijani GE, Goldberg ME, Boerner TF: Erythromycin treatment inhibits alfentanil metabolism. Anesthesiology 69:A590, 1988

309. Bartkowski RR, Goldberg ME, Huffnagle S, Epstein RH: Effect of erythromycin on sufentanil metabolism: differences from alfentanil. Anesth Analg 70:S16, 1990

Clinical Pharmacology of Partial Agonist, Mixed Agonist-Antagonist, and Antagonist Opioids

T. Andrew Bowdle and Wendel L. Nelson

Partial agonist and agonist-antagonist opioids are used relatively infrequently in clinical anesthesia practice compared with full agonist opioids. Nevertheless, they are an important class of drugs. They are historically significant, and they have proved to be clinically useful for specific purposes. Agonist-antagonist pharmacology has been crucial for understanding the family of opioid receptors. Although the full agonist opioids in current clinical use are primarily μ agonists, partial agonist and agonist-antagonist opioids have substantial effects at κ receptors and μ receptors. Therefore, these drugs are a window through which κ opioid receptor pharmacology has been observed in humans. The purposes of this chapter are (1) to review the fundamentals of opioid receptor pharmacology that are essential for understanding the partial agonist, agonist-antagonist, and antagonist opioids (see Ch. 2) and (2) to examine the clinical applications of these drugs in anesthesiology.

HISTORIC BACKGROUND

A brief review of the history of the development of agonist-antagonist opioids illustrates basic principles of opioid pharmacology. The prototype agonist-antagonist opioid, nalorphine, synthesized in the early 1940s, antagonized the effects of morphine in animals.[1]

The distinguished anesthesiologist James Eckenhoff[2] with his colleagues first reported the use of nalorphine to antagonize morphine overdosage in humans in 1951. Nalorphine precipitated an abstinence or withdrawal syndrome in morphine dependent subjects, and it was clinically useful for the treatment of opioid overdoses. Nalorphine was also a potent analgesic. However, clinical application was precluded by the prominent dysphoria and psychotomimetic effects it produced. The paradoxical combination of potent analgesic agonist properties and antagonist effects toward morphine stimulated an intense search for opioids that would produce analgesia without addiction and for explanations of the underlying pharmacologic mechanisms of action. Our knowledge of the mechanisms of action of opioids has grown tremendously as a result.

Another distinguished anesthesiologist, Arthur Keats,[3] reported with Telford in 1966 that there was a "ceiling" to the respiratory depressant effects of nalorphine in humans. The prospect of designing opioids with potent analgesic effects, but with significantly less respiratory effects than morphine-like opioids, was provocative. Research continues today in the hope of finding highly selective opioid analgesics that do not cause respiratory depression. There are reasons to believe that this goal may be attainable, for example, prototype κ receptor agonists produce analgesia but virtually no respiratory depression (see section on Kappa Receptor).

Nalorphine was used clinically as an antidote for opioid overdose until the advent of naloxone in the late 1960s. Naloxone was the first "pure" opioid antagonist with virtually no agonist effects. The anesthesiologist, Francis Foldes[4] and his colleagues performed the first studies showing that naloxone antagonized the respiratory depressant effects of opioid agonists. Naloxone sensitivity remains the essential feature defining opioid receptors.

RECEPTOR PHARMACOLOGY

Understanding agonist-antagonist opioid pharmacology requires some background knowledge of drug receptor theory and some specific information about opioid receptors. These areas are discussed in the next section.

Potency refers to the quantity of drug required to produce a particular degree of receptor occupancy and is related to the affinity of the drug for the receptor. Potency is usually expressed in terms of the dose administered, often in milligrams or milligrams per kilogram. In molecular pharmacology (in vitro), potency is considered in terms of concentration. A reduction in potency shifts the dose effect curve (to the right) but does not change its shape (Fig. 5-1).

Efficacy or *intrinsic activity* refers to the shape of the dose effect curve and is related to the molecular consequences of the interaction between the drug and the receptor. There is a spectrum of intrinsic activity ranging from a maximum to zero. Agonists are capable of producing the maximum effect possible from binding with the receptor. Antagonists bind the receptor but cause no direct effects. Between these two extremes are partial agonist drugs with intermediate activity that produce some effect but are incapable of producing the maximum effect of the full agonist (Fig. 5-1).

Partial agonists produce a dose effect curve that is less steep and has a lower maximum response (Fig. 5-1).[5] A lower maximum response does not necessarily imply a lack of potency. Hypothetically,

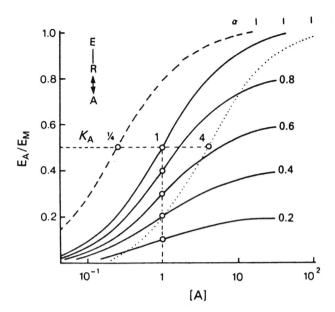

Fig. 5-1 Hypothetical dose effect curves for a series of drugs with intrinsic activity or efficacy (α) varying from 0.2 to 1. [A] is the concentration or dose of the agonist. E_A/E_M is the effect of the drug, E_A, as a fraction of maximal effect, E_M. The dashed and dotted lines illustrate the left and right shifts of the dose effect curve that occur when affinity ($1/K_A$) for the receptor is varied from $K_A = 1/4$ to $K_A = 4$, holding the intrinsic activity constant ($\alpha = 1$). (From Ariens et al.,[5] with permission.)

partial agonists may be potent, such that small quantities of the drug may produce a significant (albeit submaximal) response.

An interesting and somewhat complicated interaction occurs when a full agonist and a partial agonist are applied together (Fig. 5-2).[5] If the concentration of the full agonist is low, the introduction of the partial agonist results in an increased response. However, if the concentration of the full agonist is relatively high, introduction of the partial agonist results in a net reduction in the response.

Nalorphine is a potent analgesic that is also capable of antagonizing morphine. The dual agonist-antagonist properties of nalorphine could be explained if nalorphine were a partial agonist of the morphine receptor. However, this explanation did not account satisfactorily for certain other aspects of nalorphine pharmacology. The subjective effects of nalorphine and related drugs differed from morphine in human volunteers, and the abstinence syndrome associated with nalorphine dependence

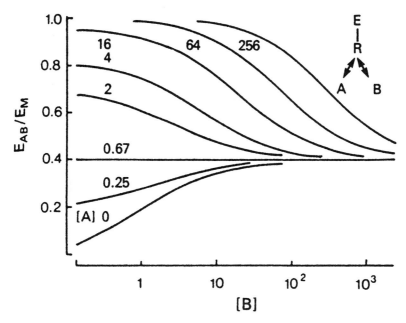

Fig. 5-2. Hypothetical log dose effect curves for a partial agonist, *B* (intrinsic activity = 0.4), in the presence of a range of concentrations of an agonist, *A*. E_{AB}/E_M is the effect of the combination of A and B as a fraction of the maximal effect E_M. As the concentration of the partial agonist increases, the effect of the combination of A and B converges on the maximum effect of the partial agonist (E_{AB}/E_M = 0.4). The partial agonist increases the response when added to a small dose of the agonist (A = 0.25) but decreases the response (behaves as an antagonist) when added to larger doses of the agonist. (From Ariens et al.,[5] with permission.)

was qualitatively different from the morphine abstinence syndrome. These observations could not be explained on the simple basis that nalorphine was a partial agonist of the morphine receptor. Thus, Martin[6] proposed in 1967 that there must be multiple opioid receptors. After almost 10 more years of study, Martin et al.[7,8] postulated a family of opioid receptors consisting of three members, i.e., μ, standing for the prototype agonist, morphine; κ, for the prototype agonist ketocyclazocine; and σ, for the prototype agonist SKF 10,047 (N-allylnormetazocine). Nalorphine and similar agonist-antagonist drugs were thought to have a variable degree of activity at each of these receptors.

Since 1967, an enormous amount of research has resulted in many changes to Martin's original proposal; however, the hypothesis of multiple opioid receptors has been confirmed. The opioid receptor family is complex, and opioid receptor pharmacology is an area of active research. However, the molecular pharmacology of opioid receptors is not as well understood as is that of some

other receptors, such as the γ-aminobutyric acid receptor. Therefore, the presentation of opioid receptor pharmacology that follows is simplified and subject to revision as new information becomes available (see Ch. 2). Recently, sequence structures for some δ,[9,10,10a,b,c] κ,[10b,c,d] and μ receptors[10a,e] have been determined based on cDNA cloning experiments. The receptors appear to comprise seven hydrophobic domains similar to those described for other G protein-linked receptors that are found on cellular membranes. the success of these experiments to determine sequences of receptors seems likely to lead rapidly to additional information about their multiplicity and their functional roles.

MULTIPLE OPIOID RECEPTORS

Opioid receptors are currently classified into three major types, based on bioassays and binding studies as follows: μ, κ, and δ (Table 5-1). There are probably additional types and subtypes of opioid receptors that are not yet identified. All three types

Table 5-1 Characteristics of μ and κ Opioid Receptors

	Receptor Type	
	μ	κ
Selective Agonists	Sufentanil	U-50,488
Selective antagonists	CTAP, β-funaltrexamine	Nor-binaltorphimine
Site of action		
Brain	+	+
Spinal cord	+	+
Periphery	+	+
Neuronal mechanism	Activation K^+ channels	Inhibition Ca^{++} channels
Tolerance	+	+
Dependence/withdrawal	+	+ (mild)
Subjective effects	Euphorigenic	Dysphoric/psychotomimetic
Abuse potential	High	Low
Side effects	Sedation, respiratory depression, constipation, nausea/vomiting, pruritus	Sedation, diuresis

(Modified from Millan,[13] with permission.)

of receptors are involved in regulating nociception through extremely complex interrelationships that are not well understood.

μ Receptor

The μ receptors appear to mediate many of the clinical effects of morphine-like drugs. Two subtypes of the μ receptor have been identified in rodents, μ_1 and μ_2.[11] The μ_1 receptors appear to mediate the supraspinal analgesic effects of morphine-like opioids; the endogenous ligands (i.e., neurotransmitters) of μ_1 receptors appear to be enkephalins. The μ_2 receptors appear to mediate respiratory depression and spinal analgesia. Significant species differences exist, but assuming different μ receptor subtypes mediate analgesia and respiratory depression in humans as well, there would be a possibility of specific μ receptor subtype agonists that would produce analgesia without respiratory depression.

κ Receptor

The κ receptors were named for the agonist-antagonist drug, ketocyclazocine.[11] The endogenous ligands of this receptor are probably the opioid peptides known as dynorphins.[12] The traditional concept was that κ receptors mediated analgesia in the spinal cord but not in the brain. Currently, it is suggested that both spinal and supraspinal κ receptors are involved in antinociception.[13] There appear to be three major κ receptor subtypes, designated κ_1, κ_2, and κ_3. The κ_1 receptors appear to mediate spinal analgesia in rodents. The κ_3 receptors have been found in the rodent brain with a density twice that of μ or δ receptors.[14] The agonist-antagonist drug, nalorphine, has been shown to produce analgesia mediated by κ_3 receptors, and this receptor has been regarded as the "original" κ receptor proposed by Martin et al.

Although both μ and κ agonists produce analgesia, the subjective effects of κ agonists are distinct from those of μ agonists. The μ agonists tend to produce euphoria; κ agonists tend to produce sedation and dysphoria. Perhaps because of these differences, experimental animals and human subjects tend to prefer self-administration of μ agonists to κ agonists. This implies that κ agonists should produce a lower potential for abuse and dependence.

κ receptors appear to mediate the psychotomimetic (hallucinations and delirium) effects[13] that are prominent with certain opioids, especially benzomorphan derivatives (e.g., pentazocine); highly selective κ receptor agonists produce naloxone sensitive dysphoria and psychotomimetic effects in humans.

An interesting neuroendocrine role of κ receptors involves the regulation of vasopressin release from the posterior pituitary.[15] The κ receptor peptide ligand, dynorphin, is contained with vasopressin in the neurosecretory vesicles of the neuron terminals in the posterior pituitary. Dynorphin appears to mediate an inhibitory feedback loop in which dynorphin released with vasopressin activates κ receptors, inhibiting further release. Thus, κ agonist drugs tend to produce a diuresis by inhibiting the release of vasopressin. This is an example of a bioassay that can be used to detect the κ agonist properties of an opioid drug.

Highly selective κ agonists have not produced respiratory depression in animals.[16,17]

δ Receptor

The opioid receptors with the greatest selectivity for the endogenous opioid peptides known as enkephalins are called δ receptors.[11] There is evidence that two δ receptor subtypes exist, designated δ_1 and δ_2. Because of their relative selectivity for enkephalins, δ receptors may not be important for the effects of exogenously administered opioids. Nevertheless, many opioid drugs bind δ receptors to some degree; thus, δ receptors may play some part in mediating the effects of opioid drugs. The δ receptors may be involved in opioid induced respiratory depression.[18]

σ Receptor

The σ receptor was one of the original triad of opioid receptors proposed by W. R. Martin[6] in 1976. Martin postulated such a receptor to explain the psychotomimetic and cardiovascular effects of SKF 10,047 and related agonist-antagonist opioids. Opioids with such properties came to be known as "σ opioids." Subsequently, an enormous effort was made to identify and characterize the σ receptor, an effort that continues presently. Although the σ receptor is not entirely understood, the results of many studies now suggest that it does not mediate the psychotomimetic effects of agonist-antagonist opioids, as originally proposed. Natural opioids (such as morphine) are levorotatory ($-$) isomers, and their dextrorotatory ($+$) enantiomers do not have opioid activity. ($\pm$) SKF 10,047 (as originally used by Martin) is a racemic mixture that is now recognized to bind (at least) three types of receptors: ($-$) SKF 10,047 binds mainly to μ and κ opioid receptors; ($+$) SKF 10,047 binds to phencyclidine receptors (ketamine also acts at this receptor, see Ch. 16) and to another receptor currently designated as σ.[19] The σ receptor shows a preference for dextrorotatory enantiomers and is not sensitive to naloxone (which is levorotatory). Because the psychotomimetic effects of agonist-antagonist opioids are mediated by levorotatory enantiomers and can be antagonized by naloxone, it appears that neither σ or phencyclidine receptors are involved, contrary to Martin's original scheme.[20] Presumably, opioid psychotomimetic effects are mediated by κ receptors[13] or by some unknown receptors. The physiologic significance, if any, of actions by dextrorotatory opioids on σ or PCP receptors is unknown.

DEFINITIONS OF AGONIST—ANTAGONIST OPIOIDS

The agonist-antagonist terminology was originally applied to nalorphine and similar drugs. These drugs were believed to be μ antagonists and κ agonists; thus, the hyphenated term, agonist-antagonist, was logical and descriptive. The term "nalorphine-like" was often used interchangeably with agonist-antagonist. The drugs most frequently classified as being nalorphine-like included pentazocine, nalbuphine, and butorphanol.

The terms agonist-antagonist and nalorphine-like have become somewhat vague and unsatisfactory as knowledge of opioid pharmacology has grown. The classification of opioid drugs will probably continue to change as the molecular pharmacology of opioid receptors evolves. A functional definition of agonist-antagonist drugs is needed that reflects our current understanding of the opioid receptor system. Perhaps a practical and broadly applicable definition of an agonist-antagonist opioid would include the following requirements: (1) agonist or partial agonist activity at one or more types of opioid receptors and (2) the ability to antagonize the effects of a full agonist at one or more types of opioid receptors. As described previously, the antagonist actions of an agonist-antagonist drug can result from partial agonist activity and true antagonist activity. Many of the so-called agonist-antagonist drugs appear to be partial agonists at more than one type of receptor, rather than a full agonist at one type of receptor and a complete antagonist at another receptor.

The classification of agonist-antagonist opioids is further complicated because some of the drugs have significant pharmacologic actions that are not mediated by opioid receptors (e.g., meptazinol and tramadol).

CLASSIFICATION OF AGONIST-ANTAGONIST OPIOIDS BY RECEPTOR TYPES

Identification of the receptors involved in the actions of particular opioids and classification of the drugs as full agonists, partial agonists, or antagonists is remarkably difficult. A combination of binding studies, bioassays, and behavioral studies have been applied to this problem. Many agonist-antagonist drugs bind with relatively high affinity to several different types of opioid receptor in vitro, but in vitro binding may not correspond to the observed in vivo pharmacologic effects of the drug in bioassays or behavioral studies. There are significant differences in the distribution and function of opioid receptors in various species. As highly selective agonists (drugs acting primarily at a single type of receptor) have become available for study, it has become apparent that drugs previously classified as acting at a single type of opioid receptor actually act at multiple types of receptors.

Table 5-2 contains a scheme for classifying agonist-antagonist drugs by their actions at various receptors. This scheme is based on an interpretation of data from many sources and from several species. It is subject to change and reinterpretation. Nevertheless, it is useful to have some system of classifying these drugs as a memory aid and as a basis for discussion.

STRUCTURE ACTIVITY RELATIONSHIPS

The understanding of structure activity relationships among opioid agonists, antagonists, and agonist-antagonist drugs is adversely affected by our incomplete knowledge of the family of opioid receptor types and subtypes and their physiologic functions. More precise knowledge of the molecular structure and function of opioid receptors in the future will probably help to elucidate the relationship between the chemical structure of opioid drugs and their interactions with receptors.

The structure of agonist-antagonist opioids can be classified based on their derivation from a basic parent structure. The major structural classes include opium alkaloids (including morphine, thebaine, and their semisynthetic derivatives), morphinans, and benzomorphans.

Morphine Series

Early investigators noted that the presence of a tertiary amine with an attached small alkyl group was required for the analgesic activity of morphine congeners (Fig. 5-3). Subsequently, a major focus of molecular modification has been on changes to the N-alkyl substituent. The change from a N-methyl group in morphine to N-ethyl produced a small decrease in analgesic potency, but larger N substituents, like pentyl and phenethyl, gave analogs with increased potency in the standard rodent antinociceptive assays.[21-23] However, the addition of some closely related N substituents, like phenacyl and cyclohexyl, resulted in analogs with decreased activity. Thus, changes in the N substituent produced somewhat unpredictable changes in analgesic activity. Remarkably, the N-allyl substituted compound, nalorphine, had significant antagonist activity; compounds with closely similar N

Table 5-2 Agonist-Antagonist and Partial Agonist Drugs Classified by Opioid Receptors[a]

	Receptor Type		
	μ	κ	Nonopioid
Nalbuphine	Partial Ag	Partial Ag	—
Butorphanol	Partial Ag	Partial Ag	—
Buprenorphine	Partial Ag	Ant?	—
Dezocine	Partial Ag	Partial Ag?	—
Meptazinol	Partial μ_1	Ant?	Antinociception partially blocked by scopolamine
Tramadol	Ag? Partial Ag?	?	Blocks monoamine reuptake

Abbreviations: Ag, agonist; Ant, antagonist.
[a] This is a hypothetical classification; see text for details.

substituents, e.g., N-propyl, N-isobutyl, and N-methylallyl, were less active antagonists.

The incorporation of nalorphine's N-allyl substituent in almost all series of synthetic opioids that contain at least three of the five rings present in morphine results in antagonist properties. Among analogous N substituted compounds in several series, general trends of agonist versus antagonist activity are observed, which are correlated with changes in N substituents.

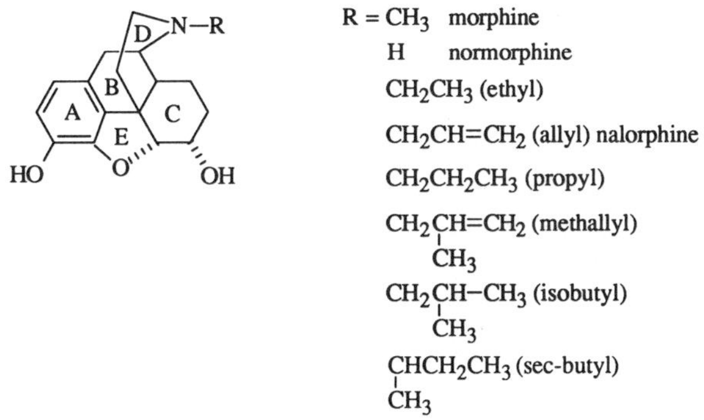

Fig. 5-3. Morphine congeners. N substituents have a marked effect on agonist or antagonist activity. Replacing the N-methyl group of morphine with a N-allyl group yields the agonist-antagonist opioid, nalorphine. Nalorphine has substantial antagonist activity.

4,5-Epoxymorphinan Series

Derivatives in the 14-hydroxy-4,5-epoxymorphinan-6-one series are closely related to morphine (Fig. 5-4). The addition of the 14-hydroxyl group increases the analgesic potency of classic 4,5-epoxymorphinan-6-one analogs. Incorporation of the N-allyl or N-cyclopropylmethyl (N-CPM) substituent has resulted in pure antagonists without analgesic activity, such as naloxone and naltrexone.[24] Incorporation of the N-cyclobutylmethyl (N-CBM) substituent in this series usually results in compounds with κ agonist and μ antagonist properties,[25,26] such as nalbuphine.

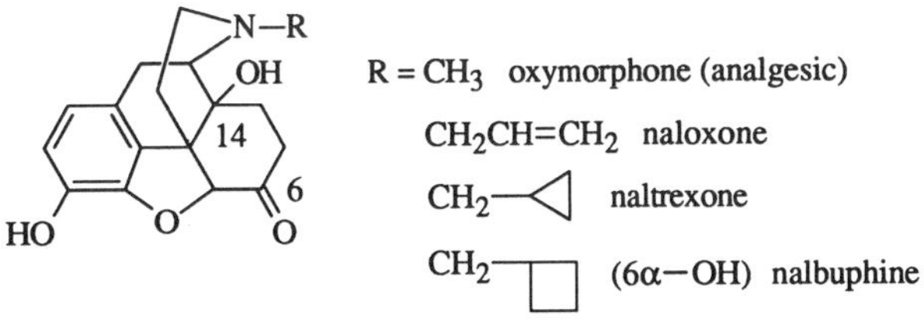

Fig. 5-4. 4,5-Epoxymorphinan series. The N-allyl congener (analogous to nalorphine in the morphine series) is the pure antagonist, naloxone. The N-cyclopropylmethyl substitution yields another pure antagonist, naltrexone. The N-cyclobutylmethyl 6-hydroxyl congener is the clinically useful agonist-antagonist drug, nalbuphine.

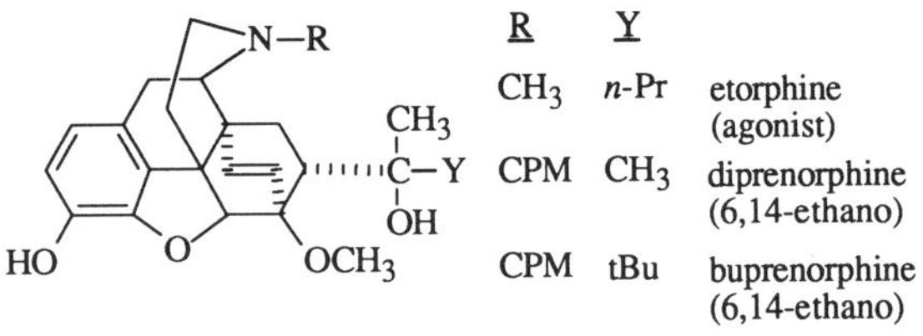

Fig. 5-5. Thebaine derivatives (etheno- and ethanotetrahydrothebaine analogs). The N-cyclopropylmethyl analog in the 6,14-ethano series is the clinically useful agonist-antagonist opioid, buprenorphine.

Thebaine Derivatives

Among the etheno- and ethanotetrahydrothebaine analogues, the N substituent and the size of the Y group in the side chain influence the balance between agonist and antagonist activity (Fig. 5-5).[27,28] Buprenorphine is the N-CPM derivative of the potent agonist, etorphine.

Morphinan Series

Morphinans are synthetic opioids (Fig. 5-6). Levorphanol, the N-methyl derivative, is a μ agonist analogous to morphine. Levallorphan, with a N-allyl substituent, is an agonist-antagonist that is analogous to nalorphine. The N-CPM and N-CBM substituents have been incorporated into several series of compounds with agonist-antagonist activity. The N-CBM analogs, such as butorphanol (analagous to nalbuphine in the 4,5-epoxy-morphinan series), are usually more potent analgesics. The N-CPM analogs, such as oxilorphan (not available for clinical use) are better antagonists (analagous to naltrexone in the 4,5-epoxy-morphinan series).[29,30] Butorphanol also has a 14-hydroxyl group incorporated, a structural modification that increases opioid activity.[31,32]

The stereochemistry of the B and C ring junction in morphinan derivatives has implications with regard to pharmacologic activity.[33] In morphinans, this ring junction is cis, and in isomorphinans, it is trans (Fig. 5-7). The geometry of the C ring with respect to the rest of the molecule is significantly different in isomorphinans than in morphinans. Antagonist activity is retained in isomorphinans, but analgesic properties are decreased.[34–36] For example, cyclorphan (N-CPM morphinan) is a much more potent analgesic (more than 200-fold) than is isocyclorphan (N-CPM isomorphinan), but the difference in antagonist potency in vivo is less than 2-fold. The isomorphinan analog of butorphanol is 100-fold less potent as an agonist but only 3-fold less potent as an antagonist compared with the morphinan.[37,38] The commercial preparation of butorphanol is entirely in the morphinan (cis) configuration.

Benzomorphan Series

The benzomorphans are also synthetic opioids. SKF 10,047 was the original benzomorphan agonist-antagonist opioid; the σ receptor was named

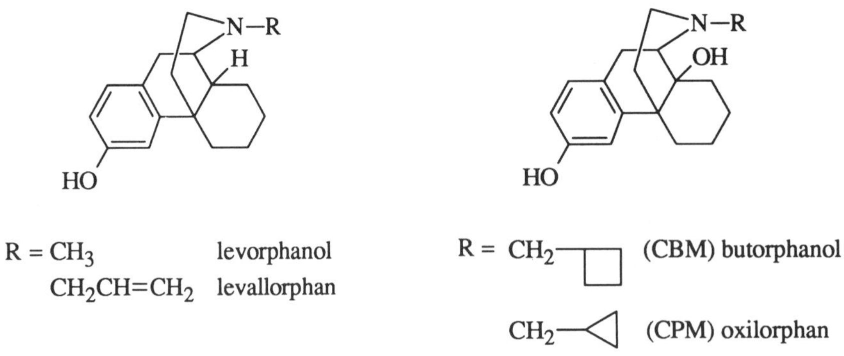

R = CH$_3$ levorphanol
CH$_2$CH=CH$_2$ levallorphan

R = CH$_2$ ▢ (CBM) butorphanol

CH$_2$ ◁ (CPM) oxilorphan

Fig. 5-6. Morphinan series. **(Left)** Levorphanol is analogous to morphine, and levallorphan is analogous to nalorphine. The N-allyl substitution produces antagonist activity, as in other series. **(Right)** The N-cyclobutylmethyl 14-hydroxylated morphinan is the clinically useful agonist-antagonist butorphanol (analogous to nalbuphine in the 4,5-epoxymorphinan series).

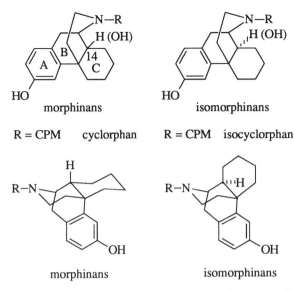

Fig. 5-7. Morphinan series. The stereochemistry of the B/C ring junction has a significant effect on pharmacologic activity, as described in the text. The morphinans have cis and the isomorphinans have trans B/C ring junctions. Each isomer is illustrated from two different perspectives to show the altered geometry of the C ring. The trans isomers (isomorphinans) have decreased analgesic activity compared with the cis isomers (morphinans).

for the "S" in SKF 10,047 (Fig. 5-8). SKF 10,047 produced notable dysphoria. Closely related derivatives produce less dysphoria.

The incorporation of the N-CPM group in the benzomorphan series produced the κ analgesic cy-

R = CH$_2$CH=CH$_2$ SKF-10047

CH$_2$—◁   cyclazocine

CH$_2$CH=C(CH$_3$)CH$_3$ pentazocine

Fig. 5-8. Benzomorphan series. Various benzomorphan congeners with agonist-antagonist activity are shown. The κ opioid receptor was named for ketocyclazocine. The illustrated compounds tend to produce dysphoria.

clazocine, and the addition of the N-dimethylallyl group led to pentazocine.[39,40] Cyclazocine produced considerable psychotomimetic effects and was not used clinically as an analgesic. Pentazocine, the only benzomorphan available for clinical use, was the result of a deliberate search for clinically valuable synthetic opioids following the observation that nalorpine had analgesic activity in humans. Pentazocine produces less dysphoria than does cyclazocine.[41–43]

Oxidation at the C1 position of the N-CPM compound yields the prototype κ agonist, ketocyclazocine (ketazocine).[44] Ketocyclazocine was an important compound in the early studies to identify multiple opioid receptors; the κ receptor was named for the "k" in ketocyclazocine. It is also a weak μ antagonist. Related substituted compounds (N-allyl and N-propyl) are also κ agonists.[45]

As with the morphinans, the stereochemical features of the benzomorphans can make a significant difference in the pharmacologic activity of certain compounds in the series. Numerous benzomorphans with various small substituents at the C6 (alkyl) and C11 (alkyl or hydroxyl) positions have been prepared to explore the structure activity relationships. With alkyl groups at C11, the cis and trans analogs are analogous to the morphinan and isomorphinan series, respectively (Fig. 5-9). Small differences in agonist and antagonist activities are observed between cis and trans pairs of these compounds, usually two- to threefold, favoring either diastereomer. An exception is the N-CBM compounds in which the analgesic activity is significantly enhanced in the cis diastereomer.[45]

The substitution of a hydroxyl group instead of an alkyl group at the C11 position produces a series of diastereomeric 11 α and 11 β-hydroxyl compounds (cis and trans) analagous to the 14-hydroxymorphinan and 14-isomorphinan series (which includes butorphanol). Compounds with the 11 β-hydroxyl group are more active than are those with the 11 α-hydroxyl group.[44–46]

Benzomorphan compounds with larger substituents on the nitrogen have also been examined (Fig. 5-10). A series of furanylalkyl and tetrahydrofuranylalkyl compounds have interesting properties.[47–50] The N-furanylethyl agent is a potent analgesic. Remarkably, the similar N-furanyl-

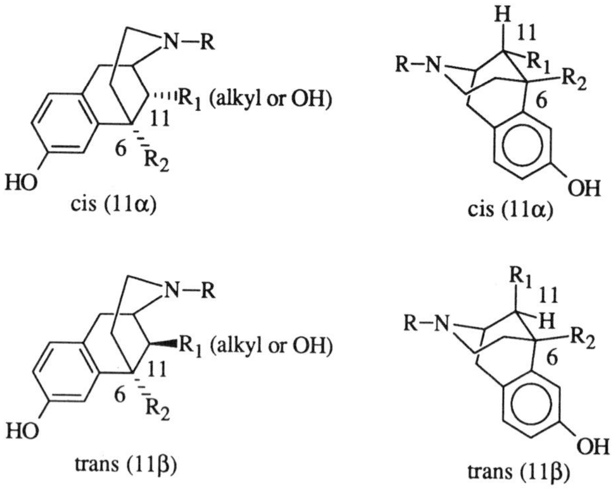

Fig. 5-9. Benzomorphan series. Stereochemistry affects the pharmacologic activity of the benzomorphans, as described in the text. The cis and trans isomers of the C11 position are each shown from two perspectives to illustrate the geometry of the ring. These benzomorphan isomers are analogous to the morphinan (cis) and isomorphinan (trans) isomers in the morphinan series (see Fig. 5-5).

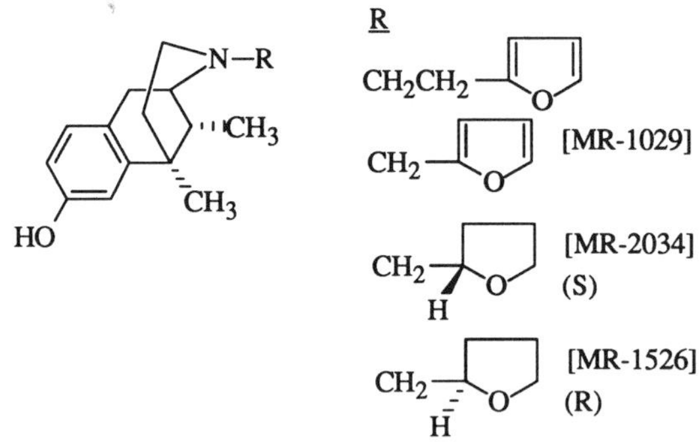

Fig. 5-10. Benzomorphan series. A series of large N substituents yields compounds with varied pharmacologic properties, as described in the text.

methyl compound (MR-1029) is a κ antagonist.[48–51] Among the tetrahydrofuranylmethyl compounds with an additional chiral center in the N substituent, the R diastereomer is a potent analgesic, but the S diastereomer is not.[49] Thus, a

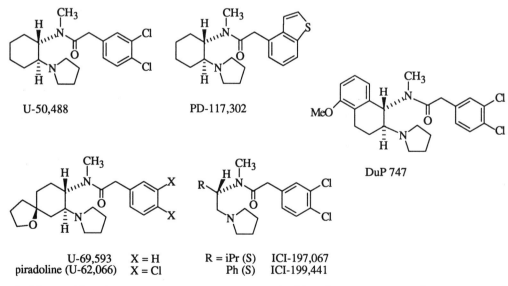

Fig. 5-11. Highly selective κ agonists. U-50,488 is a highly selective κ agonist that is structurally unrelated to previous κ receptor ligands. Several analogs are under investigation.

small structural change greatly influences the observed effects in this series.

Highly Selective κ Agonists and Antagonists

There is considerable interest in the structural aspects of κ agonists. U-50,488, a highly selective κ agonist, is structurally unrelated to most other κ receptor ligands (Fig. 5-11).[52] U-50,488 has served as a model for the development of agents with potentially useful properties.[53–55] Among the series of analogs that are being investigated are those in which the aromatic substituent of the aracylamide portion of the molecule is increased in size and those in which the six membered ring is altered to an aralkyl or alkyl side chain.[13] Two closely related ligands include U-69,593, which now serves as a radioligand for κ opioid receptor displacement assays, and spiradoline (U-62,066), which is presently under development.[56] Some examples of related analogs under study are shown in Figure 5-11.[57–62]

Recently, some selective κ antagonists have been discovered. Norbinaltorphimine and binaltorphimine are the most well known (Fig. 5-12). They antagonize ethylketocyclazocine and U-50,488.[63,64] These compounds, or other related molecules, should prove to be valuable in the characterization of κ receptors.

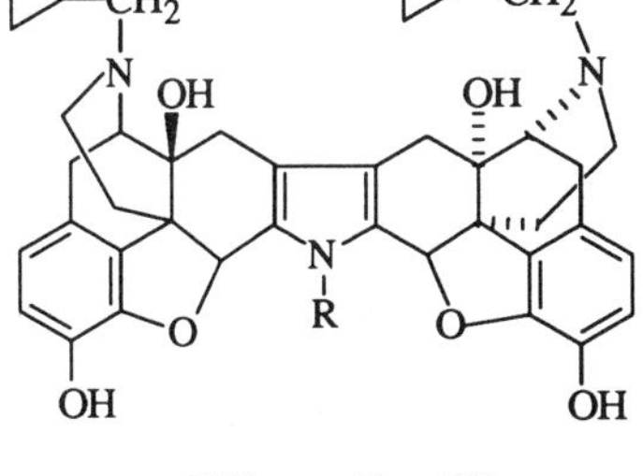

BNI   R = CH₃
norBNI   R = H

Fig. 5-12. Binaltorphimine (BNI) and norbinaltorphimine (norBNI) are recently discovered selective κ antagonists.

CLINICAL PHARMACOLOGY OF PARTICULAR DRUGS

Nalorphine-Like Drugs

The so-called nalorphine-like drugs, including pentazocine, nalbuphine, and butorphanol, were originally thought to be μ antagonists and κ agonists. These drugs are probably more accurately described as partial agonists at both μ and κ receptors, with the intensity of agonist activity varying somewhat from one drug to another.[65–68]

Some of the reasons for classifying nalorphine-like drugs as partial μ and partial κ agonists are interesting to examine. Although nalorphine-like drugs uniformly produce respiratory depression, selective κ agonists appear not to produce respiratory depression. The selective κ agonist, bremazocine, did not produce respiratory depression in dogs or rats.[16] The highly selective prototype κ agonist drug, U-50,488, did not depress ventilation when given by intrathecal or intracerebroventricular routes to rats.[17] These results imply that κ receptors do not mediate the respiratory effects of opioids and that nalorphine-like drugs mediate their respiratory depressant effects through μ receptors. The compound β-funaltrexamine is a highly selective μ receptor antagonist. It markedly shifts to the right, in a nonparallel fashion, the dose effect curves of nalorphine, nalbuphine, and butorphanol in the mouse abdominal constriction assay, a bioassay that reflects opioid mediated analgesia. This further supports the notion that nalorphine-like drugs are partial μ agonists.[66] Thus, the ability of nalorphine-like drugs to antagonize morphine-like μ agonists is probably because of μ partial agonist activity (Fig. 5-2).

The effect of κ agonists to suppress vasopressin levels and produce diuresis has been a useful bioassay for classifying κ agonist activity. The results of such studies suggest that nalorphine-like drugs are partial κ agonists; nalorphine and butorphanol supressed vasopressin levels but did not have the full efficacy of prototype κ agonists such as U-50,488.[69]

Although nalorphine-like drugs share many similarities, there are significant differences between the individual drugs that have been demonstrated in studies of human volunteers or patients. Nalorphine and pentazocine produce more intense dysphoria and psychotomimetic effects than do nalbuphine or butorphanol, and they have cardiovascular stimulating properties. Although butorphanol and nalbuphine tend not to produce as much dysphoria or cardiovascular stimulation, they do produce sedation, presumably mediated by κ receptors. Butorphanol, in particular, appears to have a marked sedative effect.[70] All the nalorphine-like drugs have antagonist activity toward full μ agonists, but nalbuphine appears to have the most prominent antagonist properties.

Buprenorphine

Buprenorphine appears to be a partial agonist at μ and κ receptors; to this extent, it resembles the nalorphine-like drugs. However, its slow dissociation from μ receptors and an unusual bell shaped dose effect curve give buprenorphine a unique pharmacologic profile.

Several studies have demonstrated that buprenorphine dissociates very slowly from opioid receptors in rat brain and guinea pig ileum. Figure 5-13 illustrates an experiment in which normorphine, pentazocine, and buprenorphine were applied to guinea pig ileum, causing contraction. The effects of normorphine and pentazocine were reversed by the addition of naloxone. Buprenorphine caused a prolonged effect that could not be antagonized by large doses of naloxone. Clinical reports suggest an analogous phenomenon in humans; naloxone does not always effectively reverse buprenorphine's effects, such as respiratory depression.

Dum and Herz[71] examined the antinociceptive effects of buprenorphine in rats and found that doses of buprenorphine up to about 0.5 mg/kg produced the expected dose related analgesia, but doses greater than 0.5 mg/kg resulted in a paradoxic reduction in antinociception (Fig. 5-14). The

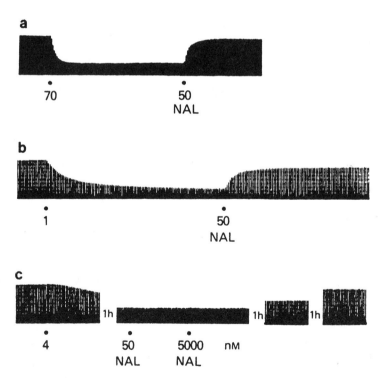

Fig. 5-13. Normorphine (*a*), pentazocine (*b*), and buprenorphine (*c*) inhibit the contraction of guinea pig ileum muscle strips. Naloxone (NAL) reverses normorphine and pentazocine promptly but not buprenorphine. The buprenorphine effect persists for several hours. The numbers refer to nanomolar concentrations. (From Schulz and Hertz,[199] with permission.)

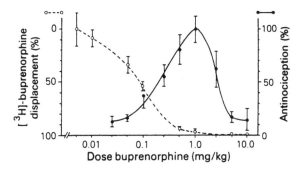

Fig. 5-14. Buprenorphine had a bell shaped dose effect curve in the rat vocalization test of antinociception. The extent of binding of buprenorphine to receptors in rat brain is shown over the same range of buprenorphine doses. (From Dum and Hertz,[71] with permission.)

opioid antagonist naltrexone shifted the buprenorphine dose effect curve symmetrically to the right, suggesting that the bell shape is related to opioid receptor activity. The explanation for the unusual buprenorphine dose effect curve is unknown, although one hypothesis suggests an interaction between μ and δ receptors.[72] Comparable dose effect studies in humans are not available; however, it is interesting to consider a case report of two patients with severe postoperative pain after balanced anesthesia with buprenorphine and nitrous oxide.[73] The anesthesiologists were aware of the bell shaped dose effect curve and reasoned that the patients had received too much buprenorphine, placing them on the downward slope of the curve (a dose related reduction in analgesia).

The administration of naloxone to these patients resulted in "total pain relief," which was consistent with a shift to the right of a bell shaped dose effect curve.

Buprenorphine binds to κ receptors in rat brain, and it antagonized the diuretic effects of the κ agonist, bremazocine, in morphine tolerant rats, suggesting buprenorphine has antagonist or partial agonist activity at κ receptors.[74]

Buprenorphine's pharmacology is complicated and not completely understood. Under some circumstances, naloxone may not completely antagonize buprenorphine's agonist effects, or naloxone may actually cause a paradoxic increase in buprenorphine's agonist effects.

Dezocine

Remotely related structurally to benzomorphans, dezocine is a partial μ agonist (Fig. 5-15). Subjective effects (sedation or dysphoria) in humans suggest dezocine has κ activity, and it did bind κ receptors in vitro.[75] Dezocine antagonized morphine effects and produced an abstinence syndrome in morphine dependent animals. Dezocine appears to be a more efficacious μ agonist than are other agonist-antagonist drugs, judging from its analgesic and respiratory effects in animals and humans. A plateau of analgesic activity and respiratory depression was demonstrated in humans, but the level of the plateau appeared higher than that for butorphanol or nalorphine.[76] The anesthetic sparing effect (reduction of the minimum alveolar concentration of enflurane) caused by dezocine in dogs was similar to that of morphine and much greater than that of nalbuphine or butorphanol.[77]

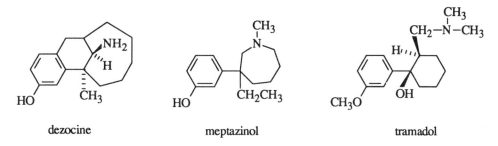

Fig. 5-15. The structures of dezocine, meptazinol, and tramadol.

Meptazinol

A compound structurally related to meperidine, meptazinol binds to μ receptors in rat brain with moderate affinity and behaves clinically as a partial μ agonist; it is moderately selective for μ_1 receptors (Fig. 5-15).[78] It has a low affinity for rat brain κ receptors and, therefore, may not have appreciable κ effects. The antinociceptive effects of meptazinol in animals are unusual because they appear to be mediated in part by a cholinergic mechanism. The antinociceptive activity of meptazinol in the mouse tail immersion test (thermal stiumulus) is antagonized by naloxone, similar to other opioids. However, scopolamine also antagonized meptazinol in this test.[79] Thus, meptazinol appears to produce analgesia by its activity in two different receptor systems.

Tramadol

The pharmacologic classification and mechanism of action of tramadol is not entirely clear (Fig. 5-15). Tramadol, with a structure only remotely related to other opioids, appears to be either a partial μ agonist or a pure μ agonist of low potency. The lack of typical morphine-like effects in humans somewhat resembles the profile of a partial agonist; however, dose effect studies of antinociceptive effects in rodents suggested that tramadol is a pure μ agonist of relatively low potency. It produced a mild withdrawal syndrome in morphine dependent monkeys but failed to precipitate or suppress the abstinence syndrome in several other animal studies.[80] Tramadol did not produce dysphoria or sedative effects in a study of nondependent human opioid abusers, suggesting that it does not have appreciable κ effects.[80] It did bind κ receptors in vitro; however, the affinity may be too low to have physiologic significance.[81] Its metabolite, O-desmethyltramadol, had greater affinity and selectivity for μ receptors and greater analgesic potency in the rat than did tramadol itself.[82]

Tramadol's antinociceptive effects in rats and mice were only partially antagonized by naloxone, suggesting an additional mechanism of analgesia not related to opioid receptors.[81] Tramadol blocked reuptake of norepinephrine and sero-tonin,[81,83] and the monoamine antagonists, yohimbine and ritanserin, blocked the antinociceptive effects of intrathecal tramadol in mice,[81] Suggesting a possible monoaminergic mechanism of analgesia.

Tramadol is not a classic agonist-antagonist drug because it appears to have little or no antagonist properties and little or no κ receptor activity; perhaps it should not be classified with the other drugs presented in this chapter. However, it may be a partial μ agonist,[80] and it produces significant analgesia while having limited respiratory effects and limited abuse potential. Therefore, regardless of its mechanism of action, it is of interest for much the same reasons as are the classic agonist-antagonist opioids.

AGONIST-ANTAGONISTS AS ANESTHETIC AGENTS

There is an interesting body of literature describing the use of agonist-antagonist opioids in various regimens of balanced anesthesia. Murphy and Hug[84] studied the enflurane sparing effect of morphine, fentanyl, butorphanol, and nalbuphine in dogs. Morphine or fentanyl reduced enflurane requirements by about 65 percent; butorphanol or nalbuphine reduced them by only 11 or 8 percent, respectively. These authors suggested that the small minimum alveolar concentration reduction with the agonist-antagonists was the result of a "ceiling" for analgesia. Hall et al.[77] studied dezocine in the same dog model and found a 58 percent reduction in enflurane requirements; the maximum dose of dezocine was limited by cardiovascular depression. These studies could be interpreted to suggest that butorphanol and nalbuphine would not be efficacious as analgesic supplements to general anesthesia. However, this conclusion may not be warranted. There are substantial differences in opioid pharmacology between various species.[85] Experiments in dogs may not apply directly to humans. The contribution of "analgesia" to general anesthesia is unclear, and many drugs that produce general anesthesia (e.g., most of the intravenous induction agents, except ketamine, and potent volatile anesthetics, except cyclopropane) do not produce analgesia in conscious subjects. Even if there is a ceiling for the antinociceptive effects, other opioid effects, such as sedation mediated by κ receptors, might contribute to the anesthetic state.

Minimum alveolar concentration reduction studies with agonist-antagonists have not been performed in humans. However, clinical studies of agonist-antagonist drugs suggest that they are efficacious as the opioid component of balanced anesthesia. Aldrete et al.[86] compared butorphanol or morphine combined with diazepam, pancuronium, and nitrous oxide in a randomized blinded study of anesthesia for coronary artery bypass surgery. The average dose of butorphanol was 25 mg compared with 127 mg of morphine. The average dose of diazepam was 22 mg in both groups. The two opioids were equally satisfactory, and there were no significant differences in hemodynamic effects during surgery. The blinded anesthesiologists were unable to discern which drug they were using. In three of four cases of patient movement, intraoperative awareness, or hemodynamic instability (in which the blinded anesthesiologist was convinced the opioid was butorphanol), the opioid was morphine.

Zsigmond et al.[87] studied nalbuphine combined with diazepam and nitrous oxide in an open study of anesthesia for cardiac surgery. No significant increases in blood pressure or circulating norepinephrine levels were found after intubation, skin incision, or sternotomy. The authors judged nalbuphine to be an effective opioid in balanced anesthesia for cardiac surgery. Lake et al.[88] gave nalbuphine in doses up to 3 mg/kg to patients undergoing cardiac surgery. They observed that none of the patients were unconscious after this dose of nalbuphine and concluded that nalbuphine was inadequate as a sole anesthetic agent. This is not surprising considering that, even full μ agonists, such as fentanyl analogs, are not generally considered adequate as sole anesthetic agents and are commonly combined with other drugs to produce complete and reliable anesthesia. Weiss et al.[89] performed a randomized, but apparently unblinded, study of anesthesia with nalbuphine or fentanyl combined with flunitrazepam for cardiac surgery. No inhaled anesthetics were used. Stress hormone concentrations were greater and more vasodilators

or other antihypertensive drugs were necessary in the nalbuphine group. Anesthesia with nalbuphine was characterized as unsatisfactory in comparison with fentanyl.

Rawal and Wennhager[90] compared nalbuphine with fentanyl in a blinded study of balanced anesthesia for gynecologic surgery. Anesthesia was induced with diazepam, thiopental, and either, nalbuphine or fentanyl. The maintenance anesthesia was 70 percent nitrous oxide plus supplemental doses of opioid, titrated to effect at the discretion of the anesthesiologist. The nalbuphine and fentanyl were provided in coded syringes of approximately equal potency on a volume basis. The total dose of nalbuphine was about 1 mg/kg (less than 10 percent of the total dose of nalbuphine used by Zsigmond et al.[87] for cardiac surgery). Anesthesia was satisfactory overall in both groups. However, there was a greater elevation of heart rate during intubation and higher blood pressure during surgery in the nalbuphine group. Patients in the nalbuphine group were more sedated following surgery. Patients in the fentanyl group had more problems with respiratory depression; 12 of 30 patients in the fentanyl group had respiratory rates less than 10/min and 4 patients required naloxone. Only 1 patient in the nalbuphine group had a respiratory rate less than 10/min. Crul et al.[91] also performed a blinded comparison of nalbuphine and fentanyl for balanced anesthesia and found results similar to those reported by Rawal et al.[90] These studies reveal some of the major differences between the agonist-antagonists and the μ agonists. Postoperative sedation was a greater problem with nalbuphine, and respiratory depression was a greater problem with fentanyl. Postoperative sedation from nalbuphine and other similar drugs is probably related to κ receptor activity, which is much more prominent than with fentanyl analogues. The lower incidence of respiratory depression with nalbuphine compared with fentanyl was probably related to a ceiling for respiratory depression.

Buprenorphine has been studied in balanced anesthesia for cardiac and noncardiac surgery. Pedersen[92] studied four doses of buprenorphine: 10, 20, 30, or 40 μg/kg in combination with diazepam and nitrous oxide. Patients receiving 10 or 20 μg/kg did not require analgesic medication within 1 hour of extubation. Remarkably, 50 percent of patients receiving the larger doses, 30 or 40μg/kg, requested an analgesic within 5 minutes. This is consistent with the bell shaped dose effect curve for buprenorphine found in animal studies. Kay[93] reported that buprenorphine, 0.3 mg (about 5 μg/kg), and nitrous oxide 75 percent produced satisfactory anesthesia for abdominal surgery in a blinded comparison with fentanyl, 0.125 mg; buprenorphine was actually superior to fentanyl in this study for suppressing the heart rate and blood pressure response to surgery. Kamal et al.[94] reported that buprenorphine combined with a propofol infusion resulted in satisfactory "total intravenous anesthesia" for cholecystectomy. They also found that an initial bolus dose of buprenorphine, 5.0 μg/kg, prevented a significant increase in heart rate and blood pressure during intubation; 2.5 μg/kg was less effective. Okutani et al.[95] combined buprenorphine with diazepam, nitrous oxide, and halothane for cardiac surgery. Buprenorphine, 12 μg/kg, was significantly more effective in controlling plasma catecholamine levels than was 6 μg/kg. Interestingly, vasopressin levels were significantly higher in the 12 μg/kg group. This is consistent with the observations from animal studies that suggest that buprenorphine has κ receptor antagonist effects[96–98] (κ agonists supress vasopressin release).

CARDIOVASCULAR EFFECTS OF AGONIST-ANTAGONIST OPIOIDS

The cardiovascular effects of agonist-antagonist opioids have not been thoroughly studied. The older agonist-antagonist drugs, nalorphine and pentazocine, have considerable cardiovascular stimulating effects. Pentazocine produces increases in blood pressure, heart rate, systemic vascular resistance, pulmonary artery pressure, and left ventricular end diastolic pressure. The newer agents (except dezocine) generally appear to have relatively minor cardiovascular effects.

Butorphanol or nalbuphine, given in large doses to patients undergoing anesthesia for cardiac surgery,[86,88] appeared to have virtually no hemodynamic effects. Butorphanol has been shown to cause a small increase in pulmonary artery pressure in some studies,[99] which is reminiscent of pentazocine; however, other studies found no change in pulmonary pressures. Buprenorphine also appeared to cause minimal hemodynamic effects.[100]

Meptazinol appeared to produce only minor hemodynamic effects when given in analgesic doses.[101] Camu and Rucquoi[102] gave larger doses of meptazinol (2, 3, or 4 mg/kg) to a small number of patients anesthetized with etomidate. The heart rates and blood pressures declined on average about 30 percent at the highest dose. Pulmonary artery pressures were unaffected. These results suggest that the hemodynamic effects of meptazinol may be of clinical importance. Additional studies are warranted.

Dezocine produced substantial cardiovascular depression in dogs.[77] Doses of 20 mg/kg in dogs anesthetized with enflurane resulted in severe hypotension; some animals died, apparently from myocardial depression. The mechanism of the cardiovascular side effects is unknown. Marked cardiovascular effects were not found in humans given analgesic doses of dezocine.[75] Additional studies are needed to elucidate the mechanism of cardiovascular depression in dogs and to determine whether similar effects are possible in humans.

Tramadol appeared to cause few hemodynamic side effects when given in analgesic doses. However, the clinical literature is sparse, and additional studies are required.[103]

RESPIRATORY EFFECTS OF AGONIST-ANTAGONIST OPIOIDS

Agonist-antagonist opioids generally produce respiratory depression, presumably mediated by μ receptors. The κ receptors do not appear to mediate respiratory depression because highly selective κ agonists have not caused respiratory depression in animals.[16,17] The agonist-antagonist opioids are generally partial μ agonists; therefore, it would not be surprising if the maximum respiratory depressant effects were less than full μ agonists. Rigorous tests of the respiratory effects of a drug should include the following features: (1) dose effect data for at least three different doses, spanning the therapeutic range of the drug; (2) tests for respiratory drive (e.g., mouth occlusion pressure or CO_2 response); (3) spirometry and blood gases; and (4) exclusion of drugs (other than the drug being tested) that affect ventilation.

Keats and associates[3,104,105] studied the respiratory effects of pentazocine, nalorphine, nalbuphine, and dezocine in human volunteers, using the ventilatory response to carbon dioxide as a measure of respiratory depression. Gal and DiFazio[76] also studied dezocine. Nalorphine, nalbuphine, and dezocine were found to have a ceiling for respiratory depression equivalent to about 30 mg/70 kg of body weight of morphine. At lower doses, the respiratory depression was dose related. Higher doses produced no additional depression of CO_2 response. The pentazocine respiratory dose effect curve was less steep than was that for morphine, but a plateau could not be demonstrated because intense dysphoria in the volunteers limited the maximum dose. Nagashima et al.[105a] found that the dose effect curve for respiratory depression for butorphanol was less steep than that for morphine, but doses large enough to establish a true ceiling were not studied. Zucker et al.[106] compared the respiratory effects of butorphanol, 0.17 mg/kg, with those of nalbuphine, 0.86 mg/kg, in a blinded randomized study of patients anesthetized with thiopental (for induction) and nitrous oxide; the authors suggested that these doses probably produced the ceiling or maximum respiratory depression. Butorphanol produced significantly greater depression of minute ventilation and the CO_2 response.

The respiratory effects of buprenorphine have not been fully characterized. de Klerk et al.[106a] studied the CO_2 response in volunteers given buprenorphine, 0.3 and 0.6 mg. The respiratory depression was similar for both doses, suggesting a flat dose effect curve for a ceiling. However, a dose effect relationship cannot be completely described with only two data points. The respiratory depression caused by buprenorphine may not always be antagonized by naloxone; doxapram, an analeptic drug that stimulates ventilation, has been suggested as an alternative antidote for buprenorphine-induced respiratory depression.[107] Unusually large doses of naloxone (5 to 10 mg) have also been tried and may be effective.[108]

The respiratory effects of meptazinol[109] and tramadol appeared to be less than morphine-like opioids, but the available data do not allow definite conclusions.

THE USE OF AGONIST-ANTAGONISTS TO ANTAGONIZE FULL AGONISTS

The agonist-antagonist opioids can antagonize full agonists under certain conditions. When there is a high degree of receptor occupancy by the full agonist, the partial agonist reduces the net effect. The partial agonist, with less efficacy than the full agonist, competes with the agonist for binding sites. When receptor occupancy by the full agonist is low, the introduction of the partial agonist may increase the net effect because the total receptor occupancy by both the agonist and partial agonist increases (Fig. 5-2). In clinical terms, agonist-antagonists may be expected to antagonize large doses of full agonist effectively, but not small doses.

The antagonist properties of nalbuphine have been studied most often. Nalbuphine (15 mg/70 kg of body weight) actually enhanced instead of antagonized the respiratory depression produced by a small dose of morphine (15 mg/70 kg), as predicted by theory.[110] However, several clinical studies have shown that nalbuphine is effective for antagonizing the respiratory depressant effects of large doses of μ agonists.[111–115] Tabatabai et al.[116] administered fentanyl, 50 to 100 μg/kg, to cats and studied the effects on medullary inspiratory neurons and the phrenic nerve. Fentanyl profoundly impaired the normal rhythmic activity of the inspiratory neurons and the phrenic nerve. Nalbuphine 0.1 mg/kg reversed these effects and restored normal neuronal activity. Bailey et al.[113] found that nalbuphine and naloxone were equally efficacious for antagonizing respiratory depression following balanced anesthesia with fentanyl in a randomized blinded comparison. Patients receiving naloxone requested analgesics significantly more often than did patients receiving nalbuphine, suggesting that nalbuphine preserved analgesia more effectively. The dose effect relationship for nalbuphine antagonist action has not been rigorously determined, and a wide range of doses have been used, from about 1 to 20 mg/70 kg IV; 2.5 to 5.0 mg is probably a reasonable starting dose in adults.

The question arises whether the antagonist properties of agonist-antagonist opioids are advantageous compared with those of naloxone. The answer to this question relates to a variety of problems associated with the clinical use of naloxone.[117–123] Naloxone has a relatively short half-life of about 1 to 1.5 hours. Because the half-lives of the commonly used opioid agonists are two to five times longer than that of naloxone, recurrence of respiratory depression is a possibility. Recurrence of pain is frequently a problem after naloxone administration. Severe hypertension, cardiac arrhythmias (including ventricular fibrillation), and pulmonary edema have been associated with naloxone administration. There are a few reports of death immediately following naloxone administration, apparently caused by pulmonary edema. Whether these adverse effects are dose related is not entirely clear, but pulmonary edema has occurred following a relatively small dose (0.1 mg).[123] The mechanism of adverse effects is not known, but there is evidence for the involvement of the sympathetic nervous system. Flacke et al.[124] showed that naloxone dramatically increased circulating catecholamine levels in unconscious unstimulated dogs anesthetized with fentanyl, nitrous oxide, and enflurane. A substantial rise in sympathetic tone would appear to be a plausible explanation for hypertension and arrhythmias. Pulmonary edema associated with naloxone is presumed to be analogous to neurogenic pulmonary edema; this mechanism has not been proved, however.

Because of the problems associated with naloxone, there is considerable interest in opioid antagonists that would preserve analgesia without elevating sympathetic tone. Mills et al.[125] found that nalbuphine did not elevate circulating catecholamines in dogs anesthetized with fentanyl and enflurane, in contrast with naloxone. Bailey et al.[113] suggested that nalbuphine preserved analgesia better than did naloxone. Zsigmond et al.[126] reported that nalbuphine antagonized fentanyl-induced respiratory depression without loss of analgesia or hemodynamic instability. However, the use of nalbuphine as an antagonist has been associated with a spectrum of naloxone-like adverse effects. Pain and cardiovascular instability[114,115,127] and pulmonary edema[128] have been reported. Nalbuphine is an interesting alternative to naloxone in the clinical setting; whether it is truly superior to naloxone is not clear.

Butorphanol has also been shown to antagonize the respiratory depression caused by fentanyl. Bowdle et al.[129] found that butorphanol, 1 mg, substantially improved ventilation and the slope of the CO_2 response curve; blood pressure, heart rate, circulating epinephrine and norepinephrine concentrations, and pain intensity were essentially unchanged. This study illustrates the importance of species differences in opioid pharmacology. In rodents, butorphanol did not have substantial antagonist properties; in humans, the antagonist properties were evident.

Boysen et al.[130] compared buprenorphine with naloxone for antagonizing the respiratory effects of fentanyl. Women undergoing abdominal hysterectomy were anesthetized with fentanyl, 25 μg/kg; midazolam, 0.2 mg/kg; and nitrous oxide. Following surgery, patients with respiratory rates of 4 breaths/min or less were randomized in a blinded fashion to receive either buprenorphine (0.6 mg in 20 ml of NaCl) or naloxone (0.4 mg in 20 ml of NaCl) at 2 ml/min until the respiratory rate exceeded 8/min or 20 ml of solution was completed. Fifteen minutes after the administration of the antagonist was begun, all patients had respiratory rates of 8/min or greater. The median dose of buprenorphine was 0.48 mg, and the median dose of naloxone was 0.16 mg. The naloxone group had a higher respiratory rate (14.5/min) compared with the nalbuphine group (10/min; $P < 0.05$) at 15 minutes; however, the naloxone group also had significantly higher pain scores. Fifty percent of patients in the naloxone group had moderate to severe pain at 15 minutes; all patients in the buprenorphine group had either no pain or mild pain. During the subsequent 3-hour study period there were no differences in $PaCO_2$, sedation, or respiratory rate. Although there were no measures of ventilatory drive in this study, the results suggest that buprenorphine may be a clinically useful antagonist of μ opioid respiratory depression. Like nalbuphine, it appeared to preserve analgesia better than did naloxone.

AGONIST-ANTAGONIST OPIOIDS FOR POSTOPERATIVE PAIN

Agonist-antagonist opioids may have a ceiling for analgesia; nevertheless, they can produce intense analgesia, which is sufficient for the treatment of postoperative pain. Numerous studies have shown that agonist-antagonist opioids produce postoperative analgesia comparable to the full μ agonists, such as morphine and meperidine.[131] There are undoubtedly subtle differences in analgesia and in the spectrum of side effects among the various opioids given for postoperative pain, but for practical purposes, several different drugs can give satisfactory results.

An argument could be made that agonist-antagonists are preferable to full μ agonists for postoperative pain, based on a consideration of their pharmacologic properties. The hypothetic advantages of agonist-antagonists would be a ceiling for respiratory depression and a lower potential for abuse. However, these advantages may not be decisive. Surgical patients are not at high risk for developing opioid addiction; therefore, a low abuse potential may not be a high priority in drug selection. Also, the dysphoria and sedation mediated by κ receptors, which probably contributes to the lower abuse potential, can also be considered an undesirable side effect. A reduced risk of respiratory depression would certainly be advantageous; however, most of the angonist-antagonist drugs appear to produce dose related respiratory depression when given in typical analgesic doses. Thus, the ceiling for respiratory depression may not be a practical advantage in many situations. However, there is some clinical evidence that differences in respiratory effects can be significant. Houmes et al.[132] performed a blinded randomized comparison of tramadol and morphine for postoperative pain control following gynecologic surgery. Under the conditions of their study, analgesia was clinically acceptable with either drug, although there was a trend for morphine to be more effective in patients with severe pain. Oxygen saturation was measured by pulse oximetry as a measure of respiratory depression (supplemental oxygen was not given during the study). In the morphine group, 13 percent of patients had an oxygen saturation less than 86 percent compared with none in the tramadol group. The authors suggested that tramadol was preferable to morphine because of this apparent difference in respiratory effects. Additional clinical studies of the respiratory effects of analgesics would be valuable to test the hypothesis that certain drugs confer a greater margin of safety with respect to respiratory depression.

The type and dose of opioid used intraoperatively as part of the anesthetic may be an important practical consideration in the choice of opioid for postoperative analgesia. If a substantial dose of a full μ agonist, such as morphine or a fentanyl analog, is used intraoperatively, an agonist-antagonist administered postoperatively may have antagonist effects. Whether this drug interaction produces desired or undesired effects will depend critically on the dose of each drug and the timing (i.e., the extent of receptor occupany by each type of opioid). This problem has not been well studied.

In addition to the standard parenteral routes of administration, butorphanol has been given transnasally[133] and buprenorphine, sublingually[134–138] (see Ch. 31). Several of the agonist-antagonists have been given by patient-controlled intravenous infusion devices.[139–144]

Postanesthetic shaking or shivering (not caused by hypothermia) has been attenuated by certain opioids. Meperidine is effective for this purpose.[145] Morphine is not effective. There is evidence that butorphanol[146,147] and tramadol[148] are also effective. The mechanisms of postanesthetic shaking and its treatment are unknown.

SPINAL ANALGESIA WITH AGONIST-ANTAGONIST OPIOIDS

Many different drugs, including agonist-antagonist opioids,[149–171] have been administered for spinal analgesia, by either the intrathecal or epidural route. The spinal administration of agonist-antagonist opioids may appear hypothetically attactive because many of these drugs are κ partial agonists and κ receptors appear to be significant for modulating nociception in the spinal cord. The ceiling for respiratory depression may be advantageous.

Before contemplating spinal administration of any drug to humans, it is probably important to test for possible spinal cord toxicity in animals.[172,173] However, this appears not to have been done for many drugs. A drug intended for epidural use also should be proved to be safe for intrathecal use because inadvertent intrathecal administration is common; the assumption should not be made that, because a drug can be given epidurally, it can be safely administered intrathecally. Ideally, toxicity studies should examine a wide range of doses, should test spinal cord function and histopathologic findings, and should consider the possible effects of vehicles and preservatives. Morphine has been the most widely used drug for spinal analgesia; intrathecal administration to animals is not associated with histopathologic changes in the spinal cord.[174,175]

Rawal et al.[173] administered butorphanol, sufentanil, and nalbuphine to sheep intrathecally. They concluded that butorphanol or large doses of sufentanil caused injury to the spinal cord. Nalbuphine or small doses of sufentanil (corresponding to therapeutic doses in humans) appeared to be nontoxic. Coombs[176] administered dezocine to dogs by intrathecal infusion for 28 to 136 days and found significant spinal cord injury. However, they were unable to separate the effects of the spinal catheter from the drug's effects.

Camann et al.[177] performed a blinded placebo controlled comparison of epidural or intravenous butorphanol 2 mg for postoperative analgesia after cesarean section. They concluded that the analgesic effects of butorphanol were similar by either route of administration. Considering that spinal butorphanol provokes spinal cord toxicity in sheep, epidural administration would not appear to be warranted if the same analgesia can be obtained by intravenous administration. Camann et al. reviewed the literature, citing evidence that the effects of lipophilic opioids (most opioids are lipophilic; morphine, which is very water soluble, is a notable exception) are substantially the same, whether given spinally or parenterally. Fox[178] made a similar argument for buprenorphine, noting that the effective epidural and parenteral dose are essentially identical; also, the toxicology of spinal buprenorphine is unknown.

Perhaps the most useful application of agonist-antagonist opioids in the area of spinal analgesia is intravenous administration to antagonize the side effects of spinal morphine, such as pruritus, nausea, and respiratory depression. Several studies suggest that nalbuphine can be used effectively for this purpose.[179–183]

ABUSE POTENTIAL FOR AGONIST-ANTAGONIST OPIOIDS

The abuse potential for agonist-antagonists is thought to be less than for μ agonists, based on studies in humans that demonstrate certain properties of agonist-antagonists (that are different from morphine-like drugs), such as (1) dysphoric subjective effects, (2) production of an abstinence syndrome (withdrawal) in opioid dependent subjects,[184,185] (3) mild physical dependence after chronic administration with an abstinence syndrome that is less severe than with morphine, and (4) the ability of subjects to distinguish agonist-antagonists for morphine in various discriminative tests. The results of abuse potential studies have been recently reviewed by Preston et al.[80,186]

The notion that agonist-antagonist opioids are less likely to be abused is reflected in the Federal drug laws of the United States. Drugs that are believed to have abuse potential are classified according to five schedules; drugs believed to have no significant abuse potential are unscheduled. Schedule I drugs have no approved medical uses and include drugs such as lysergic acid diethylamide. Full μ agonists, such as morphine, are classified as Schedule II drugs and are highly regulated. Drugs with lesser abuse potential are classified into Schedules III, IV, or V, with Schedule V relecting the least abuse potential. Pentazocine was originally unscheduled, but following an epidemic of abuse, it was classified in Schedule IV. Buprenorphine is in Schedule V. Butorphanol, nalbuphine, and dezocine are unscheduled.

Postsurgical patients or other patients with acute pain are not at high risk to develop opioid addiction. Therefore, the lower abuse potential of agonist-antagonists is probably not a critical factor in choosing analgesics for perioperative pain. However, opioid abuse is a major concern in office based medical practice and for patients with chronic pain problems. In these settings, the lower abuse potential of agonist-antagonists may be valuable. Abuse potential is relative, not absolute; drugs with supposedly low abuse potential can be abused and cause serious problems, as was shown by the abuse of pentazocine.

ANTAGONISTS

Naloxone is a pure antagonist of all three types of opioid receptors, although higher doses are required to antagonize κ and δ agonists than for μ agonists. Naloxone has a relatively short duration of action compared with many of the opioid agonists; the terminal half-life is about 1 to 1.5 hours. Thus, there may be a risk of recurrence of opioid agonist effects when naloxone is given in a small bolus dose. Longnecker et al.[187] were able to prolong the action of naloxone by giving it intramuscularly, i.e., from 80 minutes (0.35 mg/70 kg IV) to 6 hours (0.7 mg/70 kg IM).

Naloxone has been given by intravenous infusion in attempts to antagonize opioid side effects such as pruritus and ventilatory depression while preserving analgesia. Some authors have reported successful results.[188–190] However, interference with analgesia is always a possibility when naloxone is used.[191] Intramuscular naloxone partially reversed respiratory depression from epidural morphine while preserving analgesia.[192] The opioid antagonist, naltrexone, has also been used to prevent the pruritus associated with epidural morphine.[193]

The use of naloxone to antagonize opioid agonist overdosage can be associated with serious cardiovascular problems.[117–123] Severe hypertension, cardiac arrhythmias (including ventricular fibrillation), and pulmonary edema have been reported; a few deaths have been attributed to naloxone administration. These adverse effects may not be dose related; pulmonary edema has been reported following a small dose (0.1 mg).[123] The mechanism of cardiovascular side effects is believed to be a sudden increase in sympathetic tone, as demonstrated by Flacke et al.[124] in dogs. The mechanism of pulmonary edema is presumed to be similar to that for neurogenic pulmonary edema.

Naloxone has been used to treat cardiovascular shock states, stroke, spinal cord injury, and a variety of miscellaneous conditions. There is also evidence that naloxone may antagonize some anesthetic drugs that are not opioids, such as nitrous oxide, benzodiazepines, and barbiturates. However, these miscellaneous uses of naloxone are not firmly established.[194]

There are remarkably few pure opioid antagonists compared with the number of opioid agonists that are available. Naltrexone and nalmefene are pure opioid antagonists that are analogues of naloxone (Fig. 5-4). Naltrexone is the N-CPM analog of oxymorphone, whereas naloxone is the N-allyl analogue. Several antagonists have resulted from modification of the C6 keto group of naltrexone, including nalmefene (the C6 methylene analogue of naltrexone), naltrindole, and nor-binaltorphimine (Fig. 5-12). Naltrindole and nor-binaltorphimine are selective antagonists of δ and κ receptors, respectively (which are not available for clinical use).[195] Naltrexone and nalmefene, like naloxone, are most potent at the μ receptors but have significant activity at all three types of opioid receptors. They both have much longer durations of action than does naloxone (terminal half-life in excess of 8 hours) and significant oral bioavailability.[196–198] The role of the newer pure antagonists in anesthesiology is unclear.

REFERENCES

1. Martin WR: History and development of mixed opioid agonists, partial agonists, and antagonists. Br J Clin Pharmacol 7:273, 1979
2. Eckenhoff JE, Elder JD, King BD: Effect of N-allylnormorphine in treatment of opiate overdose. Am J Med Sci 222:115, 1951

3. Keats AS, Telford T: Studies of analgesic drugs X. Respiratory effects of narcotic antagonists. J Pharmacol Exp Ther 112:126, 1966

4. Foldes FF, Lunn JN, Moore J, Brown IM: N-allylnoroxymorphone: a new potent narcotic antagonist. Am J Med Sci 245:23, 1963

5. Ariens EJ, Simonis AM, Van Rossum JM: Molecular Pharmacology: The Mode of Action of Biologically Active Compounds. Academic Press, New York, 1964, pp. 140, 170

6. Martin WR: Opioid antagonists. Pharmacol Rev 19:463, 1967

7. Martin WR, Eades CG, Thompson WO et al: The effects of morphine and nalorphine-like drugs in the non-dependent chronic spinal dog. J Pharmacol Exp Ther 197:517, 1976

8. Gilbert PE, Martin WR: The effects of morphine and nalorphine-like drugs in the nondependent, morphine-dependent and cyclazocine-dependent chronic spinal dog. J Pharmacol Exp Ther 198:66, 1976

9. Evans C, Keith D, Morrison H et al: Cloning of a δ opioid receptor by functional expression. Science 258:1952, 1992

10. Kieffer B, Befort K, Gaveriaux-Ruff C, Hirth C: The δ-opioid receptor: isolation of a cDNA by expression cloning and pharmacological characterization. Proc Natl Acad Sci U S A 89:12048, 1992

10a. Fukuda A, Kato S, Mori K, Nishi M, Takeshima H: Primary structures and expression from cDNAs of rat opioid receptor δ- and μ-subtypes. FEBS Lett 327:311, 1993

10b. Yasuda K, Raynor K, Kong H et al: Cloning and functional comparison of κ and δ opioid receptors from mouse brain. Proc Natl Acad Sci USA 90:6736, 1993

10c. Chen Y, Mestek A, Liu J, Yu L: Molecular cloning of a rat kappa opioid receptor reveals sequence similarities to the μ and δ opioid receptors. Biochem J 295:625, 1993

10d. Li S, Zhu J, Chen C et al: Molecular cloning and expression of a rat κ opioid receptor. Biochem J 295:629, 1993

10e. Thompson R, Mansour A, Akil H, Watson S: Cloning and pharmacological characterization of a rat μ opioid receptor. Neuron 11:903, 1993

11. Itzhak Y: Multiple opioid binding sites. In Pasternak GW (ed): The Opiate Receptors. The Humana Press, Clifton, 1988

12. Chavkin C, James IF, Goldstein A: Dynorphin is a specific endogenous ligand of the κ opioid receptor. Science 215:413, 1982

13. Millan MJ: κ-opioid receptors and analgesia. Trends Pharmacol Sci 11:70, 1990

14. Pasternak G: Pharmacological mechanisms of opioid analgesics. Clin Neuropharmacol 16:1, 1993

15. Cox BM: Peripheral actions mediated by opioid receptors. In Pasternack GW (ed): The Opiate Receptors. The Humana Press, Clifton, 1988

16. Freye E, Hartung E, Schenk GK: Bremazocine: an opiate that induces sedation and analgesia without respiratory depression. Anesth Analg 62:483, 1983

17. Castillo R, Kissin I, Bradley E: Selective κ opioid agonist for spinal analgesia without the risk of respiratory depression. Anesth Analg 65:350, 1986

18. Pazos A, Florez J: Interaction of naloxone with μ and δ opioid agonists on the respiration of rats. Eur J Pharmacol 87:309, 1983

19. Walker J, Bowen W, Walker F et al: σ receptors: biology and function. Pharmacol Rev 42:355 1990

20. Musacchio J: The psychotomimetic effects of opiates and the sigma receptor. Neuropsychopharmacology 3:191, 1990

21. Clark R, Pessolano A, Weijlard J, Pfister K: N-substituted epoxymorphinans. J Am Chem Soc 75:4963, 1953

22. Winter C, Orahovats P, Lehman E: Analgesic activity and morphine antagonism of compounds related to nalorphine. Arch Int Pharmacodyn Ther 110:186, 1957

23. Lasagna L, Beecher H: The analgesic effectiveness of nalorphine and nalorphine-morphine combinations in man. J Pharmacol Exp Ther 112:356, 1954

24. Casy A, Parfit R: Opioid Analgesics, Chemistry and Receptors. Plenum Press, New York, 1986

25. Archer S, Harris L: Narcotic antagonists. Prog Drug Res 8:262, 1965

26. Archer S, Michne W: Recent progress in research on narcotic antagonists. Prog Drug Res 20:45, 1976

27. Lewis J: Ring C-bridged derivatives of thebaine and oripavine. Adv Biochem Psychopharmacol 8:123, 1973

28. Blane G, Boura A, Leach E et al: Dissociation of analgesic and respiratory depressant properties in N-substituted analogues of etorphine. J Pharm Pharmacol 20:796, 1968

29. Kotick M, Leland D, Polazzi J, Schut R: Analgesic narcotic antagonists. 1. 8β-alkyl-, 8β-acyl-, and 8β-(tertiary alcohol) dihydrocodeinones and -dihydromorphinones. J Med Chem 24:166, 1980

30. Leland D, Kotick M: Analgesic narcotic antagonists. 5. 7,7-dimethyldihydrocodeinones and 7,7-dimethyldihydromorphinones. J Med Chem 24:717, 1981

31. Monkovic I, Conway T, Wong H et al: Total synthesis and pharmacological activities of N-substituted 3,14-dihydroxymorphinans. J Am Chem Soc 95:7910, 1973

32. Monkovic I, Wong H, Belleau B et al: Synthetic morphinans and hasubanans, part IV. Can J Chem 53:2515, 1975

33. Gates M, Webb W: The synthesis and resolution of 3-hydroxy-N-methylisomorphinan. J Am Chem Soc 80:1186, 1958

34. Leimgruber M, Mohacsi E, Baruth H, Randall L: Levallorphan and related compounds. Adv Biochem Psychopharmacol 8:45, 1973

35. Lasagna L: Drug interaction in the field of analgesic drugs. Proc Soc Med 58:978, 1965

36. White C Jr, Megirian R, Marcus P: RO-1-7780, a potent antagonist of alphaprodine. Proc Soc Exp Biol Med 92:512, 1956

37. Belleau B, Wong H, Monkovic I, Perron Y: Total synthesis of 3, 14-dihydroxy-3-methano hasbubans. J Chem Soc Chem Commun 603, 1974

38. Lambert Y, Daris J-P, Monkovic I, Pircio A: Analgesics and narcotic antagonists in the benzomorphan and 8-oxamorphinan series 5. J Med Chem 21:423, 1978

39. Archer S, Albertson N, Harris L et al: Pentazocine. Strong analgesic and analgesic antagonists in the benzomorphinan series. J Med Chem 7:123, 1964

40. Michne W, Albertson N: Analgetic 1-oxidized-2,6-methano-3-benzoazocines. J Med Chem 15:1278, 1972

41. Lord J, Waterfield A, Hughes J, Kosterlitz H: Endogenous opioid peptides: multiple agonists and antagonists. Nature 267:495, 1977

42. Payne J: The clinical pharmacology of pentazocine. Drugs 5:1, 1973

43. Brogden R, Speight T, Avery G: Pentazocine: a review of its pharmacological properties, therapeutic efficacy and dependence liability. Drugs 5:6, 1973

44. Albertson N: Cyclazocine and congeners. Adv Biochem Psychopharmacol 8:63, 1973

45. Saucier M, Daris J-P, Lambert Y et al: 5-allyl-9-oxobenzomorphan. 3. potent narcotic antagonists on the series of substituted 2′,9β-dihydroxy-6,7-benzomorphan. J Med Chem 20:676, 1977

46. Albertson N: Effect of 9-hydroxylation on benzomorphan antagonist activity. J Med Chem 18:619, 1975

47. May E, Eddy N: Interesting pharmacological properties of the optical isomers of α-5,9-diethyl-2′-hydroxy-2-methyl-6,7-benzomorphan. J Med Chem 9:851, 1966

48. Merz H, Stockhaus K, Wick H: Stereoisomeric 5,9-dimethyl-2′-hydroxy-2-tetrahydrofurfuryl-6,7-benzomorphans, strong analgesics with non-morphine-like action profiles. J Med Chem 18:996, 1975

49. Merz H, Stockhaus K: N-[(Tetrahydrofuryl)alkyl] and N-(alkoxyalkyl) derivatives of (−)-normetazocine, compounds with differentiated opioid action profiles. J Med Chem 22:1475, 1977

50. Gordon M, Lafferty J, Tedeschi D et al: New benzomorphan analgesics. J Med Pharm Chem 5:633, 1962

51. Merz H, Langbein K, Stockhause K et al: Structure-activity relationships in narcotic antagonists by N-furylmethyl substituents. Adv Biochem Psychopharmacol 8:91, 1974

52. Rees D: Chemical structures and biological activities of non-peptide selective κ opioid ligands. Prog Med Chem 29:109, 1992

53. Szmuszkovicz J, VonVoightlander P: Benzeneacetamide amines: structurally novel non-μ opioids. J Med Chem 25:1126, 1982

54. Lahti R, VonVoightlander P, Barsuhn C: Properties of a selective κ agonist, U-50,448H. Life Sci 31:2257, 1987

55. Katz J, Woods J, Winger G, Jacobson A: Compounds of novel structure having κ-agonist behavioral effects in rhesus monkeys. Life Sci 31:2375, 1987

56. Lahti R, Nickelson M, McCall J, VonVoightlander P: [^{3}H]U-69593 a highly selective ligand for the opioid κ-receptor. Eur J Pharmacol 109:281, 1985

57. Clark C, Halfpenny P, Hill R et al: Highly selective κ opioid analgesics. Synthesis and structure-activity relationships of novel N-[(2-aminocyclohexyl)aryl]-acetamide and N-[(2-aminocyclohexyl)aryloxy]acetamide derivatives. J Med Chem 31:831, 1988

58. Clark C, Birchmore B, Sharif N et al: PD117302: a selective agonist for the κ-opioid receptor. Br J Pharmacol 618, 1988

59. Halfpenny P, Hill R, Horwell D et al: Highly selective κ-opioid analgesics. 2. Synthesis and structure activity relationships of novel N-[(2-aminocyclohexyl)aryl]acetamide derivatives. J Med Chem 32:1620, 1989

60. Costello G, Main B, Barlow J et al: A novel series of potent and selective agonists at the opioid receptor. Eur J Pharmacol 151:475, 1988

61. Costello G, James R, Shaw J et al: 2-(3,4-dichlorophenyl)-N-methyl-N-[2-(1-pyrrolindinyl)-1-substituted-ethyl]-acetamides: the use of conformational analysis in the development of a novel series

of potent opioid κ agonists. J Med Chem 34:181, 1991

62. Rajagopalan P, Scribner R, Penner P et al: DuP 747: SAR study. Biorg Med Chem Lett 2:721, 1992

63. Portoghese P, Lipkowski A, Takemori A: Binaltorphimine and nor-binaltorphimine, potent selective κ-opioid receptor antagonists. Life Sci 40:1287, 1987

64. Takemori A, Ho B, Naeseth J, Portoghese P: Nor-binaltorphimine, a highly selective κ-opioid antagonist in analgesic and receptor binding assays. J Pharmacol Exp Ther 246:255, 1987

65. Dykstra LA: Butorphanol, levallorphan, nalbuphine, and nalorphine as antagonists in the squirrel monkey. J Pharmacol Exp Ther 254:245, 1990

66. Zimmerman DM, Leander JD, Reel JK, Hynes MD: Use of β-funaltrexamine to determine μ opioid receptor involvement in the analgesic activity of various opioid ligands. J Pharmacol Exp Ther 241:374, 1987

67. Horan PJ, Ho IK: Comparative pharmacological and biochemical studies between butorphanol and morphine. Pharmacol Biochem Behav 34:847, 1989

68. Picker MJ, Negus S, Craft RM: Butorphanol's efficacy at μ and κ opioid receptors: inferences based on the schedule-controlled behavior of nontolerant and morphine-tolerant rats and on the responding of rats under a drug discrimination procedure. Pharmacol Biochem Behav 36:563, 1990

69. Leander JD, Hart JC, Zerbe RL: κ agonist-induced diuresis: evidence for stereoselectivity, strain differences, independence of hydration variables and a result of decreased plasma vasopressin levels. J Pharmacol Exp Ther 242:33, 1987

70. Dershwitz M, Rosow CE, DiBiase PM, Zaslavsky A: Comparison of the sedative effects of butorphanol and midazolam. Anesthesiology 74:717, 1991

71. Dum JE, Herz A: In vivo receptor binding of the opiate partial agonist, buprenorphine, correlated with its agonistic and antagonistic actions. Br J Pharmacol 74:627, 1981

72. Sadee W, Richards ML, Grevel J, Rosenbaum JS: In vivo characterization of four types of opioid binding sites in rat brain. Life Sci, suppl. 1:187, 1983

73. Pedersen JE, Chraemmer-Jorgensen B, Schmidt JF, Risbo A: Naloxone—a strong analgesic in combination with high-dose buprenorphine? Br J Anaesth 57:1045, 1985

74. Richards ML, Sadee W: Buprenorphine is an antagonists at the κ opioid receptor. Pharm Res 4:178, 1985

75. O'Brien JJ, Benfield P: Dezocine: a preliminary review of its pharmacodynamic and pharmacokinetic properties, and therapeutic efficacy. Drugs 38:226, 1989

76. Gal TJ, DiFazio CA: Ventilatory and analgesic effects of dezocine in humans. Anesthesiology 61:716, 1984

77. Hall RI, Murphy MR, Szlam F, Hug CC: Dezocine-MAC reduction and evidence for myocardial depression in the presence of enflurane. Anesth Analg 66:1169, 1987

78. Spiegel K, Pasternak GW: Meptazinol: a novel μ-1 selective opioid analgesic. J Pharmacol Exp Ther 228:414, 1984

79. Bill DJ, Hartley JE, Stephens RJ, Thompson AM: The antinociceptive activity of meptazinol depends on both oiate and cholinergic mechanisms. Br J Pharmacol 79:191, 1983

80. Preston KL, Jasinski DR, Testa M: Abuse potential and pharmacological comparison of tramadol and morphine. Drug Alcohol Depend 27:7 1991

81. Raffa RB, Friderichs E, Reimann W et al: Opioid and nonopioid components independently contribute to the mechanism of action of tramadol, an "atypical" opioid analgesic. J Pharmacol Exp Ther 260:275, 1992

82. Hennies H-H, Friderichs E, Schneider J: Receptor binding, analgesic and antitussive potency of tramadol and other selected opioids. Arzneim-Forsch 38:877, 1988

83. Driessen B, Reimann W: Interaction of the central analgesic, tramadol, with the uptake and release of 5-hydroxytryptamine in the rat brain in vitro. Br J Pharmacol 105:147, 1992

84. Murphy MR, Hug CC: The enflurane sparing effect of morphine, butorphanol and nalbuphine. Anesthesiology 57:489, 1982

85. Mansour A, Khachaturian H, Lewis ME et al: Anatomy of CNS opioid receptors. Trends Neurosci 11:308, 1988

86. Aldrete JA, de Campo T, Usubiaga LE et al: Comparison of butorphanol and morphine as analgesics for coronary bypass surgery: a double-blind, randomized study. Anesth Analg 62:78, 1983

87. Zsigmond EK, Winnie AP, Raza SMA et al: Nalbuphine as an analgesic component in balanced anesthesia for cardiac surgery. Anesth Analg 66:1155, 1987

88. Lake CL, Duckworth EN, DiFazio CA et al: Cardiovascular effects of nalbuphine in patients with coronary or valvular heart disease. Anesthesiology 57:498, 1982

89. Weiss BM, Schmid ER, Gattiker RI: Comparison of nalbuphine and fentanyl anesthesia for coronary artery bypass surgery: hemodynamics, hormonal response, and postoperative respiratory depression. Anesth Analg 73:521, 1991

90. Rawal N, Wennhager M: Influence of perioperative nalbuphine and fentanyl on postoperative respiration and analgesia. Acta Anaesthesiol Scand 34:197, 1990

91. Crul JF, Smets MJW, van Edmond J: The efficacy and safety of nalbuphine (Nubain) in balanced anesthesia: a double blind comparison with fentanyl in gynecological and urological surgery. Acta Anaesth Belg 41:261, 1990

92. Pedersen JE: Peroperative buprenorphine: do high dosages shorten analgesia postoperatively? Acta Anaesthesiol Scand 30:660, 1986

93. Kay B: A double-blind comparison between fentanyl and buprenorphine in analgesic-supplemented anaesthesia. Br J Anaesth 52:453, 1980

94. Kamal RS, Khan FA, Khan FH: Total intravenous anaesthesia with propofol and buprenorphine. Anaesthesia 45:865, 1990

95. Okutani R, Kono K, Kinoshita O et al: Variations in hemodynamic and stress hormonal responses in open heart surgery with buprenorphine/diazepam anesthesia. J Cardiothorac Anesth 3:401, 1989

96. Boachie-Ansah G, Sitsapesan R, Kane KA, Parratt JR: The antiarrhythmic and cardiac electrophysiological effects of buprenorphine. Br J Pharmacol. 97:801, 1989

97. Parratt JR, Sitsapesan R: Stereospecific antiarrhythmic effect of opioid receptor antagonists in myocardial ischaemia. Br J Pharmacol 87:621, 1986

98. Sitsapesan R, Parratt JR: The effects of drugs interacting with opioid receptors on the early ventricular arrhythmias arising from myocardial ischaemia. Br J Pharmacol 97:795, 1989

99. Popio K, Jackson D, Ross A et al: Hemodynamic and respiratory effects of morphine and butorphanol. Clin Pharmacol Ther 23:281, 1978

100. Heel RC, Brogden RN, Speight TM, Avery GS: Buprenorphine: a review of its pharmacological properties and therapeutic efficacy. Drugs 17:81, 1979

101. Holmes B, Ward A: Meptazinol: a review of its pharmacodynamic and pharmacokinetic properties and therapeutic efficacy. Drugs 30:285, 1985

102. Camu F, Rucquoi M: Cardiac and circulatory effects of high-dose meptazinol in anaesthetized patients. Postgrad Med J, suppl. 1:60, 1983

103. Muller B, Wilsmann K: Cardiac and hemodynamic effects of the centrally acting analgesics tramadol and pentazocine in anaesthetized rabbits and isolated guinea-pig atria and papillary muscles. Arzneimittel forschung 34:430, 1984

104. Romagnoli A, Keats AS: Ceiling effect for respiratory depression by nalbuphine. Clin Pharmacol Ther 27:478, 1980

105. Romagnoli A, Keats AS: Ceiling respiratory depression by dezocine. Clin Pharmacol Ther 35:367, 1984

105a. Nagashima H, Karmanian A, Malovany R et al: Respiratory and circulatory effects of intravenous butorphanol and morphine. Clin Pharmacol Ther 19:738, 1976

106. Zucker JR, Neuenfeldt T, Freund PR: Respiratory effects of nalbuphine and butorphanol in anesthetized patients. Anesth Analg 66:879, 1987

106a. de Klerk G, Mattie H, Spierdijk J: Comparative study on the circulatory and respiratory effects of buprenorphine and methadone. Acta Anaesthesiol Belg 32:131, 1981

107. Orwin JM: The effect of doxapram on buprenorphine induced respiratory depression. Acta Anaesth Belg 2:93, 1977

108. Gal T: Naloxone reversal of buprenorphine-induced respiratory depression. Clin Pharmacol Ther 45:66, 1989

109. Jones JG: The respiratory effects of meptazinol. Postgrad Med J, suppl. 1:72, 1983

110. Bailey PL, Clark NJ, Pace NL et al: Failure of nalbuphine to antagonize morphine: a double-blind comparison with naloxone. Anesth Analg 65:605, 1986

111. Freye E, Azevedo L, Hartung E: Reversal of fentanyl related respiratory depression with nalbuphine. Acta Anaesthesiol Belg 4:365, 1985

112. Latasch L, Teichmuller T, Dudziak R, Probst S: Antagonisation of fentanyl-induced respiratory depression by nalbuphine. Acta Anaesth Belg 40:35, 1989

113. Bailey PL, Clark NJ, Pace NL et al: Antagonism of postoperative opioid-induced respiratory depression: nalbuphine versus naloxone. Anesth Analg 66:1109, 1987

114. Jaffe RS, Moldenhauer CC, Hug CC et al: Nalbuphine antagonism of fentanyl-induced ventilatory depression: a randomized trial. Anesthesiology 68:254, 1988

115. Ramsay JG, Higgs BD, Wynands JE et al: Early extubation after high-dose fentanyl anaesthesia for aortocoronary bypass surgery: reversal of respiratory depression with low-dose nalbuphine. Can J Anaesth 32:597, 1985

116. Tabatabai M, Kitahata LM, Collins JG: Disruption

of the rhythmic activity of the medullary inspiratory neurons and phrenic nerve by fentanyl and reversal with nalbuphine. Anesthesiology 70:489, 1989

117. Michalis L, Hickey P, Clark T: Ventricular irritability associated with the use of naloxone. Ann Thorac Surg 18:608, 1974

118. Tanaka G: Hypertensive reaction to naloxone. JAMA 228:25, 1974

119. Flacke J, Flacke W, Williams G: Acute pulmonary edema following naloxone reversal of high-dose morphine anesthesia. Anesthesiology 47:376, 1977

120. Azar I, Turndorf H: Severe hypertension and multiple atrial premature contractions following naloxone administration. Anesth Analg 58:524, 1979

121. Andree R: Sudden death following naloxone administration. Anesth Analg 59:782, 1980

122. Taff R: Pulmonary edema following naloxone administration in a patient without heart disease. Anesthesiology 59:576, 1983

123. Prough D, Roy R, Bumgardner J, Shannon G: Acute pulmonary edema in healthy teenagers following conservative doses of intravenous naloxone. Anesthesiology 60:485, 1984

124. Flacke J, Flacke W, Bloor B, Olewine S: Effects of fentanyl, naloxone and clonidine on hemodynamics and plasma catecholamine levels in dogs. Anesth Analg 62:305, 1983

125. Mills CA, Flacke JW, Flacke WE et al: Narcotic reversal in hypercapnic dogs: comparison of naloxone and nalbuphine. Can J Anaesth 37:238, 1990

126. Zsigmond EK, Durrani Z, Barabas E et al: Endocrine and hemodynamic effects of antagonism of fentanyl-induced respiratory depression by nalbuphine. Anesth Analg 66:421, 1987

127. Blaise GA, Nugent M, McMichan JC, Durant PAC: Side effects of nalbuphine while reserving opioid-induced respiratory depression: report of four cases. Can J Anaesth 37:794, 1990

128. DesMarteau JK, Cassot L: Acute pulmonary edema resulting from nalbuphine reversal of fentanyl-induced respiratory depression. Anesthesiology 65:237, 1986

129. Bowdle TA, Greichen SL, Bjurstrom RL, Schoene TB: Butorphanol improves CO_2 response and ventilation after fentanyl anesthesia. Anesth Analg 66:517, 1987

130. Boysen K, Hertel S, Chraemmer-Jorgensen B et al: Buprenorphine antagonism of ventilatory depression following fentanyl anaesthesia. Acta Anaesthesiol Scand 32:490, 1988

131. Hoskin PJ, Hanks GW: Opioid agonist-antagonist drugs in acute and chronic pain states. Drugs 41:326. 1991

132. Houmes RM, Voets MA, Verkaaik A et al: Efficacy and safety of tramadol versus morphine for moderate and severe postoperative pain with special regard to respiratory depression. Anesth Analg 74:510, 1992

133. Abboud TK, Zhu J, Gangolly J et al: Transnasal butorphanol: a new method for pain relief in post-cesarean section pain. Acta Anaesthesiol Scand 35:14, 1991

134. Carl P, Crawford ME, Madsen NBB et al: Pain relief after major abdominal surgery: a double-blind controlled comparison of sublingual buprenorphine, intramuscular buprenorphine, and intramuscular meperidine. Anesth Analg 66:142, 1987

135. Bullingham RES, McQuay HJ, Dwyer D et al: Sublingual buprenorphine used postoperatively: clinical observations and preliminary pharmacokinetic analysis. Br J Clin Pharmacol 12:117, 1981

136. Bullingham RES, McQuay HJ, Porter EJB et al: Sublingual buprenorphine used postoperatively: ten hour plasma drug concentration analysis. Br J Clin Pharmacol 13:665, 1982

137. Maunuksela E, Korpela R, Olkkola KT: Comparison of buprenorphine with morphine in the treatment of postoperative pain in children. Anesth Analg 67:233, 1988

138. Moa G, Zetterstrom H: Sublingual buprenorphine as postoperative analgesic: a double-blind comparison with pethidine. Acta Anaesthesiol Scand 34:68, 1990

139. Lehmann KA, Kratzenberg U, Schroeder-Bark B, Horrichs-Haermeyer G: Postoperative patient-controlled analgesia with tramadol: analgesic efficacy and minimum effective concentrations. Clin J Pain 6:212, 1990

140. Lehmann KA, Tenbuhs B: Patient-controlled analgesia with nalbuphine, a new narcotic agonist-antagonist, for the treatment of postoperative pain. Eur J Clin Pharmacol 31:267, 1986

141. Podlas J, Breland BD: Patient-controlled analgesia with nalbuphine during labor. Obstet Gynecol 70:202, 1987

142. Woods MP, Rayburn WF, McIntosh DG et al: Nalbuphine after major gynecologic surgery: comparison of patient-controlled analgesia and intramuscular injections. J Rprod Med 36:647, 1991

143. Shah MV, Jones DI, Rosen M: "Patient demand" postoperative analgesia with buprenorphine: comparison between sublingual and i.m. administration. Br J Anaesth 58:508, 1986

144. Kay B, Krishnan A: On-demand nalbuphine for postoperative pain relief. Acta Anaesth Belg 37:33, 1986

145. Macintyre PE, Pavlin EG, Dwersteg JF: Effect of meperidine on oxygen consumption, carbon dioxide production and respiratory gas exchange in postanesthesia shivering. Anesth Analg 66:751, 1987

146. Vogelsang J, Hayes SR: Butorphanol tartrate (Stadol) relieves postanesthesia shaking more effectively than meperidine (Demerol) or morphine. J Post Anesth Nurs 7:94, 1992

147. Vogelsang J, Hayes SR: Stadol attenuates postanesthesia shivering. J Post Anesth Nurs 4:222, 1989

148. Pausawasdi S, Jirasirithum S, Phanarai C: The use of tramadol hydrochloride in the treatment of postanesthetic shivering. J Med Assoc Thai 73:16, 1990

149. Abboud TK, Moore M, Zhu J et al: Epidural butorphanol or morphine for the relief of post-cesarean section pain: ventilatory responses to carbon dioxide. Anesth Analg 66:887, 1987

150. Abboud TK, Afrasiabi A, Zhu J et al: Epidural morphine or butorphanol augments bupivacaine analgesia during labor. Reg Anesth 14:115, 1989

151. Abboud TK, Afrasiabi A, Zhu J et al: Bupivacaine/butorphanol/epinephrine for epidural anesthesia in obstetrics: maternal and neonatal effects. Reg Anesth 14:219, 1989

152. Wolff J, Carl P, Crawford ME: Epidural buprenorphine for postoperative analgesia. A controlled comparison with epidural morphine. Anaesthesia 46:77, 1986

153. Capogna G, Celleno D, Tagariello V, Loffred-Mancinelli C: Intrathecal buprenorphine for postoperative analgesia in the elderly patient. Anaesthesia 43:128, 1988

154. Celleno D, Capogna G, Sebastiani M et al: Epidural analgesia during the after cesarean delivery: comparison of five opioids. Reg Anesth 16:79, 1991

155. Bilsback P, Rolly G, Tampubolon O: Efficacy of the extradural administration of lofentanil, buprenorphine or saline in the management of postoperative pain: a double-blind study. Br J Anaesth 57:943, 1985

156. Cahill J, Murphy D, O'Brien D et al: Epidural buprenorphine for pain relief after major abdominal surgery: a controlled comparison with epidural morphine. Anaesthesia 38:760, 1983

157. Simpson KH, Madej TH, McDowell M et al: Comparison of extradural buprenorphine and extradural morphine after caesarean section. Br J Anaesth 60:627, 1988

158. Baxter AD, Laganiere S, Samson B et al: A dose-response study of nalbuphine for post-thoracotomy epidural analgesia. Can J Anaesth 38:175, 1991

159. Camann WR, Hurley RH, Gilbertson LI et al: Epidural nalbuphine for analgesia following caesarean delivery: dose-response and effect of local anaesthetic choice. Can J Anaesth 38:728, 1991

160. Lawhorn CD, McNitt JD, Fibuch EE et al: Epidural morphine with butorphanol for postoperative analgesia after cesarean delivery. Anesth Analg 72:53, 1991

161. Palacios QT, Jones MM, Hawkins JL et al: Post-caesarean section analgesia: a comparison of epidural butorphanol and morphine. Can J Anaesth 38:24, 1991

162. Etches RC: A comparison of the analgesic and respiratory effects of epidural nalburphine or morphine in postthoracotomy patients. Anesthesiology 75:9, 1991

163. Rodriguez J, Abboud TK, Reyes A et al: Continuous infusion epidural anesthesia during labor: a randomized, double-blind comparison of 0.0625% bupivacaine/0.002% butorphanol and 0.125% bupivacaine. Reg Anesth 15:300, 1990

164. Chrubasik J, Vogel W, Trotschler H, Farthmann EH: Continuous-plus-on-demand epidural infusion of buprenorphine versus morphine in postoperative treatment of pain. Arzeim-Forsch 37:361, 1987

165. Gundersen RY, Andersen R, Narverud G: Postoperative pain relief with high-dose epidural buprenorphine: a double-blind study. Acta Anaesthiol Scan 30:664, 1986

166. Celleno D, Capogna G: Spinal buprenorphine for postoperative analgesia after caesarean section. Acta Anaesthesiol Scand 33:236, 1989

167. Molke Jensen F, Jensen N-H, Holk IK, Ravnborg M: Prolonged and biphasic respiratory depression following epidural buprenorphine. Anaesthesia 42:470, 1987

168. Carol P, Crawford ME, Ravlo O, Bach V: Long term treatment with epidural opioids. Anaesthesia 41:32, 1986

169. Ackerman WE, Juneja MM, Kaczorowski DM, Colclough GW: A comparison of the incidence of pruritus following epidural opioid administration in the parturient. Can J Anaesth 36:388, 1989

170. Cohen S, Amar D, Pantuck CB et al: Epidural patient-controlled analgesia after cesarean section: buprenorphine-0.015% bupivacaine with epinephrine versus fentanyl-0.015% bupivacaine with and without epinephrine. Anesth Analg 74:226, 1992

171. Hunt CO: Epidural butorphanol-bupivacaine for analgesia during labor and delivery. Anesth Analg 68:323, 1989

172. Yaksh TL, Collins JG: Studies in animals should

precede human use of spinally administered drugs. Anesthesiology 70:4, 1989

173. Rawal N, Nuutinen L, Raj PP et al: Behavioral and histopathologic effects following intrathecal administration of butorphanol, sufentanil, and nalbuphine in sheep. Anesthesiology 75:1025, 1991

174. Abouleish E, Barmada MA, Nemoto EM et al: Acute and chronic effects of intrathecal morphine in monkeys. Br. J. Anesth. 53:1027, 1981

175. King FG, Baxter AD, Mathieson G: Tissue reaction of morphine applied to the epidural space of dogs. Can J Anaesth 31:268, 1984

176. Coombs DW: Toxicity of chronic spinal analgesia in a canine model: neuropathologic observations with dezocine lactate. 15:94, 1990

177. Camann WR, Loferski BL, Fanciullo GJ et al: Does epidural administration of butorphanol offer any clinical advantage over the intravenous route? Anesthesiology 76:216, 1992

178. Fox AW: Epidural buprenorphine. Can J Anaesth 37:273, 1990

179. Henderson SK, Cohen H: Nalbuphine augmentation of analgesia and reversal of side effects following epidural hydromorphone. Anesthesiology 65:216, 1986

180. Baxter AD, Samson B, Penning J et al: Prevention of epidural morphine-induced respiratory depression with intravenous nalbuphine infusion in postthoracotomy patients. Can J Anaesth 36:503, 1989

181. Cheng EY, May J: Nalbuphine reversal of respiratory depression after epidural sufentanil. Crit Care Med 17:378, 1989

182. Penning JP, Samson B, Baxter AD: Reversal of epidural morphine-induced respiratory depression and pruritus with nalbuphine. Can J Anaesth 35:599, 1988

183. Davies GG: A blinded study using nalbuphine for prevention of pruritus induced by epidural fentanyl. Anesthesiology 69:763, 1988

184. Preston KL, Bigelow GE, Liebson IA: Antagonist effects of nalbuphine in opioid-dependent human volunteers. J Pharmacol Exp Ther 248:929, 1989

185. Preston KL, Bigelow GE, Liebson IA: Butorphanol-precipitated withdrawal in opioid-dependent humans. J Pharmacol Exp Ther 246:441, 1988

186. Preston KL, Jasinski DR: Abuse liability studies of opioid agonist-antagonists in humans. Drug Alcohol Depend 28:49, 1991

187. Longnecker D, Grazis P, Eggers G: Naloxone antagonism of morphine induced respiratory depression. Anesth Analg 52:447, 1973

188. Dailey P, Brookshire G, Shnider S et al: The effects of naloxone associated with the intrathecal use of morphine in labor. Anesth Analg 64:658, 1985

189. Rawal N, Schott U, Dahlstrom B et al: Influence of naloxone infusion on analgesia and respiratory depression following epidural morphine. Anesthesiology 64:194, 1986

190. Johnson A, Bengtsson M, Lofstrom J et al: Influence of postoperative naloxone infusion on respiration and pain relief after intrathecal morphine. Reg Anesth 13:146, 1988

191. Geuneron J, Ecoffey C, Carli P et al: Effect of naloxone infusion on analgesia and respiratory depression after epidural fentanyl. Anesth Analg 67:35, 1988

192. Korbon G, James D, Verlander M et al: Intramuscular naloxone reverses the side effects of epidural morphine while preserving analgesia. Reg Anesth 10:16, 1985

193. Abboud T, Afrasiabi A, Davidson J et al: Prophylactic oral naltrexone with epidural morphine: effect on adverse reactions and ventilatory responses to carbon dioxide. Anesthesiology 72:233, 1990

194. Smith G, Pinnock C: Naloxone—paradox or panacea? Br J Anaesth 57:547, 1985

195. Zimmerman D, Leander J: Opioid antagonists: structure activity relationships. NIDA Res Monogr 96:50, 1990

196. Gal T, DiFazio C: Prolonged antagonism of opioid action with intravenous nalmefene in man. Anesthesiology 64:175, 1986

197. Gal T, DiFazio C, Dixon R: Prolonged blockade of opioid effect with oral nalmefene. Clin Pharmacol Ther 40:537, 1986

198. Konieczko K, Jones J, Barrowcliffe M et al: Antagonism of morphine-induced respiratory depression with nalmefene. Br J Anaesth 61:318, 1988

199. Schulz R, Hertz A: The guinea pig ileum as an in vitro model to analyse dependence liability of narcotic drugs. p. 319. In Kosterlitz HW (ed): Opioids and Endogenous Opioid Peptides. North-Holland, Amsterdam, 1976

Clinical Pharmacology and Applications of Spinal Opioids

Alan N. Sandler

The term *spinally administered opioid* includes all opioids injected into either the epidural or subarachnoid spaces surrounding the spinal cord. This practice has been adopted universally as a powerful technique for the control of acute and chronic pain. The discovery of discrete opioid receptors[1] and the demonstration of their presence in the brain[2] and spinal cord[3] was a major impetus for the introduction of the technique. Spinally administered opioids exhibit major differences in pharmacokinetic and pharmacodynamic characteristics compared with the more usual routes of administration (intramuscular, intravenous). Rational clinical use depends on an understanding of these basic aspects of this method of opioid administration.

PHARMACOKINETICS OF SPINAL OPIOID ADMINISTRATION

Important physical chemical properties for spinal opioids include molecular weight, lipid solubility, degree of ionization, and specific and nonspecific receptor binding in the spinal cord.[4] In general, these factors are of greater importance for epidural administration than for intrathecal administration as a result of the barrier imposed to access to the cerebrospinal fluid (CSF) by the dura mater. Routes of entry into the CSF from the epidural space include blood vessels around the dorsal nerve roots and the arachnoid granulations located at the entry zones of the nerve roots. Once in the CSF, penetration of the spinal cord and bulk movement of CSF circulation become the important rate limiting steps for the onset of analgesia and side effects (Fig. 6-1). Opioids with low molecular weight tend to have a high permeability through the dura in vitro.[5] Thus, the permeability of lumbar dura mater in vitro is nine times greater for morphine (molecular weight, 285) than for buprenorphine (molecular weight, 468). The pK_a of most opioids (i.e., the pH at which ionized and un-ionized forms are equal) can vary from 7.9 to 9.4 (i.e., most are weak bases). This means that, at physiologic pH (7.3 for CSF), most opioids are predominantly ionized. Alfentanil, with a pK_a of 6.5 is an exception; at pH 7.4, alfentanil has an un-ionized fraction of 89%. The un-ionized opioid is more lipid soluble and thus crosses lipid membranes more readily. Lipid solubility is expressed by the partition coefficient (P), which measures the ratio of the opioid in the hydrophobic phase (e.g., octanol) to the drug in the hydrophilic phase (water). Lipid solubility tends to promote more rapid absorption from the epidural space into the systemic circulation (epidural veins) and into the CSF.[6] Opioids with high lipid solubility, such as

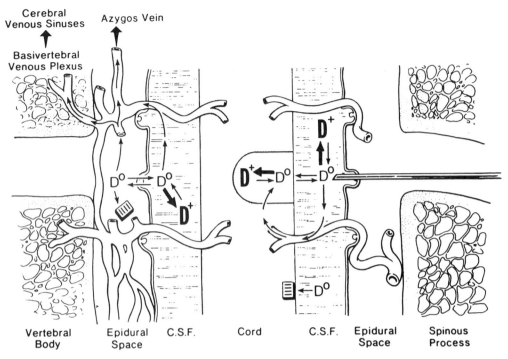

Fig. 6-1 Pharmacokinetic model of a subarachnoid injection of a hydrophilic opioid such as morphine. D^0, un-ionized drug; D^+, ionized hydrophilic drug. A spinal needle is shown delivering opioid directly to the cerebrospinal fluid (CSF). Nearby spinal arteries are in proximity to the arachnoid granulations. In the spinal cord, equilibria of D^0 and D^+ on spinal receptors are shown, with nonspecific lipid binding sites (boxes with lines). Epidural veins, in proximity to arachnoid granulations, are depicted as the major spinal route of clearance of intrathecal opioid. The two alternative routes of venous drainage are shown. (From Cousins et al.,[49] with permission.)

buprenorphine, sufentanil, lofentanil, and fentanyl, diffuse more easily across the dura than do opioids with low lipid solubility, such as morphine, dihydromorphine, hydromorphone, and ketobemidone. Conversely, hydrophilic opioids are very slowly reabsorbed from the CSF back into the systemic circulation and thus tend to have a longer duration of action. This principle probably holds true for epidural or intrathecal injections of lipid soluble and lipid insoluble opioids. Thus the onset of analgesia is slow and the duration is prolonged for morphine. The onset is much faster for a bolus of fentanyl, but analgesia is only marginally longer in duration than for an equivalent intravenous dose (Fig. 6-2).[7] When epidural opioids are administered by bolus plus infusion, the lipid soluble opioids (alfentanil, fentanyl, and sufentanil) seem to confer no advantage over intravenous adminis-

tration[8–14] because the opioid dose, plasma concentration, degree of pain relief, and side effects are similar between the two routes. In contrast, lipid insoluble opioids (morphine) are effective when given by epidural infusion at very low doses and do not tend to accumulate in the systemic circulation.

Model of Intrathecal Opioids

Most animal and human investigation has involved morphine because its long duration of analgesia makes it suitable for a single subarachnoid dose. Intrathecal injection of morphine (highly hydrophilic) produces extremely high CSF concentrations.[15,16] The morphine moves slowly into spinal cord specific and nonspecific binding sites and clearance sites (arachnoid granulations). Uptake into the systemic circulation is minimal, resulting in subanalgesic plasma concentrations.[17,18] Distribu-

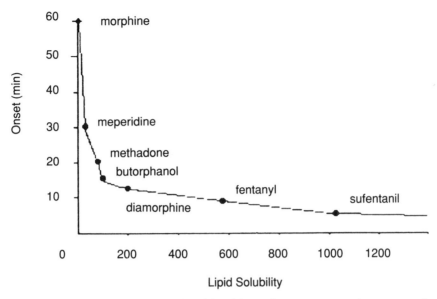

Fig. 6-2 Relationship between lipid solubility, blood-brain barrier penetration rate, and rapidity of onset for spinal opioids. Low lipid solubility and limited rate of blood-brain barrier penetration results in slow onset. Higher blood-brain barrier solubility results in a rapid onset of opioid effects. (Adapted from De Castro et al.,[188] with permission.)

tion of morphine within the CSF is related to CSF bulk flow. DiChiro[19] showed that 30 percent of lumbar intrathecal labeled albumin reaches the ventricular system within 12 hours and 100 percent within 24 hrs. The slow movement of morphine cephalad from the lumbar sac has been demonstrated pharmacodynamically in volunteer studies[20,21] in which the rostral spread of morphine (after epidural injection) was tracked by the slow cephalad progression of analgesia to ice and pin scratch and the onset of respiratory depression (depressed CO_2 response curve), nausea, pruritus, and urine retention (Fig. 6-3). Enhancement of CSF bulk flow may occur with changes in intra-abdominal and intrathoracic pressure,[22] but more importantly, the patient's position (e.g., head down) can affect CSF movement. Allinson et al.[23] demonstrated that, in the head down position, a water soluble contrast medium spreads within 10 to 15 minutes to the lateral ventricle; the same may apply to opioids that persist in the CSF (e.g., morphine). Thus, for morphine, low lipid solubility and slow uptake into the spinal cord result in a slow

onset of analgesia (although it is faster than that for epidural administration), and slow egress results in prolonged duration.

For a lipid soluble opioid such as fentanyl,[24] the onset of analgesia is rapid, but the duration (2 to 3 hours) is not as long as for morphine because of the rapid entry into and egress from the spinal cord. Agents with high μ receptor affinity (e.g., lofentanil[24]) have a longer duration of action (5 to 10 hours). Nonspecific lipid binding sites in the spinal cord tend to form a "sink" for lipid soluble opioids,[4] and this is reflected in the large doses required for intrathecal analgesia, e.g., 1/300th of the intravenous dose of morphine (0.2 to 0.5 mg) provides 12 to 24 hours of analgesia postoperatively, whereas the fentanyl dose is reduced by only 25 percent (50 to 75 μg) and sufentanil is reduced by 50 percent (25 to 50 μg).

Model of Epidural Opioids

The epidural route presents a more complicated model than does the intrathecal route, which is related to dural penetration, fat deposition, systemic

DELAYED RESPIRATORY DEPRESSION

Hours	+0.5	+3	+4.5	+5	+6–9	+16–22
Analgetic Level	0	T_{9-11}	T_5	C_{7-8}/T_1	V_1-V_3	
					Urine Retention	
				Pruritis	Nausea	
CO_2 Response		Brief↓	Sustained↓ ·····················→		Peak↓	Residual↓

Fig. 6-3 Respiratory and other side effects following epidural morphine. (Adapted from Cousins et al.,[49] with permission.)

absorption, and larger drug doses. Morphine is absorbed into the systemic circulation after epidural bolus injection with peak plasma concentrations occurring within 15 minutes.[18,25] The morphine plasma concentration curves were similar to those seen after intramuscular injection of the similar doses[18,25] (6 mg epidurally and 10 mg intramuscularly; plasma levels ~45 to 50 ng/ml; analgesic plasma concentration for morphine = 15 to 35 ng/ml[26]). Morphine is also measurable in the CSF 15 minutes after epidural injection, but peak concentrations occur 90 to 120 minutes after administration.[25,27] The peak CSF concentration (e.g., 1,575 ng/ml) is approximately 25 to 30 times that in the plasma and may reach very high concentrations.[28] In contrast, the intramuscular administration of morphine produced peak CSF levels of 10 to 20 ng/ml. Morphine's presence in the CSF is protracted with 80 percent still present 4 hours after injection and about 50 percent remaining 24 hours after injection.[27] Meperidine and heroin (diacetylmorphine), both more lipid soluble than morphine, enter the CSF faster, and the more rapid increase in CSF concentration coincides with the onset of analgesia.[27,29] Similarly, peak plasma concentrations of these moderately lipid soluble opioids also occur rapidly (within 10 to 15 minutes), and large doses can produce analgesic blood levels for a short period of time.[30,31] A dose of 30 mg of epidural meperidine produced a systemic

concentration of approximately 200 ng/ml within 15 minutes in the study by Sjostrom et al.[27] (systemic analgesic concentration for meperidine = 400 to 800 ng/ml).[32] However, like morphine, bolus doses of epidural meperidine and heroin produce analgesia that persists well beyond the time when the blood concentrations have declined below analgesic levels, suggesting a primarily spinal mode of action. Bolus doses of highly lipid soluble opioids, such as fentanyl and sufentanil, are rapidly absorbed into the CSF.[33,34] Lipophilic opioids (fentanyl, alfentanil, and sufentanil) have a significantly more rapid onset of analgesia than does morphine and a shorter duration.[35,36] Sufentanil's peak blood concentrations were lower after epidural administration compared with intravenous administration of equivalent doses.[37] After epidural bolus doses of fentanyl,[7] plasma concentrations were below analgesic levels (1 to 3 ng/ml). In addition, fentanyl blood concentrations were lower after epidural compared with intramuscular administration with longer lasting and improved analgesia after the epidural administration.[38]

Epidural opioid models become more complex when combination bolus/infusion regimens are used. The rationale for continuous epidural morphine infusion use is the reduction in analgesic requirements and thus a reduced incidence of side effects, especially respiratory depression.[39] Epidural morphine infusions are effective in producing analgesia and allow very low doses to be used (100 to 500 μg/h).[40–43] At these rates of infusion, plasma morphine concentrations are very low or undetectable (2 to 7 ng/ml)[40,42] compared with the much higher plasma concentrations seen after bolus epidural morphine doses.[25,44,45] Presumably, the CSF concentration also is markedly decreased. In contrast, most clinical studies involving lipid soluble opioids show no benefit of epidural over intravenous infusions when they are administered over 24 to 48 hours.[8–14,46,47] The plasma concentrations of lipid soluble opioids at equianalgesic epidural or intravenous doses are very similar, indicating pronounced systemic absorption.[10,12] Positioning of the epidural catheter at the precise dermatomal level of the surgery allows a decrease in the epidural dose of fentanyl and a consequent reduction in the plasma concentration, at least for post-thoracotomy pain relief.[48]

THERAPEUTIC DRUG EFFECTS

The primary therapeutic effect of using spinal opioid techniques is the production of analgesia in acute and chronic pain states.[49] However, not all acute and chronic pain situations are amenable to spinal opioids. For example, spinal opioids alone (except for meperidine) are inadequate for surgical anesthesia, and epidural opioids alone are generally inadequate for labor pain,[50–52] although intrathecal opioids are effective for the first and second stages of labor.[53,54] Similarly, in patients with cancer who have "central" pain unresponsive to oral opioids, spinal opioids are also likely to be ineffective. For pain of neoplastic origin, spinal opioids are the most predictable in their efficacy when used to treat continuous dull somatic pain from deep structures or continuous visceral pain.[55] The therapeutic advantages of spinal opioids are apparent when they are contrasted with those of local anesthetic agents, the other class of drugs that are commonly given spinally to produce regional anesthesia and analgesia. Spinal opioids are not associated with sympathetic, sensory, or motor blockade. Neuraxial opioids may also play an important role in decreasing morbidity and mortality rates after major surgery or in critically ill patients (see Acute Pain: Outcome Studies).[56–61] Spinal morphine has

been used as a treatment for bladder spasm[62] and for the short-term treatment of enuresis.[63] Spinal morphine has been shown to block polysynaptic flexion reflexes and has been used for the treatment of muscle spasms associated with spasticity[64] and multiple sclerosis.[65]

Mode of Action of Therapeutic Effects of Spinal Opioids

Opioids exert their spinal analgesic effect through opioid receptors in the substantia gelatinosa (Fig. 6-4). This is thought to produce presynaptic and postsynaptic inhibition of neuronal conduction,[66,67] most likely mediated by ion channels. Sharp, intense pain (surgical pain or labor pain conducted by A-δ fibers) is less readily blocked than is dull pain (C fibers). Of all the opioids used spinally, intrathecal meperidine is the only agent shown to be effective as a sole anesthetic agent for surgery,[68] probably because of its combined local anesthetic and opioid effects; meperidine has pronounced local anesthetic effects.

In general, opioids exert their analgesic effects predominantly at the spinal level after intrathecal administration; small doses are required, especially for morphine, resulting in high CSF levels and low blood levels. This concept is probably also correct for epidural bolus doses and infusions of lipid insoluble opioids. However, epidural infusions of lipid soluble opioids (including methadone[69]) produce analgesia by a combined spinal/systemic effect as a result of the relatively high blood concentrations that develop.

Spinal opioids have much less effect on the neuroendocrine and metabolic response to surgery[70–72] (or any trauma) than do spinally administered local anesthetic agents. The neuroendocrine/metabolic response to surgery is complex[73] and involves changes in many critical hormones and metabolic mechanisms, including glucose, glucagon, insulin, free fatty acids, nitrogen balance, cortisol, growth hormone, catecholamines, and other substances. Nonetheless, the better analgesia produced by spinal opioids compared with intramuscular or intravenous agents was associated with a reduction in neuroendocrine response, as measured by antidiuretic hormone secretion or adrenocortical and hyperglycemic responses.[70,74] These effects can also

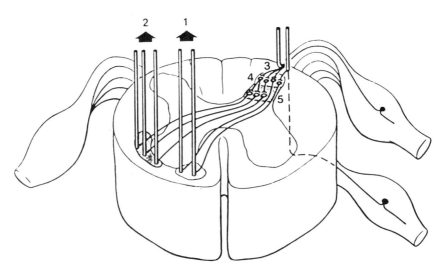

Fig. 6-4 Ascending pathways and dorsal horn region of spinal cord. Afferent fibers are shown entering the dorsal nerve root by way of dorsal root ganglion to reach Lissauer's tract (*3*). Primary afferents have their cell body in the dorsal root ganglion. The second order neuron has its cell body in the substantia gelatinosa (*4*). (*1*) and (*2*) = intermingled fibers of spinothalamic and spinoreticular tracts; (*5*) = Rexed laminae IV, V, and VI. (From Cousins et al.,[49] with permission.)

be demonstrated using high dose intravenous opioid infusion, but this requires prolonged mechanical ventilation.[75]

NONTHERAPEUTIC DRUG EFFECTS

Nontherapeutic drug effects is the term used to describe the unwanted side effects produced by spinal opioids, including nausea and vomiting, pruritus, urinary retention, and respiratory depression.

Nausea and Vomiting

Incidence

Nausea and vomiting occur frequently after surgery with reported frequencies of 20 to 50 percent.[76] Other contributory factors, apart from opioid administration, include the type of surgery, pain, hypotension, gastric distention, motion, and gender (women are two to three times more susceptible to opioid induced nausea and vomiting than are men).[76,77] Opioids administered by the spinal route do not appear to have a higher incidence of nausea and vomiting than do those administered by other routes.[78,79] Rapp et al.[77] found an incidence of approximately 20 to 30 percent after gynecologic surgery with either patient-controlled analgesia using morphine or epidural morphine. Similarly, there was no difference in the incidence associated with lipid soluble opioids (fentanyl), whether given by intravenous or epidural infusion.[8,12] The dose-response relationship for spinal opioids and nausea and vomiting is not clear, with some studies showing no relationship between nausea and vomiting and the total dose of epidural morphine,[80] although studies with intrathecal morphine demonstrate a positive dose response.[81,82]

Mechanism

Opioids cause nausea and vomiting by direct stimulation of the chemoreceptor trigger zone of the brain stem and because of delayed gastric emptying. The inhibition of gastric emptying is related to the direct action of opioids on the gastrointestinal tract, inhibiting acetylcholine induced smooth muscle contraction. The activation of opioid receptors in the fourth ventricle and spinal cord also decreases gastric emptying.[83]

Treatment

Routine prophylactic administration of antiemetics is unreliable and is associated with significant side effects.[76] For example, transdermal scopolamine has been used prophylactically before epidural morphine. A decrease in nausea and vomiting was seen, but there was an unacceptable increase in side effects (dry mouth, drowsiness, and disorientation).[84,85] Opioid antagonists (e.g., naloxone) in small doses are often useful for treating spinal opioid induced nausea and vomiting.[86] However, prophylactic naloxone infusions or oral naltrexone, when used with spinal opioids, tend to be associated with a decreased intensity and duration of pain relief.[87,88] When nausea and vomiting occur, attention should be paid to optimizing the patient's clinical condition, including correction of hypotension and treatment of excessive pain. If nausea and vomiting persist, specific intravenous antiemetic therapy should be used (see Ch. 30). Droperidol has been administered epidurally with morphine, resulting in a significant decrease in the incidence of nausea and vomiting.[89,90] The new selective serotonin 5-HT$_3$ receptor antagonists (e.g., ondansetron) may be effective in the treatment of opioid-induced nausea and vomiting.[91] Refractory cases may require treatment with scopolamine or naloxone by infusion. A change to an alternative opioid may be helpful in some cases.

Pruritus

Incidence

Pruritus is a common side effect of opioids, regardless of the route of administration. For spinally administered morphine, there is considerable evidence that the incidence and severity of pruritus is markedly increased in comparison with morphine administered either intramuscularly or by patient-controlled analgesia (Table 6-1).[78,79,92–94] Pruritus is a particularly common side effect after epidural morphine analgesia for cesarean section.[95]

Mechanism

The mechanism of pruritus after spinal opioid administration is unknown but does not seem to be mediated by histamine release. Pruritus often presents in the facial area several hours after administration of intrathecal morphine (0.1 to 0.25 mg),[54] corresponding to the demonstrated cephalad movement of morphine in the CSF.[34] The small dose and the time delay to symptoms implies a centrally mediated effect.

Table 6-1 Pruritus Following Morphine Administration[a]

| Reference | Pruritus | Route of Administration | | |
		Intramuscular	Patient-Controlled Analgesia	Epidural
Harrison et al.[93] (1988)	Present	17	38	72
	Treated	6	11	45
Eisenach et al.[79] (1988)	Present	35	60	85
	Treated	5	5	40
Daley et al.[78] (1990)	Present	46	N/A	91
	Treated	15	N/A	40
Loper and Ready[94] (1989)	Present	N/A	35	73
	Treated	N/A	17	26
Loper et al.[92] (1989)	Present	N/A	N/A	N/A
	Treated	N/A	4	33

Abbreviations: NA, not available.

[a] All values given as the percentage of the total.

(Adapted from Etches,[105] with permission.)

Treatment

Pruritus following spinal opioids is often unresponsive to antihistamines. Small doses of naloxone (40 μg IV or 100 to 200 μg IM) are generally effective without reversing analgesia. Oral naltrexone[88] or intravenous nalbuphine[97] are also effective alternative treatments.

Urinary Retention

Incidence

Urinary retention after anesthesia and surgery is common and has many contributing factors, e.g., pain, sedation, the supine position, and the anticholinergic effect of antiemetic drugs and opioids administered for analgesia. The reported incidence of urinary retention after spinal opioids is much higher than for opioids administered by other parenteral routes. For example, epidural morphine resulted in urinary retention in 90 percent of male volunteers[98] and in 48 to 62 percent of patients after orthopaedic surgery compared with 12 to 24 percent when intramuscular or intravenous opioids are used.[85,99,100] Stenseth et al.[80] found an incidence of 42 percent with epidural morphine after a variety of surgical procedures.

Mechanism

Bladder relaxation and loss of micturition reflexes have been demonstrated in animal models and in humans after spinal morphine[101–103] with an increase in external sphincter tone in humans.[67] Inhibition of primary parasympathetic afferent activity from the bladder plus inhibition of efferent parasympathetic and somatic outflow to the bladder, urethra, and pelvic floor have been suggested as possible mechanisms causing urinary retention after spinal opioids.[101]

Treatment

Autonomically active drugs (e.g., bethanechol) or α antagonists (e.g., phenoxybenzamine) are only minimally or partially effective in treating opioid induced urinary retention.[98,104] Intravenous naloxone is effective in reversing urinary retention, but large doses may be required, which may reverse analgesia.[104] A practical approach often involves "in-and-out" urethral catheterization or indwelling catheterization if necessary.[105]

Respiratory Depression

Incidence

Respiratory depression is by far the most serious side effect secondary to opioid administration by any route. The first reports of severe respiratory depression caused by spinal opioids appeared in 1979.[106] There are now numerous case reports of severe clinical respiratory depression after spinal opioids.[106] The incidence of clinically significant respiratory depression, gleaned from retrospective surveys and large scale chart reviews,[107,108] is very low, ranging from 0.25 to 0.4 percent in earlier nationwide studies in Sweden[107] (6,000 to 9,000 patients) to 0.09 percent (epidural) and 0.36 percent (intrathecal) in later surveys (11,000 patients).[108] Epidural morphine was the primary opioid used in these two surveys, and patients with chronic pain were included, who may be resistant to the respiratory depressant effects of opioids. However, a similar range of incidence has been reported in retrospective surveys of patients with acute pain who have received epidural morphine, e.g., 0.6 percent (623 patients),[109] 3.1 percent (128 patients),[110] and 0.9 percent (1,085 patients).[80] In a retrospective study of 4,880 patients who had undergone cesarian section, a single dose of epidural morphine (2 to 5 mg) was associated with 0.25 percent incidence of decreased respiratory rate but no life threatening respiratory depression.[111] However, smaller, prospective studies have found a higher incidence of respiratory depression from epidural morphine (Table 6-2).[112–120] Thus, respiratory depression after spinal opioids may be more common than indicated from retrospective surveys, but it appears to be infrequently life threatening. There are few large scale studies examining respiratory depression after lipid soluble opioids. One study of epidural fentanyl infusions (500 patients) reported an incidence of respiratory depression of 0.6 percent, which is similar to that of morphine.[121] The incidence of life threatening respiratory depression for parenteral opioids has been minimally investigated; the one survey commonly cited puts the incidence at 0.9 percent (860 patients).[122]

Table 6-2 Respiratory Depression Detected in Prospective Studies of Epidural Morphine

Reference	Incidence	Dose	Comments
Chambers et al.[114] (1981)	1/10	10 mg	Delayed emergence from anesthesia. Naloxone 0.2 mg × 1
Torda and Pybus[115] (1981)	1/130	4 mg	Respiratory depression 12 h postinjection. Not responsive to naloxone. Etiology unknown.
Modig and Paalzow[116] (1981)	1/42	5 mg + 5 mg	T8 epidural for abdominal aortic aneurysm surgery. Respiratory depression 6 h following second dose.
Weddell et al.[119] (1981)	1/34	8.4 mg	70-year-old woman. Somnolent and respiratory rate of 6, 6 h after injection. Naloxone × 4 doses at 6, 8, 10 and 12 h.
Klinck and Lindop[118] (1982)	1/10	8 mg	71-year-old fit man. Thoracic epidural. Slow respiratory rate at 8 and 14 h. Responded to naloxone × 2 doses.
Martin et al.[119] (1982)	1/12	8 mg	Respiratory rate of 8 and PCO₂ of 49, 10 h postinjection. Responded to naloxone 0.2 mg.
Ready et al.[120] (1987)	2/66	4–5 mg	Respiratory rate < 8 on one occasion. Patients in no distress. Time since injection not given.

(Adapted from Etches et al.,[106] with permission.)

Mechanism

Respiratory depression after spinal morphine is related to the movement of morphine in the CSF cephalad toward the fourth ventricle with subsequent access to the respiratory centers. The onset of respiratory depression after intrathecal morphine is extremely variable but tends to occur several hours after injection.[49,106] Respiratory depression after epidural morphine and meperidine, has occurred more quickly, within 1 hour,[123] and it may be related to early systemic absorption and redistribution to the respiratory center.[34] However, respiratory depression is usually delayed for 4 to 6 hours and may occur long after administration.[106] Several factors predisposing patients to respiratory depression after spinal opioids are listed in Table 6-3.

The mechanism of respiratory depression after spinal lipid soluble opioids is less clear but may be related to both the movement of the opioid in the CSF[124] and the systemic uptake and redistribution to the brain stem respiratory centers. This mechanism appears to apply to prolonged epidural infusions of fentanyl.[12,125,126] Early, severe respiratory depression has occurred after large bolus doses of epidural sufentanil.[33] The onset of respiratory depression may be unpredictable in some cases, as with morphine.[121]

Treatment

Naloxone in small bolus doses (100 μg) or by infusion (400 to 800 μg/h) may reverse spinal opioid induced respiratory depression without reversing

Table 6-3 Factors Predisposing to the Development of Respiratory Depression Following Epidural Opioids

Drug Factors
   Hydrophilic drug (i.e., morphine)
   Large doses
   Repeated doses
   Concomitant administration of parenteral opioids or other central nervous system depressants.

Patient Factors
   Elderly or debilitated
   Coexisting respiratory disease
   Thoracic epidural
   High sensitivity to opioids (i.e., no previous exposure to opioids)
   Intrathecal administration
   Raised intrathoracic pressure (e.g., controlled ventilation, coughing, or vomiting)

(Adapted from Etches et al.[106] with permission.)

analgesia, although this claim is controversial.[87,127–129] As the effects of naloxone are short lived (intravenous, 45 minutes; intramuscular, 2 to 3 hours), infusions are often necessary. Opioid agonist-antagonist agents (e.g., nalbuphine)[97,130] have also been used to treat or prevent respiratory depression with some degree of success (see Ch. 5). In extreme cases, mechanical ventilation may be required.

Dysphoria and Other Central Nervous System Effects

Dysphoria, sedation, and catatonia (after prolonged use in patients with cancer)[131] have been reported in both volunteer and clinical studies. Sedation can be minimized by using smaller doses.[97,132,133]

DOSE-RESPONSE RELATIONSHIPS

Dose-response relationships have been examined for postoperative opioid spinal analgesia and for some of the related side effects.[49] These have been particularly well described for morphine for postoperative analgesia,[119,134,135] postcesarean section analgesia,[136] and analgesia for labor and delivery.[51] Two, 4, or 8 mg of epidural morphine are more effective than 0.5 to 1.0 mg for postoperative analgesia after abdominal or lower limb surgery.[119] Similar results were obtained after cesarean section in which 2 mg of morphine was ineffective, but larger doses (5 to 7.5 mg) provided good analgesia.[134,137] Other studies have found little difference in the degree of analgesia after doses of epidural morphine ranging between 2 and 8 mg, but they described a graded increase in duration as the doses increased.[18,138] Increasing the dose also leads to an increase in side effects, especially respiratory depression.[106,113,132,135] The dose-response relationship for postoperative epidural morphine analgesia is strongly affected by age; decreased doses are effective in elderly patients.[139] Ready[120] described a significant negative correlation between age and effective dose per 24 hours.

DRUG INTERACTIONS

Drug interactions between spinal opioids and other agents can be divided into interactions of spinal opioids with other spinally administered drugs or with systemically administered drugs. Several different types of agents have been either mixed with spinal opioids or given concurrently through spinal or systemic routes to achieve an increase in analgesic efficacy and/or duration or a decrease in side effects. These include epinephrine, local anesthetic agents, droperidol, clonidine, and nonsteroidal analgesic agents. In addition, opioid antagonists (e.g., naloxone) or agonist-antagonist agents (e.g., nalbuphine) have been administered with spinal opioids to decrease the respiratory depressant effects.

Epinephrine

The rationale for the use of a vasoconstrictor such as epinephrine in combination with spinal opioids is to decrease the rate of systemic absorption of the opioid and thereby enhance analgesia. The results of studies in which epinephrine was added to epidurally administered morphine are controversial,[141] with some decrease in systemic absorption being demonstrated but with conflicting results regarding an improvement in analgesia. An increase in the severity of side effects, especially respiratory depression, has been claimed.[140] The addition of epinephrine to diamorphine decreased the latter's systemic absorption and prolonged analgesia,[142] prolonged epidural sufentanil analgesia in volunteers,[143] and prolonged postcesarian section analgesia with epidural fentanyl.[144]

Local Anesthetic Agents

Bupivacaine is the most common local anesthetic used in combination with spinal opioids. Low dose morphine and bupivacaine (morphine, 0.1 mg/ml; bupivacaine, 0.1 percent was effective, but no better than morphine (0.1 mg/ml) alone, after thoracotomy[41] or upper abdominal surgery.[145] Similar results were found for bupivacaine combined with fentanyl for pain relief after thoracotomy, upper abdominal surgery, or knee surgery.[146,147] Low dose bupivacaine (0.125 percent) added to heroin for posthysterectomy analgesia was only superior to heroin alone when given by such high infusion rates that a T6-T8 sensory level block and 70 percent urinary retention developed.[148] Morphine combined with higher concentrations of bupivacaine (0.5 percent) produced total analgesia after upper abdominal surgery but also produced a high sensory block (T6-T8) and a 20 percent incidence of hypotension requiring treatment.[149] However, recent studies have suggested that the synergistic effects of the two different types of analgesics acting by different mechanisms may allow decreased dosages and thus decreased side effects of both opioids and local anesthetics. Bupivacaine in concentrations between 0.125 and 0.25 percent, added to low doses of morphine or fentanyl, can provide significantly better analgesia than the opioid alone, with the 0.125 percent mixture having the least number of side effects.[150,151] Combinations of opioids and local anesthetics (usually bupivacaine) are extensively used in obstetric patients for labor analgesia because epidural opioids alone are relatively ineffective during labor. As in postoperative patients, the optimal concentration of bupivacaine lies between 0.125 and 0.25 percent, although lower concentrations have been used with effective analgesia, especially in early labor (see Obstetric Pain).

Droperidol

Droperidol, a dopamine receptor antagonist with antiemetic properties has been given epidurally with epidural morphine. A significant reduction in nausea and vomiting was seen with only a minimal increase in sedation.[89,90]

α_2 Agonists

Clonidine, an α_2 agonist, provides some degree of analgesia when given epidurally by activating postjunctional α_2 adrenoceptors in the dorsal horn and inhibiting the firing of nociceptive neurons. Conflicting results have been reported as to the degree of analgesia and the incidence of side effects (sedation, hypotension, bradycardia, and possibly respiratory depression).[152] However, recent studies of epidural clonidine combined with fentanyl,[153] sufentanil,[154] or morphine[155] have shown improved

analgesia and decreased supplemental opioid usage.

Nonsteroidal Anti-Inflammatory Drugs

Nonsteroidal anti-inflammatory drugs (e.g., indomethacin, and diclofenac) have been used in conjunction with spinal opioids or with spinal opioid/local anesthetic combinations. Excellent postoperative analgesia with a reduction in epidural opioid requirement was seen with this type of combination therapy.[156–158]

Interactions With Agents to Decrease Respiratory Depression

Several agents and techniques have been used to decrease the incidence and severity of respiratory depression from spinal opioids, with varying degrees of success. These include the systemic administration of mixed agonist-antagonist opioids, such as nalbuphine,[130] and low dose intravenous naloxone infusion.[128]

Interactions With Systemic Opioids and Sedative Agents

The interaction of systemic opioids or sedative agents with spinal opioids generally increases the risk of respiratory depression.[106–108,159,160] The clinical significance of these interactions has not been well defined.

INDIVIDUAL DRUGS

μ Agonist Opioids

Morphine

Epidural

Epidural bolus doses are typically 2 to 5 mg for peripheral surgery or 6 to 8 mg for major intracavitary surgery.[139,152,161] The peak analgesic effect is obtained after 30 to 60 minutes.[25,56,119,159] The duration of analgesia is variable but prolonged (6 to 24 hours or longer).[117] Epidural morphine enters the CSF slowly and produces high CSF concentrations that remain elevated for a prolonged period.[162] There is also a small amount of systemic uptake after each bolus dose,[163] however, plasma levels fall away fairly rapidly, supporting the concept of a primarily spinal site of action of spinal morphine. Epidural infusion of morphine (0.1 to 0.5 mg/h) after small bolus doses (2 to 5 mg) is also effective and does not produce significant systemic uptake.[41,42] However, breakthrough pain may require incremental bolus doses.

Intrathecal

Large doses of morphine were once used intrathecally, before the advent of epidural administration.[164] However, even small doses of intrathecal morphine (0.1 to 0.25 mg)[82,165] can produce intense and prolonged analgesia.[16,18] Doses of 0.25 to 0.5 mg produce higher CSF concentrations than are produced by epidural morphine 4 to 6 mg[16,18] with low plasma concentrations. A dose-response study in volunteers revealed increasing respiratory depression (hypoxemia) with 0.2 to 0.6 mg of morphine.[166] Small doses of intrathecal morphine given by infusion (200 μg/24 h) have provided effective analgesia.[167]

Meperidine

Epidural

Epidural administration of meperidine was reported shortly after morphine.[30] Meperidine has an octanol/water partition coefficient roughly 40 times that of morphine and thus penetrates the dura more rapidly.[27] The onset of analgesia is faster compared with morphine (15 to 30 minutes), but the duration of action is shorter (4 to 6 hours).[29,30] Meperidine, 30 to 50 mg following lower abdominal surgery or 50 to 100 mg for upper abdominal or thoracic surgery produces analgesia comparable to that of epidural morphine.[168,169]

Intrathecal

Meperidine given intrathecally in relatively high doses (100 mg) acts, not only as an analgesic, but also as a local anesthetic. Spinal anesthesia adequate for perineal surgery (40 to 120 minutes), a transient motor and sensory block of the lower limbs and lower abdomen, and in some cases, a sympathetic block is produced[68,170] (see Intraoperative Use). The potential for delayed respiratory depression requires close and prolonged postoperative supervision.

Fentanyl

Epidural

Fentanyl is 800 times more lipid soluble than is morphine. It has become the most popular lipid soluble spinal opioid in North America and has been the subject of extensive investigation. The reason for its popularity relates to the rapid onset of action when given epidurally and the perception that the risk of respiratory depression is low. When given as an epidural bolus dose of approximately 1 μg/kg, relatively large quantities can be found in the CSF at various levels along the neuraxis up to the cranium.[124] Very small amounts enter the blood stream following a bolus. However, when fentanyl is given by bolus plus infusion, fentanyl accumulates in the systemic circulation. Onset of action after a bolus dose occurs rapidly with a maximal effect reached after about 10 to 20 minutes, but effective analgesia is short-lived, lasting about 2 to 4 hours.[171,172] Doses of 50 to 100 μg through a lumbar epidural catheter are effective for lower abdominal procedures.[171,173,174] Following upper abdominal or thoracic surgery, larger doses (100 to 200 μg) are required.[172] Speed of onset may be related to the volume and the dose injected, with a volume of 5 ml of more producing a faster onset than volumes less than 5 ml, when the mass of fentanyl is held constant at 50 μg.[175]

The short duration of action of epidural fentanyl has led to the use of bolus plus continuous infusions. Optimal analgesia is achieved if the epidural catheter is placed adjacent to the appropriate dermatomes at which the surgery is to take place, i.e., a thoracic catheter for thoracic surgery and a lower thoracic catheter for upper abdominal surgery.[48] Fentanyl solutions with a concentration of 10 μg/ml, given at a rate of 0.5 to 1 μg/kg/h, provide effective pain relief when the catheter is close to the surgical incision,[48,135] and plasma fentanyl levels are moderate. In contrast, when a lumbar epidural catheter is used for thoracotomy/upper abdominal surgery, higher doses such as 1 to 1.5 μg/kg/h of fentanyl are necessary to provide pain relief, leading to high systemic fentanyl concentrations of 1 to 2 ng/ml.[12,126] Several studies have demonstrated that these higher infusion doses produce systemic levels that are comparable to those of intravenous infusions of fentanyl.[8,9,12] Similar results have been found for alfentanil and sufentanil.[10,13,14]

Intrathecal

Fentanyl has been given by intrathecal bolus in doses of 25 to 50 μg, usually during cesarian section (with local anesthetics) to improve intraoperative conditions and to provide early postoperative analgesia.[176–178] Fentanyl has also been administered as a continuous subarachnoid infusion using a 28 gauge spinal catheter after hip arthroplasty, but it was not superior to subarachnoid morphine.[167]

Alfentanil

Epidural

Alfentanil is less lipid soluble than is fentanyl and much more lipid soluble than is morphine. It has a rapid onset when given systemically. When used epidurally, it has properties similar to epidural fentanyl, although it seems to have a shorter duration of action. Doses of 15 to 30 μg/kg given epidurally produce effective analgesia for about 90 to 100 minutes.[37,179] Alfentanil needs to be used as an epidural infusion to obtain prolonged analgesia.[37] Prolonged epidural infusions[10,14] produce high systemic concentrations (like fentanyl) and thus offer little advantage over intravenous infusions. Alfentanil offers no apparent advantages over fentanyl.

Sufentanil

Epidural

Sufentanil has a lipid solubility, roughly twice that of fentanyl and is a highly selective μ receptor ligand. Bolus doses of 30 to 50 μg provide a rapid onset of analgesia (15 minutes) with a duration only slightly longer than fentanyl (4 to 6 hours).[33,35] Larger doses (50 to 75 μg) may lead to respiratory

depression and increased sedation.[33,35,180] Following cesarian section and orthopaedic surgery,[37,171,181,182] even lower doses (15 to 30 μg) may be effective. Although sufentanil is five to seven times as potent as fentanyl when given systemically, it is only twice as potent when given epidurally or intrathecally.[183] This may be the result of nonspecific binding to lipophilic tissues. The short duration of analgesia has led to the use of continuous infusions after thoracotomy or upper abdominal surgery (e.g., 0.15 to 0.30 μg/kg/h or 1.0 μg/ml of solution).[13,47] However, systemic absorption from continuous epidural infusion is high, and the question has been raised whether this is merely a complex method of administering the opioid intravenously, as with fentanyl.[13]

Intrathecal

Sufentanil has not been widely used intrathecally for acute pain[184,185] because of the short duration of analgesia. Intrathecal sufentanil undergoes rapid clearance from the CSF to the plasma.[184] Small doses (7.5 μg) of sufentanil combined with lidocaine provide effective intraoperative anesthesia.[186] Intrathecal sufentanil has been shown to provide short-lived but intense analgesia during labor.[187]

Several other μ agonists have been investigated for spinal use. Agents, such as hydromorphone, heroin,* or nicomorphine* do not offer significant advantages over morphine or the lipid soluble agents,[188] and others have specific disadvantages. For example, methadone has an unpredictable duration of action when administered spinally, which is not significantly different from the duration of analgesia with systemic administration. Thus, spinal methadone does not confer any advantages over intramuscular injection.[188] Lofentanil, an extremely potent opioid (500 to 1000 times the potency of morphine) with a high affinity for the μ receptor, has had limited use because of long lasting respiratory depression that is difficult to antagonize with naloxone.[189]

---

* Heroin (diacetylmorphine or diamorphine) and nicomorphine are Schedule I substances in the United States; thus, they are not available for clinical use.

Mixed Opioid Agonist-Antagonists and Partial Agonist-Antagonists

Buprenorphine

Buprenorphine is a partial agonist with a high affinity for the μ receptor. Because of its high lipid solubility, the onset of analgesia is fairly rapid (5 to 10 minutes) with a duration of action similar to morphine (6 to 10 hours). Because the duration of analgesia for buprenorphine is determined primarily by its receptor binding kinetics, the duration of analgesia is independent of the route of administration. Epidural bolus doses range from 0.15 to 0.30 mg with 0.02 mg/h used for continuous epidural infusions. Early respiratory depression has been seen with buprenorphine, which may be related to systemic absorption.[190,191] As buprenorphine dissociates very slowly from μ receptors, naloxone may be relatively ineffective in reversing respiratory depression (see Ch. 5).[192] Because buprenorphine is a partial agonist, its analgesic activity may be limited (see Ch. 5).

Nalbuphine/Butorphanol

Nalbuphine and butorphanol are partial agonists at μ and κ opioid receptors (see Ch. 5). Both of these opioids are lipid soluble and have a rapid onset of action when given epidurally. Butorphanol in epidural doses of 1 to 4 mg has a duration of analgesia of 2 to 4 hours,[193] although 10 mg of epidural nalbuphine produces analgesia for 4 to 8 hours.[194] The major advantage of these agents is the low incidence of side effects of nausea, vomiting, or pruritus.[193–195] Although these agents have been used epidurally after a variety of surgical procedures (cesarean section, upper abdominal surgery, and thoracotomy), their analgesic action is relatively weak or even absent in some studies[196] and inferior to that of μ agonists (e.g., morphine).[193,195,196] In addition, both agents produce marked sedation (50 to 90 percent of patients) and measurable respiratory depression at doses required for analgesia.[193,195] As a result, these agents are not widely used as spinal opioids.

Toxicology of Spinal Opioids

It may be advisable to test for possible spinal cord toxicity in animals before administering a drug spinally to humans.[197,198] Drugs for epidural use should also be proved to be safe for intrathecal use because inadvertent intrathecal administration is possible. Ideal toxicity studies should examine a wide range of doses, should test spinal cord function and histopathologic findings, and should consider the possible effects of vehicles and preservatives. The intrathecal administration of morphine to animals is not associated with histopathologic changes in the spinal cord.[199,200] Other drugs have not been so extensively tested (see Ch. 5).

CLINICAL APPLICATIONS AND PRACTICAL ADVICE

Preoperative Administration

Spinal opioids are often administered preoperatively when the epidural or spinal procedure is usually performed in the awake patient. Because of the slow onset of spinal morphine, the earlier the administration is done, the higher the probability will be of additive analgesia intraoperatively and decreased analgesic requirements postoperatively.[201] Epidural methadone analgesia prior to surgery in patients with hip fractures resulted in improved mobilization.[202] Pre-emptive analgesia is the concept that greater amounts of analgesics are required if administered after injury (surgery) in comparison with administration before injury because of sensitization of the spinal cord to noxious afferent input and development of the "wind-up" phenomenon.[203] The administration of epidural fentanyl as a single dose prior to thoracotomy decreased the requirement for postoperative opioids compared with epidural fentanyl given during the surgery. Although the decrease in postoperative analgesia and opioid requirement was small, it was statistically significant, lending credence to the concept of pre-emptive analgesia.[204]

Intraoperative Use

Spinal opioids have been used intraoperatively to achieve improved anesthesia/analgesia with local anesthetics (either intrathecal or epidural), to decrease analgesic requirements for intravenous or inhalational anesthetic agents, and in the case of intrathecal meperidine, to provide total spinal anesthesia. Combined epidural local anesthetic agents and opioids are used widely for cesarean section (see Obstetric Pain). Opioids are often combined with local anesthetics for surgical procedures performed under epidural blockade. Whether this provides better anesthetic conditions than the local anesthetic alone is difficult to demonstrate.[205] Epidural fentanyl has been shown to reduce volatile agent requirements during thoracotomy more effectively than does the same dose of fentanyl given intravenously.[206] Intrathecal morphine produced a greater reduction in the minimum alveolar concentration for halothane compared with the same morphine dose given intramuscularly.[207] Intrathecal meperidine is uniquely capable of producing surgical anesthesia with sympathetic, sensory, and motor block. Thus, intrathecal meperidine in doses of 1 mg/kg has been used as the sole agent for abdominal surgery.[68,170] Similar side effects to those seen with local anesthetics occur, including hypotension.[208] In addition, intubation and respiratory assistance may be necessary.

Postoperative Pain Control

Spinal opioids have been used most widely in the postoperative setting.[49]

Intrathecal

Intrathecal opioids have been used for postoperative analgesia after a wide variety of procedures (e.g., abdominal, vascular, hip, spinal, cardiac, genitourinary, and prostatic surgery) but especially when spinal local anesthesia is used. A wide variety of opioids and dosing regimens have been used (Table 6-4). Typical doses of intrathecal opioids have been drastically reduced as experience and knowledge has accumulated, thereby decreasing the potential for respiratory depression. Several studies found intrathecal opioids to be equal or superior to other methods of opioid administration.[165,209] Although long acting opioids (e.g., morphine) can provide prolonged postoperative analgesia when used intrathecally, usually only one dose is administered, limiting the duration of action. The use of microgauge intrathecal catheters for the intermittent injection of intrathecal opioids has not been extensively investigated,[167] especially regarding the potential for respiratory depression

and infection. Moreover, reports of neurotoxicity associated with local anesthetic agents and microspinal catheters has prompted their recall in North America.

Epidural

Virtually every known opioid has been used by the epidural route to provide postoperative analgesia, including opioid agonists (morphine, heroin, phenoperidine, meperidine, methadone, hydromorphone, nicomorphine, fentanyl, alfentanil, sufentanil, and lofentanil), agonist-antagonists, and partial agonists (buprenorphine, nalbuphine, butorphanol, pentazocine, meptazinol, and tramadol).[188] These agents have been used to provide epidural analgesia after virtually all types of surgery (abdominal, hip, knee, spinal, thoracic, cardiac, prostatic, anal, urogenital, and gynecologic; Table 6-4). They may be administered as a bolus, bolus plus infusions, or by patient-controlled analgesia (bolus, or bolus plus background infusion), the latter usually being reserved for rapid onset, lipid soluble opioids. There are currently hundreds of articles reporting the highly effective postoperative analgesia that is achieved by the epidural route of administration,[49,161,188,210] however, only a small number have compared epidural opioids with other routes of administration. It has been shown in controlled studies after knee surgery,[94,159] abdominal surgery,[57,145,211] thoracic surgery,[41,58,112,212] and laminectomy[211] that pain relief is superior after epidural opioids compared with intramuscular or intravenous opioids. Other benefits of spinal opioids are also apparent and are discussed under Acute Pain: Outcome Studies.

Nonsurgical Acute Pain Situations

Spinal opioids have also found an effective place in nonsurgical acute pain, including post-trauma pain and some acute medical conditions.

Post-Trauma Pain

Spinal opioids have been useful for controlling pain and improving pulmonary function after blunt chest trauma. Epidural morphine alone was an effective method of analgesia after multiple rib fractures[213] and in combination with bupivacaine for blunt chest injury.[214] Significant improvement

Table 6-4 Reported Clinical Applications of Intrathecal and Epidural Opioids

Reported Applications	Technique
Acute pain	
During surgery (and postsurgery)	
Open heart	Intrathecal
Gynecologic	Epidural
General surgery	Epidural
	Intrathecal
Orthopaedic	Intrathecal
Postsurgery	
Thoracotomy	Epidural, epidural PCA
Orthopaedic	Epidural
	Epidural-intrathecal
	Intrathecal
Prostatectomy	Epidural
Abdominal and general surgery	Epidural, epidural PCA
	Epidural infusion
Anal and urogenital	Caudal epidural
	Epidural
Gynecologic	Epidural, epidural PCA
Post-trauma pain	Epidural
Obstetrics	Epidural, epidural PCA
Labor pain[a]	Intrathecal
	Epidural
Postcesarean section	Epidural, epidural PCA
Second trimester abortion	Epidural
Complicated obstetrics	Intrathecal
Acute medical conditions	
Myocardial infarction	Epidural
	Intrathecal
Thrombophlebitis	Epidural
Herpes zoster	Epidural
Nephrolithiasis	Epidural
Chronic pain	
Cancer pain	Intrathecal (single dose)
	Intrathecal catheter with implanted pump
	Epidural top-up by percutaneous catheter
	Epidural by implanted "portal"
	Epidural infusion by implanted catheter and infusion pump
Chronic noncancer pain	
Bladder spasm	Epidural
Back pain	Epidural
Ischemic rest pain	Epidural
Causalgia	Epidural
Spasticity or muscle spasm	Epidural

Abbreviations: PCA, patient-controlled analgesia.

[a] Most studies reported unsatisfactory relief of labor pain with epidural morphine and satisfactory relief only after high dose meperidine with added epinephrine. In comparison, intrathecal opioids were more effective. The combination of opioid and local anesthetic was effective.

(Adapted from Cousins et al.,[49] with permission.)

in pulmonary function and effective analgesia was seen with the use of epidural fentanyl infusions in patients with chest trauma.[125] A trial comparing thoracic epidural morphine with systemic opioids in patients with multiple rib fractures found that the spinal opioid group had less ventilator-dependent time, decreased intensive care unit time, and a shorter hospital stay.[215]

Nonsurgical Conditions

Acute clinical pain conditions that have been effectively treated by spinal opioids include acute myocardial infarction,[216,217] thrombophlebitis,[218] herpes zoster,[115,218] and nephrolithiasis.[218] It is noteworthy that relief of myocardial infarction pain was achieved after failure of intravenous and intramuscular opioids.[216,217,219]

Pediatrics

Limited experience with caudal and lumbar epidural opioids in children has shown that the same advantages and limitations exist in the pediatric population as in adults. Caudal morphine has been administered after orthopaedic, genitourinary, abdominal, and thoracic surgery.[220,221] Lumbar epidural morphine has also been used successfully to provide analgesia after thoracotomy and laparotomy.[222,223] Morphine by caudal administration (50 to 100 μg/kg) provided prolonged analgesia (8 to 24 hours) after inguinal and genital surgery.[224,225] Krane et al.[225] compared three doses of caudal morphine (33, 67, and 100 μg/kg) after abdominal, genitourinary, or orthopaedic surgery and found little difference in the duration of action (10 to 13 hours). However, one child in the 100-μg/kg group developed delayed respiratory depression, and thus, the authors recommended 33 μg/kg as a starting dose.[226] The incidence of nausea and vomiting was similar to that in adults (approximately 40 percent), and pruritus was also common, but in contrast to the adult population, it rarely required treatment. Urinary retention also occurs, but the incidence is variable and may be no higher than that seen after caudal bupivacaine. In one study, 19 of 56 children developed urinary retention after 70 μg/kg of caudal morphine for postoperative pain.[220] Delayed respiratory depression has been reported to occur with a higher incidence than in

adults,[220] but most studies are retrospective. For example, Valley and Bailey[220] reported 11 cases of respiratory depression in 138 patients receiving caudal morphine. This represents an incidence of approximately 8 percent and occurred within 12 hours of morphine administration. However, 54 percent of this population were younger than 12 months of age, and 60 percent received intravenous opioids intraoperatively.

Obstetric Pain

Spinally administered local anesthetic agents have long been the treatment of choice for obstetric pain. It is not surprising therefore that spinally administered opioids have been intensely scrutinized in this setting. Spinally administered opioids and opioid/local anesthetic combinations are used in two different settings: labor and vaginal delivery and for cesarean section. Delivery techniques include subarachnoid bolus, epidural bolus with or without continuous infusions, and epidural bolus with patient-controlled epidural analgesia (bolus alone or bolus plus background infusion).[227]

Labor and Delivery

Subarachnoid opioids can provide effective analgesia for the first and second stages of labor. Morphine in doses of 0.5 to 1 mg is effective and safe.[54,228] The onset of analgesia is slow (45 to 60 minutes) but prolonged (8 hours). The frequent side effects are a distinct disadvantage (pruritus, nausea and vomiting, urinary retention, drowsiness, dizziness, respiratory depression, and postdural puncture headache). Subarachnoid opioids alone do not provide adequate analgesia for episiotomy or forceps delivery. The combination of fentanyl and morphine (0.25 mg of morphine with 25 μg of fentanyl) produces a faster onset of analgesia with a 4- to 5-hour duration.[229] Similarly, intrathecal sufentanil has been shown to provide brief but intense analgesia during labor.[187] Although subarachnoid opioids suffer from too many drawbacks to become widely adopted for labor and delivery at present, the technique may be useful in certain clinical situations in which regional analgesic techniques with local anesthetic agents may produce problems,[230,231] e.g., in patients with severe cardiac disease. The incidence of respiratory depression from this technique remains uncertain.

Epidural opioids alone have not produced analgesia comparable to that of subarachnoid opioids. Epidural morphine in doses of 7.5 to 10 mg provides moderate to unsatisfactory analgesia for labor and little analgesia for delivery.[51,110] Lower doses (2 to 5 mg) are ineffective. The reason for this relative lack of effectiveness may be related to the greater systemic uptake of opioids by the engorged epidural venous system.[232,233] Epidural morphine in doses of 10 mg is accompanied by a high incidence of side effects (pruritus, nausea, vomiting, and drowsiness). Meperidine (100 mg) and fentanyl (100 to 200 μg) provide a rapid onset of analgesia of short duration (1 to 2 hours), which is effective only in the early part of the first stage.[234,235] Epidural alfentanil (30 μg/kg plus infusion) was an ineffective analgesic for labor and was associated with neonatal hypotonus.[236] In contrast, epidural sufentanil alone has been reported to provide significant analgesia for labor in doses up to 50 μg without neonatal complications. The duration of analgesia is short (1 to 2 hours), as for other lipid soluble opioids.[237]

The combination of epidural opioids and local anesthetic agents has been used to avoid the disadvantages of either opioids or local anesthetic agents when each is used as a single agent for labor and delivery. Mixtures of the two types of agents have been administered by bolus dose plus or minus continuous infusions or by patient-controlled analgesia. Fentanyl in doses of 50 to 100 μg added to bupivacaine 0.125 to 0.5 percent provides better pain relief than does bupivacaine alone, decreasing the onset and increasing both the duration and intensity of analgesia.[238] Subanalgesic concentrations of bupivacaine 0.05 to 0.0625 percent are effective when combined with 1 to 2 μg/ml of fentanyl and infused at a rate of about 10 ml/h.[239] Pain thresholds vary between patients over at least a fivefold range; so higher concentrations (0.25 percent) and infusion rates (12 to 15 ml/h) may be necessary. This regimen often provides good analgesia without motor block in the first stage and often the second stage of labor. Other opioid/local anesthetic combinations for labor and delivery include:

1. Sufentanil/bupivacaine (bolus : sufentanil 20 μg with bupivacaine 0.125 percent in a 10-ml volume; infusion: sufentanil 1 μg/ml with bupivacaine 0.125 percent at a rate of 10 ml/h) provided excellent analgesia for the first and second stages of labor with minimal motor block, no adverse maternal or neonatal effects, and undetectable umbilical cord concentrations of sufentanil.[240]
2. Alfentanil/bupivacaine: (bolus : alfentanil 10 μg/ kg with bupivacaine 0.125 percent in a 10-ml bolus; infusion : alfentanil 5 to 20 μg/kg/h with bupivacaine 0.125 percent at a rate of 10 ml/h) provided good analgesia for the first and second stages of labor without the adverse neonatal effects seen when larger doses of alfentanil are used alone.[241]
3. Butorphanol/bupivacaine: (bolus: butorphanol 1 to 3 mg with bupivacaine 0.25 percent; infusion : butorphanol 0.002% with bupivacaine 0.0625 percent) was an effective analgesic combination although the 3-mg butorphanol bolus dose is associated with maternal somnolence and adverse fetal effects.[242]
4. Morphine/bupivacaine: (bolus: morphine 2 mg with bupivacaine 0.25 percent) improved the duration and intensity of labor and postpartum analgesia with decreased motor block, lower anesthetic dose requirements, and decreased side effects. However, other studies of bolus dose morphine/bupivacaine did not find any improvement over bupivacaine alone.[96,243]

Cesarean Section: Intraoperative and Postoperative Spinal Analgesia

Subarachnoid Opioids

Fentanyl, sufentanil, and morphine have been used by subarachnoid administration in conjunction with spinal anesthesia (tetracaine 1 percent or bupivacaine 0.5 and 0.75 percent) for cesarean section. Fentanyl (6.25 to 50 μg) and sufentanil 10 μg increase the duration of the block and provide postoperative analgesia lasting 4 to 6 hours. The larger doses of fentanyl increased side effects, especially pruritus.[178] Morphine (0.1 to 0.5 mg) improves intraoperative analgesia and provides prolonged postoperative pain relief.[244] Up to 0.6 mg of morphine added to hyperbaric bupivacaine has been shown to increase analgesia up to 48 hours with few side effects compared with 0.2 and 0.4 mg.[245] Although respiratory depression has not been reported with the use of these small doses of morphine combined with subarachnoid local anesthetic agents, caution should be exercised and close monitoring utilized during the postoperative period because significant CSF concentrations of morphine will be present.

Epidural Opioids

Short acting lipid soluble opioids, including fentanyl and sufentanil, have been added to intraoperatively administered local anesthetic agents (usually bupivacaine) for cesarean section to enhance the local anesthetic agent. Epidural fentanyl (50 to 100 μg) increased the speed of onset and potentiated intraoperative analgesia for cesarean section, decreased nausea and vomiting during uterine manipulation, decreased requirements for supplemental opioid medication, shortened hospital stay, and has not been associated with adverse maternal or neonatal effects.[174,246,247] Intensive studies evaluating neonatal neurobehavioral status and the pattern of breathing after 50 to 100 μg of epidural fentanyl used before delivery by cesarean section have not found adverse effects.[246–248] Nonetheless, severe maternal respiratory depression has been reported after 100 μg of epidural fentanyl used during cesarean section.[249] In this case, temporary apnea and hypoxemia developed 100 minutes after the epidural injection of 100 μg of fentanyl and required naloxone for reversal.[249] Doses between 25 and 50 μg of epidural fentanyl seem to be optimal for supplementation during cesarean section.[250]

Epidural sufentanil (20 μg) added to 0.5 percent bupivacaine with epinephrine (1 : 200,000) also improves intraoperative anesthesia and results in longer postoperative analgesia compared with bupivacaine alone, with minimal maternal and neonatal adverse effects.[251] Increased dosages of sufentanil (50 μg) have an unacceptably high incidence of side effects, including maternal somnolence, pruritus, and emesis. Increasing the dose of sufentanil from 30 to 50 μg or higher does not prolong

analgesia significantly, indicating that the optimal dose is 30 μg or less.

The use of epidural opioids has become widespread for postoperative analgesia after cesarean section. Epidural morphine is the most commonly used opioid currently. Doses of 2 mg are ineffective, but 3 to 5 mg of epidural morphine provides effective, safe, and prolonged analgesia (up to 24 hours) after cesarean delivery with relatively mild and easily treatable side effects.[78,136] In a study of 1,000 patients given 5 mg of epidural morphine, 85 percent cited good to excellent postoperative analgesia lasting 23 hours. Between 20 and 30 percent experienced moderate to severe pruritus and nausea and vomiting. One patient developed severe respiratory depression, which was treated with oxygen and intravenous naloxone.[94] Other large scale studies have confirmed these findings.[111] Studies of potential respiratory depression following the use of epidural morphine indicate that, although mild decreases in oxygen saturation occur, maternal morbidity has not been observed.[78] An unexpected problem associated with epidural morphine use in postpartum patients is the development of recurrent herpes simplex labialis 2 to 5 days after receiving epidural morphine, with an incidence ranging from 10 to 35 percent.[252] Lipid soluble opioids, such as fentanyl, have been used by continuous infusion (50 to 75 μg/h of fentanyl),[253] but there is some evidence that substantial systemic absorption occurs and the analgesic effect may be partially provided by circulating fentanyl.[9]

Epidural butorphanol in doses of 1 to 6 mg has been used to provide moderately effective dose dependent postoperative analgesia of widely varying duration (300 to 700 minutes). However, butorphanol produces marked somnolence, and doses greater than 2 mg depress the ventilatory response to CO_2.[104] Other agents, including phenoperidine, heroin, hydromorphone, and meperidine, have been used to provide postoperative epidural analgesia after cesarean section. The analgesia tends to be of shorter duration than with morphine, although hydromorphone has been shown to be effective for up to 19 hours. The expected side effects of pruritus, nausea, and vomiting occur with all these drugs, although meperidine is reported to have less side effects than do the other opioids.[254]

Acute Pain: Outcome Studies

Outcome studies have shown benefits from spinal opioids other than improved analgesia. Pulmonary function, as measured by pulmonary function tests, arterial blood gases, and the incidence of pulmonary complications, has been consistently improved by epidural opioids compared with intravenous or intramuscular opioids or epidural local anesthetics.[56,58,255–257] Rawal et al.[57] showed improved pulmonary function after epidural morphine compared with intramuscular morphine after gastroplasty in morbidly obese patients. Similar results were found for cholecystectomy (subcostal incision) when comparing epidural morphine with intercostal nerve block or intramuscular opioid.[258] Several other studies demonstrated improved pulmonary function after thoracic or abdominal surgery[36,58] or fewer complications or infections[259] with epidural opioids.

Earlier extubation in the intensive care unit after major abdominal or cardiac surgery has been shown to follow the use of intrathecal or epidural morphine.[260,261] Patients admitted to the the unit with multiple rib fractures and treated with thoracic epidural morphine infusion had a lower incidence of tracheostomy, less ventilator-dependent time, and decreased unit and hospital stays compared with patients treated with parenteral morphine.[215] Studies examining the time to return of bowel function after abdominal surgery have produced conflicting results, with epidural local anesthetic agents being associated with less postoperative ileus compared with epidural or intramuscular opioids.[262] Rawal et al.[57] demonstrated earlier passage of flatus and feces after epidural morphine, but this has not been corroborated by others.[72] The use of epidural opioids (with or without with local anesthetic agents) after major surgery in patients undergoing abdominal aneurysm surgery[59] or in patients at high risk for ischemic cardiac disease[60] was associated with an overall decrease in morbidity and mortality rates. The incidence of myocardial ischemia and hypercoagulability after abdominal aneurysm surgery was decreased by postoperative epidural opioid use.[61] However, other recent studies have not been able to confirm these findings.[263]

Chronic Pain

Cancer Pain

Cancer pain management using spinal opioids has been extensively investigated. The risk-benefit ratio would seem to be favorable because many of these patients are highly tolerant to large opioid doses; patients previously exposed to very large opioid doses are at minimal risk of respiratory depression, the most important hazard of spinal opioids. It is a basic principle in the treatment of cancer pain that the initial treatment centers on the use of oral opioids in adequate doses with, appropriate adjuvant drugs. It must be emphasized that less than 10 percent of patients with cancer pain require techniques such as spinal opioids or more permanent neuroablative procedures, and the vast majority can be managed with oral opioids and adjuvant drugs.[204] Thus, the indications for the use of spinal opioids in cancer pain include (1) patients whose pain cannot be adequately controlled with the use of oral opioids and (2) patients who achieve effective pain relief with oral opioids but in whom side effects (sedation, disorientation, nausea, and vomiting) reach unacceptable levels. The site, nature, and presence of metastatic spread of the neoplasm; the character of the pain; and the life expectancy of the patient are all important factors related to the decision to commence spinal opioid therapy. The neuropathic and "deafferentation" pain caused by neoplasms is not amenable to spinal opioids.[49] The best results from spinal opioids are obtained when the pain has a deep, constant, somatic nature, which is relatively widespread. It is often useful to carry out a trial of epidural opioid using standard techniques[265] to assess its efficacy before proceeding to more permanent implantable systems. The efficacy of spinal opioid therapy is illustrated by a report of 55 patients with cancer who were treated with spinal opioids; only 28 became pain free.[55] Morphine is usually the opioid of choice. For bolus dose administration, the starting dose may be calculated as one-tenth the dose that was effective by mouth (usually 2 to 10 mg), although considerable adjustment of dose may be necessary. Doses for infusion can vary from 5 to 100 mg/24 h.

Long-term spinal opioid delivery requires an intrathecal or epidural catheter system connected to an injection system and usually a reservoir.[266–268] Tunneling of the catheter under the skin and the use of an implantable subcutaneous injection port or a subcutaneous continuous infusion device are necessary. Both the intrathecal and epidural systems have advantages and disadvantages. The intrathecal route allows the use of much lower doses but has the potential for CSF leak, headache, meningitis, and arachnoiditis.[188] Epidural administration requires higher doses, and catheter tip fibrosis may lead to failure of analgesic effectiveness; several reports indicate that catheter failure often occurs after 3 to 6 months,[264,267] although very long-term treatment (up to 1 year) has been successful.[269] A loss of efficacy may be related to obstruction to CSF flow from fibrous or neoplastic masses, obstructed catheters, or the development of tolerance. True tolerance is difficult to diagnose and may require only an increase in dose or a change to another opioid.[270] The use of local anesthetic agents for 3 to 5 days may allow reinstitution of the opioid with effective results.

Complications of long-term spinal opioid therapy with standard percutaneous catheters (non-tunneled) include obstruction, breakage, kinking or removal of catheters, local infection, and meningitis.[269] Most catheters required replacement at least once. With subcutaneously tunneled catheters and fully implanted systems, the incidence of infection is negligible.[266,267]

Chronic Noncancer Pain

Several chronic pain conditions have also been successfully treated with spinal opioids (e.g., bladder spasm, back pain, ischemic rest pain, causalgia, and muscle spasm). The treatment of muscle spasm and pain associated with spasticity responds well to epidural opioids and has, like cancer pain, utilized implanted epidural systems.[64]

REFERENCES

1. Goldstein A, Lowney LE, Pal BK: Stereospecific and nonspecific interactions of the morphine congener levorphanol in subcellular fractions of the mouse brain. Proc Natl Acad Sci U S A 58:1742, 1971
2. Pert CB, Snyder SH: Opiate receptor: demonstration in nervous tissue. Science 179:1011, 1973
3. LaMotte C, Pert CB, Snyde SH: Opiate receptor binding in primate spinal cord: distribution and changes after dorsal root section. Brain Res 112:407, 1976
4. McQuay HJ, Sullivan AF, Smallman K, Dickenson AH: Intrathecal opioids, potency and lipophilicity. Pain 36:111, 1989
5. Moore RA, Bullingham RES, McQuay HJ et al: Dural permeability to narcotics: in vitro determination and application to extradural administration. Br J Anaesth 54:1117, 1982
6. Gourlay G, Cherry DA, Plummer JL et al: The influence of drug polarity on the absorption of opioid drugs into the CSF and subsequent cephalad migration following lumbar epidural administration: application to morphine and pethidine. Pain 31:297, 1987
7. Wolfe MJ, Davies GK: Analgesic action of extradural fentanyl. Br J Anaesth 52:357, 1980
8. Loper KA, Ready LB, Downey M et al: Epidural and intravenous fentanyl infusions are clinically equivalent after knee surgery. Anesth Analg 70:72, 1990
9. Ellis DJ, Millar WL, Reisner LS: A randomized double-blind comparison of epidural versus intravenous fentanyl infusion for analgesia after cesarean section. Anesthesiology 72:981, 1990
10. Camu F, Debucquoy F: Alfentanil infusion for postoperative pain: a comparison of epidural and intravenous routes. Anesthesiology 75:171, 1991
11. Glass PSA, Estok P, Ginsberg B et al: Use of patient-controlled analgesia to compare the efficacy of epidural to intravenous fentanyl administration. Anesth Analg 74:345, 1992
12. Sandler AN, Stringer D, Panos L et al: A randomized, double-blind comparison of lumbar epidural and intravenous fentanyl infusions for post-thoracotomy pain relief: analgesic, pharmacokinetic and respiratory effects. Anesthesiology 77:626, 1992
13. Geller E, Chrubasik J, Graf R et al: A randomized double-blind comparison of epidural sufentanil versus intravenous sufentanil or epidural fentanyl analgesia after major abdominal surgery. Anesth Analg 76:1243, 1993

14. Chauvin M, Hongnat JM, Mourgeon E et al: Equivalence of postoperative analgesia with patient-controlled intravenous or epidural alfentanil. Anesth Analg 76:1251, 1993
15. Moore RA, Bullingham RSJ, McQuay HJ et al: Spinal fluid kinetics of morphine and heroin in man. Clin Pharmacol Ther 35:40, 1984
16. Nordberg G, Hedner T, Mellstrand T et al: Pharmacokinetic aspects of intrathecal morphine analgesia. Anesthesiology 60:448, 1984
17. Chauvin M, Samii K, Schermann JM et al: Plasma pharmacokinetics of morphine after IM, extradural and intrathecal administration. Br J Anaesth 54:843, 1981
18. Nordberg G: Pharmacokinetic aspects of spinal morphine analgesia. Acta Anaesthesiol Scand 79:1, 1984
19. DiChiro G: Movement of the cerebrospinal fluid in human beings. Nature 204:290, 1964
20. Bromage PR, Camporesi E, Leslie J: Epidural narcotics in volunteers: sensitivity to pain and to carbon dioxide. Pain 9:145, 1980
21. Bromage PR, Camporesi EM, Durant PAC et al: Rostral spread of epidural morphine. Anesthesiology 56:431, 1982
22. Payne R: CSF distribution of opioids in animals and man. Acta Anaesthesiol Scand, suppl. 85:31, 1987
23. Allinson RR, Stach PE: Intrathecal drug therapy. DICP 12:347, 1978
24. Mather LE: Clinical pharmacokinetics of fentanyl and its newer derivatives. Clin Pharmacokinet 8:422, 1983
25. Nordberg G, Hedner T, Mellstrand T et al: Pharmacokinetic aspects of epidural morphine analgesia. Anesthesiology 58:545, 1983
26. Nayman J: Measurement and control of postoperative pain. Ann R Coll Surg Engl 61:419, 1979
27. Sjostrom S, Hartvig P, Persson MP et al: Pharmacokinetics of epidural morphine and meperidine in humans. Anesthesiology 67:877, 1987
28. Gustaffson LL, Ackerman S, Adamson H et al: Disposition of morphine in cerebrospinal fluid after epidural administration. Lancet 1:796, 1982
29. Cousins MJ, Mather LE, Glynn CJ et al: Selective spinal analgesia. Lancet 1:1141, 1979
30. Glynn CJ, Mather LE, Cousins MJ et al: Peridural meperidine in humans: analgetic response, pharmacokinetics and transmission into CSF. Anesthesiology 55:520, 1981
31. Watson J, Moore A, McQuay H et al: Plasma morphine concentrations and analgesic effects of lumbar extradural morphine and heroin. Anesth Analg 63:629, 1984
32. Mather LE, Meffin PJ: Clinical pharmacokinetics of pethidine. Clin Pharmacokinet 3:352, 1978
33. Whiting WG, Sandler AN, Lau LC et al: Analgesic and respiratory effects of epidural sufentanil in post-thoracotomy patients. Anesthesiology 69:36, 1988
34. Gourlay GK, Cherry DA, Cousins MJ: Cephalad migration of morphine in CSF following lumbar epidural administration in patients with cancer pain. Pain 23:317, 1985
35. Van der Auwera D, Verborgh C, Camu F: Analgesic and cardiorespiratory effects of epidural sufentanil and morphine in humans. Anesth Analg 66:999, 1987
36. Chrubasik J, Wust H, Schulte-Monting J et al: Relative analgesic potency of epidural fentanyl, alfentanil and morphine in the treatment of postoperative pain. Anesthesiology 68:929, 1988
37. Tan S, Cohen SE, White PF: Sufentanil for analgesia after cesarean section: intravenous versus epidural administration. Anesth Analg, suppl.:1, 1986
38. Justins DM, Knott C, Luthman J, Reynolds F: Epidural versus intramuscular fentanyl. Analgesia and pharmacokinetics in labour. Anaesthesia 38:937, 1983
39. Chrubasik J, Scholler KL, Wiemers K et al: Low-dose infusion of morphine prevents respiratory depression. Lancet 1:793, 1984
40. Chrubasik J, Wiemers K: Continuous-plus-on-demand epidural infusion of morphine for postoperative pain relief by means of a small, externally worn infusion device. Anesthesiology 62:263, 1985
41. Logas WG, El-Baz N, El-Ganzouri A et al: Continuous thoracic epidural analgesia for postoperative pain relief following thoracotomy: a randomized prospective study. Anesthesiology 67:787, 1987
42. El-Baz N, Goldin M: Continuous epidural infusion of morphine for pain relief after cardiac operations. J Thorac Cardiovasc Surg 93:878, 1987
43. Planner RS, Cowie RW, Babarczy AS: Continuous epidural morphine analgesia after radical operations upon the pelvis. Surg Gynecol Obstet 166:229, 1988
44. Chauvin M, Samii K, Schermann JM et al: Plasma concentration of morphine after IM, extradural and intrathecal administration. Br J Anaesth 53:911, 1981
45. Berkowitz BA, Ngai SH, Yang JC et al: The disposition of morphine in surgical patients. Clin Pharmacol Ther 17:629, 1975

46. Guinard JP, Mavrocordatos P, Chiolero R et al: A randomized comparison of intravenous versus lumbar and thoracic epidural fentanyl for analgesia after thoracotomy. Anesthesiology 77:1108, 1992
47. Cheng EY, Koebert RF, Hopwood M et al: Continuous epidural sufentanil for postoperative analgesia. Anesthesiology 67:A233, 1987
48. Salomaki TE, Laitinen JO, Nuutinen LS: A randomized double-blind comparison of epidural versus intravenous fentanyl infusion for analgesia after thoracotomy. Anesthesiology 75:790, 1991
49. Cousins MJ, Cherry DA, Gourlay GK: Acute and chronic pain: use of spinal opioids, p. 955. In Cousins MJ, Bridenbaugh PO (eds): Neural Blockade in Clinical Anesthesia and Management of Pain. 2nd Ed. JB Lippincott, Philadelphia, 1988
50. Hughes SC: Intraspinal narcotics in obstetrics. Clin Perinatol 1:167, 1982
51. Hughes SC, Rosen MA, Shnider SM et al: Maternal and neonatal effects of epidural morphine for labor and delivery. Anesth Analg 63:319, 1984
52. Husemeyer RP, O'Connor MC, Davenport HT: Failure of epidural morphine to relieve pain in labor. Anesthesia 35:161, 1980
53. Bonnardot JP, Maillet M, Calou JC et al: Maternal and fetal concentrations of morphine after intrathecal administration during labor. Br J Anaesth 54:487, 1982
54. Abboud TK, Shnider SM, Dailey PA et al: Intrathecal administration of hyperbaric morphine for the relief of pain in labour. Br J Anaesth 56:1351, 1984
55. Arner S, Arner B: Differential effects of epidural morphine in the treatment of cancer-related pain. Acta Anesthesiol Scand 29:32, 1985
56. Bromage PR, Camporesi E, Chestnut D: Epidural narcotics for postoperative analgesia. Anesth Analg 59:473, 1980
57. Rawal N, Sjostrand U, Christofferson E et al: Comparison of intramuscular and epidural morphine for postoperative analgesia in the grossly obese: influence on postoperative ambulation and pulmonary function. Anesth Analg 63:583, 1984
58. Shulman M, Sandler AN, Bradley JW et al: Post-thoracotomy pain and pulmonary function following epidural and systemic morphine. Anesthesiology 61:569, 1984
59. Yeager MP, Glass DD, Neff RK et al: Epidural anesthesia and analgesia in high-risk surgical patients. Anesthesiology 66:729, 1987
60. Beattie WS, Buckley DN, Forrest JB: Epidural morphine reduces the risk of postoperative myocardial

61. ischemia in patients with cardiac risk factors. Can J Anaesth 40:532, 1993
61. Tuman KJ, McCarthy RJ, March RJ et al: Effects of epidural anesthesia and analgesia on coagulation and outcome after major vascular surgery. Anesth Analg 73:696, 1991
62. Baxter AD, Kirulata G: Detrusor tone after epidural morphine. Anesth Analg 63:464, 1984
63. Cardan E: Spinal morphine in enuresis. Br J Anaesth 57:354, 1985
64. Erickson DL, Blacklock JB, Michaelson M et al: Control of spasticity by implantable continuous flow morphine pump. Neurosurgery 16:215, 1985
65. Struppler A, Burgmayer B, Ochs G et al: The effect of epidural application of opioids on spasticity of spinal origin. Life Sci 33:607, 1983
66. Duggan AW, Johnson SM, Morton CR: Differing distribution of receptors for morphine and met[5] enkephalinamide in the dorsal horn of the cat. Brain Res 229:379, 1981
67. Yaksh TL, Noueihed R: The physiology and pharmacology of spinal opiates. Annu Rev Pharmacol Toxicol 25:433, 1985
68. Mirceau N, Constaninescu C, Jianu C et al: Anaesthesie sous-arachnoidienne par la pethidine. Ann Fr Anesth Reanim 1:167, 1982
69. Wang J, Denson D, Knarr D et al: Continuous epidural methadone in the management of postoperative pain following lower abdominal surgery. Reg Anesth 13:58, 1988
70. Christensen P, Brandt MR, Rem J et al: Influence of extradural morphine on the adrenocortical and hyperglycaemic response to surgery. Br J Anaesth 54:23, 1982
71. Jorgensen BC, Andersen HB, Engquist A: Influence of epidural morphine on postoperative pain, endocrine-metabolic, and renal responses to surgery. A controlled study. Acta Anaesthesiol Scand 26:63, 1982
72. Hjortso NC, Neuman P, Frosig F et al: A controlled study on the effect of epidural analgesia with local anaesthetics and morphine on morbidity after abdominal surgery. Acta Anaesthesiol Scand 29:790, 1985
73. Kehlet H: The modifying effect of general and regional anesthesia on the endocrine-metabolic response to surgery. Reg Anesth 7:S39, 1982
74. Rutberg H, Hakanson E, Anderberg B et al: Effects of the extradural administration of morphine, or bupivacaine, on the endocrine response to upper abdominal surgery. Br J Anaesth 56:233, 1984

75. Mangano DT, Siliciano D, Hollenberg M et al: Postoperative myocardial ischemia: therapeutic trials using intensive analgesia following surgery. Anesthesiology 76:342, 1992

76. Palazzo MGA, Strunin L: Anesthesia and emesis. I. Etiology. Can J Anaesth 31:178, 1984

77. Rapp SE, Ready LB, Greer BE: Postoperative pain management in gynecologic patients utilizing epidural opiate analgesia and patient-controlled analgesia. Gynecol Oncol 35:341, 1989

78. Daley DM, Sandler AN, Turner KE et al: A comparison of epidural and intramuscular morphine in patients following cesarean section. Anesthesiology 72:289, 1990

79. Eisenach JC, Grice SC, Dewan DM: Patient-controlled analgesia following cesarean section: a comparison with epidural and intramuscular narcotics. Anesthesiology 68:444, 1988

80. Stenseth R, Sellevold O, Breivik H: Epidural morphine for postoperative pain: experience with 1085 patients. Acta Anaesthesiol Scand 29:148, 1985

81. Abboud TK, Dror A, Mosaad P et al: Mini-dose intrathecal morphine for the relief of post-cesarean section pain: safety, efficacy and ventilatory responses to carbon dioxide. Anesth Analg 67:137, 1988

82. Kirson LE, Goldman JM, Slover RB: Low-dose intrathecal morphine for postoperative pain control in patients undergoing transurethral resection of the prostate. Anesthesiology 71:192, 1989

83. Gilman AG, Rall W, Nies AS, Taylor P: Goodman and Gilman's The Pharmacological Basis of Therapeutics. 8th Ed. Pergamon Press, New York, 1990

84. Kotelko DM, Rottman RL, Wright WC et al: Transdermal scopolamine decreases nausea and vomiting following cesarean section in patients receiving epidural morphine. Anesthesiology 71:675, 1989

85. Loper KA, Ready LB, Dorman BH: Prophylactic transdermal scopolamine patches reduce nausea in postoperative patients receiving epidural morphine. Anesth Analg 68:144, 1989

86. Rawal N, Dahlstrom B, Inturrisi CE et al: Prevention of complications of epidural morphine analgesia by low dose naloxone infusion. Acta Anaesthesiol Scand 29:135, 1985

87. Gowan JD, Hurtig JB, Fraser RA et al: Naloxone infusion after prophylactic epidural morphine: effects on incidence of postoperative side-effects and quality of analgesia. Can J Anaesth 35:143, 1988

88. Abboud TK, Lee K, Reyes A et al: Prophylactic oral naltrexone with intrathecal morphine for cesarean section: effects on adverse reactions and analgesia. Anesth Analg 71:367, 1990

89. Bach V, Carl P, Ravlo O et al: Potentiation of epidural opioids with epidural droperidol. Anaesthesia 41:1116, 1986

90. Naji P, Farschtschian M, Wilder-Smith O, Wilder-Smith CH: Epidural droperidol and morphine for postoperative pain. Anesth Analg 70:583, 1990

91. Leeser J, Lip H: Prevention of postoperative nausea and vomiting using ondansetron, a new, selective, 5-HT$_3$ receptor antagonist. Anesth Analg 72:751, 1991

92. Loper KA, Ready LB, Nessley M et al: Epidural morphine provides greater pain relief than patient-controlled intravenous morphine following cholecystectomy. Anesth Analg 69:826, 1989

93. Harrison DM, Sinatra R, Morgese L et al: Epidural narcotic and patient-controlled analgesia for post-cesarean section pain relief. Anesthesiology 68:454, 1988

94. Loper KA, Ready LB: Epidural morphine after anterior cruciate ligament repair: a comparison with patient-controlled intravenous morphine. Anesth Analg 68:350, 1989

95. Leicht CH, Hughes SC, Dailey PA et al: Epidural morphine sulfate for analgesia after cesarean section: a prospective report of 1000 patients. Anesthesiology 65:A366, 1985

96. Abboud TK, Afrasiabi A, Zhu J et al: Epidural morphine or butorphanol augments bupivacaine analgesia during labor. Anesthesiology 69:A684, 1988

97. Penning JP, Samson B, Baxter AD: Reversal of epidural morphine-induced respiratory depression and pruritus with nalbuphine. Can J Anaesth 35:599, 1988

98. Bromage PR, Camporesi EM, Durant PAC et al: Non-respiratory side effects of epidural morphine. Anesth Analg 61:490, 1982

99. Lanz E, Kehrberger E, Theiss D: Epidural morphine: a clinical double blind study of dosage. Anesth Analg 64:786, 1985

100. Walts LF, Kaufman RD, Moreland IR et al: Total hip arthroplasty: an investigation of factors related to postoperative urinary retention. Clin Orthop 194:280, 1985

101. Durant PAC, Yaksh TL: Drug effects on urinary bladder tone during spinal morphine-induced inhibition of the micturition reflex in unanesthetized rats. Anesthesiology 68:325, 1988

102. Drenger B, Magora F: Urodynamic studies after intrathecal fentanyl and buprenorphine in the dog. Anesth Analg 69:348, 1989

103. Rawal N, Mollefors K, Axelsson K et al: An experimental study of urodynamic effects of epidural mor-

phine and naloxone reversal. Anesth Analg 62:641, 1983

104. Evron S, Magora F, Sadovsky E: Prevention of urinary retention with phenoxybenzamine during epidural morphine. BMJ 288:190, 1984
105. Etches RC: Complications of acute pain management. Anesthesiol Clin North Am 10:417, 1992
106. Etches RC, Sandler AN, Daley MD: Respiratory depression and spinal opioids. Can J Anaesth 36:165, 1989
107. Gustafsson LL, Schildt B, Jacobsen K: Adverse effects of extradural and intrathecal opiates: report of a nationwide survey in Sweden. Br J Anaesth 54:479, 1982
108. Rawal N, Arner S, Gustafsson LL et al: Present state of extradural and intrathecal opioid analgesia in Sweden. A nationwide follow-up survey. Br J Anaesth 59:791, 1987
109. Ready LB, Oden R, Chadwick HS et al: Development of an anesthesiology-based postoperative pain management service. Anesthesiology 68:100, 1988
110. Writer WDR, Hurtig JB, Edelist G et al: Epidural morphine prophylaxis of postoperative pain: report of a double-blind, multicentre study. Can J Anaesth 32:330, 1985
111. Fuller JG, McMorland GH, Douglas MJ: Epidural morphine for analgesia after cesarean section: a report of 4880 patients. Can J Anaesth 37:636, 1990
112. El-Baz NMI, Faber LP, Jensik RJ: Continuous epidural infusion of morphine for treatment of pain after thoracic surgery: a new technique. Anesth Analg 63:757, 1984
113. Sandler AN, Chovaz P, Whiting W: Respiratory depression following epidural morphine: a clinical study. Can J Anaesth 33:542, 1986
114. Chambers WA, Sinclair CJ, Scott DB: Extradural morphine for pain after surgery. Br J Anaesth 53:921, 1981
115. Torda TA, Pybus DA: Clinical experience with epidural morphine. Anaesth Intensive Care 9:129, 1981
116. Modig J, Paalzow L: A comparison of epidural morphine and epidural bupicavaine for postoperative pain relief. Acta Anaesthesiol Scand 25:437, 1981
117. Weddel SJ, Ritter RR: Serum levels following epidural administration of morphine and correlation with relief of postsurgical pain. Anesthesiology 54:210, 1981
118. Klinck JR, Lindop MJ: Epidural morphine in the elderly. Anaesthesia 37:907, 1982
119. Martin R, Salbaing J, Blaise G et al: Epidural morphine for postoperative pain relief: a dose response curve. Anesthesiology 56:423, 1982
120. Ready LB, Chadwick HS, Ross B: Age predicts effective epidural morphine dose after abdominal hysterectomy. Anesth Analg 66:1215, 1987
121. Weightman WM: Respiratory arrest during epidural infusion of bupivacaine and fentanyl. Anaesth Intensive Care 19:282, 1991
122. Miller RR: Analgesics. In Miller RR, Greenblatt DJ (eds): Drug Effects in Hospitalized Patients. p. 151. Wiley and Sons, New York, 1976
123. Scott DB, McClure J: Selective epidural analgesia. Lancet 1:1410, 1979
124. Gourlay GK, Murphy TM, Plummer JL et al: Pharmacokinetics of fentanyl in lumbar and cervical CSF following lumbar epidural and intravenous administration. Pain 38:253, 1989
125. Mackersie RC, Shackford SR, Hoyt DB et al: Continuous epidural fentanyl analgesia: ventilatory function improvement with routine use in treatment of blunt chest injury. J Trauma 27:1207, 1987
126. Badner NH, Sandler AN, Koren G et al: Lumbar epidural fentanyl infusions for post-thoracotomy patients: analgesic, respiratory, and pharmacokinetic effects. J Cardiothorac Vasc Anesth 4:543, 1990
127. Thind GS, Wells JCD, Wikes RG: The effects of continuous intravenous naloxone on epidural morphine. Anaesthesia 41:582, 1986
128. Rawal N, Schott U, Dahlstrom B et al: Influence of naloxone infusion on analgesia and respiratory depression following epidural morphine. Anesthesiology 64:194, 1986
129. Gueneron JP, Ecoffey C, Carli P et al: Effect of naloxone infusion on analgesia and respiratory depression after epidural fentanyl. Anesth Analg 67:35, 1988
130. Baxter AD, Samson B, Doran R: Prevention of epidural morphine-induced respiratory depression with intravenous nalbuphine infusion in post-thoracotomy patients. Can J Anaesth 36:503, 1989
131. Enquist A, Jorgensen BC, Anderson HB: Catatonia after epidural morphine. Acta Anaesthesiol Scand 25:445, 1981
132. Rawal N, Wattwil M: Respiratory depression following epidural morphine. An experimental and clinical study. Anesth Analg 63:8, 1984
133. Knill RL, Clement JL, Thomson WR: Epidural morphine causes delayed and prolonged ventilatory depression. Can J Anaesth 28:537, 1981
134. Crawford RD, Batra MS, Fox F: Epidural morphine dose response for postoperative analgesia. Anesthesiology 55:A150, 1981
135. Ahuja BR, Strunin L: Respiratory effects of epidural fentanyl. Anaesthesia 40:949, 1985

136. Rosen MA, Hughes SC, Shnider SM et al: Epidural morphine for relief of postoperative pain after cesarean delivery. Anesth Analg 62:666, 1983

137. Hughes SC, Rosen MA, Shnider SM et al: Epidural morphine for the relief of postoperative pain after cesarean section. Anesth Analg 61:190, 1982

138. Pybus DA, Torda TA: Dose-effect relationships of extradural morphine. Br J Anaesth 54:1259, 1982

139. Ready LB: Intraspinal opioid analgesia in the perioperative period. Anesthesiol Clin North Am 10:145, 1992

140. Bromage PR, Camporesi EM, Durant PAC, Nielsen CH: Influence of epinephrine as an adjuvant to epidural morphine. Anesthesiology 58:257, 1983

141. Nordberg G, Mellstrand T, Borg L, Hedner T: Extradural morphine: influence of adrenaline mixture. Br J Anaesth 58:598, 1986

142. Jamous MA, Hand CW, Moore RA et al: Epinephrine reduces systemic absorption of extradural diacetylmorphine. Anesth Analg 65:1290, 1986

143. Klepper ID, Sherril DL, Boetger CL et al: Analgesic and respiratory effects of extradural sufentanil in volunteers and the influence of adrenaline as an adjuvant. Br J Anaesth 59:1147, 1987

144. Robertson K, Douglas MJ, McMorland GH: Epidural fentanyl, with and without epinephrine for post-cesarean section analgesia. Can J Anaesth 32:502, 1985

145. Cullen ML, Staren ED, el-Ganzouri A et al: Continuous epidural infusion for analgesia after major abdominal operations: A randomized, prospective, double-blind study. Surgery 98:718, 1985

146. Badner NH, Reimer EJ, Komar WE, Moote CA: Low dose bupivicaine does not improve epidural fentanyl analgesia in orthopedic patients. Anesth Analg 72:337, 1991

147. Badner NH, Komar WE: Bupivicaine 0.1% does not improve postoperative epidural fentanyl analgesia after abdominal or thoracic surgery. Can J Anaesth 39:330, 1992

148. Lee A, Simpson D, Whitfield A et al: Postoperative analgesia by continuous extradural infusion of bupivacaine and diamorphine. Br J Anaesth 60:845, 1988

149. Scott NB, Mogensen T, Bigler D et al: Continuous thoracic extradural 0.5% bupivacaine with or without morphine: effect on quality of blockade, lung function and the surgical stress response. Br J Anaesth 62:253, 1989

150. Badner NH, Komar WE: 0.125% bupivacaine—the optimum concentration for postoperative epidural fentanyl: analgesic effects. Can J Anaesth 39:A71, 1992

151. Dahl JB, Rosenberg J, Hansen BL et al: Differential analgesic effects of low-dose epidural morphine and morphine-bupivacaine at rest and during mobilization after major abdominal surgery. Anesth Analg 74:362, 1992

152. Badner NH: Epidural agents for postoperative analgesia. Anesthesiol Clin North Am 10:417, 1992

153. Rostaing S, Bonnet F, Levron JC et al: Effect of epidural clonidine on epidural fentanyl analgesia and pharmacokinetics in postoperative patients. Anesthesiology 73:A779, 1990

154. Vercauteren M, Meese G, Lauwers E et al: Addition of clonidine potentiates postoperative analgesia of epidural sufentanil. Anesth Analg 70:S5, 1990

155. Motsch J, Graber E, Ludwig K: Addition of clonidine enhances postoperative analgesia from epidural morphine: a double blind study. Anesthesiology 73:1067, 1990

156. Dahl JB, Rosenberg J, Dirkes WE et al: Prevention of postoperative pain by balanced analgesia. Br J Anaesth 64:518, 1990

157. Schulze S, Roikjaer O, Hasselstrom O et al: Epidural bupivacaine and morphine plus systemic indomethacin eliminates pain but not systemic response and convalescence after cholecystectomy. Surgery 103:321, 1988

158. Schulze S, Sommer P, Bigler D et al: Effects of combined prednisolone, epidural analgesia and indomethacin on the systemic response after colonic surgery. Arch Surg 127:325, 1992

159. Gustafsson LL, Frieberg-Nielsen S, Garle M: Extradural and parenteral morphine: kinetics and effects in postoperative pain. A controlled clinical study. Br J Anaesth 54:1167, 1982

160. Cohen SE, Rothblatt AJ, Albright GA: Early respiratory depression with epidural narcotic and intravenous droperidol. Anesthesiology 59:559, 1983

161. Morgan M: The rational use of intrathecal and extradural opioids. Br J Anaesth 63:165, 1989

162. Gustafsson LL, Grell AM, Garle M et al: Kinetics of morphine in cerebrospinal fluid after epidural administration. Acta Anaesthesiol Scand 28:535, 1984

163. Drost RH, Ionescu TI, van Rossum JM et al: Pharmacokinetics of morphine after epidural administration in man. Arzneimittelforschung 36:1096, 1986

164. Wang JK: Analgesic effect of intrathecally administered morphine. Reg Anesth 2:3, 1977

165. Katz J, Nelson W: Intrathecal morphine for postoperative pain relief. Reg Anesth 61:1, 1981

166. Bailey PL, Rhondeau S, Schafer PG et al: Dose-response pharmacology of intrathecal morphine in human volunteers. Anesthesiology 79:49, 1993

167. Niemi L, Pitkanen MT, Tuominen MK et al: Comparison of intrathecal fentanyl infusion with intrathecal morphine infusion or bolus for postoperative pain relief after hip arthroplasty. Anesth Analg 77:126, 1993

168. Torda TA, Pybus DA: Comparison of four narcotic analgesics for extradural analgesia. Br J Anaesth 54:291, 1982

169. Gustafsson LL, Garle M, Johannisson J et al: Regional epidural analgesia: kinetics of pethidine. Acta Anaesthesiol Scand 26:165, 1982

170. Naguib M, Famewo CE, Absood A: Pharmacokinetics of meperidine in spinal anaesthesia. Can J Anaesth 33:162, 1986

171. Madej TH, Strunin L: Comparison of epidural fentanyl with sufentanil. Anaesthesia 42:1156, 1987

172. Melendez JA, Cirella VN, Delphin ES: Lumbar epidural fentanyl analgesia after thoracic surgery. J Cardiothorac Vasc Anesth 3:150, 1989

173. Lomessy A, Magnin C, Viale JP et al: Clinical advantages of fentanyl given epidurally for postoperative analgesia. Anesthesiology 61:466, 1984

174. Naulty JS, Datta S, Ostheimer G et al: Epidural fentanyl for postcesarean delivery pain management. Anesthesiology 63:694, 1985

175. Birnbach DJ, Johnson MD, Arcario T et al: Effect of diluent volume of analgesia produced by epidural fentanyl. Anesth Analg 68:808, 1989

176. Belzarena SD: Clinical effects of intrathecally administered fentanyl in patients undergoing cesarean section. Anesth Analg 74:653, 1992

177. Bohannon TW, Estes MD: Evaluation of subarachnoid fentanyl for postoperative analgesia. Anesthesiology 67:A237, 1987

178. Hunt CO, Naulty JS, Bader AM et al: Perioperative analgesia with subarachnoid fentanyl-bupivacaine for cesarean delivery. Anesthesiology 71:535, 1989

179. Chauvin M, Salbaing J, Perrin D et al: Clinical assessment and plasma pharmacokinetics associated with intramuscular or extradural alfentanil. Br J Anaesth 57:886, 1985

180. Stanton-Hicks MDA, Gielen M, Hasenbos M et al: High thoracic epidural with sufentanil for postthoracotomy pain. Reg Anesth 13:62, 1988

181. Donadoni R, Rolly G, Noordum H et al: Epidural sufentanil for postoperative pain relief. Anaesthesia 40:634, 1985

182. Rosen MA, Dailey PA, Hughes SC et al: Epidural sufentanil for postoperative analgesia after cesarean section. Anesthesiology 69:971, 1988

183. Cohen SE, Tan S, White PF: Sufentanil analgesia following cesarean section: epidural vesus intravenous administration. Anesthesiology 68:129, 1988

184. Hansdottir V, Hedner T, Woestenborghs CE et al: The CSF and plasma pharmacokinetics of sufentanil after intrathecal administration. Anesthesiology 74:264, 1991

185. Ionescu IT, Taverne RHT, Hovweling PL et al: Pharmacokinetic study of extradural and intrathecal sufentanil anesthesia for major surgery. Br J Anaesth 66:458, 1991

186. Donadoni R, Vermeulen H, Noorduin H et al: Intrathecal sufentanil as a supplement to subarachnoid anaesthesia with lignocaine. Br J Anaesth 59:1523, 1987

187. Camann WR, Denney RA, Holby ED et al: A comparison of intrathecal, epidural, and intravenous sufentanil for labour analgesia. Anesthesiology 77:884, 1992

188. De Castro J, Meynadier J, Zenz M: Regional Opioid Analgesia. Kluwer Academic Publishers, Dordrecht, The Netherlands, 1991

189. Bilsback P, Rolly G, Tampubolon O: Efficacy of extradural administration of lofentanil, buprenorphine or saline in the management of postoperative pain. A double-blind study. Br J Anaesth 57:943, 1985

190. Pasqualucci V, Tantucci C, Paoletti F et al: Buprenorphine vs morphine via the epidural route: a controlled comparative clinical study of respiratory effects and analgesic activity. Pain 29:273, 1987

191. Gundersen RY, Andersen R, Narverud G: Postoperative pain relief with high-dose epidural buprenorphine: a double-blind study. Acta Anaesthesiol Scand 30:664, 1986

192. Christensen FR, Andersen LW: Adverse reaction to extradural buprenorphine. Br J Anaesth 54:476, 1982

193. Abboud TK, Moore M, Zhu J et al: Epidural butorphanol or morphine for the relief of post-cesarean section pain: ventilatory responses to carbon dioxide. Anesth Analg 66:887, 1987

194. Mok MS, Lippman M, Wang JJ et al: Efficacy of epidural nalbuphine in postoperative pain control. Anesthesiology 61:A187, 1984

195. Baxter AD, Laganiere S, Samson B et al: A dose-response study of nalbuphine for post-thoracotomy epidural analgesia. Can J Anaesth 38:125, 1991

196. Etches R, Sandler AN: Analgesic effects of epidural nubain in post-thoracotomy patients. Anesthesiology 75:9, 1991

197. Yaksh TL, Collins JG: Studies in animals should precede human use of spinally administered drugs. Anesthesiology 70:4, 1989

198. Rawal N, Nuutinen L, Raj PP et al: Behavioral and histopathologic effects following intrathecal

administration of butorphanol, sufentanil, and nalbuphine in sheep. Anesthesiology 75:1025, 1991

199. Abouleish E, Barmada MA, Nemoto EM et al: Acute and chronic effects of intrathecal morphine in monkeys. Br J Anaesth 53:1027, 1981

200. King FG, Baxter AD, Mathieson G: Tissue reaction of morphine applied to the epidural space of dogs. Can J Anaesth 31:268, 1984

201. Gurel A, Unal N, Elevli M et al: Epidural morphine for postoperative pain relief in anorectal surgery. Anesth Analg 65:499, 1986

202. Nyska M, Klin B, Shapira Y et al: Epidural methadone for preoperative analgesia in patients with proximal femoral fractures. BMJ 293:1347, 1986

203. Woolf CJ, Chong MS: Preemptive analgesia—treating postoperative pain by preventing the establishment of central sensitization. Anesth Analg 77:362, 1993

204. Katz J, Kavanagh BP, Sandler AN et al: Pre-emptive analgesia: clinical evidence of neuroplasticity contributing to postoperative pain. Anesthesiology 77:439, 1992

205. Camara PB, de Salinas ADM, Guasch RG et al: Epidural fentanyl with etidocaine or bupivacaine compared in hip surgery. Rev Esp Anestesiol Reanim 31:144, 1984

206. Grant GJ, Ramanathan S, Turndorf H: Epidural fentanyl reduces isoflurane requirements during thoracotomy. Anesthesiology 71:A668, 1989

207. Drasner K, Bernards C, Ozanne GM: Intrathecal morphine reduces the minimum alveolar concentration of halothane in humans. Anesthesiology 69:310, 1988

208. Cozian A, Pinaud M, LePage JY et al: Effects of meperidine spinal anesthesia on hemodynamics, plasma catecholamines, angiotensin I, aldosterone, and histamine concentrations in elderly men. Anesthesiology 64:815, 1986

209. Gjessing J, Tomlin PJ: Postoperative pain control with intrathecal morphine. Anaesthesia 36:268, 1981

210. Sjostrand UH, Rawal N (eds): Regional opioids in anesthesiology and pain management. Int Anesthesiol Clin 24:43, 1986

211. Rechtine GR, Reinert CM, Bohlman HH: The use of epidural morphine to decrease postoperative pain in patients undergoing lumbar laminectomy. J Bone Joint Surg [Am] 66:113, 1984

212. Hasenbos M, Van Egmond J, Gielen M et al: Postoperative analgesia by epidural versus intramuscular nicomorphine after thoracotomy. Pt. 1. Acta Anaesthesiol Scand 29:572, 1985

213. Johnson JR, McCaughey W: Epidural morphine. A method of management of multiple fracture ribs. Anaesthesia 35:155, 1980

214. Rankin APN, Comber REH: Management of fifty cases of chest injury with a regimen of epidural bupivacaine and morphine. Anaesth Intensive Care 12:311, 1984

215. Ullman DA, Wimpy RE, Fortune JB et al: The treatment of patients with multiple rib fractures using continuous thoracic narcotic infusion. Reg Anesth 14:43, 1989

216. Pasqualucci V, Moricca G, Solinas P: Intrathecal morphine for the control of pain of myocardial infarction. Anaesthesia 36:68, 1981

217. Skoeld M, Gilberg L, Ohlsson O: Pain relief in myocardial infarction after continuous epidural morphine analgesia. N Engl J Med 312:650, 1985

218. Magora F, Olshwang D, Eimerl D et al: Observations of extradural morphine analgesia in various pain conditions. Br J Anaesth 52:247, 1980

219. Clemensen SE, Thaysen P, Hole P: Epidural morphine for outpatients with severe anginal pain. BMJ 294:475, 1987

220. Valley RD, Bailey AG: Caudal morphine for postoperative analgesia in infants and children: a report of 138 cases. Anesth Analg 72:120, 1991

221. Rosen KR, Rosen DA: Caudal epidural morphine for control of pain following open heart surgery in children. Anesthesiology 70:418, 1989

222. Shapiro LA, Jedeikin RJ, Shaley D et al: Epidural morphine analgesia in children. Anesthesiology 61:210, 1984

223. Glenski JA, Warner MA, Dawson B et al: Postoperative use of epidurally administered morphine in children and adolescents. Mayo Clin Proc 59:530, 1984

224. Jensen BH: Caudal block for post-operative pain relief in children after genital operations. A comparison between bupivacaine and morphine. Acta Anaesthesiol Scand 23:373, 1981

225. Krane EJ, Tyler DC, Jacobson LE: The dose response of caudal morphine in children. Anesthesiology 71:48, 1989

226. Krane EJ: Delayed respiratory depression in a child after epidural morphine. Anesth Analg 67:79, 1988

227. Lysak SZ, Eisenach JC, Dobson CE: Patient controlled analgesia during labor: a comparison of three solutions with a continuous infusion control. Anesthesiology 72:44, 1990

228. Baraka A, Noueihed R, Hajj S: Intrathecal injection of morphine for obstetric analgesia. Anesthesiology 54:136, 1981

229. Leighton BL, DeSimone CA, Norris MC et al: Intrathecal narcotics for labor revisited: the combination of fentanyl and morphine intrathecally provides rapid onset of profound, prolonged analgesia. Anesth Analg 69:122, 1989

230. Abboud TK, Raya J, Noueihed R et al: Intrathecal morphine for relief of labor pain in a parturient with severe pulmonary hypertension. Anesthesiology 59:477, 1983

231. Ahmad S, Hawes D, Dooley S et al: Intrathecal morphine in a parturient with a single ventricle. Anesthesiology 54:515, 1981

232. Husenmeyer RP, Davenport HT, Cummings AJ, Rosankiewicz JR: Comparison of epidural and intramuscular pethidine for analgesia in labour. Br J Obstet Gynaecol 88:711, 1981

233. Husemeyer RP, Cummings AJ, Rosankiewicz JR, Davenport HT: A study of pethidine kinetics and analgesia in women in labour following intravenous, intramuscular and epidural administration. Br J Clin Pharmacol 13:171, 1982

234. Baraka A, Maktabi M, Noueihed R: Epidural meperidine-bupivacaine for obstetric analgesia. Anesth Analg 61:652, 1982

235. Carrie LES, O'sullivan GM, Seegobin R et al: Epidural fentanyl in labour. Anaesthesia 36:965, 1981

236. Heytens L, Cammu H, Camu F: Extradural analgesia during labour using alfentanil. Br J Anaesth 59:331, 1987

237. Steinberg RB, Powell G, Hu XH et al: Epidural sufentanil for analgesia for labor and delivery. Reg Anesth 14:225, 1989

238. Cohen SE, Tan S, Albright GA: Epidural fentanyl/bupivacaine mixtures for obstetric analgesia. Anesthesiology 67:403, 1987

239. Chestnut DH, Owen CL, Bates JN et al: Continuous infusion epidural analgesia during labor: a randomized, double-blind comparison of 0.0625% bupivacaine/0.0002% fentanyl versus 0.125% bupivacaine. Anesthesiology 68:754, 1988

240. Philips GH: Continuous infusion epidural analgesia in labor: the effect of adding sufentanil to 0.125% bupivacaine. Anesth Analg 67:462, 1988

241. Carp H, Johnson MD, Bader AM et al: Continuous epidural infusion of alfentanil and bupivacaine for labor and delivery. Anesthesiology 69:A687, 1988

242. Hunt CO, Naulty JS, Malinow AM et al: Epidural butorphanol-bupivacaine for analgesia during labor and delivery. Anesth Analg 68:323, 1989

243. Niv D, Rudick V, Golan A et al: Augmentation of bupivacaine analgesia in labor by epidural morphine. Obstet Gynecol 67:206, 1986

244. Abouleish E, Rawal N, Fallon K et al: Combined intrathecal morphine and bupivacaine for cesarean section. Anesth Analg 67:370, 1988

245. Zakowski M, Ramanathan S, Turndorf H: Intrathecal morphine for post-cesarean section analgesia. Anesthesiology 71:A870, 1989

246. Preston PG, Rosen MA, Hughes SC et al: Epidural anesthesia with fentanyl and lidocaine for cesarean section: maternal effects and neonatal outcome. Anesthesiology 68:938, 1988

247. Gaffud MP, Bansal P, Lawton C et al: Surgical analgesia for cesarean section with epidural bupivacaine and fentanyl. Anesthesiology 65:331, 1986

248. Milon D, Bentue-Ferrer D, Noury D et al: Anesthesia peridurale pour cesarienne par association bupivacaine-fentanyl. Ann Fr Anesth Reanim 2:273, 1983

249. Brockway MS, Noble DW, Sharwood-Smith GH, McClure JH. Profound respiratory depression after extradural fentanyl. Br J Anaesth 64:243, 1990

250. Yee I, Carstoniu J, Halpern S, Pittini R: A comparison of two doses of epidural fentanyl during cesarean section. Can J Anaesth 40:772, 1993

251. Vertommen J, Vandermeulen E, Shnider SM et al: The effect of the addition of epidural sufentanil to bupivacaine 0.5% for elective cesarean section. Anesthesiology 71:A868, 1989

252. Crone LL, Conly JM, Clark KM et al: Recurrent herpes simplex virus labialis and the use of epidural morphine in obstetric patients. Anesth Analg 67:318, 1988

253. James CF, Banner TCE: High-volume fentanyl compared with other narcotics after cesarean section: analgesia and respiratory status. Anesth Analg 70:S178, 1990

254. Perriss BW, Latham BV, Wilson IH: Analgesia following extradural and i.m. pethidine in post-caesarean section patients. Br J Anaesth 64:355, 1990

255. Benhamou D, Samii K, Noviant Y: Effect of analgesia on respiratory muscle function after upper abdominal surgery. Acta Anaesthesiol Scand 27:22, 1983

256. Torda TA, Pybus DA: Extradural administration of morphine and bupivacaine. Br J Anaesth 56:141, 1984

257. Rybro L, Schurizek BA, Petersen TK et al: Postoperative analgesia and lung function: a comparison of intramuscular with epidural morphine. Acta Anaesthesiol Scand 26:514, 1982

258. Rawal N, Sjostrand UH, Dahlstrom B et al: Epidural morphine for postoperative pain relief: a

comparative study with intramuscular narcotic and intercostal nerve block. Anesth Analg 61:93, 1982

259. Cuschieri RJ, Morran CJ, Howie JC et al: Postoperative pain and pulmonary complications: comparison of three analgesic regimens. Br J Surg 72:485, 1985

260. Isaacson IJ, Weitz FI, Berry AJ et al: Intrathecal morphine's effect on the postoperative course of patients undergoing abdominal aortic surgery. Anesth Analg 66:S86, 1987

261. El-Baz N, Goldin M: Continuous epidural morphine infusion for pain relief after open heart surgery. Anesthesiology 59:A193, 1983

262. Scheinin B, Asantila R, Orko R: The effect of bupivacaine and morphine on pain and bowel function after colonic surgery. Acta Anaesthesiol Scand 31:161, 1987

263. Garnett RL, MacIntyre A, Lindsay MP: Perioperative ischemia in aortic surgery: epidural anaesthesia/analgesia vs general anaesthesia/iv analgesia. Can J Anaesth 40:A52, 1993

264. Ventafridda V, Tamburini M, DeConno F: Comprehensive treatment in cancer pain. p. 617. In Fields H, Dubner R, Cervero F (eds): Advances in Pain Research and Therapy. Vol. 9. Raven Press, New York, 1985

265. Cherry DA, Gourlay GK, McLachlan M et al: Diagnostic epidural opioid blockade and chronic pain. Preliminary report. Pain 21:143, 1985a

266. Cherry DA, Gourlay GK, Cousins MJ et al: A technique for the insertion of an implantable portal system for the long term epidural administration of opioids in the treatment of cancer pain. Anaesth Intensive Care 13:145, 1985

267. Coombs DW, Maurer LH, Saunders RL et al: Outcomes and complications of continuous intraspinal narcotic analgesia for cancer pain control. J Clin Oncol 2:1414, 1984

268. Harbaugh RE, Coombs DW, Saunders RI et al: Implanted continuous epidural morphine system. Preliminary report. J Neurosurg 36:803, 1982

269. Zenz M: Epidural opiates: long term experience in cancer pain. Klin Wochenschr 63:225, 1985

270. Carl P, Crawford ME, Ravlo O et al: Long term treatment with epidural opioids. A retrospective study comprising 150 patients treated with morphine chloride and buprenorphine. Anaesthesia 41:32, 1986

Chapter 7

Basic Pharmacology of Local Anesthetics

Toshio Narahashi

Cocaine is contained in the leaves of *Erythroxylon coca*, a shrub growing in the Andes mountains, and the leaves had long been used by people in Peru before being introduced into medicine; they chewed the leaves to get a sense of well-being. Freud and Koller introduced cocaine into ophthalmological use in 1884, and shortly thereafter, Hall used it for dental operations.

The era of synthetic local anesthetics began when Einhorn introduced procaine in 1905. Procaine almost completely replaced cocaine because of its more favorable therapeutic index. Subsequently, a number of synthetic local anesthetics were introduced into clinical use (Table 7-1). Lidocaine, introduced in 1948, is the most widely used local anesthetic.

DESIRABLE PROPERTIES

A chemical must be endowed with certain properties to become useful for local anesthesia. These properties include the following:

1. The time required for the onset of local anesthesia should be short, and the anesthesia should last long enough to allow time for the contemplated surgery.

2. The systemic toxicity should be low.
3. There should be no side effects, such as irritation or permanent damage to the nerve.
4. The compound should be soluble in water and stable in solution for storage.

CHEMISTRY

The chemical structures of some of the commonly used local anesthetics are shown in Table 7-1. Three points are worthy of note in considering structure-activity relationships:

1. Most of the local anesthetic molecules are composed of three parts, an aromatic residue (lipophilic), an intermediate chain, and an amine group (hydrophilic).
2. The terminal amino group is usually a secondary or tertiary amine and determines the pK_a value of the compound. This is important because the pK_a value affects the distribution of the compound outside and inside the cell.
3. The intermediate chain is either an amide, as in lidocaine, or an ester, as in procaine. This difference in the intermediate chain is important in connection with the metabolic degradation of local anesthetics, which will be discussed later.

179

Table 7-1 Chemical Structures, the Years When Used Clinically for the First Time, and pK$_a$ Values of Commonly Used Local Anesthetics

Type	First Clinical Use	pK$_a$	
Ester			
Procaine	1905	9.0	
Chloroprocaine	1955	8.7	
Tetracaine	1930	8.5	
Cocaine	1884	8.8	
Benzocaine	1900	2.5	
Amide			
Lidocaine	1944	7.7	
Mepivacaine	1957	7.6	
Prilocaine	1960	7.7	

(Continues)

Table 7-1 (Continued)

Type	First Clinical Use	pKa	
Bupivacaine	1963	8.1	
Dibucaine	1929	8.8	
Etidocaine	1972	7.7	

Because of the presence of a secondary or tertiary amino in the molecule, most local anesthetics exist in an uncharged molecular form (B) and a positively charged cationic form (BH$^+$):

$$B + H_2O \rightleftharpoons BH^+ + OH^- \quad (1)$$

For example, procaine is dissociated as follows:

$$NH_2C_6H_4COOCH_2CH_2N\begin{smallmatrix}C_2H_5\\\\C_2H_5\end{smallmatrix} + H_2O$$

$$\rightleftharpoons NH_2C_6H_4COOCH_2CH_2N^+H\begin{smallmatrix}C_2H_5\\\\C_2H_5\end{smallmatrix} + OH^- \quad (2)$$

The ratio of the charged to uncharged form is determined by the pKa of the compound and the pH of the medium and is given by the Henderson-Hasselbalch equation:

$$\log \frac{[BH^+]}{[B]} = pK_a - pH \quad (3)$$

where [BH$^+$] and [B] represent the concentrations of the charged and uncharged forms, respectively. The pKa values of local anesthetics are usually between 7.5 and 9.0 (Table 7-1); therefore, both forms exist in the physiologic pH range.

MODE OF ACTION OF LOCAL ANESTHETICS

Local anesthetics block nerve conduction without affecting the resting membrane potential. Sometimes the term "stabilization" is used to express this type of action, but this word is misleading and becoming obsolete. Excitation of nerve fibers takes place as a result of the opening and closing of sodium and potassium channels, which in turn, alters the ionic permeability of the nerve membrane. Local anesthetics modify ion channel activity. Therefore, to study the mechanism of action of local anesthetics on nerve fibers, it is imperative to understand how ion channels function and how their activity can be measured.

Mechanism of Nerve Excitation

The mechanism of nerve excitation had been studied for many years, but it was not until 1952 that the ionic basis of excitation was firmly established. Hodgkin and Huxley[1-4] performed extensive experiments with squid giant axons by using the improved voltage clamp technique[5] that was originally developed by Cole.[6] This ion theory of excitation was later extended to many other excitable cells with some modification, and it laid the foundation of the basic understanding of nerve excitation and drug action.[7] In the following account, squid giant axons are used as the prototype for excitable cells.

Potassium concentration is higher inside the axon than outside it; sodium concentration is higher outside than inside. In resting conditions, some of the potassium channels are open and most of the sodium channels are closed. Thus, the nerve membrane is permeable to potassium but only sparingly so to sodium. This condition creates a potential difference across the nerve membrane in an amount close to the potassium equilibrium potential (E_K) as defined by the Nernst equation (Fig. 7-1):

$$E_K = \frac{RT}{F} \ln \frac{[K^+]_o}{[K^+]_i} \qquad (4)$$

where $[K^+]_o$ and $[K^+]_i$ represent the potassium concentrations (strictly speaking, the activities) outside and inside the cell, respectively, and R, T, and F represent the gas constant, absolute temperature, and Faraday constant, respectively. Because of the slight contributions of permeabilities to sodium and other ions, and resting potential (approximately -70 mV) is usually slightly less negative than is the calculated potassium equilibrium potential (-80 mV).

On membrane depolarization, the membrane

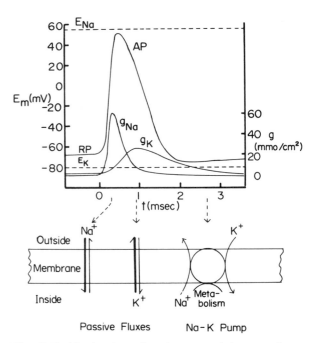

Fig. 7-1 Mechanism of action potential generation. Upper half illustrates changes in membrane sodium conductance (g_{Na}) and K conductance (g_K) during an action potential (AP). Resting potential (RP) is close to the K equilibrium potential (E_K), and the peak of the action potential approaches the sodium equilibrium potential (E_{Na}). Lower half illustrates ionic fluxes during and after the action potential. See text for further explanation. E_m, membrane potential; g, conductance. (From Narahashi,[8] with permission.)

permeability to sodium increases rapidly as a result of the opening of sodium channels, bringing the membrane potential close to the sodium equilibrium potential (E_{Na}, $\sim +50$ mV), as defined by the Nernst equation for sodium:

$$E_{Na} = \frac{RT}{F} \ln \frac{[Na^+]_o}{[Na^+]_i} \qquad (5)$$

where $[Na^+]_o$ and $[Na^+]_i$ refer to the external and internal sodium concentrations, respectively. This results in the rising phase of the action potential, and the membrane potential is reversed in polarity (Fig. 7-1). Sodium permeability soon starts to decrease as a result of closing of sodium channels (sometimes called sodium inactivation), and potassium permeability is increased beyond the resting level as a result of the opening of many potassium channels. These two processes restore the membrane potential toward the potassium equilibrium potential and result in the falling phase of the action potential. During an action potential, sodium ions enter the cell through the open sodium channels, according to their electrochemical gradient across the membrane, and potassium ions leave the cell through the open potassium channels, according to their electrochemical gradient (Fig. 7-1). All these processes, including opening and closing of ion channels and their resulting ionic fluxes, are passive phenomena that do not immediately require metabolic energy. The changes in the sodium and potassium concentrations inside the cell as a result of one action potential are very small, e.g., approximately 1/1,000 for an axon with a diameter of 1 μm. However, these small imbalances in ionic concentrations must be restored for the axon to maintain excitability. This is accomplished by the energy (adenosine triphosphate)-dependent Na-K pump, which pumps extra sodium out and potassium into the cell (Fig. 7-1).

In summary, there are three ionic permeability components of the action potential:

1. Increase in sodium permeability, responsible for the rising phase of action potential.
2. Decrease in sodium permeability.
3. Increase in potassium permeability. Steps 2 and 3 are responsible for the falling phase of the action potential.

Voltage Clamp: Principle and Technique

The voltage clamp is a powerful and straightforward technique by which ionic permeabilities can be measured.[8,9] The technique is based on two principles, Ohm's law and space clamp. Ohm's law states that electric conductance (the inverse of resistance) is current divided by electrical potential. Thus, if we can measure the currents carried by sodium (I_{Na}) and potassium (I_K), the membrane potential (E_m), and the respective equilibrium potentials, the membrane conductances to sodium (g_{Na}) and potassium (g_K) are given by:

$$g_{Na} = I_{Na}/(E_m - E_{Na}) \qquad (6)$$

$$g_K = I_K/(E_m - E_K) \qquad (7)$$

However, the complex structure of an axon causes a problem. To understand the situation, we must analyze the electrical properties of an axon. A portion of an axon can be represented by analogy to an electrical circuit as shown in Fig. 7-2. The external and internal phases of the axon have external resistance (r_o) and internal resistance (r_i), respectively. The membrane also has resistance (r_m). In addition, the membrane has capacity (c_m). Therefore, when a current is injected into the axon, the current and the resultant membrane po-

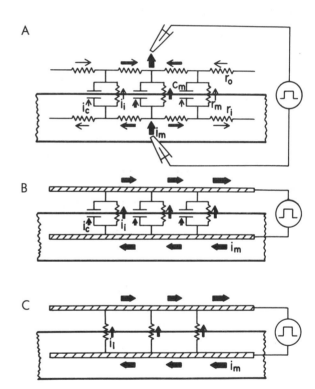

Fig. 7-2 Current flow in an axon preparation. **(A)** Current is applied to the axon through internal and external microelectrodes. The membrane current and longitudinal current are not uniform along the axon. **(B)** Current is applied through internal and external wire electrodes. The membrane current and longitudinal current are uniform along the axon (space clamp). **(C)** When the axon in the space clamp condition is voltage clamped, no capacitive current (i_c) flows while the membrane potential is maintained at a constant level, making it possible to measure the ionic current (i_i). c_m, membrane capacity i_m, total membrane current; r_o, external resistance; r_i, internal resistance; r_m, membrane resistance. (From Narahashi,[35] with permission.)

tential change are distributed along the axon in a nonuniform manner, as shown by arrows with different widths (Fig. 7-2A). The distribution of current and membrane potential change can be made uniform if the external and internal resistances are eliminated. This can be accomplished by placing a large, longitudinal metal electrode, which has a negligible resistance compared with r_i, outside the axon and by inserting a similar electrode inside (Fig. 7-2B). This establishes a space clamp condition. However, this manipulation leaves the membrane capacitance intact, still causing a complex flow of current across the membrane. The capacity current can be eliminated if the membrane current is measured while keeping the membrane potential constant by a voltage clamp (Fig. 7-2C). Thus, the space clamp is a prerequisite for the voltage clamp measurement of membrane ionic currents.

The voltage clamp arrangement for an internally perfused squid giant axon is illustrated in Figure 7-3. The membrane potential is recorded by a glass capillary electrode inserted longitudinally into the axon and another glass capillary reference electrode placed outside the axon. The recorded membrane potential is fed into a control amplifier, and a command pulse that is generated from a pulse generator is applied. The difference between the

membrane potential and the command pulse is then amplified by the control amplifier, and a current is generated from the output of the amplifier. This current flows across the membrane through a longitudinal internal wire electrode and large external metal electrodes in such a way as to make the membrane potential equal to the command pulse. Thus, with the aid of the voltage clamp feedback circuit, the membrane potential is maintained at the desired level (command pulse), and the membrane current (I_M) necessary for the voltage clamp can be recorded by a current-recording amplifier.

Membrane currents associated with a step depolarizing pulse under a voltage clamp condition are illustrated in Figure 7-4. A step depolarization generates a capacitive current (I_c), which is initially large but decays quickly. The capacitive current is followed by an inward current (downward deflection). This current attains a peak and is followed by a steady-state outward current (upward deflection). On termination of the depolarizing step, another capacitive current appears that is equal in magnitude but opposite to the capacitive current that appears at the beginning of the pulse. Then a tail current (I_{tail}) follows and declines toward the original zero current level. The transient inward current is carried largely by sodium ions; the steady-

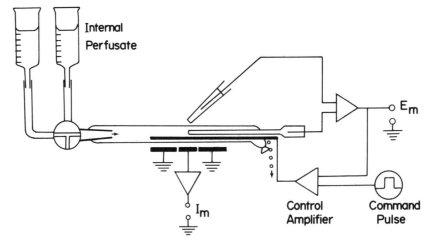

Fig. 7-3 Voltage clamp of an internally perfused squid giant axon. See text for further explanation. E_m, membrane potential; I_m, membrane current. (From Narahashi,[8] with permission).

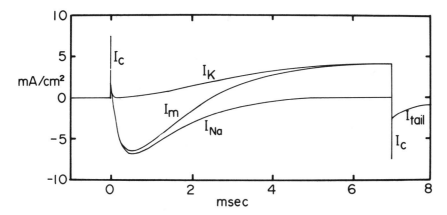

Fig. 7-4 Membrane current (I_m) and its sodium current (I_{Na}), potassium current (I_K), and capacitive current (I_c) components associated with a step depolarization of the nerve membrane under voltage clamp condition. (From Narahashi,[36] with permission.)

state outward current is carried largely by potassium ions. Thus, the peak and steady-state currents represent, as a first approximation, sodium and potassium currents, respectively.

The peak sodium current and the steady-state potassium current can be plotted as a function of the membrane potential to construct a current-voltage (I-V) relationship (Fig. 7-5). The peak inward sodium current increases in amplitude with increasing membrane depolarization up to around -25 mV. However, the amplitude of the sodium current decreases with further increasing membrane depolarization, reverses its polarity around $+35$ mV, and becomes outward with larger depolarizations. The membrane potential at which the sodium current reverses its polarity is close to the sodium equilibrium potential. The sodium conductance calculated by equation 6 increases with increasing depolarization and attains a maximum at around -25 mV. The outward potassium current also increases with depolarization.

Patch Clamp

Whereas the voltage clamp is a straightforward technique to measure the membrane conductances to various ions, the application is limited to certain forms of excitable cells as a result of the need for a space clamp. Furthermore, the ionic currents thus recorded are derived from the activity of a large number of ion channels present in the preparation. Another quantum leap was made in the ion channel field when Neher and Sakmann[10] in Germany successfully recorded tiny ionic currents passing through individual ion channels. This technique, called patch clamp, was later improved to enable the measurement of single channel currents more accurately and to measure ionic currents passing through the entire membrane of a small cell. The technique is based on applying a glass capillary

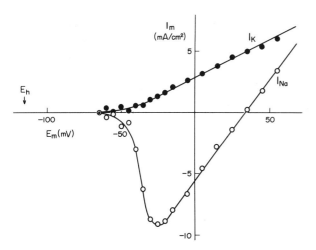

Fig. 7-5 Current-voltage (I_m-E_m) relationships for the peak sodium current (I_{Na}) and for the steady-state potassium current (I_K) in a lobster giant axon. E_h, holding membrane potential. (From Narahashi,[37] with permission.)

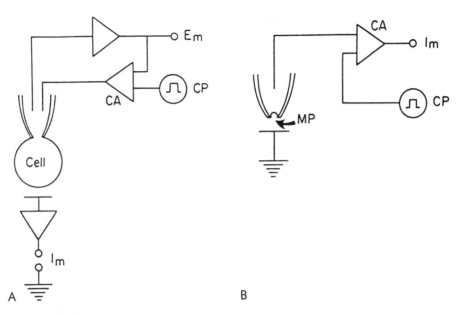

Fig. 7-6 Schematic diagram of patch clamp. **(A)** whole cell patch clamp; **(B)** single channel recording from an isolated membrane patch; *CA*, control amplifier; *CP*, command pulse; E_m, membrane potential; I_m, membrane current; *MP*, membrane patch. See text for further explanation. (From Narahashi,[9] with permission.)

electrode with a small opening onto the cell membrane and establishing a very large seal resistance (10 to 100 GΩ) at the orifice of the capillary electrode.[11] Whole cell and single channel current recording by patch clamp is illustrated in Figure 7-6. The patch clamp technique is applicable to practically any cells, including neurons, cardiac myocytes, lymphocytes, secretory cells, and red blood cells, and it is widely used for the study of the physiology, pharmacology, and toxicology of ion channels.

Internal Perfusion

Internal perfusion is not essential but may be very useful for voltage clamp experiments, especially for the study of local anesthetics. Internal perfusion allows control of the internal and the external environment, including ionic composition, pH, and test compound. For example, if sodium currents are to be measured, potassium currents can be eliminated by perfusing the axon externally and internally with media free of potassium. Certain drugs, including local anesthetics, are ionized depending on the pH of the medium and the pK_a of

the compound, and this can be controlled easily by using internal perfusion techniques. Any test compound can be applied either externally or internally. This is also important because certain chemicals act only from one side of the membrane. Therefore, internal perfusion techniques can greatly broaden the spectrum of measurements and analyses in voltage clamp experiments. Internal perfusion techniques were originally developed for squid giant axons by two groups, Baker et al.[12] in England and Oikawa et al.[13] in the United States, and they have been used extensively in various studies, including those of local anesthetics.

Local Anesthetic Action on Ionic Permeabilities

Studies of the mechanism of drug action on ion channels have become one of the most active fields in neuropharmacology. The modern era of this field began when voltage clamp techniques were first applied to the study of local anesthetics in the late 1950s. Taylor[14] and Shanes et al.[15] demonstrated that procaine and cocaine suppressed both sodium and potassium conductances in squid giant axons. Additional study was later extended to other local anesthetics applied externally or internally.[16,17] Most clinically relevant local anesthetics are tertiary amines, and they suppress both sodium and potassium conductances when applied either externally or internally to squid giant axons (Fig. 7-7). The suppression of sodium conductance is directly responsible for the conduction block.

In some nerve fibers, increasing the external calcium concentration partially antagonizes the local anesthetic block.[18] A variety of hypotheses have been put forward to account for this phenomenon. The hypothesis that calls for competition between calcium and local anesthetic for a binding site on the nerve membrane surface[19] (as described in some textbooks) is no longer accepted.[20] The most plausible explanation for the calcium antagonism of local anesthetic block is as follows. The ability of

the sodium channel to open on stimulation changes with the membrane potential, decreasing with membrane depolarization, i.e., the sodium channels become inactivated by membrane depolarization and can no longer open on stimulation.[3,7] The relationship between the ability of the sodium channels to open and the membrane potential (called the sodium inactivation curve) is shifted in the direction of more negative membrane potential by certain local anesthetics (Fig. 7-8).[21] Such a shift will result in a decrease in sodium current because local anesthetics do not change the resting potential. Calcium ions have an opposite effect on the sodium inactivation curve as a result of their ability to neutralize fixed negative charges on the surface of nerve membrane. An increase in calcium concentration shifts the curve in the direction of the less negative membrane potential.[22] Thus, high cal-

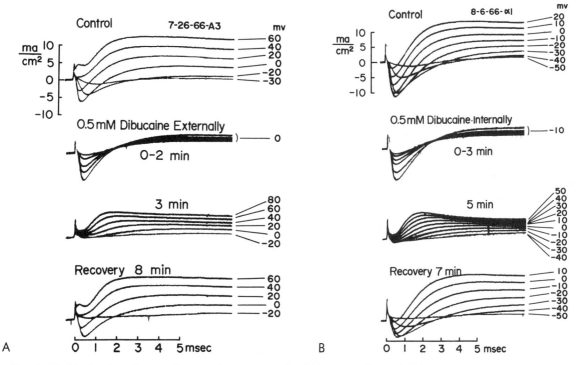

Fig. 7-7 Block of sodium and potassium currents by **(A)** externally and **(B)** internally applied 0.5 mM dibucaine in internally perfused squid giant axons. Families of ionic currents associated with step depolarizations to various levels indicated are shown before (control, top row), during application of dibucaine (second and third rows), and after washing with drug-free media (bottom row). (From Narahashi et al.,[16] with permission.)

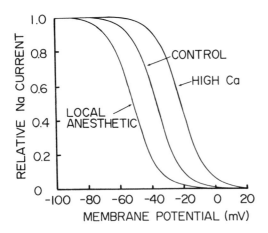

Fig. 7-8 Sodium inactivation curve as a function of the membrane potential. The curve depicts the relationship between the ability of sodium channels to open on stimulation and the membrane potential. This ability decreases with membrane depolarization (less negative potential) and is lost when the membrane is depolarized beyond a certain level. Increasing the external calcium concentration causes a shift of the curve in the direction of depolarization. Certain local anesthetics shift the curve in the direction of hyperpolarization. Thus an increase in calcium concentration antagonizes the local anesthetic-induced shift of the sodium inactivation curve, resulting in a recovery of action potential.

cium concentration restores the local anesthetic shift of the sodium inactivation curve, thereby causing a recovery from the local anesthetic block.

Tetrodotoxin Block of Sodium Channel

Tetrodotoxin (TTX) (Fig. 7-9) is contained in the ovary and liver of the puffer fish. It is a potent nerve and muscle blocking agent and kills animals and humans by respiratory paralysis. The LD_{50} value in mice is estimated to be 10 μg/kg. Although various attempts to develop TTX into a useful local anesthetic have failed for a number of reasons (including severe side effects, such as hypotension and the lack of antidotes), it has been used as a powerful chemical tool in the laboratory since the discovery of TTX's potent and selective blocking action on the sodium channel.[23,24] The mechanism of action of TTX is crucial in understanding the mechanism of action of local anesthetics; therefore, a brief account is given here.

TTX blocks the action potentials of nerve and

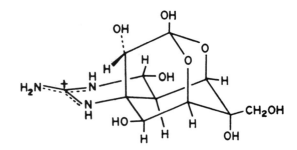

Fig. 7-9. Chemical structure of tetrodotoxin.

skeletal muscle without changing the resting potential. Voltage clamp experiments clearly demonstrated that it blocks the sodium current without any effect on the potassium current (Fig. 7-10).[24] This discovery ignited a widespread interest in using specific chemicals as probes for the study of ion

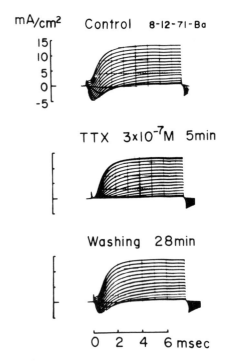

Fig. 7-10. Families of membrane currents associated with step depolarizations (10-mV steps) in a squid giant axon before and during external applications of 3×10^{-7} M tetrodotoxin (*TTX*) and after washing with toxin-free medium. Note that TTX blocks transient sodium currents without any effect on steady-state potassium currents. (From Narahashi,[38] with permission.)

channels.[25,26] TTX reversibly blocks the sodium channel only when applied to the external membrane surface. There is a one-to-one stoichiometric relationship between sodium channels and TTX, with a K_d value in the nanomolar range. One of the most remarkable uses of TTX as a tool is to estimate the density of sodium channels in the nerve membrane. By using a bioassay technique to measure TTX concentration, the density of sodium channels in lobster walking leg nerves was estimated to be $13/\mu m^2$ of the membrane.[27] Additional study was later extended to several other preparations by using [³H]TTX or [³H]saxitoxin, another toxin that exerts a sodium channel blocking effect similar to that of TTX. The most accurate estimates of sodium channel density include: $90/\mu m^2$ for lobster walking leg nerves, 300 to $500/\mu m^2$ for squid giant axons, $110/\mu m^2$ for rabbit vagus nerves, $80/\mu m^2$ for mouse neuroblastoma cells, $380/\mu m^2$ for frog sartorius muscle, $420/\mu m^2$ for rat diaphragm muscle, and $12,000/\mu m^2$ for rabbit sciatic nerve nodes of Ranvier.[26] With the exception of the node of Ranvier, these represent fairly low densities. For example, a density of 100 channels/ μm^2 of membrane means that two sodium channels having dimensions of 3×5Å are separated by a distance of 1,000Å.

Site of Action and Active Form of Local Anesthetics

Because most local anesthetics exist in both charged and uncharged forms at neutral pH, a question arises as to which form is responsible for nerve block. This problem has been studied by a number of investigators, but it was not until 1970 that a definitive answer was obtained to account for a variety of seemingly controversial observations.[28,29]

The active form of a local anesthetic can be determined by comparing its blocking potency at different pH values because the ratio [BH⁺]/[B] is pH dependent. Earlier studies showed that increasing the pH increased the local anesthetic potency. From such observations, it was concluded that the uncharged molecular form was responsible for nerve block. However, data suggesting that the charged cationic form is active started accumulating after 1960. For example, the blocking potency was higher at high pH values if the isolated intact

nerve preparation was used, whereas the reverse was true if the desheathed nerve was used. This and several other experiments led Ritchie and Greengard[30] to conclude that the nerve sheath was a substantial barrier to diffusion and that local anesthetics penetrated the nerve sheath in the uncharged form and exerted the blocking action in the charged form. However, there were many observations that could not be accounted for by this model.

One important factor that had drawn little attention in this analysis was the site of action in a nerve fiber. If the site of action were located on the internal surface of the nerve membrane, local anesthetic molecules would have to penetrate two diffusion barriers: the nerve sheath and the nerve membrane before exerting their blocking action. Therefore, the effect of pH on the local anesthetic potency was reexamined with internally perfused squid giant axons.[28,29] In short, local anesthetics were applied either outside or inside of the perfused squid axon at various controlled pH levels, and the blocking potency was compared at high and low pH values.

Two tertiary lidocaine analogs were chosen for this purpose because of their unusually low and high pK_a values. One analog was 6211 (2-[N-(2-methoxyethyl)-methylamino]-2′,6′-acetoxylidide) with a pK_a of 6.3, and the other was 6603 (4-diethylamino-2′,6′-butyroxylidide) with a pK_a of 9.8. Changes in pH in these experiments were limited to seven to eight for the internal solution and seven to nine for the external solution in order to avoid the direct effect of pH change on the channel activity. Thus, the two extreme pK_a values allowed us to change the ratio [BH⁺]/[B] present in the external or internal phase. An example of such an experiment is illustrated in Figure 7-11. All the data on 6211 or 6603 applied internally or externally at varying pH values are compatible only with the scheme that calls for the cationic form to block the channel from inside. The compound 6211 blocked the action potential to the same extent when the 6211 concentration and internal pH were altered simultaneously in such a way as to maintain the internally present 6211 cation concentration at a constant (Fig. 7-12).[31] These observations have clearly demonstrated that local anesthetic molecules penetrate the nerve sheath and the nerve

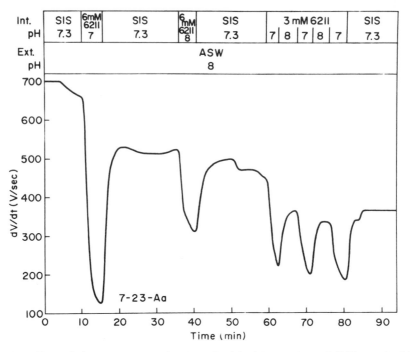

Fig. 7-11 The effect of changing internal pH on the blocking action of 6211 applied internally to a squid giant axon. *ASW,* artificial sea water (extrnal solution); *SIS,* standard internal solution. The compound 6211 blocks more strongly at internal pH 7 than pH 8. (From Narahashi et al.,[28] with permission.)

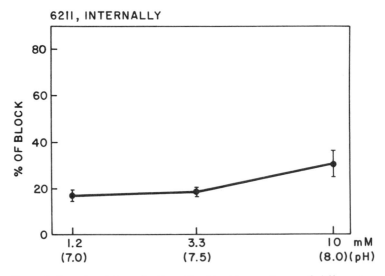

Fig. 7-12 The effect of changing internal pH on the blocking potency of different concentrations of 6211 applied inside a squid axon. Both pH and concentration were changed to make the internally present 6211 cation concentration constant. Each point represents the mean of four experiments with the standard error indicated by the bars. There are no significant differences among the three measurements. (From Frazier et al.,[31] with permission.)

membrane in the uncharged form and block the sodium and potassium channels from inside of the nerve membrane in the charged cationic form (Fig. 7-13). In support of this notion, the quaternary local anesthetics, QX-314 (N-[2,6-dimethylphenyl-carbamoylmethyl] triethylammonium bromide), QX-572 (N,N-bis(phenylcarbamoylmethyl) dimethylammonium chloride), and hemicholinium-3, could block the action potential only when applied to the internal surface of the nerve membrane.[29] Benzocaine is an exception. It exists only in the uncharged form at normal physiologic pH and, therefore, blocks the channels in that form.

TTX and the local anesthetic block of sodium channels is illustrated in Figure 7-14. At the resting potential, in the absence of drug, the activation (m) gate is closed while the inactivation (h) gate is kept open (Fig. 7-14Aa). On membrane depolarization, the m gate quickly opens allowing sodium ions to flow in (Fig. 7-14Ab). When the depolarization is maintained, the h gate slowly closes while the m gate is kept open causing sodium current inactivation (Fig. 7-14Ac). The TTX molecule contains a guanidinium group (Fig. 7-9), which has a dimension enabling penetration of the sodium channel, but the remainder of the molecule is too large to

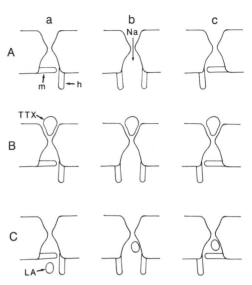

Fig. 7-14 Gating activity of sodium channel and block by tetrodotoxin (TTX) and local anesthetic cation (LA$^+$). **(A)** Control. **(B)** Channel occlusion by TTX without changing the gating mechanism. **(C)** Channel block by LA$^+$. See text for further explanation.

penetrate. Thus, TTX occludes the sodium channel at its external orifice, causing a block of the sodium current, despite the fact that m and h gates function normally (Fig. 7-14B). The local anesthetic cation that is present inside the cell cannot penetrate the sodium channel at rest because the m gate is closed (Fig. 7-14Ca). On depolarization, the local anesthetic cation enters the channel when the m gate opens, causing channel block (Fig. 7-14Cb). During maintained depolarization the h gate closes while m gate is kept open, trapping the local anesthetic cation inside the channel (Fig. 7-14Cc). In some preparations, certain local anesthetic cations can somehow escape from the sodium channel while the h gate is closed.

Mechanism of Channel Block: Use-Dependent Block

The local anesthetic block is greatly enhanced by repetitive stimulation of the nerve. This phenomenon, called use-dependent block, frequency-dependent block, or phasic block, was known for a long time, but it was not until 1973 that the underlying mechanism was investigated using advanced electrophysiologic techniques.[32] The enhanced lo-

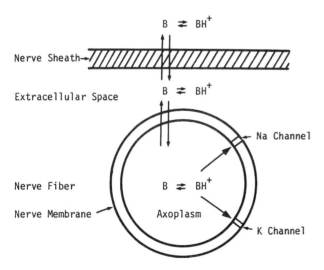

Fig. 7-13 Penetration of local anesthetic in its molecular form (*B*) to the nerve sheath and nerve membrane and block of sodium and potassium channels in its cationic form (*BH$^+$*) from inside the channel.

cal anesthetic block during repetitive stimuli can be explained by the ability of the charged cationic species of local anesthetic molecule to reach the binding site within the sodium channel only when the channel gate located near the internal surface is open. Repetitive excitation increases the chance for the local anesthetic cation to enter the channel, thereby causing an enhanced block. The uncharged local anesthetic molecule can also reach the binding site through the lipid phase of the membrane by virtue of its lipid solubility, representing the secondary or minor pathway to reach the site.[33] Thus, benzocaine, which is in the uncharged form, does not exhibit frequency-dependent block.

Mechanism of Single Channel Block

The open channel block by local anesthetics as described earlier can be directly observed at the single channel level by using patch clamp techniques. An example of an experiment with nicotinic acetylcholine receptor channels is shown in Figure 7-15.[34] Under normal conditions, a single channel is kept open for about 50 ms. When QX-222, a quaternary lidocaine derivative, was applied at a concentration of 5 μM, current flickered while a channel was open because the QX-222 cation entered the open channel and repetitively bound and unbound at an intrachannel site. More intense flickerings are observed with QX-222 concentrations of 10 and 50

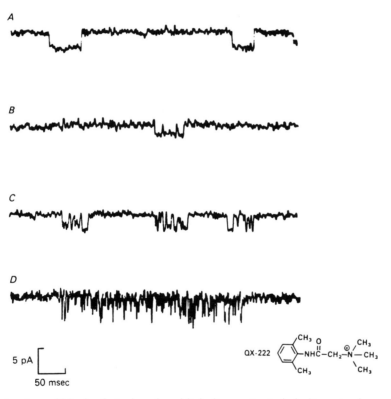

Fig. 7-15 Mechanism of block of single suberyldicholine-activated cholinergic channels by QX-222, a quaternary lidocaine derivative. (A) Control. (B, C, and D) In the presence of 5 μM, 10 μM, and 50 μM QX-222, respectively. See text for further explanation. (From Neher and Steinbach,[34] with permission.)

μM. QX-314, another quaternary lidocaine derivative, produces a flickering too high to be recorded, and the channel current may be seen to be simply suppressed in amplitude. The sodium channel has been found to behave similarly to the acetylcholine channel in response to various local anesthetics and their derivatives.

REFERENCES

1. Hodgkin AL, Huxley AF: Currents carried by sodium and potassium ions through the membrane of giant axon of *Loligo*. J Physiol (Lond) 116:449, 1952
2. Hodgkin AL, Huxley AF: The components of membrane conductance in the giant axon of *Loligo*. J Physiol (Lond) 116:473, 1952
3. Hodgkin AL, Huxley AF: The dual effect of membrane potential on sodium conductance in the giant axon of *Loligo*. J Physiol (Lond) 116:497, 1952
4. Hodgkin AL, Huxley AF: A quantitative description of membrane current and its application to conduction and excitation in nerve. J Physiol (Lond) 117:500, 1952
5. Hodgkin AL, Huxley AF, Katz B: Measurement of current-voltage relations in the membrane of the giant axon of *Loligo*. J Physiol (Lond) 116:424, 1952
6. Cole KS: Dynamic electrical characteristics of the squid axon membrane. Arch Sci Physiol 3:253, 1949
7. Hille B: Ionic Channels of Excitable Membranes. Sinauer Associates, Sunderland, MA, 1992
8. Narahashi T: Drug-ionic channel interactions: single-channel measurements. Ann Neurol 16:S39, 1984
9. Narahashi T: Mechanisms of neurotoxicity. Electrophysiological studies. Cellular electrophysiology. p. 155. In Abou-Donia MB (ed): Neurotoxicology. CRC Press, Boca Raton, FL, 1992
10. Neher E, Sakmann B: Single-channel currents recorded from membrane of denervated frog muscle fibres. Nature 260:779, 1976
11. Hamill OP, Marty A, Neher E et al: Improved patch-clamp techniques for high-resolution current recording from cells and cell-free membrane patches. Pflügers Arch 391:85, 1981
12. Bakere PF, Hodgkin AL, Shaw TI: Replacement of the protoplasm of a giant nerve fibre with artificial solutions. Nature 190:885, 1961
13. Oikawa T, Spyropoulous CS, Tasaki I, Teorell T: Methods for perfusing the giant axon of *Loligo pealii*. Acta Physiol Scand 52:195, 1961
14. Taylor RE: Effect of procaine on electrical properties of squid axon membrane. Am J Physiol 196:1071, 1959
15. Shanes AM, Freygang WH, Grundfest H, Amatniek E: Anesthetic and calcium action in the voltage clamped squid giant axon. J Gen Physiol 42:793, 1959
16. Narahashi T, Moore JW, Poston RN: Anesthetic blocking of nerve membrane conductances by internal and external applications. J Neurobiol 1:3, 1969
17. Narahashi T, Frazier DT, Moore JW: Comparison of tertiary and quaternary amine local anesthetics in their ability to depress membrane ionic conductances. J Neurobiol 3:267, 1972
18. Aceves J, Machne X: The action of calcium and of local anesthetics on nerve cells and their interaction during excitation. J Pharmacol Exp Ther 140:138, 1963
19. Blaustein MP, Goldman DE: Competitive action of calcium and procaine on lobster axon. J Gen Physiol 49:1043, 1966
20. Narahashi T, Frazier DT, Takeno K: Effects of calcium on the local anesthetic suppression of ionic conductances in squid giant axon membranes. J Pharmacol Exp Ther 197:426, 1976
21. Strichartz G: Molecular mechanisms of nerve block by local anesthetics. Anesthesiology 45:421, 1976
22. Frankenhaeuser B, Hodgkin AL: The action of calcium on the electrical properties of squid axons. J Physiol (Lond) 137:217, 1957
23. Narahashi T, Deguchi T, Urakawa N, Ohkubo Y: Stabilization and rectification of muscle fiber membrane by tetraodotoxin. Am J Physiol 198:934, 1960
24. Narahashi T, Moore JW, Scott WR: Tetrodotoxin blockage of sodium conductance increase in lobster giant axons. J Gen Physiol 47:965, 1964
25. Narahashi T: Chemicals as tools in the study of excitable membranes. Physiol Rev 54:813, 1974
26. Narahashi T: Mechanism of tetrodotoxin and saxitoxin action. p. 185. In Tu AT (ed): Handbook of Natural Toxins. Vol. 3. Marcel Dekker, New York, 1988
27. Moore JW, Narahashi T, Shaw TI: An upper limit to the number of sodium channels in nerve membrane? J Physiol (Lond) 188:99, 1967
28. Narahashi T, Frazier DT, Yamada M: The site of action and active form of local anesthetics. I. Theory and pH experiments with tertiary compounds. J Pharmacol Exp Ther 171:32, 1970
29. Frazier DT, Narahashi T, Yamada M: The site of action and active form of local anesthetics. II. Experi-

ments with quaternary compounds. J Pharmacol Exp Ther 171:45, 1970

30. Ritchie JM, Greengard P: On the mode of action of local anesthetics. Annu Rev Pharmacol 6:405, 1966

31. Frazier D, Murayama K, Narahashi T: Comparison of the blocking potency of local anesthetics applied at different pH values. Experientia 27:419, 1971

32. Strichartz GR: The inhibition of sodium currents in myelinated nerve by quaternary derivatives of lidocaine. J Gen Physiol 62:37, 1973

33. Hille B: Local anesthetics: hydrophilic and hydrophobic pathways for the drug-receptor reaction. J Gen Physiol 69:497, 1977

34. Neher E, Steinbach JH: Local anaesthetics transiently block currents through single acetylcholine-receptor channels. J Physiol (Lond) 277:153, 1978

35. Narahashi T: Effects of insecticides on excitable tissues. p. 1. In Beament JWL, Treherne JE, Wigglesworth VB (eds): Advances in Insect Physiology. Vol. 8. Academic Press, New York, 1971

36. Narahashi T: Mode of action of chlorinated hydrocarbon pesticides on the nervous system. p. 222. In Khan MAQ (ed): Halogenated Hydrocarbons: Health and Ecological Effects. Pergamon Press, Elmsford, NY, 1981

37. Narahashi T: Excitable membrane and calcium. Seibutsu Butsuri (Biophysics) 4:101, 1964

38. Narahashi T: Mode of action of dinoflagellate toxins on nerve membranes. p. 395. In LoCicero VR (ed): Proceedings of the First International Conference on Toxic Dinoflagellate Blooms. Massachusetts Science and Technology Foundation, Wakefield, MA, 1975

Chapter 8

Pharmacokinetics of Local Anesthetics

Anton G. L. Burm and Jack W. van Kleef

In contrast to general anesthetics, local anesthetics are deposited close to the target nerve structures and therefore do not depend on the systemic circulation for transport to their targets. Instead, transport occurs by local distribution processes. Uptake of local anesthetic into venous blood vessels and subsequent transfer into the general circulation (systemic absorption) reduces the amount of local anesthetic at and near the site of injection, thereby reducing the concentration gradient for diffusion and, ultimately, lowering the concentration in the nerves. Consequently, systemic absorption limits the duration of nerve blockade. In addition, the uptake of local anesthetics into the systemic circulation is of importance in view of their systemic effects. Generally, the systemic effects produced by concentrations of local anesthetics in the blood that are associated with correctly performed nerve blocks have little, if any, clinical significance. However, the administration of excessive doses or inadvertent intravascular injection can result in adverse effects, including central nervous system toxicity and cardiotoxicity (see Ch. 9). Therefore, knowledge of the toxicity of local anesthetics and an appreciation of their pharmacokinetics are essential

requirements when using local anesthetics in clinical practice.

LOCAL ANESTHETIC AGENTS

The most widely used local anesthetic agents are amino-amides (Fig. 8-1). Amino-esters are less frequently used. Examples of amino-esters are procaine, chloroprocaine, and tetracaine. Lidocaine, prilocaine, mepivacaine, bupivacaine, and etidocaine are the most commonly used amino-amides. Other agents that have found clinical application are cocaine and benzocaine, both ester type agents, and dibucaine, an amino-amide. Articaine, a thiophene derivative, is used in dentistry in some countries and has also been examined for use in epidural anesthesia.[1]

The molecules of prilocaine, mepivacaine, bupivacaine, and etidocaine all possess a chiral center (Fig. 8-1) and, therefore, exist in two optically active stereoisomeric forms or enantiomers that may have different local anesthetic activity, pharmacokinetics, and toxicity.[2-4] Clinically used solutions contain equal amounts of both enantiomers (racemic mixtures). Ropivacaine, the n-propyl homo-

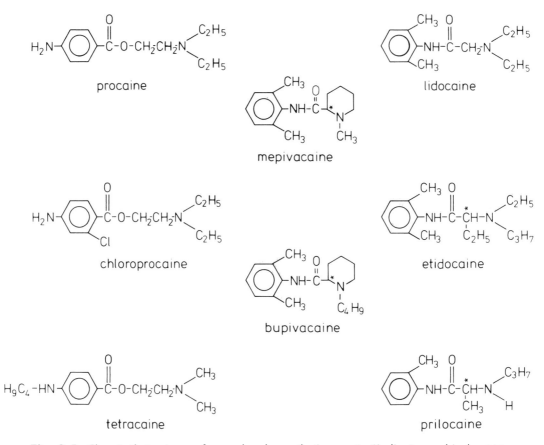

Fig. 8-1 Chemical structures of some local anesthetic agents. *Indicates a chiral center.

log of mepivacaine and bupivacaine, also possesses a chiral center (Fig. 8-2). However, this agent, which is currently under clinical investigation, is made available as the pure S-(−)-enantiomer.

Because of the presence of an amino group in their molecules, all commonly used local anesthetics are weak bases with pK_a values varying from 7.9 for mepivacaine to 9.3 for chloroprocaine (Table 8-1). Consequently, these agents are predominantly ionized in the commercially available acidic aqueous solutions that are used in clinical practice. Major differences exist in the lipophilicity and protein binding of the agents, and these are reflected in the blood/plasma concentration ratios and in the pharmacokinetics.

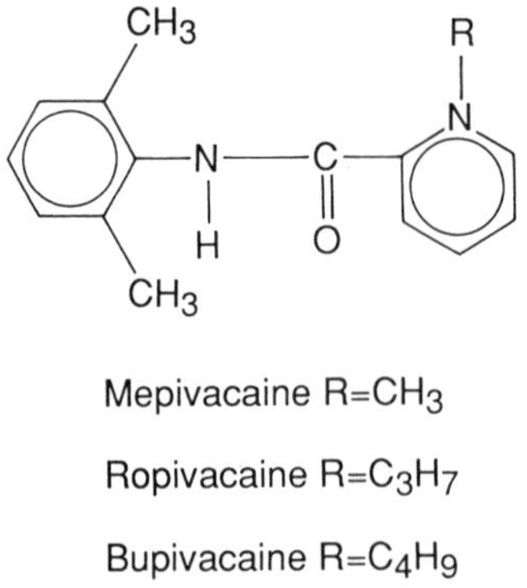

Mepivacaine R=CH₃

Ropivacaine R=C₃H₇

Bupivacaine R=C₄H₉

Fig. 8-2 The chemical structures of mepivacaine, ropivacaine, and bupivacaine are closely related.

Table 8-1 Physicochemical Properties of the Major Local Anesthetic Agents

Agent	pK$_a$ (25°C)	Partition Coefficient^a (25°C)	Serum Protein Binding (%)	Blood/Plasma Concentration Ratio
Esters				
Procaine	9.1	1.7	—	—
Chloroprocaine	9.3	9.0	—	—
Tetracaine	8.6	221	—	—
Amides				
Prilocaine	8.0	25	40	1.0
Lidocaine	8.2	43	70	0.84
Etidocaine	8.1	800	95	0.58
Mepivacaine	7.9	21	75	0.92
Ropivacaine	8.2	115	95	0.69
Bupivacaine	8.2	346	95	0.73

^{a}Octanol/buffer (pH = 7.4).
(Modified from Arthur and Covino,[5] with permission. Data from Strichartz et al.,[6] Arthur et al. (unpublished data), Tucker and Mather,[7] and Lee et al.[8].)

LOCAL DISTRIBUTION AND ONSET OF ACTION

Nerve blockade is the clinical manifestation of an interaction of local anesthetic molecules with the sodium channels in excitable membranes (see Ch. 7). Binding to and dissociation from the sodium channels are fast processes; therefore, the intensity of the effect is dependent on the concentration of local anesthetic near the channels. Another factor of importance is the proportion of the drug that is uncharged (free base). Although both the cation and free base forms are involved in the blockade of sodium channels, these forms are not equipotent, and consequently, the effect depends on the degree of ionization, i.e., on the pK$_a$ of the local anesthetic and the pH of the axoplasm.

Local Disposition

Current knowledge on local distribution is mainly theoretic, based on in vitro and clinical observations. Chemical data, which could enhance our understanding of local distribution, are scarce and difficult to interpret. For example, concentrations of bupivacaine have been determined in cerebrospinal fluid (CSF) after epidural and subarachnoid administration.[9] However, because local anesthetics are not homogeneously distributed within the CSF, the concentration-time profiles in the CSF, collected from a single sampling site, should be interpreted with caution and cannot be used for formal pharmacokinetic analysis.

Processes involved in local drug distribution include physical spreading of the solution by bulk flow, diffusion, and vascular transport. These have been considered in detail by Tucker and Mather.[10] Bulk flow of the solution during and immediately after the injection is a major determinant of the number of nerves or spinal segments or the length of nerve that is exposed to local anesthetic. Once deposited, further transport of local anesthetic to the target axons occurs mainly by passive diffusion. In addition, vascular transport may contribute to the local drug transport. For example, it has been postulated that drugs may be transported from the epidural and subarachnoid spaces to the spinal cord after uptake into the spinal radicular arteries.[11]

Binding of local anesthetics to tissues at the site of injection or on their way to the target axons delays diffusion and, consequently, the onset of action. At the same time, the slow dissociation of the local anesthetic from local binding sites maintains the concentration gradient for diffusion and will delay egress of local anesthetic out of the nerves, thereby prolonging the duration of action.

Removal of drug by systemic absorption lowers the amount of drug at the site of injection, thereby reducing the concentration gradient for diffusion and, ultimately, lowering the concentration in the nerves.

Onset of Neural Blockade

The onset of neural blockade varies markedly with the anesthetic procedure.[12] Major anatomic factors that affect the rate of onset include the site of injection, the size and location of individual fibers within the nerves, and the presence and thickness of diffusion barriers, such as the myelin sheath, endoneurium, perineurium, and epineurium, or with central blocks, the pia mater, arachnoid mater, and dura mater. The deposition of a local anesthetic solution very close to the target nerve structures results in an almost immediate onset of sensory blockade, irrespective of the agent used.[12] In contrast, deposition at a more remote site results in a much slower onset, taking up to 30 minutes or longer, depending on the local anesthetic agent and its concentration. Administration of a local anesthetic for brachial plexus block usually results in blockade that progresses from the upper arm to the lower arm, to the hand, reflecting more rapid diffusion into mantle fibers that innervate proximal regions than into core fibers, which innervate more distal regions.[13] The initial onset of spinal anesthesia following injection of a local anesthetic into the CSF, bathing the intradural spinal nerves and the spinal cord, usually occurs within 1 to 2 minutes. The initial onset of epidural anesthesia following injection outside the dura mater usually takes much longer, even though epidural doses are 5- to 10-fold higher than are subarachnoid doses. The full development of spinal and epidural anesthesia usually takes up to 20 or 30 minutes, respectively,[12] because higher spinal segments are exposed to considerably lower amounts of local anesthetic.

Different modalities of nerve function are not blocked at the same rate. In general, sympathetic blockade precedes sensory blockade, which in turn, precedes motor blockade, reflecting the different degrees of myelinization of different fibers.[14] How-ever, the sequence of blockade may vary with the local anesthetic and the site of injection. For example, following an injection of lidocaine for brachial plexus block, motor blockade precedes or occurs simultaneously with sensory blockade.[13] This may be explained by the more peripheral location of the motor nerves in the mantle bundles and/or a greater sensitivity of motor fibers to local anesthetics.[15,16] In contrast, following epidural administration, sensory blockade usually precedes motor blockade, but marked differences exist between agents in the relative onset times of sensory and motor blockade. Thus, for comparable degrees of sensory blockade, motor block in the legs is much faster and usually is more profound following epidural administration of etidocaine compared with bupivacaine.[17] This difference in sensory-motor dissociation between bupivacaine and etidocaine in part may be caused by a slower diffusion of bupivacaine into motor fibers, as a result of its higher pK_a and lower lipid solubility,[18] although other factors are also involved.[19]

In view of the role of diffusion in the transport of local anesthetics from the site of injection to the target axons, the rate of onset may be expected to vary with the physicochemical properties of the agents, in particular lipophilicity and pK_a. In vitro, good correlations have been found between these properties and the onset of conduction block.[12] However, in vivo, these correlations are largely obscured by other factors, including extraneural binding and systemic absorption.

A slow onset can, within limits, be compensated for by administration of more concentrated solutions (higher doses). For example, chloroprocaine has low lipid solubility and a high pK_a, and consequently, it is predominantly ionized in strongly acidic solutions. However, the low systemic toxicity of this agent allows the administration of concentrated solutions.[20] Alkalinization of strongly acidic solutions, such as those of the ester-type agents and commercial solutions containing epinephrine, enhances the fraction of unionized diffusible drug and, thereby, may speed the onset of action, but the effect varies between studies.[21–23] The injection of carbonated local anesthetics, instead of the commonly used hydrochloride salt solutions, may result in a faster onset and/or a better quality of block because of a direct effect of carbon dioxide on the axons, enhanced diffusion, and a decrease in intraneural pH, but this too remains controversial.[23–25]

SYSTEMIC ABSORPTION

The uptake of a local anesthetic into blood vessels in the area where it has been deposited and its subsequent transfer into the systemic circulation is generally referred to as systemic absorption. The main factors controlling the rate of systemic absorption are (1) binding to tissues at and near the site of injection and (2) local perfusion. Both vary considerably between injection sites. Furthermore, local anesthetics may alter local perfusion,[26] both directly by affecting vasomotor tone and indirectly by producing sympathetic blockade. To reduce local perfusion, epinephrine is often added to local anesthetic solutions. Factors that can affect the systemic absorption rate include the effects of the local anesthetic, added vasoconstrictors, and other drugs; cardiovascular changes caused by central sympathetic blockade; and pathophysiologic features.[10]

Absorption Kinetics

The absorption characteristics of local anesthetics injected into the epidural space cannot be determined directly from resulting plasma concentrations because absorption, distribution, and elimination occur simultaneously. The solution to this problem is to determine the distribution and elimination kinetics from intravenous administration and deduce the absorption kinetics by deconvoluting the kinetic profile obtained from epidural administration. Intravenous and epidural profiles can be obtained at the same time by labeling the intravenous drug with a stable isotope (e.g. deuterium) to obtain an analog that has a pharmacokinetic behavior identical to that of the unlabeled drug but can be analyzed separately by mass spectrometry. A biphasic absorption pattern has been found for epidural lidocaine, bupivacaine, and etidocaine in healthy volunteers[7] and for epidural lidocaine and bupivacaine in surgical patients (Table 8-2).[27,28] The rapid initial absorption following epidural administration is most likely related to the high con-

Table 8-2 Mean Pharmacokinetic Data, Characterizing the Absorption of Lidocaine and Bupivacaine After Epidural and Subarachnoid Injection in Surgical Patients

Parameter	Epidural Lidocaine	Epidural Bupivacaine	Subarachnoid Lidocaine	Subarachnoid Bupivacaine
F_1	0.38	0.28	—	0.35
$t_{1/2a1}$ (h)	0.16	0.12	—	0.83
F_2	0.58	0.66	—	0.61
$t_{1/2a2}$ (h)	1.4	6.0	1.2	6.8
F	0.96	0.94	1.03	0.96
MAT (h)	1.8	8.6	1.7	8.8

Abbreviations: F, estimated total fraction of the dose ultimately absorbed into the general circulation; F_1 and F_2, fractions of the dose characterizing the fast and slow absorption phases; MAT, mean absorption time; $t_{1/2a1}$ and $t_{1/2a2}$, half-lives characterizing the fast and slow absorption phases.
(Modified from Burm,[31] with permission. Data from Burm et al.[27,29])

centration gradient between the drug in the solution and in the blood. In addition, profound increases in epidural blood flow, as observed during epidural administration of bupivacaine,[26] may contribute to the fast initial absorption rate. Later on, after the local anesthetic has been taken up into local tissues such as epidural fat, absorption will become dependent on tissue-blood partitioning, resulting in a marked slowing of the absorption.

The initial absorption rates of lidocaine, bupivacaine, and etidocaine following epidural administration appear to be similar. However, the absorption rates of bupivacaine and etidocaine during the slower secondary absorption phase are much slower than that of lidocaine (Fig. 8-3). This is in keeping with the greater tissue affinity of bupivacaine and etidocaine and is consistent with their longer duration of action and with the observation that significant concentrations of etidocaine were still present in epidural fat 12 hours after epidural injection in sheep, whereas corresponding lidocaine concentrations were much lower.[10]

A biphasic absorption pattern has also been observed after subarachnoid injection of bupivacaine (Table 8-2).[29–31] However, compared with absorption after epidural administration, the initial ab-

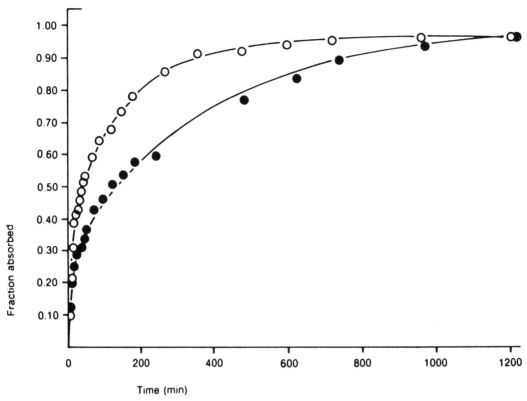

Fig. 8-3 The fractions of lidocaine (○) and bupivacaine (●) absorbed into the circulation following epidural administration as a function of time, which was determined by a stable isotope method in young healthy patients. (From Burm,[31] with permission.)

sorption rate is much slower. Factors that may contribute to the slower absorption from the subarachnoid space are the immediate dilution of the solution on injection into the CSF, poor perfusion of the subarachnoid space, and perhaps, lesser vasodilatation associated with the smaller dose of bupivacaine. The absorption of lidocaine after subarachnoid injection appears to be monophasic. The absorption rate of lidocaine and the secondary absorption rate of bupivacaine following subarachnoid injection are similar to the slow absorption rates of these agents after epidural injection. This suggests that secondary absorption occurs from a common tissue, probably epidural fat.

Absorption kinetics following other routes of administration have not been determined. Inspection of the concentration-time profiles suggests a biphasic absorption pattern following most procedures.

DISTRIBUTION AND PLASMA PROTEIN BINDING

Lipophilic local anesthetics should readily cross diffusion barriers, such as cell membranes, the blood-brain barrier, and the placenta. Consequently, the tissue distribution of these drugs is likely to be highly dependent on tissue perfusion. This hypothesis is supported by the fact that a physiologic perfusion model, which assumed no diffusion limitations, closely predicted measured arterial blood concentrations in humans.[32]

Plasma Protein Binding

The degree of binding to plasma proteins varies considerably between local anesthetic agents (Table 8-1). Binding occurs predominantly to high affinity, low capacity sites on α_1-acid glycoprotein (AAG) and to a lesser extent to low affinity, high capacity sites, probably on albumin.[33,34] At higher concentrations, binding to AAG approaches saturation, resulting in higher free fractions.[33,35] Changes in plasma protein concentrations are often accompanied by changes in the protein binding of the local anesthetics.[36] AAG concentrations vary widely because it is an acute phase reactant protein (see Ch. 4, Table 4-8). Furthermore, the degree of protein binding is very sensitive to changes in plasma pH and hemodilution.[33,37,38] With local anesthetics possessing a chiral center, the protein binding may differ between enantiomers, as has been demonstrated in plasma of sheep.[39] However, in humans, the binding of mepivacaine and bupivacaine did not appear to be stereoselective.[35]

The role of protein binding in relation to the pharmacokinetics and the systemic toxicity of local anesthetics will be considered in the following sections. Briefly, it is important to consider protein binding when interpreting plasma concentrations in relation to systemic toxicity because toxic effects are probably more closely related to free than to total plasma concentrations.[40,41]

Uptake Into the Lung

After uptake into the venous circulation, local anesthetics are subject to uptake in the lung before entering the arterial circulation. The first-pass pulmonary uptake of local anesthetics may be substantial, as with many other basic drugs. For example, the first-pass lung uptake of lidocaine in humans given a small intravenous bolus dose averaged approximately 60 percent of the dose.[42,43] Studies in pigs and rabbits showed that pulmonary uptake was increased by alkalemia[44] and decreased by acidemia.[45] Other studies in pigs indicated that the pulmonary uptake of lidocaine is saturable.[46] Saturability is also suggested by the displacement of mepivacaine from binding sites in the lung in humans following administration of an intravenous bolus dose of lidocaine.[43]

The implications of pulmonary uptake vary with the input rate. When the drug input is rapid, such as after inadvertent intravenous injections or following cuff release after administration for intravenous regional anesthesia,[47] the peak arterial blood concentration will be delayed and may be markedly lower than that in the pulmonary arterial blood, entering the lung. When the drug input is slower,

such as after correctly administered regional blocks, the difference between systemic arterial and pulmonary arterial concentration profiles will be minimal.

Uptake Into the Brain and Heart

The main target organs for systemic toxicity, the brain and heart, receive relatively large fractions of the cardiac output and proportional fractions of the amount of local anesthetic in the arterial circulation. Rich perfusion, moderate tissue/blood partition coefficients,[32,48,49] and the lack of serious diffusion limitations ensure rapid equilibration between these tissues and the blood. For example, a study of the uptake of lidocaine into the brain following rapid intravenous infusion in dogs showed that pseudoequilibrium between brain and blood was attained in less than 10 minutes.[50]

The free drug hypothesis suggests that only the drug in plasma that is not bound to plasma proteins (free drug) is available to reach sites of action outside of the circulation.

The free drug hypothesis suggests that only the drug in plasma that is not bound to plasma protein (free drug) is available to reach sites of action outside of the circulation. However, the brain's uptake of drug and hormones exceeded the free fraction in some animal experiments. A portion of the AAG bound pool of lidocaine was available for uptake into the brain following intracarotid injection in rats.[51] Similar findings were reported for bupivacaine.[52] These findings suggest rapid (within one brain transit time) dissociation of local anesthetic from AAG.

Clinical reports of continuous epidural anesthesia or intravenous antiarrhythmic therapy have suggested that under pseudoequilibrium conditions, central nervous system toxicity from lidocaine or bupivacaine correlates better with the concentration of free drug in the plasma than with total drug (bound plus free drug) in the plasma.[40,41] Subsequent studies by Marathe et al.[50] using an animal model supported these clinical reports. Lidocaine was administered to dogs by intravenous bolus and plasma protein binding, and lidocaine entry into the CSF and brain tissue were sampled during a 1-hour period. Lidocaine brain/serum partitioning was found to be limited by its binding to AAG. The correlation between the ratio of brain/serum lidocaine and the lidocaine free fraction in the plasma was r = 0.92 (*P* = 0.003, Fig. 8-4). The correlation between the ratio of CSF/serum lidocaine and plasma free fraction was r = 0.90 (*P* = 0.01).

Tissue uptake may be affected by changes in plasma or tissue pH, because local anesthetics are weak bases with pK_a values close to physiologic pH.

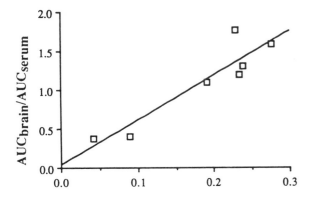

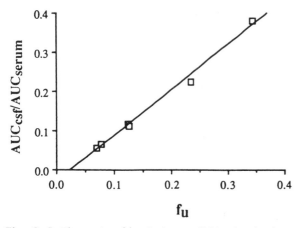

Fig. 8-4 The ratio of brain/serum lidocaine (*top*) was highly correlated to the lidocaine free fraction (r = 0.92, *P* = 0.003). A higher brain/serum ratio indicates greater partitioning of lidocaine into the brain. The correlation between the brain/serum ratio and lidocaine free fraction shows that plasma protein binding limits the partitioning of lidocaine into the brain. The ratio of cerebrospinal fluid (CSF)/serum lidocaine (*bottom*) was also highly correlated to the lidocaine free fraction (r = 0.90, *P* = 0.01), indicating that plasma protein binding limits partitioning of lidocaine into the CSF. (From Marathe et al.,[50] with permission.)

In rabbits, respiratory acidosis did not alter the heart/blood partitioning of lidocaine and bupivacaine,[53] suggesting similar changes in tissue and blood pH. Metabolic acidosis would be expected to increase the uptake into the tissues where the acid is generated because of larger decreases in intracellular pH than in blood pH, resulting in increased ion trapping. Thus, increased brain/blood concentration ratios have been observed following drug induced status epilepticus in rats.[54] Metabolic acidosis may increase local anesthetic effects as a result of a decrease in intracellular pH and an increase in the fraction of ionized local anesthetic, which is probably the most pharmacologically active form.[55]

Volume of Distribution

Volumes of distribution based on total blood concentrations of the amide-type local anesthetics, as derived from the concentration time profiles following rapid intravenous infusion in volunteers,[7] are presented in Table 8-3. The volumes of distribution based on the plasma concentrations will be somewhat lower than for blood concentrations because the plasma concentrations are usually higher than the blood concentrations, as a result of plasma protein binding (Table 8-1). Volumes of distribution based on free (unbound) drug concentrations in plasma water vary considerably between agents, reflecting the marked differences in the physicochemical properties of the agents (Table 8-1). Volumes distribution based on total blood concentration vary little between agents because the more extensive tissue binding of agents, such as bupivacaine and etidocaine (tending to promote a large volume of distribution), is largely offset by more extensive binding to plasma proteins (tending to promote a smaller volume of distribution).

Until recently, the possibility of stereoselective distribution has received little attention. It should be emphasized that the data on prilocaine, mepivacaine, bupivacaine, and etidocaine, which are presented in Table 8-3, have been derived after the administration of the racemates and are based on the measurement of the total concentrations of the mixed enantiomers. Recent studies involving the administration of individual enantiomers to sheep demonstrated differences in the volumes of distri-

Table 8-3 Pharmacokinetic Data[a] Characterizing the Disposition Kinetics of Amide-Type Local Anesthetics in Adult Male Volunteers

	Lidocaine	Prilocaine	Etidocaine	Mepivacaine	Ropivacaine	Bupivacaine
V_{ss} (L)	91	191	134	84	59	73
Vu_{ss} (L)	253	—	1478	382	678	1028
CL (L/min)	0.95	2.37	1.11	0.78	0.73	0.58
E_H	0.65	—	0.74	0.52	—	0.38
$t_{1/2}$ (h)	1.6	1.6	2.7	1.9	1.9	2.7
MBRT (h)	1.6	1.3	2.0	1.8	—	2.1

Abbreviations: CL, systemic clearance; E_H, estimated hepatic extraction ratio; MBRT, mean body residence time; $t_{1/2}$, terminal half-life; V_{ss}, volume of distribution at steady state based on total blood concentrations; Vu_{ss}, volume of distribution at steady state based on unbound drug concentrations in plasma water.

[a]Data are specified with respect to arterial blood drug concentration, with the exception of prilocaine data, which are specified with respect to peripheral venous blood drug concentrations.

(Modified from Tucker,[56] with permission. Data from Tucker and Mather,[7] Arthur et al.,[57] and Lee et al.[8])

bution of the enantiomers of mepivacaine but not in those of bupivacaine.[2]

Little is known of the distribution of ester-type local anesthetics. The mean volume of distribution following high-dose infusions of procaine in humans was highly dose dependent, varying from 0.23 L/kg (dose, 1.5 mg/kg/min) to 0.79 L/kg (dose, 1 mg/kg/min).[58]

CLEARANCE AND BIOTRANSFORMATION

Local anesthetics are removed from the body mainly by biotransformation. Renal excretion of unchanged drug accounts only for a small fraction of the dose, at least in adults.[10] Biotransformation of the ester-type drugs involves ester hydrolysis, both by plasma pseudocholinesterases and red cell esterases in the blood, and by esterases in the liver. Amide-type agents are predominantly metabolized in the liver, although prilocaine may also undergo substantial metabolism elsewhere in the body because the estimated total body clearance considerably exceeds the hepatic blood flow (Table 8-3).

The total body clearances of various amide-type agents, determined after rapid intravenous infusion in volunteers, are presented in Table 8-3. Clearances vary from 0.58 L/min for bupivacaine up to 2.37 L/min for prilocaine. Corresponding half-lives range from 1.6 to 2.7 hours. Again, the

clearances and half-lives of prilocaine, mepivacaine, bupivacaine, and etidocaine are based on the measurements of the mixed enantiomers. In volunteers, plasma concentrations of the S-(+)-isomer of prilocaine have been shown to be markedly higher than those of the R-(−)-isomer after oral administration of racemic prilocaine,[4] reflecting a difference in intrinsic clearance. Marked differences have been observed in the clearances of the individual enantiomers following administration of racemic mepivacaine for combined psoas compartment/sciatic nerve block.[59] In addition, the same study demonstrated a marked interindividual variability in the stereoselectivity, i.e., the ratios of the clearances of R-(+)-mepivacaine and S-(−)-mepivacaine among the 10 studied patients varied from 1.2 to 2.9 (mean ratio, 1.9). Differences in the clearances of the enantiomers of bupivacaine have also been observed after prolonged interpleural infusion of racemic bupivacaine (K. Groen, personal communication, 1993). Furthermore, the stereoselective clearance of bupivacaine, but not mepivacaine, has been observed following intravenous bolus injections of individual enantiomers or racemic bupivacaine in sheep.[2,3]

In vitro hydrolysis rates of ester-type agents in human plasma decrease in the order: chloroprocaine > procaine > tetracaine.[60] The in vitro half-lives in normal human plasma are less than 1 minute for both chloroprocaine and procaine.[61] In vivo, a marked dose dependency of the clearance of procaine has been observed during procaine infusion; the total body clearance varied from 0.04 L/kg/min (dose, 1.5 mg/kg/min) to 0.08 L/kg/min (dose, 1.0 mg/kg/min);[58] because the volume of distribution was dose related in the same direction (see Volume of Distribution), corresponding half-lives were similar, 7.1 and 8.3 minutes, respectively. Significant slowing of the rate of hydrolysis can occur when esterases become saturated, by substrate inhibition, or if the enzymes are atypical.[60]

Metabolic Pathways

The principal pathway for the metabolism of ester-type agents is ester hydrolysis. The main pathways involved in the biotransformation of amide-type agents are N-dealkylation, aromatic hydroxylation, and amide hydrolysis; an example showing the biotransformation pathways of lidocaine is shown in Fig. 8-5. For a more complete description of biotransformation pathways of other local anesthetics, the reader is referred to a previous publication by Tucker and Mather.[10]

Active Metabolites

Although biotransformation most often results in the formation of more polar or hydrophilic products that lack pharmacologic activity, the formation of active metabolites does occur. Within the amide series, metabolic products that have been shown or are suspected to possess pharmacologic activity include, mainly, dealkylation products and some hydroxylation products. Monoethylglycine xylidide,

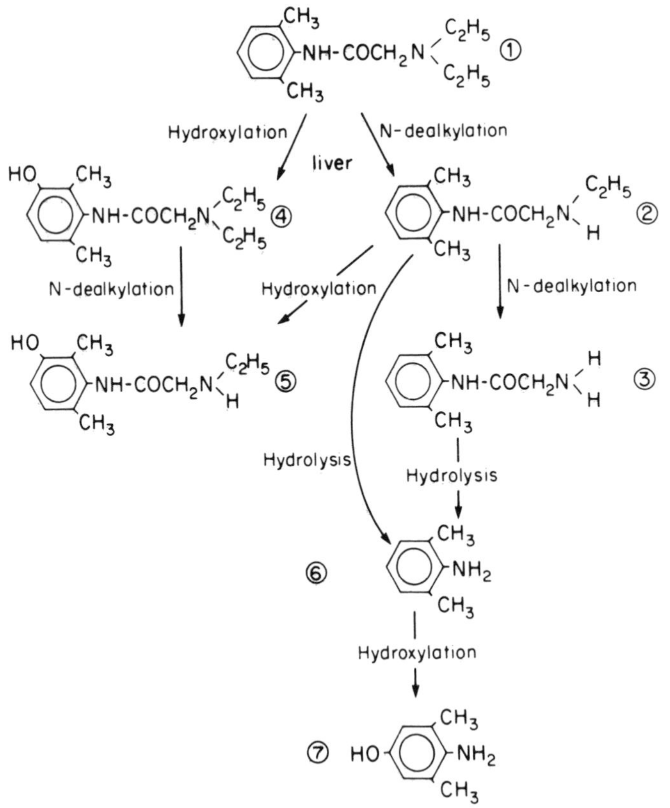

Fig. 8-5 Metabolic pathway of lidocaine. (1) Lidocaine; (2) monoethylglycine xylidide; (3) glycine xylidide; (4) 3-hydroxylidocaine; (5) 3-hydroxymonoethylglycine xylidide; (6) 2,6-xylidine; (7) 4-hydroxy-2,6-xylidine. (From Arthur and Covino,[5] with permission.)

formed by N-dealkylation of lidocaine, possesses antiarrhythmic and convulsant activity similar to lidocaine and a somewhat longer half-life, and it contributes to the antiarrhythmic effects and toxicity during lidocaine infusion in cardiac patients.[62] This should also hold during continuous epidural infusions. Glycine xylidide, another metabolic product of lidocaine, possesses weak antiarrhythmic effects, but it lacks convulsant activity.[63]

2,6-Pipecoloxylidide, a dealkylation product of both mepivacaine, bupivacaine, and presumably, ropivacaine, also possesses significant pharmacologic activity. However, its plasma concentrations following continuous administration of bupivacaine are low compared with those of the parent drug.[64,65] N-dealkylation products have also been identified following administration of etidocaine.[66] However, little is known about their toxicologic profile.

The hydroxylation of o-toluidine, formed by the amide hydrolysis of prilocaine, is believed to be responsible for the methemoglobinemia that is associated with higher doses of this local anesthetic.[67] The aminobenzoic acid derivatives that are formed by hydrolysis of the ester-type agents are probably involved in the rare allergic reactions that occur following the administration of these agents.

PLASMA CONCENTRATION-TIME PROFILES

Plasma or blood concentration profiles of local anesthetics following perineural administration reflect the net result of systemic absorption, distribution, and elimination. In comparing concentration-time profiles of local anesthetics following different routes of administration, it is often assumed that the route has little effect on the systemic disposition and differences in the profiles are usually interpreted as being the consequence of differences in the systemic absorption. This may not always be justified. For example, significant decreases in hepatic blood flow have been observed during high epidural anesthesia in humans[68] and during high spinal anesthesia in monkeys,[69] and this may affect the clearance of flow-dependent drugs, such as lidocaine, etidocaine, and prilocaine.

On the other hand, studies in sheep indicated that volume loading may attenuate this effect.[70] High spinal anesthesia in monkeys also resulted in a marked reduction in cardiac output and blood flow to several other organs.[69] The volume of distribution of lidocaine was larger in patients receiving spinal anesthesia (mean sensory level, T5) than in unanesthetized volunteers;[29] the clearance of lidocaine did not differ between the patients and volunteers. Epidural blocks up to T6 did not influence the pharmacokinetics of lidocaine, bupivacaine, or etidocaine.[7,27]

Marked arteriovenous concentration differences in the arm have been observed during epidural anesthesia in volunteers.[7] These were attributed to reduced perfusion of the arm as a result of compensatory vasoconstriction in the upper limbs caused by vasodilatation in the lower limbs from sympathetic blockade. Differences in sampling sites (arterial or venous) may contribute significantly to the variability between studies in plasma or blood concentrations after epidural administration.

Concentrations Following Single Injections

Following single injections, the peak concentrations, relative to the toxic threshold, may be considered a reasonable measure of safety. Peak plasma or blood concentrations of different agents following various routes of administration, and the corresponding peak times, have been tabulated by Tucker and Mather.[10] Examples that illustrate the differences between local anesthetic agents and the influence of the route of administration are presented in Figures 8-6 and 8-7. Peak concentrations generally occur within 5 to 60 minutes, depending predominantly on the route of administration. The highest concentrations are usually attained after intercostal administration, irrespective of the agent. However, bupivacaine concentrations following interpleural injection have exceeded those after intercostal administration.[73] The peak plasma concentrations in the latter study exceeded the threshold generally assumed to be associated with toxicity in 6 of 12 patients; however, toxicity was not observed in any patients.

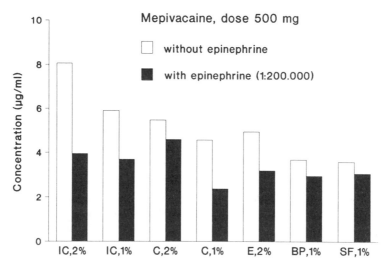

Fig. 8-6 Mean peak plasma concentrations of mepivacaine, measured after injection of solutions with or without epinephrine for various regional block procedures. IC, intercostal block; C, caudal block; E, epidural block; BP, brachial plexus block; SF, sciatic/femoral block. (Modified from Tucker et al.,[71] with permission.)

Concentrations Following Repeated Injections and During Continuous Infusion

Predictions of the plasma concentration profiles for repeated epidural injections of lidocaine (study period, 5 hours) or etidocaine (10 hours), based on pharmacokinetic data obtained after single injections, corresponded reasonably well with actually measured concentration-time profiles.[74] These predictions and measurements indicated that systemic accumulation tends to be faster with the

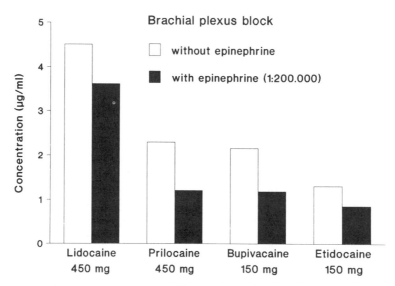

Fig. 8-7 Mean peak plasma concentrations of lidocaine, prilocaine, bupivacaine, and etidocaine measured after injection of solutions with or without epinephrine for brachial plexus block. (Modified from Arthur and Covino,[5] with permission. Data from Wildsmith et al.[72])

shorter acting agent lidocaine than with the longer acting agent etidocaine.

Long-term infusion of bupivacaine into the brachial plexus sheath, and long-term intercostal, epidural, and interpleural infusions of bupivacaine or lidocaine for the relief of postoperative pain, have been shown to result in continuously increasing plasma concentrations,[65,75–77] probably because of changes in plasma protein binding. AAG increases substantially in the postoperative period, increasing total, but not unbound drug concentrations. This may explain why toxic reactions did not occur in most studies, even though total bupivacaine or lidocaine concentrations exceeded the threshold concentration normally assumed to be associated with toxicity.

Plasma concentrations after repeated injection or infusion of procaine or chloroprocaine should be very low because of the rapid elimination by ester hydrolysis.[78]

Addition of Epinephrine, Phenylephrine, or Clonidine

Epinephrine is often added to local anesthetic solutions to slow the systemic absorption. A comparison of the absorption kinetics of lidocaine and etidocaine following the epidural injection of plain and epinephrine containing solutions showed that epinephrine decreased the *fraction* absorbed during the initial fast absorption phase, without appreciably altering the initial absorption *rate*.[7] This is in keeping with other observations that peak plasma concentrations of these and other agents after epidural injection are generally reduced by the use of epinephrine, whereas the peak times are usually little affected.

Epinephrine may also affect the plasma concentrations of local anesthetics because of its cardiovascular effects. These are generally β-adrenergic in nature. For example, the addition of epinephrine to epidural bupivacaine solutions resulted in a significant increase in cardiac output.[79] Overall, the effect of the addition of epinephrine (usually, $1:200,000$, or less) on the total blood or plasma concentrations following single injections varies markedly with the type of regional block and the type, dose, and concentration of the local anesthetic.[10] Examples are presented in Figures 8-6 and 8-7. In general, lidocaine, prilocaine, and mepivacaine concentrations tend to be reduced more by the addition of epinephrine than do those of the longer acting agents. The largest reductions in peak plasma concentrations by epinephrine are generally seen with intercostal block.

During continuous infusion, the steady-state concentrations depend only on the infusion rate and the systemic clearance. Slowing of the absorption of local anesthetics should not affect the steady-state concentration, but systemic effects of epinephrine may potentially alter steady-state levels by affecting clearance. However, in a recent study, lidocaine concentrations during continuous epidural infusion were not significantly altered by epinephrine.[80]

The addition of phenylephrine does not reduce lidocaine plasma concentrations to the same extent as does the addition of epinephrine,[81] probably because of differences in the systemic effects of those agents. Low dose intravenous infusions of phenylephrine after epidural injection of bupivacaine were associated with considerably higher plasma bupivacaine concentrations than were low dose intravenous infusions of epinephrine.[82] Epidural injection or intravenous infusion of phenylephrine reduced the cardiac output, whereas epidural injection or intravenous infusion of epinephrine increased the cardiac output.[81,82]

Addition of clonidine to epidural lidocaine solutions tended to result in higher plasma concentrations compared with plain solutions.[83] Also, addition of clonidine to lidocaine solutions for brachial plexus block was associated with markedly higher peak lidocaine concentrations compared with addition of epinephrine.[84]

Other Factors Altering the Plasma Concentration Profiles

Peak plasma concentrations following injections of local anesthetics generally tend to be proportional to the dose but independent of the concentration in the solution.[85,86] However, the use of more concentrated (1 versus 0.5 percent) lidocaine solutions for intravenous regional anesthesia,[47] the intercostal or caudal administration of more concentrated mepivacaine solutions (2 versus 1 percent),[71] and lumbar epidural injection of more concentrated etidocaine solutions (1.5 versus 1 percent)[86,87] tended to result in greater blood or plasma concentrations. Also, although peak etidocaine concentrations appeared to be proportional to the dose up to 300 mg, the injection of larger doses resulted in disproportionally larger plasma concentrations.[86] The higher plasma concentrations with more concentrated solutions and the disproportionate increases with higher etidocaine doses are most likely the result of the saturation of local binding sites or increased vasodilatation.

The speed of injection appears to have little or no influence on the peak plasma concentrations.[85] Alkalinization[21] or carbonation[88–90] do not alter the achieved plasma concentrations.

PHARMACOKINETIC DRUG INTERACTIONS

Most of the current knowledge about the effects of other drugs on the pharmacokinetics of local anesthetics has been derived from studies after intravenous administration, and it may not always be possible to extrapolate the findings to patients receiving regional anesthesia. This is especially a problem if the co-administered drug produces cardiovascular effects.[56]

General anesthesia with halothane and nitrous oxide reduced the clearance of intravenously administered lidocaine compared with a balanced technique, involving thiopental, fentanyl, and nitrous oxide.[91] This reflects a reduction in hepatic blood flow and/or inhibition of mixed function oxidase enzymes by halothane. More detailed studies in sheep confirmed the depressing effect of halothane on the total body clearance of lidocaine, but they were inconclusive with respect to the effect on the hepatic clearance.[92]

Pretreatment with propranolol reduced the clearance and prolonged the half-lives of intravenously administered lidocaine[93,94] and bupivacaine,[95] mainly by enzyme inhibition, and in part, by decreasing hepatic blood flow. The influence of metoprolol on lidocaine clearance is smaller than that of propranolol.[96] Plasma concentrations of bupivacaine following intercostal administration were not significantly increased by coadministration of β-blockers.[97]

Pretreatment with cimetidine for 1 to 4 days consistently decreased the systemic clearance of intravenously administered lidocaine.[98–100] Some studies also showed a decrease in the volume of distribution, such that the elimination half-life of lidocaine was not affected.[99,100] However, in another study, the volume of distribution was not changed, whereas the elimination half-life was increased with cimetidine.[98] Previous administration of cimetidine decreased the total body clearance of intravenous bupivacaine, increased the elimination half-life, and did not change the volume of distribution.[101] However, in another study, cimetidine did not alter the pharmacokinetics of intramuscularly administered bupivacaine.[102]

Plasma concentrations of lidocaine and bupivacaine in parturients undergoing cesarean section under epidural anesthesia were not affected by previous administration of cimetidine in most studies.[103–107] However, one study showed a marked increase in peak lidocaine concentrations in parturients given prophylactic cimetidine.[108] Pretreatment with ranitidine did not significantly alter the pharmacokinetics of intravenously administered lidocaine or bupivacaine,[101,109] and it did not significantly affect the plasma concentrations of lidocaine following epidural administration.[105–108]

Phenytoin has been shown to increase the total body clearance of intravenously administered lidocaine by enzyme induction.[110] Intravenous injection of ephedrine increases the clearance of lidocaine,[111] but it may also promote the absorption of local anesthetics.[112]

The influence of sedative premedication preceding regional anesthetic procedures is largely unknown. A recent study showed that premedication with diazepam increased the peak plasma concentration and the area under the plasma concentration-time curve of bupivacaine, but not lidocaine, following caudal injection of a mixture of these agents in children.[113]

Bupivacaine may inhibit the hydrolysis of chloroprocaine.[114,115]

GERIATRICS

Studies on the effects of aging on the pharmacokinetics of intravenously administered lidocaine are partially confounded by complicating disease states and in some cases, concomitant drug therapy. Compared with young subjects, elderly patients generally had unchanged[116] or somewhat prolonged[117-118] elimination half-lives of intravenous lidocaine, unchanged[116,118] or a somewhat decreased total body clearances, and unchanged[116-117] or increased[118] volumes of distribution. One study comparing healthy elderly and young patients demonstrated a marked dependency on gender; in elderly men, the total body clearance was increased and the elimination half-life markedly prolonged, whereas in women, the pharmacokinetics were essentially independent of age.[119] Studies on the disposition of intravenously administered deuterium-labeled bupivacaine in surgical patients receiving epidural anesthesia indicated a decrease in the clearance of bupivacaine and a prolongation of the elimination half-life with increasing age.[28,30]

The total body clearance of lidocaine[120] and bupivacaine[121] calculated from the area under the plasma concentration-time curves after single epidural injections or from the steady-state concentration during continuous epidural infusion of bupivacaine[122] decreased consistently with increasing age. Peak plasma concentration following caudal[123] or epidural[120-121,124] injection of lidocaine or bupivacaine were virtually independent of age. One study reported a significantly shortened time to peak plasma concentration following epidural injection of lidocaine in older patients,[124] but this was not confirmed by the other studies.

Recent studies of the absorption kinetics after epidural and subarachnoid injection of bupivacaine showed a somewhat faster absorption rate in older patients.[28,30] However, this was statistically significant only after subarachnoid administration. The protein binding of bupivacaine does not appear to change with increasing age.[125]

OBSTETRICS

Regional procedures, in particular epidural blocks, are increasingly used in obstetrics. Single injection techniques are commonly used for elective cesarean section, whereas continuous block techniques are frequently used for the relief of labor pain. The most commonly used local anesthetic is bupivacaine.

Epidural dose requirements are reduced in pregnant women, possibly because of a greater sensitivity and/or enhanced diffusion related to hormonal changes.[126,127] Peak plasma concentrations and areas under the concentration-time curves of etidocaine and bupivacaine following single epidural injections in pregnant women appear to be similar to or somewhat greater than those in healthy nonpregnant women.[128,129] During continuous blocks, bupivacaine concentrations accumulate slowly.[130-132] Epidural administration of bupivacaine for emergency cesarean section in women that had previously received epidural bupivacaine during labor may result in plasma concentrations that approach toxic levels.[133,134]

Plasma chloroprocaine concentrations following epidural administration for cesarean section or for labor were very low.[78]

Placental Transfer

Placental transfer of local anesthetics is likely to be perfusion limited.[135] Equilibration between bupivacaine concentrations in the umbilical vein and those in maternal blood occurs very rapidly, possibly within one circulation time.[134] In addition, bupivacaine concentrations in the umbilical artery approach umbilical venous concentrations in approximately 30 minutes, indicating rapid tissue/blood partitioning in the fetus.

Even though plasma concentrations in the fetus equilibrate rapidly with maternal plasma concentrations, total umbilical venous/maternal venous plasma concentrations ratios may be considerably less than unity; for example, ratios of bupivacaine at delivery generally are in the range of 0.2 to 0.4. This low ratio reflects a considerably lower degree of protein binding of bupivacaine in the fetal plasma than in the maternal plasma. Unbound bupivacaine concentrations at equilibrium are likely to be similar on either side of the placenta, or possibly somewhat higher in the acidotic fetus, as a result of ion trapping.[136] This also holds for other local anesthetics.[56]

Neonatal Drug Disposition

Knowledge of the disposition of various local anesthetics in neonates is still incomplete. In general, local anesthetics are eliminated from newborns much more slowly than they are from adults.[137]

Estimated elimination half-lives of mepivacaine, lidocaine, etidocaine, and bupivacaine were approximately two- to fourfold longer than in adults. The longer half-lives in neonates reflect a larger volume of distribution and/or a smaller clearance. Volumes of distribution (corrected for body weight) of mepivacaine and lidocaine were twofold larger in newborns compared with adults. Plasma or blood clearance of mepivacaine, but not lidocaine, was less than one-half the adult value. The renal clearance of lidocaine and mepivacaine was significantly larger in newborns compared with adults.

PEDIATRICS

Peak plasma or blood concentrations in infants and children following caudal injection of lidocaine,[138,139] mepivacaine,[139] or bupivacaine,[139–142] or epidural[143] or intercostal[144,145] injection of bupivacaine appear to be broadly comparable to those in adults, given a similar dose on a milligram per kilogram basis.

The clearance (normalized for body weight) of lidocaine calculated from the area under the plasma concentration-time curve after caudal injection also appears to be similar to the clearance in adults.[138] However, studies of bupivacaine found a consistently higher clearance in infants and children compared with adults.[141–145] This may be a result of a lower degree of plasma protein binding in infants and children. The plasma protein binding of bupivacaine in infants increased gradually from 1 to 6 months of age in parallel with increasing AAG concentrations (Fig. 8-8).[142]

SPECIFIC DISEASE STATES

Cardiovascular Disease

Plasma lidocaine and monoethylglycine xylidide concentrations following intravenous administration of lidocaine in patients with congestive heart failure were markedly increased.[146,147] These increases may be attributed to a decreased volume of distribution and a decreased clearance.[147] Analogous changes in the pharmacokinetics of lidocaine have been found in patients with orthostatic hypotension[148] and during cardiopulmonary resuscitation.[149]

Hepatic Disease

Because amide-type agents are highly dependent on hepatic metabolism for their elimination,

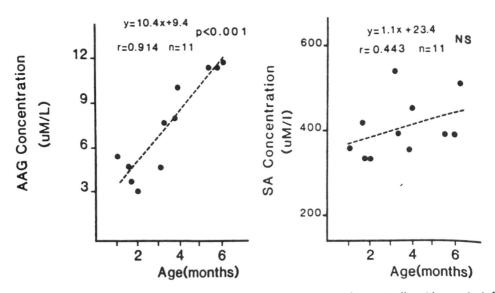

Fig. 8-8 The concentration of α_1-acid glycoprotein (AAG) increases dramatically with age in infants. The free fraction of bupivacaine (not shown) declined significantly as a result. Serum albumin (SA) did not change significantly. (From Mazoit et al.,[142] with permission.)

changes in hepatic function or hepatic blood flow may have significant consequences. Lidocaine elimination half-lives were prolonged during acute hepatitis[150] but not during chronic hepatitis.[151] The clearance of lidocaine was markedly reduced by hepatic cirrhosis; in addition, the volume of distribution was considerably increased such that the half-life was more than doubled.[147]

High bupivacaine concentrations, extending into the putative toxic range, have been measured in patients after liver transplantation, but no adverse effects attributable to bupivacaine were observed.[152]

Renal Disease

Because local anesthetics are mainly eliminated by biotransformation, their pharmacokinetics should not be markedly altered by renal disease.[147] However, metabolites that are excreted by the kidneys may accumulate if renal function is impaired. For example, considerable accumulation of glycine xylidide has been observed during continuous intravenous infusion of lidocaine in patients with renal failure.[153]

Pulmonary Disease

First-pass lung uptake of lidocaine was not altered in ventilated intensive care patients compared with normal volunteers.[43]

REFERENCES

1. Brinkløv MM: Clinical effects of carticaine, a new local anesthetic. A survey and a double-blind investigation comparing carticaine with lidocaine in epidural analgesia. Acta Anaesthesiol Scand 21:5, 1977
2. Mather LE: Disposition of mepivacaine and bupivacaine enantiomers in sheep. Br J Anaesth 67:239, 1991
3. Rutten AJ, Mather LE, McLean CF: Cardiovascular effects and regional clearances of i.v. bupivacaine in sheep: enantiomeric analysis. Br J Anaesth 67:247, 1991
4. Tucker GT, Mather LE, Lennard MS, Gregory A: Plasma concentrations of the stereoisomers of prilocaine after administration of the racemate: implications for toxicity? Br J Anaesth 65:333, 1990
5. Arthur GR, Covino BG: Pharmacokinetics of local anaesthetics. p. 635. In: White PF: Kinetics of Anesthetic Drugs in Clinical Anaesthesiology. Vol. 5. Baillère Tindall, London, 1991
6. Strichartz GR, Sanchez V, Arthur GR et al: Fundamental properties of local anesthetics. II. Measured octanol:buffer partition coefficients and pKa values of clinically used drugs. Anesth Analg 71:158, 1990
7. Tucker GT, Mather LE: Pharmacokinetics of local anaesthetic agents. Br J Anaesth 47:213, 1975
8. Lee A, Fagan D, Lamont M et al: Disposition kinetics of ropivacaine in humans. Anesth Analg 69:736, 1989
9. Meyer J, Nolte H: Liquorkonzentration von Bupivacain nach subduraler Applikation. Reg Anaesth 1:38, 1978
10. Tucker GT, Mather LE: Properties, absorption, and disposition of local anesthetic agents. p. 47. In Cousins MJ, Bridenbaugh PO (eds): Neural Blockade in Clinical Anesthesia and Management of Pain. 2nd Ed. JB Lippincott, Philadelphia, 1988
11. Cousins MJ, Mather LE: Intrathecal and epidural administration of opioids. Anesthesiology 61:276, 1984
12. Covino BG, Vassallo HG: Local Anesthetics. Mechanisms of Action and Clinical Use. Grune and Stratton, New York, 1976
13. Winnie AP, Tay C-H, Patel KP et al: Pharmacokinetics of local anesthetics during plexus blocks. Anesth Analg 56:852, 1977
14. Wildsmith JAW: Peripheral nerve and local anaesthetic drugs. Br J Anaesth 58:692, 1986
15. Gissen AJ, Covino BG, Gregus J: Differential sensitivities of mammalian nerve fibers to local anesthetic agents. Anesthesiology 53:467, 1980
16. Wildsmith JAW, Gissen AJ, Gregus J, Covino BG: Differential nerve blocking activity of amino-ester local anaesthetics. Br J Anaesth 57:612, 1985
17. Bromage PR: Epidural Analgesia. WB Saunders, Philadelphia, 1978
18. Gissen AJ, Covino BG, Gregus J: Differential sensitivity of fast and slow fibers in mammalian nerve: III. Effect of etidocaine and bupivacaine on fast/slow fibers. Anesth Analg 61:570, 1982
19. Raymond SA, Gissen AJ: Mechanisms of differential nerve block. p. 95. In Strichartz GR (ed): Local Anesthetics. Springer-Verlag, Berlin, 1987
20. Covino BG: Pharmacology of local anaesthetic agents. Br J Anaesth 58:701, 1986
21. DiFazio CA, Carron H, Grosslight KR et al: Comparison of pH-adjusted lidocaine solutions for epidural anesthesia. Anesth Analg 65:760, 1986
22. McMorland GH, Douglas MJ, Jeffery WK et al: Effect of pH adjustment of bupivacaine on onset and

duration of epidural analgesia in parturients. Can J Anaesth 33:537, 1986

23. Liepert DJ, Douglas MJ, McMorland GH et al: Comparison of lidocaine CO_2, two per cent lidocaine hydrochloride and pH adjusted lidocaine hydrochloride for caesarian section anaesthesia. Can J Anaesth 37:333, 1990

24. Nickel PM, Bromage PR, Sherrill DL: Comparison of hydrochloride and carbonated salts of lidocaine for epidural analgesia. Reg Anesth 11:62, 1986

25. Sukhani R, Winnie AP: Clinical pharmacokinetics of carbonated local anesthetics II: interscalene brachial block model. Anesth Analg 66:1245, 1987

26. Dahl JB, Simonsen L, Mogensen T et al: The effect of 0.5% ropivacaine on epidural blood flow. Acta Anaesthesiol Scand 34:308, 1990

27. Burm AGL, Vermeulen NPE, Van Kleef JW et al: Pharmacokinetics of lignocaine and bupivacaine in surgical patients following epidural administration. Simultaneous investigation of absorption and disposition kinetics using stable isotopes. Clin Pharmacokinet 13:191, 1987

28. Veering BTh, Burm AGL, Vletter AA et al: The effect of age on the systemic absorption, disposition and pharmacodynamics of bupivacaine after epidural administration. Clin Pharmacokinet 22:75, 1992

29. Burm AGL, Van Kleef JW, Vermeulen NPE et al: Pharmacokinetics of lidocaine and bupivacaine following subarachnoid administration in surgical patients: simultaneous investigation of absorption and disposition kinetics using stable isotopes. Anesthesiology 69:584, 1988

30. Veering BTh, Burm AGL, Vletter AA et al: The effect of age on systemic absorption and systemic disposition of bupivacaine after subarachnoid administration. Anesthesiology 74:250, 1991

31. Burm AGL: Clinical pharmacokinetics of epidural and spinal anaesthesia. Clin Pharmacokinet 16:283, 1989

32. Benowitz N, Forsyth RP, Melmon KL, Rowland M: Lidocaine disposition kinetics in monkey and man: I. Prediction by a perfusion model. Clin Pharmacol Ther 16:87, 1974

33. Denson D, Coyle D, Thompson G, Myers J: Alpha$_1$-acid glycoprotein and albumin in human serum bupivacaine binding. Clin Pharmacol Ther 35:409, 1984

34. Routledge PA, Barchowsky A, Bjornsson TD et al: Lidocaine plasma protein binding. Clin Pharmacol Ther 27:347, 1980

35. Tucker GT, Boyes RN, Bridenbaugh PO, Moore DC: Binding of anilide-type local anesthetics in human plasma: I. Relationships between binding, physicochemical properties, and anesthetic activity. Anesthesiology 33:287, 1970

36. Wood M: Plasma drug binding: implications for anesthesiologists. Anesth Analg 65:786, 1986

37. Remmel RP, Copa AK, Angaran DM: The effects of hemodilution, pH, and protamine on lidocaine protein binding and red blood-cell uptake in vitro. Pharm Res 8:127, 1990

38. Bachman B, Biscoping J, Violka T et al: Pharmakokinetische Untersuchungen zur Plasmaproteinbindung von Bupivacain nach akuter präoperativer Hämodilution. Reg Anaesth 14:32, 1991

39. Rutten AJ, Mather LE, Plummer JL, Henning EC: Postoperative course of plasma protein binding of lignocaine, ropivacaine and bupivacaine in sheep. J Pharm Pharmacol 44:355, 1992

40. Pieper JA, Wyman MG, Goldreyer BN et al: Lidocaine toxicity: effect of total versus free lidocaine concentrations. Circulation 62: Suppl. III-181, 1980

41. Denson DD, Myers JA, Hartrick CT et al: The relationship between free bupivacaine concentration and central nervous system toxicity. Anesthesiology, suppl. 3A:A211, 1984

42. Jorfeldt L, Lewis DH, Löfström JB, Post C: Lung uptake of lidocaine in healthy volunteers. Acta Anaesthesiol Scand 23:567, 1979

43. Jorfeldt L, Lewis DH, Löfström JB, Post C: Lung uptake of lidocaine in man as influenced by anaesthesia, mepivacaine infusion or lung insufficiency. Acta Anaesthesiol Scand 27:5, 1983

44. Post C, Andersson RG, Ryrfeldt A et al: Physicochemical modification of lidocaine uptake in rat lung tissue. Acta Pharmacol Toxicol 44:103, 1979

45. Palazzo MGA, Kalso EA, Argiras E et al: First pass lung uptake of bupivacaine: effect of acidosis in an intact rabbit lung model. Br J Anaesth 67:759, 1991

46. Bertler Å, Lewis DH, Löfström JB, Post C: In vivo lung uptake of lidocaine in pigs. Acta Anaesthesiol Scand 22:530, 1978

47. Tucker GT, Boas RA: Pharmacokinetic aspects of intravenous regional anesthesia. Anesthesiology 34:538, 1971

48. Nancarrow C, Runciman WB, Mather LE et al: The influence of acidosis on the distribution of lidocaine and bupivacaine into the myocardium and brain of the sheep. Anesth Analg 66:925, 1987

49. Nakazono T, Murakami T, Higashi Y, Yata N: Study on brain uptake of local anesthetics in rats. J Pharmacobiodyn 14:605, 1991

50. Marathe PH, Shen DD, Artru AA, Bowdle TA: Effect of serum protein binding on the entry of lido-

caine into brain and cerebrospinal fluid in dogs. Anesthesiology 75:804, 1991

51. Pardridge WM, Sakiyama R, Fierer G: Transport of propranolol and lidocaine through the rat blood-brain barrier. J Clin Invest 71:900, 1983

52. Terasaki T, Pardridge WM, Denson DD: Differential effect of plasma protein binding of bupivacaine on its in vivo transfer into the brain and salivary gland of rats. J Pharmacol Exp Ther 239:724, 1986

53. Halpern SH, Eisler EA, Shnider SM et al: Myocardial tissue uptake of bupivacaine and lidocaine after intravenous injection in normal and acidotic rabbits. Anesthesiology, suppl. 3A:A208, 1984

54. Simon RP, Benowitz NL, Culala S: Motor paralysis increases brain uptake of lidocaine during status epilepticus. Neurology 34:384, 1984

55. Englesson S, Grevsten S: The influence of acid-base changes on central nervous system toxicity of local anaesthetic agents II. Acta Anaesthesiol Scand 18:88, 1974

56. Tucker GT: Pharmacokinetics of local anaesthetics. Br J Anaesth 58:717, 1986

57. Arthur GR, Scott DHT, Boyes RN, Scott DB: Pharmacokinetic and clinical pharmacological studies with mepivacaine and prilocaine. Br J Anaesth 51:481, 1979

58. Seifen AB, Ferrari AA, Seifen EE et al: Pharmacokinetics of intravenous procaine infusion in humans. Anesth Analg 58:382, 1979

59. Vree TB, Beumer EMC, Lagerwerf AJ et al: Clinical pharmacokinetics of R(+)- and S(−)-mepivacaine after high doses of racemic mepivacaine with epinephrine in the combined psoas compartment/sciatic nerve block. Anesth Analg 75:75, 1992

60. Foldes FF, Davidson GM, Duncalf D, Kuwabara S: The intravenous toxicity of local anesthetic agents in man. Clin Pharmacol Ther 6:328, 1965

61. Reidenberg MM, James M, Dring LG: The rate of procaine hydrolysis in serum of normal subjects and diseased patients. Clin Pharmacol Ther 13:279, 1972

62. Drayer DE, Lorenzo B, Werns S, Reidenberg MM: Plasma levels, protein binding, and elimination data of lidocaine and active metabolites in cardiac patients of various ages. Clin Pharmacol Ther 34:14, 1983

63. Blumer J, Strong JM, Atkinson AJ: The convulsant potency of lidocaine and its n-dealkylated metabolites. J Pharmacol Exp Ther 186:31, 1973

64. Kuhnert PM, Kuhnert BR, Stitts JM, Gross TL: The use of a selected ion monitoring technique to study the disposition of bupivacaine in mother, fetus, and neonate following epidural anesthesia for cesarean section. Anesthesiology 55:611, 1981

65. Rosenberg PH, Pere P, Hekali R, Tuominen M: Plasma concentrations of bupivacaine and two of its metabolites during continuous interscalene brachial plexus block. Br J Anaesth 66:25, 1991

66. Thomas J, Morgan D, Vine J: Metabolism of etidocaine in man. Xenobiotica 6:39, 1976

67. Hjelm M, Holmdahl MH: Biochemical effects of aromatic amines: II. Cyanosis, methaemoglobinaemia and Heinz-body formation induced by a local anaesthetic agent (prilocaine). Acta Anaesthesiol Scand 9:99, 1965

68. Kennedy WF, Everett GB, Cobb LA, Allen GD: Simultaneous systemic and hepatic hemodynamic measurements during high peridural anesthesia in normal man. Anesth Analg 50:1069, 1971

69. Sivarajan M, Amory DW, Lindbloom LE, Schwettmann RS: Systemic and regional blood-flow changes during spinal anesthesia in the rhesus monkey. Anesthesiology 43:78, 1975

70. Runciman WB, Mather LE, Ilsley AH et al: A sheep preparation for studying interactions between blood flow and drug disposition. III: Effects of general and spinal anaesthesia on regional blood flow and oxygen tensions. Br J Anaesth 56:1247, 1984

71. Tucker GT, Moore DC, Bridenbaugh PO et al: Systemic absorption of mepivacaine in commonly used regional block procedures. Anesthesiology 37:277, 1972

72. Wildsmith JAW, Tucker GT, Cooper S et al: Plasma concentrations of local anaesthetics after interscalene brachial plexus block. Br J Anaesth 49:461, 1977

73. Van Kleef JW, Burm AGL, Vletter AA: Single-dose interpleural versus intercostal blockade: nerve block characteristics and plasma concentration profiles after administration of 0.5% bupivacaine with epinephrine. Anesth Analg 70:484, 1990

74. Tucker GT, Cooper S, Littlewood D et al: Observed and predicted accumulation of local anaesthetic agents during continuous extradural analgesia. Br J Anaesth 49:237, 1977

75. Safran D, Kuhlman G, Orhant EE et al: Continuous intercostal blockade with lidocaine after thoracic surgery. Anesth Analg 70:345, 1990

76. Ross RA, Clarke JE, Armitage EN: Postoperative pain prevention by continuous epidural infusion. A study of the clinical effects and the plasma concentrations obtained. Anaesthesia 35:663, 1980

77. Van Kleef JW, Logeman EA, Burm AGL et al: Continuous interpleural infusion of bupivacaine for

postoperative analgesia after surgery with flank incisions: a double-blind comparison of 0.25% and 0.5% solutions. Anesth Analg 75:268, 1992

78. Kuhnert BR, Kuhnert PM, Prochaska AL, Gross TL: Plasma levels of 2-chloroprocaine in obstetric patients and their neonates after epidural anesthesia. Anesthesiology 53:21, 1980

79. Salevsky FC, Whalley DG, Kalant D, Crawhall J: Epidural epinephrine and the systemic circulation during peripheral vascular surgery. Can J Anaesth 37:160, 1990

80. Takasaki M, Kajitani H: Plasma lidocaine concentrations during continuous epidural infusion of lidocaine with and without epinephrine. Can J Anaesth 37:166, 1990

81. Stanton-Hicks M, Berges PU, Bonica JJ: Circulatory effects of peridural block: IV. Comparison of the effects of epinephrine and phenylephrine. Anesthesiology 39:308, 1973

82. Sharrock NE, Go G, Mineo R: Effect of low-dose adrenaline and phenylephrine infusions on plasma concentrations of bupivacaine after lumbar extradural anaesthesia in elderly patients. Br J Anaesth 67:694, 1991

83. Nishikawa T, Dohi S. Clinical evaluation of clonidine added to lidocaine solution for epidural anesthesia. Anesthesiology 73:853, 1990

84. Gaumann D, Forster A, Griessen M et al: Comparison between clonidine and epinephrine admixture to lidocaine in brachial plexus block. Anesth Analg 75:69, 1992

85. Scott DB, Jebson PJR, Braid DP et al: Factors affecting plasma levels of lignocaine and prilocaine. Br J Anaesth 44:1040, 1972

86. Lund PC, Bush DF, Covino BG: Determinants of etidocaine concentration in the blood. Anesthesiology 42:497, 1975

87. Lund PC, Cwik JC, Pagdanganan RT: Etidocaine—a new long-acting local anesthetic agent: a clinical evaluation. Anesth Analg 52:482, 1973

88. Sukhani R, Winnie AP: Clinical pharmacokinetics of carbonated local anesthetics: III. Interscalene brachial block model. Anesth Analg 68:90, 1989

89. Appleyard TN, Witt A, Atkinson RE, Nicholas ADG: Bupivacaine carbonate and bupivacaine hydrochloride: a comparison of blood concentrations during epidural blockade for vaginal surgery. Br J Anaesth 46:530, 1974

90. Cousins MJ, Bromage PR: A comparison of the hydrochloride and carbonated salts of lignocaine for caudal analgesia in out-patients. Br J Anaesth 43:1149, 1971

91. Bentley JB, Glass S, Gandolfi AJ: The influence of halothane on lidocaine pharmacokinetics in man. Anesthesiology, suppl. :A246, 1983

92. Mather LE, Runciman WB, Carapetis RJ et al: Hepatic and renal clearances in conscious and anesthetized sheep. Anesth Analg 65:943, 1986

93. Bax NDS, Tucker GT, Lennard MS, Woods HF: The impairment of lignocaine clearance by propranolol—major contribution from enzyme inhibition. Br J Clin Pharmacol 19:597, 1985

94. Tucker GT, Bax NDS, Lennard MS et al: Effects of β-adrenoceptor antagonists on the pharmacokinetics of lignocaine. Br J Clin Pharmacol, suppl. :21S, 1984

95. Bowdle TA, Freund PR, Slattery JT: Propranolol reduces bupivacaine clearance. Anesthesiology 66:36. 1987

96. Conrad KA, Byers JM, Finley PR, Burnham L: Lidocaine elimination: effects of metoprolol and propranolol. Clin Pharmacol Ther 33:133, 1983

97. Ponten J, Biber B, Henriksson B-A, Jonsteg C: Bupivacaine for intercostal nerve blockade in patients on long-term beta-receptor blocking therapy. Acta Anaesthesiol Scand, suppl. :70, 1982

98. Bauer LA, Edwards WAD, Randolph FP et al: Cimetidine-induced decrease in lidocaine metabolism. Am Heart J 108:413, 1984

99. Feely J, Wilkinson GR, McAllistor CB, Wood AJJ: Increased toxicity and reduced clearance of lidocaine by cimetidine. Ann Intern Med 96:592, 1982

100. Wing LMH, Miners JO, Birkett DJ et al: Lidocaine disposition—sex differences and effects of cimetidine. Clin Pharmacol Ther 35:695, 1984

101. Noble DW, Smith KJ, Dundas CR: Effects of H-2 antagonists on the elimination of bupivacaine. Br J Anaesth 59:735, 1987

102. Pihlajamäki KK, Lindberg RLP, Jantunen ME: Lack of cimetidine on the pharmacokinetics of bupivacaine in healthy subjects. Br J Clin Pharmacol 26:403, 1988

103. Kuhnert BR, Zuspan KJ, Kuhnert PM et al: Lack of influence of cimetidine on bupivacaine levels during parturition. Anesth Analg 66:986, 1987

104. Flynn RJ, Moore J, Collier PS, Howard PJ: Effect of intravenous cimetidine on lignocaine disposition during extradural caesarean section. Anaesthesia 44:739, 1989

105. Flynn RJ, Moore J, Collier PS, McClean E: Does pretreatment with cimetidine and ranitidine affect the disposition of bupivacaine. Br J Anaesth 62:87, 1989

106. O'Sullivan GM, Smith M, Morgan B et al: H₂ antag-

onists and bupivacaine clearance. Anaesthesia 43:93, 1988

107. Brashear WT, Zuspan KJ, Lazebnik et al: Effect of ranitidine on bupivacaine disposition. Anesth Analg 72:369, 1991

108. Dailey PA, Hughes SC, Rosen MA et al: Lidocaine levels during cesarean section after pretreatment with ranitidine and cimetidine. Anesthesiology, suppl. :A444, 1985

109. Feely J, Guy E: Lack of effect of ranitidine on the disposition of lignocaine. Br J Clin Pharmacol 16:378, 1983

110. Perucca E, Richens A: Reduction of oral bioavailability of lignocaine by induction of first pass metabolism in epileptic patients. Br J Clin Pharmacol 8:21, 1979

111. Wiklund L, Tucker GT, Engberg G: Influence of intravenously administered ephedrine on splanchnic haemodynamics and clearance of lidocaine. Acta Anaesthesiol Scand 21:275, 1977

112. Mather LE, Tucker GT, Murphy TM et al: Hemodynamic drug interaction: peridural lidocaine and intravenous ephedrine. Acta Anaesthesiol Scand 20:207, 1976

113. Giaufre E, Bruguerolle B, Morisson-Lacombe G, Rousset-Rouviere B: The influence of diazepam on the plasma concentrations of bupivacaine and lignocaine after caudal injection of a mixture of the local anaesthetics in children. Br J Clin Pharmacol 26:116, 1988

114. Lalka D, Vicuna N, Burrow SR et al: Bupivacaine and other amide local anesthetics inhibit the hydrolysis of chloroprocaine in human serum. Anesth Analg 57:534, 1978

115. Raj PP, Ohlweiler D, Hitt BA, Denson DD: Kinetics of local anesthetic esters and the effects of adjuvant drugs on 2-chloroprocaine hydrolysis. Anesthesiology 53:307, 1980

116. Cusson J, Nattel S, Matthews C et al: Age-dependent lidocaine disposition in patients with acute myocardial infarction. Clin Pharmacol Ther 37:381, 1985

117. Cusack B, O'Malley K, Lavan J et al: Protein binding and disposition of lignocaine in the elderly. Br J Clin Pharmacol 29:323, 1985

118. Nation RL, Triggs EJ, Selig M: Lignocaine kinetics in cardiac patients and aged subjects. Br J Clin Pharmacol 4:439, 1977

119. Abernethy DR, Greenblatt DJ: Impairment of lidocaine clearance in elderly male subjects. J Cardiovasc Pharmacol 5:1093, 1983

120. Bowdle TA, Freund PR, Slattery JT: Age-depen-

dent lidocaine pharmacokinetics during lumbar peridural anesthesia with lidocaine hydrocarbonate and lidocaine hydrochloride. Reg Anesth 11:123, 1986

121. Veering BTh, Burm AGL, Van Kleef JW et al: Epidural anesthesia with bupivacaine: effect of age on neural blockade and pharmacokinetics. Anesth Analg 66:589, 1987

122. Concilus RR, Denson DD, Knarr D et al: Bupivacaine clearance in continuous epidural infusions for postoperative pain relief. Reg Anesth, suppl. 25:69, 1988

123. Freund PR, Bowdle TA, Slattery JT, Bell LE: Caudal anesthesia with lidocaine or bupivacaine: plasma local anesthetic concentration and extent of sensory spread in old and young patients. Anesth Analg 63:1017, 1984

124. Finucane BT, Hammonds WD, Welch MB: Influence of age on vascular absorption of lidocaine from the epidural space. Anesth Analg 66:843, 1987

125. Veering BTh, Burm AGL, Gladines MPRR, Spierdijk J; Age does not influence the serum protein binding of bupivacaine. Br J Clin Pharmacol 32:501, 1991

126. Datta S, Lambert DH, Gregus J et al: Differential sensitivities of mammalian nerve fibers during pregnancy. Anesth Analg 62:1070, 1983

127. Flanagan HL, Datta S, Lambert DH et al: Effect of pregnancy on bupivacaine-induced conduction blockade in the isolated rabbit vagus nerve. Anesth Analg 66:123, 1987

128. Morgan DJ, Cousins MJ, McQuillan D, Thomas J: Disposition and placental transfer of etidocaine in pregnancy. Eur J Clin Pharmacol 12:359, 1977

129. Pihlajamäki K, Kanto J, Lindberg R et al: Extradural administration of bupivacaine: pharmacokinetics and metabolism in pregnant and non-pregnant women. Br J Anaesth 64:556, 1990

130. Reynolds F, Hargrove RL, Wyman JB: Maternal and fetal plasma concentrations of bupivacaine after epidural block. Br J Anaesth 45:1049, 1973

131. Glover DJ: Continuous epidural analgesia in the obstetric patient: a feasibility study using a mechanical infusion pump. Anaesthesia 32:499, 1977

132. Pierce ET, Denson DD, Essell SK et al: The effect of rate of infusion on continuous epidural analgesia for labor and delivery. Reg Anesth 14:31, 1989

133. Thompson EM, Wilson CM, Moore J, McLean E: Plasma bupivacaine levels associated with extradural anaesthesia for caesarean section. Anaesthesia 40:427, 1985

134. Reynolds F, Laishley R, Morgan B, Lee A: Effect of

time and adrenaline on the feto-maternal distribution of bupivacaine. Br J Anaesth 62:509, 1989

135. Hamshaw-Thomas A, Rogerson N, Reynolds F: Transfer of bupivacaine, lignocaine and pethidine across the rabbit placenta: influence of maternal protein binding and fetal flow. Placenta 5:61, 1984

136. Kennedy RL, Erenberg A, Robillard JE et al: Effects of changes in maternal-fetal pH on the transplacental equilibrium of bupivacaine. Anesthesiology 51:50, 1979

137. Kanto J: Obstetric analgesia. Clinical pharmacokinetic considerations. Clin Pharmacokinet 11:283, 1986.

138. Ecoffey C, Desparmet J, Berdeaux A et al: Pharmacokinetics of lignocaine in children following caudal anaesthesia. Br J Anaesth 56:1399, 1984

139. Takasaki M: Blood concentrations of lidocaine, mepivacaine and bupivacaine during caudal analgesia in children. Acta Anaesthesiol Scand 28:211, 1984

140. Bertrix L, Foussat C, Moussa et al: Anesthesie caudale en chirurgie pediatrique. Étude pharmacokinetique et interet clinique. Chir Pediatr 30:47, 1989

141. Ecoffey C, Desparmet J, Maury M et al: Bupivacaine in children: pharmacokinetics following caudal anesthesia. Anesthesiology 63:447, 1985

142. Mazoit JX, Denson DD, Samii K: Pharmacokinetics of bupivacaine following caudal anesthesia in infants. Anesthesiology 68:387, 1988

143. Murat I, Montay G, Delleur MM et al: Bupivacaine pharmacokinetics during epidural anaesthesia in children. Eur J Anaesthesiol 5:113, 1988

144. Rothstein P, Arthur GR, Feldman HS et al: Bupivacaine for intercostal nerve block in children: blood concentrations and pharmacokinetics. Anesth Analg 65:625, 1986

145. Bricker SRW, Telford RJ, Booker PD: Pharmacokinetics of bupivacaine following intraoperative intercostal nerve block in neonates and in infants aged less than 6 months. Anesthesiology 70:942, 1989

146. Halkin H, Meffin P, Melmon KL, Rowland M: Influence of congestive heart failure on blood levels of lidocaine and its active monodeethylated metabolite. Clin Pharmacol Ther 17:669, 1975

147. Thomson PD, Melmon KL, Richardson JA et al: Lidocaine pharmacokinetics in advanced heart failure, liver disease and renal failure in humans. Ann Intern Med 78:499, 1973

148. Feely J, Wade D, McAllister CB et al: Effect of hypotension on liver blood flow and lidocaine disposition. N Engl J Med 307:866, 1982

149. Chow MSS, Ronfeld RA, Ruffett D et al: Lidocaine pharmacokinetics during cardiac arrest and external cardiopulmonary resuscitation. Am Heart J 102:799, 1981

150. Williams RL, Blaschke TF, Meffin PG et al: Influence of viral hepatitis on the disposition of two compounds with high hepatic clearance: lidocaine and indocyanine green. Clin Pharmacol Ther 20:290, 1976

151. Huet P-M, Lelorier J: Effects of smoking and chronic hepatitis B on lidocaine and indocyanine green kinetics. Clin Pharmacol Ther 28:208, 1980

152. Bodenham A, Park GR: Plasma concentrations of bupivacaine after intercostal block in patients after orthotopic liver transplantation. Br J Anaesth 64:436, 1990

153. Collinsworth KA, Strong JM, Atkinson AJ et al: Pharmacokinetics and metabolism of lidocaine in patients with renal failure. Clin Pharmacol Ther 18:59, 1975

Chapter 9

Clinical Pharmacology and Applications of Local Anesthetics

Per H. Rosenberg

The use of local anesthetics differs from many other drugs in that they are typically applied at, or near the site of their action; most drugs require transportation in the blood after various routes of administration to the site of action. Certain clinical pharmacologic aspects, such as penetration through various tissue layers and direct vascular effects of the local anesthetics, become particularly important in the characterization of these drugs.

A major practical problem with the presently available local anesthetics is that they are not very specific or selective in their action. All nerve axons are eventually blocked by most local anesthetics without a clear selection between the type or function of the axons. Furthermore, most local anesthetics have nontherapeutic or toxic effects. Therefore, one of the most important goals in local anesthetic drug development is to find nerve-specific, pain fiber-selective, and nontoxic local anesthetics.

THERAPEUTIC LOCAL ANESTHETIC EFFECTS

Nerve Blocking Action

Anatomic and chemical factors determine the susceptibility of nerve fibers to become blocked by local anesthetics, the rate of onset, maximum block-
ing effect, and the duration of nerve blocks. Organ-specific and drug molecule-related factors also determine the differential actions of local anesthetics on the various kinds of excitable tissues.

The molecular mechanisms of local anesthetics are presented in Chapter 7. Local anesthetics inhibit transmission of nerve impulses by preventing increases in the permeability of nerve membranes to sodium ion, slowing the rate of depolarization such that threshold potential is not reached and an action potential is not propagated.[1] Local anesthetics do not alter the resting transmembrane or threshold potentials. Potassium and calcium channels are also affected by local anesthetics,[2] but for the mechanism of nerve block, these actions are of secondary importance.

In vitro, isolated thin nerves are easily blocked by concentrations of local anesthetics in the 100 μM range.[3] However, in clinical regional anesthesia, local anesthetic solutions in the 10 to 30 mM (0.5 to 1 percent) range are commonly used. This is necessary to compensate for the loss of a substantial portion of the local anesthetic in the process of diffusion from the site of injection to the target. Because diffusion is a slow process, the local anesthetic solution is continually being diluted with tissue fluids. At the same time, drug is continuously absorbed by blood and lymphatic vessels. Also, much of the drug is bound to various non-neural structures.

Because this uptake is essentially the result of hydrophobic (lipophilic) absorption, generally, the more lipid soluble agents exhibit a slow onset of nerve block. The local anesthetic should be deposited as close to the nerve as possible in order to produce anesthesia without undue delay.

Although proximity to the nerve is important, a regional anesthetic block can often be enhanced by restricting the vascular absorption of the local anesthetic. Absorption may be slowed (and the block prolonged) by including epinephrine or other vasoconstrictor in the local anesthetic solution.[4] Clinically, there is no benefit in using epinephrine that is more concentrated than 5 μg/ml when major regional blocks (e.g., epidural or brachial plexus blocks) are performed.

Drugs injected into highly perfused tissues, e.g., the intercostal nerve space, epidural space, and interpleural space, are absorbed much faster than drugs injected into less well perfused regions.

Differential Nerve Block

Different nerve fibers require different minimum concentrations of local anesthetic to disrupt neural transmission. A clinically demonstrable block of the thin A-δ and the thin unmyelinated C-fibers (i.e., pain fibers) may be achieved, while leaving most of the thickest myelinated fibers (e.g., A-α and A-β fibers, i.e., motor function and touch fibers) relatively unaffected. Traditionally, this phenomenon is believed to be associated with the differences in nerve fiber thickness; a minimum blocking concentration of the local anesthetic is more easily achieved in thin than in thick fibers.[5] In myelinated nerve fibers, the length of fiber exposed to the local anesthetic must involve at least three consecutive nodes of Ranvier for the interruption of impulse propagation.[6] Recently, the "three-node" principle has been applied to the mechanism of action of differential epidural and spinal block (see Differential Epidural Block).[7]

The minimum effective local anesthetic concentration remains the same independent of the anatomic location; it is the same whether the axon is located in a spinal nerve root or in a peripheral nerve. Hypothetically, blockade of specific types of nerve fibers could be obtained by injecting just the minimum effective concentration corresponding to

a particular nerve to be blocked. However, as mentioned, the local anesthetic solutions injected into the vicinity of the nerve are subject to a variety of concentration reducing and dilutional factors that determine the actual concentration finally reaching the interior of the nerve axon.

Clinically, differential block is most clearly and reproducibly obtained in obstetric epidural analgesia and in postoperative epidural analgesia with the use of dilute bupivacaine solutions (0.06 to 0.25 percent).

Antiarrhythmic Action of Local Anesthetics

Local anesthetics slow the maximum rate of depolarization (phase 0). The general term for this property is membrane stabilizing activity, which may contribute to stopping dysrhythmias by limiting the responsiveness to excitation of cardiac cells in general. Procainamide belongs to class IA (prolongs refractoriness) and lidocaine (and tocainide) to class IB (shortens refractoriness).[8]

The effect of procainamide on the heart is essentially the same as that of quinidine (i.e., reduced automaticity, prolongation of cardiac refractory period, and anticholinergic effect). Procainamide is usually administered by mouth (250 mg every 4 to 6 hours). It may also be given intravenously at 25 to 50 mg/min, with electrocardiogram monitoring (maximum dose, 1 g). Hypotension results from too rapid administration. Allergic reactions of various types may occur, and there is allergic cross reactivity with procaine.[9]

Lidocaine, like quinidine, possesses membrane stabilizing (class I) effects, but unlike quinidine, it reduces the cardiac refractory period. It is probably because of this difference that lidocaine can sometimes terminate a dysrhythmia when quinidine and procainamide fail. Lidocaine is used by the intravenous route or occasionally by the intramuscular route. Dosing by mouth is unsatisfactory because the elimination half-life (approximately 90 minutes) is too short to maintain a stable plasma concentration by repeated administration. Lidocaine is well absorbed from the gastrointestinal tract, but it undergoes substantial first-pass clearance in the liver. The intravenous route is safe to use, and the short elimination half-life facilitates the adjustment of plasma levels. Lidocaine is almost entirely metabolized in the liver, and the rate at which it is cleared from the blood depends on hepatic blood flow.

Lidocaine is used primarily for the treatment of ventricular arrhythmias, especially those complicating myocardial infarction. In the presence of acute myocardial infarction, the prophylactic administration of lidocaine reduces the incidence of primary ventricular fibrillation.[10] The therapeutic blood concentration is 2 to 5 μg/ml (plasma concentrations approximately, 2.5 to 6 μg/ml). The acute treatment can start with an intravenous loading dose of 1 to 2 mg/kg followed by a continuous infusion of 15 to 30 μg/kg/min. If necessary to suppress arrhythmias, an initial 1 mg/kg bolus may be followed by 0.5 mg/kg boluses every 8 to 10 minutes if needed, up to a total of 3 mg/kg. In an emergency situation outside the hospital, 4 to 5 mg/kg of lidocaine may be administered by intramuscular injection. Endotracheal administration of 2 mg/kg of lidocaine will also result in therapeutic blood concentrations, at least in patients with an adequate pulmonary and systemic circulation.[11] In patients with decreased cardiac output, elderly patients (older than 70 years) and those with hepatic dysfunction, the dose of lidocaine for arrhythmia treatment should be reduced.

Anticonvulsive Action of Local Anesthetics

In general, the anticonvulsant activity of local anesthetic agents occurs at doses and blood levels considerably lower than those associated with seizure activity. In experimental animals, a marked anti-epileptic effect was observed at lidocaine plasma levels of 0.5 to 4.0 μg/ml; at levels greater than 7.5 μg/ml, seizure activity became evident.[12] For the treatment of seizures in newborns, a bolus of 2 mg/kg IV, followed by an infusion of 6 mg/kg/h has been recommended.[13] However, as a result of its relatively narrow therapeutic range for anticonvulsive action, lidocaine is not a primary choice in the treatment of epileptic seizures. Because local anesthetics are additive in their toxic effects,[14] lidocaine should not be used for the treatment of local anesthetic induced seizures.

Local Anesthetics in Treatment of Central Pain

Intravenous local anesthetic administration has been found beneficial in relieving neuralgia, deafferentation pain, and other central pain problems. Both intravenous lidocaine and tocainide (a lidocaine-like, antiarrhythmic drug) are able to depress C-afferent fiber-evoked activity in the spinal cord selectively.[15] In addition, 2-chloroprocaine intravenous infusions have been used and found to be beneficial in certain central pain conditions. This ester-type local anesthetic is infused at 1 to 1.5 mg/kg/min to a total dose of 10 to 20 mg/kg.[16]

Study reports suggest that about one-half of the patients with chronic pain who benefit from intravenous local anesthetic therapy require four to six treatments; the other half require additional treatment at intervals of 2 to 3 weeks.[17]

Anti-Inflammatory Effect of Local Anesthetics

Amide local anesthetics have been found to inhibit several steps involved in the pathophysiology of inflammation.[18] Intravenous infusion of lidocaine almost completely abolishes the delivery of polymorphonuclear granulocytes to the inflammatory site in aseptic peritonitis in rabbits, and this effect has been found to be more than 10-fold greater than the effect of methylprednisolone.[19]

As formulated for clinical use, local anesthetics are either bacteriostatic or bacteriocidal.[20,21] Bupivacaine at 5 mg/ml inhibits the growth of most common infectious bacteria (with the exception of *Pseudomonas aeruginosa*) when isolates are exposed to the local anesthetic for 18 hours.[22]

PLACENTAL TRANSFER OF LOCAL ANESTHETICS
Ester-Type Local Anesthetics

After injection of 2-chloroprocaine to mothers, the plasma concentrations in both maternal and umbilical cord blood are very low.[23] Elimination half-lives of 2-chloroprocaine and procaine are about twice as long in neonatal plasma as in maternal plasma (Table 9-1), and pregnancy is associated

Table 9-1 In Vitro Plasma Half-Lives of 2-Chloroprocaine and Procaine[a]

	Normal	Pregnant	Neonate
2-Chloroprocaine	21 ± 2	21 ± 1	43 ± 2
Procaine	39 ± 8		84 ± 30

[a] In seconds ± standard deviation.
(Modified from Tucker and Mather,[145] with permission.)

with a decrease in pseudocholinesterase activity.[24,25] However the absolute rate of hydrolysis in the mother remains fast enough to prevent intoxication of the fetus.

Depending on the scoring method for neonatal neurobehavior, it has been suggested that 2-chloroprocaine epidural anesthesia for cesarean section may result in long-term (up to 3 days) neurobehavioral deficits.[26] There is no explanation for this finding at the present time, although a late action of metabolites of 2-chloroprocaine have been suggested.

Amide-Type Local Anesthetics

At delivery by cesarean section, umbilical vein/maternal vein plasma concentration ratios of the various local anesthetics vary considerably. Except in the case of prilocaine, the umbilical blood (plasma) concentrations are lower (Table 9-2). The different ratios reflect differences in plasma protein binding between maternal blood and fetal blood. The fetal blood contains relatively low concentrations of

Table 9-2 Umbilical Vein/Maternal Vein Plasma Concentration Ratios at the Time of Delivery by Cesarean Section Under Epidural Anesthesia

Drug	Concentration Ratio
Prilocaine	1.0–1.2
Lidocaine	0.5–0.7
Mepivacaine	0.7
Bupivacaine	0.3–0.4
Etidocaine	0.1–0.4

(Modified from Covino and Vassallo,[146] with permission.)

plasma α_1-acid glycoprotein.[27,28] Thus these ratios are not directly predictive of fetal toxicity because they are based on measurements of the total plasma concentrations of the local anesthetics. Concentration ratios of free (unbound) drug across the placenta are close to unity for all agents; in the case of fetal acidosis, the ratio exceeds unity as a result of ion trapping.[29,30]

EFFECTS OF DISEASES ON PHARMACOKINETICS OF LOCAL ANESTHETICS

Any condition that influences hepatic blood flow can alter the pharmacokinetic parameters of the amide-type local anesthetics. Lidocaine has been studied the most because of its intravenous use as an antiarrhythmic agent. In patients with heart failure (reduced cardiac output), lidocaine clearance is significantly reduced.[31]

In patients with cirrhosis of the liver caused by alcoholism, the clearance of lidocaine is also reduced.[32] There is an increase in the volume of distribution and in the elimination half-life. In renal insufficiency, lidocaine clearance has been found to be normal.[33] However, there is accumulation of the metabolite, glycine xylidide. The potential toxicity of this primary amine is not known. After an intramuscular injection of lidocaine, peak plasma concentrations of glycine xylidide did not occur until 6 hours, and the peak urinary concentrations occurred between 10 and 24 hours.[32] The main metabolite of lidocaine, monoethylglycine xylidide, has been shown to occur at normal concentrations after lidocaine administration in patients with renal failure.

The metabolic complications of renal failure may be greater risk factors predisposing to local anesthetic toxicity than are the effects on local anesthetic pharmacokinetics. Such known factors are metabolic acidosis and hyperkalemia.[33]

The duration of sensory analgesia during brachial plexus block[34] and bupivacaine spinal block[35] has been found to be shorter in patients with renal failure than in those with normal renal function.

In patients with orthostatic hypotension, the volume of distribution and the clearance of lidocaine are significantly reduced during hypotensive conditions (e.g., sitting).[36] This is probably a result of reduced hepatic perfusion caused by hypotension.

It is unlikely that disease states will greatly affect the quality and duration of local anesthetic blocks, and thus, for practical clinical purposes, such influences are hard to predict. In the case of amide-type local anesthetics, plasma protein binding is promoted by disease and trauma-stimulated synthesis of α_1-acid glycoprotein,[37] which affords some protection against local anesthetic toxicity. Because all ester-type local anesthetics are metabolized by blood esterases, an inherited or acquired reduction of esterase activity may lead to enhanced toxicity. The incidence of the atypical $E_1^a E_1^a$ gene for plasma esterase 1 : 4,000 to 1 : 30,000 and that of the so-called silent $E_1^s E_1^s$ gene is approximately 1 : 170,000.[38]

EFFECT OF PREGNANCY ON PHARMACOKINETICS OF LOCAL ANESTHETICS

Although engorgement of the vertebral veins and a hyperkinetic circulation may result in an increased vascular absorption of local anesthetics after epidural anesthesia in pregnant patients, the plasma drug concentrations versus time profiles seem to be similar to those in nonpregnant patients.[39] Plasma concentrations of bupivacaine after epidural administration in pregnant patients were slightly higher than those in nonpregnant patients,[40] but the absorption rate and terminal half-life in the serum were similar. The pregnant women had significantly more desbutylbupivacaine (pipecoloxylidine) in the serum than did the nonpregnant women.

In pre-eclampsia, higher plasma concentrations of lidocaine than normal have been observed, probably as a result of a lower clearance of the drug in this condition.[41]

A major reason for smaller dose requirements for a local anesthetic in a spinal or epidural block in a pregnant patient is probably progesterone-induced increase in nervous system sensitivity to local anesthetics.[42] Progesterone also enhances the cardiotoxicity of bupivacaine.[43]

CLINICAL USE OF LOCAL ANESTHETICS IN NERVE BLOCKS

Local Infiltration

In principle, any of the available local anesthetics may be used for local infiltration, the choice and concentration being determined by the extent of the area to be blocked and the duration of the painful procedure. Lidocaine is by far the most popular local anesthetic for local infiltration. Lidocaine solutions of 0.25 to 2 percent may be used, considering maximum recommended doses (Table 9-3). The dose of local anesthetic can be increased, and the duration of the block prolonged (almost doubled with lidocaine) by the addition of epinephrine, 5 μg/ml (1 : 200,000). Because of the risk of ischemia and necrosis, such epinephrine-containing solutions should not be injected into tissues supplied by end arteries (i.e., fingers, nose, earlobe, penis, or toes).

Peripheral Nerve Block

A peripheral nerve block can be achieved by injecting local anesthetic in the vicinity of individual nerves or nerve plexuses. After injection, the local

Table 9-3 Recommended Maximum Single Dose of the Local Anesthetic[a]

	Without Epinephrine	With Epinephrine
Lidocaine	300 mg (Spinal 100 mg)	500 mg
Prilocaine	600 mg	900 mg[b]
Mepivacaine	400 mg (Spinal 100 mg)	500 mg
Bupivacaine	200 mg (Spinal 20 mg)	200 mg
Etidocaine	300 mg	400 mg
Dibucaine	Spinal 10 mg	
Procaine	1,000 mg (Spinal 200 mg)	
Chloroprocaine	800 mg	1,000 mg
Tetracaine	Spinal 20 mg	
Cocaine	Topical 150 mg	

[a] The patient is assumed to be a healthy adult; time limit is 4 hours. (Modified from Covino,[147] with permission.)
[b] Recommended by the author.

anesthetic will diffuse from the outer surface toward the center of the nerve, according to the concentration gradient. Nerve fibers located in the periphery of a mixed nerve are blocked first, and these "mantle" nerve fibers are usually distributed to more proximal anatomic structures, in contrast to distal structures innervated by nerve fibers near the "core" of the nerve.

Skeletal muscle paralysis may precede the onset of sensory blockade when motor nerve fibers are distributed peripheral to sensory fibers in the mixed peripheral nerve.[44]

The duration of peripheral nerve blocks depends on the dose of local anesthetic, its lipid solubility, the degree of tissue binding, and the concomitant use of a vasoconstrictor (usually epinephrine). In general, the duration is more safely prolonged by adding epinephrine than by increasing the dose. When epinephrine is added to bupivacaine for brachial plexus blocks, the duration may sometimes extend to 24 hours.

Intravenous Regional Anesthesia (Bier's Block)

Intravenous regional anesthesia (IVRA) is performed by injecting local anesthetic into the veins of an extremity isolated by a tourniquet. The block lasts as long as the tourniquet is kept inflated. Normal sensation and skeletal muscle tone usually return rapidly on deflation of the tourniquet. Approximately 30 percent of the total dose of the local anesthetic used for the block is flushed into the systemic circulation immediately when the cuff is deflated.[45] Therefore, symptoms of mild central nervous system toxicity occur frequently, independent of the agent used.

The mechanism of IVRA is multifactorial. It includes an initial peripheral nerve ending (and small nerve) block followed by a block of the major nerve trunks (in the proximal part) that is supplemented by ischemia (asphyxia) and nerve compression (by tourniquet).

Both ester- and amide-type local anesthetics have been used for IVRA. At the present, lidocaine (0.5 percent) and prilocaine (0.5 percent) are the most popular drugs used. The low (negligible) incidence of thrombophlebitis and rapid distribution and metabolism (low degree of toxicity) of prilo-

caine following tourniquet deflation makes this agent a good choice for use in IVRA. The dose of prilocaine (200 to 225 mg in adults) is well below the dose likely to produce clinically detectable methemoglobinemia, i.e., 600 mg.[46]

Lidocaine is commonly used for IVRA. It does not cause venous irritation and the slightly more frequent occurrence of mild central nervous system (CNS) toxicity symptoms after tourniquet cuff deflation, in comparison with the use of prilocaine,[47] cannot be considered a restrictive contraindication.

The use of 2-chloroprocaine for IVRA has occasionally been associated with thrombophlebitis.[48] This side effect was thought to be related to the preservative (methylparaben) and the antioxidant (sodium bisulfite), in addition to the formulation's low pH (3.1). Recently, a preservative-free 2-chloroprocaine solution has been tested for IVRA.[49] Unfortunately, this solution was also found to be irritating to veins.

The frequent clinical recommendation not to deflate the tourniquet cuff before 20 minutes is based on the clinical impression that there are more often symptoms of central nervous system toxicity when the "tourniquet-inflation time" is short. On the other hand, peak local anesthetic plasma concentrations were not significantly different whether the inflation time was short or long.[49] The peak concentrations tended to occur later when the inflation time was long. The dose flushed out from the extremity can be regulated, as needed (e.g., when the patient is at a higher than normal risk of encountering toxic reactions), by deflating and reinflating the tourniquet cuff in cycles.

Epidural Analgesia and Anesthesia

Local anesthetics injected into the epidural space (peridural space) may reach spinal nerve structures by different routes. The most important one is a relatively rapid diffusion of local anesthetic into the cerebrospinal fluid at the dural cuff region. Peak local anesthetic concentrations are reached within 10 to 20 minutes after epidural injection, and the concentrations are high enough to produce blockade of nerve impulse propagation in spinal nerve roots and their branches. Diffusion into the intradural spinal nerve roots also plays a major role during the early stages of epidural block. This is clearly associated with a rapid onset of a segmental pattern of the block. Subsequently, local anesthetic seepage through intervertebral foramina may contribute to the block by producing multiple paravertebral nerve blocks.

Almost all available local anesthetics have been used for epidural analgesia and anesthesia (Table 9-4). A great flexibility of sensory and motor block can be obtained when needed. For example, 0.25 percent bupivacaine may provide satisfactory analgesia for acute pain with little motor block; 0.5 percent etidocaine may cause a moderate to good degree of motor block but minimal analgesia.

If more potent analgesia with moderate motor block is required, 0.4 to 0.5 percent bupivacaine or 1.5 to 2 percent lidocaine without epinephrine may be chosen. Bupivacaine is preferred for continuous analgesic techniques. The need for profound sensory and motor block is best met by 2 percent lidocaine with epinephrine (5 μg/ml). If a long duration is required, suitable choices are 1.5 percent etidocaine or 0.75 percent bupivacaine.

Table 9-4 Agents for Epidural Block

Applications	Agent	Characteristics
Surgical anesthesia (medium to long duration)	2% lidocaine (HCl or CO_2)($\pm$ epi)[a]	Rapid onset, good sensory and motor block, medium duration
	3% 2-Chloroprocaine	For brief procedures only, rapid onset
	1.0–1.5% Etidocaine ($\pm$ epi)[a]	Rapid onset, profound analgesia and motor block (analgesia may be shorter than motor block), long duration
	0.5–0.75% Bupivacaine (0.75% bupivacaine should not be used for obstetric epidural blocks)	Slow onset, good analgesia, moderate motor block, long duration
	0.75–1.0% Ropivacaine	Slow onset, good analgesia, moderate motor block, medium or long duration
Postoperative pain (long duration)	0.125–0.5% Bupivacaine (often combined with low doses of opioids)	Slow onset, long duration of sensory analgesia with little motor block
	0.125–0.5% Ropivacaine	Slow onset, medium or long duration of sensory analgesia with little motor block
Obstetric analgesia (long duration)	0.06–0.5% Bupivacaine (− epi)[a]	Slow onset, dose-dependent duration, little motor block
	1% Lidocaine (HCl or CO_2; + epi)[a]	Rapid onset, medium duration
Obstetric surgery (medium to long duration)	0.5% Bupivacaine	Slow onset, good analgesia, moderate motor block
	2% Lidocaine (+ epi)[a]	Rapid onset, good analgesia, good motor block
	3% 2-Chloroprocaine ($\pm$ epi)[a]	Rapid onset, good analgesia, good motor block, short duration
Diagnostic and therapeutic sympathetic blocks	0.5–1% Lidocaine	Rapid onset, moderate duration
	0.125–0.5% Bupivacaine	Slow onset, long duration

[a] + epi, with epinephrine; − epi, without epinephrine; ± epi, with or without epinephrine.

2-Chloroprocaine is a useful agent for short obstetric procedures (e.g., cesarean section). The onset of epidural anesthesia is fast with a 2 to 3 percent solution, and the clinically useful duration of action is usually less than 1 hour after a single dose.

Differential Epidural Block

Selective blockade of sensory nerves, so-called "differential block," depends on several factors. The physical characteristics of the agent and the concentration of the solution play a role in the rate of block development in sensory and motor fibers. In an in vivo situation, the nerve blocking sensitivity does not correlate simply with fiber thickness but also with the distance of the fibers exposed to local anesthetic.[7] At the thoracic and lumbar level, the portion of a spinal nerve from the end of the dural cuff to the exit of the nerve from the intervertebral foramen is no more than a few millimeters. The distance is hardly long enough to accommodate the block of three consecutive nodes of Ranvier in the A-β skeletal motor fibers, but it may be more than enough for a three-node block of conduction in A-δ and C pain fibers. Epidural block with an appropriate dose of a relatively weak concentration of a local anesthetic tends to limit the block to this portion of the spinal nerves because it is this portion that is most directly accessible to the epidural solution.[7]

Plasma Concentrations of Local Anesthetics

A major difference between epidural block and spinal block is the large dose of local anesthetic required to produce epidural block. This results in substantial absorption of local anesthetic into the systemic circulation. Typically, peak plasma concentrations of lidocaine after epidural injection of 400 mg of lidocaine in adults are 3 to 4 μg/ml. Peak plasma concentrations after the administration of 150 mg of bupivacaine epidurally average approximately 1 μg/ml.

The addition of epinephrine (5 μg/ml) to the solutions decreases the systemic absorption by about one-third. The systemic absorption of epinephrine may cause β_2 adrenergic stimulation, resulting in a decrease in peripheral vascular resistance and a fall in blood pressure, even though cardiac output is increased by the inotropic and chronotropic effects.[4] Enhancement of the block

duration by epinephrine is minimal with the longer-acting agents, bupivacaine and etidocaine. The addition of epinephrine in a concentration of 5 μg/ml may enhance the intensity of the motor block, the quality of the sensory block, and the duration of blockade at least for the medium-long acting agents: lidocaine, mepivacaine, and prilocaine.

Alkalinized or carbonated local anesthetic solutions are without any significant influence on the pharmacokinetics of these drugs.

Continuous Infusion Epidural Analgesia

Elevated concentrations of the acute phase reactant protein, α_1-acid glycoprotein[50] will provide some protection against toxicity from amide-type local anesthetics. Generally, toxic reactions have not been observed, despite a marked accumulation of plasma bupivacaine up to 4 μg/ml, or even higher, in postoperative patients receiving continuous infusion epidural analgesia.[51,52] Although the total drug concentration in the plasma may exceed an assumed "minimal toxic concentration," the free drug concentration remains within acceptable limits because of increased plasma protein binding. Patients with chronic renal failure, recent myocardial infarction, and cancer may also have increased plasma levels of α_1-acid glycoprotein.[37]

Some of the bupivacaine metabolites, 4-hydroxybupivacaine and desbutylbupivacaine have been assessed after single[40] and repeated epidural administration,[53] but their concentrations are so low that no pharmacologic or toxicologic effects are expected. This has been verified also in continuous brachial plexus blocks; the accumulation of bupivacaine, desbutylbupivacaine, and 4-hydroxybupivacaine in plasma has not been associated with toxicity.[54,55]

Spinal Anesthesia

Spinal anesthesia is produced by the injection of a local anesthetic into the lumbar subarachnoid space at a level below the second lumbar vertebra. During spinal anesthesia, the local anesthetic is found both in the nerve roots and within the substance of the spinal cord.[56] The major cause of loss of sensation and muscle relaxation during spinal anesthesia is, however, the presence of local anes-

Table 9-5 Local Anesthetics Used in Spinal Anesthesia

Bupivacaine	
0.5% plain (saline)	5–20 mg
0.5% hyperbaric (8% glucose)	5–20 mg
0.75% hyperbaric (8.25% glucose)	3.75–15 mg
Lidocaine	
2% plain (saline)	20–100 mg
5% hyperbaric (6.8% glucose)	20–100 mg
Mepivacaine	
4% hyperbaric (9.5% glucose)	20–80 mg
Dibucaine	
0.5% plain (saline)	2–10 mg
0.25% hyperbaric (5% glucose)	2–10 mg
Procaine	
5% plain (saline)	50–200 mg
Tetracaine	
0.5% isobaric (with cerebral spinal fluid)	5–20 mg
0.5% hyperbaric (5% glucose)	5–20 mg

thetic in the spinal nerve roots and in dorsal root ganglia.

Many of the clinically available local anesthetics are used for spinal anesthesia (Table 9-5). For the production of hyperbaric spinal anesthetic solutions, glucose is added. The concept of baricity in the understanding of the spread of spinal anesthesia is important. The dose of local anesthetic and the baricity (i.e., the ratio between the density of the solution and that of the cerebrospinal fluid) of the solution are probably the major determinants of spread of a spinal block. By adjustment of the posture of the patient in relation to the baricity of the local anesthetic solution, the final spread of a spinal block can usually be predicted with sufficient accuracy. In principle, all solutions can be made hypobaric with the addition of distilled water. Tetracaine is hypobaric in concentrations less than 0.33 percent (Fig. 9-1). The baricities of local anesthetic solutions are listed in Table 9-6.

The duration of anesthesia of the ester-type local anesthetics can be prolonged considerably by the addition of epinephrine (maximum, 0.2 mg) to the solution. Epinephrine presumably acts by delaying vascular absorption of the local anesthetics, but an antinociceptive action of epinephrine at the spinal level has also been suggested (α-adrenergic agonist action, see Ch. 27). Epinephrine increased the intensity and effectiveness of tetracaine spinal anesthesia.[57] Conflicting results have been reported for

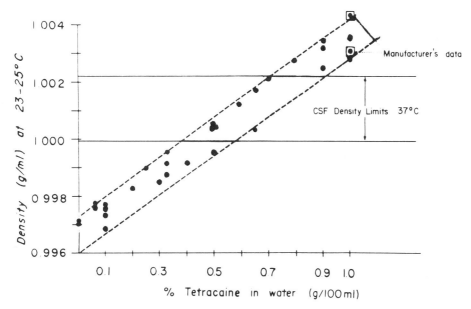

Fig. 9-1 The effect on density of the dilution of 1 percent tetracaine with water at 23 to 25°C. Cerebrospinal fluid (CSF) density limits are ± three standard deviations. (From Rosenberg,[148] with permission.)

Table 9-6 Densities and Baricities of Local Anesthetic Solutions at 37°C

Solution	Density g/ml	Baricity[a]
Distilled water	0.993	0.992
Tetracaine 1%	0.995	0.994
Procaine 1%	0.995	0.994
Tetracaine 1% in 0.09% saline	0.995	0.994
Dibucaine 0.066% in 0.5% saline	0.997	0.996
Mepivacaine 4%	0.998	0.997
Procaine 2.5% in water	0.999	0.998
Bupivacaine 0.5%	0.999	0.998
Epinephrine 0.1%	0.999	0.998
Procaine 5% in 0.05% epinephrine and 0.2% sodium bisulfite	1.000	0.999
Saline, normal	1.000	0.999
Phenylephrine 0.2%	1.001	1.000
Cerebrospinal fluid, mean	1.001	1.000
Tetracaine 0.5% in 4.5% saline and 5% glucose	1.014	1.013
Bupivacaine 0.5% in 8% glucose	1.021	1.020
Lidocaine 5% in 5% glucose	1.027	1.026

[a] Calculated by dividing density of anesthetic solution at 37°C by density of cerebrospinal fluid at 37°C.
(Modified from Greene;[149] with permission.)

the effects of epinephrine on amide-type local anesthetic spinal block, with some investigators reporting a prolongation of the block and others not. Phenylephrine added to the local anesthetic solution increased the duration of spinal anesthesia produced by lidocaine and tetracaine[58,59] but not bupivacaine.[60] The addition of phenylephrine resulted in a longer duration of tetracaine anesthesia compared with epinephrine.[61] The optimal dose of phenylephrine for use in spinal anesthesia appears to be 5 mg. Clonidine (an α_2-adrenergic agonist) added to bupivacaine spinal anesthetic solution has been shown to prolong sensory and motor block.[62]

The elimination of the local anesthetic from the spinal region occurs through vascular absorption, both in the subarachnoid space and in the epidural space (after diffusion). However, the amounts absorbed into the circulation are clinically insignificant.

Topical Local Anesthesia

Local anesthetics are used for topical anesthesia of the skin, conjunctiva, and mucous membranes (nose, mouth, respiratory tract, esophagus, genitourinary tract, and anus).

Lidocaine, 2 to 10 percent formulations (liquid, spray, gel, and cream), is commonly used for topical anesthesia of the various mucosal membranes. The absorption is rapid in vascular areas; the absorption of lidocaine from the tracheobronchial tree is so rapid and extensive that the kinetic behavior resembles that of lidocaine after intravenous administration.[11,63] If the oral mucosa is dry as a result of anticholinergic drug administration, the absorption of topically applied lidocaine has been found to be greater than that during normal mucosal wetness.[64] A smaller loss of local anesthetic in the saliva (and swallowed) is the probable explanation for the greater absorption; analgesia was also more effective.

A eutectic mixture of lidocaine and prilocaine is effective for topical skin analgesia. Its greatest benefit has been in providing local anesthesia for vascular cannulations in children.[65] For effective skin analgesia, the application time of this cream has to be 60 to 90 minutes. The cream has also been applied on mucosal membranes in the mouth and nose.[66,67] The application of 200 mg of the cream (100 mg of lidocaine + 100 mg of prilocaine) on the gingivae resulted in mean maximum plasma concentrations of 0.2 μg/ml of lidocaine and 0.09 μg/ml of prilocaine.[66]

Lidocaine is absorbed sparingly from the mucosa of the urinary bladder. After doses of lidocaine (gel) up to 1,200 mg, plasma concentrations were negligible.[68] Application of lidocaine, 400 mg, into the urethra of male patients resulted in mean maximum plasma concentrations of 0.06 μg/ml.[69]

Tetracaine is an effective topical local anesthetic agent. It is used for conjunctival anesthesia as 0.5 or 1 percent solutions, and a 5 percent tetracaine cream is effective for skin analgesia.[70] An interesting mixture of 0.5 percent tetracaine, 0.05 percent epinephrine, and 11.8 percent cocaine has been used as a topical anesthetic for skin lacerations in children.[71] Some concern has been expressed regarding the absorption of the cocaine, which seems to be unpredictable.

Several local anesthetic agents that are not otherwise used in anesthesiology are used in ophthalmology to produce topical conjunctival anesthesia. Examples include oxybuprocaine, proparacaine, piperocaine, and benoxinate.

COMBINATIONS OF LOCAL ANESTHETICS

An ideal local anesthetic drug with a fast onset and long duration of action has not been devised. Etidocaine has the desired properties of fast onset and long duration; however, the profound, prolonged motor block associated with etidocaine has limited its applications. Local anesthetics have been combined mainly in attempts to quicken the slow onset of the long-acting drug, bupivacaine, or conversely, to prolong the action of the fast onset drug, lidocaine. Combinations that have been widely used include tetracaine and lidocaine, bupivacaine and lidocaine, and bupivacaine and chloroprocaine. Generally, combinations have properties that are intermediate between the properties of the component drugs,[72] rather than having the ideal properties of fast onset and long duration; whether the properties of the combination are advantageous compared with the component drugs depends on the clinical circumstances. However, chloroprocaine appears to be an exception to this

generalization. The combination of chloroprocaine, 1.5 percent, and bupivacaine, 0.5 percent, produced epidural block resembling chloroprocaine alone.[73] When epidural administration of chloroprocaine preceded bupivacaine, the effects of subsequent doses of bupivacaine were attenuated.[74] Interestingly, chloroprocaine was also reported to attenuate analgesia from subsequent administration of epidural opioids.[75]

4-Amino-2-chlorobenzoic acid, a metabolite of chloroprocaine, has been implicated as an antagonist of bupivacaine neural blockade.[76]

The systemic toxicity of local anesthetics appears to be at most additive; therefore, mixtures of local anesthetics are no more toxic than are those of the components.[77]

CARBONATED LOCAL ANESTHETICS AND ADDITION OF SODIUM BICARBONATE

The local anesthetics are weak bases with pK_a ranging from 7.6 to 9.1. The commercially available formulations are usually acidified with hydrochloric acid to protonate the amine nitrogen, forming a cation. This is necessary because the un-ionized (free base) forms of the local anesthetics are insoluble in aqueous solution. However, it is the un-ionized molecule that is best able to cross lipid barriers and penetrate the neuron. In an attempt to increase the availability of the un-ionized local anesthetic, two different approaches have been tried. Carbonic acid has been substituted for hydrochloric acid, and sodium bicarbonate has been added, just before use, to standard formulations containing hydrochloric acid.

Carbonic acid is in equilibrium with carbon dioxide in solution. Thus, these solutions are often referred to as "carbonated" or "fizzy" because bubbles of CO_2 may be evident on opening the vials, as with a carbonated beverage. The rationale for carbonated local anesthetic solutions is that, on injection, the CO_2 will diffuse away from the site of injection, raising the pH and the percentage of local anesthetic in the un-ionized form. CO_2 may also enter the nerve cell, lowering the intracellular pH, favoring the formation of the cationic form of the local anesthetic, which is the most active in blocking the sodium channel. Whether carbonation actually accomplishes this is controversial. Double-blind trials of epidural anesthesia have not found significant differences between carbonated and standard local anesthetic solutions,[78–80] although more intense anesthesia of the L5-S1 dermatomes has been reported.[81] Carbonation did not alter the pharmacokinetics of epidural lidocaine.[82] Carbonation has been reported to improve variously the speed of onset, spread, or intensity of brachial plexus blocks.

Although local anesthetic solutions must be acidified to prevent precipitation of local anesthetic during storage, the addition of sodium bicarbonate sufficient to raise the pH to 7.0 to 7.4, just prior to use, does not cause obvious precipitation. The adjustment of the pH appears to result in a faster onset and longer duration of bupivacaine brachial plexus[83] and sciatic nerve block,[84] although others have not confirmed these results.[85] The adjustment of the pH also appeared to increase the speed of onset and the duration of lidocaine[86] or bupivacaine[87] epidural block. Plasma levels of the local anesthetic appeared not to be affected by pH adjustment.

CLINICAL TOXICITY OF LOCAL ANESTHETICS

Regional anesthesia that is properly performed does not usually result in toxic blood or tissue concentrations of local anesthetics. The systemic effects of local anesthetic intoxication generally become manifest most dramatically in the central nervous system (CNS) and in the cardiovascular system. Allergic reactions are unusual, and they are associated with the use of ester-type local anesthetics, with some rare exceptions.

The most common reason for toxic reactions is inadvertent intravascular (usually intravenous) injection of a local anesthetic. Toxicity resulting from properly performed regional blocks is uncommon, although symptoms of mild central nervous system toxicity may be observed with the maximum recommended doses in epidural or brachial plexus blocks. Recommended doses (Table 9-3) are often exceeded when an epidural or brachial plexus block is immediately followed by a continuous local

anesthetic infusion for the prolongation of the block or for postoperative analgesia.[88]

In acute local anesthetic intoxication, the arterial blood concentrations correspond to drug effects better than do the venous blood concentrations. The lungs play a major role in determining the peak arterial concentration of intravenously injected local anesthetic by temporarily binding a substantial amount of drug on the first pass through the pulmonary circulation. Pulmonary uptake of lidocaine in volunteers receiving 0.5 mg/kg IV as a bolus, was 60 percent of the administered dose over a period of 15 to 20 seconds.[89] However, the drug is then released rapidly. The protective ("buffering") effect of the pulmonary uptake is saturable and, therefore, reduced as the dose of the local anesthetic is increased. Pulmonary uptake of prilocaine in humans exceeds that of lidocaine and many other amide-type local anesthetics, and it may be a significant factor favoring the greater systemic safety of prilocaine.[90] Theoretically, local anesthetics may displace each other from lung binding sites according to their individual binding affinity, i.e., bupivacaine > etidocaine > lidocaine.[91] Basic drugs, such as propranolol and meperidine, may also compete for lung binding sites with local anesthetics.[37] The clinical significance of this kind of interaction is unknown.

Central Nervous System Toxicity

CNS toxicity is proportional to local anesthetic potency, but the correlation between plasma concentrations and symptoms is surprisingly poor.[37,92] During slow intravenous infusion the signs and symptoms progress from the initial phase of minor symptoms, such as lightheadedness and tinnitus, to a phase of drowsiness and muscular twitching and, finally, to generalized convulsions, unconsciousness and coma. In the case of lidocaine, CNS effects are thought to develop progressively with a rise in lidocaine plasma concentration up to approximately 20 to 25 μg/ml. In the case of bupivacaine, the corresponding plasma concentrations would be about 50 percent lower.

When an inadvertent intravascular injection of local anesthetic occurs, the milder premonitory CNS symptoms may be bypassed, and convulsions and unconsciousness may occur directly. This has been reported in several case presentations.[93-95] In one of the patients, bupivacaine, 45 mg, was injected into the vertebral artery, and the patient developed instantaneous unconsciousness without other symptoms.[95]

Injection of local anesthetics in the head and neck area may produce central nervous system side effects in the absence of toxic systemic blood levels of the local anesthetic. This occurs when the local anesthetic reaches the brain by direct injection into the arteries, such as the carotid or vertebral arteries, or by retrograde spread along the nerves or veins or in the subarachnoid space. A high concentration of local anesthetic may reach a localized area of the brain. A common example is retrobulbar block. The spread of local anesthetic from the orbit by intravascular or perineural pathways may result in confusion, convulsions, brain stem nerve palsies, apnea, cardiovascular instability, or loss of consciousness.[96]

Studies in pregnant ewes have indicated that thresholds for severe CNS toxicity (e.g., convulsions) are not affected by pregnancy.[97]

The cardiovascular changes associated with local anesthetic induced convulsions can alter the pharmacokinetic profile of amide-type local anesthetics.[98] A significant increase in the volume of distribution and elimination half-lives and a reduction in the clearance of clinically used local anesthetics were demonstrated during the convulsive phase of intoxication in dogs.[98]

Cardiovascular Toxicity

The cardiovascular side effects of local anesthetics are much more likely to produce morbidity or mortality than are the CNS effects. Fortunately, higher doses of local anesthetics are required to produce cardiovascular toxicity. The dose of lidocaine producing cardiovascular toxicity in sheep is about seven times greater than the dose producing CNS toxicity.[99] Thus, for lidocaine at least, there is a large margin of cardiovascular safety.

The main direct cardiovascular effects of local anesthetics are decreased myocardial contractility, decreased rate of conduction of impulses through the cardiac conduction system, and peripheral vasodilation. Local anesthetics may also have indirect effects on the cardiovascular system that are mediated by the sympathetic nervous system. Relatively low doses of local anesthetics produce increased sympathetic tone and cardiovascular stimulation. As the local anesthetic concentration rises, cardiovascular depression and collapse supervene.

The negative inotropic effects of local anesthetics are generally related to their anesthetic potency (Fig. 9-2). However, there are significant quantitative and qualitative differences in cardiovascular toxicity between specific drugs. Bupivacaine and etidocaine, in particular, appear to have a pronounced tendency to produce cardiovascular toxicity, out of proportion to their anesthetic potency. Thus, the dose of bupivacaine in sheep that produced cardiovascular toxicity was only about 4 times greater than the dose that produced CNS toxicity (compared with a ratio of 7 for lidocaine).[99] Bupivacaine was approximately 70 times more potent than lidocaine in its effects on cardiac conduction; it was only about 4 times more potent than lidocaine in producing nerve conduction block.[100]

Bupivacaine and etidocaine also produce ventricular arrhythmias, in contrast to lidocaine. Clinically, severe ventricular arrhythmias and cardiovas-

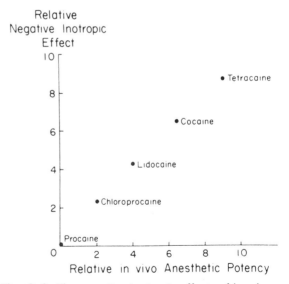

Fig. 9-2 The negative inotropic effects of local anesthetics are proportional to nerve blocking potency for the agents shown. By contrast, the cardiovascular toxicity of bupivacaine and etidocaine are relatively greater than would be expected from their nerve blocking potencies. (From Covino[147] with permission.)

cular collapse from bupivacaine toxicity have been difficult or impossible to treat.[101] The mechanism of local anesthetic induced arrhythmias may be related to direct prolonged sodium channel binding and consequent cardiac electrophysiologic effects.[100] However, CNS mechanisms may also be involved. Heavner[102] and Bernards and Artru[103] demonstrated that intracerebroventricular bupivacaine administration to animals produced ventricular arrhythmias that were blocked by hexamethonium (a ganglionic blocker) or midazolam. Bernards and Artru[103] proposed a model of bupivacaine induced cardiovascular toxicity involving γ-aminobutyric acid pathways in the brain stem (Fig. 9-3). The relative importance of direct and indirect (CNS) mechanisms of local anesthetic cardiovascular toxicity is unknown.

Cardiovascular toxicity of local anesthetics is markedly exacerbated by hypoxia and acidosis. The myocardial depressant effect of bupivacaine in sheep was greater during pregnancy,[97] perhaps as a result of reduced plasma protein binding of bupivacaine.[104] However, isolated cardiac tissue from animals treated with progesterone was more sensitive to bupivacaine.[105]

Treatment of Local Anesthetic Toxicity

Local anesthetic induced seizures are typically short in duration and would seldom be life-threatening, except that the hypoxemia and acidosis pro-

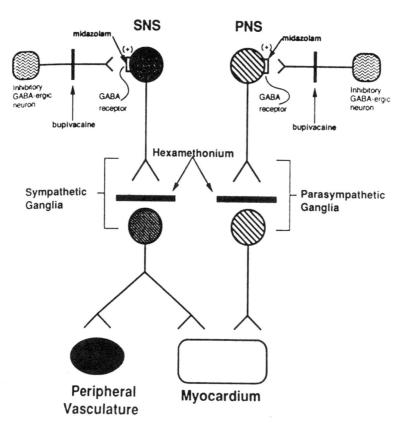

Fig. 9-3 Postulated mechanism by which intracerebroventricular bupivacaine produces dysrhythmias and hypertension. Bupivacaine blocks γ-aminobutyric acidergic (GABA) neurons that normally inhibit autonomic nervous system outflow from the brain stem. Increased sympathetic nervous system (*SNS*) and parasympathetic nervous system (*PNS*) activity mediate some of the cardiovascular effects of bupivacaine. Midazolam or hexamethonium prevent these effects. Midazolam increases inhibitory γ-aminobutyric acid activity. Hexamethonium blocks autonomic ganglia. (From Bernards and Artru;[103] with permission.)

duced by the seizure may substantially worsen local anesthetic induced cardiovascular toxicity.[106] The cardiovascular toxicity induced by bupivacaine or etidocaine may be fatal. Therefore, seizures should be terminated by the use of muscle relaxants (e.g., succinylcholine) or anticonvulsant drugs (e.g., midazolam or thiopental). The possible cardiovascular depressant effects of anticonvulsant drugs should be considered prior to use. Oxygen should be administered, and respiratory and/or metabolic acidosis should be corrected. Arrhythmias and cardiovascular depression should be treated by standard protocols (e.g., American Heart Association advanced cardiac life support), except that lidocaine should probably not be used to treat ventricular arrhythmias; studies of animals have suggested that bretylium should be substituted for lidocaine.[107] Animal studies have also suggested that larger than usual doses of epinephrine may be necessary for effective treatment of the cardiac arrest.[108,109] Profound cardiac depression from bupivacaine in pigs was effectively treated by amrinone.[110] Pretreatment with the calcium channel blocker, nicardipine, significantly reduced the cardiovascular effects of bupivacaine in rats.[111] Whether calcium channel blockers play a role in the treatment of bupivacaine toxicity in humans is unknown. Cardiovascular collapse from bupivacaine or etidocaine may be prolonged and refractory to conventional therapies. The successful use of cardiopulmonary bypass for the treatment of bupivacaine induced cardiac arrest has been reported.[112] The rationale for this treatment is to re-establish perfusion and, thereby, facilitate the redistribution and elimination of bupivacaine.

ALLERGIC REACTIONS

True allergic reactions to local anesthetics are probably rare, although many patients will recount a history of adverse experiences associated with local anesthetic administration for dental procedures. It may be virtually impossible to document such a history, and immunologic testing, such as provocative skin testing, may not be conclusive. Also, patients may be allergic to the preservatives contained in some local anesthetic solutions, such as methylparaben. Among patients truly allergic to local anesthetics, the vast majority are allergic to ester-type local anesthetics. A true allergy to amide-type local anesthetics appears to be extremely rare. Thus, in situations in which the possibility of a true allergy to local anesthetics cannot be excluded and the administration of local anesthetics is highly desirable, many clinicians proceed by cautiously administering an amide-type local anesthetic.

OTHER TOXIC REACTIONS

Methemoglobinemia, to an extent compromising oxygen transport in blood, may occur after the administration of large doses of prilocaine.[46] The oxidation of oxyhemoglobin (the ferrous form) to methemoglobin (the ferric form) is accomplished by the o-toluidine metabolite of prilocaine. Also benzocaine, sulfonamides, nitrates, and nitrites may cause methemoglobinemia. Methylene blue (1 to 2 mg/kg IV slowly) reduces methemoglobin back to oxyhemoglobin.

Skeletal myotoxicity may result from the injection of local anesthetic into muscle tissue[113] or even into nearby tissues.[114] Recovery (regeneration) occurs normally in 1 to 2 weeks.

Nerve tissue damage may occur if a local anesthetic injection is made intraneurally,[115] or if concentrated forms of the local anesthetics are applied directly on a nerve.[115,116] The latter mechanism may explain the cauda equina syndromes described after the administration of large doses of hyperbaric local anesthetic solutions through intrathecal catheters.[117,118]

2-Chloroprocaine was associated with neurologic injury following accidental subarachnoid injection of large doses. Animal studies suggested that the preservative, sodium bisulfite, was neurotoxic in the presence of a low pH, but that chloroprocaine itself was not toxic in clinically relevant concentrations.[119] A newer formulation of chloroprocaine without preservatives is available.

DRUG INTERACTIONS
Local Anesthetics

The combined effect of two local anesthetics on a nerve block and various toxic end points (convulsions and asystole) is clearly additive.[14]

Plasma protein binding interactions may occur, and it has been shown that, at clinically relevant concentrations, bupivacaine may displace lidocaine[120] and mepivacaine[121] from their binding sites.

The hydrolysis of 2-chloroprocaine may be inhibited by 10 to 40 percent by clinically relevant concentrations of bupivacaine.[122]

General Anesthetics

A lower clearance of lidocaine (34 percent reduction) and a smaller volume of distribution at steady state have been reported in patients anesthetized with halothane plus nitrous oxide compared with patients anesthetized with fentanyl, thiopental, and nitrous oxide.[123] The pharmacokinetic parameters in the latter group were similar to those of unanesthetized subjects. Such results are consistent with the effect of halothane in decreasing both hepatic and renal blood flow,[124] renal tubular secretory activity, and mixed function oxidase activity.[125]

General anesthesia also lowers the first-pass extraction of lidocaine by the lungs, to a small extent.[126]

Intravenous administration of lidocaine or procaine produce analgesia. A continuous low dose infusion of lidocaine, to maintain a plasma concentration at 1 to 2 μg/ml, has been shown to reduce the need for additional analgesics in postoperative patients.[127] The halothane minimum alveolar concentration was significantly reduced by lidocaine, 1 μg/ml or higher.[128]

Premedication Drugs

Meperidine binds to α_1-acid glycoprotein in the plasma; however at clinically relevant concentrations of meperidine, there was no change in the free fraction of bupivacaine.[129]

Benzodiazepines, which are often used for anxiolysis prior to regional anesthesia, are known to raise the seizure threshold, thereby providing protection against the central nervous system toxicity of local anesthetics in animals.[130,131] In studies of pigs, benzodiazepine premedication did not affect the dose or blood concentration of bupivacaine that produced cardiovascular collapse.[132] A clinically relevant observation in these studies was that

almost all animals premedicated with the benzodiazepine progressed directly to cardiovascular collapse without first manifesting seizures.[132] However, premedication with normal sedative doses of a benzodiazepine or morphine did not abolish the mild central nervous system toxicity from rapid intravenous injection of lidocaine in human volunteers. Also, the subjects were able to distinguish the various signs and symptoms of mild toxicity.[92]

Sympathomimetic Drugs

The inclusion of epinephrine in the local anesthetic solutions used in major regional anesthetic blocks (e.g., epidural) may lead to a significant increase in cardiac output and a fall in peripheral vascular resistance.[4] These effects, together with an increase in hepatic blood flow (mediated also in part by intrahepatic β_2-adrenergic receptors), could influence the systemic disposition of local anesthetics. Studies in humans showed that epinephrine absorbed from the epidural space offset temporarily the lowering of hepatic blood flow caused by the sympathetic blockade.[133]

Intravenous injection of 20 mg (a large dose) of ephedrine has been found to increase the clearance of lidocaine through a stimulating effect on hepatic blood flow.[134]

β-Adrenergic Blocking Agents

In therapeutic doses, propranolol lowers the clearance of lidocaine in humans by about 40 percent. The mechanisms are several, mainly a direct inhibition of mixed-function oxidase activity, a decrease of hepatic blood flow, a lowering of cardiac output and an intrahepatic β_2-receptor blockade.[135] Propranolol does not impair the plasma protein binding of lidocaine at clinically relevant concentrations.[120]

Calcium Channel Blocking Agents

Verapamil binds strongly to α_1-acid glycoprotein and to albumin in the plasma. At clinical concentrations, verapamil may displace lidocaine, diazepam, propranolol, and salicylate from their plasma protein binding sites.[136] The clinical significance of these interactions is unknown. Experimental studies in rats have shown a protective effect of pretreatment with calcium channel blockers on the cardiotoxicity of bupivacaine.[137,138]

Histamine H$_2$-Receptor Antagonists

Cimetidine is an inhibitor of the hepatic mixed-function oxidase system, and it also decreases hepatic blood flow. Thus, therapeutic doses of cimetidine lowered the clearance of lidocaine in humans by 20 to 30 percent.[139] In contrast, ranitidine did not affect the disposition of lidocaine.[140]

Enzyme-Inducing Agents

The systemic clearance of free lidocaine was shown to be approximately 25 percent greater in epileptic patients receiving phenytoin than in control subjects.[141] Long-term therapy with phenytoin also leads to the induction of α_1-acid glycoprotein synthesis, enhancing plasma protein binding of lidocaine and lowering of its erythrocyte/plasma concentration ratio.[142] The synthesis of α_1-acid glycoprotein is not stimulated by all drugs that induce the synthesis of drug metabolizing enzymes. For example, rifampin did in not affect α_1-acid glycoprotein concentrations or the plasma protein binding of lidocaine.[143]

Anticholinesterases

Inhibitors of plasma pseudocholinesterase, such as neostigmine and echothiophate at clinical concentrations may block the metabolism of ester-type local anesthetics and increase their toxicity. Also the carbonic anhydrase inhibitor, acetazolamide, inhibited erythrocyte esterase and slowed the hydrolysis of procaine.[144]

REFERENCES

1. Ritchie JM, Greengard P: On the mode of action of local anesthetics. Annu Rev Pharmacol 6:405, 1966
2. Strichartz GR, Ritchie JM: The action of local anesthetics on ion channels of excitable tissues. p. 21. In Strichartz GR (ed): Local Anesthetics, Handbook of Experimental Pharmacology. Vol. 81. Springer-Verlag, New York, 1987
3. Rosenberg PH, Heavner JE: Temperature dependent nerve blocking action of lidocaine and halothane. Acta Anaesthesiol Scand 24:314, 1980
4. Bonica JJ, Akamatsu TJ, Berges PU et al: Circulatory effects of peridural block: II. Effects of epinephrine. Anesthesiology 34:514, 1971
5. Gasser HS, Erlanger J: Role of fiber size in establishment of nerve block by pressure and cocaine. Am J Physiol 88:581, 1929
6. Tasaki I: Nervous Transmission. p. 164. Charles C Thomas, Springfield, IL, 1953
7. Fink BR: Mechanisms of differential axial blockade in epidural and subarachnoid anesthesia. Anesthesiology 70:851, 1989
8. Laurence DR, Bennett PN: Clinical Pharmacology. 6th Ed. Churchill Livingstone, New York, 1987
9. De Jong RH: Local Anesthetics. Charles C Thomas, Springfield, IL, 1977
10. Koster RW, Dunning AJ: Intramuscular lidocaine for prevention of lethal arrhythmia in the prehospital phase of acute myocardial infarction. N Engl J Med 313:1105, 1985
11. Prengel AW, Lindner KH, Hähnel J, Ahnefeld FW: Endotracheal and endobronchial lidocaine administration: effects on plasma lidocaine concentration and blood gases. Crit Care Med 19:911, 1991
12. Julien RM: Lidocaine in experimental epilepsy. Correlation of anticonvulsant effect with blood concentrations. Electroencephalogr Clin Neurophysiol 34:639, 1973
13. Hällström-Westas L, Westergren U, Rosén I, Svenningsen I: Lidocaine for treatment of severe seizure in newborn infants. Acta Paediatr Scand 77:79, 1988
14. Kyttä J, Heavner JE, Badgwell JM, Rosenberg PH: Cardiovascular and central nervous system effects of coadministered lidocaine and bupivacaine. Reg Anesth 16:89, 1991
15. Wiesenfeld-Hallin Z, Lindblom U: The effect of systemic tocainide, lidocaine and bupivacaine on nociception in the rat. Pain 23:357, 1985
16. Schnapp M, Mays KS, North WC: Intravenous 2-chloroprocaine in treatment of chronic pain. Anesth Analg 60:844, 1981
17. Boas RA, Cousins MJ: Diagnostic neural blockade. p. 885. In Cousins MJ, Bridenbaugh PO (eds): Neural Blockade in Clinical Anesthesia and Management of Pain. 2nd Ed. JB Lippincott, Philadelphia, 1988
18. Rimbäck G, Cassuto J, Wallin G, Westlander G: Inhibition of peritonitis by amide local anesthetics. Anesthesiology 69:881, 1988
19. MacGregor RR, Thorner RE, Wright DM: Lidocaine inhibits granulocyte adherence and prevents

granulocyte delivery to inflammatory sites. Blood 56:203, 1980

20. Kleinfeld J, Ellis PP: Effects of topical anesthetics on growth of microorganisms. Arch Ophthalmol 76:712, 1966
21. Schmidt RM, Rosenkranz HS: Antimicrobial activity of local anesthetics: lidocaine and procaine. J Infect Dis 121:597, 1970
22. Rosenberg PH, Renkonen OV: Antimicrobial activity of bupivacaine and morphine. Anesthesiology 62:178, 1985
23. Abboud TK, Kim KC, Noueihed R et al: Epidural bupivacaine, chloroprocaine or lidocaine for cesarean section—maternal and neonatal effects. Anesth Analg 62:914, 1983
24. O'Brian JE, Abbey V, Hinsvark O et al: Metabolism and measurement of chloroprocaine, an ester-type local anesthetic. J Pharm Sci 68:75, 1979
25. Kuhnert BR, Kuhnert PM, Prochaska AL, Gross TL: Plasma levels of 2-chloroprocaine in obstetric patients and their neonates after epidural anesthesia. Anesthesiology 53:21, 1980
26. Kuhnert BR, Kennard MJ, Linn PI: Neonatal neurobehavior after epidural anesthesia for cesarean section: a comparison of bupivacaine and chloroprocaine. Anesth Analg 67:64, 1988
27. Mather LE, Long GJ, Thomas J: The binding of bupivacaine to maternal and foetal plasma proteins. J Pharm Pharmacol 23:359, 1971
28. Wood M, Wood AJJ: Changes in plasma drug binding and alpha₁-acid glycoprotein in mother and newborn infant. Clin Pharmacol Ther 29:522, 1981
29. Teramo K, Rajamäki A: Foetal and maternal plasma levels of mepivacaine and foetal acid-base balance and heart rate after paracervical block during labour. Br J Anaesth 43:300, 1971
30. Philipson EH, Kuhnert BR, Syracuse CD: Maternal, fetal, and neonatal lidocaine levels following local perineal infiltration. Am J Obstet Gynecol 149:403, 1984
31. Bax NDS, Tucker GT, Woods HF: Lignocaine and indocyanine green kinetics following myocardial infarction. Br J Clin Pharmacol 10:353, 1980
32. Collinsworth KA, Stron JM, Atkinson AJ et al: Pharmacokinetics and metabolism of lidocaine in patients with renal failure. Clin Pharmacol Ther 18:59, 1975
33. Gould DB, Aldrete JA: Bupivacaine cardiotoxicity in a patient with renal failure. Acta Anaesthesiol Scand 27:18, 1983
34. Bromage PR, Gertel M: Brachial plexus anesthesia in chronic renal failure. Anesthesiology 35:488, 1972

35. Orko R, Pitkänen M, Rosenberg PH: Subarachnoid anaesthesia with 0.75% bupivacaine in patients with chronic renal failure. Br J Anaesth 58:605, 1986
36. Feely J, Wade D, McAllister CB et al: Effect of hypotension on liver blood flow and lidocaine disposition. N Engl J Med 307:866, 1982
37. Tucker GT: Pharmacokinetics of local anaesthetics. Br J Anaesth 58:717, 1986
38. Foldes FF: Enzymes in Anesthesiology. Springer-Verlag, New York, 1978
39. Morgan DJ, Koay BB, Paull GT: Plasma protein binding of etidocaine during pregnancy and labour. Eur J Clin Pharmacol 22:451, 1982
40. Pihlajamäki K, Kanto J, Lindberg R et al: Extradural administration of bupivacaine:pharmacokinetics and metabolism in pregnant and non-pregnant women. Br J Anesth 64:556, 1990
41. Ramanathan J, Bottorf M, Sibai BM: Maternal and neonatal effects of epidural lidocaine in preeclamptic women undergoing cesarean section. Anesth Analg 64:268, 1985
42. Flanagan HL, Datta S, Lambert DH, Gissen AJ: Effects of pregnancy on bupivacaine-induced conduction blockade in the isolated rabbit vagus nerve. Anesth Analg 66:123, 1987
43. Moller RA, Datta S, Fox J et al: Effects of progesterone on the cardiac electrophysiological action bupivacaine and lidocaine. Anesthesiology 76:604, 1992
44. Winnie AP, Tay C-H, Patel KP et al: Pharmacokinetics of local anesthetics during plexus blocks. Anesth Analg 56:852, 1977
45. Tucker GT, Boas RA: Pharmacokinetic aspects of intravenous regional anesthesia. Anesthesiology 34:538, 1971
46. Hjelm M, Holmdahl MH: Clinical chemistry of prilocaine and clinical evaluation of methaemoglobinaemia induced by this agent. Acta Anaesthesiol Scand, suppl. 16:161, 1965
47. Kerr JH: Intravenous regional analgesia. Anaesthesia 22:562, 1967
48. Harris WH: Choice of anesthetic agents for intravenous regional anesthesia. Acta Anaesthesiol Scand, suppl. 36:47, 1969
48a. Pitkänen M, Kyttä J, Rosenberg PH: Comparison of 2-chloroprocaine and prilocaine for intravenous regional anaesthesia of the arm: a clinical study. Anaesthesia 48:1091, 1993
49. Kalso E, Tuominen M, Rosenberg PH, Alila A: Bupivacaine blood levels after intravenous regional anesthesia of the arm. Regional-Anaesthesie 5:81, 1982
50. Aronsen K-F, Ekelung G, Kindmark C-O, Laurell

C-B: Sequential changes of plasma proteins after surgical trauma. Scand J Clin Lab Invest, suppl. 124:127, 1972

51. Renck H, Edströrm H, Kinnberger B, Brandt G: Thoracic epidural analgesia: II. Prolongation in the early postoperative period by continuous injection of 1.0% bupivacaine. Acta Anaesthesiol Scand 20:47, 1976

52. Ross RA, Clarke JE, Armitage EN: Postoperative pain prevention by continuous epidural infusion. Anaesthesia 35:663, 1980

53. Reynolds F, Taylor G: Maternal and neonatal blood concentrations of bupivacaine. A comparison with lignocaine during continuous extradural analgesia. Anaesthesia 25:14, 1970

54. Rosenberg PH, Pere P, Tuominen M: Plasma concentrations of bupivacaine and two of its metabolites during continuous interscalene brachial plexus block. Br J Anaesth 66:25, 1991

55. Pere P, Tuominen M, Rosenberg PH: Cumulation of bupivacaine, desbutylbupivacaine and 4-hydroxybupivacaine during and after continuous interscalene brachial plexus block. Acta Anaesthesiol Scand 35:647, 1991

56. Cohen EN: Distribution of local anesthetic agents in the neuraxis of the dog. Anesthesiology 29:1002, 1968

57. Carpenter RL, Smith HS, Bridenbaugh LD: Epinephrine increases the effectiveness of spinal anesthesia. Anesthesiology 71:33, 1989

58. Armstrong IR, Littlewood DG, Chambers WA: Spinal anesthesia with tetracaine-effect of added vasoconstrictors. Anesth Analg 62:793, 1983

59. Vaida GT, Moss P, Capan LM, Turndorf H: Prolongation of lidocaine spinal anesthesia with phenylephrine. Anesth Analg 65:781, 1986

60. Chambers WA, Littlewood DG, Scott DB: Spinal anesthesia with hyperbaric bupivacaine. Effect of added vasoconstrictors. Anesth Analg 61:49, 1982

61. Caldwell C, Nielsen C, Baltz T et al: Comparison of high-dose epinephrine and phenylephrine in spinal anesthesia with tetracaine. Anesthesiology 62:804, 1985

62. Racle JB, Benkhadra A, Poy JY, Gleizal B: Prolongation of isobaric bupivacaine spinal anesthesia with epinephrine and clonidine for hip surgery in the elderly. Anesth Analg 66:442, 1987

63. McDonald JL: Serum lidocaine levels during cardiopulmonary resuscitation after intravenous and endotracheal administration. Crit Care Med 13:914, 1985

64. Watanabe H, Lindgren L, Rosenberg PH, Randell T: Glycopyrronium prolongs topical anaesthesia of oral mucosa and enhances adsorption of lignocaine. Br J Anaesth 70:94, 1993

65. Hallén B, Carlsson P, Uppfeldt A: Clinical study of a lignocaine-prilocaine cream to relieve the pain of venepuncture. Br J Anaesth 57:326, 1985

66. Haasio J, Jokinen T, Numminen M, Rosenberg P: Topical anaesthesia of gingival mucosa by 5% eutectic mixture of lignocaine and prilocaine or by 10% lignocaine spray. Br J Oral Maxillofac Surg 28:99, 1990

67. Randell T, Yli-Hankala A, Valli H, Lindgren L: Topical anaesthesia of the nasal mucosa for fiberoptic airway endoscopy. Br J Anaesth 68:164, 1992

68. Trasher JB, Peterson NE, Donatucci CF: Lidocaine as a topical anesthetic for bladder biopsies. J Urol 145:1209, 1991

69. Axelsson K, Jozwiak H, Lingårdh G et al: Blood concentration of lignocaine after application of 2% lignocaine gel in the urethra. Br J Urol 55:64, 1983

70. Mazumdar B, Tomlinson AA, Faulder GC: Preliminary study to assay plasma amethocaine concentrations after topical application of a new local anaesthetic cream containing amethocaine. Br J Anaesth 67:432, 1991

71. Terndrup TE, Walls HC, Mariani PJ et al: Plasma cocaine and tetracaine levels following application of topical anesthesia in children. Ann Emerg Med 21:162, 1992

72. Seow LT, Lips FJ, Cousins, MJ, Mather, LE: Lidocaine and bupivacaine mixtures for epidural blockade. Anesthesiology 56:177, 1982

73. Cohen S, Thurlow A: Comparison of a chloroprocaine-bupivacaine mixture with chloroprocaine and bupivacaine used individually for obstetric epidural analgesia. Anesthesiology 51:288, 1979

74. Hodgkinson R, Husain FJ, Bluhm C: Reduced effectiveness of bupivacaine 0.5% to relieve labor pain after prior injection of chloroprocaine 2%. Anesthesiology 57:3A201, 1982

75. Eisenach J, Schlairet T, Dobson C, Hood D: Effect of prior anesthetic solution on epidural morphine analgesia. Anesth Analg 73:112, 1991

76. Corke BC, Carlson CG, Dettbarn W-D: The influence of 2-chloroprocaine on the subsequent analgesic potency of bupivacaine. Anesthesiology 60:25, 1984

77. de Jong RH, Bonin JD: Mixtures of local anesthetics are no more toxic than the parent drugs. Anesthesiology 54:177, 1981.

78. Cole CP, McMorland GH, Axelson JE, Jenkins LC: Epidural blockade for cesarean section comparing lidocaine hydrocarbonate and lidocaine hydrochloride. Anesthesiology 62:348, 1985

79. Brown DT, Morison DH, Covino BG, Scott DB: Comparison of carbonated bupivacaine and bupivacaine hydrochloride for extradural anaesthesia. Br J Anaesth 52:419, 1980

80. Morison DH: A double-blind comparison of carbonated lidocaine and lidocaine hydrochloride in epidural anaesthesia. Can J Anaesth 28:387, 1981

81. Martin R, Lamarche Y, Tetreault L: Comparison of the clinical effectiveness of lidocaine hydrocarbonate and lidocaine hydrochloride with and without epinephrine in epidural anaesthesia. Can J Anaesth 28:217, 1981

82. Bowdle T, Freund P, Slattery J: Age-dependent lidocaine pharmacokinetics during lumbar peridural anesthesia with lidocaine hydrocarbonate or lidocaine hydrochloride. Reg Anesth 11:123, 1986

83. Hilgier M: Alkalinization of bupivacaine for brachial plexus block. Reg Anesth 8:59, 1985

84. Coventry DM, Todd JG: Alkalinisation of bupivacaine for sciatic nerve blockade. Anaesthesia 44:467, 1989

85. Bedder MD, Kozody R, Craig DB: Comparison of bupivacaine and alkalinized bupivacaine in brachial plexus anesthesia. Anesth Analg 67:48, 1988

86. DiFazio CA, Carron H, Grosslight KR et al: Comparison of pH-adjusted lidocaine solutions for epidural anesthesia. Anesth Analg 65:760, 1986

87. McMorland GH, Douglas JM, Jeffery WK et al: Effect of pH-adjustment of bupivacaine on onset and duration of epidural analgesia in parturients. Can J Anaesth 33:537, 1986

88. Scott DB; Test dose in extradural block. Br J Anaesth 61:129, 1988

89. Jorfeldt L, Lewis DH, Löfström B, Post C: Lung uptake of lidocaine in healthy volunteers. Acta Anaesthesiol Scand 23:567, 1979

90. Arthur GR: Distribution and Elimination of Local Anaesthetic Agents: The Role of Lung, Liver and Kidney (thesis). University of Edinburgh, Edinburgh, 1981

91. Post C, Andersson RGG, Ryrfeldt A, Nilsson E: Physicochemical modification of lidocaine uptake of lidocaine in rat lung tissue. Acta Pharmacol Toxicol 51:136, 1979

92. Haasio J, Hekali R, Rosenberg PH: Influence of premedication on lignocaine-induced acute toxicity and plasma concentrations of lignocaine. Br J Anaesth 61:131, 1988

93. Moore DC, Thompson GE, Crawford RD: Long-acting local anesthetic drugs and convulsions with hypoxia and acidosis. Anesthesiology 56:230, 1982

94. Rosenberg PH, Kalso EA, Tuominen MK, Lindén HB: Acute bupivacaine toxicity as a result of venous leakage under the tourniquet cuff curing a Bier block. Anesthesiology 58:95, 1983

95. Tuominen MK, Pere P, Rosenberg PH: Unintentional arterial catheterization and bupivacaine toxicity associated with interscalene brachial plexus block. Anesthesiology 75:356, 1991

96. Hamilton RC: Brainstem anesthesia as a complication of regional anesthesia for ophtholmic surgery. Can J Ophthalmol 27:323, 1992

97. Morishima G, Pedersen H, Finster K et al: Bupivacaine toxicity in pregnant and nonpregnant ewes. Anesthesiology 63:134, 1985

98. Arthur GR, Feldman HS, Covino BG: Alterations in the pharmacokinetic properties of amide local anaesthetics following local anaesthetic induced convulsions. Acta Anaesthesiol Scand 32:522, 1988

99. Morishima HO, Pedersen H, Finster M et al: Is bupivacaine more cardiotoxic than lidocaine? Anesthesiology 59:A409, 1983

100. Clarkson CW, Hondeghem LM: Mechanism for bupivacaine depression of cardiac conduction: fast block of sodium channels during the action potential with slow recovery from block during diastole. Anesthesiology 62:396, 1985

101. Albright GA: Cardiac arrest following regional anesthesia with etidocaine or bupivacaine. Anesthesiology 51:285, 1979

102. Heavner JE: Cardiac dysrhythmias induced by infusion of local anesthetics into the lateral cerebral ventricle of cats. Anesth Analg 65:133, 1986

103. Bernards C, Artru AA: Hexamethonium and midazolam terminate dysrhythmias and hypertension caused by intracerebroventricular bupivacaine in rabbits. Anesthesiology 74:89, 1991

104. Santos AC, Pedersen H, Harmon TW et al: Does pregnancy alter the systemic toxicity of local anesthetics? Anesthesiology 70:991, 1989

105. Moller RA, Covino BG: Effect of progesterone on the cardiac electrophysiologic alterations produced by ropivacaine and bupivacaine. Anesthesiology 77:735, 1992

106. Rosen MA, Thigpen JW, Shnider SM et al: Bupivacaine-induced cardiotoxicity in hypoxic and acidotic sheep. Anesth Analg 64:1089, 1985

107. Kasten GW, Martin ST: Bupivacaine cardiovascular toxicity: comparison of treatment with bretylium and lidocaine. Anesth Analg 64:911, 1985

108. Chadwick HS: Toxicity and resuscitation in lidocaine- or bupivacaine-infused cats. Anesthesiology 63:385, 1985

109. Bernards CM, Carpenter RL, Kenter ME et al: Effect of epinephrine on central nervous system and cardiovascular toxicity of bupivacaine in pigs. Anesthesiology 71:711, 1989

110. Lingren L, Randell T, Suzuki N et al: The effect of amrinone on recovery from severe bupivacaine intoxication in pigs. Anesthesiology 77:309, 1992

111. Matsuda F, Kinney W, Wright W, Kambam JR: Nicardipine reduces the cardio-respiratory toxicity of intravenously administered bupivacaine in rats. Can J Anaesth 37:920, 1990

112. Long WB, Rosenblum S, Grady IP: Successful resuscitation of bupivacaine-induced cardiac arrest using cardiopulmonary bypass. Anesth Analg 69:403, 1989

113. Parris WCV, Dettbarn WD: Muscle atrophy following bupivacaine trigger point injection. Anesth Rev 16:50, 1989

114. Benoit PW, Belt WD: Destruction and regeneration of skeletal muscle after treatment with a local anaesthetic, bupivacaine (Marcaine®). J Anat 107:547, 1970

115. Selander D, Brattsand R, Lundborg G et al: Local anesthetics: importance of mode of application, concentration and adrenaline for the appearance of nerve lesion. Acta Anaesthesiol Scand 23:127, 1979

116. Kyttä J, Rosenberg PH, Wahlström T, Olkkola K: Histopathological changes in rabbit spinal cord caused by bupivacaine. Regional-Anaesthesie 5:85, 1982

117. Lambert DH, Hurley RJ: Cauda equina syndrome and continuous spinal anesthesia. Anesth Analg 72:817, 1991

118. Ross BK, Coda B, Heath CH: Local anesthetic distribution in a spinal model: a possible mechanism of neurologic injury after continuous spinal anesthesia. Reg Anesth 17:69, 1992

119. Gissen AJ, Datta S, Lambert D: The chloroprocaine controversy: II. Is chloroprocaine neurotoxic? Reg Anesth 9:135, 1984

120. Goolkasian DL, Slaughter RL, Edwards DJ, Lalka D: Displacement of lidocaine from serum alpha₁-acid glycoprotein binding sites by basic drugs. Eur J Clin Pharmacol 25:413, 1983

121. Hartrick CT, Raj PP, Dirkes WE, Denson DD: Compounding of bupivacaine and mepivacaine for regional anesthesia. A safe practice? Reg Anesth 9:94, 1984

122. Raj PP, Ohlweiler D, Hitt BA, Denson DD: Kinetics of local anesthetic esters and adjuvant drugs on 2-chloroprocaine hydrolysis. Anesthesiology 53:307, 1980

123. Bentley JB, Glass S, Gandolfi AJ: The influence of halothane on lidocaine pharmacokinetics in man. Anesthesiology 59:A246, 1983

124. Runciman WB, Mather LE, Ilsley AH et al: A sheep preparation for studying interactions between blood flow and drug dispositions: II. Experimental applications. Br J Anesth 56:1117, 1984

125. Denson DD, Myers JA, Watters C, Raj PP: Selective inhibition of the aromatic hydroxylation of bupivacaine by halothane. Anesthesiology 57:A242, 1982

126. Jorfeldt L, Lewis DH, Löfström B, Post C: Lung uptake of lidocaine in man as influenced by anaesthesia, mepivacaine infusion or lung insufficiency. Acta Anaesthesiol Scand 27:5, 1983

127. Cassuto J, Wallin G, Högström S, Faxén A, Rimbäck G: Inhibition of postoperative pain by continuous low-dose intravenous infusion of lidocaine. Anesth Analg 64:971, 1985

128. DiFazio CA, Niederlehner JR, Burney RG: The anesthetic potency of lidocaine in the rat. Anesth Analg 55:818, 1976

129. Denson DD, Myers JA, Coyle DE: The clinical relevance of the drug displacement interaction between meperidine and bupivacaine. Res Commun Chem Pathol Pharmacol 45:323, 1984

130. De Jong RH, Heavner JE: Diazepam prevents local anesthetic seizures. Anesthesiology 34:523, 1971

131. Ausinsch B, Malagodi MH, Munson ES: Diazepam in the prophylaxis of lignocaine seizures. Br J Anaesth 48:309, 1976

132. Bernards CM, Carpenter RL, Rupp SM et al: Effect of midazolam and diazepam premedication on central nervous system and cardiovascular toxicity of bupivacaine in pigs. Anesthesiology 70:318, 1989

133. Kennedy WF, Everett GB, Cobb LA, Allen GD: Simultaneous systemic and hepatic hemodynamic measurements during high peridural anesthesia in normal man. Anesth Analg 50:1069, 1971

134. Wiklund L, Tucker GT, Engberg G: Influence of intravenously administered epinephrine on splanchnic haemodynamics and clearance of lidocaine. Acta Anaesthesiol Scand 21:275, 1977

135. Bax NDS, Tucker GT, Lennard MS, Woods HF: The impairment of lignocaine clearance by propranolol—major contribution from enzyme inhibition. Br J Clin Pharmacol 19:597, 1985

136. Edouard A, Froidevaux R, Berdeaux A et al: Verapamil-bupivacaine interaction in conscious dogs. Anesthesiology 63:A257, 1985

137. Kinney WW, Kambam JR, Matsuda F et al: Bupivacaine cardiotoxicity is reduced by verapamil pretreatment in rats. Anesthesiology 71:A1145, 1989

138. Hyman SA, Kinney WW, Horn JL et al: Nimodipine reduces the cardiorespiratory toxicity of intravenous bupivacaine in rats. Anesthesiology 75:A677, 1991
139. Bauer LA, Edwards WAD, Randolph FP, Blouin RA: Cimetidine-induced decrease in lidocaine metabolism. Am Heart J 108:413, 1984
140. Robson RA, Wing LMH, Miners JO et al: The effect of ranitidine on the disposition of lignocaine. Br J Clin Pharmacol 20:170, 1985
141. Perucca E, Richens A: Reduction of oral bioavailability of lignocaine by induction of first-pass metabolism in epileptic patients. Br J Clin Pharmacol 8:21,1979
142. Routledge PA, Stargel WW, Finn AL et al: Lignocaine disposition in blood in epilepsy. Br J Clin Pharmacol 12:663, 1981
143. Feely J, Clee M, Pereira L, Guy E: Enzyme inhibition with rifampicin: lipoproteins and drug binding to alpha$_1$-acid glycoprotein. Br J Clin Pharmacol 16:195, 1983
144. Calvo R, Carlos R, Erill S: Effects of disease and acetazolamide on procaine hydrolysis by red cell enzymes. Clin Pharmacol Ther 27:175, 1980
145. Tucker GT, Mather LE: Clinical pharmacology of local anesthetic agents. Clin Pharmacokinet 4:241, 1979
146. Covino BG, Vassallo HG: Local Anesthetics. Mechanisms of Action and Clinical Use. Grune & Stratton, New York, 1976
147. Covino BG: Clinical pharmacology of local anesthetics. p. 112. In Cousins MJ, Bridenbaugh PO (eds): Neural Blockade in Clinical Anesthesia and Management. 2nd Ed. JB Lippincott, Philadelphia, 1988
148. Rosenberg H: Density of tetracaine-water mixtures and the effectiveness of 0.33 per cent tetracaine in hypobaric spinal anesthesia. Anesthesiology 45:682, 1976
149. Greene NM: Physiology of Spinal Anesthesia. 3rd Ed. Williams & Wilkins, Baltimore, 1981

Chapter 10

Basic Pharmacology of Benzodiazepines

Linda D. McCauley, Kelvin W. Gee, and Henry I. Yamamura

The discovery of the therapeutically useful benzodiazepines in the 1950s is attributed to the search for an orally active muscle relaxant. Systematic pharmacologic screening resulted in an observation that these compounds produced a "taming" effect on various test animals, including primates.[1,2] Because the taming effect on animals occurred at doses less than those that produce ataxia or sedation, the clinical application of these compounds as antianxiety agents was suggested. Benzodiazepines became commercially available in the early 1960s with the introduction of chlordiazepoxide as an antianxiety agent. In the period following the entrance of benzodiazepines onto the commercial market, this class of compounds has become one of the most commonly prescribed drugs. Their widespread use is in part attributable to their effectiveness on the central nervous system and to their relative safety. The therapeutically useful effects of the benzodiazepines include their anticonvulsant, anxiolytic, muscle relaxant, and sedative-hypnotic activities. Among those less desirable effects are tolerance, interactions with other drugs (e.g., alcohol), and anterograde amnesia. The benzodiazepines gained such widespread use so rapidly that published opinions speculated on the possible misuse of them in clinical practice.[3–6] This surge of popularity would not have been likely without the high therapeutic index enjoyed by the benzodiazepines. Despite their prevalence, more than 10 years passed before scientists made major advances in the elucidation of their mechanism of action. In the middle to late 1970s, evidence began to accumulate that linked benzodiazepine action to the inhibitory neurotransmitter γ-aminobutyric acid (GABA).[7–9] The first demonstration of specific benzodiazepine binding sites in the brain was published by Squires and Braestrup[10] in 1977. Their report was followed shortly thereafter and supported by Mohler and Okada.[11] Using the initial reports as a springboard, our understanding of the mechanism of action of benzodiazepines exploded during subsequent years.

Benzodiazepine receptors are typically divided into two classes that are distinguished on the basis of their anatomic localization. The "central" benzodiazepine receptor is associated with a GABA-gated chloride ionophore on the neuronal membrane, and the "peripheral" benzodiazepine receptor resides on the outer mitochondrial membrane. Each receptor has different ligand specificities. Currently, none of the common central nervous system effects observed in the clinical use of benzodiazepines has been attributed to a mechanism of action involving the peripheral benzodiazepine receptor. Most of these diverse effects can, however, be explained based on the function of the central benzodiazepine receptor and its modulation of the associated chloride channel.

THE BENZODIAZEPINE RECEPTOR

The benzodiazepines interact primarily with a specific neurotransmitter system that uses GABA, which is the principal inhibitory neurotransmitter in the mammalian central nervous system. GABA binds to two types of receptors, $GABA_A$ and $GABA_B$, which are differentiated on the basis of agonist-antagonist selectivity.[12,13] The $GABA_B$ receptor, which has not been shown to be involved in benzodiazepine action, appears to be linked to ion channels through guanine nucleotide binding proteins (G-proteins). GABAergic neurons are distributed extensively throughout the brain[14] and exert either presynaptic (axoaxonic synapses) or postsynaptic (all others, e.g., axodendritic) inhibition. The high affinity, central benzodiazepine receptor is coupled to the $GABA_A$ receptor, which gates a postsynaptic chloride channel and comprises the majority of GABAergic synapses in the central nervous system.[15] Laboratory results suggest that all benzodiazepine receptors are associated with a $GABA_A$ receptor, but not all $GABA_A$ receptors are coupled to a benzodiazepine receptor.[16,17] In presynaptic inhibition, the physiologic result is depolarization of the nerve terminal, which results in a diminished release of excitatory transmitter, whereas in postsynaptic inhibition, it is a hyperpolarization of the postsynaptic cell that results in a state less sensitive to the excitatory transmitter. Both responses are mediated by the intrinsic chloride channel; however, the direction of ion flow depends on the relative chloride ion concentrations within the neuron and the membrane potential (i.e., the electrochemical gradient) and, thus, determines the ultimate membrane polarity.[15,18] Generally, benzodiazepines have been shown to enhance the effects of GABA regardless of the pre- or postsynaptic receptor location. Together, the $GABA_A$ and benzodiazepine receptors along with the chloride channel form the multisubunit $GABA_A$/benzodiazepine receptor complex (GBRC). GABA exerts its inhibitory neuronal effects by opening the chloride channel, allowing chloride ions to flow down their electrochemical gradient into the neuron. The resultant effect is a hyperpolarization of the neuronal membrane and a decrease in the likelihood that the neuron will conduct an action potential. The distribution of benzodiazepine receptors was initially shown to be highly correlated with that of $GABA_A$ receptors.[19] Subsequent studies that combined receptor autoradiography and immunohistochemical analysis strongly supported the colocalization of benzodiazepine and $GABA_A$ receptors at both the light and electron microscopic levels.[20–24] Investigators have since purified a macromolecule that contains both the benzodiazepine and $GABA_A$ receptors,[25,26] further supporting the existence of benzodiazepine receptors in association with the $GABA_A$ receptor-gated chloride ionophore.

The effect of GABA on chloride flux can be allosterically modulated by several classes of compounds acting at distinct but interacting sites on the receptor complex. These sites include those for the centrally acting benzodiazepines, the barbiturates, picrotoxin or t-butylbicyclophosphorothionate, and the more recently identified neuroactive steroids.[27–32] The presence of more than one binding site on the GBRC creates the potential for cooperativity among them. Generally, the interaction between any two different binding sites on the receptor complex is defined as either positive or negative heterotropic cooperatively, depending on how one site affects the binding affinity of the other.[30] Furthermore, if the binding of one compound to its recognition site enhances the binding of another compound to its respective binding site (i.e., positive heterotropic cooperativity), then the binding of the second compound must enhance the binding of the first compound in exactly the same manner.[31] Benzodiazepine cooperativity is diagrammed in Figure 10-1. It is currently believed that the central nervous system effects of the benzodiazepines are mediated by the central benzodiazepine receptor on the GBRC and is subject to the influence of the other sites on the receptor complex. Biochemical and pharmacologic evidence supports a mechanism of action whereby the classic benzodiazepines positively modulate the $GABA_A$ receptor by enhancing GABA's affinity for the receptor and, thus, influence the degree to which

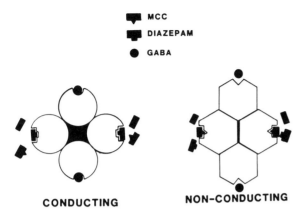

Fig. 10-1 A model for the conducting and non-conducting conformations of the GABA/benzodiazepine receptor complex. The open circles represent the channel in the open conformation activated by the binding of GABA and enhanced by benzodiazepine (diazepam) binding. The open hexagons represent the channel in the closed, non-conducting conformation. Inverse agonists, such as β-CCM (MCC), cause the channel to close, thus inhibiting chloride ion currents. (From Gee,[106] with permission.)

GABA can modify chloride ion permeability. Facilitation of GABA effects by benzodiazepines leads to an increase in the frequency of chloride channel opening (as opposed to the barbiturate effect of an increased duration of channel open time) and consequent changes in neuronal membrane excitability. Benzodiazepine binding in vivo correlates well with the clinical and pharmacologic potencies of these drugs.[32–37] Furthermore, studies have shown that a greater fraction of benzodiazepine receptors must be occupied to elicit the muscle relaxant effects than to produce the anxiolytic effects.[38–40] Accordingly, both the intrinsic efficacy and receptor occupancy of a ligand determine the response in a biologic system.

ENDOGENOUS AGONISTS

Traditionally, we like to think of evolution as an efficient way to screen for the necessities of life. At the present time, the benzodiazepine receptor is still somewhat of an enigma. Extensive data have been collected by numerous laboratories attesting to the efficacy of altering brain excitability through the benzodiazepine receptor. However, it remains

open to debate whether an endogenous ligand for the benzodiazepine receptor exists. As is the case with the opioid receptors whose existence led to the discovery of its endogenous ligands, the endorphins, the existence of the benzodiazepine receptors obliges us to question the existence of their naturally occurring ligands. Initial hopes were pinned on ethyl-β-carboline-3-carboxylate (β-CCE), extracted from human urine, which was found to inhibit [³H]diazepam binding,[41] the screen commonly used for benzodiazepine ligands. Subsequently, β-CCE was found to be an artifact of the extraction process. Others have proposed purines,[42,43] nicotinamide,[44] and large molecular weight peptides ranging up to 70 kD[45–48] as endogenous agents for the benzodiazepine receptor. One laboratory has demonstrated that benzodiazepine-like compounds are formed in the rat brain.[49] It has not yet been determined whether these molecules are actually synthesized de novo by mammalian tissues or if they are absorbed from ingested foods and retained in tissues. Recently, Rothstein et al.[50] described additional nonpeptide agents with the ability to displace tritiated benzodiazepines and function as positive allosteric modulators at the GBRC.

One candidate that has nurtured scientific interest for a relatively long period is a 10-kD peptide termed diazepam binding inhibitor (DBI) because it was found to displace [³H]diazepam binding in brain membranes.[51] In primary cultures of spinal cord neurons taken from mouse embryos, DBI produced negative modulatory effects on GABA-mediated chloride conductance.[52,53] This type of action is reminiscent of the β-carbolines, which are inverse agonists at the benzodiazepine receptor. As described earlier, β-CCE was the first β-carboline that exhibited high affinity binding to the benzodiazepine receptor. However, when administered to animals (and later to humans), it produced effects opposite to those of the benzodiazepines, namely anxiogenic, proconflict (as opposed to anticonflict), proconvulsant, and convulsant activities. These pharmacologic effects were associated with decreased GABA binding to its receptor (i.e., negative modulation) with a consequent decrease in chloride conductance. Thus, the term "inverse agonist" was applied to these drugs that exhibited high affinity binding to the benzodiazepine receptors, but whose pharmacologic effects were opposite to those of the benzodiazepines. The action of DBI on these receptors was further supported by electrophysiologic studies using flumazenil, a true antagonist of the benzodiazepine receptor, to block the DBI-mediated inhibition of chloride currents induced by GABA.[52] For a prospective endogenous ligand to remain in contention, it should be present, not only in the brain, but also in sufficient concentrations for biologic activity. Interestingly, DBI has been found to reach concentrations of 10 to 50 μM in certain brain areas and some peripheral tissues.[51,54–57] The question of whether DBI and/or fragments of DBI are physiologically relevant ligands for the central benzodiazepine receptor is of primary interest at the present time. DBI can be cleaved post-translationally into biologically active fragments by brain specific endopeptidases.[51,58] At least three neuropeptides derived from DBI have been identified in the rat brain and share amino acid 50 of DBI as their carboxy terminus.[51,59] Three of these are triakontatetraneuropeptide (DBI 17-50), octadecaneuropeptide (DBI 33-50), and eicosapentaneuropeptide (DBI 26-50). Their primary sequences are shown in Table 10-1.

Octadecaneuropeptide and eicosapentaneuropeptide appear to have greater potency in displacing [³H]flumazenil or [³H]flunitrazepam binding from central benzodiazepine sites, whereas triakontatetraneuropeptide has greater potency on the benzodiazepine site associated with the outer mitochondrial membrane.[51,58,59] Laboratory studies using a behavioral test to determine the in vivo activity of DBI show that DBI, octadecaneuropep-

Triazolopyridazine

CL 218,872

Isoquinoline

PK 11195

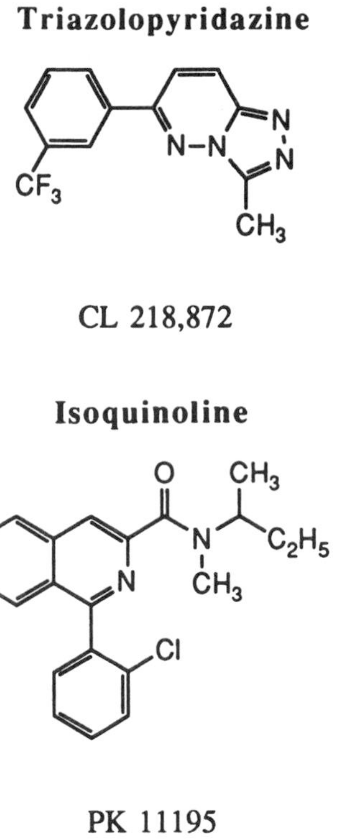

Fig. 10-2 Structures of the isoquinoline PK 11195 and the triazolopyridazine CL 218,872.

tide, and triakontatetraneuropeptide all produced a proconflict (inverse agonist) effect.[59,60] Furthermore, the effect of both DBI and octadecaneuropeptide was antagonized following pretreatment with flumazenil, whereas that of triakontatetraneuropeptide was not changed by flumazenil but was decreased by PK 11195, an isoquinoline carboxamide derivative (Fig. 10-2) with high affinity

Table 10-1 Amino Acid Sequences of Diazepam Binding Inhibitor and Its Three Fragments

Peptide Name	Primary Sequence
DBI (1-86)	SQADFDKAAEEVKRLKTQPTDEEMLFIYSH FKQATVGDVNTDRPGLLDLKGKAKWDSW NKLKGTSKENAMKTYVEKVEELKKKYGI
TTN (17-50)	TQPTDEEMLFIYSHFKQATVGDVNTDRPGL LDLK
EPN (26-50)	FIYSHFKQATVGDVNTDRPGLLDLK
ODN (33-50)	QATVGDVNTDRPGLLDLK

Abbreviations: DBI, diazepam binding inhibitor; EPN, eicosapentaneuropeptide; ODN, octadecaneuropeptide; TTN, triakontatetraneuropeptide.

for the peripheral benzodiazepine site. The significance of these findings remains unclear because it is difficult to replicate exactly in vivo conditions in an in vitro experiment. Although DBI has been shown to be present in the brain in quantities seemingly sufficient to elicit a response, it is still not universally accepted as an endogenous ligand for the benzodiazepine receptor.

STRUCTURE-ACTIVITY RELATIONSHIPS

The clinically useful 1,4-benzodiazepines are descendants of the first synthesis of chlordiazepoxide by the chemist, Sternbach, at Hoffmann-La Roche in 1955. They are a class of heteroring compounds consisting of two six-membered and one seven-membered rings. One benzene ring (ring *a*) is fused to the seven-membered 1,4-diazepine ring (ring *b*), hence the name 1,4-benzodiazepines. A selection of some of the more common benzodiazepines of this type is shown in Figure 10-3. Only compounds that contain a substituent at position 7 of ring a are highly active. Furthermore, the most important structure-activity relationship for this class of compounds involves the nature of the substituent at this position. The electron-withdrawing properties of some of the heavier halogens and nitro groups tend to increase the biologic potency, whereas electron-releasing substituents significantly decrease the activity. In addition, the character of the substituent at the ortho position of ring c can have profound effects. Substitutions in the meta or para positions generally had negative results.

The benzodiazepine receptor represents a unique protein through which a full spectrum of pharmacologic actions is mediated, ranging from the anxiolytic, sedative, and anticonvulsant effects of the full agonists (e.g., diazepam) to the anxiogenic, proconflict, and convulsant effects of the inverse agonists, such as β-CCE. The wide range of actions is displayed in Figure 10-4. The neurochemical correlates of these responses are readily apparent in the different efficacies of the various benzodiazepines and β-carbolines on muscimol (a GABA agonist)-stimulated chloride uptake as shown in Table 10-2.[61] Some of the clinically useful

benzodiazepines exhibit a full agonist profile (i.e., they produce a leftward shift of the GABA dose-response curve in a concentration dependent manner) as a result of increasing the affinity of GABA for its receptor. The functional result of this change in affinity is an enhancement of GABA-mediated chloride conductance. In the absence of GABA, the classical benzodiazepines have no functional efficacy. Examples of full agonists include diazepam, midazolam, and flunitrazepam. Those compounds that retain agonist profiles but demonstrate less intrinsic efficacy are classified as partial agonists. Partial agonists still enhance GABA-stimulated chloride flux; however, the extent to which this effect occurs is reduced. Partial agonists represent an interesting basis for novel drug development in that they do not produce a maximal effect on the benzodiazepine receptor, even when all receptors are fully occupied, and they antagonize the effects of full agonists.[62–65] Examples of partial agonists include the well known benzodiazepine clonazepam, chlordiazepoxide, CL 218,872 (3-methyl-6-[3-trifluoromethylphenyl]-1,2,4-triazolo-[4,3-b] pyridazine) (Fig. 10-2), and more recently, Ro 16-6028 (bretazenil). Weak intrinsic efficacy is characteristic of partial agonists and tends to decrease the muscle relaxant and sedative properties of benzodiazepines, which require full benzodiazepine receptor stimulation. Benzodiazepine antagonists have very weak or no inherent efficacy but retain affinity for the receptor, thereby conferring the ability to interfere or prevent the interaction of agonists with the receptors. The classic benzodiazepine antagonist is flumazenil. In laboratory animals, this antagonist has been observed to block the effects of ethanol,[66] and it has been suggested that it may prove useful in the clinic to reverse ethanol overdosage.[67,68] The 50 percent inhibitory concentrations of many benzodiazepines derived from the inhibition of [^{3}H]diazepam are listed in Table 10-3.

Continuing to the other side of the spectrum, the partial inverse agonists act as noncompetitive antagonists of the $GABA_A$ receptor and include the photoaffinity label Ro 15-4513 (ethyl-8-azido-6-dihydro-5-methyl-6-oxo-4H-imidazo[1,5a]-[1,4]benzodiazepine-3-carboxylate). Full inverse agonists often exhibit proconvulsant activity. This results directly from the tendency of inverse ago-

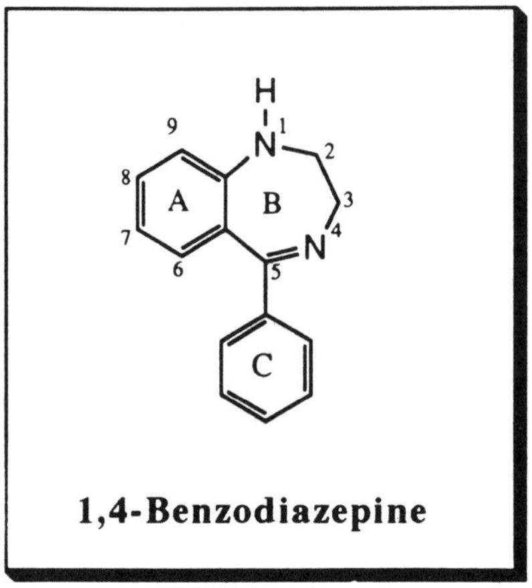

1,4-Benzodiazepine

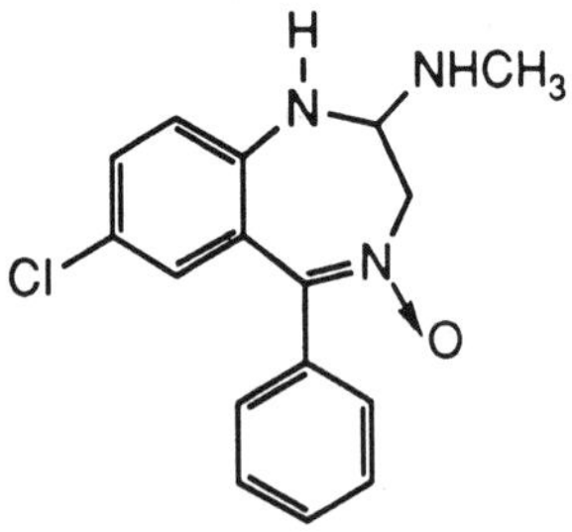

Chlorodiazepoxide

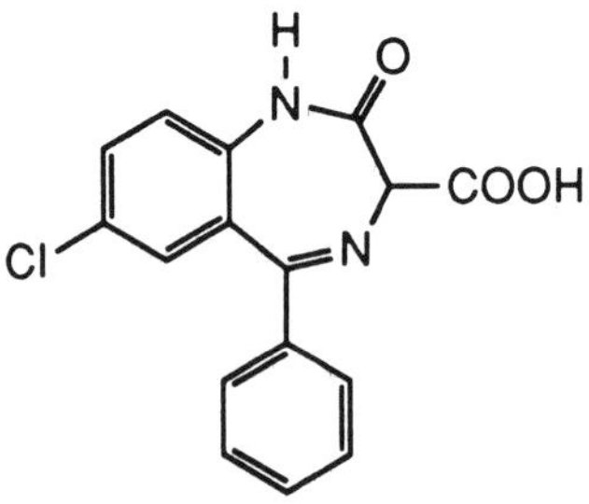

Clorazepate

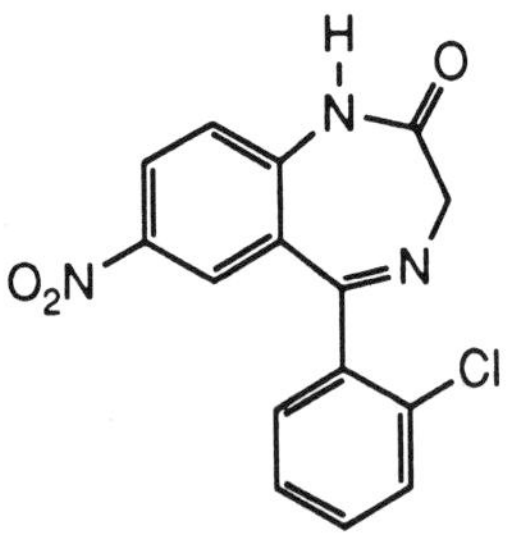

Clonazepam

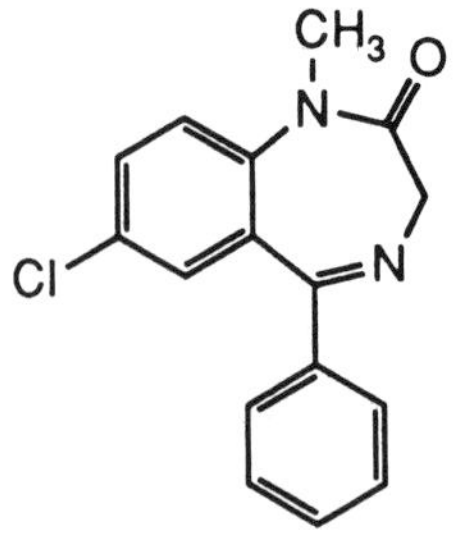

Diazepam

Fig. 10-3 Structures of some of the classic 1,4-benzodiazepines. Compounds of this class are often full or partial agonists. (*Figure continues.*)

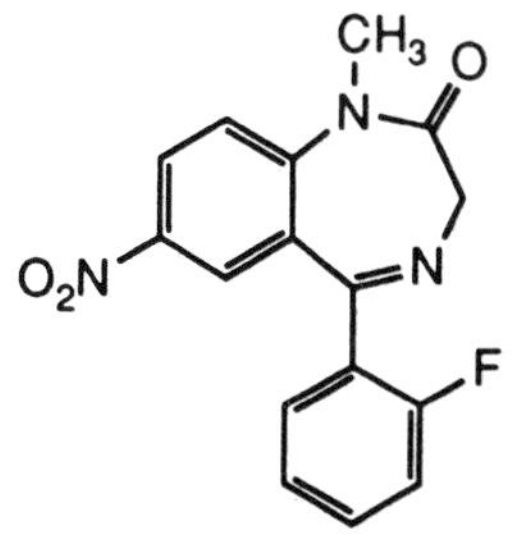

Flunitrazepam

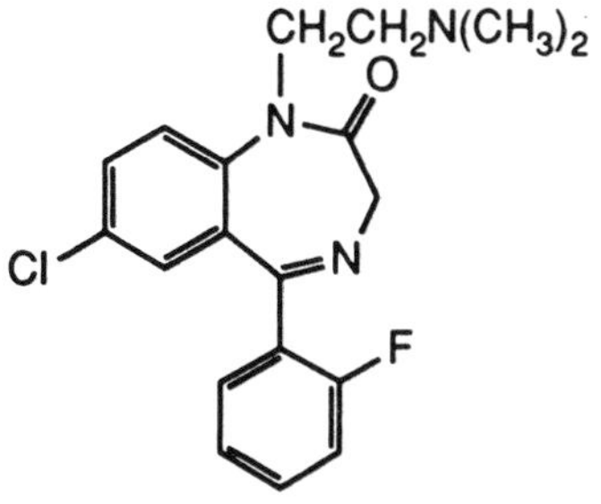

Flurazepam

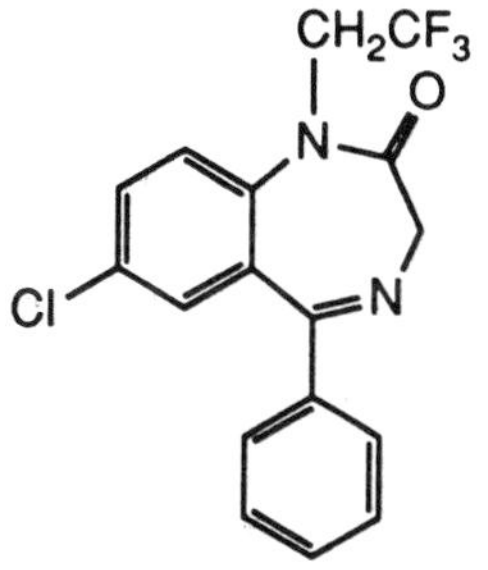

Halazepam

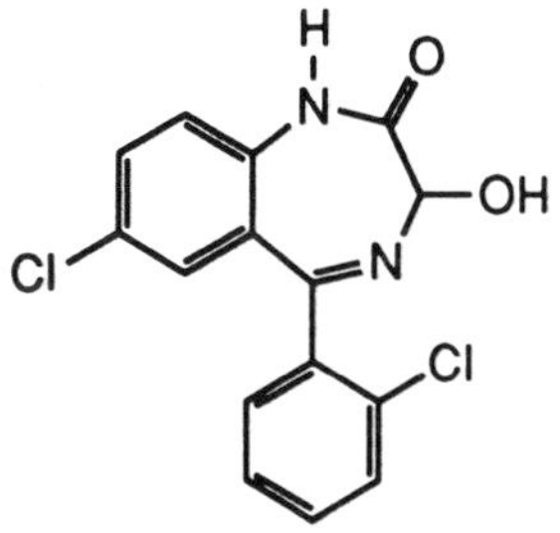

Lorazepam

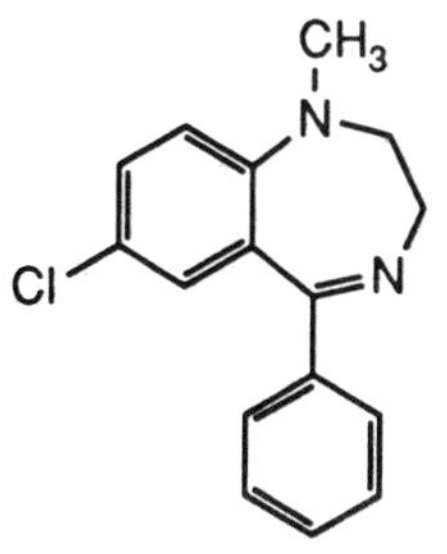

Medazepam

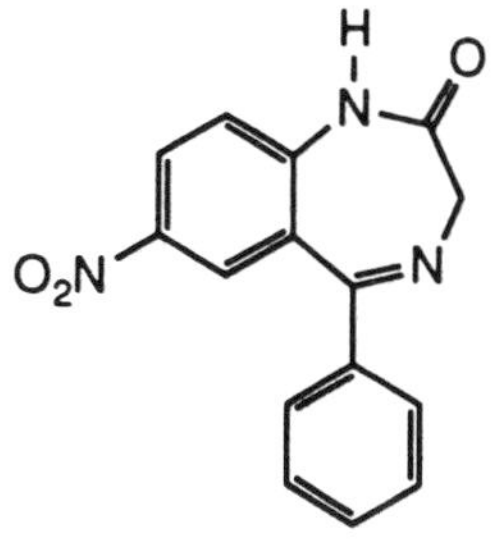

Nitrazepam

Fig. 10-3 (*Continues*).

nists to close the chloride channel, rendering the neuron especially vulnerable to excitation. Often, inverse agonists belong to the β-carboline class of compounds, which bind to benzodiazepine receptors with high affinity. Examples of this class of compounds are shown in Figure 10-5. They include β-CCE (and also the methyl and propyl esters), norharmane, and 3-hydroxymethyl-β-carboline, which have been shown to antagonize the anxiolytic,[69,70] anticonvulsant,[69,71] and sedative-

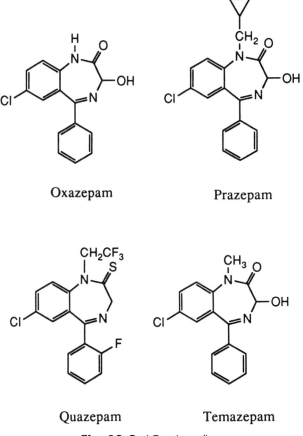

Oxazepam   Prazepam

Quazepam   Temazepam

Fig. 10-3 (Continued).

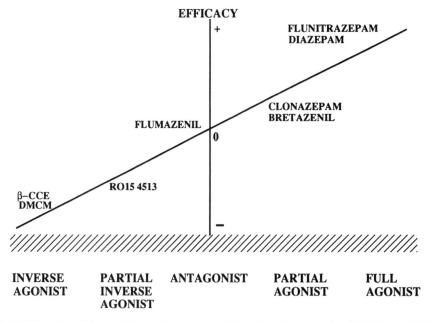

Fig. 10-4 Diversity of benzodiazepine receptor ligands effects on the GABA-gated chloride ionophore.

Table 10-2 Effect of Benzodiazepine Agonists, Antagonists, and Inverse Agonists on Muscimol-Stimulated Chloride Uptake

Drug	Change in $^{36}Cl^-$ Uptake (nmol/mg of protein)	Percent Change
Diazepam (1 μM)	5.81 ± 0.51	59
Flurazepam (10 μM)	4.76 ± 0.37	49
Clonazepam (1 μM)	3.64 ± 0.54	37
Flurazepam (1 μM)	2.43 ± 0.26	25
Flumazenil (2 μM)	0.9 ± 0.17	9
Flurazepam (10 μM) + Flumazenil (2 μM)	0.5 ± 0.22	5
β-CCE (5 μM)	-3.51 ± 0.26	-36
DMCM (5 μM)	-4.92 ± 0.24	-50

Abbreviations: β-CCE, ethyl-β-carboline-3-carboxylate; DMCM, 6,7-dimethoxy-4-ethyl-β-carboline-3-carboxylic acid methyl ester.
(Adapted from Morrow et al.,[61] with permission.)

hypnotic[72,73] actions of classic benzodiazepines. Elucidation of structure-activity relationships for the β-carbolines pointed to certain positions as being important determinants for their activity. Skolnick et al.[74] found substitutions at the C1 posi-

Table 10-3 Binding Affinities of Benzodiazepine Receptor Ligands[a]

Benzodiazepine	IC_{50} (nM)
Alprazolam	20
Chlordiazepoxide	350
Clonazepam	2
Clorazepate	59
Diazepam	8
Flunitrazepam	4
Flurazepam	15
Lorazepam	4
Medazepam	870
Midazolam	5
Nitrazepam	10
Oxazepam	18
Prazepam	110
Temazepam	16
Triazolam	4

Abbreviations: IC_{50}, 50 percent inhibitory concentration.
[a] IC_{50}s are derived from the inhibition of [^{3}H]diazepam.
(Data from Haefely et al.[104])

tion decreased the drug's affinity for the receptor; substitutions at the C3 position tended to increase the affinity. For example, 3-carbomethoxy-β-carboline has more than a 1,000-fold higher affinity compared with the unsubstituted norharmane. Further studies by the same laboratory demonstrated that a methyl substitution at position N9 resulted in an almost total loss of activity, whereas substituents at position C9 had a minimal effect.

RECEPTOR HETEROGENEITY

Like the GABA$_A$ receptor, pharmacologic data suggest that the benzodiazepine receptor population is also heterogeneous. Initial studies probing the binding properties of classic benzodiazepines with labeled ligands, such as flunitrazepam and diazepam, indicated a homogeneous population of receptors.[11,75,76] Several years later, the re-examination and addition of new binding data suggested the presence of at least two benzodiazepine subtypes.[77–80] The most compelling evidence for benzodiazepine receptor heterogeneity derives from concurrent biochemical studies that demonstrate complex interactions between a compound belonging to the triazolopyridazine class, CL 218,872, and the receptor. This ligand was the first compound

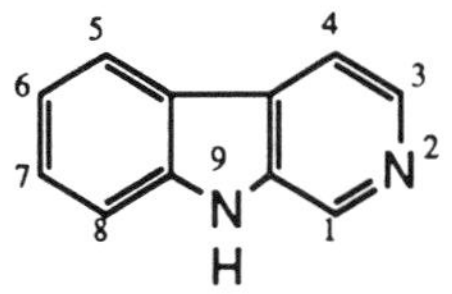

β-Carboline

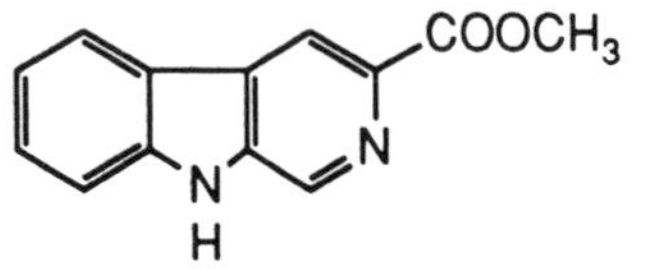

Methyl β-carboline-3-carboxylate

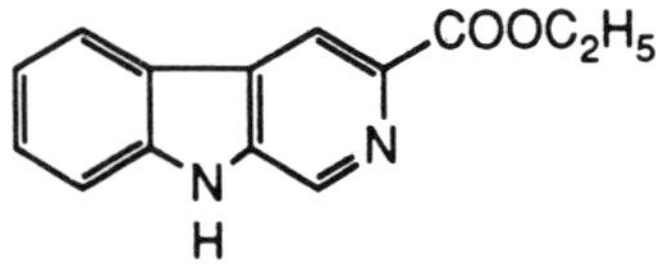

Ethyl β-carboline-3-carboxylate

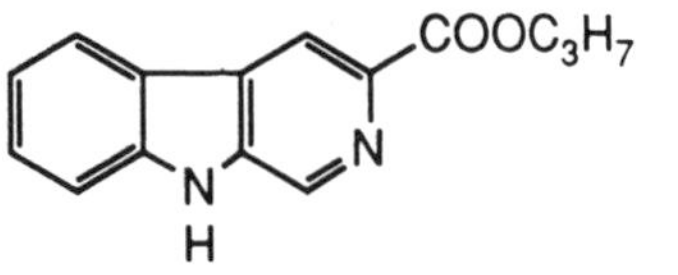

Propyl β-carboline-3-carboxylate

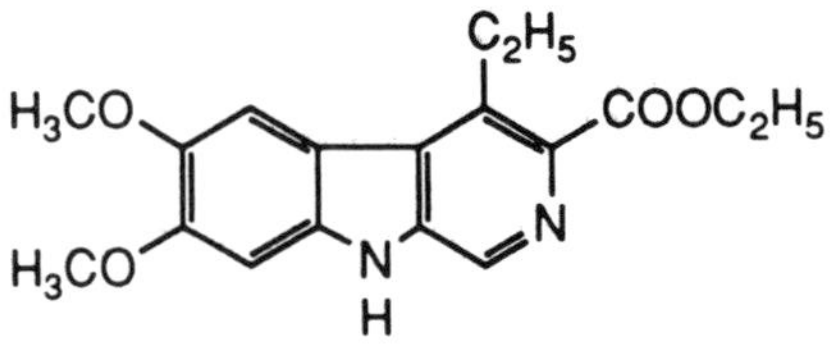

6,7-Dimethoxy-4-ethyl- β-carboline-3-carboxylic acid methyl ester

Fig. 10-5 Structures of some β-carbolines. Those shown here are inverse agonists at the benzodiazepine receptor.

reported to discriminate between two subtypes of benzodiazepine receptors. The Hill coefficient derived from the inhibition of [³H]flunitrazepam by the triazolopyridazine, CL 218,872, was less than unity, indicating the presence of more than one recognition site.[77,81–84] In contrast, the classic benzodiazepines displaced [³H]benzodiazepines that yielded competition curves the Hill slopes of which did not significantly differ from unity.[84]

On the basis of the CL 218,872 discrimination between benzodiazepine receptors, those sites for which it had high affinity (i.e., affinity similar to that of the 1,4-benzodiazepines for the benzodiazepine receptor) were designated type 1 while those for which it has low affinity were called type 2.[85] The authors of that study proposed that the type 1 receptors mediated the anxiolytic effects of benzodiazepine ligands, whereas the other pharmaco-

Table 10-4 Percentage of Type 1 Benzodiazepine Receptors in Various Regions of the Brain

Region	Percent of Type 1 Benzodiazepine Receptors[a]
Cerebellum	100
Medial cortex	84
Pons	81
Occipital cortex	81
Thalamus	80
Frontal cortex	78
Bulbus olfactorius	78
Whole forebrain	69
Corpus striatum	62
Hippocampus	59
Nucleus accumbens	57
Hypothalamus	57

[a] Percentage of type 1 benzodiazepine receptors based on the cerebellum being assigned the value of 100 percent.
(Data from Braestrup and Nielsen.[105])

logic effects were attributed to type 2 receptors. This hypothesis was supported by the observation that, although CL 218,872 was as potent in anticonvulsant and anxiolytic tests, it did not produce the muscle relaxant and sedative effects found with classic benzodiazepines, such as diazepam.[86,87] This claim was disputed by subsequent studies that showed that, at 37°C, the physiologically relevant temperature, CL 218,872 did not discriminate between benzodiazepine receptors, except in the cerebellum.[88] The controversy remains, not as to the existence, but as to the physiologic significance of the subtypes of benzodiazepine receptors. The relative proportion of type 1 receptors in various regions of the brain is shown in Table 10-4. More recently, it has been proposed that the sedative-hypnotic effects of benzodiazepine agonists were induced by type 1 receptors, and the type 2 receptors mediated the anticonvulsant and anxiolytic effects.[89,90] The growing body of molecular biologic evidence overwhelmingly supports benzodiazepine receptor heterogeneity and may ultimately resolve the physiologic significance of type 1 versus type 2 subtypes.

MOLECULAR BIOLOGY OF THE γ-AMINOBUTYRIC ACID/BENZODIAZEPINE RECEPTOR COMPLEX

The first hint of the complexity of the GBRC came from preliminary attempts to purify the benzodiazepine receptor by using flunitrazepam in photoaffinity labeling experiments. Initially, these studies identified at least four proteins associated with the central benzodiazepine site.[91] The major polypeptide subunit, α, 50 to 53 kD molecular weight, contained the benzodiazepine binding site, whereas the other major polypeptide subunit, β, 56 to 58 kD molecular weight, held the binding site for GABA.[92] Advances in the field of molecular biology have facilitated the isolation of the individual subunits that comprise the GBRC. Similarities between the nicotinic cholinergic receptor, the glycine receptor-gated channel, and the GBRC primary sequences led to the proposal that they all are members of a superfamily of ligand-gated channel receptors.[12,93] To date six α, four β, three γ, one δ, and one ρ subunit of the GBRC have been identified. These statistics change often. Amino acid sequences of two subunits of the same type (e.g., α_1 and α_2) share 60 to 70 percent sequence homology, whereas sequence identity between subunits of two different types (e.g., α and β) is approximately 30 percent. Sequence analyses of the α, β, γ, and δ subunits suggested that they all contain four putative α-helical membrane spanning regions[93,94] and potential sites for N-linked glycosylation in the extracellular domain. Figure 10-6 presents a possible arrangement of the individual subunits in the neuronal membrane and how they form the ion channel. Although the precise subunit stoichiometry is unknown, studies using recombinantly expressed receptors reveal that an α, β, and γ_2 subunit are required to reconstitute the correct pharmacology of the native receptor complex, including high affinity benzodiazepine binding.[94] Moreover, the distinction between type I and II benzodiazepine receptors described by Sieghart and Karobath[91] was pharmacologically reproduced in recombinantly expressed receptors based upon the α subunit.[95–97] The cotransfection of α_1, γ_2, and a β subunit conferred to the expressed receptors a type I profile

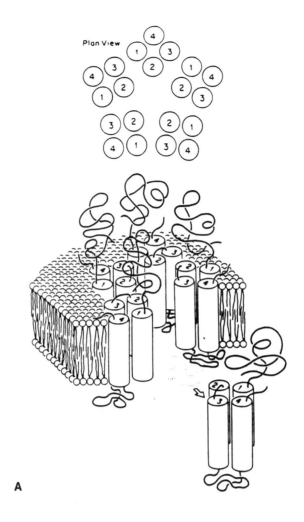

Plan View

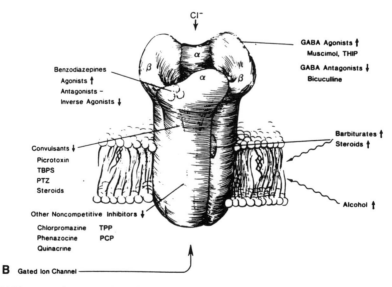

GABA Receptor Complex

Fig. 10-6(A) Hypothetic model of how the individual subunits of the GABA/benzodiazepine receptor complex unite to form a ligand-gated ion channel. (From Olsen and Tobin,[107] with permission.) **(B)** Proposed model of the GABA/benzodiazepine receptor complex in the neuronal membrane. (From Schwartz,[108] with permission.)

exhibiting a 10-fold higher affinity for CL 218,872 compared with receptors derived from an α_2, α_3,[96] or α_5[94] in combination with a β and γ_2 subunit, which exhibited type II pharmacology. It has been shown that the α subunit contributes significantly to the diversity of the pharmacologic activities observed in GBRCs,[98] but a β and γ_2 subunit are always required to maintain the reproducibility of native receptor function. These studies shed the first light on how the heterogeneity of subunit composition influences benzodiazepine receptor pharmacology. Of considerable interest was the discovery that a single histidine residue in the α subunit is instrumental for the activity of the clinically useful benzodiazepines.[99] Ligand selectivity for specific subunits may be observed even with benzodiazepine compounds that are classified as subtype nonselective. For instance, diazepam binds receptors coexpressing the α_3, a β, and the γ_2 subunits with much higher affinity than those that contain other α subunits.[96] Recent studies have shown that the γ_3 subunit may replace the γ_2 subunit and impart the same properties of bidirectional modulation of the GABA$_A$ receptor by benzodiazepines.[100] Subsequently, Xenopus oocytes injected with only either α or β subunits were found to reconstitute GABA-sensitive ion channels with normal pharmacologic properties.[101] This suggests that the multiple conductance states (i.e., the permeability of the GBRC to chloride ions) observed with GABA$_A$ receptors may be intrinsic to the receptor subunits. Not only has the heterogeneous composition of GBRCs been well established, but evidence has also been reported to suggest the heterogeneity of the allosteric interaction between GABA$_A$ and benzodiazepine receptors.[102] Exciting new data have been published on the use of immunofluorescence staining to identify some of the likely combinations of GBRC subunits in various regions of the brain.[103] These types of studies hold the promise of defining neuronal sensitivity to GABA and its modulators on the basis of subunit composition. More extensive studies on both hetero- and homo-oligomeric receptors are in order to elucidate the underlying mechanism for the apparent heterogeneity among GABA-mediated responses and the physiologic significance of benzodiazepine receptor heterogeneity.

REFERENCES

1. Randall LO: Pharmacology of methaminodiazepoxide. Dis Nerv Syst 21:7, 1960
2. Randall LO, Schallek W, Heise GA et al: The psychosedative properties of methaminodiazepoxide. J Pharmacol Exp Ther 129:163, 1960
3. Lader M: Benzodiazepines, the opium of the masses? Neuroscience 3:159, 1978
4. Rickels K: Benzodiazepines: use and misuse. p. 1. In Klein DF, Rabkin J (eds): Anxiety: New Research and Changing Concepts. Raven Press, New York, 1981
5. Tyrer PF: Benzodiazepines on trial. BMJ 288:1101, 1984
6. Catalan J, Gath DH: Benzodiazepines in general practice: time for a decision. BMJ 290:1374, 1985
7. Costa E, Guidotti A, Mao CC: Evidence for involvement of GABA in the action of benzodiazepines: studies on rat cerebellum. p. 113. In Costa E, Greengard P (eds): Mechanism of Action of Benzodiazepines. Raven Press, New York, 1975
8. Fuxe K, Agnatil LF, Bolme P et al: The possible involvement of GABA mechanisms in the action of benzodiazepines on central catecholamine neurons. p. 45. In Costa E, Greengard P (eds): Mechanism of Action of Benzodiazepines. Raven Press, New York, 1975
9. Haefely W, Kulcsar A, Mohler H et al: Possible involvement of GABA in the central actions of benzodiazepines. p. 131. In Costa E, Greengard P (eds): Mechanism of Action of Benzodiazepines. Raven Press, New York, 1975
10. Squires RF, Braestrup C: Benzodiazepine receptors in rat brain. Nature 266:732, 1977
11. Mohler H, Okada T: Benzodiazepine receptor: demonstration in the central nervous system. Science 198:849, 1977
12. Olsen RW, Venter JC: Benzodiazepine/GABA receptors and chloride channels: structural and functional properties. In Olsen RW, Venter JC (eds): Receptor Biochemistry and Methodology. Vol. 5. Alan R. Liss, New York, 1986
13. Bormann J: Electrophysiology of GABA$_A$ and GABA$_B$ receptor subtypes. Trends Neurosci 11:112, 1988
14. Mugnani E, Oertel WH: An atlas of the distribution of GABAergic neurons and terminals in the rat CNS as revealed by GAD immunohistochemistry. p. 436. In Bjorklund A, Hokfelt T (eds): Handbook of Chemical Neuroanatomy. Vol. 4, Elsevier, Amsterdam, 1985

15. Simmonds MA: Physiological and pharmacological characterization of the actions of GABA. p. 27. In Bowery NG (ed): Actions and Interactions of GABA and Benzodiazepines. Raven Press, New York, 1984

16. Briley MS, Langer SZ: Influence of GABA receptor agonists and antagonists on the binding of ^{3}H-diazepam to the benzodiazepine receptor. Eur J Pharmacol 52:129, 1978

17. Reisine TD, Overstreet D, Gale K et al: Benzodiazepine receptors: the effect of GABA on their characteristics in human brain and their alteration in Huntington's disease. Brain Res 199:79, 1980

18. Snodgrass SR: Receptors for amino acid transmitters. p. 167. In Iversen LL, Iversen SD, Snyder SH (eds): Handbook of Psychopharmacology. Vol. 17. Plenum, New York, 1983

19. Braestrup C, Albrechtsen E, Squires RF: High densities of benzodiazepine receptors in human cortical areas. Nature 269:702, 1977

20. Young WS III, Kuhar MJ: Autoradiographic localization of benzodiazepine receptors in the brains of humans and animals. Nature 280:393, 1979

21. Placheta P, Karobath M: Regional distribution of Na$^+$-independent GABA and benzodiazepine binding sites in rat CNS. Brain Res 178:550, 1979

22. Young WS III, Kuhar MJ: Radiohistochemical localization of benzodiazepine receptors in rat brain. J Pharmacol Exp Ther 212:337, 1980

23. Kuhar MJ: Radiohistochemical localization of benzodiazepine receptors. p. 149. In Usdin E, Skolnick P, Tallman JF et al (eds): Pharmacology of Benzodiazepines. Verlag Chemie, Weinheim, 1983

24. Mohler H, Richards JG: Benzodiazepine receptors in the central nervous system. p. 93. In Costa E (ed): The Benzodiazepines From Molecular Biology to Clinical Practice. Raven Press, New York, 1983

25. Schoch P, Haring P, Takacs B et al: A GABA/benzodiazepine receptor complex from bovine brain: purification, reconstitution and immunological characterization. J Recept Res 4:189, 1984

26. Haring P, Stahli C, Schoch P et al: Monoclonal antibodies reveal structural homogeneity of γ-aminobutyric acid/benzodiazepine receptors in different brain regions. Proc Natl Acad Sci U S A 82:4837, 1985

27. Majewska MD, Harrison NL, Schwartz RD et al: Steroid metabolites are barbiturate-like modulators of the GABA receptor. Science 232:1004, 1986

28. Harrison NL, Majewska MD, Harrington JW, Barker JL: Structure-activity relationships for steroid interaction with the γ-aminobutyric acid-A receptor complex. J Pharmacol Exp Ther 241:346, 1987

29. Gee KW, Brinton RE, Chang WC, McEwen BS: γ-Aminobutyric acid-dependent modulation of the chloride ionophore by steroids in rat brain. Eur J Pharmacol 136:419, 1987

30. Monod J, Wyman J, Changeux J-P: On the nature of allosteric transitions: a plausible model. J Mol Biol 12:88, 1965

31. Weber G: Energetics of ligand binding to proteins. p. 1. In Anfinsen CB, Edsall JT, Richards FM (eds): Advances in Protein Chemistry. Vol. 29. Academic Press, New York, 1975

32. Chang RS, Snyder SH: Benzodiazepine receptors: labelling in intact animals with ^{3}H-flunitrazepam. Eur J Pharmacol 48:213, 1978

33. Tallman JF, Paul SM, Skolnick P, Gallager DW: Receptors for the age of anxiety: pharmacology of the benzodiazepines. Science 270:274, 1980

34. Paul SM, Marangos PJ, Skolnick P: the benzodiazepine-GABA-chloride ionophore receptor complex: common site of minor tranquilizer action. Biol Psychiatry 16:213, 1981

35. Mennini T, Cotecchia S, Caccia S, Garattini S: Benzodiazepines: relationship between pharmacological activity in the rat and *in vivo* receptor binding. Pharmacol Biochem Behav 16:529, 1982

36. Olsen RW: Drug interactions at the GABA receptor ionophore complex. Annu Rev Pharmacol Toxicol 22:245, 1982

37. Skolnick P, Paul SM: Benzodiazepine receptors in the central nervous system. Int Rev Neurobiol 23:103, 1982

38. Brown CL, Martin IL, Jones B, Oakely N: *In vivo* determination of efficacy of pyrazoloquinolinones at the benzodiazepine receptor. Eur J Pharmacol 103:139, 1984

39. Haefely W: Molecular aspects of benzodiazepine receptors and their ligands. p. 658. In Racagni G, Paoletti R, Kielholz P (eds): Clinical Neuropharmacology. Raven Press, New York, 1984

40. Mennini T, Barone D, Gobbi M: *In vivo* interactions of premazepam with benzodiazepine receptors: relation to its pharmacological effects. Psychopharmacology 86:464, 1985

41. Braestrup C, Nielsen M, Olsen CF: Urinary and brain β-carboline-3-carboxylates as potent inhibitors of brain benzodiazepine receptors. Proc Natl Acad Sci U S A 77:2288, 1980

42. Marangos PJ, Paul SM, Greenlaw P et al: Demonstration of an endogenous, competitive inhibitor(s)

of [^{3}H]diazepam binding in bovine brain. Life Sci 22:1893, 1978

43. Skolnick P, Marangos PJ, Goodwin FK et al: Identification of inosine and hypoxanthine as endogenous inhibitors of [^{3}H]diazepam binding in the central nervous system. Life Sci 23:1473, 1978

44. Mohler H, Polc P, Cumin R et al: Nicotinamide is a brain constituent with benzodiazepine-like action. Nature 278:563, 1979

45. Colello GD, Hockenberry DM, Bosmann HB et al: Competitive inhibition of benzodiazepine binding by fractions from porcine brain. Proc Natl Acad Sci U S A 75:6319, 1978

46. Davis LC, Cohen RK: Identification of an endogenous peptide-ligand for the benzodiazepine receptor. Biochem Biophys Res Commun 92:141, 1980

47. Woolf JH, Nixon JC: Endogenous effector of benzodiazepine binding sites: purification and characterization. Biochemistry 20:4263, 1981

48. Massotti M, Guidotti A, Costa E: Characterization of benzodiazepine and γ-aminobutyric acid recognition sites and their endogenous modulators. J Neurosci 1:409, 1981

49. Piva MA, Medina JH, de Blas AL, Pena C: Formation of benzodiazepine-like molecules in rat brain. Biochem Biophys Res Commun 180:972, 1991

50. Rothstein JD, Garland W, Puia G et al: Purification and characterization of naturally occurring benzodiazepine receptor ligands in rat and human brain. J Neurochem 58:2102, 1992

51. Guidotti A, Forchetti CM, Corda MG et al: Isolation, characterization and purification to homogeneity of an endogenous polypeptide with agonistic action on benzodiazepine receptors. Proc Natl Acad Sci U S A 80:3531, 1983

52. Bormann J, Ferrero P, Guidotti A, Costa E: Neuropeptide modulation at GABA receptor Cl$^-$ channels. Regul Pept 4:33, 1985

53. Bormann J: Electrophysiological characterization of diazepam binding inhibitor (DBI) on GABA$_A$ receptors. Neuropharmacology 30:1387, 1991

54. Alho H, Costa E, Ferrero P et al: Diazepam-binding inhibitor: a neuropeptide located in selected neuronal populations of rat brain. Science 229:179, 1985

55. Costa E, Guidotti A: Neuropeptides are cotransmitters: modulatory effects at GABAergic synapses. p. 425. In Meltzer HY (ed): Psychopharmacology, the Third Generation of Progress. Raven Press, New York, 1987

56. Ferrarese C, Appollonio I, Frigo M et al: Distribution of a putative endogenous modulator of the GABAergic system in human brain. Neurology 39:443, 1989

57. Bovolin P, Schlichting M, Miyata C et al: Distribution and characterization of diazepam binding inhibitor (DBI) in peripheral tissues of rat. Regul Pept 29:267, 1990

58. Guidotti A, Alho H, Berkovich A et al: DBI processing: allosteric modulation at different GABA/benzodiazepine receptor subtypes. p. 100. In Barnard EA, Costa E (eds): Allosteric Modulation of Amino Acid Receptors: Therapeutic Implications. Raven Press, New York, 1989

59. Ferero P, Santi MR, Conti-Tronconi B et al: Study of an octadecaneuropeptide derived from diazepam binding inhibitor (DBI): biological activity and presence in rat brain. Proc Natl Acad Sci U S A 83:827, 1986

60. Slobodyansky E, Guidotti A, Wambebe C et al: Isolation and characterization of a rat brain triakonta-tetraneuropeptide, a posttranslational product of diazepam binding inhibitor: specific action at the Ro5-4864 recognition site. J Neurochem 53:1276, 1989

61. Morrow AL, Paul SM: Benzodiazepine enhancement of γ-aminobutyric acid-mediated chloride ion flux in rat brain synaptoneurosomes. J Neurochem 50:302, 1988

62. Gee KW, Yamamura HI: Selective anxiolytics: are the actions related to partial "agonist" activity or a preferential affinity for benzodiazepine receptor subtypes. p. 1. In Biggio G, Costa E (eds): Benzodiazepine Recognition Site Ligands: Biochemistry and Pharmacology. Raven Press, New York, 1983

63. Keim KL, Sullivan JW, Anderson C et al: Neuropharmacologic and anticonflict benzodiazepine agonist effects of CGS 9896: possible rat/mouse species differences. Fed Proc 43:930, 1984

64. Bernard PS, Bennett DA, Paster G et al: CGS 9896: agonist-antagonist benzodiazepine receptor activity revealed by anxiolytic, anticonvulsant and muscle relaxation assessment in rodents. J Pharmacol Exp Ther 235:98, 1985

65. Morel E, Perrault G, Sanger DJ, Zivkovic B: Diazepam antagonist effects of the pyrazoloquinoline CGS 9896. Br J Pharmacol 88:295P, 1986

66. Suzdak PD, Glowa JR, Crawley JN et al: A selective imidazobenzodiazepine antagonist of ethanol in the rat. Science 234:1243, 1986

67. Boast CA, Bernard PS, Barbaz BS, Bergen KM: The neuropharmacology of various diazepam antagonists. Neuropharmacology 22:1511, 1983

68. Flumazenil (editorial). Lancet 2:828, 1988
69. Skolnick P, Paul S, Crawley J et al: 3-Hydroxymethyl-β-carboline antagonizes some pharmacologic effects of diazepam. Eur J Pharmacol 69:525, 1981
70. Cain M, Weber RW, Guzman F et al: β-Carbolines: synthesis and neurochemical and pharmacological actions on brain benzodiazepine receptors. J Med Chem 25:1081, 1982
71. Morin A, Tanaka I, Wasterlain C: Norharmane inhibition of [³H]diazepam binding in mouse brain. Life Sci 28:2257, 1981
72. Cowen P, Green A, Nutt D, Martin I: Ethyl-β-carboline-3-carboxylate lowers seizure threshold and antagonizes flurazepam-induced sedation in rats. Nature 290:54, 1981
73. Mendelson WB, Cain M, Cook JM et al: Do benzodiazepine receptors play a role in sleep regulation? Studies with the benzodiazepine antagonist, 3-hydroxymethyl-β-carboline (3-HMC). p. 253. In: Proceedings of a workshop held at The Salk Institute organized by Floyd Bloom, Jack Barchas, Merton Sandler, Earl Usdin: Beta-Carbolines and Tetrahydroisoquinolones. Alan R. Liss, New York, 1982
74. Skolnick P, Williams EF, Cook JM et al: β-Carbolines and benzodiazepine receptors: structure-activity relationships and pharmacologic activity. p. 233. In: Proceedings of a workshop held at The Salk Institute organized by Floyd Bloom, Jack Barchas, Merton Sandler, Earl Usdin: Beta-Carbolines and Tetrahydroisoquinolones. Alan R, Liss, New York, 1982
75. Braestrup C, Squires RF: Specific benzodiazepine receptors in rat brain characterized by high affinity [³H]diazepam binding. Proc Natl Acad Sci U S A 74:3805, 1977
76. Braestrup C, Squires RF: Brain specific benzodiazepine receptors. Br J Psychiatry 133:249, 1978
77. Squires RF, Benson DI, Braestrup C et al: Some properties of brain specific benzodiazepine receptors: new evidence for multiple receptors. Pharmacol Biochem Behav 10:825, 1979
78. Costa T, Rodbard D, Pert C: Is the benzodiazepine receptor coupled to a chloride anion channel? Nature 277:315, 1979
79. Squires RF, Naquet R, Riche D, Braestrup C: Increased thermolability of benzodiazepine receptors in cerebral cortex of a baboon with spontaneous seizures: a case report. Epilepsia 20:215, 1979
80. Chiu TH, Dryden DM, Rosenberg HC: Kinetics of [³H]flunitrazepam binding to membrane-bound benzodiazepine receptors. Mol Pharmacol 21:57, 1982
81. Speth RC, Wastek GJ, Johnson PC, Yamamura HI: Benzodiazepine binding in human brain: characterization using ³H-flunitrazepam. Life Sci 22:859, 1978
82. Nielsen M, Braestrup C: Ethyl β-carboline-3-carboxylate shows differential benzodiazepine receptor interaction. Nature 286:606, 1980
83. Ehlert FJ, Roeske WR, Yamamura HI: Multiple benzodiazepine receptors and their regulation by γ-aminobutyric acid. Life Sci 29:235, 1981
84. Nielsen M, Schou H, Braestrup C: [³H]Propyl β-carboline-3-carboxylate binds specifically to brain benzodiazepine receptors. J Neurochem 36:276, 1981
85. Klepner CA, Lippa AS, Benson DI et al: Resolution of two biochemically and pharmacologically distinct benzodiazepine receptors. Pharmacol Biochem Behav 11:457, 1979
86. Lippa AS, Coupet J, Greenblatt EN et al: A synthetic non-benzodiazepine ligand for benzodiazepine receptors: a probe for investigating neuronal substrates of anxiety. Pharmacol Biochem Behav 11:99, 1979
87. Lippa AS, Critchett DJ, Sano MC et al: Benzodiazepine receptors: cellular and behavioral characteristics. Pharmacol Biochem Behav 10:831, 1979
88. Gee KW, Yamamura HI: Regional heterogeneity of benzodiazepine receptors at 37°C: an *in vitro* study in various regions of the rat brain. Life Sci 31:1939, 1982
89. Dennis T, Dubois A, Benavides J, Scatton B: Distribution of central ω1 (benzodiazepine₁) and ω2 (benzodiazepine₂) receptor subtypes in the monkey and human brain. An autoradiographic study with [³H]flunitrazepam and the ω1 selective ligand [³H]zolpidem. J Pharmacol Exp Ther 247:309, 1988
90. Perrault G, Morel E, Sanger DJ, Zivkovic B: Differences in pharmacological profiles of a new generation of benzodiazepine and non-benzodiazepine hypnotics. Eur J Pharmacol 187:487, 1990
91. Sieghart W, Karobath M: Molecular heterogeneity of benzodiazepine receptors. Nature 286:285, 1980
92. Sigel E, Stephenson RA, Mamalaki C, Barnard EA: A γ-aminobutyric acid/benzodiazepine receptor complex of bovine cerebral cortex. Purification and partial characterization. J Biol Chem 258:6965, 1983
93. Schofield PR, Darlison MG, Fujita N et al: Sequence and functional expression of the GABA_A receptor

shows a ligand-gated receptor superfamily. Nature 328:221, 1987

94. Pritchett DB, Sontheimer H, Shivers B et al: Importance of a novel GABA$_A$ receptor subunit for benzodiazepine pharmacology. Nature 338:582, 1989

95. Levitan ES, Schofield PR, Burt DR et al: Structural and functional basis for GABA$_A$ receptor heterogeneity. Nature 335:76, 1988

96. Pritchett DB, Luddens H, Seeburg PH: Type I and type II GABA$_A$-benzodiazepine receptors produced in transfected cells. Science 245:1389, 1989

97. Pritchett DB, Seeburg PH: γ-Aminobutyric acid$_A$ receptor α5-subunit creates novel type II benzodiazepine receptor pharmacology. J Neurochem 54:1802, 1990

98. Luddens H, Wisden W: Function and pharmacology of multiple GABA$_A$ receptor subunits. Trends Pharmacol Sci 12:49, 1991

99. Weiland HA, Luddens H, Seeburg PH: A single histidine in GABA$_A$ receptor is essential for benzodiazepine agonist binding. J Biol Chem 267:1426, 1992

100. Knoflach F, Rhyner T, Villa M et al: The γ3-subunit of the GABA$_A$-receptor confers sensitivity to benzodiazepine receptor ligands. FEBS Lett 293:191, 1991

101. Blair LAC, Levitan ES, Marshall J et al: Single subunits of the GABA$_A$ receptor form ion channels with properties of the native receptor. Science 242:577, 1988

102. Ruano D, Vizuete M, Cano J et al: Heterogeneity in the allosteric interaction between the γ-aminobutyric acid (GABA) binding site and three different benzodiazepine binding sites of the GABA$_A$/benzodiazepine receptor complex in the rat nervous system. J Neurochem 58:485, 1992

103. Fritschy J-M, Benke D, Mertens S et al: Five subtypes of type A γ-aminobutyric acid receptors identified in neurons by double and triple immunofluorescence staining with subunit-specific antibodies. Proc Natl Acad Sci U S A 89:6727, 1992

104. Haefely W, Kyburz E, Gerecke M, Mohler H: Recent advances in the molecular pharmacology of benzodiazepine receptors and in the structure-activity relationships of their agonists and antagonists. Adv Drug Res 14:165, 1985

105. Braestrup C, Nielsen M: Benzodiazepine receptors. p. 285. In Iversen LL, Inversen SD, Snyder SH (eds): Handbook of Psychopharmacology. Vol. 17. Plenum, New York, 1983

106. Gee KW: Steroid modulation of the GABA/benzodiazepine receptor-linked chloride ionophore. Mol Neurobiol 2:291, 1988

107. Olsen RW, Tobin AJ: Molecular biology of GABA$_A$ receptors. FASEB J 4:1469, 1990

108. Schwartz RD: The GABA$_A$ receptor-gated ion channel: biochemical and pharmacological studies of structure and function. Biochem Pharmacol 37:3369, 1988

Chapter 11

Pharmacokinetics of Benzodiazepines

Randall B. Smith, Sharon E. Corey, and Patricia D. Kroboth

Benzodiazepines are among the most frequently prescribed drugs. Alprazolam, for instance, ranks third in the number of new and refill prescriptions and fifth overall on the list of top 200 drugs compiled by IMS America.[1] Currently, there are fifteen benzodiazepines marketed in the United States. All of the benzodiazepines have pharmacologic effects caused by depression of central nervous system (CNS) activity: reduction of anxiety, increased sedation, anterograde amnesia, anticonvulsant effects, and muscle relaxation. Despite the commonality of pharmacologic effects, the benzodiazepines differ in their pharmacokinetic and pharmacodynamic profiles. These differences have resulted in the development of benzodiazepines for different indications. Of the available benzodiazepines, a few predominate in importance for anesthesiology. Thus, the focus of this chapter is on diazepam, lorazepam, and midazolam.

Benzodiazepine effects appear to result almost entirely from reversible interactions with the γ-amino butyric acid (GABA)$_A$ benzodiazepine receptor complex in the CNS. The time course of benzodiazepine binding to the GABA receptor complex is determined by the time course of benzodiazepine concentration in the CNS, the number of receptor units, and the affinity of the benzodiazepine for the receptor. A good correlation between the dose required for anxiolysis and the GABA receptor affinity of various benzodiazepines has been reported.[2] Very little is known about receptor changes due to age, disease states, or other patient factors. There is some evidence of increased concentration of GABA$_A$ benzodiazepine receptors in severe hepatic disease based on ^{11}C-flumazenil binding measured by positron emission tomography (PET).[3] Animal studies have demonstrated both increases and decreases in benzodiazepine binding during chronic administration that could account for observations of development of tolerance and for withdrawal symptoms.[4-6]

Factors affecting benzodiazepine plasma concentrations have been studied more extensively than either pharmacodynamics or receptor pharmacology in humans. Benzodiazepine plasma concentrations are linearly related to dose over the clinically relevant range of doses. Benzodiazepines are bound to plasma proteins to a variable extent, ranging from 40 to 97 percent bound, and the binding is independent of concentration. All benzodiazepines are eliminated from the body by metabolism and subsequent elimination in the urine. With the exception of lorazepam, the benzodiazepines discussed herein undergo oxidative metabolism; lorazepam is metabolized by conjugation with glucuronic acid.

Benzodiazepine pharmacokinetics can be affected by patient characteristics such as age, body habitus, disease states such as cirrhosis, and interactions with concomitantly administered medications. Almost all these alterations are a result of effects on oxidative drug metabolism. Lorazepam is less susceptible to many of these effects because it does not undergo oxidative metabolism.

Drug concentration is generally a better predictor of extent of response than is drug dose since it provides a better estimate of drug available to interact with receptors. Establishing a relationship between drug concentration and pharmacologic effect also permits a better understanding of the time course of drug effects. The effect-concentration relationships have been evaluated in many different ways, ranging from simple observations of drug concentrations as an event occurs to complex pharmacokinetic-pharmacodynamic models.[7-10]

In contrast to the time course of plasma concentrations, the time course of benzodiazepine anxiolytic or hypnotic effects are relatively difficult to study. Most attention has been directed at measuring CNS depression. These effects can be detected by changes in psychomotor test performance, observer-rated sedation, self-rated sedation, various memory tests, critical flicker fusion threshold, saccadic eye velocity, driving simulator results, and electroencephalogram (EEG). In some cases such as psychomotor performance tests, saccadic eye velocity, and others, the measurements are surrogates for the clinical end point of interest (e.g., anxiolysis) and it is sometimes difficult to relate the results to clinical situations. Other tests such as

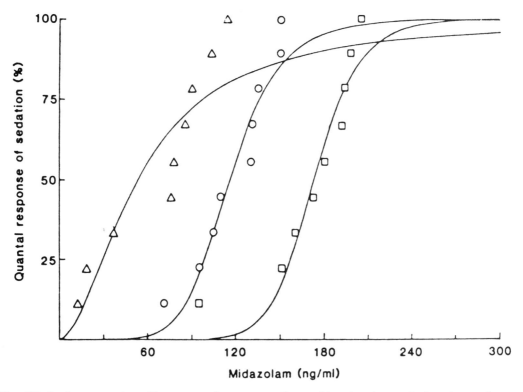

Fig. 11-1 Concentration-effect curves for recovery from midazolam in surgical patients who received midazolam to induce and maintain sleep during epidural anesthesia. *Squares,* ability to give name and birth date; *circles,* the step from arousable to drowsy, *triangles,* the step from drowsy to awake. (From Persson et al.,[12] with permission.)

memory tests may relate directly to the clinical use of the drugs to reduce recall of noxious procedures.

PHARMACOKINETIC AND PHARMACODYNAMIC RELATIONSHIPS

Some investigators have suggested that the time course of benzodiazepine plasma concentrations may not always correspond to the time course of drug effects. For example, ex vivo studies of benzodiazepine receptor binding in rats suggested that the relatively long duration of action of lorazepam might be due to slow dissociation from benzodiazepine receptors.[3] However, other evidence supports a close relationship between plasma concentrations and pharmacologic effects, especially for midazolam and diazepam. Miller et al.[11] studied benzodiazepine receptor occupancy in mice and con-

cluded that brain concentrations of clonazepam and lorazepam declined in parallel with plasma concentrations and that receptor occupancy was related to brain concentrations by a sigmoidal function. Persson et al.[12] studied surgical patients and found a close relationship between sedation or amnesia and midazolam plasma concentrations (Figs. 11-1 and 11-2). Studies of volunteers, utilizing EEG as a measure of benzodiazepine effect, found relationships between midazolam and diazepam plasma concentrations and EEG effects that could be fit to sigmoid E_{max} pharmacodynamic models, further supporting a close relationship between plasma concentrations and drug effects.[13,14]

Effect of Plasma Protein Binding

Lorazepam, diazepam, and midazolam are highly bound to plasma protein, primarily albumin. The "free drug hypothesis" predicts that drug effects should be related to the concentration of unbound

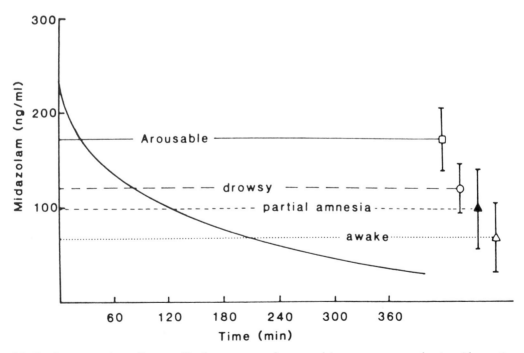

Fig. 11-2 Concentration-effect profile for recovery from total intravenous anesthesia with continuous infusions of midazolam and alfentanil. The mean (±SD) concentrations associated with various end points are shown. (From Persson et al.,[12] with permission.)

drug in plasma, because the unbound drug is able to diffuse into the central nervous system, while the bound drug is restricted to the plasma. Several studies have provided evidence that the free drug hypothesis applies to benzodiazepines[15] (Fig. 11-3). In a study of particular relevance to the use of benzodiazepines as induction agents, Reves et al.[16] demonstrated a statistically significant positive correlation between serum albumin concentration and the time required for loss of lid reflex following a bolus dose of midazolam.

Effect of Metabolites

The relationship between plasma drug concentrations and drug effects becomes more complex when there are active metabolites. Midazolam is metabolized in humans primarily to α-hydroxymidazolam (1-hydroxymidazolam), which is nearly as

potent as midazolam itself[17,18] (Fig. 11-4) when comparisons are based on total plasma concentrations (plasma protein bound plus unbound). When potency is determined from unbound plasma concentrations, midazolam is about five times more potent than the metabolite, but a lesser degree of plasma protein binding of the metabolite compensates almost exactly for the difference in absolute potency.[18] Following bolus intravenous administration of midazolam, plasma concentrations of the metabolite are relatively low and the effects attributable to α-hydroxymidazolam appear to be small, perhaps 10 percent of total benzodiazepine activity. However, after oral administration of midazolam, the substantial first pass clearance results in relatively higher concentrations of α-hydroxymidazolam, and under this circumstance, the activity of the metabolite is substantial.[18] The major metabo-

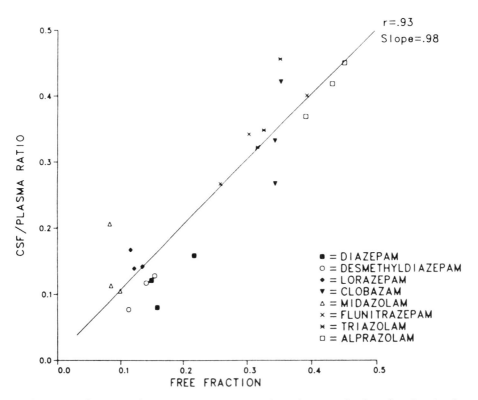

Fig. 11-3 The ratio of CSF to plasma concentration is plotted versus the free fraction in plasma for various benzodiazepines, following intravenous administration to cats. Lesser plasma protein binding (higher free fraction) is associated with enhanced entry of drug into CSF (higher CSF/plasma ratio). (From Arendt et al.,[15] with permission.)

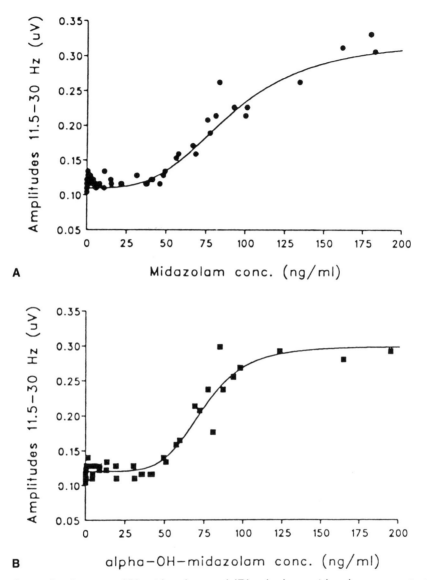

Fig. 11-4 Relationship between **(A)** midazolam and **(B)** α-hydroxymidazolam concentrations and EEG effects after intravenous administration of either drug to a single volunteer. The concentration-effect curve for the metabolite is virtually identical to that of the parent drug. (From Mandema et al.,[18] with permission.)

lite of diazepam is nordiazepam, which has pharmacologic activity comparable to diazepam itself. Following administration of an intravenous bolus of diazepam the concentrations of nordiazepam are relatively low, and Greenblatt et al.[14] found that effects attributable to nordiazepam were insignifi-

cant in a pharmacodynamic model of EEG effects. However, under circumstances of multiple or continuous dosing, steady-state desmethyldiazepam concentrations are equal to or greater than those of diazepam.[19] Lorazepam probably has no active metabolites.

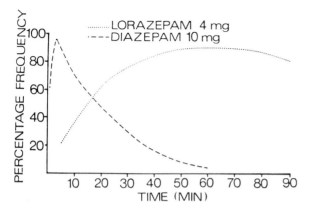

Fig. 11-5 Prevalence of loss of the ability to recall objects at time intervals following intravenous administration of lorazepam or diazepam. Lorazepam has a very slow onset of action relative to diazepam, requiring as long as 1 hour to produce amnesia. (From Dundee et al.,[20] with permission.)

Speed of Onset

Pharmacodynamic studies utilizing EEG effects have shown that diazepam has a speed of onset two to three times faster than midazolam, although both drugs have a rapid onset, with peak effects occurring within a few minutes of intravenous administration. Lorazepam has a much slower speed of onset, based on studies of the onset of amnestic effects[20] (Fig. 11-5). Peak effects of lorazepam may

be delayed for as long as 1 hour following intravenous administration. The explanation for the differences in speed of onset between the drugs is uncertain. Lorazepam is less lipid-soluble (octanol:buffer partition coefficient = 240) than midazolam (475) or diazepam (820), however Arendt et al.[15] found that lipophilicity was not significantly correlated to the rate of entry of benzodiazepines into the brains of cats.[15] However, Arendt et al.[21] did find a correlation between HPLC retention index (a measure of lipophilicity that is an alternative to the octanol:buffer partition coefficient) and entry of benzodiazepines into rat brain. Jack et al.[3] have suggested that slow association with benzodiazepine receptors may explain the slow speed of onset of lorazepam.

The diazepine ring of midazolam opens in acidic solution with pH less than 4, greatly enhancing water solubility (Fig. 11-6). At physiologic pH of 7.4 and temperature of 37°C the diazepine ring closes, resulting in a highly lipid soluble moiety (n-octanol:pH 7.5 buffer partition coefficient = 475) that will rapidly traverse the blood-brain barrier. However, ring closure is slow, with a half-life of about 10 minutes.[22] It is interesting to speculate whether the rate-limiting step in onset of midazolam after intravenous injection is diazepine ring closure. This might explain the relatively slower onset of midzolam relative to diazepam.

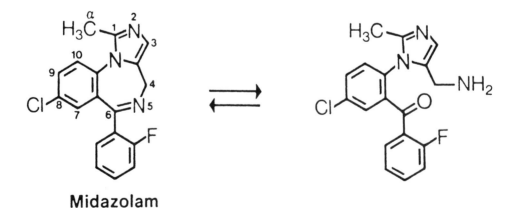

Midazolam

Fig. 11-6 At pH less than about 4, midazolam exists primarily in the ring-opened form (*right*), which is quite water soluble. At physiologic pH, the ring closes (*left*), yielding a highly lipid-soluble molecule with an n-octanol:phosphate buffer partition coefficient of 475 (pH = 7.5). (From Pieri et al.,[22] with permission.)

Duration of Action

The duration of effects is longest for lorazepam, intermediate for diazepam, and shortest for midazolam. The duration of effect of midazolam and diazepam following intravenous bolus administration is determined primarily by distribution, as with thiopental and other lipid-soluble intravenous anesthetics. The distribution of diazepam is considerably slower than midazolam and probably accounts for its relatively longer duration of action. Diazepam has a rapid distribution phase with a half-life of 10 to 15 minutes, but this is followed by a slower distribution phase with a half-life of 1 to 2 hours. Although diazepam has a very long terminal elimination half-life of at least 20 hours, this is not particularly relevant to the duration of action following an intravenous bolus dose. The longer duration of action of lorazepam is not readily explained by pharmacokinetic properties. Distribution of lorazepam is rapid with a half-life similar to that of midazolam. The elimination half-life is relatively long (10 to 20 hours) but shorter than that of diazepam. Arendt et al.[15] observed that duration of EEG effects were longest for less lipophilic benzodiazepines with smaller volumes of distribution[15]; however, the mechanistic basis for this observation is unclear. Slow dissociation of lorazepam from benzodiazepine receptors has been proposed as the explanation for the longer duration of action,[3] but this has been disputed.[11]

PHARMACOKINETICS OF INDIVIDUAL BENZODIAZEPINES

Midazolam

Among the major characteristics that distinguish midazolam from other benzodiazepines are its pH-dependent water solubility (pH $\leq$ 4),[22] which obviates the need for propylene glycol to solubilize the drug in the injectable formulation. This results in less irritation after intravenous administration than occurs with diazepam. At physiologic pH, midazolam is extremely lipid soluble and thus easily passes through lipid membranes,[23] this property contributes to its rapid onset of action and large volume of distribution.

Midazolam has a short distribution half-life,[24]

high plasma clearance short elimination half-life, and correspondingly short duration of action after a single intravenous dose.[25] Representative values for midazolam pharmacokinetic parameter estimates in healthy subjects are shown in Table 11-1.[26,27]

Midazolam is cleared almost exclusively by metabolism, primarily to 1-hydroxy-, 4-hydroxy-, and 1,4-dihydroxy-midazolam; less than 1 percent is excreted in urine as unchanged drug.[25] These hydroxylated metabolites are then conjugated and subsequently eliminated in urine. The 1-hydroxy metabolite is detectable in plasma at concentrations 40 to 100 percent of those of parent drug and is pharmacologically active at the GABA-benzodiazepine receptor complex. Thus, 1-hydroxy-midazolam concentrations exceeding 60 ng/ml must be taken into account when examining concentration-effect relationships.[18,28]

Midazolam pharmacokinetics have been studied in numerous special populations. Pharmacokinetic parameter estimates for these populations are provided in Table 11-2. The volume of distribution (V_d) is increased in pregnancy, renal insufficiency, age, and obesity; women tend to have a greater volume of distribution than men. Clearance is reduced in both elderly men and women after intramuscular or intravenous injections and elimination half-life is increased.[29–31] In obese subjects, the half-life of midazolam was prolonged from a mean of 2.7 to 8.4 hours, due to a decreased clearance (normalized for body weight) and an increased volume of distribution. In subjects with cirrhosis of

Table 11-1 Benzodiazepine Pharmacokinetic Parameter Estimates in Young Healthy Subjects

	$t_{1/2}$ (h)	V_d (l/kg)	Cl (ml/min/kg)	% Bound
Midazolam	1–5	0.4–2.0	4.0–8.0	95
Diazepam	20–40	0.7–1.2	0.25–0.5	97
Lorazepam	10–20	0.7–1.0	0.80–1.3	88–92
Triazolam	1–5	0.6–0.9	2.3–4.1(IV) 6.2–8.0(PO)	85–90
Alprazolam	9–15	0.5–0.9	0.5–2.0	70
Flumazenil	0.7–1.3	0.6–1.6	8.0–16.0	54–64

Table 11-2 Pharmacokinetics of Midazolam

Patient Population	Dose of Midazolam	$t_{1/2}$ h	Cl ml/min/kg	V_d l/kg	Reference
Young					
Men	5 mg IV	2.1	7.75	1.34	29
Women	5 mg IV	2.6	9.39	2.00	29
Elderly					
Men	5 mg IV	5.6	4.41	1.64	29
Women	5 mg IV	4.0	7.5	2.11	29
Adult					
Normal	5 mg IV	2.73	8.06	1.74	29
Obese	5 mg IV	8.40	4.21	2.66	29
Adult					
Normal	0.2 mg/kg	4.93	6.74	2.18	30
Chronic renal Failure	0.2 mg/kg	4.58	11.40	3.79	30
Young					
Men	7.5 mg IM	1.4	5.74	0.72	31
Women	7.5 mg IM	1.8	6.73	1.5	31
Elderly					
Men	7.5 mg IM	3.3	3.88	1.7	24
Women	7.5 mg IM	3.6	5.59	1.9	24
Adult					
Normal	0.075 mg/kg	1.6	10.4	1.3	32
Cirrhotics	0.075 mg/kg	3.9	5.4	1.5	32

the liver clearance is decreased.[32] Since midazolam is metabolized by the liver, chronic renal failure does not alter midazolam elimination half-life. Midazolam clearance is reduced by cimetidine, which inhibits hepatic metabolic enzymes.

Midazolam is 94 to 96 percent bound to proteins in plasma. The unbound fraction has been reported to increase in chronic renal failure without an increase in the clearance of unbound midazolam. Smoking, age, obesity, and gender do not affect the fraction of midazolam bound to plasma proteins.

Several studies have examined midazolam pharmacokinetics in surgical patients. In general, surgery has little effect on the distribution and elimination of midazolam.[27] When midazolam kinetics were affected elimination half-life was generally increased. There have been reports that a small percentage of surgical patients (5 to 8 percent) have $t_{1/2}$ greater than 8 hours, suggesting polymorphic metabolism with a group of poor metabolizers. Subse-

quent studies in sparteine (CYP2D6) phenotyped subjects failed to support this hypothesis.

The hepatic clearance of midazolam is approximately 50 percent of hepatic blood flow; thus, factors such as body position that alter hepatic flow may alter midazolam clearance. This high hepatic clearance is associated with a significant first pass presystemic metabolism of midazolam after oral administration and consequently only 35 to 40 percent of an oral midazolam dose is systemically available.

Table 11-3 summarizes reported EC_{50} values for midazolam using psychomotor performance tests or EEG parameters as the effect measure. Buhrer and co-workers[33] report that the EC_{50} values determined by these surrogate end points are very similar to concentrations reported for clinically relevant events on emergence from anesthesia.[12] There are no reports of pharmacodynamic modeling of midazolam effects and concentrations in elderly or other special populations.

Table 11-3 Midazolam EC_{50} Estimates From Pharmacodynamic Modeling of EEG and Psychomotor Performance Measures and Midazolam Plasma Concentrations

Pharmacologic Parameter	EC_{50} (ng/ml)	Reference
EEG %13–30 hz	35.2	26
EEG power α band	42.6	29
EEG av. amplitude (11.5 to 30 hz)	77	49
EEG voltage (uV)	152	28
Reaction time test	104	30
Tracing test	171	30
Saccadic eye measures	40	49

Diazepam

The pharmacokinetics of diazepam have been the subject of numerous reviews.[34,35] Representative values for diazepam Cl, volume of distribution (V_d) and elimination $t_{1/2}$ are shown in Table 11-4. After intravenous administration there is rapid distribution of diazepam to the CNS, as evidenced by the fast onset of CNS effects, which then decline due to redistribution of diazepam on other tissues. Diazepam concentrations decline by 50 percent during this distribution phase. Postdistribution diazepam concentration decline with a relatively long half-life. During chronic oral administration, diazepam clearance is the primary determinant of diazepam steady-state concentrations and the extent and duration of CNS effects.

Table 11-4 Diazepam Pharmacokinetic Parameter Estimates

Population	$t_{1/2}$ (h)	V_d (l/kg)	Cl (ml/min/kg)
Young, healthy	20–60	0.7–1.2	0.5
Elderly			
Men	98	1.8	0.24
Women	71	2.64	0.48
Hepatic disease	>100	1.74	0.25

(Data from Greenblatt et al.[34] and Kaplan and Jack.[35])

Diazepam is eliminated by hepatic oxidative metabolism. It undergoes direct N-demethylation to form nordiazepam, its major metabolite. After multiple doses of diazepam or continuous diazepam administration, nordiazepam plasma concentrations are very similar to diazepam concentrations; both parent and metabolite contribute to the observed pharmacologic effects.[19]

Diazepam clearance is decreased when hepatic metabolic capacity is diminished due to age, hepatic disease, or drug interactions with inhibitors of drug metabolism such as cimetidine (Table 11-4). The decrease in clearance can result in much higher steady-state diazepam plasma concentrations. The elimination half-life of diazepam increases linearly with age primarily because volume of distribution increases linearly with age. Greenblatt and co-workers[34] have shown that diazepam binding to plasma proteins decreases in elderly subjects and that the clearance of unbound diazepam is about one-half that of young subjects. Thus, unbound diazepam concentrations will be higher at steady state in elderly subjects. Diazepam elimination half-life is also prolonged in obese subjects due to an increase in volume of distribution; clearance is not changed. In obese subjects, therefore, steady-state concentrations will not be significantly different but will be achieved much later than in normal weight subjects. It will also take longer for diazepam levels to decline after dosing is discontinued.

After oral administration, diazepam is rapidly and completely absorbed with peak concentrations occurring about 1 hour after administration. Although intramuscular administration of diazepam has been described, absorption is erratic.

Several studies have examined the relationship between diazepam anxiolytic effects and plasma concentrations. Dasberg and co-workers[36] suggested that the anxiolytic effects are directly related to diazepam steady-state concentrations and that about 400 ng/ml is a minimum effective level. Other workers have reported EEG changes with diazepam concentrations of 100 ng/ml.[37] Diazepam levels of 400 to 500 ng/ml have been recommended as the minimum effective concentration range in convulsive disorders.[38] Effects of diazepam on psychomotor performance and other surrogate measures of CNS depression have not shown a clear relationship to diazepam or diazepam plus nordiazepam plasma concentrations.[39,40]

Diazepam effects on EEG after intravenous administration have been related to diazepam plasma concentrations using pharmacodynamic models.[14] The EC_{50} for diazepam effects on EEG power in the 13 to 30 Hz range was found to be 269 ng/ml.[14] Midazolam was also studied and found to be approximately seven times more potent than diazepam with an EC_{50} of 35 ng/ml, reflecting differences in GABA receptor affinity. Buhrer and co-workers[33,41] found the EC_{50} of diazepam to be 958 ± 200 ng/ml, using a different EEG endpoint. The significantly higher EC_{50} in their study was most likely due to the evaluation of a greater degree of CNS depression than was reported in wakeful subjects. Buhrer and co-workers[33] reported a similar difference between diazepam and midazolam, with midazolam being about 5 times more potent.

Jack and co-workers[3] have used a pharmacokinetic-pharmacodynamic model to describe the relationship between amnestic effects and plasma concentrations of diazepam and lorazepam. They found that the EC_{50} for diazepam and lorazepam were 235 ng/ml and 3.1 ng/ml, respectively. The approximately seven times greater EC_{50} for diazepam is partially due to the difference in the Ki inhibition constants for inhibition of flunitrazepam binding to benzodiazepine receptor sites, 27.4 nM and 1.1 nM for diazepam and lorazepam, respectively. Based on the model, Jack et al.[3] concluded that the duration of action of benodiazepines with high receptor affinity, such as lorazepam, would be longer than predicted based on plasma concentrations. The duration of action of benzodiazepines with affinities equal or less than diazepam would be adequately predicted by plasma concentrations.

Lorazepam

Lorazepam is qualitatively similar to diazepam in its pharmacologic effects but differs in pharmacokinetic properties. Lorazepam is not oxidately metabolized to a significant extent. It is metabolized by conjugation and subsequently eliminated in urine. Its pharmacokinetics have been included in numerous reviews of benzodiazepine kinetics[40,41] and its pharmacokinetic parameters are shown in Table 11-1.

Lorazepam has a relatively short distribution half-life after intravenous administration, with plasma concentrations falling to 50 percent of the peak concentration in the first hour after administration. Lorazepam plasma concentrations then decline during the elimination phase, with a half-life of 10 to 20 hours. The metabolism and elimination of lorazepam is little affected by hepatic disease, renal disease, or concomitant drugs that inhibit drug metabolism. There are no active metabolites.

Lorazepam is well absorbed after intramuscular injection and oral administration with peak plasma concentrations occurring 1 to 1.5 hours after dosing.

Onset of activity after intravenous administration of lorazepam is much slower than that of diazepam.[43] Lorazepam effects do not reach their peak until about 30 to 60 minutes after dosing. This is apparently a result of slower distribution of lorazepam into the CNS due to lower lipid solubility. The effects of lorazepam are longer lasting than those of diazepam as discussed above. There have been few reports of pharmacodynamic modeling of lorazepam CNS effects and concentrations. Examination of plots of changes in EEG (percent 13 to 30 Hz activity) and lorazepam concentrations after intravenous administration suggest that the EC_{50} for lorazepam is about one-tenth that of diazepam or about 25 to 35 ng/ml for lorazepam.[44] This value is very similar to that reported in a previous study, which concluded that a concentration of 30 ng/ml is required for amnestic, sedative, and anxiolytic effects after oral administration in surgical patients.

Flumazenil

Flumazenil is a specific benzodiazepine antagonist that selectively reverses benzodiazepine-induced CNS depression. Its pharmacokinetic properties and potential uses have recently been reviewed.[45,46] Flumazenil interacts with the GABA-benzodiazepine receptor complex and competitively displaces agonist benzodiazepines. Flumazenil probably has some partial agonist activity; however, this has not been apparent in clinical use.[47] Flumazenil has nu-

Table 11-5 Duration of the Antagonistic Activity of Flumazenil on the Effect of Some Benzodiazepine Derivatives in Healthy Subjects

Agonist	Dose of flumazenil	Duration of antagonistic activity (hrs)
3-Methylclonazepam 6 mg orally	200 mg orally	2.5
3-Methylclonazepam 12 mg orally	200 mg orally	2.5
3-Methylclonazepam 35 mg orally	20 mg IV	3–4
Diazepam 40 mg orally	200 mg orally	6
Flunitrazepam 2 mg/70 kg IV	0.15 mg/kg IV	2
Steady-state midazolam concentration 55 ± 11 μg/L	2.5 mg IV	2–3
Steady-state midazolam concentration mean 0.6 mg/L	10 mg IV	2–2.5

merous potential uses including treatment of benzodiazepine intoxication, differential diagnosis of intoxications and coma, and reversal of excessive postoperative sedation from benzodiazepines.

Flumazenil has a very rapid onset, reversing benzodiazepine effects in minutes, but a short duration of effect, which is a result of its pharmacokinetic profile. Representative pharmacokinetic parameter estimates for flumazenil are shown in Table 11-1. Flumazenil is oxidatively metabolized by N-demethylation and hydrolysis of the ester with subsequent glucuronidation and excretion in urine. It has a relatively high total plasma clearance and subsequently is subject to extensive first-pass presystemic metabolism after oral administration; only about 15 percent of an oral dose is systemically available. A large volume of distribution indicates a rapid and extensive tissue uptake after flumazenil administration. Rapid uptake of flumazenil in the brain has been demonstrated with PET scans after dosing with ^{11}C-flumazenil. Flumazenil has a short elimination half-life of about 1 hour.

Flumazenil pharmacokinetic parameters would be expected to be affected by liver disease, age, and concomitment administration of enzyme inhibitors in a manner similar to diazepam and other oxidatively metabolized benzodiazepines. Studies in patients with liver disease have shown a significant decrease in flumazenil clearance.[46,48] Flumazenil is apparently free of any serious adverse effects and there is little need to reduce dosage in these pa-

tients. Concomitant administration of flumazenil with benzodiazepine agonists or alcohol does not alter flumazenil pharmacokinetic parameters.[45]

In original reports on the safety of flumazenil, oral doses of 20 to 600 mg or up to 100 mg IV did not affect psychomotor test performance, sedation rating, EEG parameters, or other measures of effects on the CNS. Continuing research has suggested that in certain situations there are partial agonist or weak inverse agonist effects. In general, these effects are very weak and have not been studied in relation to flumazenil plasma concentration. The duration of antagonistic activity of flumazenil on the effect of some benzodiazepine derivatives is shown in Table 11-5.

REFERENCES

1. Simonsen LL: Top 200 drugs of 1991: What are pharmacists dispensing most often? Pharmacy Times 58:47, 1992
2. Soderpalm B: Pharmacology of the benzodiazepines with special emphasis on alprazolam. Acta Psychiatr Scand 76(suppl 335):39, 1987
3. Jack ML, Colburn WA, Spirt NM et al: A pharmacokinetic/pharmacodynamic receptor binding model to predict the onset and duration of pharmacological activity of the benzodiazepines. Prog Neuropsychopharmacol Biol Psychiatry 7:5, 1983
4. Miller LG, Greenblatt DJ, Barnhill JG, Shader RI: Chronic benzodiazepine administration. I. Tolerance is associated with benzodiazepine receptor down-

regulation and decreased γ aminobutyric acid$_A$ receptor function. Pharm Exper Ther 246:170, 1988

5. Miller LG, Greenblatt DJ, Roy RB et al: Chronic benzodiazepine administration. II. Discontinuation syndrome is associated with upregulation of γ-aminobutyric acid$_A$ receptor complex binding and function. Pharm Exper Ther 246:177, 1988

6. Miller LG, Greenblatt DJ, Barnhill JG et al: Benzodiazepine receptor binding of triazolobenzodiazepines in vivo: increased receptor number with low-dose alprazolam. Neurochem 49:1595, 1987

7. Sheiner LB, Stanski DR, Vozeh S et al: Simultaneous modeling of pharmacokinetics and pharmacodynamics: Application to d-tubocurarine. Clin Pharmacol Ther 25:358, 1979

8. Campbell DB: The use of kinetic-dynamic interactions in the evaluation of drugs. Psychopharmacol 100:433, 1990

9. Dingemanse J, Danhof M, Breimer DD: Pharmacokinetic-pharmacodynamic modeling of CNS drug effects: an overview. Pharmacol Ther 38:1, 1988

10. Stanski D: Pharmacodynamic modeling of anesthetic EEG drug effects. Annu Rev Pharmacol Toxicol 32:423, 1992

11. Miller LG, Greenblatt DJ, Paul SM, Shader RI: Benzodiazepine receptor occupancy in vivo: correlation with brain concentrations and pharmacodynamic actions. J Pharmacol Exp Ther 240:516, 1987

12. Persson MP, Nilsson A, Hartvig P: Relation of sedation and amnesia to plasma concentrations of midazolam in surgical patients. Clin Pharmacol Ther 43:324, 1988

13. Buhrer M, Maitre PO, Crevoisier C, Stanski DR: Electroencephalographic effect of benzodiazepines. II. Pharmacodynamic modeling of the electroencephalographic effects of midazolam and diazepam. Clin Pharmacol Ther 48:555, 1990

14. Greenblatt DJ, Ehrenberg BL, Gunderman J et al: Pharmacokinetic and electroencephalographic study of intravenous diazepam, midazolam, and placebo. Clin Pharmacol Ther 45:356, 1989

15. Arendt RM, Greenblatt DJ, deJong RH et al: In vitro correlates of benzodiazepine cerebrospinal fluid uptake, pharmacodynamic action and peripheral distribution. J Pharmacol Exp Ther 227:98, 1983

16. Reves JG, Newfield P, Smith LR: Influence of serum protein, serum albumin concentrations and dose on midazolam induction times. Can Anaesth Soc J 28:556, 1981

17. Ziegler WH, Schalch E, Leishman B, Eckert M: Comparison of the effects of intravenously administered midzolam, triazolam and their hydroxy metabolites. Br J Clin Pharmac 16:63S, 1983

18. Mandema JW, Tuk B, van Steveninck AL et al: Pharmacokinetic-pharmacodynamic modeling of the central nervous system effects of midazolam and its main metabolite alpha-hydroxymidazolam in healthy volunteers. Clin Pharmacol Ther 51:715, 1992

19. Greenblatt DJ, Laughren TP, Allen MD et al: Plasma diazepam and desmethyldiazepam concentrations during long-term diazepam therapy. Br J Clin Pharmacol 11:35, 1981

20. Dundee JW, McGowan AW, Lilburn JK et al: Comparison of the actions of diazepam and lorazepam. Br J Anesth 51:439, 1979

21. Arendt RM, Greenblatt DJ, Liebisch DC et al: Determinants of benzodiazepine brain uptake: lipophilicity versus binding affinity. Psychopharmacology 93:72, 1987

22. Pieri L, Schaffner R, Scherschlicht R et al: Pharmacology of midazolam. Arzneim-Forsch/Drug Res 31:2180, 1981

23. Greenblatt DJ, Shader RI: Physicochemical and pharmacokinetic properties of midazolam in humans. Anesthesiol 13:7, 1986

24. Allonen H, Ziegler G, Klotz U: Midazolam kinetics. Clin Pharmacol Ther 30:653, 1981

25. Smith MT, Eadie MJ, O'Rourke-Brophy T: The pharmacokinetics of midazolam in man. Eur J Clin Pharmacol 19:271, 1981

26. Kanto JH: Midazolam: the first water-soluble benzodiazepine pharmacology, pharmacokinetics and efficacy in insomnia and anesthesia. Pharmacother 5:138, 1985

27. Garzone PD, Kroboth PD: Pharamcokinetics of the newer benzodiazepines. Clin Pharamcokin 16:337, 1989

28. Crevoisier C, Ziegler WH, Cano JP: Relation between pharmacokinetics and pharmacodynamics of intravenously administered midazolam, triazolam and their hydroxy-metabolites. II Congress of International American Society for Clinical Pharmacology and Therapy and XI Congress of the Latin American Association of Pharmacology. Buenos Aires, Argentina, Abstract 47

29. Greenblatt DJ, Abernethy DR, Locniskar A et al: Effect of age, gender, and obesity on midazolam kinetics. Anesthesiology 61:27, 1984

30. Vinik HR, Reves JG, Greenblatt DJ et al: The pharmacokinetics of midazolam in chronic renal failure patients. Anesthesiology 59:390, 1983

31. Holazo AA, Winkler MB, Patel IH: Effects of age,

gender and oral contraceptives on intramuscular midazolam pharmacokinetics. J Clin Pharmacol 28:1040, 1988

32. Macgilchrist AJ, Birnie GG, Cook A et al: Pharmacokinetics and pharmacodynamics of intravenous midazolam in patients with severe alcoholic cirrhosis. Gut 27:190, 1986

33. Buhrer M, Maitre PO, Crevoisier C, Stanski DR: Electroencephalographic effects of benzodiazepines. II. Pharmacodynamic modeling of the electroencephalographic effects of midazolam and diazepam. Clin Pharmacol Ther 48:555, 1990

34. Greenblatt DJ, Allen MD, Harmatz JS, Shader RI: Diazepam disposition determinants. Clin Pharmacol Ther 27:301, 1980

35. Kaplan SA, Jack ML: Pharmacokinetics and metabolism of anxiolytics, p. 321. In Hoffmeister F, Stille G (eds): Psychotropic Agents. Part II: Anxiolytics, Gerontopsychopharmacological Agents, and Psychomotor Stimulants, Springer-Verlag, Berlin, 1980

36. Dasberg HH, van der Kleijn E, Guelen PJR, van Praag HM: Plasma concentration of diazepam and of its metabolite N-desmethyldiazepam in relation to anxiolytic effects. Clin Pharmacol Ther 15:473, 1974

37. Fink M, Irwin P, Weinfeld RE et al: Blood levels and electroencephalographic effects of diazepam and bromazepam. Clin Pharmacol Ther 20:184, 1976

38. Dasta JF, Brier KL, Kidwell GA et al: Diazepam infusion in tetanus: correlation of drug levels with effect. Southern Med J 74:278, 1981

39. Linnoila M, Erwin CW, Brendle BA, Simpson D: Psychomotor effects of diazepam in anxious patients and healthy volunteers. J Clin Psychopharmacol 3:88, 1983

40. McLeaod DR, Hoehn-Saric R, Labib S, Greenblatt DJ: Six weeks of diazepam treatment in normal women: effects on psychomotor performance and psychophysiology. J Clin Psychopharmacol 8:83, 1988

41. Buhrer M, Maitre PO, Hung O, Stanski DR: Electroencepholographic effects of benzodiazepines. I. Choosing an electroencephalographic parameter to measure the effect of midazolam on the central nervous system. Clin Pharmacol Ther 48:544, 1990

42. Kaplan SA, Jack ML: Metabolism of the benzodiazepines: pharmacokinetic and pharmacodynamic considerations. In Costa E (ed): Benzodiazepines: From Molecular Biology to Clinical Practice. Raven Press, New York, 1983

43. Swerdlow BN, Holley FO: Intravenous anaesthetic agents. Pharmacokinetic-pharmacodynamic relationships. Clin Pharmacokin 12:79, 1987

44. Greenblatt DJ, Ehrenberg BL, Gunderman J et al: Kinetic and dynamic study of intravenous lorazepam: comparison with intravenous diazepam. J Pharmacol Exp Ther 250:134, 1989

45. Klotz U, Kanto J: Pharmacokinetics and clinical use of flumazenil (Ro 15-1788). Clin Pharmacokin 14:1, 1988

46. Janssen U, Walker S, Maier K et al: Flumazenil disposition and elimination in cirrhosis. Clin Pharmacol Ther 46:317, 1989

47. Haefely W, Hunkeler W: The story of flumazenil. Eur J Anaesthesiol 52:3, 1988

48. Pomier-Layrargues G, Giguere JF, Lavoie J et al: Pharmacokinetics of benzodiazepine antagonist Ro 15-1788 in cirrhotic patients with moderate or severe liver dysfunction. Hepatology 10:969, 1989

49. Gupta SK, Ellinwood EH, Nikaido AM, Heatherly DG: Simultaneous modeling of the pharmacokinetic and pharmacodynamic properties of benzodiazepines. II. Triazolam. Pharmaceutical Res 7:570, 1990

Chapter 12

Clinical Pharmacology and Applications of Benzodiazepine Agonists and Antagonists

Joseph J. Quinlan and Leonard L. Firestone

The essential components of clinical anesthesia are amnesia (unconsciousness), analgesia, muscle relaxation, and blunting of autonomic reflexes. Anesthesiologists may use a "complete," volatile-type anesthetic (e.g., isoflurane) to provide all of these components or may administer a mixture of drugs, each of which provides one or more of the elements of anesthesia. The latter approach is termed *balanced anesthesia*. Benzodiazepines are widely used by anesthesiologists to provide the amnestic component of balanced anesthesia as well as for sedation throughout the perioperative period. The recent advent of a benzodiazepine antagonist has improved the safety and versatility of these agents.

The benzodiazepines used by anesthesiologists are not identical (Fig. 12-1 and Table 12-1) and are chosen for use on the basis of their formulations (Table 12-2), pharmacokinetics, and pharmacodynamics. This chapter surveys these properties, reviews the conventional perioperative clinical use and clinical pharmacology of benzodiazepine agonists, and evaluates the emerging role of the recently approved benzodiazepine antagonist, flumazenil.

PERIOPERATIVE USES FOR BENZODIAZEPINES

Insomnia Before Surgery

Sedating drugs are often prescribed by anesthesiologists to avoid insomnia on the night before surgery. Because anxiety frequently contributes to preoperative insomnia, and benzodiazepines possess anxiolytic as well as sedative effects, they are a logical choice for this indication. Although they have not been rigorously evaluated for this use, any of the benzodiazepines available for oral administration would seem acceptable. Flurazepam may be particularly appropriate because of its rapid absorption after oral administration and consequent short sleep latency.[1]

Premedication

The goal of premedication in the immediate preoperative period is to render the patient calm, cooperative, and without recall of unpleasant events before induction of anesthesia. Because of their anxiolytic, sedative, and amnestic actions, benzodiazepines have gained wide acceptance as premedicants. Compared with other choices such as

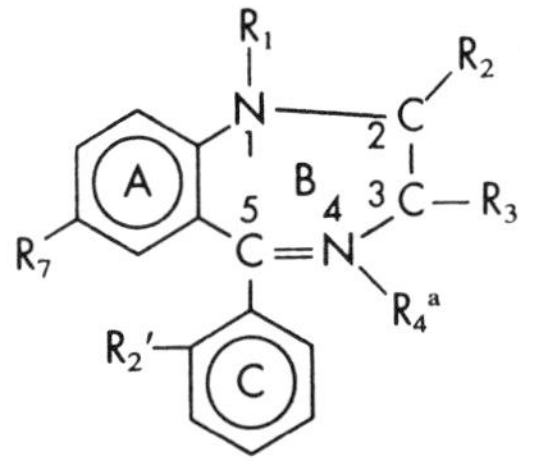

Fig. 12-1 Benzodiazepine chemical structure (see Table 12-1).

narcotics, hydroxyzine, scopolamine, and α_2-adrenergic agonists, the many benzodiazepines offer the advantages of multiple routes of administration, a relative lack of cardiorespiratory effects at the doses commonly used, a variety of durations of action, and a specific pharmacologic antagonist should antagonism prove necessary.

Diazepam

Diazepam may be administered by the intravenous, intramuscular, and oral routes. Oral diazepam is rapidly absorbed, with a bioavailability that averaged 94 percent.[2] Absorption of intramuscular diazepam was slow and incomplete in some subjects, suggesting that the intramuscular route is less reliable.[2] Although 10 mg of oral diazepam produces a satisfactory anxiolytic and sedative effect in adults,[3,4] this dose is poorly amnestic, impairing recall at 90 minutes in only 20 to 30 percent of pa-

tients.[3,5] Larger oral doses (e.g., 20 mg) must be used to abolish recall in 50 percent of patients.[5] The effect of the same doses intramuscularly is qualitatively similar.[6] In contrast, intravenous administration will produce transient (generally less than 10 minutes) anterograde amnesia in approximately 60 percent of healthy patients.[7]

Lorazepam

Compared with diazepam, lorazepam is a more efficacious amnestic that has a more gradual onset and a longer duration of sedative action. Amnesia occurs more frequently in patients given lorazepam (4 mg) than in those given diazepam (10 to 20 mg) by the same route.[6,7] A 4-mg dose of lorazepam produces satisfactory sedation, which peaks about 90 minutes after oral ingestion and persists for several hours.[5,8] When the same dose of lorazepam is given intravenously, the peak time to sedation remains delayed (approximately 30 to 40 minutes),[8] and anterograde amnesia persists for up to 4 hours.[7] Lorazepam is also better absorbed by the intramuscular route than is diazepam, and causes minimal pain at the site of injection. A 4 mg IM dose produces excellent anxiolysis, profound, long-lasting anterograde amnesia (abolishing recall in 60 percent of patients for up to 6 hours), and a peak sedative effect approximately 90 minutes after injection in healthy adult patients.[6,8] Intramuscular lorazepam has no effect on blood pressure or heart rate in adult preoperative patients.[6,8]

Table 12-1 Benzodiazepine Chemical Structure

	R_1	R_2	R_3	R_7	$R_{2'}$
Diazepam	$-CH_3$	$= O$	$-H$	$-Cl$	$-H$
Flumazenil[a,b]	(fused imidazo ring)		$-H$	$-F$	(no ring C)
Flunitrazepam	$-CH_3$	$= O$	$-H$	$-NO_2$	$-F$
Flurazepam	$-CH_2CH_2N(C_2H_5)_2$	$= O$	$-H$	$-Cl$	$-F$
Lorazepam	$-H$	$= O$	$-OH$	$-Cl$	$-Cl$
Midazolam	(fused imidazo ring)		$-H$	$-Cl$	$-F$
Oxazepam	$-H$	$= O$	$-OH$	$-Cl$	$-H$
Temazepam	$-CH_3$	$= O$	$-OH$	$-Cl$	$-H$
Triazolam	(fused triazolo ring)		$-H$	$-Cl$	$-Cl$

[a]R_4 is $-CH_3$ in flumazenil; otherwise no substituent.
[b]No double bond between positions 4 and 5.

Table 12-2 Benzodiazepine Formulations

Drug Name	Route	Typical Dose[a] (form)
Anti-insomnia		
Flurazepam	PO	15–30 mg (capsule)
Oxazepam	PO	15–30 mg (capsule, tablet)
Sedating Premedication		
Diazepam	PO, IM	5–15 mg (tablet, liquid)
Lorazepam	PO, IM	2–6 mg (tablet)
Midazolam	IM (nasal)	2–6 mg (0.3 mg/kg)
Flunitrazepam[b]	PO	1 mg
Temazepam	PO	15–30 mg (capsule)
Triazolam	PO	0.25 mg (tablet)
Induction of Anesthesia[c]		
Diazepam	IV	5–30 mg (injection)
Midazolam	IV	1–10 mg (injection)
Lorazepam	IV	2–12 mg (injection)
Flunitrazepam	IV	2–3 mg (injection)
Postoperative Sedation		
Midazolam	IV infusion	0.05–2 mg/h
Antagonism		
Flumazenil	IV	1–4 mg

[a]For full-sized adult.
[b]Not available in the United States.
[c]Intermittent dosing for maintenance of anesthesia.
(Adapted from Gilman et al.,[200] with permission.)

Midazolam

In healthy adults oral midazolam has a reasonably rapid onset of action (generally within 30 minutes) and provides superior anxiolysis, equivalent amnesia and sedation, but slower recovery than does intravenous diazepam (10 mg).[9] Oral midazolam is also an effective premedicant in children, with a peak effect observed 30 to 45 minutes after oral ingestion.[10] For example, 30 minutes after ingestion of 0.5 to 0.75 mg/kg PO, 90 percent of children are calm and willing to separate from their parents.[11] Moreover, such doses generally do not delay emergence or discharge from the recovery room in children as young as 1 year of age after short surgical procedures.[10,11] Although an oral preparation of midazolam is not available in the United States, several "recipes" have been developed to make the intravenous form palatable for children.[12,13]

Midazolam is also widely used as an intramuscular and intravenous premedicant for adults. Intramuscular midazolam (0.07 to 0.1 mg/kg or about 5 mg for healthy adults) produces satisfactory sedation, amnesia, and anxiolysis, and was rated superior to hydroxyzine (1 to 1.5 mg/kg).[14–16] These doses of midazolam did not delay recovery, even in ambulatory patients after short procedures, although the population tested was generally young and healthy.[16] In children aged 1 to 15 years, intramuscular midazolam (0.08 mg/kg) was judged to produce better sedation and smoother induction conditions than morphine (0.15 mg/kg), as well as a shorter length of stay in the recovery room after halothane and nitrous oxide by mask for various ambulatory surgical procedures.[17] A reduced dose of midazolam, 2 to 3 mg IM, has been recommended for patients aged 60 to 69 years because the elderly are more sensitive to the effects of benzodiazepines; these patients should probably be observed continuously following drug administration.[18] Even greater caution is recommended for patients older than 70 years, because they may become obtunded, even with reduced doses.[19] Intravenous midazolam can also produce satisfactory anxiolysis, sedation, and profound anterograde amnesia in adults, and it is particularly useful if sedation is required immediately before a procedure.[20]

Midazolam has also been given as a premedicant by less conventional routes. For preoperative sedation in children, intranasal midazolam (0.2 to 0.3 mg/kg) provides rapid and effective anxiolysis (onset in 5 to 10 minutes) without respiratory compromise or delayed emergence.[21] Compared with intranasal sufentanil (2 μg/kg), midazolam (0.2 mg/kg) was associated with more crying on administration, but with comparable sedation and less chest wall stiffness during subsequent inhalation induction.[22] The intranasal route has not been evaluated rigorously in adults, but anecdotal reports indicate that it has been successful in patients who had no available intravenous access.[23] Like the barbiturates, midazolam can also be administered rectally for premedication and induction in children. In patients as young as 8 months of age, a dose of 1 mg/kg rectally produces sedation and calm separation from parents within about 10 minutes, without inducing unconsciousness, impairing gas exchange, or delaying discharge from the postanesthesia care unit.[24]

Other Benzodiazepines

Several other benzodiazepines have been used as premedicants. Intravenous flunitrazepam (1 mg) has pharmacologic effects very similar to those of intravenous diazepam (10 mg) in that it produces adequate sedation and anxiolysis, but the amnestic effect is complete in only 60 to 70 percent of patients and lasts for only approximately 20 minutes.[7] When administered orally, 1 mg of flunitrazepam has effects equivalent to 20 mg of oral diazepam.[5] Oral temazepam, a diazepam metabolite, in doses of 20 to 40 mg provides comparable sedation and anxiolysis but possibly inferior amnesia when compared with intravenous diazepam (10 to 20 mg).[25,26] Finally, oral triazolam (0.25 mg) produces satisfactory sedation and amnesia comparable to that found with 10 mg of oral diazepam, but inadequate anxiolysis.[4] This shortcoming seemed to be a function of an inadequate dose, since 0.5 mg produced anxiolysis comparable to that observed with 10 mg of oral diazepam.[3] A dose of 0.5 mg triazolam abolished recall in approximately 40 percent of cases.[27]

Induction of Anesthesia

Because of their relative lack of adverse cardiovascular effects, benzodiazepines frequently have been recommended as induction agents either alone or in combination, especially in patients with compromised cardiovascular status.

Diazepam

Diazepam has been used for anesthetic induction for almost three decades. Doses of 0.2 to 0.6 mg/kg IV provide a smooth loss of consciousness in approximately 2 minutes.[28–30] By comparison with thiopental (2.5 mg/kg), diazepam (0.3 to 0.45 mg/kg) induces anesthesia more gradually, and is associated with a longer emergence time after a halothane anesthetic in young women.[29] Diazepam (0.3 mg/kg) induced unconsciousness in a mean time of 64 seconds, versus 44.5 seconds for thiopental (4 mg/kg). Return to consciousness after a subsequent brief halothane or nitrous oxide anesthetic was approximately twice as long as that with thiopental (22 versus 13 minutes) in a large group of patients undergoing cystoscopy.[31] Nonetheless, because of its relative lack of harmful cardiac effects (see Clinical Effects), diazepam is widely used for induction of anesthesia, particularly in patients with cardiac disease. For example, diazepam (0.5 mg/kg) induced loss of consciousness with minimal changes in hemodynamics in patients presenting for elective coronary artery bypass graft (CABG) surgery[32]; others have reported decreases of up to 20 percent in mean systemic arterial pressure after induction with up to 0.6 mg/kg in patients scheduled for a variety of cardiac procedures.[33] Diazepam alone does not abolish the response to laryngoscopy and intubation.[32,33] Thus, it is often combined with opioids or other intravenous anesthetics, such as ketamine (see Maintenance of Anesthesia, below).

Midazolam

Midazolam similarly induces anesthesia without excitatory phenomena. Its major advantage over diazepam for induction is its lack of venous irritation.[20] Induction also is slower than with barbiturates, with peak action at about 3 minutes after intravenous injection.[34] The incidence of transient apnea during induction may be less with midazolam than with thiopental.[18] As with diazepam, induction with midazolam leads to a more prolonged emergence than with thiopental.[18] The major disadvantage of midazolam for induction, however, is the wide variation in response to an induction dose of up to 0.5 mg/kg IV in healthy, unpremedicated patients.[34] Up to 25 percent of healthy adult patients younger than 50 years will remain conscious 3 minutes after injection of a standard induction dose of 0.3 mg/kg of midazolam.[35] Failure of doses as high as 0.4 to 0.5 mg/kg to induce unconsciousness in healthy adult patients has been reported.[18,20] Midazolam is even less reliable as an intravenous induction agent in children. The time to disappearance of the eyelid reflex after a large induction dose of midazolam (0.6 mg/kg) was four times that observed after a bolus of thiopental (5 mg/kg), and one-third of young children did not lose consciousness.[36] In constrast, elderly patients (age greater than 50 years) tend to respond in a more predictable manner, and an induction dose of 0.3 mg/kg is uniformly effective.[34,35] A dose reduced to 0.15 mg/kg remains effective for patients aged 70 to 90 years.[37] Despite these reports of relative unreliability in inducing unconsciousness, midazolam alone (0.3 mg/kg) or in combination (0.15 mg/kg) with ketamine (0.75 mg/kg) has been reported to be a safe and effective induction agent for rapid-sequence induction of anesthesia in otherwise healthy adult patients requiring emergency surgery.[38] Like diazepam, midazolam has also become a popular induction agent in patients with heart disease,[39] even though midazolam produces a somewhat greater decrease in blood pressure.[40] Midazolam alone does not abolish the hemodynamic response to laryngoscopy and endotracheal intubation.[40]

Flunitrazepam

Flunitrazepam (0.036 mg/kg) has also been used as an induction agent in cardiac patients, providing induction conditions and hemodynamic responses similar to those produced by diazepam (0.32 mg/kg).[33] Flunitrazepam shares with midazolam a slow, unreliable onset of action and a prolonged recovery in young children.[41]

Maintenance of Anesthesia

Benzodiazepines are often integrated into the anesthetic maintenance regimen because of their sedative-hypnotic and amnestic properties. They decrease the requirement for volatile agents[42,43] and thus can provide the hypnotic component of a balanced anesthetic technique. Compared with other hypnotics such as thiopental (3 mg/kg), less inhalational agents or opioids are required with diazepam (0.45 mg/kg) or midazolam (0.2 mg/kg) combined with nitrous oxide and succinylcholine in healthy patients undergoing short procedures.[29,44,45] However, recovery after ambulatory surgical procedures may be slightly longer with midazolam than with thiopental.[45]

Benzodiazepines are often combined with high-dose opioids (e.g., fentanyl 35 to 75 μg/kg) to provide additional amnesia and hypnosis. However, in patients undergoing CABG surgery, induction with opioids plus midazolam (0.075 to 0.15 mg kg IV) or diazepam (0.125 to 0.5 mg/kg IV) produces substantially greater decreases in mean arterial pressure, systemic vascular resistance, cardiac filling pressures, cardiac index, and stroke index than do opioids alone (see Clinical Effects of Benzodiazepines).[45,47]

Adjunctive Use During Anesthesia

Benzodiazepines may be combined with ketamine and reduce many of ketamine's undesirable side effects, including sympathetic stimulation. For example, diazepam (0.4 mg/kg) and ketamine (2 mg/kg) provided smooth induction of anesthesia in cardiac surgical patients, without change in heart rate, mean arterial pressure, or systemic vascular resistance.[48] The combination of midazolam (0.15 mg/kg) and ketamine (0.75 mg/kg) provided satisfactory rapid-sequence induction of anesthesia in otherwise healthy patients for emergency procedures, with a smaller increase in heart rate than that produced by either drug alone or a standard induction dose of thiopental, without altering mean arterial pressure.[38] Diazepam (0.2 mg/kg), flunitrazepam (0.02 mg/kg), midazolam (0.15 mg/kg), and lorazepam (4 mg) all reduce the incidence of unpleasant dreams and emergence delirium frequently encountered with ketamine; lorazepam is probably the most efficacious in this regard, possibly because of its longer duration of action.[38,49,50] However, benzodiazepines do not prevent the increases in intracranial pressure caused by ketamine, so this combination may not be appropriate in patients with abnormal intracranial compliance.[51]

Benzodiazepines are often used as adjuncts to regional anesthetic techniques. Both midazolam and diazepam can be used to sedate patients undergoing procedures with spinal anesthesia, without affecting hemodynamics or airway reflexes.[52] However, sedation to the point of unresponsiveness has been implicated in cases of unexpected cardiac arrest during spinal anesthesia[53]; more than one-half of those patients had received diazepam in doses commonly used for clinical sedation. Thus, a high degree of vigilance for individual variation in response is recommended when using benzodiazepines in this setting, particularly in the presence of a high level of autonomic blockade.[53] Benzodiazepines have also been used in combination with ketamine to provide sedation during major conduction anesthesia. Diazepam (0.15 mg/kg) and ketamine (0.5 mg/kg) produced acceptable sedation without significantly altering hemodynamics or causing unpleasant dreaming or emergence excitation in healthy young and middle-aged patients.[54] Midazolam has also been combined with fentanyl to provide patient-controlled sedation during regional anesthesia.[55]

"Conscious Sedation" for Invasive Procedures

Conscious sedation is defined as the administration of sedative-hypnotic drugs to patients in doses that do not abolish consciousness or protective airway reflexes. Benzodiazepines are widely used to produce conscious sedation during invasive procedures or minor surgery under local anesthesia. In recent years, midazolam has replaced diazepam as the preferred benzodiazepine for conscious sedation because of its shorter duration and lower incidence of venous irritation and phlebitis. A double-blind comparison of midazolam and diazepam for conscious sedation during endoscopy found that midazolam induced sedation faster and provided superior amnesia, with comparable recovery times.[56] Orally administered benzodiazepines have also been used for procedures such as endoscopy and oral surgery, when intravenous access is typically not available. For example, oral temazepam (20 to 40 mg) provided conditions comparable to those achieved with intravenous diazepam.[25,26]

Postoperative Sedation

Sedation is often necessary for patients supported by mechanical ventilation in the postanesthesia care unit or intensive care unit (ICU). Benzodiazepines provide excellent sedation in this setting, and may reduce the need for vasodilators in patients after CABG surgery.[57] One factor limiting their use is slow awakening, possibly because the benzodiazepines (especially diazepam) and their metabolites may accumulate after repeated administration.[58,59] Continuous infusion regimens have been developed for sedation in the ICU. For example, a bolus of midazolam (0.3 mg/kg over 30 minutes) followed by an infusion (0.06 mg/kg/h for up to 180 hours) provided satisfactory sedation with prompt return (within 1 to 2 hours) to an alert mental state in adult patients requiring mechanical ventilation for a variety of diseases.[60] Prompt awakening has been confirmed by other authors,[61] who used titrated midazolam infusions (0.1 to 20.3 μg/kg/h) to facilitate ventilation in adult patients. After CABG surgery performed with an opioid technique, midazolam infusion (2 mg/h) decreased the requirements for supplemental morphine and vasodilators.[57] Although the midazolam infusion delayed the time to recovery of spontaneous movement, eye opening, and onset of spontaneous respiration, it did not delay the time to tracheal extubation or prolong the ICU stay.[57] Midazolam infusions, both alone and combined with opioids, have also been used in children who require ventilatory support. After a loading dose of 0.2 mg/kg, an infusion of 0.4 to 0.6 μg/kg/min provided sedation in both children and neonates while still allowing spontaneous ventilation.[62] In conjunction with a morphine infusion at 0.33 μg/kg/min, the same midazolam loading dose with a higher mean infusion rate (3 μg/kg/min) provided satisfactory sedation in children (6 months to 8 years of age) who had undergone cardiac surgical repair, and a state of wakefulness compatible with extubation was achieved within 2 hours of discontinuing the infusion.[63] Notably, recovery may be delayed in children who develop renal, and especially hepatic, insufficiency.[63] Another infusion combination that has been suggested for pediatric postoperative analgesia and sedation consists of midazolam (0.4 to 4 μg/kg/min) and ketamine (10 to 70 μg/kg/min).[64]

Self-administration protocols similar to those used for opioids in patient-controlled analgesia have been applied to benzodiazepines. One such "patient-controlled anxiolysis" regimen, consisting of incremental doses of midazolam starting at 0.25 mg with a lockout interval of 10 minutes, was used in an adult population to control ICU-related stress and anxiety.[65]

CLINICAL EFFECTS OF BENZODIAZEPINES

Central Nervous System Effects

Sedation and Amnesia

In young, healthy volunteers, rapid injection of 10 mg of midazolam induced unconsciousness in 30 to 97 seconds that lasted 3 to 6 minutes.[66] Although patients who have awakened after receiving benzodiazepines may seem alert, sensitive tests of psychometric ability indicate impairment of fine motor responses and reaction time for at least 5 hours after intravenous midazolam (15 mg) and 10 hours after intravenous triazolam (1 mg).[67] Sensitivity to the obtunding effect of benzodiazepines increases with age. The time to loss of consciousness after an intravenous dose of midazolam (0.3 mg/kg) is correlated negatively with age.[35]

Obtundation with midazolam is associated with a shift in the electroencephalogram (EEG) to widespread β activity at 15 and 22 Hz, with disappearance of α rhythm.[66] EEG activity during deep sedation with lorazepam is characterized by a similar loss of α activity and activity at 15 Hz.[68] An increase in the $\beta 1/\alpha$ power ratio of the EEG correlates with the degree of amnesia induced by an infusion of midazolam.[69] Midazolam increases the latency but has no effect on the amplitude of somatosensory evoked signals.[70]

Memory and the effects of benzodiazepines on memory processes recently have been reviewed.[71] Benzodiazepines cannot produce retrograde amnesia, but do produce reliable anterograde amnesia.[5,6,8] Lorazepam provides the most consistent and longest lasting amnestic effect of the benzodiazepines (up to 4 to 6 hours after 4 mg intramuscularly), whereas the amnestic actions of diazepam are short-lived and unreliable unless large doses (20 mg or more) are given.[5,6] Midazolam's amnestic action appears to be equivalent to that of diazepam.[9] Benzodiazepine-induced amnesia occurs at subhypnotic doses. Midazolam doses that are generally considered unreliable for induction (0.15 mg/kg) produced anterograde amnesia for approximately 40 minutes.[72]

Benzodiazepines exhibit complex interactions with a number of other anesthetic drugs. For example, diazepam and midazolam decrease the minimum alveolar concentration (MAC) of volatile anesthetics. The maximum reduction in the MAC of halothane caused by diazepam is about 34 percent for diazepam doses of 0.2 mg/kg,[44] whereas midazolam decreases MAC in a dose-dependent manner, with midazolam, 0.6 mg/kg, decreasing the MAC of halothane by approximately 50 percent.[73] Nitrous oxide enhanced the anxiolytic effects but not the sedative effect of diazepam in mice assessed with a staircase test.[74] Midazolam synergistically interacts with the barbiturates thiopental and pentobarbital to ablate the righting reflex in rats.[75] This should not be surprising given the effects of these drugs on the γ aminobutyric acid (GABA) ionophore (see Chapter 10).

Acute oral coadministration of diazepam (5 to 10 mg) and ethanol (0.5 to 0.8 g/kg) dramatically impaired psychomotor skills (as assessed by tests of choice reaction and coordination), whereas administration of either drug alone did not impair such skills.[76] The exact length of time after administration of benzodiazepines during which patients are at risk for interactions with ethanol is unknown, but probably depends on the dose and pharmacokinetic properties of the benzodiazepine. However, healthy volunteers who consumed 0.7 g/kg of ethanol (equivalent to approximately 1 L of wine) 4 hours after administration of a sedating dose of intravenous midazolam (0.1 mg/kg) were no more impaired than those who were injected with placebo and ingested alcohol, suggesting that ambulatory surgical patients sedated with midazolam can safely consume alcohol after arrival at home.[77] Chronic alcohol intake that is sufficient to produce tolerance to the effects of acute alcohol intake induces cross-tolerance to the obtunding effect of diazepam in rats, suggesting that alcoholic patients might have a higher benzodiazepine requirement to produce a given level of sedation.[78]

The sedative-hypnotic interaction of benzodiazepines and opioids depends greatly on the method by which it is measured. The interaction is highly synergistic with regard to hypnosis, measured by loss of the righting reflex in animals or lack of response to verbal stimulus in humans.[79-81] Subanalgesic doses of alfentanil (3 μg/kg) reduced by one-half the EC_{50} at which midazolam induced unconsciousness in adult women (Fig. 12-2).[84] Strictly additive effects of these drugs are observed in producing sedation, as measured by inhibition of locomotor activity in animals or a visual analog scale in humans.[82,83] However, the interaction between benzodiazepines and opioids is less than additive if the measure of effect is a noxious stimulus.[84,85] This difference may be due to antagonism by benzodiazepines of opioid analgesia (see Antinociception, below).

Anxiolysis

All the benzodiazepines induce anxiolysis, and there is little data to suggest that one benzodiazepine is superior to another in this regard. Anxioly-

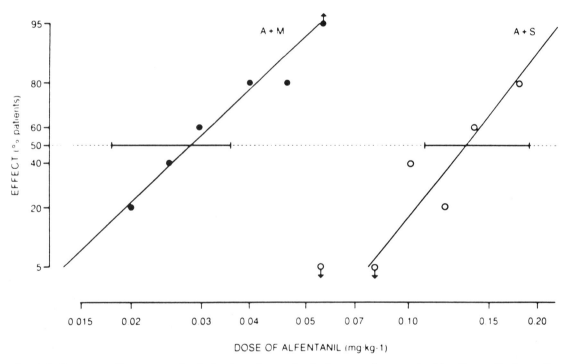

Fig. 12-2 Dose-effect curves for induction of anesthesia (unconsciousness) with alfentanil plus saline (*right*) or alfentanil plus midazolam (*left*) in unpremedicated patients. Data are plotted on a log-log scale. Midazolam (0.07 mg/kg IV) reduced the alfentanil ED_{50} for unconsciousness by about 80 percent. These data demonstrate the synergistic interaction of opioids and benzodiazepines with respect to hypnotic effects. (From Vinik et al.,[80] with permission.)

tic effects are observed with doses of benzodiazepines that are mildly sedative, but less than those required to produce amnesia.[3] This suggests that anxiolytic effects are mediated at low levels of receptor occupancy by benzodiazepine agonists.

Anticonvulsive Effects

Benzodiazepines are very efficacious anticonvulsants. Although not the drugs of choice for chronic treatment of epilepsy, they are often used in acute treatment of seizures. Benzodiazepines will control status epilepticus in approximately 80 percent of patients.[86] Although some evidence exists that midazolam may be effective when diazepam and lorazepam have failed,[87] the choice of benzodiazepine is largely based on pharmacokinetic considerations: lorazepam provides long-lasting control, whereas diazepam and midazolam may require continuous infusion to maintain a therapeutic effect.[86]

Benzodiazepines may be useful in preventing convulsions due to toxic levels of local anesthetics. Intramuscular diazepam (0.25 mg/kg) increased the median convulsant dose for lidocaine by two-thirds in monkeys.[88] This protective effect is shared by the other benzodiazepines as well. At a dose of 1 mg/kg IM, diazepam, lorazepam, and midazolam all decreased the incidence of seizures induced by lidocaine, etidocaine, or bupivacaine from 95 percent in control mice to 5 to 50 percent in treated animals, and decreased the mortality rate by two-thirds or more.[89] Flunitrazepam may be superior to diazepam in preventing mortality from local anesthetic overdose, because flunitrazepam eliminated the 20 to 40 percent mortality observed with an equivalent dose of diazepam in mice.[90] Although the decrease in frequency of seizures has been very reproducible for all the benzodiazepines, the decrease in mortality was not observed with midazolam in rats.[91] This protective effect of benzodiazepines may not apply to the heart, as a sedating dose of diazepam (0.2 mg/kg IV) did not mitigate the effects of a subsequent injection of a cardiotoxic dose of intravenous bupivacaine. On the contrary, rats treated with diazepam developed more than twice the incidence of serious arrhythmias encountered in control animals.[92] Bupivacaine cardiac toxicity may be mediated through the central nervous system, at least in part, because intracerebroventricular injection of bupivacaine induces hypertension and dysrhythmias in rabbits. Interestingly, these effects can be terminated by intracerebroventricular midazolam.[93] Thus, benzodiazepines may still be of theoretic value in the treatment of cardiac manifestations of local anesthetic toxicity. Further experiments are necessary to provide definitive data.

Cerebral Metabolism

Benzodiazepines have potent effects on cerebral metabolism. Whereas barbiturates decrease cerebral blood flow and metabolism proportionately, benzodiazepines in clinically relevant doses generally have a greater effect on cerebral blood flow than on metabolism. Anesthetic doses of diazepam (up to 0.3 mg/kg) and and midazolam (0.2 mg/kg) decrease cerebral blood flow approximately 30 to 60 percent, without changing the cerebral metabolic rate for oxygen ($CMRO_2$) in rats and dogs.[94,95] Large doses of lorazepam in the monkey (4 mg/kg) decreased both cerebral blood flow and $CMRO_2$ by 30 percent.[96] Data in humans are limited, but intravenous midazolam (0.15 mg/kg) decreased cerebral blood flow by more than 30 percent in healthy volunteers.[97] No data exist regarding the effect of benzodiazepines on $CMRO_2$ in humans.

Decreases in both cerebral blood flow (to as low as 30 percent of control) and $CMRO_2$ (to as low as 55 percent of control) have been reported with supratherapeutic concentrations of diazepam (3 to 7.5 mg/kg) or midazolam (0.57 to 10 mg/kg).[95,98] The magnitude of the effect of midazolam on cerebral blood flow and metabolism increases with age in rats.[99] Even with large doses of benzodiazepines, cerebral blood flow is still 50 percent greater than the nadir achieveable with barbiturates.[95] Thus benzodiazepines have not been used as cerebral protective agents in the same way as barbiturates.

Benzodiazepines also interact with other anesthetics to alter cerebral metabolism. Although nitrous oxide alone had no effect on cerebral blood flow, when added to diazepam (0.3 mg/kg) nitrous oxide reportedly decreased $CMRO_2$ by approximately 40 percent.[94] However, not all studies have confirmed such a synergistic effect of nitrous oxide with diazepam or midazolam.[95,100] Doses of ethanol that by themselves have no effect on $CMRO_2$, double the decrease in cerebral blood flow and $CMRO_2$ produced by midazolam (0.57 mg/kg) in rats.[98] Midazolam decreased cerebral blood flow and metabolism to control levels in rats undergoing alcohol withdrawal.[101]

Cardiovascular Control

The cardiovascular actions of benzodiazepines are mediated predominantly through central nervous system (CNS) cardiovascular control centers, rather than directly at peripheral cardiovascular sites. Intravenous infusion of midazolam (0.2 mg/kg/h) blunted the increase in systolic blood pressure induced by electrical stimulation of control centers in the hypothalamus and reticular formation of cats, but did not change peripherally mediated increases in infrarenal aortic blood flow.[102] This finding is consistent with a selective action of midazolam at CNS control sites with little effect on peripheral cardiovascular reflex pathways.

Small doses of diazepam given to adults for conscious sedation during coronary angiography (5 to 8.5 mg) produced no change in heart rate, a mild decrease in systemic blood pressure, and a significant decrease in left ventricular end-diastolic pressure.[103] Coronary blood flow and coronary resistance did not change, but myocardial oxygen consumption decreased.[103] Thus, the hemodynamic effects of diazepam resembled those of nitroglycerin in this setting.

Compared with thiopental, induction doses of midazolam (0.25 mg/kg) given to healthy patients produced a smaller decrease in mean arterial pressure.[104] Similarly, induction doses of benzodiazepines (diazepam 0.5 mg/kg or midazolam 0.2 mg/kg) given to patients with known coronary artery disease produced only mild hemodynamic alterations. Diazepam induced no significant change in heart rate and a mild (approximately 10 percent) decrease in blood pressure, associated with a decrease in systemic vascular resistance and mild decreases in mean pulmonary artery pressure, stroke index, and right ventricular stroke work index.[32,40] Midazolam produced a minimal (approximately 10 percent) increase in heart rate and a somewhat greater (approximately 15 to 25 percent) decrease in blood pressure, with no significant decrease in

systemic vascular resistance, as well as decreases in pulmonary artery pressure, pulmonary capillary wedge pressure, stroke index, and right and left ventricular stroke-work indexes.[40,105] Global and regional myocardial function, as assessed by radionuclide angiography, is unaffected by doses of benzodiazepines approaching those used for induction of anesthesia (diazepam or midazolam 0.2 mg/kg, flunitrazepam 0.02 mg/kg) in patients with coronary artery disease.[106]

Although administration of benzodiazepines alone is associated with minimal hemodynamic changes, combining benzodiazepines with opioids can produce significant cardiovascular depression. When given to patients with coronary artery disease immediately before high doses of fentanyl (50 μg/kg), diazepam (0.125 to 0.5 mg/kg IV) caused significant decreases in mean arterial blood pressure and systemic vascular resistance, whereas fentanyl or diazepam alone caused no change (Fig. 12-3).[47,107] Patients with mitral stenosis given intravenous diazepam after fentanyl (50 μg/kg) exhibited decreases in stroke volume, cardiac output, mean arterial pressure, and peripheral resistance, as well as an increase in central venous pressure.[108] The profound vasodilation is probably caused by a decrease in sympathetic nervous system outflow, because doses of diazepam up to 1 mg/kg caused no hemodynamic change when coadministered with fentanyl (100 μg/kg) to dogs whose autonomic tone was ablated with a total spinal anesthetic.[110] Interestingly, the combination of lorazepam (0.05 mg IV) with sufentanil (15 μg/kg) did not produce cardiovascular depression.[109]

The effects of benzodiazepines on coronary blood flow and its regulation vary according to the specific agent. Diazepam and flunitrazepam are potent coronary vasodilators. Sedating doses of flunitrazepam (15 μg/kg) decreased coronary resistance by 10 percent while decreasing myocardial oxygen consumption in patients undergoing coronary angiography.[111] Sedating doses of intravenous diazepam (0.1 mg/kg) increased myocardial blood flow by 22.5 percent in patients with normal coronary arteries and 73 percent in patients with diseased coronary arteries,[112] whereas similar doses decreased myocardial oxygen consumption by approximately 15 percent.[103] These data are consis-

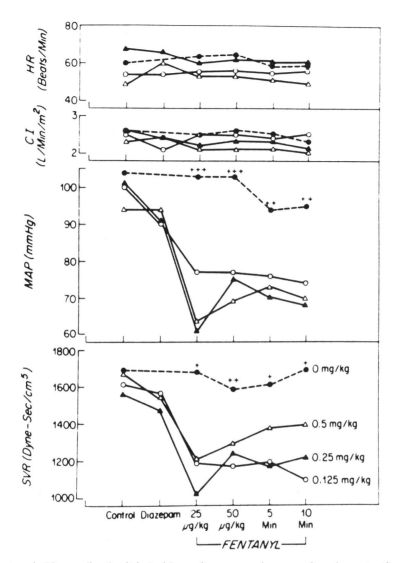

Fig. 12-3 Fentanyl, 50 mcg/kg (*solid circle*), or diazepam alone produced no significant changes in (from top of figure) heart rate (HR), cardiac index (CI), mean arterial pressure (MAP) or systemic vascular resistance (SVR) when administered to cardiac surgery patients for induction of anesthesia. The combination of fentanyl and diazepam (0.5 [*open triangle*], 0.25 [*solid triangle*], or 0.125 mg/kg [*open circle*]) resulted in substantial reductions in mean arterial blood pressure and systemic vascular resistance. (From Tomicheck et al.,[107] with permission.)

tent with mild to moderate disruption of normal coronary autoregulation. In contrast, induction doses of midazolam (0.2 mg/kg) decreased both coronary sinus blood flow and myocardial oxygen consumption by about one-quarter with no change in lactate extraction or coronary vascular resitance, indicating that midazolam has minimal effects on

coronary autoregulation and metabolism.[105] These data suggest that midazolam would be the benzodiazepine least likely to cause "coronary steal" because of coronary vasodilatation, although none of the other benzodiazepines has been implicated in a clinical case of coronary steal.

Benzodiazepines interfere with peripheral autonomic reflexes to only a limited degree. Induction doses of diazepam and midazolam decrease the slope of the pressor baroreflex response approximately 40 percent, a degree of depression less than that seen with inhalational agents.[105]

Respiratory Control

Benzodiazepines depress central respiratory drive. Normal intravenous induction doses of diazepam (0.3 to 0.4 mg/kg) and midazolam (0.15 to 0.2 mg/kg) decrease the ventilatory response to carbon dioxide (CO_2) (approximately 50 to 65 percent for diazepam and 25 to 65 percent for midazolam) in healthy adults.[113–116] The 25 percent decrease seen with midazolam (0.2 mg/kg IV) is comparable to that produced by an induction dose of thiopental (3.5 mg/kg IV).[115] The degree of respiratory depression induced by midazolam is the same whether the drug is given by rapid intravenous push or by infusion over 5 minutes.[117] Respiratory drive is impaired for at least 30 minutes after diazepam[114] and for at least 15 minutes after midazolam.[115] Midazolam-induced respiratory depression is exaggerated in patients with chronic obstructive pulmonary disease, since the decrease in the slope of the CO_2 response curve (one-third of the control value at 15 minutes after administration) is more drastic, and the time to recovery is longer than that in healthy adults.[115]

Sedating doses of midazolam (up to 0.2 mg/kg) decrease tidal volume by approximately 40 percent but increase respiratory rate, such that the change in resting minute ventilation is nil.[118] Doses of midazolam that would commonly be used in conscious sedation (0.1 mg/kg) decrease the slope of the CO_2 response curve less than induction doses (approximately 25 percent), but a slightly lower dose (0.075 mg/kg) does not significantly change the ventilatory response to CO_2 in healthy, young volunteers.[119]

Doses of diazepam that would commonly be used for sedation (0.1 to 0.2 mg/kg) have induced a more variable ventilatory response to CO_2. Most healthy subjects given intravenous diazepam (0.1 mg/kg) exhibited an occlusion pressure response to CO_2 that was less than control, although approximately 20 percent of the subjects actually exhibited values greater than control.[120] The mean slope of

the ventilatory response to CO_2 is unchanged in healthy subjects at this dose, whether the drug is given intravenously or intramuscularly.[120,121] Studies at a slightly higher dose (0.15 mg/kg) have produced conflicting results. One study found no effect on the CO_2 ventilatory response curve at this dose,[119] while another study found that one-half of the healthy adult patients exhibited significant decreases in the slope of their CO_2 ventilatory response curve.[122] A third study noted a 20 percent decrease in the slope of the CO_2 ventilatory response.[123] Doses of 0.2 mg/kg uniformly decrease the slope of the CO_2 response curve by up to approximately 50 percent[124]; interestingly, these authors reported that respiratory depression induced by diazepam could be reversed with extremely high doses of naloxone (30 mg).[124]

Lorazepam (0.05 mg/kg IV) actually increased the slope of the CO_2 response curve and shifted it to the left, consistent with an *increase* in respiratory drive, and attenuated the respiratory depression associated with meperidine.[125] Variable responses of the CO_2 response curve to sedating (5 to 7.5 mg) doses of intravenous lorazepam have been reported by others.[126]

Although sedating doses of benzodiazepines do not consistently alter the ventilatory response to CO_2, sedating doses of intramuscular diazepam (10 mg) and intravenous midazolam (0.1 mg/kg) substantially blunt the response to hypoxia, depressing the slope of the ventilatory response to hypoxia approximately 50 percent in healthy adults.[121,127] Furthermore, the tachycardia usually seen with hypoxia may be masked in the presence of midazolam.[127]

Although sedating doses of benzodiazepines have minimal or no effect on respiratory drive, respiratory depression is perhaps the most dangerous side effect of conscious sedation with the benzodiazepines. A notable number of deaths occurred in patients given midazolam for conscious sedation within the time period shortly after its introduction. Although it is unclear how many of these deaths may have been associated with relative overdosage or inadequate monitoring of respiratory function, many of these patients received midazolam in combination with opioids, which are potent respiratory depressants by themselves. The addition of intravenous midazolam (0.05 mg/kg), which alone has no effect on the ventilatory response to CO_2 and does not cause hypoxia or apnea in healthy volunteers, to intravenous fentanyl (2 μg/kg) increased the incidence of hypoxia from 50 percent with fentanyl alone to over 90 percent, and the incidence of apnea from 0 percent to 50 percent.[120] The combined use of benzodiazepines and opioids should occur only in the presence of adequate respiratory monitoring, supplemental oxygen, and personnel skilled in airway management.[120]

Muscle Tone

Benzodiazepines exhibit central muscle relaxant properties that have been postulated to be secondary to an effect at glycine receptors in the spinal cord[128,129] or at supraspinal sites.[130] They do not directly affect neuromuscular transmission. Although some early studies claimed that diazepam increased the action of depolarizing muscle relaxants and decreased the action of nondepolarizing agents,[131] later studies both in humans and with isolated muscle preparations indicated that only supratherapeutic doses of diazepam interacted with neuromuscular blocking drugs.[132,133] Midazolam does not interact with depolarizing or nondepolarizing neuromuscular blockers.[134]

Antinociception

Determining whether a drug has an antinociceptive effect can be very complex. For example, different methods of applying painful stimuli and different methods of testing for analgesia may elicit different responses to the same drug.[135–137] Additionally, rigorous examination should include a placebo group. Reports that benzodiazepines possess[136,138] or lack[139,140] antinociceptive properties can be found in the literature, but some studies with positive findings failed to include placebo controls.[138] Although benzodiazepines may possess an antinociceptive effect, it appears to be weak.[138] Benzodiazepines have also been variously reported to potentiate, antagonize, or have no effect on morphine-induced antinociception.[136–141]

Spinally administered benzodiazepines definitely have a spinal antinociceptive action. Intrathecal diazepam depresses C-fiber-evoked ascending no-

ciceptive activity in the spinal cord,[142] and midazolam (0.5 to 1 mg) markedly decreases the sympathetic responses induced by direct neural stimulation in the dog.[143] Intrathecal midazolam (1 mg) significantly suppressed the sympathoadrenal catecholamine response to painful stimulation of the sciatic nerve in cats.[144] Intrathecal doses of midazolam (10 μg) exhibit analgesic effects in rats, whereas an intraperitoneal dose of 1 to 10 mg/kg produces hyperalgesia, suggesting that the analgesic effect of benzodiazepines may be mediated at the spinal cord, whereas sedative and hyperalgesic effects are mediated at a supraspinal level.[145] This hypothesis is supported by the finding that diazepam or midazolam injected into the cerebral ventricles of rats antagonized the antinociceptive effect of parenterally administered morphine.[146]

The antinociceptive effect of intrathecal benzodiazepines is mediated via benzodiazpine binding sites on $GABA_A$ receptors, because the analgesia resulting from intrathecally administered midazolam can be blocked by flumazenil and by the $GABA_A$ antagonist, bicuculline.[147] However, spinal antinociception probably also involves an interaction with spinal opioid receptors. Low doses of intrathecal midazolam (10 μg) and intrathecal morphine (10 μg) promote antinociception synergistically, and naloxone can antagonize midazolam-induced antinociception in rats.[148] The nature of this interaction between spinal opioid and benzodiazepine receptors is complex, since doses of either midazolam or morphine exceeding 20 μg antagonize the antinociceptive effect of the other. This antagonism may be due to inhibition of opioid receptor binding by benzodiazepines.[148] Thus far, benzodiazepine-induced spinal antinociception has had no clinical application, perhaps because of concerns about the potential neurotoxicity of intrathecal midazolam.[149]

Peripheral Effects on Myocardial Performance

Large doses of midazolam and diazepam directly decrease myocardial contractility, decreasing the maximum change in pressure with respect to time (dp/dt_{max}) in the dog[150] and the isolated rat heart.[151] Midazolam 1 to 10 mg/kg and diazepam 1 to 2.5 mg/kg decreased canine left ventricular (LV) dp/dt$_{max}$ by approximately 15 percent, whereas the usual induction doses of 0.25 mg/kg of midazolam or 0.5 mg/kg of diazepam had no effect.[150] More pronounced decreases (approaching 70 percent below baseline) in LV dP/dt$_{max}$ were found in the isolated rat heart with microgram concentrations of midazolam or diazepam, an order of magnitude above the therapeutic range.[151] Because these drugs produce sedation with concentrations in the nanogram per milliliter range and the EC$_{50}$ of midazolam for cardiovascular effects in humans is 50 to 60 ng/ml,[152] the clinical importance of direct myocardial depression with supratherapeutic concentrations is questionable.

SIDE EFFECTS AND CONTRAINDICATIONS

The most dangerous side effect of benzodiazepine use is respiratory depression, as discussed above in detail. Serious hemodynamic compromise after administration of benzodiazepines alone is unusual in the absence of extremely high levels of sympathetic tone but may be more apparent when benzodiazepines are administered together with opioids (see Clinical Effects of Benzodiazepines).

A common side effect of intravenous benzodiazepine administration is venous irritation and thrombophlebitis, especially with diazepam. The incidence of thrombophlebitis in patients receiving current formulations of intravenous diazepam ranges from 15 to 39 percent.[153,154] Development of compartment syndrome after intravenous injection, and loss of limb after inadvertent arterial injection of diazepam, have also been reported.[155,156] Thrombophlebitis is far less common with the aqueous-based form of midazolam, with a reported incidence of 0 to 10 percent.[34,42,72]

Hiccups also occur rather frequently after high induction doses of midazolam in unpremedicated healthy patients, but do not seem to presage vomiting or aspiration.[34] Other rare complications of benzodiazepine use include dystonic reactions[157] and disinhibitory reactions characterized by aggressive behavior.[158]

Teratogenesis can be a concern when agents are given to women of childbearing age. Benzodiazepines appear to be safe for the developing fetus.

Concentrations of midazolam in the clinical range had no adverse effect on in vitro development of mouse embryos, or on subsequent in vivo fertilization and cell division.[159]

Midazolam has proved safe in patients at risk for malignant hyperthermia, when combined with sufentanil and nitrous oxide.[160]

ANTAGONISM OF BENZODIAZEPINE EFFECTS

Before the discovery of the receptor-specific benzodiazepine antagonist flumazenil, nonspecific partial reversal of benzodiazepine sedative effects had been reported with physostigmine (0.4 mg/kg)[161] or aminophylline (2 mg/kg IV),[162–165] although the latter did not reverse the amnestic or psychomotor effects of the benzodiazepine agonists.[162] In the course of a search for a partial benzodiazepine agonist, flumazenil was discovered to be a specific benzodiazepine antagonist. Flumazenil is one of several such antagonist compounds, that possess high in vitro binding affinities to the benzodiazepine receptor, but low in vivo agonist activity, thus antagonizing the effects of a normal dose of an agonist.[166] Flumazenil is the only drug of this category to have reached clinical use.

The most common clinical use of flumazenil is the reversal of benzodiazepine agonist effects. For example, flumazenil has been shown to reverse residual sedation after midazolam-fentanyl-nitrous oxide anesthesia for gynecologic surgery.[167] A mean (± standard deviation) flumazenil dose of 0.83 mg ± 0.04 mg reversed a mean midazolam dose of 12.4 ± 2.4 mg, producing calm wakefulness in patients for up to 2 hours.[167] Flumazenil has been used to reverse benzodiazepine-induced obtundation intraoperatively during spinal fusion[168] or immediately postoperatively after craniotomy,[169] thereby facilitating immediate evaluation of neurologic status. Flumazenil has also been used to reverse obtundation caused by overdosage of benzodiazepines.[170]

Another role for flumazenil may be the pharmacologic reversal of hepatic encephalopathy. Altered synaptic transmission at central GABAergic synapses may contribute to the development of hepatic encephalopathy, possibly through the action of an endogenous benzodiazepine ligand.[171] A benzodiazepine-like immunoreactivity is more than fourfold greater in patients with hepatic encephalopathy relative to controls or patients with nonhepatic encephalopathy.[172,173] Anecdotal reports and small series of patients with hepatic encephalopathy indicate that flumazenil can transiently reverse hepatic encephalopathy,[174] but full-scale clinical trials have yet to be undertaken. A related benzodiazepine antagonist (CGS 8216) reversed the behavioral and electrophysiologic signs of hepatic encephalopathy in a rat model of fulminant hepatic failure.[175]

Flumazenil is not useful in reversing intoxication or obtundation due to ethanol[176,177] or volatile anesthetics,[178,179] drugs that also may act via central $GABA_A$ receptors.

Clinical Pharmacology of Flumazenil

Although flumazenil is not a pure antagonist, when given alone it is practically devoid of pharmacologic effects. For example, 0.1 mg/kg IV (i.e., a dose well above the usual therapeutic dose) does not affect performance on psychometric tests,[180] nor does it produce retrograde amnesia, alter the EEG, or change cerebral blood flow.[181] This same dose of flumazenil does not change mean arterial pressure and produces only a minimal decrease in heart rate in healthy adults.[181] A lower dose of 0.04 mg/kg IV (at the upper end of the typical clinical dose range) had no significant effect on blood pressure, heart rate, pulmonary capillary wedge pressure, cardiac index, or vascular resistance in a series of patients with ischemic heart disease.[182] Even higher doses fail to affect respiratory variables such as end-tidal CO_2 concentration,[181] tidal volume, respiratory rate, minute ventilation, or mean inspiratory flow.[181]

Flumazenil competitively antagonizes *all* effects of benzodiazepine agonists to some degree. For example, diazepam-induced amnesia is partially, but not completely, reversed by flumazenil (up to 1 mg) in healthy patients.[183] Healthy adults obtunded with a continuous infusion of midazolam awaken within 1 to 2 minutes of administration of flumazenil, (10 mg) and their performance on a psychometric tracing test returns to baseline.[184] Healthy volunteers given diazepam to the point of slurred speech become awake and alert within 2

minutes after administration of flumazenil (0.001 to 0.014 mg/kg IV), whereas subjects given placebo remain drowsy.[185] Flumazenil's duration of action in reversing sedation is dose-dependent (e.g., 15 minutes after 0.003 mg/kg, but up to 75 minutes after 0.014 mg/kg).[185] Greater doses (0.007 mg/kg or higher) may be required to reverse the amnestic effects of diazepam than to reverse obtundation.[185] Larger doses (0.014 mg/kg or more) may be required to reverse equivalent levels of sedation produced by lorazepam, presumably because the latter has a higher binding affinity to the benzodiazepine receptor than does diazepam (see Dosage below).[185] Flumazenil antagonizes the decrease in cerebral blood flow produced by midzolam[181] and thus may increase intracranial pressure in patients with altered intracranial compliance who have previously received benzodiazepines.[186] This change in intracranial pressure is not due to any effect of flumazenil on cerebrospinal fluid formation or reabsorption.[187] Despite this association, flumazenil has been used successfully to awaken patients after craniotomy without adversely affecting cerebral blood flow or metabolic rate.[169] Flumazenil antagonizes the decrease in motor tone (as assessed by electromyography) and the EEG changes (increase in frequency and decrease in amplitude) accompanying benzodiazepine administration.[181] Flumazenil also effectively reverses the respiratory depression induced by benzodiazepine agonists as measured by tidal volume, minute ventilation, and inspiratory flow.[180,188] However, doses of flumazenil that reverse sedation after diazepam may not reverse benzodiazepine-induced depression of the slope of the CO_2 ventilatory response[188] or hypoxic ventilatory drive.[189]

Reversal of benzodiazepine sedation and psychomotor impairment occurs in the relative absence of hemodynamic changes. Patients sedated with diazepam for coronary angiography who were then given flumazenil (0.2 mg) exhibited no change in pulse, systemic or pulmonary pressures or resistances, LV filling pressures, or cardiac output.[190–192] Similar results were observed when flumazenil was used to reverse benzodiazepine sedation after regional anesthesia,[193] and after cardiac surgery, although the latter group of patients experienced greater levels of anxiety than those given placebo.[194] Reversal of benzodiazepine sedation by flumazenil does not change catecholamine, vasopressin, or β-endorphin levels in patients undergoing procedures with local anesthesia.[195]

Dosage

In principle, because flumazenil's therapeutic effect in reversing benzodiazepine agonists results from competitive antagonism at the benzodiazepine receptor, the specific effective dose is a consequence of three factors.

1. *The relative receptor binding affinities of the agonist and flumazenil.* For an agonist with greater affinity (e.g., lorazepam), a greater dose of flumazenil would be necessary. Because flumazenil has a binding affinity that is equivalent to or greater than that of the most potent benzodiazepine agonists, this is rarely an important consideration.
2. *The concentration of agonist.* Since the interaction at the benzodiazepine receptor is competitive, a greater concentration of flumazenil will be required to reverse a greater concentration of agonist.
3. *The degree of reversal desired.* In general, low receptor occupancy by agonists suffices for anticonvulsive and anxiolytic actions, whereas higher receptor occupancy is required to produce obtundation. Thus, a higher flumazenil dose is required to reverse anxiolysis than to reverse obtundation.

To antagonize the sedative effects of benzodiazepine agonists, an initial dose of flumazenil of 0.2 mg IV with subsequent additional doses titrated up to a total of 1 mg have proved effective.[196] If resedation is a concern, an infusion of 0.1 to 0.4 mg/h should suffice.[196]

Side Effects

An important side effect that has been associated with the administration of flumazenil is the onset of seizures.[197] Benzodiazepine agonists act as anticonvulsants, and in known epileptic patients treated with benzodiazepines, or perhaps in untreated latent epileptic patients, flumazenil may unmask a propensity for convulsions. However, the evidence for the latter mechanism is far from clear. A review of 43 cases of seizures temporally related to the administration of flumazenil found no relation between the dose of flumazenil and the development of seizures.[197] In addition, many patients who exhibited flumazenil-associated seizures had ingested overdoses of tricyclic antidepressants, had been treated chronically with benzodiazepines, were undergoing other drug withdrawal, or had a history of seizures.[197] Interestingly, flumazenil alone has been used successfully as an anticonvulsant.[198] Local anesthetic-induced seizures are not influenced by flumazenil, but flumazenil does reverse the protective effect of benzodiazepine agonists against such seizures.[199]

REFERENCES

1. Greenblatt DJ, Shader RI, Abernethy DR: Current status of benzodiazepines. N Engl J Med 309:410, 1983
2. Divoll M, Greenblatt DJ, Ochs HR, Shader RI: Absolute bioavailability of oral and intramuscular diazepam: effects of age and sex. Anesth Analg 62:1, 1983
3. Stallworth JM, Martino-Saltzmann D: Comparison of benzodiazepine premedications triazolam and diazepam: amnesia, anxiolysis, and sedation, abstracted. Anesth Analg 66:S165, 1987
4. Pinnock CA, Fell D, Hunt PCW et al: A comparison of triazolam and diazepam as premedication agents for minor gynaecological surgery. Anaesthesia 40:324, 1985
5. McKay AC, Dundee JW: Effect of oral benzodiazepines on memory. Br J Anaesth 52:1247, 1980
6. Fragen RJ, Caldwell N: Lorazepam premedication: lack of recall and relief of anxiety. Anesth Analg 55:792, 1976
7. George KA, Dundee JW: Relative amnesic actions of diazepam, flunitrazepam, and lorazepam in man. Br J Clin Pharmac 4:45, 1977
8. Dundee JW, Lilburn JK, Nair SG, George KA: Studies of drugs given before anaesthesia XXVI: lorazepam. Br J Anaesth 49:1047, 1977
9. O'Boyle CA, Harris D, Barry H et al: Comparison of midazolam by mouth and diazepam I.V. in outpatient oral surgery. Br J Anaesth 59:746, 1987
10. Weldon BC, Watcha MF, White PF: Oral midazolam in children: effect of time and adjunctive therapy. Anesth Analg 75:51, 1992
11. Feld LH, Negus JB, White PF: Oral midazolam preanesthetic medication in pediatric outpatients. Anesthesiology 73:831, 1990

12. Rosen DA, Rosen KR: A palatable gelatin vehicle for midazolam and ketamine. Anesthesiology 75:914, 1991
13. Peterson MD: Making oral midazolam palatable for children. Anesthesiology 73:1053, 1990
14. Fragen RJ, Funk DI, Avram MJ et al: Midazolam versus hydroxyzine as intramuscular premedicant. Can Anaesth Soc J 30:136, 1983
15. Vinik HR, Reves JG, Wright D: Premedication with intramuscular midazolam: a prospective randomized double-blind controlled study. Anesth Analg 61:933, 1982
16. Shafer A, White PF, Urquhart ML, Doze VA: Outpatient premedication: use of midazolam and opioid analgesics, Anesthesiology 71:495, 1989
17. Rita L, Seleny FL, Mazurek A, Rabins S: Intramuscular midazolam for pediatric preanesthetic sedation: a double-blind controlled study with morphine. Anesthesiology 63:528, 1985
18. Kanto J, Sjövall S, Vuori A: Effect of different kinds of premedication on the induction properties of midazolam. Br J Anaesth 54:507, 1982
19. Wong HY, Fragen RJ, Dunn K: Dose-finding study of intramuscular midazolam preanesthetic medication in the elderly. Anesthesiology 74:675, 1991
20. Conner JT, Katz RL, Pagano RR, Graham CW: RO 21-3981 for intravenous surgical premedication and induction of anesthesia. Anesth Analg 57:1, 1978
21. Wilton NCT, Leigh J, Rosen DR, Pandit UA: Preanesthetic sedation of preschool children using intranasal midazolam. Anesthesiology 69:972, 1988
22. Karl HW, Keifer AT, Rosenberger JL et al: Comparison of the safety and efficacy of intranasal midazolam or sufentanil for preinduction of anesthesia in pediatric patients. Anesthesiology 76:209, 1992
23. Cheng ACK: Intranasal midazolam for rapidly sedating an adult patient. Anesth Analg 76:904, 1993
24. Spear RM, Yaster M, Berkowitz ID et al: Preinduction of anesthesia in children with rectally administered midazolam. Anesthesiology 74:670, 1991
25. O'Boyle CA, Harris D, Barry H: Sedation in outpatient oral surgery: comparison of temazepam by mouth and diazepam I.V. Br J Anaesth 58:378, 1986
26. Douglas JG, Nimmo WS, Wanless R et al: Sedation for upper gastro-intestinal endoscopy: a comparison of oral temazepam and I.V. diazepam. Br J Anaesth 52:811, 1980
27. Baughmann VL, Becker GL, Ryan CM et al: Effectiveness of triazolam, diazepam, and placebo as preanesthetic medications. Anesthesiology 71:196, 1989
28. McClish A: Diazepam as an intravenous induction agent for general anaesthesia. Can Anaesth Soc J 13:562, 1966
29. Wyant GM, Studney LJ: A study of diazepam (Valium®) for induction of anaesthesia. Can Anaesth Soc J 17:166, 1970
30. Baker AB: Induction of anaesthesia with diazepam. Anaesthesia 24:388, 1969
31. Fox GS, Wynands JE, Bhambhami M: A clinical comparison of diazepam and thiopentone as induction agents to general anesthesia. Can Anaesth Soc J 15:281, 1968
32. Samuelson PN, Lell WA, Kouchokos NT et al: Hemodynamics during diazepam induction of anesthesia for coronary artery bypass grafting. Southern Med J 73:332, 1980
33. Clarke RSJ, Lyons SM: Diazepam and flunitrazepam as induction agents for cardiac surgical operations Acta Anaesth Scand 21:282, 1977
34. Gamble JAS, Kawar P, Dundee JW et al: Evaluation of midazolam as an intravenous induction agent. Anaesthesia 36:868, 1981
35. Dundee JW, Halliday NJ, Loughran PG, Harper KW: The influence of age on the onset of anaesthesia with midazolam. Anaesthesia 40:441, 1985
36. Salonen M, Kanto J, Iisalo E, Himberg J-J: Midazolam as an induction agent in children: a pharmacokinetic and clinical study. Anesth Analg 66:625, 1987
37. Kanto J, Aaltonen L, Himberg J-J, Hovi-Viander M: Midazolam as an intravenous induction agent in the elderly. Anesth Analg 65:15, 1986
38. White PF: Comparative evaluation of intravenous agents for rapid sequence induction—thiopental, ketamine, and midazolam. Anesthesiology 57:279, 1982
39. Schulte-Sasse U, Hess W, Tarnow J: Haemodynamic responses to induction of anaesthesia using midazolam in cardiac surgical patients. Br J Anaesth 54:1053, 1982
40. Samuelson PN, Reves JG, Kouchoukos NT et al: Hemodynamic responses to anesthetic induction with midazolam or diazepam in patients with ischemic heart disease. Anesth Analg 60:802, 1981
41. Iisalo E, Kanto J, Aaltonen L, Mäkelä J: Flunitrazepam as an induction agent in children: a clinical and pharmacokinetic study. Br J Anaesth 56:899, 1984
42. Melvin MA, Johnson BH, Quasha AL, Eger EI II: Induction of anesthesia with midazolam decreases halothane MAC in humans. Anesthesiology 57:238, 1982
43. Perisho JA, Buechel DR, Miller RD: The effect of

diazepam (Valium®) on minimum alveolar anesthetic requirement (MAC) in man. Can Anaesth Soc J: 18:536, 1971

44. Reves JG, Vinik R, Hirschfeld AM et al: Midazolam compared with thiopentone as a hypnotic component in balanced anaesthesia: a randomized, double-blind study. Can Anaesth Soc J 26:42, 1979

45. Crawford ME, Carl P, Anderson RS, Mikkelsen BO: Comparison between midazolam and thiopentone-based balanced anaesthesia for day-case surgery. Br J Anaesth 56:165, 1984

46. Heikkilä H, Jalonen J, Arola M et al: Midazolam as adjunct to high-dose fentanyl anaesthesia for coronary artery bypass grafting operation. Acta Anaesthesiol Scand 28:683, 1984

47. Tomicheck RC, Rosow CE, Schneider RC et al: Cardiovascular effects of diazepam-fentanyl anesthesia in patients with coronary artery disease. Anesth Analg 61:217, 1982

48. Jackson APF, Dhadphale PR, Callaghan ML, Alseri S: Haemodynamic studies during induction of anaesthesia for open-heart surgery using diazepam and ketamine. Br J Anaesth 50:375, 1978

49. Lilburn JK, Dundee JW, Nair SG et al: Ketamine sequelae: evaluation of the ability of various premedicants to attenuate its psychic actions. Anaesthesia 33:307, 1978

50. Kothary SP, Zsigmond EK: A double-blind study of the effective antihallucinatory doses of diazepam prior to ketamine anesthesia. Clin Pharmacol Ther 21:108, 1977

51. Belopavlovic M, Buchtal A: Modification of ketamine-induced intracranial hypertension in neurosurgical patients by treatment with midazolam. Acta Anaesth Scand 26:458, 1982

52. McClure JH, Brown DT, Wildsmith JAW: Comparison of the I.V. administration of midazolam and diazepam as sedation during spinal anesthesia. Br J Anaesth 55:1089, 1983

53. Caplan RA, Ward RJ, Posner K, Cheny FW: Unexpected cardiac arrest during spinal anesthesia: a closed claims analysis of predisposing factors. Anesthesiology 68:5, 1988

54. Korttila K, Levänen J: Untoward effects of ketamine combined with diazepam for supplementing conduction anaesthesia in young and middle-aged adults. Acta Anaesth Scand 22:640, 1978

55. Park WY, Watkins PA: Patient-controlled sedation during epidural anesthesia. Anesth Analg 72:304, 1991

56. Cole SG, Brozinsky S, Isenberg JI: Midazolam, a new more potent benzodiazepine, compared with diazepam: a randomized, double-blind study of pre-endoscopic sedatives. Gastrointest Endosc 29:219, 1983

57. Westphal LM, Cheng EY, White PF et al: Use of midazolam infusion for sedation following cardiac surgery. Anesthesiology 67:257, 1987

58. Gamble JAS, Dundee JW, Gray RC: Plasma diazepam concentrations following prolonged administration. Br J Anaesth 48:1087, 1976

59. Byatt CM, Lewis LD, Dawling S, Cochrane GM: Accumulation of midazolam after repeated dosage in patients receiving mechanical ventilation in an ICU. Br Med J 289:799, 1984

60. Michalk S, Moncorge C, Fichelle A et al: Midazolam infusion for basal sedation in intensive care: absence of accumulation. Intensive Care Med 15:37, 1988

61. Shapiro JM, Westphal LM, White PF et al: Midazolam infusion for sedation in the ICU: effect on adrenal function. Anesthesiology 64:394, 1986

62. Silvasi DL, Rosen DA, Rosen KR: Continuous intravenous midazolam infusion for sedation in the pediatric ICU. Anesth Analg 67:286, 1988

63. Lloyd-Thomas AR, Booker PD: Infusion of midazolam in paediatric patients after cardiac surgery. Br J Anaesth 58:1109, 1986

64. Rosen DA, Rosen KR: Pain control for pediatric cardiac and thoracic surgery. p. 125. In Gravlee GP, Rauck RL (eds): Pain Management in Cardiothoracic Surgery. Lippincott, Philadelphia, 1993

65. Loper KA, Ready LB, Brody M: Patient-controlled anxiolysis with midazolam. Anesth Analg 67:1118, 1988

66. Brown CR, Sarnquist FH, Canup CA, Pedley TA: Clinical electroencephalographic, and pharmacokinetic studies of a water-soluble benzodiazepine, midazolam maleate. Anesthesiology 50:467, 1979

67. Ziegler WH, Schalch E, Leishman B, Eckert M: Comparison of the effects of intravenously administered midazolam, triazolam, and their hydroxy metabolites. Br J Clin Pharmacol 16:63S, 1983

68. Elliott HW, Nomof N, Navarro G et al: Central nervous system and cardiovascular effects of lorazepam in man. Clin Pharmacol Ther 12:468, 1971

69. Veselis RA, Reinsel R, Alagesan R et al: The EEG as a monitor of midazolam amnesia: changes in power and topography as a function of amnesic state. Anesthesiology 74:866, 1991

70. Koht A, Schütz W, Schmidt G et al: Effects of etomidate, midazolam, and thiopental on median nerve somatosensory evoked potentials and the additive effects of fentanyl and nitrous oxide. Anesth Analg 67:435, 1988

71. Ghoneim MM, Mewaldt SP: Benzodiazepines and human memory: a review. Anesthesiology 72:926, 1990

72. Forster A, Gardaz JP, Suter PM, Gemperle M: I.V. midazolam as an induction agent for anaesthesia: a study in volunteers. Br J Anaesth 52:907, 1980

73. Melvin MA, Johnson BH, Quasha AL, Eger EI II: Induction of anesthesia with midazolam decreases halothane MAC in humans. Anesthesiology 57:238, 1982

74. Pruhs RJ, Quock RM: Interaction between nitrous oxide and diazepam in the mouse staircase rest. Anesth Analg 68:501, 1989

75. Kissin I, Mason JO III, Bradley EL Jr: Pentobarbital and thiopental anesthetic interactions with midazolam. Anesthesiology 67:26, 1987

76. Linnoila M, Mattila MJ: Drug interaction on psychomotor skills related to driving: diazepam and alcohol. Eur J Clin Pharmacol 5:186, 1973

77. Lichtor JL, Zacny J, Korttila K et al: Alcohol after midazolam sedation: does it really matter? Anesth Analg 72:661, 1991

78. Newman LM, Curran MA, Becker GL: Effects of chronic alcohol intake on anesthetic responses to diazepam and thiopental in rats. Anesthesiology 65:196, 1986

79. Kissin I, Brown PT, Bradley EL Jr et al: Diazepam-morphine hypnotic synergism in rats. Anesthesiology 70:689, 1989

80. Vinik HR, Bradley EL Jr, Kissin I: Midazolam-alfentanil synergism for anesthetic induction in patients. Anesth Analg 69:213, 1989

81. Kissin I, Vinik HR, Castillo R, Bradley EL Jr: Alfentanil potentiates midazolam-induced unconsciousness in subanalgesic doses. Anesth Analg 71:65, 1990

82. Tverskoy M, Fleyshman G, Ezry J et al: Midazolam-morphine sedative interaction in patients. Anesth Analg 68:282, 1989

83. Kissin I, Brown PT, Bradley EL Jr: Sedative and hypnotic midazolam-morphine interaction in rats. Anesth Analg 71:137, 1990

84. Kissin I, Brown PT, Bradley EL Jr: Morphine and fentanyl anesthetic interactions with diazepam: relative antagonism in rats. Anesth Analg 71:236, 1990

85. Schweiger IM, Hall RI, Hug CC Jr: Less than additive antinociceptive interaction between midazolam and fentananyl in enflurane-anesthetized dogs. Anesthesiology 74:1060, 1991

86. Treiman DM: The role of benzodiazepines in the management of status epilepticus. Neurology 40:32, 1990

87. Kumar A, Bleck TP: Intravenous midazolam for the treatment of refractory status epilepticus. Crit Care Med 20:483, 1992

88. de Jong RH, Heavner JE: Diazepam prevents and aborts lidocaine convulsions in monkeys. Anesthesiology 41:226, 1974

89. de Jong RH, Bonin JD: Benzodiazepines protect mice from local anesthetic convulsions and deaths. Anesth Analg 60:385, 1981

90. Vatashsky E, Aronson HB: Flunitrazepam protects mice against lidocaine and bupivacaine-induced convulsions. Can Anaesth Soc J 30:32, 1983

91. Torbiner ML, Yagiela JA, Mito RS: Effect of midazolam pretreatment on the intravenous toxicity of lidocaine with and without epinephrine in rats. Anesth Analg 68:744, 1989

92. Gregg RV, Turner PA, Denson DD et al: Does diazepam really reduce the cardiotoxic effects of intravenous bupivacaine? Anesth Analg 67:9, 1988

93. Bernards CM, Artru AA: Hexamethonium and midazolam terminate dysrhythymias and hypertension caused by intracerebroventricular bupivacaine in rabbits. Anesthesiology 74:89, 1991

94. Carlsson C, Hägerdal M, Kaasik AE, Siesjö BK: The effects of diazepam on cerebral blood flow and oxygen consumption in rats and its synergistic interaction with nitrous oxide. Anesthesiology 45:319, 1976

95. Nugent M, Artru AA, Michenfelder JD: Cerebral metabolic, vascular and protective effects of midazolam maleate. Anesthesiology 56:172, 1982

96. Rockoff MA, Naughton KVH, Shapiro HM et al: Cerebral circulatory and metabolic responses to intravenously administered lorazepam. Anesthesiology 53:215, 1980

97. Forster A, Juge O, Morel D: Effects of midazolam on cerebral blood flow in human volunteers. Anesthesiology 56:453, 1982

98. Van Gorder PN, Hoffman WE, Baughman V et al: Midazolam-ethanol interactions and reversal with a benzodiazepine antagonist. Anesth Analg 64:129, 1985

99. Baughman VL, Hoffman WE, Albrecht RF, Miletich DJ: Cerebral vascular and metabolic effects of fentanyl and midazolam in young and aged rats. Anesthesiology 67:314, 1987

100. Hoffman WE, Miletich DJ, Albrecht RF: The effects of midazolam on cerebral blood flow and oxygen consumption and its interaction with nitrous oxide. Anesth Analg 65:729, 1986

101. Newman LM, Hoffman WE, Miletich DJ, Albrecht RF: Regional blood flow and cerebral metabolic

changes during alcohol withdrawal and following midazolam therapy. Anesthesiology 63:395, 1985

102. Poterack KA, Kampine JP, Schmeling WT: Effects of isoflurane, midazolam, and etomidate on cardiovascular responses to stimulation of central nervous system pressor sites in chronically instrumented cats. Anesth Analg 73:64, 1991

103. Cote P, Gueret P, Bourassa MG: Systemic and coronary hemodynamic effects of diazepam in patients with normal and diseased coronary arteries. Circulation 50:1210, 1974

104. Lebowitz PW, Cote ME, Daniels AL et al: Comparative cardiovascular effects of midazolam and thiopental in healthy patients. Anesth Analg 61:771, 1982

105. Marty J, Gauzit R, Lefevre P et al: Effects of diazepam and midazolam on baroreflex control of heart rate and on sympathetic activity in humans. Anesth Analg 65:113, 1986

106. Lepage J-Y, Blanloeil Y, Pinaud M et al: Hemodynamic effects of diazepam, flunitrazepam, and midazolam in patients with ischemic heart disease: assessment with a radionuclide approach. Anesthesiology 65:678, 1986

107. Tomicheck RC, Rosow CE, Philbin DM et al: Diazepam-fentanyl interaction—hemodynamic and hormonal effects in coronary artery surgery. Anesth Analg 62:881, 1983

108. Stanley TH, Webster LR: Anesthetic requirements and cardiovascular effects of fentanyl-oxygen and fentanyl-diazepam-oxygen anesthesia in man. Anesth Analg 57:411, 1978

109. Benson KT, Tomlinson DL, Goto H, Arakawa K: Cardiovascular effects of lorazepam during sufentanil anesthesia. Anesth Analg 67:996, 1988

110. Flacke JW, Davis LJ, Flacke WE et al: Effects of fentanyl and diazepam in dogs deprived of autonomic tone. Anesth Analg 64:1053, 1985

111. Nitenberg A, Marty J, Blanchet F et al: Effects of flunitrazepam on left ventricular performance, coronary haemodynamics and myocardial metabolism in patients with coronary artery disease. Br J Anaesth 55:1179, 1983

112. Ikram H, Rubin AP, Jewkes RF: Effect of diazepam on myocardial blood flow of patients with and without coronary artery disease. Br Heart J 35:626, 1973

113. Forster A, Gardaz JP, Suter PM, Gemperle M: Respiratory depression by midazolam and diazepam. Anesthesiology 53:494, 1980

114. Gross JB, Smith L, Smith TC: Time course of ventilatory response to CO_2 after intravenous diazepam. Anesthesiology 57:18, 1982

115. Gross JB, Zebrowski ME et al: Time course of ventilatory depression after thiopental and midazolam in normal subjects and in patients with chronic obstructive pulmonary disease. Anesthesiology 58:540, 1983

116. Spaulding BC, Choi SD, Gross JB et al: The effect of physostigmine on diazepam-induced ventilatory depression: a double blind study. Anesthesiology 61:551, 1984

117. Alexander CM, Teller LE, Gross JB: Slow injection does not prevent midazolam-induced ventilatory depression. Anesth Analg 74:260, 1992

118. Forster A, Morel D, Bachmann M, Gemperle M: Respiratory depressant effects of different doses of midazolam and lack of reversal with naloxone—a double blind study. Anesth Analg 62:920, 1983

119. Power SJ, Morgan M, Chakrabarti MK: Carbon dioxide response curves following midazolam and diazepam. Br J Anaesth 55:837, 1983

120. Bailey PL, Pace NL, Ashburn MA et al: Frequent hypoxemia and apnea after sedation with midazolam and fentanyl. Anesthesiology 73:826, 1990

121. Lakshminarayan S, Sahn SA, Hudson LD, Weil JV: Effect of diazepam on ventilatory responses. Clin Pharmacol Ther 20:178, 1976

122. Catchlove RFH, Kafer ER: The effects of diazepam on the ventilatory response to carbon dioxide and on steady state gas exchange. Anesthesiology 34:9, 1971

123. Clergue F, Desmonts JM, Duvaldestin P et al: Depression of respiratory drive by diazepam as premedication. Br J Anaesth 53:1059, 1981

124. Jordan C, Lehane JR, Jones JG: Respiratory depression following diazepam: reversal with high-dose naloxone. Anesthesiology 53:293, 1980

125. Paulson BA, Becker LD, Way WL: The effects of intravenous lorazepam alone and with meperidine on ventilation in man. Acta Anaesthesiol Scand 27:400, 1983

126. Elliot HW, Nomof N, Navarro G et al: Central nervous system and cardiovascular effects of lorazepam in man. Clin Pharmacol Ther 12:468, 1971

127. Alexander CM, Gross JB: Sedative doses of midazolam depress hypoxic ventilatory responses in humans. Anesth Analg 67:377, 1988

128. Snyder SH, Enna SJ, Young AB: Brain mechanisms associated with therapeutic actions of benzodiazepines: focus on neurotransmitters. Am J Psychiatry 134:662, 1977

129. Snyder SH, Enna SJ: The role of central glycine receptors in the pharamcologic actions of benzodiazepines. Adv Biochem Psychopharmacol 14:81, 1975

130. Ngai SH, Tseng DTC, Wang SC: Effect of diazepam and other central nervous system depressants on spinal reflexes in cats: a study of site of action. J Pharmacol Exp Ther 153:344, 1966

131. Feldman SA, Crawley BE: Interaction of diazepam with the muscle-relaxant drugs. Br Med J 2:336, 1970

132. Hunter AR: Diazepam (Valium) as a muscle relaxant during general anaesthesia: a pilot study. Br J Anaesth 39:633, 1967

133. Dretchen K, Ghoneim MM, Long JP: The interaction of diazepam with myoneural blocking agents. Anesthesiology 34:463, 1971

134. Cronnely R, Morris RB, Miller RD: Comparison of thiopental and midazolam on the neuromuscular responses to succinylcholine or pancuronium in humans. Anesth Analg 62:75, 1983

135. Robson JG, Davenport HT, Sugiyama R: Differentiation of two types of pain by anesthetics. Anesthesiology 26:31, 1965

136. Morichi R, Pepeu G: A study of the influence of hydroxyzine and diazepam on morphine antinociception in the rat. Pain 7:173, 1979

137. Abbott FV, Franklin KBJ: Noncompetitive antagonism of morphine analgesia by diazepam in the formalin test. Pharmacol Biochem Behavior 24:319, 1986

138. Singh PN, Sharma P, Gupta PK, Pandey: Clinical evaluation of diazepam for relief of postoperative pain. Br J Anaesth 53:831, 1981

139. Daghero AM, Bradley EL Jr., Kissin I: Midazolam antagonizes the analgesic effect of morphine in rats. Anesth Analg 66:944, 1987

140. Rosland JH, Hole K: 1,4-Benzodiazepines antagonize opiate-induced antinociception in mice. Anesth Analg 71:242, 1990

141. Shannon HE, Holtzman SG, Davis DC: Interactions between narcotic analgescis and benzodiazepine derivatives on behavior in the mouse. J Pharmacol Exp Ther 199:389, 1976

142. Jurna I: Depression of nociceptive sensory activity in the rat spinal cord due to the intrathecal administration of drugs: effect of diazepam. Neurosurgery 15:917, 1984

143. Niv D, Whitwam JG, Loh L: Depression of nociceptive sympathetic reflexes by the intrathecal administration of midazolam. Br J Anaesth 55:541, 1983

144. Gaumann DM, Yaksh TL, Tyce GM: Effects of intrathecal morphine, clonidine, and midazolam on the somato-sympathoadrenal reflex response in halothane-anesthetized cats. Anesthesiology 73:425, 1990

145. Niv D, Davidovich S, Geller E, Urca G: Analgesic and hyperalgesic effects of midazolam: dependence on route of administration. Anesth Analg 67:1169, 1988

146. Mantegazza P, Parenti M, Tammiso R, et al: Modification of the antinociceptive effect of morphine by centrally administered diazepam and midazolam. Br J Pharmacol 75:569, 1982

147. Edwards M, Serrao JM, Gent JP, Goodchild CS: On the mechanism by which midazolam causes spinally mediated analgesia. Anesthesiology 73:273, 1990

148. Rattan AK, McDonald JS, Tejwani GA: Differential effects of ontrathecal midazolam on morphine-induced antinociception in the rat: role of spinal opioid receptors. Anesth Analg 73:124, 1991

149. Malinovsky J-M, Cozian A, Lepage J-Y et al: Ketamine and midazolam neurotoxicity in the rabbit. Anesthesiology 75:91, 1991

150. Jones DJ, Stehling LC, Zauder HL: Cardiovascular responses to diazepam and midazolam maleate in the dog. Anesthesiology 51:430, 1979

151. Reves JG, Kissin I, Fournier S: Negative inotropic effects of midazolam. Anesthesiology 60:517, 1984

152. Sunzel M, Paalzow L, Berggren L, Eriksson I: Respiratory and cardiovascular effects in relation to plasma levels of midazolam and diazepam. Br J Clin Pharmac 25:561, 1988

153. Mikkelsen H, Hoel TM, Bryne H, Krohn CD: Local reactions after I.V. injections of diazepam, flunitrazepam and isotonic saline. Br J Anaesth 52:817, 1980

154. Hegarty JE, Dundee JW: Sequelae after the intravenous injection of three benzodiazepines—diazepam, lorazepam, and flunitrazepam. Br Med J 2:1384, 1977

155. Bortolussi ME, Hunter JG, Handal AG: Forearm compartment syndrome after diazepam administration. Anesthesiology 75:159, 1991

156. Schneider S, Mace JW: Loss of limb following intravenous diazepam. Pediatrics 53:112, 1974

157. Stolarek IH, Ford MJ: Acute dystonia induced by midazolam and abolished by flumazenil. Br Med J 300:614, 1990

158. Van der Bijl P, Roelofse JA: Disinhibitory reactions to benzodiazepines: a review. J Oral Maxillofacial Surg 49:519, 1991

159. Swanson RJ, Leavitt MG: Fertilization and mouse embryo development in the presence of midazolam. Anesth Analg 75:549, 1992

160. Tuman KJ, Spiess BD, Wong CA, Ivankovich AD: Sufentanil-midazolam anesthesia in malignant hyperthermia. Anesth Analg 67:405, 1988

161. Vatashsky E, Beilin B, Razin M, Weinstock M: Mechanism of antagonism by physostigmine of acute flunitrazepam intoxication. Anesthesiology 64:248, 1986

162. Gürel A, Elevli M, Hamulu A: Aminophylline reversal of flunitrazepam sedation. Anesth Analg 66:333, 1987

163. Wangler MA, Kilpatrick DS: Aminophylline is an antagonist of lorazepam. Anesth Analg 64:834, 1985

164. Meyer BH, Weis OF, Muller FO: Antagonism of diazepam by aminophylline in healthy volunteers. Anesth Analg 63:900, 1984

165. Stirt JA: Aminophylline is a diazepam antagonist. Anesth Analg 60:767, 1981

166. Haefely W, Hunkeler W: The story of flumazenil. Eur J Anaesth (suppl 2):3, 1988

167. Philip BK, Simpson TH, Hauch MA, Mallampati SR: Flumazenil reverses sedation after midazolam-induced general anesthesia in ambulatory surgery patients. Anesth Analg 71:371, 1990

168. Eldar I, Lieberman N, Shiber R et al: Use of flumazenil for intraoperative arousal during spine fusion. Anesth Analg 75:580, 1992

169. Knudsen L, Cold GE, Holdgard HO et al: Effects of flumazenil on cerebral blood flow and oxygen consumption after midazolam anesthesia for craniotomy. Br J Anaesth 67:277, 1991

170. The Flumazenil in Benzodiazepine Intoxication Multicenter Study Group: Treatment of benzodiazepine overdose with flumazenil. Clin Ther 14:978, 1992

171. Mullen KD, Mendelson WB, Martin JV et al: Could an endogenous benzodiazepine ligand contribute to hepatic encephalopathy? Lancet X:457, 1988

172. Olasmaa M, Guidotti A, Costa E et al: Endogenous benzodiazepines in hepatic encehalopathy. Lancet X:491, 1989

173. Mullen KD, Szauter KM, Kaminsky-Russ K: "Endogenous" benzodiazepine activity in body fluids of patients with hepatic encephalopathy. Lancet 336:81, 1990

174. Grimm G, Ferenci P, Katzenschlager R et al: Improvement of hepatic encephalopathy treated with flumazenil. Lancet 2:1392, 1988

175. Baraldi M, Zeneroli ML, Ventura E: Supersensitivity of benzodiazepine receptors in hepatic encephalopathy due to fulminant hepatic failure in the rat: reversal by a benzodiazepine antagonist. Clin Sci 67:167, 1984

176. Lheureux P, Askenasi R: Efficacy of flumazenil in acute alcohol intoxication: double blind placebo-controlled evaluation. Human Exp Toxicol 10:235, 1991

177. Clausen TG, Wolff J, Carl P, Theilgaard A: The effect of the benzodiazepine antagonist, flumazenil, on psychometric performance in acute ethanol intoxication in man. Eur J Clin Pharmacol 38:233, 1990

178. Schweiger IM, Szlam F, Hug CC Jr: Absence of agonistic or antagonistic effect of flumazenil (RO 15-1788) in dogs anesthetized with enflurane, isoflurane, or fentanyl-enflurane. Anesthesiology 70:477, 1989

179. Greiner AS, Larach DR: The effect of benzodiazepine receptor antagonism by flumazenil on the MAC of halothane in the rat. Anesthesiology 70:644, 1989

180. Forster A, Crettenand G, Morel DR: Absence of ventilatory agonist or inverse agonist effects of an overdose of RO 15-1788, a specific benzodiazepine antagonist, abstracted. Anesthesiology 67:A144, 1987

181. Forster A, Juge O. Louis M, Nahory A: Effects of a specific benzodiazepine antagonist (RO 15-1788) on cerebral blood flow. Anesth Analg 66:309, 1987

182. Croughwell ND, Reves JG, Will CJ et al: Safety of flumazenil in patients with ischaemic heart disease. Eur J Anaesthesiol 2:177, 1988

183. Ghoneim MM, Dembo JB, Block RI: Time course of antagonism of sedative and amnesic effects of diazepam by flumazenil. Anesthesiology 70:899, 1989

184. Lauven PM, Schwilden H, Stoeckel H, Greenblatt DJ: The effects of a benzodiazepine antagonist RO 15-1788 in the presence of stable concentrations of midazolam. Anesthesiology 63:61, 1985

185. Dunton AW, Schwamm E, Pitman V et al: Flumazenil: US clinical pharmacology studies. Eur J Anaesthesiol 2:81, 1988

186. Chiolero RL, Ravussin P, Anderes JP et al: The effects of midazolam reversal by RO 15-1788 on cerebral perfusion pressure in patients with severe head injury. Intensive Care Med 14:196, 1988

187. Artru AA: The rate of CSF formation, resistance to reabsorption of CSF, and aperiodic analysis of the EEG following administration of flumazenil to dogs. Anesthesiology 72:111, 1990

188. Gross JB, Weller RS, Conard P: Flumazenil antago-

nism of midazolam-induced ventilatory depression. Anesthesiology 75:179, 1991

189. Mora CT, Torjman M, White PF: Effects of diazepam and flumazenil on sedation and hypoxic ventilatory response. Anesth Analg 68:473, 1989

190. Geller E, Niv D, Rudick V, Vidne B: The use of RO 15-1788, a benzodiazepine antagonist, in the diagnosis and treatment of benzodiazepine overdose, abstracted. Anesthesiology 61:A135, 1984

191. Geller E, Chernilas J, Halpern P et al: Hemodynamics following reversal of benzodiazepine sedation with RO 15-1788 in cardiac patients, abstracted. Anesthesiology 65:A49, 1986

192. Geller E, Halpern P, Cherilas J et al: Cardiorespiratory effects of antagonsim of diazepam sedation with flumazenil in patients with cardiac disease. Anesth Analg 72:207, 1991

193. Sage DJ, Close A, Boas RA: Reversal of midazolam sedation with Anexate. Br J Anaesth 59:459, 1987

194. Louis M, Forster A, Suter PM, Gemperle M: Clinical and hemodynamic effects of a specific benzodiazepine antagonist (RO 15-1788) after open heart surgery, abstracted. Anesthesiology 61:A61, 1984

195. White PF, Shafer A, Boyle WA, Doze VA: Stress response following reversal of benzodiazepine-induced sedation. Eur J Anaesthesiol 2:173, 1988

196. Amrein R, Hetzel W, Hartmann D, Lorscheid T: Clinical pharamacology of flumazenil. Eur J Anaesth 2:65:188

197. Spivey WH: Flumazenil and seizures: analysis of 43 cases. Clin Therapeutics 14:292, 1992

198. Scollo-Lavizzari G: The clinical anti-convulsant effects of flumazenil, a benzodiazepine antagonist. Eur J Anaesthesiol 2:129, 1988

199. Yokoyama M, Benson KT, Arakawa K, Goto H: Effects of flumazenil on intravenous lidocaine-induced convulsions and anticonvulsant property of diazepam in rats. Anesth Analg 75:87, 1992

200. Gilman AG, Goodman LS, Gilman A (eds): Goodman and Gilman's The Pharmacological Basis of Therapeutics. 6th Ed. Macmillan, New York, 1980

Chapter 13

Basic Pharmacology of Intravenous Induction Agents

Tim G. Hales and Richard W. Olsen

There is an extraordinary diversity of molecular structures capable of inducing general anesthesia. Ignoring the volatile agents and the alcohols, where is the similarity in the structures of the intravenous agents illustrated in Figure 13-1? Do these agents act through a common site, or is there more than one site involved? Considering solely the molecular architecture of these compounds, it seems inconceivable that they act through a single site.

The site of action of general anesthetics is the subject of a seemingly endless debate (see Ch. 23). The most fundamental and recurrent theme of this debate has been focused on whether the site of action is lipid or protein. This discussion began in 1899 when Meyer and Overton demonstrated a striking correlation between an anesthetic's potency and its oil/water partition coefficient.[1] The log-log plot of the potency of an anesthetic versus its lipid solubility has a slope of −1, implying that the potency of an agent is exclusively related to its lipid solubility. This led to the suggestion that anesthetics in some way produce anesthesia by partitioning into cell membranes.

A number of mechanisms have been proposed in which a molecule might cause anesthesia through an interaction with a lipid membrane. A widely held belief is that general anesthetics partition into cell membranes and disrupt the activity of ion channels. Whether or not lipid is the primary site through which disruption occurs (and we will consider evidence to the contrary later), there are compelling data that implicate ion channels in the actions of intravenous anesthetics.

ION CHANNELS AND NEURONAL EXCITABILITY

The membranes of neurons contain a variety of channels that allow the passage of specific ions from one side of a cell membrane to another, the direction of travel of an ion through a channel being dictated by the concentration gradient and the membrane potential. The direction an ion will travel at a particular membrane potential can be predicted by using the Nernst equation when the intracellular and extracellular concentrations of the ion are known.[2]

Broadly speaking, ion channels can be divided into three categories: (1) voltage-activated ion channels, (2) ligand-activated ion channels, and (3) metabotropic receptor-regulated ion channels. Among the latter are included the intracellular messenger-regulated ion channels and the G-protein-regulated ion channels (Table 13-1). Channels control the electrical excitability of a neuron by controlling the permeability of its membrane to

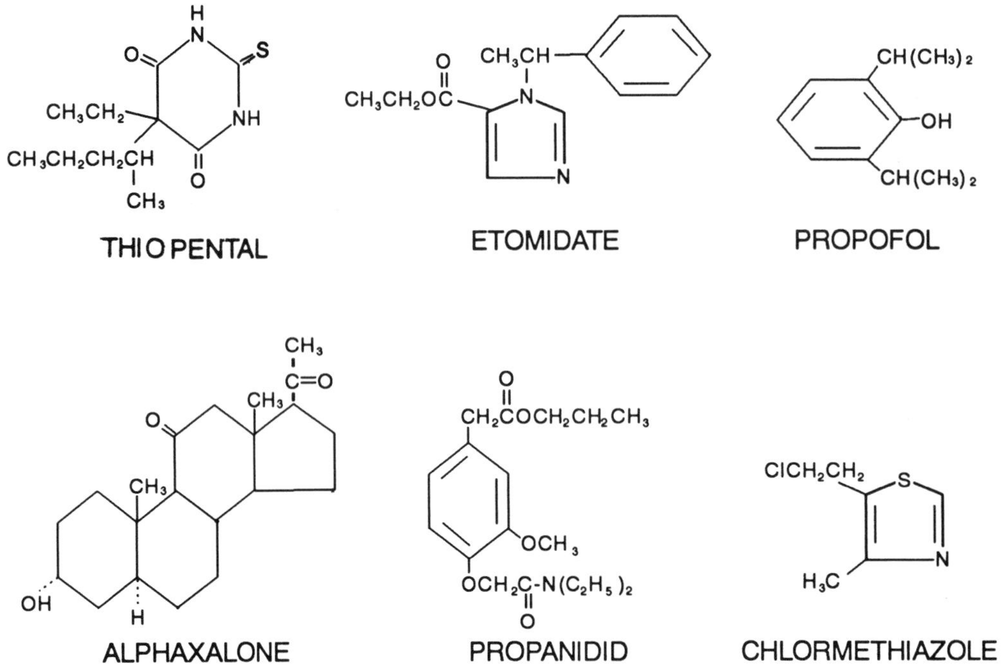

Fig. 13-1 Structures of various compounds that possess general anesthetic properties. These compounds have been used clinically as induction agents.

Table 13-1 Classes of Ion Channels

Channel Class	Examples	Permeant Ion(s)
Voltage activated	Calcium channel	Ca^{++}
	Sodium channel	Na^+
	$K(Ca^{++}, V)$	K^+
Ligand activated	$GABA_A$ receptor	Cl^-
	Glycine receptor	Cl^-
	Glutamate receptor	Na^+/Ca^{++}
	Nicotinic (Ach) receptor	Na^+/K^+
Intracellular messenger regulated	$K(Ca^{++}, V)$ channel	K^+
	K(ATP) channel	K^+
G-protein regulated	Potassium channel	K^+
	Calcium channel	Ca^{++}

Abbreviations: Ach, acetylcholine; $GABA_A$ receptor, γ-aminobutyric acid type A receptor; G-protein, guanosine triphosphate-binding protein; K(ATP) channel, adenosine triphosphate-blocked potassium channel; $K(Ca^{++}, V)$ channel, calcium and voltage-activated potassium channel.

ions such as potassium, sodium, calcium, and chloride. Activation or inhibition of one or more of these categories of channel can profoundly influence neuronal excitability. An example of this is illustrated in Figure 13-4, and this will be discussed in detail.

ION CHANNELS MODULATED BY BARBITURATES

The barbiturates are the best studied class of intravenous induction agents. Electrophysiologic investigation exposed the actions of barbiturates on a number of ion channels.[3] Pentobarbital abolishes action potentials recorded from squid axons, possibly by the blockade of voltage-dependent sodium channels,[4] and thiopental reduces potassium permeability in the axons of the lobster and squid.[5,6] These effects require relatively high doses of barbiturates. However, lower concentrations were demonstrated to block potassium conductance in small diameter fibers.[7] Pentobarbital, at doses within the anesthetic dose range, does not completely block voltage-activated sodium channels, although it was reported to reduce the open time of sodium channels in lipid bilayers prepared from the human brain.[8] Adenosine triphosphate (ATP)-sensitive potassium channels in pancreatic β cells are blocked by clinically relevant doses of thiopental, pentobarbital, and secobarbital.[9] In addition to their prevalence in the endocrine pancreas, ATP-sensitive potassium channels are also expressed by cortical neurons,[10] in which their blockade by barbiturates could contribute to the central actions of this class of anesthetic.

Some barbiturates increase the opening of calcium-activated potassium channels.[11] The resulting increase of potassium flux leads to hyperpolarization of central neurons.[12] This action may be secondary to an increase in intracellular calcium concentration,[13] although pentobarbital does not affect resting calcium levels in mouse whole brain synaptosomes.[14] Interestingly, the ability of a number of general anesthetics (e.g., phenobarbital, pentobarbital, and halothane) to hyperpolarize neurons by an increase in potassium permeability correlates well with their anesthetic potency.[12] The anesthetic-induced increase in neuronal membrane permeability to potassium ions may stabilize the membrane potential around the reversal potential for potassium ions and prevent depolarization to the threshold for firing action potentials.[15]

Barbiturates also block voltage-gated calcium channels, leading to a reduction of calcium uptake into synaptosomal preparations.[16] In dorsal root ganglion neurons, pentobarbital and phenobarbital block the activation of L-type calcium channels. In addition, both barbiturates appear to increase the inactivation rate of N-type calcium current under certain conditions.[17] There are two consequences of reduced calcium channel entry into neurons: (1) a reduction of presynaptic neurotransmitter release and (2) a shortening of calcium-dependent action potentials (e.g., mouse spinal neurons).[18] Both would be expected to disrupt neuronal communication. However, significant effects of pentobarbital and phenobarbital on calcium-dependent action potentials are only seen at the upper end of the anesthetic dose range.[18] Barbiturates, at concentrations within the anesthetic range, also depress current through human neuronal calcium channels expressed in Xenopus oocytes.[19] The order of potency of calcium channel blockade by barbiturates in this study does not correlate with their order of potency as anesthetics.[20,21]

Some ligand-gated ion channels are modulated by barbiturates. Considerable effort has been devoted to studying the effects of anesthetics on nicotinic receptors. This member of the ligand-activated ion channel family (physiologically activated by acetylcholine, Table 13-1) is the most fully characterized. The nicotinic receptor mediates vertebrate neuromuscular transmission and is found in autonomic ganglia and in certain central nervous system (CNS) regions. A rich source of the ion channel is the electric organ of *Torpedo californica*. The channel was first cloned in 1982[22] and is known to consist of five subunits, each having four plasma membrane spanning regions, which combine to form the passage through which sodium and potassium ions travel.[23] Pentobarbital inhibits acetylcholine-stimulated cation flux through the nicotinic acetylcholine receptor's ion channel[24] and barbiturates also block excitatory postsynaptic potentials through nicotinic receptors in skeletal muscle and autonomic ganglia.[25] Pentobarbital decreases acetylcholine binding to nicotinic receptors of *T. californica* in a saturable, dose-dependent, and stereoselective fashion, at clinically relevant concentrations;[26] however, the relative potencies of a series of compounds do not correlate well with their anesthetic efficacy. Our knowledge of the distribution of nicotinic receptors and their physiologic role within the mammalian brain is still rudimentary. Therefore, it is not possible to determine whether any of the central actions of barbiturates can be explained by their effects on these ion channels. However, studies of nicotinic receptors in electric organ and muscle have provided considerable information in regard to the mechanisms by which anesthetics modulate ion channels.[27]

The excitatory amino acid receptors represent another potential site for the action of the barbiturates. Receptors for the excitatory neurotransmitter glutamate are widely distributed throughout the CNS. Barbiturates have been shown to inhibit currents activated by agonists for subtypes of glutamate receptors, as recorded from voltage-clamped hippocampal neurons.[28] However, relatively high concentrations of pentobarbital are required, and the inhibition is only partial. A number of barbiturates also inhibit the sodium flux evoked by activation of non-N-methyl-D-aspartate subtypes of glutamate receptors in brain slices.[29] A mechanism by which anesthetics can functionally antagonize glutamate responses is discussed subsequently (see also Fig. 13-4).

When considering whether a particular ion channel represents an appropriate site through which anesthetics exert their actions, a number of factors should be considered:

1. Is the ion channel located in a suitable site to contribute to general anesthesia (i.e., on central neurons)?
2. Are the actions of anesthetics on the ion channel likely to cause a sufficient reduction in neuronal excitability to produce anesthesia?
3. Is the channel modulated by a clinically relevant dose of a given anesthetic?
4. Is there a correlation between the potency of general anesthetics as channel modulators and their potency as anesthetics?
5. Do many (most and/or all) general anesthetics act on the channel?

Many of the ion channels discussed earlier fail to fulfill one or more of these criteria, but they may contribute to the central and/or peripheral actions of barbiturates. However, there is a growing body of evidence that supports a primary role for the major inhibitory neurotransmitter receptor in the actions of these intravenous induction agents.

MODULATION OF γ-AMINOBUTYRIC ACID-A RECEPTORS BY GENERAL ANESTHETICS

γ-Aminobutyric acid (GABA) is the major inhibitory neurotransmitter in the brain. The transmitter is released from presynaptic neurons and binds to postsynaptic GABA$_A$ receptors, opening the associated chloride ion channel. Like the nicotinic acetyl-choline receptor, GABA$_A$ receptors are members of the ligand-activated class of ion channel (Table 13-1) and are thought to be composed of five subunits. Each subunit is believed to contain four membrane spanning domains, which contribute to the formation of the chloride channel (Fig. 13-2).[30] Many different varieties of subunits have been cloned, including α_1 to α_6, β_1 to β_3, γ_1, γ_{2S}, γ_{2L}, γ_3, and δ.[30,31] This subunit diversity provides the potential for numerous GABA$_A$ receptor subtypes.[31] There is evidence for multiple subtypes in the mammalian nervous system based on ligand binding, protein chemistry, and immunoblotting studies.[32,33] In situ hybridization has provided information as to the distribution of GABA$_A$ receptor polypeptide encoding messenger RNAs (mRNAs) within the CNS.[34,35] However, because of the difficulties associated with obtaining the large numbers of pure neuronal populations required for biochemical analysis, there is little information available in regard to the subunit composition of GABA$_A$ receptors in specific types of neurons. This problem can be overcome by studying immortalized (self-replicating) neurons known to express GABA$_A$ receptors.[36] In addition, techniques are being developed for analyzing mRNA encoding GABA$_A$ receptors in small numbers of cells.

Regardless of the diversity of GABA$_A$ receptor subtypes, a variety of compounds with depressant actions, including the anesthetic barbiturates, etomidate, and propofol, modulate GABA$_A$ receptors in a variety of different preparations.[37,38] The barbiturates, etomidate, and propofol all increase the binding of the GABA$_A$ receptor agonist [^{3}H]muscimol to, and displace the binding of the convulsant [^{35}S]-t-butylbicyclophosphorothionate from rat brain membranes.[39,40] Electrophysiologically, the anesthetic barbiturates, etomidate, and propofol have remarkably similar effects on the GABA$_A$ receptor. This is also true of the other compounds that have been used as intravenous induction agents, such as the steroid anesthetic alfaxalone, propanidid, and clomethiazole (Fig. 13-1). All these intravenous induction agents have two distinct actions on GABA$_A$ receptors with different concentration thresholds as described subsequently.

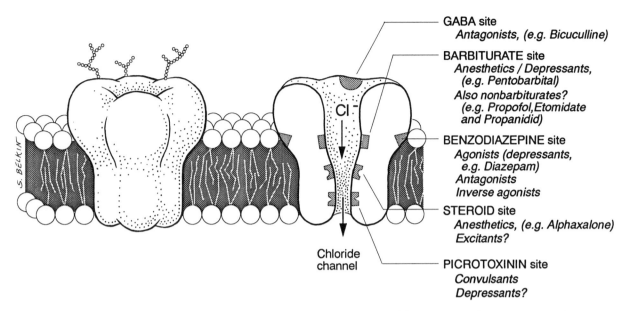

GABA site
Antagonists, (e.g. Bicuculline)

BARBITURATE site
*Anesthetics / Depressants,
(e.g. Pentobarbital)
Also nonbarbiturates?
(e.g. Propofol,Etomidate
and Propanidid)*

BENZODIAZEPINE site
*Agonists (depressants,
e.g. Diazepam)
Antagonists
Inverse agonists*

STEROID site
*Anesthetics, (e.g. Alphaxalone)
Excitants?*

PICROTOXININ site
*Convulsants
Depressants?*

Chloride channel

Fig. 13-2 Schematic representation of GABA$_A$ receptor with modulatory sites. The target sites of a number of agonists, antagonists, anesthetics, and benzodiazepines are listed. This is not intended to give an accurate representation of their location within the receptor complex. GABA$_A$, γ-aminobutyric acid-A. (Adapted from Delorey and Olsen,[74] with permission.)

Modulation of γ-Aminobutyric Acid-A Receptors by Low Doses of Intravenous Induction Agents

Barbiturates enhance the inhibitory synaptic transmission known to be mediated by GABA$_A$ receptors.[41–43] In addition, studies using the patch-clamp technique[44] demonstrated that GABA-activated chloride currents are potentiated by barbiturates (e.g., pentobarbital[18,45]), propofol,[38] etomidate,[37] clomethiazole (chlormethiazole),[46] propanidid,[47] and anesthetic steroids.[48,49] Examples of propofol-evoked modulation of GABA-activated currents recorded from a bovine chromaffin cell and a rat cortical neuron are illustrated in Figure 13-3. Currents activated by transiently applied GABA are potentiated in a reversible and dose-dependent manner by propofol administered to the recording chamber (Fig. 13-3).[38] Barbiturates and anesthetic steroids potentiate GABA-activated ^{36}Cl$^-$ flux in brain slices[39,50] and membrane vesicles.[51,52] The barbiturates and other anesthetics also were shown

to modulate allosterically the binding of radioactively labeled GABA, picrotoxin, and benzodiazepine ligands to their recognition sites on the GABA$_A$ receptor complex.[39,53]

In addition to the intravenous induction agents, the benzodiazepines also modulate GABA$_A$ receptors[54] (see Ch. 10). The binding site for the benzodiazepines associated with the GABA$_A$ receptor is well characterized. Benzodiazepine antagonists, such as flumazenil, which reversibly inhibit potentiation of GABA-evoked whole cell currents by diazepam or flunitrazepam,[49,38] have no effect on the potentiation elicited by the intravenous induction agents.[38,46,47,49] This suggests that these agents bind to a site (or sites) distinct from that of the benzodiazepines (Fig. 13-3).

Potentiation of GABA responses by the intravenous induction agents may contribute to their mechanism of action. As the major inhibitory neurotransmitter receptor in the brain, the GABA$_A$ receptor provides an appropriate site of action for these drugs. Moreover, the blood levels attained

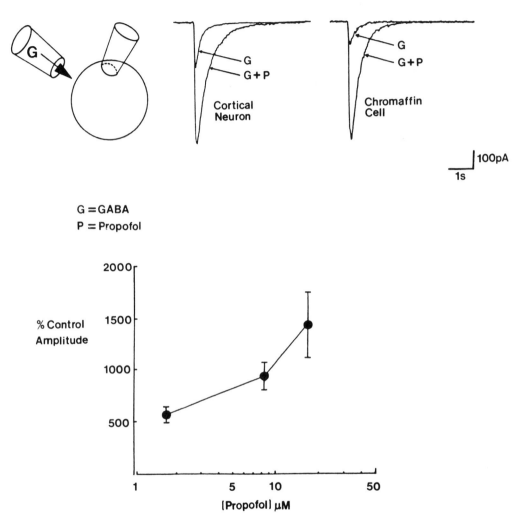

Fig. 13-3 Potentiation of GABA-activated currents by propofol. GABA (100 μM)-activated currents were recorded from a cortical neuron and a chromaffin cell voltage clamped at -60 mV, using the whole cell configuration of the patch-clamp technique[44] (schematically represented top left). GABA (G) was applied for 20 ms from a micropipette by pressure ejection. Bath application of propofol (8.4 μM, P) increased the amplitude and duration of the GABA-activated current. The dose dependency of propofol potentiation of GABA-evoked currents recorded from chromaffin cells is also illustrated. The data are plotted as a percentage of the control response amplitude against the concentration of propofol in the bath solution. The data points are the mean of at least four experiments with different cells, and the vertical bars indicate the standard error of mean. GABA$_A$, γ-aminobutyric acid-A. (Adapted from Hales and Lambert,[38] with permission.)

after administration of anesthetic doses of these drugs are commensurate with the concentrations that potentiate GABA responses.

γ-Aminobutyric Acid-A Receptor Activation by General Anesthetics

Electrophysiologic studies have uncovered an agonist action of pentobarbital,[55] etomidate,[37] propofol,[38] alfaxalone (alphaxalone),[49] and clomethiazole[46] at the GABA_A receptor. Application of these agents to voltage-clamped neurons and chromaffin cells directly activates whole cell currents in the absence of GABA. The holding potential at which these activated currents reverse (i.e., change direction from outward to inward or vice versa) is dependent on the concentration gradient for chloride ions across the cell membrane. At the single channel level, on outside-out patches, the intravenous anesthetics activate channels with similar properties to those activated by GABA. These evoked currents are abolished by the GABA_A receptor antagonist, bicuculline, and the channel blocker, picrotoxin. In addition, in neurochemical assays, barbiturates and steroid anesthetics activate $^{36}Cl^-$ flux in the absence of added GABA.[3,50-52] Taken together, these observations indicate that the intravenous induction agents directly activate GABA_A receptors.

Direct activation of the GABA_A receptor has profound effects on neuronal excitability. Figure 13-4 illustrates diagramatically how postsynaptic activation of GABA_A receptors can lead to a reduction in the excitability of neurons by opening the associated chloride ion channels. The continued presence of the drug causes chloride to enter the neuron down a concentration gradient. In this representation, the intracellular chloride concentration is taken to be 13 mM; the concentration of extracellular chloride is 145 mM (Fig. 13-4). The influx of chloride ions will continue until the driv-

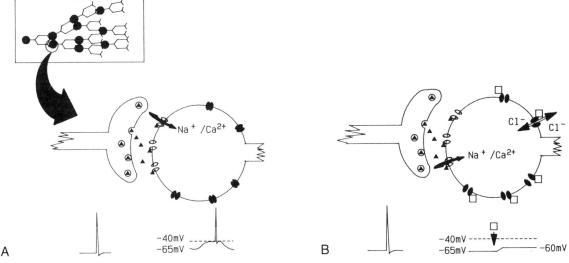

Fig. 13-4 Diagram depicting a mechanism for the functional antagonism of glutamate responses by intravenous anesthetics. **(A)** The inset is a diagramatic representation of synaptically coupled neurons. The synapse has been expanded to illustrate how transmission by the neurotransmitter glutamate (▲) communicates excitation from the nerve terminal of one neuron (on the left) to the next, the postsynaptic neuron. **(B)** An intravenous anesthetic (□) activates GABA_A receptor chloride ion channels. The postsynaptic neuron depolarizes slightly until the equilibrium potential for Cl⁻ is reached[2] (−60 mV, assuming 13 mM [Cl⁻] inside and 145 mM [Cl⁻] outside). In the presence of the anesthetic, the GABA_A receptor-mediated chloride channels remain open, and the postsynaptic neuron is clamped at −60 mV and cannot depolarize in response to glutamate. GABA_A, γ-aminobutyric acid-A. (Adapted from Bloor and Hales,[75] with permission.)

ing force on the ions, by virtue of the concentration gradient, is balanced by the outward driving force on the ions caused by the cell's negative potential. Under these conditions, the point at which chloride flow reaches equilibrium is calculated (by using the Nernst equation[2]) to be approximately −60 mV. This chloride equilibrium potential, the potential at which there is no driving force on chloride ions, will be maintained while the drug continues to open sufficient chloride channels. This shunting ("shorting-out") effect of the drug will effectively clamp the membrane potential at the reversal potential for chloride, in this example, at −75 mV. Under such conditions, stimulation of the postsynaptic neuron by the excitatory neurotransmitter, glutamate, will be functionally antagonized. Although glutamate will still bind to its postsynaptic receptors and open their associated sodium and calcium ion channels, the influx of sodium and calcium will not depolarize the neuron, provided that sufficient Cl^- channels are opened by the anesthetic. The cell will not reach the threshold potential required for firing action potentials and will therefore not communicate the signal to its synaptically coupled neighbors. This result will only apply if the drug increases membrane chloride conductance sufficiently to reduce the cell's input resistance profoundly. Current clamp recordings from neurons support the hypothesis that intravenous induction agents functionally antagonize glutamate-evoked depolarization by activation of $GABA_A$ receptors. In these experiments, the neuronal membrane potential is allowed to vary, more closely reproducing the physiologic activity of the neuron. Transient application of glutamate depolarizes neurons, leading to action potentials. In the presence of the steroid anesthetic alfaxalone, glutamate no longer depolarizes neurons, and action potentials are abolished. In contrast, under voltage-clamp conditions, alfaxalone has no effect on the amplitude of glutamate-evoked whole cell currents recorded from the same cells.[28] This suggests that, rather than acting as an antagonist at glutamate receptors, alfaxalone is functionally antagonizing the glutamate excitatory response by activating $GABA_A$ receptor associated chloride ion channels. Similar results have been obtained with propofol (Hales TG, Lambert JJ, unpublished observations) and pentobarbital.[55] Direct $GABA_A$ receptor activation by these agents requires higher concentrations than for their GABA potentiating effects. The threshold concentration of propofol to activate $GABA_A$ receptors directly is less than 8 μM.[38] Because concentrations of propofol in the blood during anesthesia have been reported to exceed 30 μM,[56] direct activation of $GABA_A$ receptors may therefore contribute to its anesthetic actions.

ACTIONS OF INTRAVENOUS INDUCTION AGENTS ON SPECIFIC SUBUNITS OF γ-AMINOBUTYRIC ACID-A RECEPTORS

As discussed earlier, $GABA_A$ receptors can be composed of many different types of subunits.[30,31] Since the first two $GABA_A$ receptor polypeptides were cloned,[57] there have been many attempts to determine the pharmacologic properties of known $GABA_A$ receptor subunit combinations.[31] Two approaches have generally been used to force cells to express known $GABA_A$ receptor subunits as follows: (1) oocytes from the frog *Xenopus laevis* have been injected with mRNAs encoding specific $GABA_A$ receptor polypeptides; and (2) peripheral tumor cells have been transfected with complementary DNAs for specific $GABA_A$ receptor polypeptides. Using these approaches, cells have been engineered that simultaneously express up to three different varieties of $GABA_A$ receptor subunits. The subunit stoichiometry of receptors in cells expressing more than one variety of $GABA_A$ receptor polypeptide is unknown. With this limitation in mind, all combinations of $GABA_A$ receptor polypeptides that form functional bicuculline-sensitive receptors in oocytes or tumor cells were modulated by the intravenous anesthetics tested to date.[58,59] The potencies of anesthetic steroids as GABA potentiators varies with the different $GABA_A$ receptor subunit combinations in functional[60] and binding assays.[61] Moreover, the degree of barbiturate and steroid modulation of $GABA_A$ receptor binding varies with different regions of the brain[53,62,63] and different subunit polypeptides.[32]

Although potentiation of GABA appears to be a feature of all functional $GABA_A$ receptors, this may not be the case for direct activation of the GABA$_A$ receptor by intravenous anesthetics. Recent reports suggest that some GABA$_A$ receptor subtypes are not directly activated by barbiturates[64] and propofol.[65]

DO INTRAVENOUS INDUCTION AGENTS ACT ON γ-AMINOBUTYRIC ACID-A RECEPTORS THROUGH PROTEIN OR LIPID?

Modulation and direct activation of GABA$_A$ receptors are properties of all intravenous anesthetics discussed thus far (Fig. 13-1). These effects occur at blood concentrations recorded during total intravenous anesthesia. Hence, the GABA$_A$ receptor may be a primary site of action for these agents. If perturbation of GABA$_A$ receptors by anesthetics leads to general anesthesia, what effect does this have on the protein and lipid hypotheses of anesthesia?

Various attempts have been made to determine whether the intravenous anesthetics affect GABA$_A$ receptors through the lipid membrane or through the receptor protein itself. Given the variety of structures (Fig. 13-1) capable of having similar actions on the GABA$_A$ receptor, it seems unlikely that they have a common recognition site within the receptor. However, structural requirements for GABA$_A$ receptor modulation within individual classes of drugs can be rigorous. For example, although alfaxalone is an anesthetic steroid that modulates the GABA receptor, its inactive stereoisomer betaxalone, lacks this property.[49] These relationships support the view that the GABA$_A$ receptor is the site of action of the anesthetic steroids and suggests that they interact with a classic recognition site within the receptor-channel complex. On the other hand, differential scanning calorimetry, small angle x-ray diffraction, and solid state nuclear magnetic resonance can detect a greater disruption of model membrane bilayers by alfaxalone than by another of its anesthetically inactive isomers Δ^{16}-alfaxalone,[66] suggesting a possible lipid site of action.

Electrophysiologic studies in which the barbiturates, anesthetic steroids,[67] and propofol[38] were applied to the intracellular face of cells suggest that these compounds are unable to access their site of GABA$_A$ receptor modulation from within the cells. In these experiments, GABA$_A$ receptors were unaffected by high intracellular concentrations of anesthetics, which argues against a simple lipid interaction accounting for the GABA$_A$ receptor activation and modulation. Also, despite the similarities between glycine and GABA$_A$ receptors, anesthetic steroids and barbiturates are ineffective in modulating the chloride ion channel associated with the glycine receptor. In contrast, propofol and clomethiazole do cause modest potentiation of glycine-activated currents recorded from spinal neurons.[38,46] If lipid perturbation by intravenous anesthetics is responsible for modulation of these inhibitory neurotransmitter receptors, then it is difficult to account for the difference in potencies of these agents at the two sites. Furthermore, the evidence that the activation of GABA$_A$ receptors by pentobarbital[64] and propofol[65] are subtype dependent suggests that this effect requires interactions with specific receptor subunits. Finally, stereospecific modulation of GABA$_A$ receptor binding by anesthetics is retained in detergent-solubilized, purified protein samples.[32,53] Although these proteins may contain a few molecules of annular lipids, they are clearly not part of a lipid membrane structure, but they are nonetheless modulated by anesthetics.

The intravenous anesthetics discussed here all have dramatic effects on GABA$_A$ receptors. At low concentrations, these compounds markedly potentiate GABA-evoked responses. At higher concentrations, but within the blood levels reached during total intravenous anesthesia, they activate GABA$_A$ receptors directly. These are not the only actions of the intravenous induction agents. Other ion channels and, perhaps, other cellular loci are affected at the upper end of the anesthetic dose range. However, the GABA$_A$ receptor appears to be an appropriate primary site of action for the agents listed in Figure 13-1. This chapter has not discussed other sedative and anesthetic agents that probably do not act through GABA$_A$ receptors. For example, only relatively high concentrations of the dissociative anesthetic ketamine have been reported to potentiate GABA responses.[68] At one-tenth of the dose required to potentiate GABA, ketamine antagonizes responses mediated by the N-methyl-D-aspartate subtype of glutamate receptor (see Ch. 16).[69]

Recently, there have been a number of reports of GABA$_A$ receptor modulation by clinically relevant concentrations of the volatile anesthetics (see Ch. 23). Like the intravenous anesthetics, the volatile agents not only potentiate GABA-evoked responses[70–73] but also directly activate receptors in the absence of GABA.[73] The demonstration that clinically relevant doses of a variety of anesthetic compounds modulate and activate GABA$_A$ receptors supports the hypothesis that these receptors are involved in the mechanism of general anesthesia.

Our increasing understanding of the heterogeneity of the GABA$_A$ receptor has also uncovered the intriguing possibility that the actions of intravenous anesthetics on this receptor may in part be subtype specific. Perhaps, by mapping the distribution of GABA$_A$ receptor subtypes, we will better understand which regions of the brain are affected by the intravenous induction agents.

REFERENCES

1. Miller KW: The nature of the site of general anesthesia. Int Rev Neurobiol 27:1, 1985
2. Hille B: Ionic Channels of Excitable Membranes. Sinauer Associates, Sunderland, MA, 1984
3. Olsen RW: Barbiturates. Int Anesthesiol Clin 26:254, 1988
4. Roth SH, Tan K-S, MacIver MB: Selective and differential effects of barbiturates on neuronal activity. p. 43. In Roth SH, Miller KW (eds): Molecular and Cellular Mechanisms of Anesthetics. Plenum, New York, 1986
5. Blaustein MP: Barbiturates block sodium and potassium conductance increases in voltage-clamped lobster axons. J Gen Physiol 51:293, 1968
6. Sevcik C: Differences between the actions of thiopental and pentobarbital in squid giant axons. J Pharmacol Exp Ther 214:657, 1980
7. Seeman P: Membrane actions of anaesthetics and tranquilizers. Pharmacol Rev 24:583, 1972
8. Frenkel C, Duch DS, Recio-Pinto E, Urban BW: Pentobarbital suppresses human brain sodium channels. Mol Brain Res 6:211, 1989
9. Kozlowski RZ, Ashford MLJ: Barbiturates inhibit ATP-K$^+$ channels and voltage-activated currents in

CRI-G1 insulin-secreting cells. Br J Pharmacol 103:2021, 1991
10. Ashford MLJ, Sturgess NC, Trout NJ et al: Adenosine-5′-triphosphate-sensitive ion channels in neonatal rat cultured central neurones. Pflugers Arch 412:297, 1988
11. Krnjevic K: Cellular and synaptic effects of general anesthetics. p. 3. In Roth SH, Miller KW (eds): Molecular and Cellular Mechanisms of Anesthetics. Plenum, New York, 1986
12. Nicoll RA, Madison DV: General anesthetics hyperpolarize neurons in the vertebrate central nervous system. Science 217:1055, 1982
13. Carlen PL, Gurevich N, Durand D: Ethanol in low doses augments calcium-mediated mechanisms measured intracellularly in hippocampal neurons. Science 215:306, 1982
14. Daniell LC, Harris RA: Neuronal intracellular calcium concentrations are altered by anesthetics: relationship to membrane fluidization. J Pharmacol Exp Ther 245:1, 1988
15. Hodgkin AL: The Conduction of the Nervous Impulse. Liverpool University Press, Liverpool, 1964
16. Blaustein MP, Ector AC: Barbiturate inhibition of calcium uptake by depolarized nerve terminals in vitro. Mol Pharmacol 11:369, 1975
17. Gross RA, Macdonald RL: Differential actions of pentobarbitone on calcium current components of mouse sensory neurones in culture. J Physiol (Lond) 405:187, 1988
18. Macdonald RL, Skerritt JH, Werz MA: Barbiturate and benzodiazepine actions on mouse neurons in cell culture. p. 17. In Roth SH, Miller KW (eds): Molecular and Cellular Mechanisms of Anesthetics. Plenum, New York, 1986
19. Gundersen CB, Umbach JA, Swartz BE: Barbiturates depress currents through human brain calcium channels studied in *Xenopus* oocytes. J Pharmacol Exp Ther 247:824, 1988
20. Ho IK, Harris RA: Mechanism of action of barbiturates. Annu Rev Pharmacol Toxicol 21:83, 1981
21. Richter JA, Holtman JR: Barbiturates: their in vivo effects and potential biochemical mechanisms. Prog Neurobiol 18:275, 1982
22. Noda M, Takahashi H, Tanabe T et al: Primary structure of the α-subunit precursor of *Torpedo californica* acetylcholine receptor deduced from cDNA sequence. Nature 299:793, 1982
23. Unwin N: The structure of ion channels in membranes of excitable cells. Neuron 3:665, 1989
24. Roth SH, Forman SA, Braswell LM, Miller KW: Actions of pentobarbital enantiomers on nicotinic cholinergic receptors. Mol Pharmacol 36:874, 1989

25. Miller KW, Braswell LM, Firestone LL et al: General anesthetics act both specifically and nonspecifically on acetylcholine receptors. p. 125. In Roth SH, Miller KW (eds): Molecular and Cellular Mechanisms of Anesthetics. Plenum, New York, 1986

26. Miller KW, Sauter JF, Braswell LM: A stereoselective pentobarbital binding site in cholinergic membranes from *Torpedo californica*. Biochem Biophys Res Commun 105:659, 1982

27. Forman SA, Miller KW: Molecular sites of anesthetic action in postsynaptic nicotinic membranes. Trends Pharmacol Sci 10:447, 1989

28. Lambert JJ, Hill-Venning CH, Peters JA et al: The actions of anesthetic steroids on inhibitory and excitatory amino acid receptors. p. 219. In Barnard EA, Costa E (eds): Transmitter Amino Acid Receptors: Structures, Transduction and Models for Drug Development. Fidia Research Foundation Symposium Series. Vol. 6. Thieme, New York, 1991

29. Luini A, Goldberg O, Teichberg VI: Distinct pharmacological properties of excitatory amino acid receptors in the rat striatum: study by Na^+ efflux assay. Proc Natl Acad Sci U S A 78:3250, 1981

30. Olsen RW, Tobin AJ: Molecular biology of $GABA_A$ receptors. FASEB J 4:1469, 1990

31. Burt DR, Kamatchi GL: $GABA_A$ receptor subtypes: from pharmacology to molecular biology. FASEB J 5:2916, 1991

32. Bureau M, Olsen RW: Multiple distinct subunits of the γ-aminobutyric acid-A receptor protein show different ligand-binding affinities. Mol Pharmacol 37:497, 1990

33. Whiting P, McKernan RM, Iversen LL: Another mechanism for creating diversity in γ-aminobutyrate type A receptors: RNA splicing directs expression of two forms of $\gamma2$ subunit, one of which contains a protein kinase C phosphorylation site. Proc Natl Acad Sci U S A 87:9966, 1990

34. Wisden W, Laurie DJ, Monyer H, Seeburg PH: The distribution of 13 $GABA_A$ receptor subunit mRNAs in the rat brain. I. Telencephalon, diencephalon, mesencephalon. J Neurosci 12:1040, 1992

35. Laurie DJ, Seeburg PH, Wisden W: The distribution of 13 $GABA_A$ receptor subunit mRNAs in the rat brain. II. Olfactory bulb and cerebellum. J Neurosci 12:1063, 1992

36. Hales TG, Kim H, Longoni B et al: Immortalized hypothalamic GT1-7 neurons express functional γ-aminobutyric acid type A receptors. Mol Pharmacol 42:197, 1992

37. Robertson B: Actions of anaesthetics and avermectin on $GABA_A$ chloride channels in mammalian dorsal root ganglion neurones. Br J Pharmacol 98:167, 1989

38. Hales TG, Lambert JJ: The actions of propofol on inhibitory amino acid receptors of bovine adrenomedullary chromaffin cells and rodent central neurones. Br J Pharmacol 104:619, 1991

39. Olsen RW, Fischer JB, Dunwiddie TV: Barbiturate enhancement of γ-aminobutyric acid receptor binding and function as a mechanism of anesthesia. p. 165. In Roth SH, Miller KW (eds): Molecular and Cellular Mechanisms of Anesthetics. Plenum, New York, 1986

40. Concas A, Santoro G, Serra M et al: Neurochemical action of the general anesthetic propofol on the chloride ion channel coupled with $GABA_A$ receptors. Brain Res 542:225, 1991

41. Nicoll RA, Eccles JC, Oshima T, Rubia F: Prolongation of hippocampal inhibitory postsynaptic potentials by barbiturates. Nature 258:625, 1975

42. Haefely W, Polc P, Keller HH et al: Facilitation of GABAergic transmission by drugs. p. 357. In Krogsgaard-Larsen P, Scheel-Kruger J, Kofod G (eds): GABA-Neurotransmitters. Munksgaard, Copenhagen, 1979

43. Dunwiddie TV, Worth TS, Olsen RW: Facilitation of recurrent inhibition in rat hippocampus by barbiturate and related nonbarbiturate depressant drugs. J Pharmacol Exp Ther 238:564, 1986

44. Hamill OP, Marty A, Neher E et al: Improved patch-clamp recording from cells and cell free membrane patches. Pflugers Arch 391:85, 1981

45. Owen DG, Barker JL, Segal M, Study RE: Postsynaptic actions of pentobarbital in cultured mouse spinal neurons and rat hippocampal neurons. p. 27. In Roth SH, Miller KW (eds): Molecular and Cellular Mechanisms of Anesthetics. Plenum, New York, 1986

46. Hales TG, Lambert JJ: Modulation of $GABA_A$ and glycine receptors by chlormethiazole. Eur J Pharmacol 210:239, 1992

47. Peters JA, Lambert JJ, Cottrell GA: An electrophysiological investigation of the characteristics and function of $GABA_A$ receptors on bovine chromaffin cells. Pflugers Arch 415:95, 1989

48. Harrison NL, Majewska MD, Harrington JW, Barker JL: Structure-activity relationships for steroid interaction with the γ-aminobutyric $acid_A$ receptor complex. J Phamacol Exp Ther 241:346, 1987

49. Cottrell GA, Lambert JJ, Peters JA: Modulation of $GABA_A$ receptor activity by alphaxalone. Br J Pharmacol 90:491, 1987

50. Wong EHF, Leeb-Lundberg LMF, Teichberg VI, Olsen RW: γ-Aminobutyric acid activation of $^{36}Cl^-$

flux in rat hippocampal slices and its potentiation by barbiturates. Brain Res 303:267, 1984

51. Huidobro-Toro JP, Bleck V, Allan AM, Harris RA: Neurochemical actions of anesthetic drugs on the γ-aminobutyric acid receptor-chloride channel complex. J Pharmacol Exp Ther 242:963, 1987

52. Schwartz RD, Jackson JA, Weigert D et al: Characterization of barbiturate-stimulated chloride efflux from rat brain synaptoneurosomes. J Neurosci 5:2963, 1985

53. Olsen RW, Sapp DM, Bureau MH et al: Allosteric actions of central nervous system depressants including anesthetics on subtypes of the inhibitory γ-aminobutyric acid$_A$ receptor-chloride channel complex. Ann NY Acad Sci 625:145, 1991

54. Polc P, Möhler H, Haefely W: The effect of diazepam on spinal cord activities: possible sites and mechanisms of action. Naunyn Schmeidebergs Arch Pharmacol 284:319, 1974

55. Mathers DA, Barker JL: (−)Pentobarbital opens ion channels of long duration in cultured mouse spinal neurons. Science 209:507, 1980

56. Kanto J, Gepts E: Pharmacokinetic implications for the clinical use of propofol. Clin Pharmacokinet 17:308, 1989

57. Schofield PR, Darlison MG, Fujita N et al: Sequence and functional expression of the GABA$_A$ receptor shows a ligand-gated receptor super-family. Nature 328:221, 1987

58. Puia G, Santi MR, Vicini S et al: Neurosteroids act on recombinant human GABA$_A$ receptors. Neuron 4:759, 1990

59. Hill-Venning C, Lambert JJ, Peters JA, Hales TG: The actions of neurosteroids on inhibitory amino acid receptors. p. 77. In Costa E, Paul SM (eds): Neurosteroids and Brain Function. Fidia Research Foundation Symposium Series. Vol. 8. Thieme, New York, 1991

60. Shingai R, Sutherland ML, Barnard EA: Effects of subunit types of cloned GABA$_A$ receptor on the response to a neurosteroid. Eur J Pharmacol 206:77, 1991

61. Lan NC, Gee KW, Bolger MB, Chen JS: Differential responses of expressed recombinant human γ-aminobutyric acid$_A$ receptors to neurosteroids. J Neurochem 57:1818, 1991

62. Carlson BX, Mans AM, Hawkins RA, Baghdoyan HA: Pentobarbital-enhanced [^{3}H]flunitrazepam binding throughout the rat brain: an autoradiographic study. J Pharmacol Exp Ther 263:1401, 1992

63. Sapp DW, Witte U, Turner DM et al: Regional variation in steroid anesthetic modulation of [^{35}S]TBPS

binding to γ-aminobutyric acid$_A$ receptors in rat brain. J Pharmacol Exp Ther 262:801, 1992

64. Cruciani RA, Valayev AY, Mahan LC et al: Pharmacological characterization of the GABA$_A$ receptor channel complex composed or rat brain α$_1$ and β$_2$ subunits. Soc Neurosci. Abstr 17:79, 1991

65. Hales TG: Direct activation of GABA$_A$ receptors by propofol may be subunit specific. Anesthesiology 77:A695, 1992

66. Makriyannis A, Yang D-P, Mavromoustakos T: The molecular features of membrane perturbation by anesthetic steroids: a study using differential scanning calorimetry, small angle x-ray diffraction and solid state ^{2}H NMR. p. 172. In Chadwick D, Widdows K (eds): Steroids and Neuronal Activity. Ciba Foundation Symposium 153. Wiley, Chichester, 1990

67. Lambert JJ, Peters JA, Sturgess NC, Hales TG: Steroid modulation of the GABA$_A$ receptor complex: electrophysiological studies. p. 56. In Chadwick D, Widdows K (eds): Steroids and Neuronal Activity. Ciba Foundation Symposium 153. Wiley, Chichester, 1990

68. Gage PW, Robertson B: Prolongation of inhibitory postsynaptic currents by pentobarbitone, halothane and ketamine in CA1 pyramidal cells in rat hippocampus. Br J Pharmacol 85:675, 1985

69. Martin D, Lodge D: Ketamine acts as a non-competitive N-methyl-D-aspartate antagonist on frog spinal cord. Neuropharmacology 24:999, 1985

70. Mody I, Tanelian DL, MacIver MB: Halothane enhances tonic neuronal inhibition by elevating intracellular calcium. Brain Res 538:319, 1991

71. Jones MV, Brooks PA, Harrison NL: Enhancement of γ-aminobutyric acid-activated Cl$^-$ currents in cultured rat hippocampal neurones by three volatile anaesthetics. J Physiol (Lond) 449:279, 1992

72. Longoni B, Olsen RW: Studies on the mechanism of interaction of anesthetics with GABA-A receptors. p. 365. In Biggio G, Concas A, Costa E (eds): GABAergic Synaptic Transmission. Advances in Biochemical Psychopharmacology. Vol. 47. Raven Press, New York, 1992

73. Hales TG, Jones MV, Harrison NL: Evidence for subunit dependent direct activation of the GABA$_A$ receptor by isoflurane. Anesthesiology 77:A698, 1992

74. Delorey TM, Olsen RW: GABA and glycine. p. 389. In Segal GI, Agranoff BW, Albers RW, Molinoff PB (eds): Basic Neurochemistry. 5th Ed. Raven Press, New York, 1994

75. Bloor BC, Hales TG: Sedatives and analgesics: from opioids to α$_2$-adrenergic agonists and beyond. Semin Anesth 11:96, 1992

Chapter 14

Pharmacokinetics of Intravenous Induction Agents

Thomas K. Henthorn

Thiopental was introduced into clinical practice in 1929. It was initially thought that the short duration of action of thiopental following a single dose resulted from rapid metabolism. However, it was discovered that distribution lowers plasma and brain concentrations before a significant degree of metabolism occurs. The kinetics of distribution is of prime importance for understanding the clinical behavior of the intravenous induction agents. This chapter discusses the pharmacokinetics of thiopental, methohexital, etomidate, and propofol. The reader is also directed to Chapter 33 for additional information.

THIOPENTAL

Thiopental is the prototypic lipid soluble intravenous induction agent. Many barbiturates share its mechanism of action, but its unique pharmacokinetic properties make it useful as an anesthetic agent. Its rapid traversal of lipid capillary membranes greatly enhances its diffusion surface area and the delivery of thiopental to the brain's effect sites occurs rapidly. The rapidity of the rise to peak effect is also related to the apparent distribution volume of the effect compartment or biophase. For thiopental, this volume is relatively small; therefore, equilibration of the biophase with plasma occurs rapidly.

Drug delivery to tissues other than the brain is also rapid. However, the apparent volumes of these tissues are much larger than that of the brain, and the equilibration process can take up to approximately 2 hours (see Fig. 33-4). Tissue distribution drives thiopental brain and plasma concentrations down, accounting for the rapid offset of effect of thiopental.

Elimination Mechanisms

The renal excretion of thiopental is negligible. Hepatic oxidative metabolism through the P-450 system to a carboxylic acid derivative accounts for the majority of thiopental elimination.[1] This process is not highly efficient; the hepatic extraction is low, on the order of 10 to 20 percent.[2] At high therapeutic concentrations, thiopental exhibits Michaelis-Menten elimination kinetics.[3] The Michaelis-Menten equation states

$$\text{Elimination rate} = V_{max} \cdot C/(K_m + C) \quad (1)$$

where C is the drug concentration, V_{max} is the maximum elimination or metabolic rate, and K_m is the Michaelis constant (the concentration at which the elimination rate is one-half maximal).

As the concentration decreases below K_m, the relationship between the elimination rate and concentration becomes increasingly first order (i.e., the clearance is constant, and the elimination rate is proportional to the concentration). As the concentration approaches and exceeds K_m, the relationship becomes nonlinear (equation 1) and eventually becomes zero order at high concentrations (i.e., the elimination rate is constant regardless of the concentration).

During a prolonged infusion of thiopental for cerebral resuscitation, a nonlinear elimination profile was observed[3] (Fig. 14-1), such that the elimination half-life gradually decreased as the concentration fell. The K_m varied among patients, from 8.1 to 67.5 μg/ml. In most patients, the K_m was closer to approximately 50 μg/ml, a concentration that produces electroencephalographic (EEG) burst suppression (Table 14-1).

It was thought that thiopental could undergo desulfuration (with an oxygen substitution) to pentobarbital, another active barbiturate.[3] However, Dundee showed that the conversion of thiopental to pentobarbital was an artifact that occurs under the alkaline conditions of plasma sample preparation for high performance liquid chromatography.

Table 14-1 Thiopental Concentration-Effect Relationships

End Point	EC_{50} (μg/ml)	Reference
Hypnosis (syringe drop)	11.3	11
Verbal command	15.6	10
Spectral edge	17.9–19.4	8, 23, 25
Tetanus response	30.3	10
EEG burst suppression	33.9	11
Trapezius squeeze	39.8–42.4	10, 12
Laryngoscopy	50.7	10
EEG silence	> 50	10
Intubation	78.8	10

Avram and Krejcie,[4] using a different preparation procedure, did not find any pentobarbital in plasma samples that contained thiopental.

Protein Binding

Thiopental binds to plasma albumin in a concentration-dependent fashion; the percentage bound varies between 60 and 97 percent in normal subjects for thiopental plasma concentrations between 15.0 μg/ml and 0.2 μg/ml, respectively.[2] Concentrations of unbound (free) thiopental were negatively correlated with plasma albumin concentrations ($r^2 = 0.71$).[5] Thiopental clearance is directly related to free thiopental and, thus, can be influenced by albumin levels and agents that displace thiopental from albumin, such as aspirin.[6] Aspirin given intravenously at the time of the return of the eyelash reflex, following an induction dose of thiopental, caused reinduction of hypnosis, despite lower thiopental plasma concentrations, because the free concentrations were increased following aspirin.[7] Plasma protein binding has a reciprocal relationship to the steady-state volume of distribution (V_{ss}). However, there is no evidence that tissue distribution rates are affected by protein binding, perhaps because of similar offsetting effects on intercompartmental clearance and distribution volumes, leaving tissue equilibration times unaffected.

The clinical relevance of pharmacokinetic data (Table 14-2) is fully realized only when coupled with appropriate pharmacodynamic information. Using a variety of experimental techniques,[8–10] es-

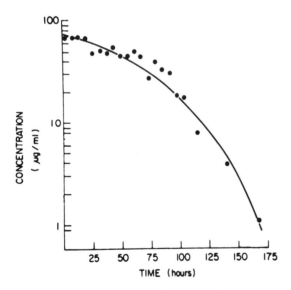

Fig. 14-1 Plasma thiopental concentrations in a patient following a 42-hour thiopental infusion (total dose, 40 g), revealing Michaelis-Menten elimination. Note the difference in shape between the elimination phase in this case and that in Figure 14-6, illustrating "normal" first-order elimination kinetics. (Modified from Stanski et al.,[3] with permission.)

Table 14-2 Thiopental Pharmacokinetics and Pharmacodynamics

Parameter	Value (Healthy 70-kg Adult)
V_1	7 L
V_2	25 L
V_3	90 L
V_{SS}	1.7 L/kg
Cl_2	4.7 L/min
Cl_3	0.6 L/min
Cl_E	250 ml/min
k_{e0}	0.6 min^{-1}
t_{max}[a]	1.6 min
V_{pe}	20 L
EC[b]	10–15 μg/ml

[a] Estimated following a simulated intravenous bolus dose.

[b] Effective concentration range for hypnosis; other agents needed for analgesia.

timates of thiopental plasma or effect site concentrations that produce various responses were obtained (Table 14-1). For loss of consciousness, a thiopental concentration of approximately 11 μg/ml[11] is required. A concentration of approximately 40 μg/ml was needed to suppress the response to a standard painful stimulus.[10,12] The latter concentration was found to be slightly higher than that producing EEG burst suppression.[11] However, much higher concentrations are needed to blunt the cardiovascular response to intubation, suggesting that deeper brain levels mediate such responses and are less affected by thiopental than is the cortex.[10]

Interindividual Differences in Pharmacokinetics and Pharmacodynamics

Advanced age,[13,14] pregnancy,[15] renal failure,[16] obesity,[17] and cirrhosis[5] all affect distribution volumes and/or elimination clearance. Neonates have reduced clearance,[18,19] and children have increased clearance.[18,20] Decreased protein binding, such as that found in neonates and patients with renal failure, increases the free fraction in the plasma and may cause an increased sensitivity to thiopental. Patients with heavy alcohol usage, but without evidence of hepatic disease, were found not to

have altered pharmacokinetics[21,22] or pharmacodynamics.[22]

Women and elderly patients have reduced requirements for thiopental for induction of anesthesia and to produce EEG burst suppression.[9,23] The increased sensitivity of the elderly patient to thiopental, originally ascribed to a marked reduction in the initial distribution volume (V_1),[23] more recently has been ascribed to reduced intercompartmental clearance to the rapidly equilibrating compartment (see Fig. 33-11).[24,25] Whether such a change explains the diminished dose requirements in elderly patients is still debatable.[24,25]

Context-Sensitive Offset Curves

The computer-generated curves in Figure 14-2 predict the time required for thiopental plasma concentrations to fall by 25, 50, and 75 percent as a function of the duration of the infusion at constant plasma concentration. Note that the time to fall to 50 percent is not always twice that of the fall by 25 percent, indicating that the decay is multiexponential, even after prolonged infusions. How we use such data depends on the relationship of the target concentration of the infusion to the concentration associated with an offset of the effect. For example, if concentrations are kept near the hypnotic threshold, a 25 percent reduction in effect site concentration will occur within 35 minutes and result in awakening.

METHOHEXITAL

Pharmacokinetics

The pharmacokinetics of methohexital appear to be similar to those of thiopental except for a much greater elimination clearance (Table 14-3).[26–28] Methohexital is a moderately high to high extraction drug with extraction ratio estimates varying from 0.5 to 0.87.[29,30] Thus, the elimination of methohexital is dependent on hepatic blood flow, unlike that of thiopental. However, under most circumstances, elimination clearance is secondary to tissue distribution for terminating the effects of methohexital; so, hepatic blood flow considerations should also remain secondary.

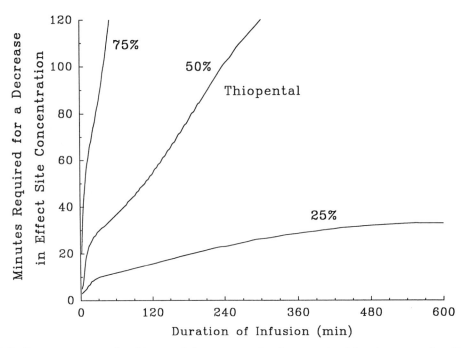

Fig. 14-2 Recovery curves for thiopental that present the time required for decreases in effect site concentrations of 25, 50, and 75 percent from the effect site concentration maintained by a computer-controlled infusion after the termination of the infusion.

Table 14-3 Methohexital Pharmacokinetics and Pharmacodynamics

Parameter	Value (Healthy 70-kg Adult)
V_1	7 L
V_2	25 L
V_3	90 L
V_{SS}	1.7 L/kg
Cl_2	4.7 L/min
Cl_3	0.6 L/min
Cl_E	690 ml/min
k_{e0}	0.6 min^{-1}
t_{max}[a]	1.6 min
V_{pe}	20 L
EC_{50}[b]	3–5 μg/ml

[a] Estimated following a simulated intravenous bolus dose.

[b] Effective concentration range for hypnosis; other agents needed for analgesia.

Figure 14-3 indicates that, for infusions of any duration, the time to decay by 25, 50, and 75 percent of the constant plasma concentration is shorter than that for thiopental (Fig. 14-2). Note that, even after infusions of up to 10 hours, recovery by a decrease of 25 percent is only 6 minutes and by 50 percent is 20 minutes, a huge improvement over the times needed for thiopental. This is consistent with data suggesting that postoperative recovery is more rapid when methohexital is used compared with thiopental.[29,30] Therefore, methohexital is a more logical selection for use in continuous infusion regimens compared with thiopental.[31-34]

Pharmacodynamics

Lauven et al.[34] found that the plasma methohexital concentration that produces hypnosis was 3.4 μg/ml and the concentration that produces burst

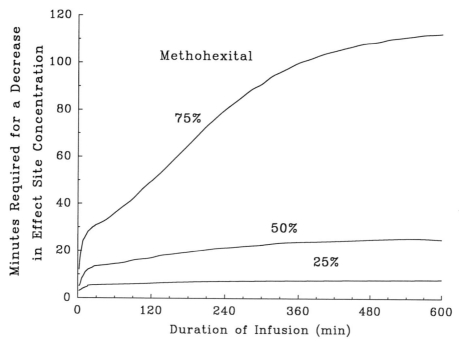

Fig. 14-3 Recovery curves for methohexital that present the time required for decreases in effect site concentrations of 25, 50, and 75 percent from the effect site concentration maintained by a computer-controlled infusion after the termination of the infusion.

suppression was 10.7 μg/ml. The ratio of these concentrations is the same as that found for thiopental (Table 14-1).[11] Crankshaw et al.[32] found that a target concentration of 5 μg/ml for a methohexital infusion was optimal, which is consistent with the general recommendation of selecting a target 15 to 50 percent more than the EC_{50} for hypnosis to ensure that the vast majority of patients will be unconscious and that most will awaken between the 25 and 50 percent predicted recovery times (Fig. 14-3).

Infusions can be classified as open or closed loop. The closed-loop type requires a measure of effect that can be used as a variable in a controller algorithm that automatically adjusts the infusion rate in a feedback control manner.[35] Schwilden et al.[31,37] designed closed-loop infusion protocols for methohexital with the median frequency of the EEG as the measure of effect. The controller algorithm was designed to maintain the median frequency

between 2 and 3 Hz. The performance of this infusion system is shown in Figure 14-4.

Interindividual Differences

There have been only a few studies of methohexital pharmacokinetics or dose requirements among patient groups. Lange et al.[30] found a significant correlation between hepatic blood flow (estimated by indocyanine green clearance) and methohexital clearance. Ghoneim et al.[28] showed that anesthesia prolongs the elimination half-life from 2.2 hours in awake controls to approximately 3.5 hours, consistent with the known effect of enflurane anesthesia to decrease hepatic blood flow. They also found that age did not affect methohexital kinetics. Duvaldestin et al.[29] found that the type of surgery (orthopedic versus abdominal) did not have any significant effect on methohexital kinetics. Neither did cirrhosis affect methohexital kinetics.

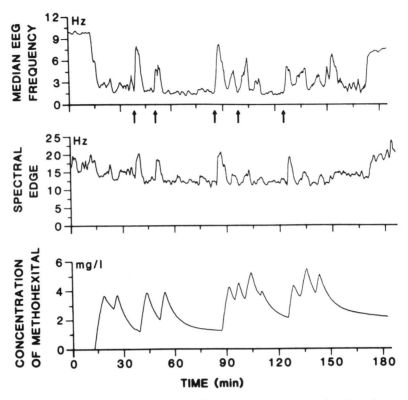

Fig. 14-4 Three panels showing the electroencephalographic response (median frequency and spectral edge) and predicted methohexital concentrations for a volunteer given no stimulation and a closed-loop methohexital infusion. The arrows under the top trace indicate times of subject awareness. (From Schwilden et al.,[31] with permission.)

ETOMIDATE

Pharmacokinetics

Etomidate has slightly larger distribution volumes than do the barbiturates and a higher elimination clearance (Table 14-4).[36,38,39] The hepatic metabolism of etomidate is mainly by ester hydrolysis.[40] The hepatic extraction ratio has been reported to be near 1.0, suggesting extrahepatic sites of metabolism (e.g., plasma esterases) as possibly contributing to plasma clearance.[36,38] High extraction ratio drugs have a direct correlation between hepatic blood flow and their elimination clearances. A reduction in hepatic blood flow during enflurane anesthesia is the probable cause of the elimination clearance estimate of only 820 ml/min reported by Van Hamme et al.[41]

Table 14-4 Etomidate Pharmacokinetics and Pharmacodynamics

Parameter	Value (Healthy 70-kg Adult)
V_1	10 L
V_2	30 L
V_3	150 L
V_{SS}	2.7 L/kg
Cl_2	1.8 L/min
Cl_3	0.5 L/min
Cl_E	1,400 ml/min
k_{e0}	0.4 min^{-1}
t_{max}[a]	1.8 min
V_{pe}	36 L
EC_{50}[b]	0.3–0.5 μg/ml

[a] Estimated following a simulated intravenous bolus dose.
[b] Effective concentration range for hypnosis; other agents needed for analgesia.

Figure 14-5 shows the favorable recovery profile even with rather lengthy infusions. The terminal half-life for etomidate is 3 to 5 hours.[36,38] Note that the prominent distribution of this drug keeps the context-sensitive offset time (the 50 percent curve, Fig. 14-5) well below the elimination half-life.

Pharmacodynamics

The etomidate EC_{50} for reducing the EEG median frequency has been reported to be 0.31 μg/ml by one group[38] and 0.43 μg/ml by another.[39] The plasma level during total intravenous anesthesia that included supplemental fentanyl but not an inhalation agent was 0.58 μg/ml, and the plasma concentration corresponding with awakening was 0.31 μg/ml.[36] These results were used to define the target concentration range (Table 14-4).

Interindividual Variability

A strong correlation ($r^2 = 0.68$) was reported for the relationship between the etomidate dose required to induce anesthesia and age (ages, 20 to 80 years).[38] As was the case for thiopental,[23] these investigators found no effect of age on the effect site equilibration rate constant (k_{e0}) or the measure of brain sensitivity, EC_{50}. A significant negative correlation was found between V_1 and age.

PROPOFOL

Pharmacokinetics

The pharmacokinetics of propofol are remarkable in that all aspects of disposition are increased compared with other intravenous hypnotics. Comparing the peripheral distribution volumes in Table 14-5 with those of the other agents, it is readily apparent that they are larger, especially V_3. Also of note are the larger intercompartmental clearance to V_3 and the elimination clearance that is greater than the hepatic blood flow. These differences translate into a remarkably different concentration-time profile compared with that of thiopental. Figure 14-6 shows that the larger volumes of distri-

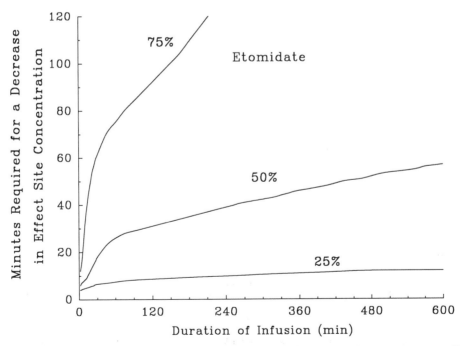

Fig. 14-5 Recovery curves for etomidate that present the time required for decreases in effect site concentrations of 25, 50, and 75 percent from the effect site concentration maintained by a computer-controlled infusion after the termination of the infusion.

Table 14-5 Propofol Pharmacokinetics and Pharmacodynamics

Parameter	Value (Healthy 70-kg Adult)
V_1	10 L
V_2	30 L
V_3	435 L
V_{SS}	6.8 L/kg
Cl_2	1.8 L/min
Cl_3	2.1 L/min
Cl_E	1,800 ml/min
k_{e0}	0.7 min^{-1}
t_{max}[a]	1.6 min
V_{pe}	20 L
EC_{50}[b]	2–3 μg/ml

[a] Estimated following a simulated intravenous bolus dose.

[b] Effective concentration range for hypnosis; other agents needed for analgesia.

bution result in a much greater drop in propofol concentration during the distribution phase compared with that of thiopental. The ratio of the distribution volumes for propofol and thiopental is approximately the same as the ratio of their elimination clearances; thus, the slopes of the terminal phases are similar. The terminal half-life, estimated at 6 hours[42] and 11 hours,[43] has little clinical relevance.

The metabolism of propofol is primarily by conjugation to glucuronides and sulfates, resulting in inactive metabolites that are readily excreted in the urine. Propofol elimination clearance (Table 14-5) exceeds the hepatic blood flow (1,500 ml/min). Lange et al.[44] used hepatic vein catheterization to estimate hepatic clearance at only 1,060 ml/min, approximately one-half the total elimination clearance. Glucuronide formation was nearly unchanged during the anhepatic phase of liver transplantation.[45,46] These studies suggest that

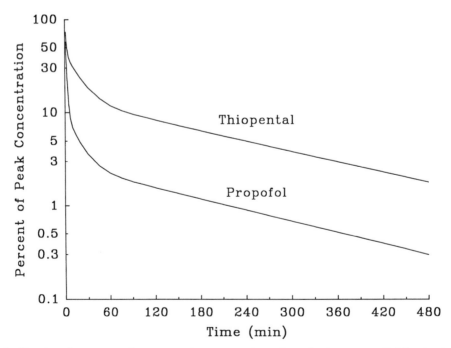

Fig. 14-6 Simulated concentration versus time curves based on the kinetics in Tables 14-2 and 14-5 for thiopental and propofol following intravenous bolus administration. Note that the rapid fall in plasma propofol concentrations predict a fivefold lower relative concentration at the end of the distribution phase. The terminal slopes are nearly identical.

approximately one-half of the metabolism of propofol is extrahepatic.

Prolonged propofol infusions in patients in intensive care units[47–50] and prolonged plasma level sampling following intraoperative infusions[51,52] yield markedly increased estimates of distribution volume and half-lives, suggesting that the tissue distribution processes are more extensive than originally thought. However, these findings are of little clinical consequence for intraoperative anesthesia and so are not reflected in Table 14-5 or Figures 14-6 and 14-7.

The importance of tissue distribution for the pharmacokinetics of propofol is evident in the context-sensitive recovery curves in Figure 14-7. Even after 10 hours of continuous infusion, a 25 percent decrease in plasma propofol concentrations can be expected in only 3 minutes.

Pharmacodynamics

Most of the data describing the pharmacodynamics of propofol concern blood levels obtained during the offset of effect. Patients regain consciousness with blood propofol levels of approximately 1.0 μg/ml.[47,53,54] Propofol blood levels of 2 to 3 μg/ml are needed intraoperatively when propofol is used for the maintenance of anesthesia in conjunction with an analgesic drug such as nitrous oxide[53,54] or an opioid.[55] Vuyk et al.[56] used a computer-controlled propofol infusion to increase propofol blood concentrations in a stepwise manner with 12-minute plateaus, a method similar to that of Bührer et al.[57] (see Fig. 33-7). They found that levels between 2.7 and 5.4 μg/ml were needed to produce loss of consciousness without other centrally acting drugs being given. Marsh et al.[58] estimated that levels twice this high may be required in children aged 3 to 10 years.

Interindividual Variability

In a comparison of 12 patients 65 to 80 years of age and 12 patients 18 to 35 years of age, Kirkpatrick et al.[43] found that mean propofol blood concentrations were higher in elderly patients during the first 2 minutes, despite a 20 percent lower dose, indicating that mixing and early tissue distribution

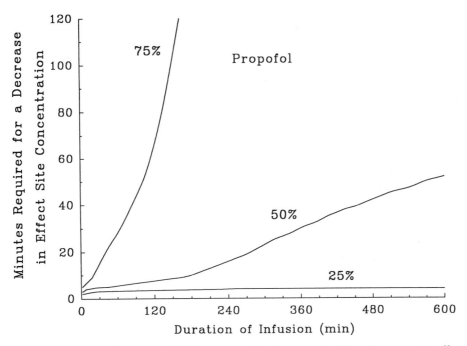

Fig. 14-7 Recovery curves for propofol that present the time required for decreases in effect site concentrations of 25, 50, and 75 percent from the effect site concentration maintained by a computer-controlled infusion after the termination of the infusion.

of propofol are reduced in such patients. They also found a 20 percent lower elimination clearance in elderly patients but no difference in V_{ss}.

Servin et al.[59] found that cirrhosis did not significantly affect the pharmacokinetics of propofol nor its protein binding. Propofol is extensively (98 percent) protein bound. Uremic patients also were found not to have significant differences in propofol pharmacokinetics compared with healthy patients.[60]

Using a computer-controlled infusion pump programmed with previously published adult pharmacokinetic values,[61] Marsh et al.[58] found that the computer systematically produced lower than expected blood propofol concentrations in children aged 3 to 10 years. They found that these children had a 50 percent greater V_1 and a 25 percent greater elimination clearance compared with adults. They also concluded that the pharmacokinetic parameters from a bolus administration study of children[62] would have produced higher than expected propofol concentrations during a computer-controlled infusion.

REFERENCES

1. Mark LC, Brand L, Kamvyssi S et al: Thiopental metabolism by human liver in vivo and in vitro. Nature 206:1117, 1965
2. Morgan DJ, Blackman GL, Paull JD, Wolf LJ: Pharmacokinetics and plasma binding of thiopental. I: Studies in surgical patients. Anesthesiology 54:468, 1981
3. Stanski DR, Mihm FG, Rosenthal MH, Kalman SM: Pharmacokinetics of high-dose thiopental used in cerebral resuscitation. Anesthesiology 53:169, 1980
4. Avram MJ, Krejcie TC: Determination of sodium pentobarbital and either sodium methohexital or sodium thiopental in plasma by high performance liquid chromatography with ultraviolet detection. J Chromatogr 414:484, 1987
5. Pandele G, Chaux F, Salvadori C et al: Thiopental pharmacokinetics in patients with cirrhosis. Anesthesiology 59:123, 1983
6. Chaplin MD, Roszkowski AP, Richards RK: Displacement of thiopental from plasma proteins by nonsteroidal anti-inflammatory agents. Proc Soc Exp Biol Med 143:667, 1973
7. Hu OY-P, Chu KM, Liu HS et al: Reinduction of the hypnotic effects of thiopental with NSAIDs by de-creasing thiopental plasma protein binding in humans. Acta Anaesthesiol Scand 37:258, 1993
8. Stanski DR, Hudson RJ, Homer TD et al: Pharmacodynamic modeling of thiopental anesthesia. J Pharmacokinet Biopharm 12:223, 1984
9. Avram MJ, Sanghvi R, Henthorn TK et al: Determinants of thiopental induction dose requirements. Anesth Analg 76:10, 1993
10. Hung OR, Varvel J, Shafer S, Stanski DR: Quantitation of thiopental anesthetic depth with clinical stimuli. Can J Anaesth 37:S18, 1990
11. Shanks CA, Avram MJ, Krejcie TC et al: A pharmacokinetic-pharmacodynamic model for quantal responses with thiopental. J Pharmacokinet Biopharm 21:309, 1993
12. Becker KE: Plasma levels of thiopental necessary for anesthesia. Anesthesiology 49:192, 1978
13. Christensen JH, Andreasen F, Jansen JA: Influence of age and sex on the pharmacokinetics of thiopentone. Br J Anaesth 53:1189, 1981
14. Jung D, Mayerson M, Perrier D et al: Thiopental disposition as a function of age in female patients undergoing surgery. Anesthesiology 56:263, 1982
15. Morgan DJ, Blackman GL, Paull JD, Wolf LJ: Pharmacokinetics and plasma binding of thiopental. II: Studies at cesarean section. Anesthesiology 54:474, 1981
16. Christensen JH, Andreasen F, Jansen J: Pharmacokinetics and pharmacodynamics of thiopental in patients undergoing renal transplantation. Acta Anaesthesiol Scand 27:513, 1983
17. Crankshaw DP, Edwards NE, Blackman GL et al: Evaluation of infusion regimens for thiopentone as a primary anaesthetic agent. Eur J Clin Pharmacol 28:543, 1985
18. Demarquez JL, Galperine R, Billeaud C, Brachet-Liermain A: High-dose thiopental pharmacokinetics in brain-injured children and neonates. Dev Pharmacol Ther 10:292, 1987
19. Bach V, Carl P, Ravlo O et al: A randomized comparison between midazolam and thiopental for elective cesarean section anesthesia: III. Placental transfer and elimination in neonates. Anesth Analg 68:238, 1989
20. Sorbo S, Hudson RJ, Loomis JC: The pharmacokinetics of thiopental in pediatric surgical patients. Anesthesiology 61:666, 1984
21. Couderc E, Ferrier C, Haberer JP et al: Thiopentone pharmacokinetics in patients with chronic alcoholism. Br J Anaesth 56:1393, 1984
22. Swerdlow BN, Holley FO, Maitre PO, Stanski DR: Chronic alcohol intake does not change thiopental

anesthetic requirement, pharmacokinetics, or pharmacodynamics. Anesthesiology 72:455, 1990

23. Homer TD, Stanski DR: The effect of increasing age on thiopental disposition and anesthetic requirement. Anesthesiology 62:714, 1985

24. Avram MJ, Krejcie TC, Henthorn TK: The relationship of age to the pharmacokinetics of early drug distribution: the concurred disposition of thiopental and indocyanine green. Anesthesiology 72:403, 1990

25. Stanski DR, Maitre PO: Population pharmacokinetics and pharmacodynamics of thiopental: the effect of age revisited. Anesthesiology 72:403, 1990

26. Breimer DD: Pharmacokinetics of methohexitone following intravenous infusion in humans. Br J Anaesth 48:643, 1976

27. Hudson RJ, Stanski DR, Burch PG: Pharmacokinetics of methohexital and thiopental in surgical patients. Anesthesiology 59:215, 1983

28. Ghoneim MM, Chiang CK, Schoenwald RD et al: The pharmacokinetics of methohexital in young and elderly subjects. Acta Anaesthesiol Scand 29:480, 1985

29. Duvaldestin P, Chauvin M, Lebrault C et al: Effect of upper abdominal surgery and cirrhosis upon the pharmacokinetics of methohexital. Acta Anaesthesiol Scand 35:159, 1991

30. Lange H, Stephan H, Brand C et al: Hepatic disposition of methohexitone in patients undergoing coronary bypass surgery. Br J Anaesth 69:478, 1992

31. Schwilden H, Schüttler J, Stoeckel H: Closed-loop feedback control of methohexital anesthesia by quantitative EEG analysis in humans. Anesthesiology 67:341, 1987

32. Crankshaw DP, Boyd MD, Bjorksten AR: Plasma drug efflux—a new approach to optimization of drug infusion for constant blood concentration of thiopental and methohexital. Anesthesiology 67:32, 1987

33. Le-Normand Y, De Villepoix C, Athouel A et al: Quantitative analysis of serum methohexital by GLC using capillary column and nitrogen-selective detection. Fundam Clin Pharmacol 2:551, 1988

34. Lauven PM, Schwilden H, Stoeckel H: Threshold hypnotic concentration of methohexitone. Eur J Clin Pharmacol 33:261, 1987

35. Avram MJ, Henthorn TK: What's new in pharmacokinetics and pharmacodynamics. Anesthesiol Clin North Am 6:251, 1988.

36. Fragen RJ, Avram MJ, Henthorn TK, Caldwell NJ: A pharmacokinetically designed etomidate infusion regimen for hypnosis. Anesth Analg 62:654, 1983

37. Schwilden H, Stoeckel H: Effective therapeutic infusions produced by closed-loop feedback control of methohexital administration during total intravenous anesthesia with fentanyl. Anesthesiology 73:225, 1990

38. Arden JR, Holley FO, Stanski DR: Increased sensitivity to etomidate in the elderly: initial distribution versus altered brain response. Anesthesiology 65:19, 1986

39. Schüttler J, Schwilden H, Stoeckel H: Quantitation of the EEG and pharmacodynamic modelling of hypnotic drugs: etomidate as an example. Eur J Anaesthesiol 2:121, 1985

40. van Beem H, Manger FW, van Boxtel C, van Bentem N: Etomidate anaesthesia in patients with cirrhosis of the liver: pharmacokinetic data. Anaesthesia 38:S61, 1983

41. Van Hamme MJ, Ghoneim MM, Ambre JJ: Pharmacokinetics of etomidate, a new intravenous anesthetic. Anesthesiology 49:274, 1978

42. Gepts E, Camu F, Cockshott ID, Douglas EJ: Disposition of propofol administered as constant rate intravenous infusions in humans. Anesth Analg 66:1256, 1987

43. Kirkpatrick T, Cockshott ID, Douglas EJ, Nimmo WS: Pharmacokinetics of propofol (Diprivan) in elderly patients. Br J Anaesth 60:146, 1988

44. Lange H, Stephan H, Rieke H et al: Hepatic and extrahepatic disposition of propofol in patients undergoing coronary bypass surgery. Br J Anaesth 64:563, 1990

45. Gray PA, Park GR, Cockshott ID et al: Propofol metabolism in man during the anhepatic and reperfusion phases of liver transplantation. Xenobiotica 22:105, 1992

46. Veroli P, O'Kelly B, Bertrand F et al: Extrahepatic metabolism of propofol in man during the anhepatic phase of orthotopic liver transplantation. Br J Anaesth 68:183, 1992

47. Barr J, Egan TD, Feeley T, Shafer S: The pharmacokinetics and pharmacodynamics of computer-controlled propofol infusions in ICU patients. Clin Pharmacol Ther 53:185, 1993

48. McMurray TJ, Collier PS, Carson IW et al: Propofol sedation after open heart surgery. A clinical and pharmacokinetic study. Anaesthesia 45:322, 1990

49. Albanese J, Martin C, Lacarelle B et al: Pharmacokinetics of long-term propofol infusion used for sedation in ICU patients. Anesthesiology 73:214, 1990

50. Bailie GR, Cockshott ID, Douglas EJ, Bowles BJ: Pharmacokinetics of propofol during and after long-term continuous infusion for maintenance of sedation in ICU patients. Br J Anaesth 68:486, 1992

51. Campbell GA, Morgan DJ, Kumar K, Crankshaw DP: Extended blood collection period required to define distribution and elimination kinetics of propofol. Br J Clin Pharmacol 26:187, 1988

52. Morgan DJ, Campbell GA, Crankshaw DP: Pharmacokinetics of propofol when given by intravenous infusion. Br J Clin Pharmacol 30:144, 1990

53. Cockshott ID, Briggs LP, Douglas EJ, White M: Pharmacokinetics of propofol in female patients. Studies using single bolus injections. Br J Anaesth 59:1103, 1987

54. Shafer A, Doze VA, Shafer SL, White PF: Pharmacokinetics and pharmacodynamics of propofol infusions during general anesthesia. Anesthesiology 69:348, 1988

55. Gepts E, Jonckheer K, Maes V et al: Disposition kinetics of propofol during alfentanil anaesthesia. Anaesthesia 8:13, 1988

56. Vuyk J, Engbers FHM, Lemmens HJM et al: Pharmacodynamics of propofol in female patients. Anesthesiology 77:3, 1992

57. Bührer M, Maitre PO, Hung OR et al: Thiopental pharmacodynamics: I. Defining the pseudo-steady-state serum concentration-EEG effect relationship. Anesthesiology 77:226, 1992

58. Marsh B, White M, Morton N, Kenny GN: Pharmacokinetic model driven infusion of propofol in children. Br J Anaesth 67:41, 1991

59. Servin F, Cockshott ID, Farinotti R et al: Pharmacokinetics of propofol infusions in patients with cirrhosis. Br J Anaesth 65:177, 1990

60. Kirvela M, Olkkola KT, Rosenberg PH et al: Pharmacokinetics of propofol and haemodynamic changes during induction of anaesthesia in uraemic patients. Br J Anaesth 68:178, 1992

61. White M, Kenny GN: Intravenous propofol anaesthesia using a computerised infusion system. Anaesthesia 45:204, 1990

62. Saint-Maurice C, Cockshott ID, Douglas EJ et al: Pharmacokinetics of propofol in young children after a single dose. Br J Anaesth 63:667, 1989

Chapter 15

Clinical Pharmacology and Applications of Intravenous Anesthetic Induction Agents

Robert J. Fragen

Although thiopental, thiamylal, methohexital, etomidate, and propofol are most commonly used for the induction of general anesthesia, they have other uses also, including maintaining the hypnotic portion of "balanced anesthesia" or "total intravenous anesthesia." Balanced anesthesia is an anesthetic technique involving intravenous injection of a hypnotic, an analgesic, and when necessary, a skeletal muscle relaxant while the patient inhales nitrous oxide or small concentrations of a potent volatile agent; total intravenous anesthesia eliminates the inhaled anesthetic. Anesthesiologists also use barbiturates for premedication, for brain protection, and as anticonvulsants. Etomidate provides brain protection and propofol, in a low dose continuous infusion, produces light sleep during local or regional anesthesia.

Thiopental, the first barbiturate used clinically,[1] was introduced separately by Ralph Waters at the University of Wisconsin and John Lundy at the Mayo Clinic in 1934, although the first barbiturate with hypnotic activity, diethylbarbituric acid, was synthesized by von Mering and Fisher in 1903. Weese and Charpf introduced hexobarbital in 1932. Thiamylal became available for clinical use in 1952 and methohexital, the oxybarbiturate, in 1957. Because the pharmacology of thiamylal is so close to that of thiopental, the information on

thiopental is this chapter is also applicable to thiamylal. Much of the pharmacology of thiopental also applies to methohexital, and differences will be noted.

The development of etomidate was the culmination of deliberate efforts to produce an anesthetic induction agent to replace thiopental and improve on its disadvantages. However, as will be discussed, it has its own disadvantages. It was first used clinically in 1973[2] and is notable for a relative lack of cardiovascular side effects.

Propofol was introduced in 1977,[3] dissolved in Cremophor EL because of its water insolubility. Then, propofol[4] and other water-insoluble intravenous hypnotics dissolved in Cremophor EL, althesin, and propanidid, were withdrawn from clinical use because of an unacceptable incidence of anaphylactoid reaction on injection. An adequate solvent was found for propofol, and clinical research resumed in 1983, leading to later worldwide approval.

THERAPEUTIC DRUG EFFECTS

The barbiturates, etomidate, and propofol are hypnotics that cause "light sleep" to deep coma, depending on the dose. They are most frequently used to induce general anesthesia, causing the patient to lose consciousness. Given by intermittant bolus injections or continuous infusion, they maintain unconsciousness. A lower dose continuous infusion can maintain light sleep while the surgery takes place under local anesthesia.

Antegrade amnesia is an important component of general anesthesia. Patients rendered unconscious from the effects of barbiturates, etomidate, or propofol are also amnesic for events in the operating room. Benzodiazepines can produce antegrade amnesia in the conscious patient. One study showed partial amnesia in volunteers with a propofol infusion that only produced sedation. Amnesia was correlated with the amount of electroencephalographic (EEG) power in the β_1 and β_2 frequencies. Whether results will be similar with the usual operating room stimuli is unknown.[5]

In addition, barbiturates may help a patient sleep during the night preceding surgery, protect the brain from focal ischemia when given in large doses, or stop seizures.

COMMERCIAL FORMULATIONS

Thiopental, thiamylal, and methohexital are prepared as sodium salts, mixed with 6 percent (by weight) anhydrous sodium carbonate to act as a buffer and maintain alkalinity in the presence of atmospheric CO_2. They are reconstituted with either water or 0.9 percent sodium chloride to produce 2.5 percent (thiopental), 2.0 percent (thiamylal), or 1.0 percent (methohexital) solutions. Their pH is alkaline, 10 to 11.

Thiopental comes as a powder in multiple dose bottles or in a ready to use syringe with the powder and diluent. A decrease in alkalinity can cause barbiturates to precipitate as free acids; therefore, they should not be reconstituted with Ringer's lactate solution or be mixed with other acidic drugs. Refrigerated, they are stable for 1 week. More concentrated solutions of thiopental were formerly used but were toxic to tissues if extravasated or injected intra-arterially, often causing gangrene of tissues and occasionaly loss of fingers.[6] Such dire consequences are no longer reported with the currently recommended concentrations.

Etomidate, a carboxylated imidazole, is prepared as a stable 2 percent solution dissolved in propyl-

ene glycol. Propofol also requires an organic solvent. The solvent is an Intralipid-like substance consisting of 10 percent soybean oil, 2.25 percent glycerol, and 1.2 percent purified egg phosphatide.[7] Patients allergic to eggs should be able to tolerate propofol as egg allergies usually arise from the egg albumen. Because propofol contains no preservative or bacteriostatic agent, it can easily grow bacteria if contaminated. It is important to use an aseptic technique when transferring propofol from the vial to a syringe. It is also intended for single patient use; any unused portion should be discarded at the end of the operation. When given by continuous infusion, these drugs can be delivered by commercially available infusion pumps in the concentrations provided by the pharmaceutical company, or in the case of barbiturates, as reconstituted by the anesthesiologist.

PREMEDICATION

Formerly, secobarbital and pentobarbital were prescribed orally for sleep the night before surgery. Now, most surgical patients arrive in the hospital the day of surgery and those in the hospital who require a nighttime sedative usually receive oral benzodiazepines before bedtime.

Barbiturates can be given orally, rectally, or intramuscularly for preoperative sedation. They produce drowsiness with minimal cardiovascular or respiratory depression and have minimal emetic effects. However, they can cause dysphoria in elderly patients and prolonged awakening after short anesthetics. Secobarbital and pentobarbital produce dose-related drowsiness over a 50- to 150-mg dose range without relieving anxiety or producing analgesia. Anesthetic induction is no easier in patients premedicated with barbiturates than with unpremedicated patients.[8]

Rectal, oral, or parenteral routes are options for premedicating children with barbiturates. Children premedicated with pentobarbital were less cooperative before surgery and more excitable in the recovery room than those given opioid premedication.[9] Variable rates of absorption, onset of effect, and duration of action have made rectal administration of barbiturates relatively unpopular.[10] Intramuscular administration of barbiturates is a seldom used option because injection is painful and oral premedication is easier.

Neither etomidate or propofol are available in other than parenteral form. They are not used for premedication.

DOSE-EFFECT RELATIONSHIPS

The recommended doses of intravenous induction agents were derived from studies of relatively small numbers of subjects (Table 15-1). They are recommendations for healthy patients who are not at the extremes of age. About 2.5 percent of the population will be particularly sensitive or resistant to a given dose of these drugs. Therefore, despite the dose recommendations, the drugs should be titrated to effect. Particularly sensitive individuals can be detected if about 25 percent of the recommended anesthetic induction dose is injected and the patient is observed for an exaggerated response. If this occurs, the calculated dose should be reduced. The recommended doses are for injection times of about 20 to 30 seconds. The speed of injection is an important, but complex variable.[11] For a specified dose, a faster injection should result in higher peak plasma concentrations and greater peak effects (and side effects) compared with a slower injection. However, in elderly adults (premedicated with temazepam, 20 mg orally, 1 hour before surgery and fentanyl, 0.075 μg/kg IV, 5 minutes before anesthetic induction), a 0.82-mg/kg dose of propofol given as a 5-second bolus caused

unconsciousness in about 40 seconds and caused no more hypotension or apnea than the same dose given over 2.5 minutes.[12]

These induction agents act in one arm-brain circulation time, producing peak brain concentrations in about 30 seconds and maximum effects in about 1 minute.[13] The central nervous system (CNS) concentration and the effects related to it will lag behind the serum concentration because the transfer of drug from the blood to the effect site is not instantaneous. The half-time for blood-brain equilibrium is estimated to be 1 to 2 minutes.[14] The duration of effect of a single anesthetic induction dose is about 5 to 8 minutes because these induction agents are rapidly distributed from the brain to other tissues of the body.

The patient's age, general state of health, and premedication can affect the dose requirement for induction of anesthesia. Generally, elderly patients require a smaller dose because there is decreased clearance of drug from the brain to the rapidly equilibrating peripheral compartment (at least in the case of thiopental).[15,16] Drug effects also last longer in elderly patients in part because clearance is slower. Geriatric patients required about two-thirds of the induction dose of thiopental needed by younger patients.[17]

There are correlations between thiopental dose requirements and patient weight, lean body mass, and cardiac output.[18] Some studies suggest that drug doses should be based on lean body mass[19] rather than actual body weight because fat tissue plays a minor role in the initial drug distribution. The calculated ED$_{95}$, based on the lean body tissue mass, was 2.56 mg/kg for propofol and 3.2 mg/kg for thiopental.[20]

Medical conditions that may reduce the dose requirement of anesthetic induction agents include shock, intestinal obstruction, malnutrition, anemia, burns, advanced malignancy, ulcerative colitis, and uremia. The acutely inebriated patient requires less drug to induce anesthesia, and the chronic alcoholic patient requires more drug than does a sober patient.

The effect of premedication depends on how it is administered. Given in appropriate doses before the patient comes to the operating room, the benzodiazepines and barbiturates have little to no ef-

Table 15-1 Induction Doses of Intravenous Anesthetics in Different Age Groups^a

	Infants	Children	Young Adults	Older Adults
Thiopental	7–8	5–6	3–5	2–4
Methohexital	2–3	1–2	1–1.5	0.75–1
Etomidate	No data	0.2–0.35	0.2–0.3	0.15–0.2
Propofol	2.8–4.5	2.2–3	1.5–2.5	1–2

^{a} Average doses (in milligrams per kilogram) that may need adjustment, depending on the medical condition of the patient and other medication they may have received.

fect on induction dose requirements. Opiods reduce the required dose slightly. Clonidine, given 15 minutes before induction of anesthesia, decreased the amount of thiopental needed by 25 percent when 2.5 mg was injected and 37 percent when 5 mg was given; the blood pressure was also lower.[21]

If premedication is given intravenously in the preoperative holding area or in the operating room shortly before anesthetic induction, anesthetic induction dose requirements may be reduced depending on which premedicants and doses are used. Synergistic interactions between anesthetic induction agents and previously administered benzodiazepines or opioids may occur.[22,23] For example, when 0.13 mg/kg of midazolam was given intravenously first, the ED_{50} of propofol to achieve anesthetic induction decreased from 1.93 mg/kg to 0.93 mg/kg.

Methohexital or propofol, given by continuous infusion, can maintain unconsciousness either in balanced anesthesia or in total intravenous anesthesia. After administering the loading (induction) dose, an infusion is initiated at a rate of 50 to 150 μg/kg/min. The infusions should be stopped at least 5 minutes before the patient should awaken. The longer the methohexital infusion lasts, the longer it will take for the plasma concentration to decrease by 50 percent, and the longer the time to awakening will be. There is a dramatic prolongation of the recovery time as the duration of a thiopental infusion increases. Recovery time after propofol is less affected by the duration of the infusion (Fig. 15-1).[24] After a 1- to 1.5-mg/kg dose of propofol, an infusion rate of 50 to 100 μg/kg/min will maintain light sleep during local or regional anesthesia for most patients. In outpatients premedicated with fentanyl, a 0.5-mg/kg initial dose and a 50-μg/kg/min infusion of propofol maintained adequate anesthesia and led to a quicker recovery than an alfentanil-midazolam technique.[25] In patients premedicated with oral benzodiazepines undergoing subarachnoid anesthesia, light sleep was maintained with a mean propofol dose of 3 mg/kg/h in patients age 65 years or older and 4.1 mg/kg/h in younger patients.[26] Midazolam, 2 mg IV, did not affect the propofol dose requirements for sedation, but amnesia and anxi-

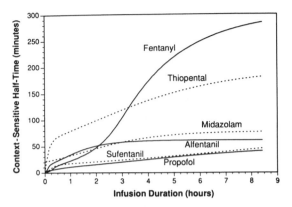

Fig. 15-1 Context-sensitive half-times as a function of infusion duration for each of the pharmacokinetic models simulated. The time needed for the plasma concentration to decrease 50 percent after stopping the infusion is shown. The line for methohexital would fall between those for thiopental and propofol. Solid and dashed line patterns are used only to permit overlapping lines to be distinguished. (From Hughes et al.,[24] with permission.)

olysis improved; recovery time was not affected.[27] Infusion rates must be titrated to obtain the desired effect. When computer controlled infusion pumps become available, the infusion pump will be programmed to achieve a given plasma concentraton (Table 15-2). That concentration will be adjustable in either direction to fulfill the patient's needs and responses. When patients show signs of light anesthesia, bolus doses of about 25 percent of the initial induction dose may be given to augment the continuous infusion.

Table 15-2 Target Plasma Concentrations for Intravenous Anesthetic Agents[a]

	Light Sleep	Anesthesia	Awake
Thiopental	—	≥ 10	4.4–7.8
Methohexital	2–5	5–15	1–3
Propofol	1–3	2–7.5	0.8–1.8
Etomidate	≥ 0.31	0.58 ± 0.2	0.31 ± 0.7

[a] In micrograms per milliliter.

Depth of anesthesia cannot be precisely quantified. The effects of individual anesthetic agents has been quantified using the EEG under laboratory conditions.[28] However, this is not a practical approach in the clinical setting in which several anesthetic drugs are typically used simultaneously. There is a biphasic relationship between serum thiopental concentrations and the number of EEG waves per second (Fig. 15-2). Higher thiopental concentrations cause a marked slowing of the EEG, leading to an isoelectric EEG.[29] The surface EEG measures cortical activity in the brain, but the sleep centers and other vital centers in the thalamus and hypothalamus are not accessible to this technique. Auditory evoked potential measurements were correlated with depth of anesthesia in a small group of patients.[30] The minimum infusion rate is the dose of an intravenous anesthetic necessary to prevent movement in response to a painful stimulus, roughly analogous to the minimum alveolar concentration concept for inhaled anesthetics.[37] However, this end point may not be appropriate for drugs with no analgesic properties. Therefore, to evaluate depth of anesthesia for intravenous anesthetics, we currently use clinical signs of the depth of anesthesia, such as hemodynamic changes, autonomic signs (tearing or diaphoresis), and movement.

When attempting to judge the depth of anesthesia from clinical signs, it is important to use muscle relaxants only when necessary and to avoid excessive neuromuscular blockade. Movement may then be used as the main sign of light anestehsia. If movement occurs, more anesthetic agent, not more muscle relaxant, should be given so the patient will remain unaware of intraoperative events. There is a report of awareness under anesthesia in a paralyzed patient who was receiving theoretically adequate infusion rate of propofol.[32]

INDUCTION SIDE EFFECTS

A urticarial rash of the face, neck, and upper chest that fades after a few minutes sometime follows injection of barbiturates. Anaphylactoid reactions consisting of hives, facial edema, bronchospasm, and/or shock occur on rare occasions after barbiturate,[33,34] or propofol injection.[35,36] Treatment of anaphylactoid reactions usually includes epinephrine and intravenous fluids. Histamine release was

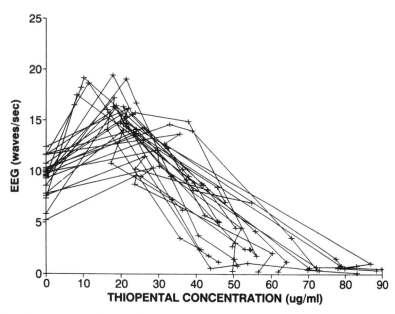

Fig. 15-2 The electroencephalographic waves per second versus measured constant serum thiopental concentrations in 26 subjects. (From Hung et al.,[29] with permission.)

reported after rapid injection of thiopental but not after other intravenous anesthetic drugs.[37,38]

Pain on injection can occur with any of the intravenous induction agents, but is most common with etomidate (because of its solvent, propylene glycol) and propofol.[39] Pain is more frequent after methohexital than after either thiopental or thiamylal. Injection pain can be decreased by slow injection into large veins rather than small hand veins and by first injecting an opioid or local anesthetic. A modified Bier block technique has been used to prevent pain from propofol.[40]

Neither etomidate nor propofol cause serious problems if injected intra-arterially.[41] However, if thiopental concentrations greater than 2.5 percent are injected intra-arterially or subcutaneously, severe tissue injury can result.[42,43] Treatment of vascular spasm caused by intra-arterial injection of thiopental may include the following: diluting the thiopental by injecting saline; injecting papaverine 40 to 80 mg in 10 to 20 ml of saline or 5 to 10 ml of 1 percent lidocaine into the involved artery; performing a stellate ganglion block on the affected side; and injecting heparin to prevent thrombosis.

Myoclonus can occur after injection of the barbiturates, propofol or etomidate. Involuntary movement from propofol is more frequent and of greater intensity in children than in adults[44] and appears coincident with slowing of the EEG.[45] Methohexital produces more severe tremors than does thiopental, especially if more than 1.5 mg/kg is injected.[46] Myoclonus can occur after rapid injection of etomidate, especially to an unpremedicated patient. This myoclonus is not associated with seizure activity on the EEG. Patients are not aware of these brief excitement phenomenon because they usually occur after loss of consciousness.

NONTHERAPEUTIC EFFECTS
Central Nervous System

Barbiturates, etomidate, and propofol cause changes in the EEG, cerebral blood flow (CBF), cerebral metabolic rate for oxygen ($CMRO_2$), cerebral vascular resistance, intracranial pressure (ICP), and intraocular pressure. These changes are particularly pertinent for patients with intracranial pathologic conditions or ophthalmologic disease.

These agents generally depress cerebral cortical function and change the EEG from its normal α rhythm to slower δ and θ waves as the dose is increased. Large doses produce burst suppression, then EEG isoelectricity (flat line),[47] associated with a 55 percent decrease in $CMRO_2$. A thiopental infusion rate of 4 mg/kg/h can maintain a flat EEG.[48] Thus, thiopental may be useful for brain protection for focal ischemia because it decreases $CMRO_2$ and decreases both CBF and ICP. High doses of etomidate might also be used for brain protection but this use of etomidate is unproved. Propofol causes less effect on $CMRO_2$ than comparable doses of barbiturates and would not be a logical choice for brain protection. Propofol offered no cerebral protection after experimentally produced focal ischemia and reprofusion in rats.[49]

Propofol and methohexital sometimes produce CNS excitation, possibly as a result of glycine antagonism at subcortical sites.[50] There are rare reports of seizures after methohexital,[51,52] etomidate,[53,54] and propofol.[55,56] Patients receiving etomidate by continuous infusion for maintenance of general anesthesia were noticed to awaken in an agitated, restless state.[57]

The intravenous induction agents possess anticonvulsant effects and can be used for patients with seizure disorders. Propofol may not be the best choice for patients undergoing electroconvulsive therapy (ECT).[58,59] In one report, the seizure duration after the ECT was about 18 seconds after induction of anesthesia with propofol and about 31 seconds after methohexital induction. However, patients receiving propofol experienced less hypotension.[60] The efficacy of ECT was unaffected by the choice of propofol or methohexital in another study.[61]

Barbiturates, etomidate,[62,63] and propofol[64,65] decrease intracranial pressure in a dose-related fashion. Cerebral perfusion pressure is better maintained after etomidate than after the other agents because etomidate has less effect on systemic arterial pressure. All these drugs are appropriate to induce and maintain anesthesia for neurosurgical procedures. The cerebrovascular re-

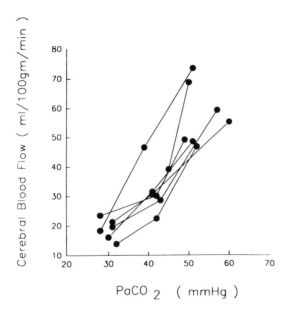

Fig. 15-3 The relationship between PaCO₂ and cerebral blood flow is shown for seven patients anesthetized with propofol and nitrous oxide. (From Fox et al.,[66] with permission.)

sponse to carbon dioxide is preserved under intravenous anesthesia (Fig. 15-3).[66]

These agents cause dose-related decreases in intraocular pressure, making them safe for intraocular surgical procedures, including operations in which the globe is opened.[67,68] Succinylcholine can cause intraocular pressure to rise above preoperative control values, and vitreous humor can be lost from an open eye. A second dose of propofol, 1 mg/kg, given just before succinylcholine administration, attenuated the rise in intraocular pressure, but a second dose of thiopental did not.[69]

Evoked potential monitoring may be affected by intravenous induction agents. Barbiturates are appropriate during both somatosensory evoked potential monitoring (SSEP) and motor evoked potential monitoring. Evoked potential components are observable even when thiopental produces a flat EEG. However, after administration of thiopental, dose-dependent changes in median nerve SSEP and brain stem auditory evoked potential signals can occur[70,71] Although propofol infusions have been used successfully during SSEP

monitoring for spinal cord surgery, the amplitude of the early components of SSEPs may be decreased.[72] Propofol does not appear to alter brain stem auditory evoked potentials, but it produces a dose-dependent prolongation of latency and a decrease in the amplitude of cortical middle latency auditory potentials.[73] Propofol produced a longer duration and greater depression of motor evoked potentials generated by electrical or magnetic stimulators compared with etomidate (Fig. 15-4).[74] Etomidate has the least depressant effect on evoked potentials. In one report, etomidate caused a dose-dependent increase in latency and a decrease in amplitude of early cortical components.

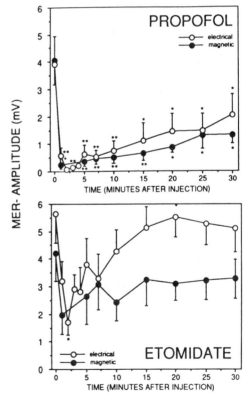

Fig. 15-4 Amplitudes (millivolts, mean ± standard error of the mean) of motor evoked responses to transcranial electrical or magnetic stimulation versus time after injection of propofol, 2 mg/kg, or etomidate, 0.3 mg/kg. *P = 0.05. **P = 0.01. (Modified from Kalkman et al.,[74] with permission.)

However, brain stem evoked responses were unaltered after etomidate injection.[75] SSEPs actually increased in amplitude and latency after etomidate administration.[76]

Respiratory System

Equivalent induction doses of etomidate cause less respiratory depression than do either propofol or the barbiturates. The degree of respiratory depression varies with the choice of premedication, dose, and rate of injection. Opioids, compared with other types of premedication, result in greater respiratory depression. The effects of these agents on airway reflexes, bronchial smooth muscle tone, rate and depth of breathing, response to elevated CO_2, and response to hypoxemia are important.

Etomidate and methohexital sometimes cause brief periods of coughing or hiccoughing.[77] Thiopental[78] and other induction agents may relax the muscles of the upper airway leading to uper airway obstruction. Laryngospasm or bronchospasm occurring after thiopental induction is more likely caused by premature insertion of oral airways or endotracheal tubes in inadequately anesthetized patients rather than increased airway reactivity. Airway reactivity is less after propofol than after other intravenous induction agents.[79] None of these agents normally cause histamine release[80] or increased airway resistance, and they can be administered safely to patients with bronchospastic diseases. However, they do not have the bronchodilating properties of ketamine or volatile anesthetics.[81]

In unpremedicated patients, induction with etomidate or propofol produces a brief period of hyperventilation, sometimes followed by apnea; the duration of apnea is longer after propofol.[82,83] Apnea is less frequent after etomidate compared with ketamine or midazolam. Apnea from intravenous induction agents lasts longer after opioid premedication and in elderly patients. The barbiturates and propofol decrease the tidal volume and respiratory rate to a similar degree.[84–86] If either methohexital or propofol is given by a continuous infusion in lower doses for light sleep during local or regional anesthesia, spontaneous ventilation can be maintained. The intravenous induction agents

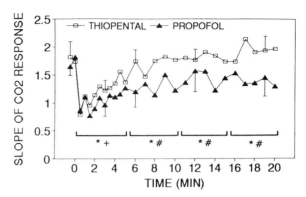

Fig. 15-5 Slope of ventilatory response to CO_2 (in liters per minute per millimeters of mercury) after propofol or thiopental. The values are means ± standard error of the mean. $*P < 0.05$ versus preinjection values for propofol; $+P < 0.05$ versus preinjection values for thiopental; $\#P < 0.05$ for propofol versus thiopental during the same time period. (From Blouin et al.,[88] with permission.)

do not inhibit hypoxic pulmonary vasoconstriction.[87]

All these agents can depress the ventilatory response to hypercarbia or hypoxia. The ventilatory response to CO_2 was depressed by thiopental and propofol in healthy volunteers; the effect of propofol, but not thiopental, persisted after the subjects regained consciousness (Fig. 15-5).[88]

Cardiovascular System

All the intravenous induction agents depress the cardiovascular system to a degree that varies with the particular agent. Many factors can influence the cardiovascular response, including the effects of anesthetic premedication, cardiovascular drug therapy, cardiovascular disease, and the patient's intravascular volume status.

The primary cardiovascular effect of the barbiturates is venodilation with pooling of blood in the periphery.[89] Barbiturates decrease myocardial contractility but to a lesser extent than do volatile anesthetics.[90] The heart rate usually increases.[91] There is more tachycardia after methohexital than after thiopental because methohexital inhibits cardiac vagal activity. The cardiac output is decreased. The systemic vascular resistance is virtually unchanged.

Barbiturates do not sensitize the heart to catecholamines. Barbiturates inhibit the sympathetic nervous system activity but do not prevent its augmentation by stimuli such as laryngoscopy and tracheal intubation.[92,93] Myocardial oxygen demand increases, but there is normally a proportional increase in myocardial blood flow and a decrease in coronary vascular resistance.[94] However, if aortic pressure is low enough, coronary blood flow will decrease. Therefore, barbiturates should be used with caution as anesthetic induction agents in situations in which tachycardia or a decreased preload could be detrimental (e.g., pericardial tamponade, congestive heart failure, heart block, hypovolemia, myocardial ischemia, or when baseline sympathetic tone is increased).

Barbiturates increase blood flow to the extremities but decrease renal plasma flow, hepatic blood flow, and cerebral blood flow. These changes do not cause clinically significant problems in healthy patients.

Propofol did not alter diastolic cardiac function in chronically instrumented dogs with autonomic nervous system blockade. However, it decreased cardiac output, systemic vascular resistance, and both systolic and diastolic arterial pressure. There was also a concentration-dependent decrease in regional myocardial contractility.[95,96] In humans, propofol decreases preload and afterload by a direct effect on vascular smooth muscle[97] (decreased systemic vascular resistance) and a decreased level of sympathetic activity. In patients with artificial hearts and a fixed cardiac output, propofol produced more venous and arterial dilation than did thiopental when equipotent doses were administered.[98] Propofol depressed myocardial contractility; both cardiac output and stroke volume decreased.[99,100] Hypotension results from vasodilation, myocardial depression, sympathetic nervous system inhibition, and impaired baroreflex function.[101] Previous reports suggested that propofol, unlike barbiturates, resets rather than depresses the baroreflex,[102] permitting slower heart rates at a given blood pressure. When isoflurane is added to a propofol infusion, there is a dose-related decrease in mean arterial pressure as a result of afterload reduction, but there is no further change in

cardiac output or stroke volume.[103] Hypotension is at least as severe after induction of anesthesia with propofol as after barbiturate induction. Systolic blood pressure usually decreases 25 to 40 percent, and left ventricular stroke work decreases by a similar amount.[104] When propofol is given by infusion, plasma concentrations are lower, and there is less hypotension than after anesthetic induction doses. Surgical stimulation returns blood pressure toward control values.

Propofol decreases myocardial oxygen demand, myocardial blood flow, and coronary vascular resistance, tending to keep supply and demand in balance.[105,106] The heart rate usually decreases, but it may increase slightly or remain unchanged.

Propofol is the most potent cardiovascular depressant of the drugs discussed here. Although it has been used successfully in patients with good ventricular function undergoing cardiac surgery,[107] it should be used with caution in patients with cardiovascular compromise. Propofol is more likely to cause more hypotention in elderly than in younger patients.[108]

The main advantage of etomidate as an anesthetic induction agent is that it causes minimal hemodynamic changes. Etomidate, 0.3 mg/kg, causes minor increases in cardiac index and slight decreases in heart rate, systemic vascular resistance, and arterial blood pressure. These changes are maximal about 3 minutes after injection and return toward preinjection values over the next 5 minutes.[109] This dose of etomidate causes a nitroglycerin-like effect on the coronary circulation. Coronary blood flow increases without an increase in myocardial metabolism. Coronary vascular resistance decreases with no change in coronary perfusion pressure.[110] Etomidate causes only minor hemodynamic changes in patients with valvular heart disease[111] and causes less hypotension than thiopental when either drug is given to patients with mild hypovolemia.[112] Etomidate does not sensitize the heart to catecholamines. Severe bradycardia has occurred following etomidate, an opioid, and succinylcholine because all three drugs tend to slow the heart rate.[113] There are also reports of severe bradycardia after a propofol-succinylcholine sequence in healthy patients.[114,115] Table 15-3 sum-

Table 15-3 Cardiovascular Effects in Healthy Adults[a]

	MAP	HR	CO	SVR	Venodilation	dP/dT
Thiopental	↓	+	↓	0 to ↑	↑	↓
Methohexital	↓	++	↓	NR	↑	↓
Etomidate	0	0	0	0	0	0
Propofol	↓	↓, 0, or sl ↑	0 to ↓	↓	↑	↓

Abbreviations: CO, cardiac output; dP/dT, myocardial contractility; HR, heart rate; MAP, mean arterial pressure; NR, not reported; SVR, systemic vascular resistance.
[a] ↑ ↑ to ↓ ↓ is a five-point scale qualitatively describing the relative increase (↑) or decrease (↓) or virtually no effect (0) among the intravenous anesthetic induction agents for each cardiovascular effect.
(Data from Fragen and Avram.[139])

marizes the cardiovascular effects of the intravenous induction agents.

Endocrine System

The intravenous anesthetics have essentially no effects on the pituitary gland, thyroid gland, parathyroid gland, pancreas, or adrenal medulla. A report of increased mortality rates in an intensive care unit in Scotland was associated with a "sedation" regimen of etomidate and morphine.[116] This finding led to studies that showed adrenal cortical suppression for at least 5 hours after induction doses of etomidate and for a longer time after an infusion of etomidate.[117,118] Thus, etomidate should not be given as a long-term continuous infusion. However there is no evidence that etomidate causes any increase in morbidity or mortality rates when it is used to induce anesthesia or when given in a short infusion during surgery. Etomidate causes a decrease in cortisol, 11-hydroxyprogesterone, aldosterone, and corticosterone production by inhibiting adrenal 11-a- and 11-b-hydroxylase and the cholesterol side chain cleavage enzymes.

Neither thiopental nor propofol, in anesthetic doses, suppresses the adrenocortical response to stress or adrenocorticotrophic hormone stimulation (Fig. 15-6),[119] but large doses of propofol in vitro inhibit the first stage of cholesterol synthesis, and large doses of thiopental inhibit 11-b-hydroxylase.[120]

Other Systems

These agents probably have no important direct effects on other systems of the body, including the gastrointestinal, hepatic, renal, or reproductive system. However, if cardiovascular depression occurs, blood flow to the liver, kidney, and uterus may decrease.

Both thiopental and propofol in high doses can affect the immune response, causing more than 50 percent inhibition of neutrophil polarization in vitro (Fig. 15-7). This could raise concerns about prolonged infusion of thiopental or propofol in intensive care units.[121]

PHYSICOCHEMICAL DRUG INTERACTIONS

Physicochemical incompatibility occurs when a drug with a high pH, such as thiopental, is mixed with drugs or solutions with an acidic pH, causing precipitation. Therefore, thiopental should not be mixed with other anesthetic drugs or injected into an intravenous line when other drugs are present. Other drugs should be injected into the line after thiopental only after the line is flushed. Atracurium could be inactivated by mixing with thiopental because the Hofmann reaction is activated at basic pH.

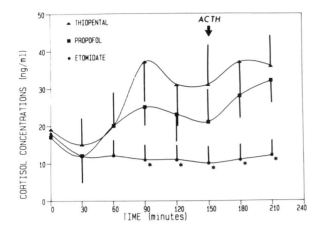

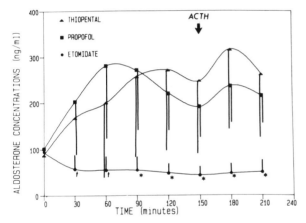

Fig. 15-6 Blood cortisol (**A**) and aldosterone (**B**) concentrations before and after induction of anesthesia with thiopental, 4 mg/kg; propofol, 2.5 mg/kg; or etomidate, 0.3 mg/kg. ACTH was administered 150 minutes after induction. *$P < 0.05$ blood cortisol or aldosterone concentrations after etomidate compared with propofol or thiopental. + $P < 0.05$ blood aldosterone concentrations after etomidate and compared with propofol at the same time. ACTH, adrenocorticotrophic hormone. (From Fragen et al.,[119] with permission.)

SPECIAL SITUATIONS

Inducible porphyria (acute intermittent or variegate porphyria or hereditary coproporphyria), may be activated by barbiturates, resulting in an acute neurologic syndrome of variable severity, ranging from abdominal pain (that may mimic an acute abdomen) to paralysis and death. Barbiturates induce

δ-aminolevulinic acid synthetase, which catalyzes the rate limiting step in the biosynthesis of porphyrins,[122] thus, all barbiturates are contraindicated. There is limited clinical experience to indicate which anesthetic drugs are safe. Nitrous oxide, opioids, and muscle relaxants appear to be safe. Propofol has been used successfully in patients with porphyria.[123,124]

The intravenous induction agents do not act as triggering agents for malignant hyperpyrexia; all are safe to use for patients susceptible to this condition.[125]

The pharmacology of these drugs in infants and children is similar to that in adults, but the pharmacokinetics may be different because of immature organs of elimination in early infancy. Induction doses tend to be larger relative to weight in children. Because children react more to pain, pain on injection may be more problematic with etomidate, propofol, and methohexital than in adults. Children in the younger age groups often prefer inhalation induction of anesthesia because they fear venipuncture. The lower incidence of nausea and vomiting after propofol than other anesthetics may recommended it for pediatric outpatient anesthesia despite the pain on injection. Propofol infusions with or without analgesics can be used for pediatric

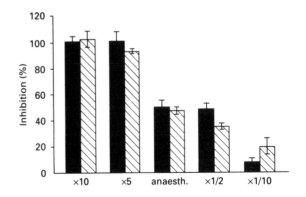

Fig. 15-7 Percent in vitro inhibition of neutrophil polarization produced by propofol (■) and thiopental (□) at concentrations likely to be required for surgical anesthesia (anaesth) (propofol, 6 μg/ml; thiopental, 40 μg/ml) and multiples or fractions of this concentration (mean ± standard error of the mean). (From O'Donnell et al.,[121] with permission.)

patients for cardiac catheterization[126] or for procedures outside the operating room.[127]

Nursing mothers can receive any of these drugs for anesthetic induction but should realize that, if they nurse on the day of surgery, trace amounts of drugs will be present in their milk and, theoretically, could cause some drowsiness in their infants. Propofol is rapidly cleared from the neonatal circulation.[128] The amount of drug in the milk the following day usually presents no problem.

A pregnant woman preferably should avoid any drugs during the first trimester of pregnancy. If general anesthesia is necessary during this time, any of these drugs can be administered because none of them cause mutagenic or teratogenic effects in humans. They all cross the placenta to depress the fetus, but they are safe when used in normal induction doses for cesarian section. When a cesarian section is performed for hemorrhage, the same precautions should be used as for any other hypovolemic patient; barbiturates and propofol in normal doses may cause profound hypotension.

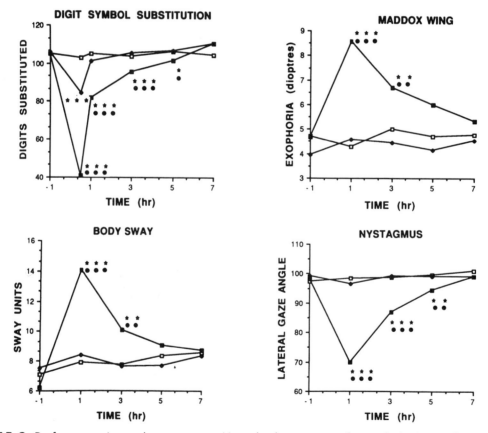

Fig. 15-8 Performance in psychomotor tests. Mean body sway on a force platform; number of digits correctly substituted for symbols in digit substitution test; exophoria in Maddox wing test; and angle for lateral gaze end point nystagmus before and after intravenous injection of propofol, 2.5 ± 1 mg/kg (◇); thiopental, 5.0 ± 2.0 mg/kg (■); and control (□) in 12 healthy volunteers. $*P < 0.05$; $** P < 0.01$, $*** P < 0.001$ versus control. $•P < 0.05$; $••P < 0.01$; $•••P < 0.001$ versus propofol. (Modified from Korttila et al.,[137] with permission.)

RECOVERY FROM ANESTHESIA

Recovery from general anesthesia should be rapid and free of side effects, but residual analgesia is beneficial. Many comparative studies show minor (5- to 10-minute) differences in recovery after induction with any of these intravenous anesthetic agents when the rest of the anesthesia is the same.[53,129,130] After propofol, recovery is more rapid, and side effects are less frequent than after etomidate or the barbiturates.[131,132] Some patients may awaken after propofol but unable to open their eyes for up to 20 minutes. The reason is unknown, but it requires no treatment.[133] Patients generally awaken with a clearer head and recovery is associated with less nausea and vomiting after propofol than after other intravenous or inhalation anesthetics. Subhypnotic doses of propofol have antiemetic properties.[134] Recovery after propofol is as rapid as after desflurane (recovery is faster after desflurane than after other volatile anesthetics).[135] Propofol used by continuous infusion with other intravenous agents or with nitrous oxide, provides rapid recovery if the propofol infusion rate is tapered toward the end of surgery and stopped about 5 minutes before the desired awakening. The same pleasant recovery occurs whether propofol is given as a maintenance infusion or only for induction of anesthesia, making it the intravenous hypnotic of choice for outpatient anesthesia. In a comparative study of outpatient anesthesia, psychomotor performance was impaired for 30 minutes after propofol injection, 60 to 90 minutes after methohexital, and up to 2 hours or longer after thiopental.[136] In volunteers given equivalent doses, psychomotor function was impaired for 1 hour after propofol and up to 5 hours after thiopental (Fig. 15-8).[137]

Venous thrombosis, phlebitis, or thrombophlebitis caused by intravenous induction agents may occur up to the 10th postoperative day. The incidence is usually less than 5 percent, but it can approach 10 to 20 percent after etomidate as a result of the osmolality of its solvent, propylene glycol. A new emulsion solvent that changes the osmolality from 4,900 to 307 and the pH from 5.1 to 6.4 is under investigation.[138] Venous reactions usually involve only a small segment of vein, rarely result in permanent damage, and are treated symptomatically.

REFERENCES

1. Pratt TW, Tatum AL, Hathaway HR et al: Sodium ethyl (1-methyl butyl) thiobarbiturate, preliminary experimental and clinical study. Am J Surg 31:464, 1935
2. Doenicke A: Etomidate, a new intravenous hypnotic. Acta Anaesthesiol Belg 25:307, 1974
3. Kay B, Rolly G: ICI 35,868, a new intravenous induction agent. Acta Anaesthesiol Belg 28:303, 1977
4. Briggs LP, Clarke RSJ, Watkins J: An adverse reaction to the administration of disoprofol (Diprivan). Anaesthesia 37:1099, 1982
5. Veselis RA, Reinsel PA, Wronski M et al: EEG and memory effects of low-dose infusions of propofol. Br J Anaesth 69:246, 1992
6. Dundee JW, Wyant GM: Intravenous Anaesthesia. 2nd Ed. Churchill Livingstone, New York, 1988
7. Sebel PS, Lowden JD: Propofol: a new intravenous anesthetic. Anesthesiology 71:260, 1989
8. Forrest WH Jr, Brown CR, Brown BW: Subjective response to six common preoperative medications. Anesthesiology 47:241, 1977
9. Eger EI II, Kraft ID, Keasling HH: A comparison of atropine or scopolamine, plus pentobarbital, meperidine, or morphine preanesthetic medication. Anesthesiology 22:962, 1961
10. Liu LMP, Gaudreault P, Friedman PA et al: Methohexital plasma concentrations in children following rectal administration. Anesthesiology 62:567, 1985
11. Goodman NW, Black AMS: Rate of injection of propofol for induction of anesthesia. Anesth Analg 74:938, 1992
12. Peacock JE, Spiers SPW, McLauchlan GA et al: Infusion of propofol to identify smallest effective doses for induction of anaesthesia in young and elderly patients. Br J Anaesth 69:363, 1992
13. Price HL: A dynamic concept of the distribution of thiopental in the human body. Anesthesiology 21:40, 1960
14. Stanski DR, Hudson TJ, Homer TD et al: Pharmacodynamic modeling of thiopental anesthesia. J Pharmacokinet Biopharm 12:223, 1984
15. Avram MJ, Krecjie TC, Henthorn TK: The relationship of age to the pharmacokinetics of early drug distribution. The concurrent disposition of thiopental and indocyanine green. Anesthesiology 72:403, 1990

16. Stanski DR, Maitre PO: Population pharmacokinetics and pharmacodynamics of thiopental: the effect of age revisited. Anesthesiology 72:412, 1990

17. Muravchick S: Effect of age and premedication on thiopental sleep dose. Anesthesiology 61:333, 1984

18. Avram MJ, Sanghvi R, Henthorn TK et al: Determinants of thiopental induction dose requirements. Anesth Analg 76:10, 1993

19. Wulfsohn NL, Joshi CW: Thiopental dosage based on lean body mass. Br J Anaesth 41:516, 1969

20. Leslie K, Crankshaw DP: Potency of propofol for loss of consciousness after a single dose. Br J Anaesth 64:734, 1990

21. Leslie K, Mooney PH, Silbert BS: Effect of intravenous clonidine on the dose of thiopental required to induce anesthesia. Anesth Analg 75:530, 1992

22. Tverskoy M, Fleyshman G, Bradley EL Jr, Kissin I: Midazolam-thiopental interaction in patients. Anesth Analg 67:342, 1988

23. Short TG, Chiu PT: Propofol and midazolam act synergistically in combination. Br J Anaesth 67:539, 1991

24. Hughes MA, Glass PSA, Jacobs JR: Context-sensitive half-time in multicompartment pharmacokinetic models for intravenous anesthetic drugs. Anesthesiology 76:334, 1992

25. Monk TG, Boure B, White PF et al: Comparison of intravenous sedative-analgesic techniques for outpatient immersion lithotripsy. Anesth Analg 72:616, 1991

26. MacKenzie N, Grant IS: Propofol for intravenous sedation. Anaesthesia 42:3, 1987

27. Taylor E, Ghouri AF, White PF: Midazolam in combination with propofol for sedation during local anesthesia. J Clin Anesth 4:213, 1992

28. Buhrer M, Maitre PO, Hung OR et al: Thiopental pharmacodynamics I. Defining the pseudo-steady state serum concentrations-EEG effect relationship. Anesthesiology 77:226, 1992

29. Hung OR, Varvel JR, Shafter SL, Stanski DR: Thiopental pharmacodynamics: II. Quantitation of clinical and encephalographic depth of anesthesia. Anesthesiology 77:237, 1992

30. Kenny GNC, McFadzean W, Mantzaridis H: Closed-loop control of anesthesia. Anesthesiology 77:A320, 1992

31. Sear JW: Pharmacokinetic and pharmacodynamic aspects of continuous infusion anaesthesia. Concept of minimum infusion rate as an index of equipotency for intravenous drugs. p. 234. In Sear JW (ed): Intravenous Anaesthesiology. Clinics in Anaesthesiology. WB Saunders, London, 1984

32. Kelly JS, Roy RC: Intraoperative awareness with propofol-oxygen total intravenous anesthesia for microlaryngeal surgery. Anesthesiology 77:207, 1992

33. Thompson DS, Eason CN, Flacke JW: Thiamylal anaphylaxis. Anesthesiology 39:556, 1973

34. Westacott P, Ramachandran PR, Jancelewicz Z: Anaphylactic reaction to thiopentone: a case report. Can J Anaesth 31:434, 1984

35. Lein-Casasola OA, Weiss A, Lema MJ: Anaphylaxis due to propofol. Anesthesiology 77:384, 1992

36. Laxenaire M, Mata-Bermejo E, Moneret-Vautrin DA, Gueant J: Life threatening anaphylactoid reactions to propofol (Diprivan). Anesthesiology 77:375, 1992

37. Doenicke A, Lorenz W, Beigl R: Histamine release after intravenous application of short-acting hypnotics. Br J Anaesth 45:1097, 1973

38. Doenicke A, Lorenz W, Stenworth D et al: Effects of propofol "Diprivan" on histamine release, immunoglobulin levels and activation of complement in healthy volunteers. Postgrad med J, suppl. 3:15, 1985

39. Hynynen M, Korttila K, Tammisto T: Pain on IV injection of propofol (ICI 35868) in emulsion formulation. Acta Anesthesiol Scand 29:651, 1985

40. Mangar D, Holak EJ: Tourniquet at 50 mmHg followed by intravenous lidocaine diminishes hand pain associated with propofol injection. Anesth Analg 74:250, 1992

41. MacPherson RD, Rasiah RL, McLeod LJ: Intraarterial propofol is not directly toxic to vascular endothelium. Anesthesiology 76:967, 1992

42. Stone HH, Donnelly CC: The accidental intra-arterial injection of thiopental. Anesthesiology 22:995, 1961

43. Clarke RSJ: Adverse effects of intravenously administered drugs used in anesthetic practice. Drugs 22:26, 1981

44. Hannallah RS, Baker SB, Casey W et al: Propofol: effective dose and induction characteristics in unpremedicated children. Anesthesiology 74:217, 1991

45. Borgeat A, Dessibourg C, Popovic V et al: Propofol and spontaneous movements: an EEG study. Anesthesiology 74:24, 1991

46. Whitwam JG: Methohexitone. Br J Anaesth 48:641, 1976

47. Kiersey DK, Bickford RG, Faulkner A: Electroencephalographic patterns produced by thiopental sodium during surgical operations: descriptions and classification. Br J Anaesth 23:141, 1951

48. Turcant A, Delhumeau A, Premel-Cabic A et al: Thiopental pharmacokinetics under conditions of long-term infusions. Anesthesiology 63:50, 1985

49. Ridenour TR, Warner DS, Todd MM, Gionet TX: Comparative effects of propofol and halothane on outcome from temporary middle cerebral artery occlusion in the rat. Anesthesiology 76:807, 1992

50. Dolin SJ, Smith MB, Soar J, Morris PJ: Does glycine antagonism underlie the excitatory effects of methohexital and propofol? Br J Anaesth 68:523, 1992

51. Gumpert J, Paul R: Activation of the electroencephalogram with intravenous Brietal (methohexitone): the findings in 100 cases. J Neurol Neurosurg Psychiatry 34:646, 1971

52. Rockoff MA, Goudsouzian NG: Seizures produced by methohexital. Anesthesiology 54:333, 1981

53. Lees NW, Hendry JCB: Etomidate in urological outpatient anaesthesia. Anaesthesia 32:592, 1977

54. Gancher S, Laxer KD, Krieger W: Activation of epileptogenic activity by etomidate. Anesthesiology 61:616, 1984

55. Victosy RA, Magee D: A case of convulsions after propofol anaesthesia. Anaesthesia 43:904, 1988

56. DeFriez CB, Wong HC: Seizures and opisthotonos after propofol anesthesia. Anesth Analg 75:630, 1992

57. Fragen RJ, Avram MJ, Henthorn TK et al: A pharmacokinetically designed etomidate infusion regimen for hypnosis. Anesth Analg 62:654, 1983

58. Simpson KH, Halsall PJ, Carr CME, Stewart KG: Propofol reduces seizure duration in patients having anaesthesia for electroconvulsive therapy. Br J Anaesth 61:343, 1988

59. Dwyer R, McCaughey W, Lavery J et al: Comparison of propofol and methohexitone as anaesthetic agents for electroconvulsive therapy. Anaesthesia 43:459, 1988

60. Rampton AJ, Griffin RM, Stuart CS et al: Comparison of methohexital and propofol for electroconvulsive therapy: effects on hemodynamic responses and seizure duration. Anesthesiology 70:412, 1989

61. Malsch E, Gratz I, Mani S: Efficacy of electroconvulsive therapy after propofol (P) or methohexital (M) anesthesia. Anesth Analg 74:S192, 1992

62. Moss E, Powell D, Gibson RM et al: Effect of etomidate on intracranial pressure and cerebral perfusion pressure. Br J Anaesth 51:347, 1979

63. Renou AM, Vernheit J, Macrez P et al: Cerebral blood flow and metabolism during etomidate anaesthesia in man. Br J Anaesth 50:1047, 1978

64. Stephan H, Sonntag H, Schenk HD et al: Einfluss von Disoprivan (propofol) auf die durchblutung

und den sauerstoffverbrauch des gehirns und die CO_2-reactivitat der hirngefasse bein menschen. Anaesthesist 36:60, 1987

65. Hartung HJ: Beeinflussung des intrakrahieliendrukes durch propofol (Disoprivan). Anaesthesist 36:66, 1987

66. Fox J, Gelb AW, Enns J et al: The responsiveness of cerebral blood flow to changes in arterial carbon dioxide is maintained during propofol-nitrous oxide anesthesia in humans. Anesthesiology 77:453, 1992

67. Famewo CE, Adugbesian CO, Osuntakum OD: Effects of etomidate on intraocular pressure. Can J Anaesth 24:712, 1977

68. Calla S, Gupta A, Sen N et al: Comparison of the effects of etomidate and thiopentone on intraocular pressure. Br J Anaesth 59:437, 1987

69. Mirakhur RK, Shepherd WFL, Darrah WC: Propofol or thiopentone: effects on intraocular pressure associated with induction of anaesthesia and tracheal intubation (facilitated with suxamethonium). Br J Anaesth 59:431, 1987

70. Drummond JC, Todd MM, U HS: The effect of high dose sodium thiopental in brain stem auditory and median nerve somatosensory evoked responses in humans. Anesthesiology 63:249, 1985

71. McPherson RW, Sell B, Traystman RJ: Effects of thiopental, fentanyl, and etomidate in upper extremity somatosensory evoked potentials in humans. Anesthesiology 65:584, 1986

72. Maurette P, Simeon F, Castagnera L et al: Propofol anaesthesia alters somatosensory evoked cortical potentials. Anaesthesia 43:44, 1988

73. Savoia G, Esposito C, Belfiore F et al: Propofol infusion and auditory evoked potentials. Anaesthesia 43:46, 1988

74. Kalkman C, Drummond JC, Ribberlink AA et al: Effects of propofol, etomidate, midazolam and fentanyl on motor evoked responses to transcranial electrical or magnetic stimulation in humans. Anesthesiology 76:502, 1992

75. Thornton C, Heneghan CPM, Navaratnarajah M et al: Effect of etomidate on the auditory evoked response in man. Br J Anaesth 57:554, 1985

76. Sloan TB, Ronai AK, Toleikis JR, Koht A: Improvement of intraoperative somatosensory evoked potentials by etomidate. Anesth Analg 67:582, 1985

77. Nimmo WS, Miller M: Pharmacology of etomidate. Contemp Anesth Pract 7:274, 1978

78. Drummond GB: Influence of thiopentone on upper airway muscles. Br J Anaesth 63:12, 1989

79. Barber P, Langton JA, Wilson IG, Smith G: Movement of the vocal cords on induction of anaesthesia

with thiopentone or propofol. Br J Anaesth 69:23, 1992

80. Guldager H, Sodergaard I, Hensen PM, Cold G: Basophil histamine release in asthma patients after in vitro provocation with althesin and etomidate. Acta Anaesthesiol Scand 29:352, 1985

81. Huber FC, Reves JG, Gutierrez J, Corsson G: Ketamine: its effect on airway resistance in man. South Med J 65:1176, 1972

82. Morgan M, Lumley J, Whitwam JG: Respiratory effects of etomidate. Br J Anaesth 49:233, 1977

83. Streisand JB, Nelson P, Bubbers S et al: The respiratory effect of propofol with and without fentanyl. Anesth Analg 66:S171, 1987

84. Taylor MB, Grounds RM, Dulroony PD, Morgan M: Ventilatory effects of propofol during induction of anesthesia. Anaesthesia 41:816, 1986

85. Goodman NW, Black AMS, Carter JA: Some ventilatory effects of propofol as sole anaesthetic agent. Br J Anaesth 59:1497, 1987

86. Grounds RM, Maxwell DL, Taylor MB et al: Acute ventilatory changes during IV induction of anaesthesia with thiopentone or propofol in man. Studies using inductance plethysmography. Br J Anaesth 59:1098, 1987

87. Van Keer L, Van Aken H, Vandermeersch E et al: Propofol does not inhibit hypoxic pulmonary vasoconstriction in humans. J Clin Anesth 1:284, 1989

88. Blouin RT, Conard PF, Gross JB: Time course of ventilatory depression following induction doses of propofol and thiopental. Anesthesiology 75:940, 1991

89. Ecksten JW, Hamilton WK, McCammond JM: The effect of thiopental on peripheral venous tone. Anesthesiology 22:525, 1961

90. Frankle WS, Pool-Wilson PA: Effects of thiopental on tension development, action potential, and exchange of calcium and potassium in rabbit ventricular myocardium. J Cardiovasc Pharmacol 3:354, 1981

91. Bristow JD, Prys-Roberts C, Fisher A et al: Effects of anesthesia on baroreflex control of heart rate in man. Anesthesiology 31:422, 1969

92. Skovsted P, Price ML, Price HL: The effects of short-acting barbiturates on arterial pressure, preganglionic sympathetic activity and barostatic reflexes. Anesthesiology 33:10, 1970

93. Ebert TJ, Kanitz DD, Kampine JP: Inhibition of sympathetic neural outflow during thiopental anesthesia in humans. Anesth Analg 71:319, 1990

94. Kettler D, Sonntag H, Wolfram-Donath U et al: Haemodynamics, myocardial function, oxygen re-

quirements, and supply of the human heart after administration of etomidate. p. 81. In Doenicke A (ed): Anaesthesiology and Resuscitation. Etomidate: An Intravenous Hypnotic Agent. Springer-Verlag, Berlin, 1977

95. Coetzee A, Fourie P, Coetzee J et al: Effects of various propofol plasma concentrations on regional myocardial contractility and left ventricular afterload. Anesth Analg 69:473, 1989

96. Pagel PS, Schmeling WT, Kampine JP, Warltier DC: Alteration of canine left ventricular diastolic function by intravenous anesthesia in vivo. Ketamine and propofol. Anesthesiology 76:419, 1992

97. Muzi M, Berens RA, Kampine JP, Ebert TJ: Venodilation contributes to propofol-mediated hypotension in humans. Anesth Analg 74:877, 1992

98. Rouby J, Andreev A, Leger P et al: Peripheral vascular effects of thiopental and propofol in humans with artificial hearts. Anesthesiology 75:32, 1991

99. Grounds RM, Twigley AJ, Carli F et al: The haemodynamic effects of thiopentone and propofol. Anaesthesia 40:735, 1985

100. Coates DP, Monk CR, Prys-Roberts C, Turtle M: Hemodynamic effects of infusions of the emulsion formulation of propofol during nitrous oxide anesthesia in humans. Anesth Analg 66:84, 1987

101. Ebert TJ, Muzi M, Berens R et al: Sympathetic responses to induction of anesthesia in humans with propofol or etomidate. Anesthesiology 76:725, 1992

102. Cullen PM, Turtle M, Prys-Roberts C et al: Effect of propofol anesthesia on baroreflex activity in humans. Anesth Analg 66:1115, 1987

103. Verborgh C, Verbessem K, Camu F: Haemodynamic effects of isoflurane during propofol anaesthesia. Br J Anaesth 69:36, 1992

104. Claeys MA, Gepts E, Camu F: Haemodynamic changes during anaesthesia induced and maintained with propofol. Br J Anaesth 60:3, 1983

105. Larson R, Rathgeber J, Bagdahn A et al: Effects of propofol on cardiovascular dynamics and coronary blood flow in geriatric patients. A comparison with etomidate. Anaesthesia 43:25, 1988

106. Stephan H, Sonntag H, Schenk HD et al: Effects of propofol on cardiovascular dynamics, myocardial blood flow, and myocardial metabolism in patients with coronary vascular disease. Br J Anaesth 58:969, 1986

107. Lippman M, Paicius R, Gingerich S et al: A controlled study of hemodynamic effects of propofol vs. thiopental during anesthesia induction. Anesth Analg 65:S89, 1986

108. Dundee JW, Robinson FP, McCollum JSC et al: Sen-

sitivity to propofol in the elderly. Anaesthesia 41:482, 1986

109. Bruckner JB: Investigations in the effects of etomidate in the human circulation. Anaesthesist 23:322, 1974

110. Kettler D, Sonntag H, Donath V et al: Haemodynamics, myocardial function, oxygen requirements and oxygen supply to the human heart after administration of etomidate. Anaesthesist 23:116, 1974

111. Reves JG, Kissen I: Intravenous anesthetics. p. 3. In Kaplan J (ed): Cardiac Anesthesia. Grune & Stratton, New York, 1983

112. Colvin MP, Savege TM, Newland PE et al: Cardiorespiratory changes following induction of anesthesia with etomidate in patients with cardiac disease. Br J Anaesth 51:551, 1979

113. Booij LHDJ: The role of hypnotic agents in intravenous anaesthesia-benzodiazepines and non-barbiturate hypnotic drugs used for induction or maintenance of anaesthesia. p. 76. In Sear JW (ed): Intravenous Anaesthesiology. Clinics in Anaesthesiology. WB Saunders, London, 1984

114. Baraka A: Severe bradycardia following propofol-suxamethonium sequence. Br J Anaesth 61:482, 1988

115. Egan TD, Brock-Utne JG: Asystole after anesthesia induction with a fentanyl, propofol, succinylcholine sequence. Anesth Analg 73:818, 1991

116. Ledingham IA, Watt I: Influence of sedation on mortality in critically ill multiple trauma patients. Lancet 1:1270, 1973

117. Wagner RL, White PF: Etomidate inhibits adrenocortical function in surgical patients. Anesthesiology 61:647, 1984

118. Fragen RJ, Shanks CA, Molteni A, Avram MJ: Effects of etomidate on hormonal responses to surgical stress. Anesthesiology 61:652, 1984

119. Fragen RJ, Weiss HW, Molteni A: The effect of propofol on adrenocortical steroidogenesis: a comparative study with etomidate and thiopental. Anesthesiology 66:839, 1987

120. Robertson WR, Reader SCJ, Davidson B et al: On the biopotency and site of action of drugs affecting endocrine tissues with specific reference to the antisteroidogenic effect of anesthetic agents. Postgrad Med J, suppl. 3:145, 1985

121. O'Donnell NG, McSharry CP, Wilkinsin PC, Asbury AJ: Comparison of the inhibitory effect of propofol, thiopentone and midazolam on neutrophil polarization in vitro in the presence or absence of human serum albumin. Br J Anaesth 69:70, 1992

122. Remmer H: The role of the liver in drug metabolism. Am J Med 49:617, 1970

123. Meissner PN, Harrison GG, Hift RJ: Propofol as an IV anaesthetic agent in variegate porphyria. Br J Anaesth 66:60, 1991

124. Tidmarsh MA, Bargent DF: Propofol in acute intermittent porphyria. Br J Anaesth 68:230, 1992

125. Mathews EL, Dhamee MS: Propofol in patients susceptible to malignant hyperpyrexia: a case report and review of the literature. J Clin Anesth 4:331, 1992

126. Lebovic S, Reich DL, Steinberg LG et al: Comparison of propofol versus ketamine for anesthesia in pediatric patients undergoing cardiac catheterization. Anesth Analg 74:490, 1992

127. Martin LD, Pasternak LR, Pudimat MA: Total intravenous anesthesia with propofol in pediatric patients outside the operating room. Anesth Analg 74:609, 1992

128. Daillard P, Cockshot ID, Lirzim JD et al: Intravenous propofol during cesarian section: placental transfer, concentrations in breast milk and neonatal effects. A preliminary study. Anesthesiology 71:827, 1989

129. Fragen RJ, Caldwell NJ: Comparison of a new formulation of etomidate with thiopental-side effects and awakening times. Anesthesiology 50:242, 1979

130. Jessup E, Grounds RM, Morgan M et al: Comparison of infusions of propofol and methohexitone to provide light general anaesthesia during surgery with regional block. Br J Anaesth 57:1173, 1985

131. Doze VA, Westphal LM, White PF: Comparison of propofol with methohexital for outpatient anesthesia. Anesth Analg 65:1189, 1986

132. Heath PJ, Kennedy DJ, Ogg TW et al: Which intravenous induction agent for day surgery? A comparison of propofol, thiopental, methohexital and etomidate. Anaesthesia 43:365, 1988

133. Marsch SCU, Schaefer HG: Problems with eye opening after propofol anesthesia. Anesth Analg 70:115, 1990

134. Borgeat A, Wilder-Smith OHG, Saiah M, Rifat K: Subhypnotic doses of propofol possess direct antiemetic properties. Anesthesiology 74:539, 1992

135. Rapp SE, Conahan TJ, Pavlin DJ et al: Comparison of desflurane with propofol in outpatients undergoing peripheral orthopedic surgery. Anesth Analg 75:65, 1992

136. Mackenzie N, Grant IS: Comparison of the new emulsion formulation of propofol with methohexitone and thiopentone for induction of anaesthesia in day cases. Br J Anaesth 57:725, 1985

137. Korttila K, Nuotto EJ, Lichtor JL et al: Clinical recovery and psychomotor function after brief anesthesia with propofol or thiopental. Anesthesiology 76:676, 1992

138. Doenicke A, Nebauer AE, Hoernecke R et al: Osmolalities of propylene glycol-containing drug formulations for parenteral use. Should propylene glycol be used for a solvent? Anesth Analg 75:431, 1992

139. Fragen RJ, Avram MJ: Comparative pharmacology of drugs used for the induction of anesthesia. p. 103. In Stoelting RK, Barash PG, Gallagher TJ (eds): Advances in Anesthesia. Year Book Medical Publishers, Chicago, 1986

Chapter 16

Basic Pharmacology of Ketamine

Thomas F. Murray

Phencyclidine (PCP), 1-(1-phenylcyclohexyl) piperidine HCl, the parent compound of ketamine, is an intravenous anesthetic agent that exhibits remarkable psychotomimetic activity in humans when administered in subanesthetic doses.[1] PCP was originally developed as part of a preanesthetic analgesic screening program. During the course of this development, it was discovered that PCP produced profound calming and anesthetic effects in monkeys. In 1957, PCP was introduced for clinical trials as an intravenous general anesthetic.[2] Although PCP was found to be generally effective as an anesthetic and preanesthetic analgesic, its use was associated with a high incidence of postoperative emergence reactions. These emergence reactions consisted of marked agitation, excitement, disorientation, hallucinations, echolalia, and logorrhea.[3] The incidence of these emergence phenomena was generally in the range of 4 to 16 percent, which was clinically unacceptable. The search for a PCP analog with a reduced propensity to produce emergence phenomena led to the development of ketamine, 2-(O-chlorophenyl)-2-methylamino cyclohexanone HCl. The structures of PCP and ketamine are depicted in Fig. 16-1.

GENERAL PHARMACOLOGY

Ketamine was synthesized by Stephens in 1963, and the initial preclinical pharmacology was investigated by McCarthy et al.[4] in 1965. The drug produced a spectrum of pharmacologic effects, including motor stimulation, ataxia, catalepsy (state of maintained waxy flexibility), and anesthesia. This spectrum of pharmacologic effects as a function of ketamine dose is depicted in Fig. 16-2. Although the relative position of a given pharmacologic action may vary as a function of the route of administration, species, and experimental paradigm, this figure illustrates the general progression of ketamine's effects. Although less potent than PCP in preclinical experimentation, ketamine caused less central stimulation and convulsive behavior and displayed a more favorable margin of safety.[4]

Based on these promising preclinical data, ketamine was advanced to clinical trials, with the first results reported by Corssen and Domino[5] in 1966. These authors introduced the term dissociative anesthesia to describe the unique state of anesthesia produced by ketamine in which the subject is profoundly analgesic while appearing disconnected

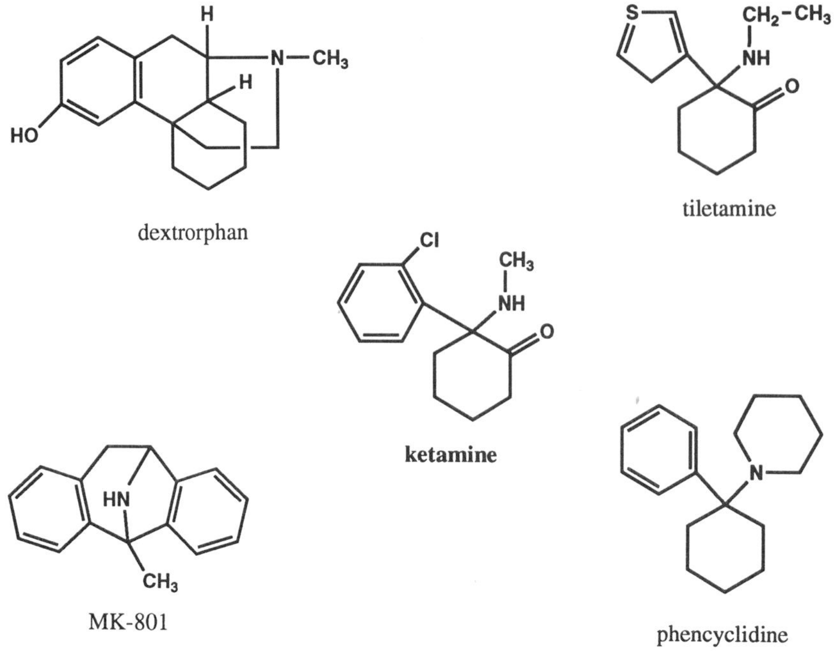

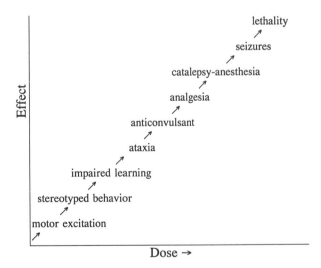

Fig. 16-1 Structures of ketamine, phencyclidine, and related noncompetitive antagonists of NMDA N-methyl-D-aspartate receptors.

Fig. 16-2 Dose-dependent spectrum of pharmacologic effects of ketamine in laboratory animals. This figure depicts the general progression of pharmacologic responses to increasing dose and is not intended to define the relative position of a given effect precisely. The relative position of an effect and the absolute dose of ketamine required to produce the effect will vary as a function of route of administration and species.

from the surroundings.[6] Domino's[6,7] group attributed the unique state of ketamine anesthesia to a drug-induced dissociation of the electroencephalographic (EEG) activity between the thalamoneocortical and the limbic systems. It was demonstrated that the cataleptic anesthetic state induced by intravenous ketamine (4 mg/kg) in cats was associated with an alternating pattern of hypersynchronous δ wave bursts and low voltage, fast wave activity in the neocortex and thalamus. Subcortically, the δ wave bursts were observed prominently in the thalamus and caudate nucleus, and the EEG patterns of thalamic nuclei were closely related phasically to the δ waves of the neocortex.[7] In contrast to the marked δ wave bursts in the neocortex, thalamus, and caudate nucleus, prominent δ waves were not observed in the cat hippocampus, hypothalamus, or midbrain reticular formation. The hippocampus showed θ "arousal" waves in spite of the appearance of high voltage, hypersynchronous δ wave bursts in the thalamus and neocortex. Thus, ketamine was demonstrated to produce a functional dissociation of the EEG activity between the hippocampus and the thalamoneocortical system. From these and related findings, it was concluded that the diffuse thalamoneocortical projecting systems may be a primary site for the anesthetic action of ketamine; the EEG dissociation between the neocortex and limbic system may contribute to the emergent and psychotomimetic effects of the drug.[6,7] These pioneering studies of Domino's group were subsequently confirmed when ketamine (25 mg/kg IM) anesthesia in cats was shown to be associated with bursts of high amplitude δ wave activity in the centromedian area of the thalamus in a hypersynchronous relationship with the neocortex. Again this hypersynchronous δ wave activity was independent of θ activity of the ventral hippocampus and amygdala, reflecting a ketamine-induced dissociation of limbic and neocortical systems of the cat brain.[8] It is noteworthy that deep ketamine anesthesia did induce bursts of hypersynchronous activity in the septum and dorsal hippocampus; thus, ketamine differentially affected the dorsal and ventral hippocampus of the cat.[8]

The unique EEG and anesthetic effects of PCP and ketamine have been incorporated into a multidirectional scheme of the progression of states of central nervous system (CNS) excitation and depression produced by various anesthetics.[9] This multidirectional scheme classifies PCP and ketamine as anesthetics that induce a continuum of CNS excitation, progressing from motor excitability of stage I anesthesia to hallucinatory and then cataleptoid components of stage II anesthesia. During stage I, the EEG is characterized by an activated pattern with high frequency and low voltage.[9] The EEG of stage II progresses from an initial phase of intermittent hypersynchronous high amplitude bursts (2.5 Hz) associated with hallucinoid behavior to a sustained hypersynchronous EEG (2.5 Hz) and, finally, to a phase in which the animals lose the righting reflex and become cataleptoid with EEG patterns of slow waves (1.5 Hz) and occasional spiking.[9] Higher doses would cause more profound CNS excitation characterized by myoclonus and EEG patterns of spike bursts and interictal periods, which may culminate in a generalized tonic/clonic seizure. Ketamine in doses of 25 and 40 mg/kg given intraperitoneally produced catalepsy in cats that was characterized by loss of the righting reflex, immobility, and a lack of responsiveness to noxious stimuli. A salient feature of these investigations was the appearance of a seizure discharge during catalepsy in the dorsal hippocampus following the 25- and 40-mg/kg doses of ketamine. This ketamine-induced seizure discharge conflicts with the characterization of this drug as a dissociative anesthetic inasmuch as the hippocampal EEG was reported to be unaffected during ketamine anesthesia in earlier studies. These discordant results are presumably related to the use of different ketamine dosing protocols and/or different coordinates for stereotaxic placement of the electrodes within the hippocampal formation. The ability of intraperitoneal ketamine (3 to 5 mg/kg) to elicit bursts of spike and wave complexes in the cortical and dorsal hippocampal EEG of freely moving cats has been reported.[10] Consequently, the anesthetic state produced by ketamine is currently designated as either dissociative anesthesia or cataleptic anesthesia.[9,11]

The aforementioned studies of the effects of ketamine on the EEG of cats used commercially available racemic ketamine solutions, containing equivalent amounts of the S(+) and R(−) enantiomers. The potential stereoselectivity of ketamine isomers was initially addressed in rats with S(+) ketamine being approximately three times more potent than R(−) ketamine as a hypnotic.[12] Similar stereoselective differences in potency were shown for the induction of behavioral and EEG effects in the cat[13] and the EEG response in humans.[14] In all cases, the S(+) isomer of ketamine was approximately two to three times more potent than the R(−) isomer. The demonstration of stereoselectivity of the anesthetic effect of ketamine enantiomers is consistent with an interaction with specific receptors rather than a generalized perturbation of membrane structure as postulated for volatile and gaseous anesthetics.

THE N-METHYL-D-ASPARTATE RECEPTOR AS A TARGET FOR KETAMINE

Ketamine is now known to act as a postsynaptic antagonist at specific excitatory synapses in the CNS. Glutamate is the principal excitatory neurotransmitter in the brain, and this acidic amino acid activates cation-selective receptor channels in neurons and glia.[15] Most synapses in the CNS are excitatory and are believed to utilize L-glutamate as a neurotransmitter to produce neuronal excitation. Glutamate neurotransmission participates in various forms of neuronal plasticity, including an activity-dependent change of synaptic efficacy, thought to underlie learning, memory, and development. Conversely, excessive glutamate neurotransmission contributes to pathologic processes, such as epilepsy and neuronal degeneration following ischemia and hypoglycemia.[16]

Glutamate receptors are classified into two major groups termed ionotropic and metabotropic receptors.[15,17] The ionotropic receptors possess integral cation-specific ion channels, whereas the metabotropic receptors are coupled to G-protein transduction elements, which in turn, modulate the production of cytoplasmic second messenger substances. The ionotropic receptors have traditionally been classified according to pharmacologic criteria; the selective agonists N-methyl-D-aspartate (NMDA), kainate (KA), and α-amino-3-hydroxy-5-methyl-4-isoxazole propionate (AMPA) have been particularly useful in this classification.[18] This rich pharmacologic literature has been complimented and extended in recent years with the cloning of numerous glutamate receptor subtypes.[17,19,20] Although investigation of the properties of recombinant receptor subtypes in some cases has blurred the distinction between AMPA and KA receptors, a classification scheme based on sequence comparisons and functional properties is depicted in Fig. 16-3.[17,19,20] Characterization of the AMPA receptor subfamily has yielded many insights into the novel

properties and functional determinants of glutamate receptors.[17,20] The AMPA receptor family comprises four closely related subunits (GluR-1 to GluR-4 or GluR-A to GluR-D), and these receptors mediate rapid excitatory postsynaptic currents at CNS synapses.[21] The KA receptor subfamily is composed of two groups of glutamate receptor channel subunits (GluR-5 to GluR-7 and KA1 and 2); the combined expression of these subunits generates KA-sensitive glutamate receptor channels with unique properties.[20]

Most germane to the pharmacology of ketamine is the NMDA receptor subfamily of glutamate receptor channels. The NMDA receptor is the most thoroughly characterized of glutamate receptors with respect to pharmacology and physiology; however, the cloning of the first NMDA-gated channel was not accomplished until 1992.[22] Activation of NMDA receptors leads to a slowly developing, long lasting excitatory postsynaptic current. The NMDA receptor has a central role in many functions associated with glutamate neurotransmission in the CNS. It is essential for inducing long-term potentiation (LTP), which is an activity-dependent enhancement of the synaptic efficacy that is most pronounced in the hippocampus and may underlie learning and memory.[23] Thus, NMDA receptors subserve hebbian synapses (type of synaptic learning mechanism originally proposed by Hebb) associated with synaptic plasticity. NMDA receptors are also involved in the processing of sensory information, including the sensation of pain.[24,25] The expression cloning of the NMDA receptor subunit NMDAR-1 revealed prominent structural similarities with AMPA and KA receptors.[22] The deduced amino acid sequence of the cloned receptor shows significant sequence similarity (22 to 26 percent) to the members of the AMPA receptor subfamily and has four putative transmembrane domains. Homomeric expression of NMDAR-1 exhibited several properties that are characteristic of NMDA receptors in mammalian neurons. These distinguishing features include Ca^{++} permeability, voltage-dependent block by Mg^{++}, positive modulation by the coagonist glycine, and positive modulation by polyamines. A schematic of the NMDA receptor with associated agonist, coagonist, and modulatory sites is shown

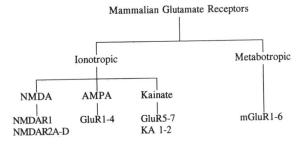

Fig. 16-3 Classification of mammalian glutamate receptor subtypes.

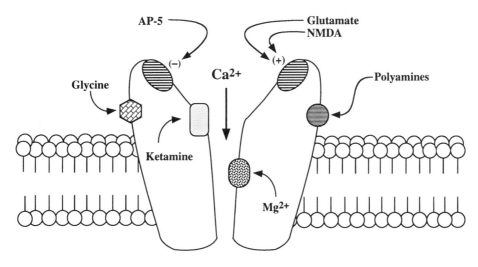

Fig. 16-4 The NMDA receptor-cation channel complex. In addition to the transmitter recognition site activated by glutamate or NMDA, the complex possesses a coagonist site for glycine, such that glycine occupancy is an absolute requirement for receptor activation. AP-5 is a competitive antagonist of the transmitter recognition site with binding mutually exclusive to that of glutamate or NMDA. Also depicted are the positive modulatory site for polyamines and the site within the channel domain at which Mg^{++} exerts its voltage-dependent block. A recognition site for ketamine and related dissociative anesthetics depicted in the vestibule of the ion channel is the site at which these compounds exert a noncompetitive antagonism of the NMDA receptor. This latter site has been historically, and is commonly, referred to as the PCP receptor.

in Fig. 16-4. When NMDAR-1 was activated by NMDA, the competitive and noncompetitive NMDA receptor antagonists D(−)-2-amino-5-phosphonovalerate (AP-5) and dizocilpine (originally designated MK-801), respectively, completely inhibited the NMDA-evoked current. Thus NMDAR-1 exhibits the pharmacologic signature characteristic of the native NMDA receptor in mammalian CNS. Since the initial cloning of NMDAR-1, four additional NMDA receptor subunits (NMDAR-2A to NMDAR-2D) have been identified.[26,27] The individual NMDAR-2 subunits exhibit distinct and more restricted expression in rat brain than does NMDAR-1. Although individual NMDAR-2 subunits do not exhibit appreciable conductance in response to glutamate exposure, combined expression of NMDAR-1 with NMDAR-2 subunits markedly augments responses to NMDA or glutamate.[26,27]

The discovery by Lodge et al.[28–30] of the capacity for ketamine and related arylcyclohexylamines to antagonize specifically the neuronal excitation me-

diated by NMDA provided a pivotal advance in our understanding of the mechanism of action of dissociative anesthetics. Based on the earlier observation that ketamine selectively reduced polysynaptic reflexes in which excitatory amino acids were the transmitters, Lodge et al. investigated the action of ketamine on the excitation of cat dorsal horn interneurons by amino acids used in the classification of excitatory amino acid receptors, namely N-methyl-DL-aspartate (NMA), quisqualate, and KA. The microionotophoretic or intravenous administration of ketamine selectively reduced the increased firing rate of dorsal horn neurons evoked by focal application of NMA.[29,30] The excitatory responses elicited by quisqualate and KA remained little affected. The selective NMA-blocking effect was not restricted to ketamine inasmuch as the dissociative anesthetics, PCP and tiletamine, had similar actions that paralleled their relative anesthetic potencies.[30,31] The NMA antagonist actions of ketamine displayed appropriate stereoselectivity; on cat Renshaw cells, the S(+) isomer of ketamine was found to be three times as potent as the R(−) isomer as an NMA antagonist.[28] Thus, the stereoselectivity of ketamine enantiomer antagonism of NMA is in accordance with that of the anesthetic effects of these isomers (vide supra).

In addition to these dissociative anesthetics, opioid compounds from structurally diverse classes, such as the morphinans, levorphanol, and dextrorphan, and the benzomorphan, cyclazocine, were shown to antagonize NMA-induced excitatory responses selectively.[32,33] The NMA antagonist potencies of dissociative anesthetics, morphinans, and benzomorphans correlated well with their respective affinities for the [³H]PCP receptor.[34,35] In addition, these compounds with affinity for the [³H]PCP receptor produced PCP-like interoceptive effects in drug discrimination studies; their relative NMA-blocking potency closely paralleled both their affinity for the [³H]PCP receptor and potency to produce PCP-like interoceptive cues.[36,37] A correlation between the 50 percent inhibitory concentration (IC_{50}) values obtained from electrophysiologic studies of NMDA antagonism in rat cortical preparations[36] and the IC_{50} values for binding to the NMDA receptor labeled with [³H]dextrorphan in rat cortical membranes[38] is depicted in Fig. 16-5. The congruence of these pharmacologic profiles indicates that the receptor mediating this drug antagonism of NMA-evoked responses is a recognition site on the NMDA-operated cation channel (i.e., the PCP receptor).

The mechanism of dissociative anesthetic antagonism of NMDA receptors has been demonstrated to be noncompetitive with respect to agonists.[36,39,40] The noncompetitive nature of the antagonism is not surprising inasmuch as dissociative anesthetics and glutamate and its analogs are structurally dissimilar. The noncompetitive antagonism of NMDA receptors by ketamine is typically revealed by concentration-dependent nonparallel displacements of NMDA dose-response curves to the right.[36,40] Moreover, in the presence of a sufficient concentration of ketamine, the maximum response to NMDA is reduced. The noncompetitive nature of the antagonism of NMDA receptor function by ketamine and related compounds is consistent with an interaction with the NMDA receptor-operated ion channel.[41] Consonant with an interaction with

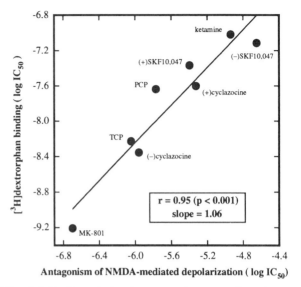

Fig. 16-5 Correlation between the potencies of compounds in competing for high-affinity [³H]dextrorphan binding to the NMDA receptor-ion channel complex of rat forebrain membranes and their reported potencies as inhibitors of NMDA-evoked depolarization in rat cerebral cortex. The data for binding to the [³H]dextrorphan-labeled NMDA receptor on the ordinate are from Franklin and Murray,[38] whereas the potencies for antagonism of the functional response to NMDA on the abscissa are from Martin and Lodge.[36] The significance of the correlation was evaluated by the *t* test of the probability of r = 0.

a site within the domain of the ion channel of the NMDA receptor, the antagonism by ketamine and PCP of NMDA-evoked currents has been found to be highly voltage dependent.[42,43] The voltage-dependent antagonism of NMDA responses by ketamine manifests as a more effective reduction of evoked currents at hyperpolarized than depolarized potentials in voltage-clamped neurons.

One explanation for the voltage dependence of NMDA receptor blockade by ketamine and related dissociative anesthetics is that the binding site is within the ion channel; hence, the drug must move through the membrane electric field to reach the site. As a consequence, the association rate constant for binding of the blocker to the channel site would be voltage dependent. This mechanism is analogous to that originally developed by Woodhull[44] to explain the voltage dependence of the blockade of Na^+ channels by protons. Woodhull showed that the steepness of the voltage dependence of channel block increases with increasing electrical distance (δ) of the binding site from the outside of the membrane. It is therefore theoretically possible to estimate the distance a blocking substance must move into the channel pore to interact with its binding site. Application of the Woodhull model to the voltage dependence of the ketamine block of the NMDA-activated ion channel yielded somewhat discrepant values for the electrical distance, δ. One group reported a δ value for ketamine of 0.55, suggesting that the drug interacts with a site halfway through the channel.[45] Another group calculated a δ value of 1, indicating a ketamine site close to the cytoplasmic side of the membrane.[46] However, the validity of the application of the Woodhull model to dissociative anesthetic blockade of the NMDA receptor ion channel more recently came under scrutiny. MacDonald et al.[45,47] proposed that the guarded receptor model can be used to explain the dissociative anesthetic effect on NMDA receptor channels. This model accounts for the use dependence of dissociative anesthetic blockade. The use dependence of the blockade results in a requirement for agonist activation of the NMDA receptor-ion channel complex for the development of full antagonism. Thus, in the presence of ketamine, the peak inward currents evoked by repeated applications of NMDA, L-aspartate, or L-glutamate progressively declined to a steady-state level of block.[45] A similar use-dependent block of NMDA receptors was demonstrated for the selective, high-affinity PCP receptor ligand dizocilpine.[48] Additional evidence for use dependence was provided by studies of the binding of radiolabeled dissociative anesthetic analogs, which indicated that NMDA agonists, such as L-glutamate, increased the rates of association and dissociation of the blocker with the NMDA receptor ion channel.[49] An extensive body of literature, derived from both biochemical and electrophysiologic investigations, unequivocally established the use dependence of the dissociative anesthetic blockade of NMDA receptors.

An additional inconsistency with the application of the Woodhull[44] model to dissociative anesthetic interaction with the NMDA receptor ion channel is that the association rate constants for blockade by PCP,[45] dizocilpine,[50] or tiletamine[51] were not dependent on the membrane potential. Most of the voltage dependence of dissociative anesthetic blockade in neurons maintained in cell culture was attributed to an increase of the dissociation rate by depolarization.[45,47] Moreover, the outward movement of ions through the NMDA receptor channel at positive potentials enhanced the dissociation rate of ketamine and PCP, presumably by electrostatic repulsion of the drug molecules from their channel binding site.[47] Based on these and additional data, MacDonald et al.[47] recently proposed that the dissociative anesthetic site (PCP receptor) may be localized in the NMDA channel mouth or vestibule; the NMDA channel must be gated open before this binding site is exposed. Channel closure subsequent to the binding of a dissociative anesthetic leads to the trapping of the blocker within the channel. This suggests that the channel mouth or vestibule area of the NMDA receptor channel is of sufficient size to accommodate ketamine and related compounds of this class.[47,52]

These investigations of the molecular mechanisms of dissociative anesthetic interaction with the NMDA receptor led to the classification of these compounds as either noncompetitive or uncompetitive antagonists. Ketamine and other dissociative anesthetics are noncompetitive NMDA receptor antagonists in that they produce an insurmountable blockade that is noncompetitive with respect to agonists such as glutamate and NMDA. These drugs may alternatively be termed uncompetitive antagonists in that the blockade displays an antecedent requirement for agonist activation of the NMDA receptor (i.e., use dependence).

ROLE OF NMDA RECEPTOR ANTAGONISM IN KETAMINE-INDUCED ANESTHESIA

Given the participation of NMDA receptors in the processing of information in the CNS, it is reasonable to posit a role for NMDA receptor antagonism in the mediation of ketamine anesthesia. The intravenous administration of both ketamine and dizo-cilpine in rats was shown to reduce synaptic responses in the ventrobasal thalamus to sensory stimulation, suggesting that some of the anesthetic action of ketamine may be caused by antagonism of thalamic NMDA receptors.[53] These intravenous ketamine doses (2.25 to 10.0 mg/kg) that were associated with a reduction in synaptic responses to sensory stimulation are similar to the hypnotic ED_{50} for ketamine in the rat (5.6 mg/kg IV).[12] Similarly, intravenous doses of 2 to 5 mg/kg in the rat largely eliminated responses to NMDA on spinal neurones.[31] Marietta et al.[12] demonstrated that ketamine plasma levels of 20 to 40 μM, following an intravenous dose of 30 mg/kg, are associated with a loss of righting reflex, whereas brain levels were 113 μM at the time of regaining the righting reflex. Although these results indicate that brain levels greater than 113 μM are required for hypnosis, the partitioning of the lipophilic ketamine into membranes would result in a substantially lower free concentration of the drug in the synaptic compartment. The IC_{50} values for ketamine's antagonism of NMDA responses in rat cortical preparations range from approximately 6 to 12 μM.[36,54] These values are comparable to the plasma concentrations (20 to 40 μM) obtained in rats following an intravenous anesthetic dose of ketamine (30 mg/kg).[12] It therefore appears likely that a large fractional occupancy of NMDA receptors may be required for induction of the anesthetic state.

Further evidence for the involvement of NMDA receptor antagonism in the mechanism of action of dissociative anesthetics comes from the demonstration that dizocilpine reduced the minimum alveolar concentration for halothane and isoflurane in the rabbit.[55] The determination of reduction in the minimum alveolar concentration by drug pretreatments represents a standard method for measurement of anesthetic potency.[56] Similarly, dizocilpine and PCP reduced the minimum alveolar concentration of halothane and ether in mice.[57] A modulation of the general anesthetic potency by the polyamine regulatory site of NMDA receptor also was observed.[58]

Given the primacy of dizocilpine as a selective, high-affinity noncompetitive antagonist of NMDA

receptors, a critical issue in asserting the involvement of NMDA receptors in ketamine anesthesia is the ability of dizocilpine to produce a dissociative anesthetic state. This question was addressed in rhesus monkeys. Dizocilpine in subcutaneous doses of 0.18 to 0.32 mg/kg produced ketamine-like anesthetic effects in rhesus monkeys.[59] The dizocilpine-induced anesthesia was characterized by the absence of eye closure or respiratory depression and by the presence of profuse salivation; these anesthetic effects resemble those of ketamine and PCP and differ from those of pentobarbital.[59] Dizocilpine also was reported to produce ketamine-like dissociative anesthesia in pigs.[60] The intravenous administration of dizocilpine in doses of 0.1 to 1.6 mg/kg in pigs produced immobilization characterized by lateral recumbency, profuse salivation, increased muscle tone, and increased respiratory rates. The most prominent difference to ketamine was a marked catalepsy associated with dizocilpine-induced immobilization in pigs. Additional evidence in support of NMDA receptor antagonism subserving the production of anesthesia resides in the ability of the competitive NMDA receptor antagonist CGS 19755 to induce anesthesia in rhesus monkeys.[61] Following intravenous administration of 56 mg/kg of CGS 19755, monkeys displayed salivation, lateral recumbency, and a lack of responsiveness to pinch or pin pricks. The CGS 19755-induced anesthesia was not associated with eye closure or loss of muscle tone. It is noteworthy that doses of CGS 19755 (cis-4-phosphonomethyl-2-piperidine-carboxylic acid) required to produce behavioral effects and anesthesia were considerably larger than doses that attenuated the effects of NMDA in rhesus monkeys.[62] It was therefore inferred that greater receptor occupancy is required to exert direct behavioral-anesthetic effects than to antagonize the effects of exogenously administered NMDA receptor agonists.[61] Thus, the similarity in the anesthetic state produced by competitive NMDA antagonists and both ketamine and dizocilpine supports the proposition that the anesthetic effect of these compounds derives from their interaction with the NMDA receptor-ion channel complex. This proposition does not exclude other actions not related to NMDA blockade contributing to the anesthesia produced by ketamine.

KETAMINE-INDUCED ANALGESIA

The analgesic action of ketamine in subanesthetic doses was originally observed in early studies in human volunteers.[63] Subsequently, ketamine was shown to produce dose-dependent analgesia in laboratory animals. The antinociceptive actions of ketamine manifested at subanesthetic doses and were documented in the phenylquinone writhing test,[64] tail flick test,[65,66] and the hot plate test.[67]

The neuroanatomic substrates for ketamine-induced analgesia are likely to include both spinal and supraspinal sites. One potential locus for the analgesic action of ketamine is the nucleus reticularis gigantocellularis in the brain stem. This nucleus receives input from spinoreticular somatosensory projections with cell bodies in lamina V of the spinal cord. Intravenous doses of ketamine (1 to 2.5 mg/kg) suppress spontaneous and evoked neuronal activity in the cat nucleus reticularis gigantocellularis, suggesting that this site may participate in its analgesic actions.[68] In regard to the spinal actions of ketamine, intravenous administration has been shown to suppress the neuronal activity of cells in Rexed laminae I and V preferentially, which are associated with nociception.[69] The depressant action of ketamine on lamina V neurons of the dorsal horn involves both a supraspinal site producing an activation of descending inhibitory system originating in the brain stem and a direct depressant action at the level of the spinal cord.[70]

The extent to which opioid systems are involved in the antinociceptive actions of ketamine has received considerable attention. Ketamine was shown to possess modest affinity for μ opioid receptors with IC_{50} values ranging from 20 to 130 μM.[66,71,72] The affinity of ketamine for δ and κ opioid receptors is approximately three to four fold lower than that for μ receptors.[72] The achievement of ketamine brain levels in excess of 100 μM following the administration of behaviorally active doses suggests that these modest affinities may be pharmacologically relevant. Moreover, several reports of a naloxone-induced antagonism of ketamine analgesia have appeared.[64,66,73] The doses of naloxone required to reverse ketamine analgesia are typically 10 to 1,000 times greater than are those required to

reverse morphine-induced analgesia.[64,73] Given the μ opioid receptor selectivity of ketamine, the requirements of large doses of naloxone for reversal is unlikely to be associated with a preferential interaction of ketamine with δ or κ opioid receptors. Moreover the pA_2 (negative logarithm of the molar concentration of antagonist that produces an equiactive agonist dose ratio of 2) values for naloxone typically vary by less than one log unit between opioid receptor subtypes.[74] In addition, an inability to reverse the antinociceptive effects of ketamine with naloxone was reported.[75,76] Thus, although opioid receptors are likely to contribute to the analgesia following high doses of ketamine, the modest affinity of this compound for opioid receptors and the requirement for large doses of naloxone to antagonize antinociceptive effects argue against a singular role for opioid systems in the analgesic action of ketamine.

Additional potential targets for the analgesic effects of ketamine include spinal NMDA receptors. Headley et al.[77,78] demonstrated that spinal motor neuron nociceptive responses to both mechanical and thermal stimuli were equally affected by NMDA receptor blocking doses of ketamine; however, non-nociceptive responses were largely unaffected. From these data, it was inferred that NMDA receptors on motor neurons participate in the processing of nociceptive information. In contrast, ketamine had no consistent effect on sensory responses in dorsal horn neurons.[77] Although NMDA receptors appear to contribute little to fast synaptic transmission in the dorsal horn, they may underlie some forms of synaptic plasticity, such as the phenomenon of wind-up.[79] Wind-up is a property of a population of nociceptive neurons in the dorsal horn of the rat that displays a progressive increase in the number of spikes evoked by repeated electrical stimulation of primary afferent C-fibers. Intravenous doses (2 to 4 mg/kg) of ketamine eliminate wind-up in the rat but have little effect on the initial response to the incoming afferent volley.[79] Thus, ketamine affects nociceptive transmission in dorsal horn neurons by attenuating this sensitization to excitatory amino acid neurotransmission.

Further evidence for the involvement of NMDA receptors in nociception is the demonstration that ketamine and related noncompetitive NMDA antagonists, that is, PCP, dextrorphan, dizocilpine, and (+) SKF 10,047 (n-allyl-normetazocine) produce analgesia in rhesus monkeys.[80] The analgesic potencies of these compounds were correlated with their relative affinity for PCP binding sites and potency in producing discriminative stimulus effects. Moreover the analgesic effects of ketamine, PCP, dextrorphan, dizocilpine, and (+)SKF 10,047 were not blocked by an opioid receptor antagonist. From these data, it was inferred that the analgesic effects of ketamine and related compounds were mediated by the PCP binding site on the NMDA receptor-ion channel and did not involve opioid systems. In accordance with these results, the relative analgesic potency of ketamine enantiomers in humans was correlated with their relative affinity for PCP binding sites in human brain membranes.[81] The same authors showed that the analgesic effect of subanesthetic doses of ketamine in humans was not antagonized by naloxone.[82] Considered together, these data support the notion that, to a large extent, ketamine-induced analgesia is a consequence of inhibition of excitatory amino acid transmission at NMDA synapses at both spinal and supraspinal sites.

ADDITIONAL PHARMACOLOGIC CONSEQUENCES OF NMDA RECEPTOR ANTAGONISM

Anticonvulsant Action

The anticonvulsant action of ketamine was first described by McCarthy et al.[4] Ketamine suppressed both electroshock and chemically induced convulsions in mice at subanesthetic doses. Subsequent studies demonstrated the efficacy of ketamine in kindled seizures.[83,84] The kindling model of epilepsy involves daily administration of single trains of electrical stimuli (typically 1 to 2 seconds at 60 Hz). Initially, this stimulation evokes only local afterdischarge at the site of stimulation. This is followed by a progressive generalization and increase in the duration of afterdischarge and the production of behavioral seizures. In kindling models, ketamine decreases the afterdischarge duration and behavioral responses in cortical kindled seizures[83] and in amygdaloid-kindled seizures.[84] The latter

study noted a ketamine-induced paradoxic increase in elicited afterdischarge spiking frequency in the amygdaloid kindled rats, which was hypothesized to result in an acceleration of mechanisms that terminate seizures.

It is now known that, in addition to ketamine, an array of noncompetitive antagonists of the NMDA receptor possesses anticonvulsant efficacy in a wide range of experimental seizure models.[54,85,86] In vitro studies of rat neocortical slices showed that ketamine and related noncompetitive antagonists reduced spontaneous and stimulus-evoked epileptiform bursts and afterpotentials.[54] Moreover, there was a good correlation between their potencies against NMDA-evoked depolarizations and against epileptiform bursts. The rank order of potency obtained was dizocilpine > PCP > cyclazocine > dextrorphan > SKF 10,047 > ketamine > dextromethorphan ≥ pentazocine. In accordance with these in vitro results, in vivo experimentation revealed that noncompetitive NMDA antagonists exerted anticonvulsant efficacy against sound-induced seizures in DBA/2 mice.[85] The anticonvulsant effects of ketamine and other noncompetitive antagonists were manifested at subanesthetic doses that produced mild to moderate behavioral excitation. Again, for dizocilpine, PCP, dextrorphan, SKF 10,047, and ketamine, there was a close correlation between relative anticonvulsant potencies and affinities for the PCP site on the NMDA receptor cation channel. These results imply that noncompetitive antagonism of NMDA receptors underlies the anticonvulsant action of these compounds.

Neuroprotective Action

The neurotoxic properties of the excitatory neurotransmitter glutamate have been proposed to contribute to the central neuronal cell loss associated with several neurologic disease states in which an excessive release of glutamate results in overactivation of NMDA receptors.[87,88] The high calcium permeability of the NMDA class of glutamate receptors provides support for the hypothesis that glutamate neurotoxicity is largely mediated by calcium influx.[88] Given the pivotal role of NMDA receptors in glutamate neurotoxicity, it is not unexpected that noncompetitive antagonists of the NMDA receptor exhibit neuroprotective actions.[88,89] The neuroprotective properties of ketamine were originally described by Olney et al.[90] using the in vitro chick embryo retina. Ketamine and PCP antagonized the NMA-induced neuronal degeneration in this system. These results were confirmed in murine cortical cells in primary culture in which ketamine afforded complete protection from glutamate neurotoxicity.[88] Ketamine has additionally been shown to mitigate the neuronal injury associated with hypoxia[91] or glucose deprivation[92] in cortical cell cultures. In primary cultures of mouse spinal cord, ketamine prevented neuronal death produced by impact injury.[93] In all cases, the neuroprotection afforded by ketamine was a consequence of NMDA receptor antagonism. Evaluation of the concentration-dependence of ketamine antagonism of NMDA-induced neuronal toxicity in cortical neurons indicated an EC_{50} value of 10 μM,[94] which is less than the plasma concentration associated with anesthesia in rats.[12] Similarly, ketamine, (+)SKF 10,047, dizocilpine, and PCP totally inhibited NMDA-induced Ca^{++} influx in cerebellar granule cells in culture with a rank order of potency in agreement with their respective affinities for the noncompetitive antagonist binding site of the NMDA receptor ion channel.[95] These findings are compatible with glutamate activation of NMDA receptors and the subsequent calcium influx as events underlying glutamate neurotoxicity. The neuroprotective properties of ketamine and related noncompetitive antagonists of the NMDA receptor may eventually be therapeutically useful in certain types of acute brain injury, such as focal ischemia.

Disruption of Learning and Memory

The pivotal role of NMDA receptors in various forms of CNS plasticity, including memory formation, renders such phenomena susceptible to NMDA antagonists. One form of synaptic plasticity that exhibits the characteristics of a "hebbian" mechanism is LTP, that is, a long-lasting enhancement of synaptic efficacy that follows a brief period of high-frequency stimulation applied to afferent fibers.[96] Inasmuch as LTP persists for several days after a rapid induction, it is postulated to be a neural mechanism for memory. The administration of

ketamine prior to high-frequency stimulation in rat hippocampus prevents the induction of LTP,[97,98] suggesting that dissociative anesthetics may impair learning and memory. Indeed, behavioral studies demonstrated that intraperitoneal doses (6 to 25 mg/kg) of ketamine attenuate short-term memory and spatial learning in rats.[99] Similarly, the order of potency of a series of noncompetitive NMDA receptor antagonists in producing deficits in the retention of a learned task was positively correlated with their respective affinities for the PCP receptor (dizocilpine > PCP > (+)SKF 10,047 > ketamine).[100] Doses of ketamine as low as 5 mg/kg given intraperitoneally disrupt a concept learning task in rats, indicating that impairment of learning and memory is one of the more potent behavioral effects of ketamine.[101] These results (derived from studies involving laboratory rodents) are consistent with reports of amnesia in PCP users and patients receiving ketamine.[102]

Phencyclidine-Like Psychoactive Effects

Patients intoxicated with PCP may present with a spectrum of subjective and psychotic effects, including distortions in body image, hallucinations, delusions, and paranoid ideation.[103] Intoxication may be associated with either a clear sensorium or disorientation, agitation, stupor, lethargy, or coma. Similarly, the medical or nonmedical use of ketamine may result in changes in body imagery, confusion, dizziness, dreams, and hallucinations.[104] The ensemble of subjective and psychotomimetic effects of PCP and ketamine may be a consequence of NMDA receptor antagonism. Studies of the discriminative stimulus properties of ketamine and PCP show that these drugs produce similar interoceptive cues in that they cross-generalize.[105,106] The use of drugs as discriminative stimuli represents a sensitive method for establishing similarities among various classes of psychoactive agents. A significant correlation between the rank order of potency of a series of drugs, including ketamine, PCP, dizocilpine, and SKF 10,047, as NMDA antagonists and their relative ability to produce PCP-like discriminative stimulus properties was reported.[36] This correlation is consistent with the involvement of NMDA receptors in the psychoactive effects of ketamine and related dissociative anesthetics. The discriminative stimulus properties of ketamine stereoisomers in PCP-trained rats is also consonant with NMDA receptor mediation, inasmuch as (+)ketamine is approximately twice as potent as (−)ketamine in producing PCP-appropriate responding.[107]

Similar to amphetamine and other indirect acting dopaminergic agents, PCP and ketamine produce hyperactivity and stereotyped behavior in laboratory rodents. Thus, a role for dopaminergic mechanisms in the behavioral effects of dissociative anesthetics has been considered. Both PCP and ketamine inhibit the high-affinity uptake of [^{3}H]dopamine into rat striatal synaptosomes with IC$_{50}$ values of 0.58 μM and 24 μM, respectively.[108] In addition, the affinities of PCP and ketamine for the dopamine transporter were found to be 1.59 μM and 84.2 μM.[109] Thus, the affinities of PCP and ketamine for the dopamine transporter are approximately 10 to 20-fold lower than their respective affinities for the PCP site on the NMDA receptor-ion channel. The observation that PCP, ketamine, and dizocilpine dose-dependently generalize to rats trained to discriminate cocaine from saline appears to support dopamine uptake blockade in the behavioral effects of these dissociative anesthetics.[110] However, the order of potency of these drugs to produce cocaine-like behavioral effects (dizocilpine > PCP > ketamine) did not correlate with their potency at the dopamine transporter. Rather, this order of potency agrees with their relative affinities for the PCP receptor. It has therefore been suggested that both the unique behavioral effects of dissociative anesthetics and those behavioral effects that PCP and ketamine share with indirect dopamine agonists may be mediated by noncompetitive antagonism of NMDA receptors. Although the primary target for the behavioral effects of ketamine and PCP appears to be the NMDA receptor, the fact that micromolar concentrations of ketamine in the brain are achieved after subanesthetic doses implies that an interaction with the dopamine[109] and possibly serotonin transporters[111] contributes to the complex constellation of dissociative anesthetic effects.

CARDIOVASCULAR EFFECTS OF KETAMINE

Ketamine is a unique intravenous anesthetic agent in that it displays cardiostimulatory effects. When administered to an animal with an intact autonomic nervous system, ketamine elicits marked increases in heart rate, cardiac output, and left ventricular systolic pressure.[112] These effects of ketamine are eliminated by prior treatment with propranolol, indicating that the cardiostimulatory effect of ketamine is a consequence of increased sympathetic discharge. The administration of ketamine directly into the cerebral circulation evoked an immediate increase in mean systemic blood pressure, cardiac output, and heart rate in goats.[113] These cardiostimulatory effects of ketamine were abolished in pentobarbital-anesthetized animals. It was therefore concluded that ketamine produced peripheral sympathomimetic effects primarily by direct stimulation of CNS structures.

Ketamine also exhibits direct effects on the myocardium that may differ with species. For example, ketamine exerts a positive inotropic effect on the isolated ferret ventricular papillary muscle, which is a consequence of ketamine's inhibition of neuronal catecholamine uptake.[114] This effect of ketamine manifests in the 30 to 100 μM concentration range. Ketamine inhibits both neuronal and extraneuronal catecholamine uptake processes, and the predominating effect on catecholamine transport in any tissue will depend on the morphology of the adrenergic innervation of the tissue.[115] Interestingly, inhibition of extraneuronal uptake of catecholamines by racemic ketamine is solely the result of an action of the (+) isomer, whereas both isomers appear capable of inhibiting neuronal uptake.[116]

Both direct positive inotropic and negative inotropic effects of ketamine on isolated myocardial preparations have been reported. In isolated guinea pig papillary muscles, ketamine causes a negative chronotropic response.[117] At concentrations of 50 to 300 μM, ketamine reduced the transsarcolemma Ca^{++} current and the action potential duration, which accounted for the negative inotropic effect. In contrast, ketamine elicited a positive inotropic effect in the rat left atria, which was attributed to a decrease in the Ca^{++}-insensitive transient outward current, leading to a prolongation of the action potential duration. Thus, species and tissue differences in the qualitative nature of the inotropic response to relatively high concentrations of ketamine may be related to differences of membrane ionic currents in various tissues.

In regard to the neuroanatomic substrate for the centrally mediated cardiostimulatory actions of ketamine, recent studies have implicated the nucleus tractus solitarii.[118] Local injection of NMDA into this area produces hypotension and bradycardia. The reduction in mean arterial pressure produced by microinjection of NMDA into the nucleus tractus solitarii was significantly antagonized by 9 mg/kg of intravenous ketamine; the attenuation of the effects of NMDA on heart rate was not significant. These provocative findings suggest that NMDA receptor antagonism in the nucleus tractus solitarii, an area receiving primary afferent fibers from the carotid sinus, may subserve the pressor response to systemically administered ketamine.

ADDITIONAL PHARMACOLOGIC ACTIONS OF KETAMINE

The effects of ketamine and PCP on various brain neurotransmitter systems has been extensively studied in an attempt to understand further the neurochemical mechanisms underlying the behavioral and anesthetic effects of these drugs.[119,120] The interactions of dissociative anesthetics with dopamine transporters and opioid receptors were described earlier in this chapter.

As a result of the involvement of the inhibitory neurotransmitter γ-aminobutyric acid (GABA) in the mechanism of action of barbiturates and general anesthetics, the influence of ketamine on GABAergic transmission was assessed. Anesthetic doses of ketamine produce modest elevations of whole brain GABA content and ketamine concentrations of 100 to 1,000 μM reduce in vitro GABA uptake in neurons and astrocytes.[121] Unlike pentobarbital, however, ketamine does not augment the inhibition of spinal reflexes or dorsal root potentials in cats following intravenous anesthetic doses

of 2.5 to 10 mg/kg;[122] the intravenous anesthetic dose in cats is 4 to 8 mg/kg. Inasmuch as both the prolonged inhibition of reflexes and dorsal root potentials are thought to be mediated by GABA, it was concluded that enhancement of GABA-mediated transmission does not contribute to the anesthetic action of ketamine. Ketamine may have functional GABA antagonist properties; concentrations of 5 to 50 μM inhibit NMDA-stimulated [^{3}H]GABA release from cultured mouse cortical neurons.[123] In contrast, ketamine was shown to potentiate the responses of rat superior cervical ganglion to GABA by an action not involving GABA transport.[124] Although reports on the effects of ketamine on GABAergic mechanisms have not been entirely consistent, it is clear that the most potent effect was to reduce NMDA-evoked GABA release and, further, that ketamine does not share with pentobarbital the ability to augment GABAergic transmission in the spinal cord.

The potential role of antimuscarinic activity in the psychotomimetic effects of PCP[125] led to an assessment of the influence of ketamine on cholinergic transmission. The affinity of ketamine for muscarinic cholinergic receptors of rat brain is 28 to 30 μM,[126] which is approximately 20-fold lower than that of PCP. Moreover, both PCP[127] and ketamine[128] alter the turnover rate of acetylcholine in various areas of the rat brain. Subanesthetic doses of PCP increase the turnover rate of acetylcholine in the cerebral cortex and diencephalon but not in the hippocampus and striatum, whereas anesthetic doses of ketamine decrease acetylcholine turnover in the hippocampus and striatum. Halothane anesthesia resulted in reduced acetylcholine turnover rates in all parts of the brain. Ketamine and PCP also interact with the ion channel domain of the nicotinic cholinergic receptor;[126] a functional consequence of this interaction may manifest as a reduction in the acetylcholine-activated channel lifetime.[129] An additional effect of ketamine on cholinergic dynamics in the CNS is the ability to antagonize NMDA-evoked release of acetylcholine from rat cerebral cortex[130] and striatum.[119] Thus, the previously described influence of ketamine and PCP on acetylcholine dynamics in the CNS could result from either an interaction with muscarinic cholinergic, nicotinic cholinergic, or NMDA receptors. The relevance of these effects on cholinergic systems to the actions of dissociative anesthetics remains to be established.

Ketamine effects on other biogenic amine neurotransmitter systems have been addressed. As previously mentioned, ketamine does inhibit serotonin uptake into synaptosomes with an IC_{50} value of 76 μM, which was reported to be lower than the IC_{50} values for the inhibition of norepinephrine, dopamine, or GABA transport, respectively, 330 μM, 290 μM, and 1,300 μM.[131] Moreover, in vivo studies indicated that ketamine (50 and 100 mg/kg, given intraperitoneally) increased serotonin turnover in the rat brain; however, this effect was not temporally correlated with ketamine-induced anesthesia. It was therefore inferred that central serotonin function is not essential for the anesthetic or analgesic response of ketamine because these effects of ketamine not only were maintained but were also potentiated by depletion of serotonin or the administration of a serotonin receptor antagonist.[67] Similarly, depletion of rat brain norepinephrine content did not affect ketamine-induced anesthesia.[132] This latter finding serves to distinguish ketamine further from barbiturates, inasmuch as barbiturate anesthesia was markedly potentiated by depletion of norepinephrine. Thus, there is presently no compelling evidence for the involvement of either serotonin or norepinephrine in ketamine-induced anesthesia.

Additional posited targets for dissociative anesthetics are the voltage-gated K^+ channels. An inhibition of voltage-regulated noninactivating presynaptic K^+ channels by PCP concentrations between 0.1 and 10 μM was demonstrated.[133] Furthermore, it was proposed that such an antagonism by PCP presynaptically would result in an increased action potential duration and Ca^{++} entry. This, in turn, would augment Ca^{++}-dependent neurotransmitter release. In contrast, the PCP and ketamine antagonism of voltage-gated K^+ currents in cultured rat hippocampal neurons requires concentrations of 100 to 3,000 μM.[134] Therefore, it appears that the concentrations of dissociative anesthetics required to inhibit voltage-gated K^+ channels in cultured hippocampal neurons are not pharmacologically relevant. Similar potencies for ketamine's antagonism of Na^+ channels have been documented; the IC_{50} values for ketamine's interaction with veratridine-stimulated Na^+ channels range from 12 to 100 μM.[135,136]

Thus, although NMDA receptors appear to represent the primary target for dissociative anesthetics, a myriad of interactions with neurotransmitter receptors and transporters, and voltage-regulated ion channels, may underlie the complex constellation of behavioral and anesthetic actions of these compounds.

REFERENCES

1. Luby ED, Cohen BD, Rosenbaum G et al: Study of a new schizophrenomimetic drug—Sernyl. Arch Neurol Psychiatry 81:363, 1959
2. Greifenstein FE, DeVault M, Yoshitake J, Gajewski JR: A study of 1-arylcyclohexyl amine for anesthesia. Anesth Analg 37:283, 1958
3. Lear E, Suntay R, Pallin IM, Chiron AE: Cyclohexamine (CI-400): a new intravenous agent. Anesthesiology 20:330, 1959
4. McCarthy DA, Chen G, Kaump DH, Ensor C: General anesthetic and other pharmacological properties of 2-(O-chlorophenyl)-2-methylaminocyclohexanone HCl (CI-581). J New Drugs 5:21, 1965
5. Corssen G, Domino EF: Dissociative anesthesia: further pharmacologic studies and first clinical experience with the phencyclidine derivative CI-581. Anesth Analg 45:29, 1966
6. Corssen G, Miyasaka M, Domino EF: Changing concepts in pain control during surgery: dissociative anesthesia with CI-581. Anesth Anal 47:746, 1968
7. Miyasaka M, Domino EF: Neuronal mechanisms of ketamine-induced anesthesia. Int J Neuropharmacol 7:557, 1968
8. Weingarten SM: Dissociation of limbic and neocortical EEG patterns in cats under ketamine anesthesia. J Neurosurg 37:429, 1972
9. Winters WD, Ferrar-Allado T, Gazman-Flores C, Alcaraz M: The cataleptic state induced by ketamine: a review of the neuropharmacology of anesthesia. Neuropharmacology 11:303, 1972
10. Kayama Y, Iwama K: The EEG, evoked potentials and single unit activity during ketamine anesthesia in cats. Anesthesiology 36:316, 1972
11. Winters WD: Neuropharmacological effects of ketamine: gross behavior, EEG, unit activity, wake-sleep, kindling and interactions with diazepam and

propranolol. In Domino EF (ed): Status of Ketamine in Anesthesiology p. 261. NPP Books, Ann Arbor, 1990

12. Marietta M, Way WL, Castagonoli N, Trevor AJ: On the pharmacology of the ketamine enantiomorphs in the rat. J Pharmacol Exp Ther 202:157, 1977

13. Benthuysen JL, Hance AJ, Quam DD, Winters WD: Comparison of isomers of ketamine on catalepsy in the rat and electrical activity of the brain and behavior in the cat. Neuropharmacology 28:1003, 1989

14. Schütter J, Stanski DR, White PF et al: Pharmacodynamic modeling of the EEG effects of ketamine and its enantiomers in man. J Pharmacokinet Biopharm 15:241, 1987

15. Monaghan DT, Bridges RJ, Cotman CW: The excitatory amino acid receptors: their classes, pharmacology, and distinct properties in the function of the central nervous system. Annu Rev Pharmacol Toxicol 29:365, 1989

16. Choi DW, Rothman SM: The role of glutamate neurotoxicity in hypoxic-ischemic neuronal death. Annu Rev Neurosci 13:171, 1990

17. Gasic GP, Hollman M: Molecular neurobiology of glutamate receptors. Annu Rev Physiol 54:507, 1992

18. Watkins JD, Krogsgaardlarsen P, Honore T: Structure activity relationships in the development of excitatory amino acid receptor agonists and competitive antagonists. Trends Pharmacol 11:25, 1990

19. Henneberry RD: Cloning of the genes for excitatory amino acid receptors. Bioessays 14:465, 1992

20. Sommer B, Seeburg PH: Glutamate receptor channels: novel properties and new clones. Trends Pharmacol Sci 13:291, 1992

21. Keinänen K, Wisden W, Sommer B et al: A family of AMPA-sensitive glutamate receptors. Science 249:556, 1990

22. Moriyoshi K, Masu M, Ishii T et al: Molecular cloning and characterization of the rat NMDA receptor. Nature 354:31, 1992

23. Collingridge GL, Singer W: Excitatory amino acid receptors and synaptic plasticity. Trends Pharmacol Sci 11:290, 1990

24. Headley PM, Parsons CG, West DC: The role of N-methylaspartate receptors in mediating responses of rat and cat spinal neurones to defined sensory stimuli. J Physiol (Lond) 385:169, 1987

25. Dickenson AH, Aydar E: Antagonism at the glycine site on the NMDA receptor reduces spinal nociception in the rat. Neurosci Lett 121:263, 1991

26. Kutsuwada T, Kashiwabuchi N, Mori H et al: Molecular diversity of the NMDA receptor channel. Nature 358:36, 1992

27. Nakanishi S: Molecular diversity of glutamate receptors and implications for brain function. Science 258:597, 1992

28. Lodge D, Anis NA: Effects of phencyclidine on excitatory amino acid activation of spinal interneurons in the cat. Eur J Pharmacol 77:203, 1982

29. Lodge D, Anis NA, Burton NR: Effects of optical isomers of ketamine on excitation of cat and rat spinal neurons by amino acids and acetycholine. Neurosci Lett 29:282, 1982

30. Lodge D, Anis NA, Berry SC, Burton NR: Arylcyclohexylamines selectively reduce excitation of mammalian neurons by aspartate like amino acids. In Kamenka J-M, Domino EF, Geneste P (eds): Phencyclidine and Related Arylcyclohexylamines: Present and Future Applications. p. 595. NPP Books, Ann Arbor, 1983

31. Anis NA, Berry SC, Burton NR, Lodge D: The dissociative anaesthetics, ketamine and phencyclidine, selectively reduce excitation of central mammalian neurones by N-methyl-aspartate. Br J Pharmacol 79:565, 1983

32. Church J, Lodge D, Berry SC: Differential effects of dextrophan and levorphanol on the excitation of rat spinal neurons by amino acids. Eur J Pharmacol 111:185, 1985

33. Thomson AM, Lodge D: Selective blockade of an excitatory synapse in rat cerebral cortex by the sigma opiate cyclazocine: an intracellular in vitro study. Neurosci Lett 54:21, 1985

34. Hampton RY, Medzihradsky F, Woods JH, Dahlstrom PJ: Stereospecific binding of [^{3}H]phencyclidine in brain membranes. Life Sci 30:2147, 1982

35. Murray TF, Leid ME: Interaction of dextrorotatory opioids with phencyclidine recognition sites in rat brain membranes. Life Sci 34:1899, 1984

36. Martin D, Lodge D: Phencyclidine receptors and N-methyl-D-aspartate antagonism: electrophysiological data correlates with known behaviors. Pharmacol Biochem Behav 31:279, 1988

37. Lodge D, Aram JA, Church J et al: Sigma opiates and excitatory amino acids. In Lodge D (ed): Excitatory Amino Acids in Health and Disease. p. 237. John Wiley and Sons, Chichester, 1988

38. Franklin PH, Murray TF: High affinity [^{3}H]dextrorphan binding in rat brain is localized to a noncompetitive antagonist site of the activated N-methyl-D-aspartate receptor-cation channel. Mol Pharmacol 41:131, 1992

39. Harrison NL, Simmonds MA: Quantitative studies

on some antagonists of N-methyl-D-aspartate in slices of rat cerebral cortex. Br J Pharmacol 84:381, 1985

40. Martin D, Lodge D: Ketamine acts as a non-competitive N-methyl-D-aspartate antagonist on frog spinal cord in vitro. Neuropharmacology 24:999, 1985

41. Lacey MG, Henderson G: Actions of phencyclidine on rat locus coeruleus neurones in vitro. Neuroscience 17:485, 1986

42. Honey R, Miljkovic Z, MacDonald JF: Ketamine and phencyclidine cause a voltage-dependent block of responses to L-aspartic acid. Neurosci Lett 61:135, 1985

43. Davies SN, Alford ST, Coan EJ et al: Ketamine blocks an NMDA receptor-mediated component of synaptic transmission in rat hippocampus in a voltage-dependent manner. Neurosci Lett 92:213, 1988

44. Woodhull AM: Ionic blockage of sodium channels in nerve. J Gen Physiol 61:687, 1973

45. MacDonald JF, Miljkovic Z, Pennefather P: Use-dependent block of excitatory amino acid currents in cultured neurons by ketamine. J Neurophysiol 58:251, 1987

46. Mayer ML, Westbrook GL, Vyklicky L Jr: Sites of antagonist action on N-methyl-D-aspartic acid receptors studied using fluctuation analysis and a rapid perfusion technique. J Neurophysiol 60:645, 1988

47. MacDonald JF, Bartlett MC, Mody I et al: Actions of ketamine, phencyclidine and MK-801 on NMDA receptor currents in cultured mouse hippocampal neurones. J Physiol (Lond) 432:483, 1991

48. Wong EHF, Kemp JA, Priestley T et al: The anticonvulsant MK-801 is a potent N-methyl-D-aspartate antagonist. Proc Natl Acad Sci USA 83:7104, 1986

49. Kloog Y, Haring R, Sokolovsky M: Kinetic characterization of the phencyclidine-N-methyl-D-aspartate receptor interaction: evidence for a steric blockade of the channel. Biochemistry 27:843, 1988

50. Huettner JE, Bean BP: Block of N-methyl-D-aspartate activated current by the anticonvulsant MK-801: selective binding to open channels. Proc Natl Acad Sci U S A 85:1307, 1988

51. Nowak LM, Wright JM: Factors influencing voltage dependence on N-methyl-D-aspartate (NMDA) channel block by tiletamine, abstracted. Biophys J 57:127a, 1990

52. MacDonald JF, Nowak LM: Mechanisms of blockade of excitatory amino acid receptor channels. Trends Pharmacol Sci 11:167, 1990

53. Salt TE, Wilson DG, Prasad SK: Antagonism of N-methylaspartate and synaptic responses of neurones in the rat ventrobasal thalamus by ketamine and MK-801. Br J Pharmacol 94:443, 1988

54. Aram JA, Martin D, Tomczyk M et al: Neocortical epileptogenesis in vitro: studies with N-methyl-D-aspartate, phencyclidine, sigma and dextromethorphan receptor ligands. J Pharmacol Exp Ther 248:320, 1989

55. Scheller MS, Zornow MH, Fleischer JE et al: The noncompetitive N-methyl-D-aspartate receptor antagonist, MK-801 profoundly reduces volatile anesthetic requirements in rabbits. Neuropharmacology 28:677, 1989

56. Eger EI, Saidman LJ, Brandstater B: Minimum alveolar anesthetic concentration: a standard of anesthetic potency. Anesthesiology 26:756, 1965

57. Daniell LC: The noncompetitive N-methyl-D-aspartate antagonists, MK-801, phencyclidine and ketamine increase the potency of general anesthetics. Pharmacol Biochem Behav 36:111, 1990

58. Daniell LC: Alteration of general anesthetic potency by agonists and antagonists of the polyamine binding site of the N-methyl-D-aspartate receptor. J Pharmacol Exp Ther 261:304, 1992

59. Koek W, Woods JH, Winger GD: MK-801, a proposed noncompetitive antagonist of excitatory amino acid neurotransmission, produces phencyclidine-like behavioral effects in pigeons, rats and rhesus monkeys. J Pharmacol Exp Ther 245:969, 1988

60. Löscher W, Fredow G, Ganter M: Comparison of pharmacodynamic effects of non-competitive NMDA receptor antagonists MK-801 and ketamine in pigs. Eur J Pharmacol 192:377, 1991

61. France CP, Winger GD, Woods JH: Analgesic, anesthetic and respiratory effects of the competitive N-methyl-D-aspartate (NMDA) antagonist CGS 19755 in rhesus monkeys. Brain Res 526:355, 1990

62. France CP, Woods JH, Ornstein P: The competitive N-methyl-D-aspartate (NMDA) antagonist CGS 19755 attenuates the rate-decreasing effects of NMDA in rhesus monkeys without producing ketamine-like discriminative stimulus effects. Eur J Pharmacol 159:133, 1989

63. Domino EF, Chodoff P, Corssen G: Pharmacologic effects of CI-581, a new dissociative anesthetic in man. Clin Pharmacol Ther 6:279, 1965

64. Ryder S, Way W, Trevor AJ: Comparative pharmacology of the optical isomers of ketamine in mice. Eur J Pharmacol 49:15, 1978

65. Smith DJ, Pekoe GM, Martin LL, Coalgate B: The interaction of ketamine with the opiate receptor. Life Sci 26:789, 1980

66. Lawrence D, Livingston A: Opiate-like analgesic activity in general anesthetics. Br J Pharmacol 73:435, 1981

67. Vargiu L, Stefanini E, Musinu C, Saba G: Possible role of brain serotonin in the central effects of ketamine. Neuropharmacology 17:405, 1978

68. Uhtani M, Kikuchi H, Kitahata LM et al: Effects of ketamine on nociceptive cells in the medial medullary reticular formation of the cat. Anesthesiology 51:414, 1979

69. Kitahata LM, Taub A, Kosaka Y: Lamina-specific suppression of dorsal-horn unit activity by ketamine hydrochloride. Anesthesiology 38:4, 1973

70. Okuda T: Comparison of direct and indirect depressant actions of ketamine on dorsal horn cells in rabbits. Neuropharmacology 25:433, 1986

71. Finck AD, Ngai SH: Opiate receptor mediation of ketamine analgesia. Anesthesiology 56:291, 1982

72. Smith DJ, Bouchal RL, DeSanctis CA et al: Properties of the interactions between ketamine and opiate binding sites in vivo and in vitro. Neuropharmacology 26:1253, 1987

73. Winters WD, Hance AJ, Cadd GG et al: Ketamine- and morphine-induced analgesia and catalepsy. I. Tolerance, cross-tolerance, potentiation, residual morphine levels and naloxone action in the rat. J Pharmacol Exp Ther 244:51, 1988

74. Ward SJ, Portoghese PS, Takemori AE: Improved assays for the assessment of κ- and δ-properties of opioid ligands. Eur J Pharmacol 85:163, 1982

75. Fratta W, Casa M, Balestrieri A et al: Failure of ketamine to interact with opiate receptors. Eur J Pharmacol 61:389, 1980

76. Wiley JN, Downs DA: Lack of antagonism by naloxone of the analgesic and locomotor stimulant actions of ketamine. Life Sci 31:1071, 1982

77. Headley PM, Parsons CG, West DC: The role of N-methylaspartate receptors in mediating responses of rat and cat spinal neurones to defined sensory stimuli. J Physiol (Lond) 385:169, 1987

78. Headley PM, Grillner S: Excitatory amino acids and synaptic transmission: the evidence for a physiological function. Trends Pharmacol Sci 11:205, 1990

79. Davies SN, Lodge D: Evidence for involvement of N-methylaspartate receptors in "wind-up" of class 2 neurones in the dorsal horn of the rat. Brain Res 424:402, 1987

80. France CP, Snyder AM, Woods JH: Analgesic effects of phencyclidine-like drugs in rhesus monkeys. J Pharmacol Exp Ther 250:197, 1989

81. Klepstad P, Maurset A, Moberg ER, Øye I: Evidence of a role of NMDA receptors in pain perception. Eur J Pharmacol 187:513, 1990

82. Maurset A, Skoglund LA, Hustveit O, Øye I: Comparison of ketamine and pethidine in experimental and postoperative pain. Pain 36:37, 1989

83. Bowyer JF, Albertson TE, Winters WD: Cortical kindled seizures: modification by excitant and depressant drugs. Epilepsia 24:356, 1983

84. Bowyer JF, Albertson TE, Winters WD, Baselt RC: Ketamine-induced changes in kindled amygdaloid seizures. Neuropharmacology 22:887, 1983

85. Chapman AG, Meldrum BS: Non-competitive N-methyl-D-aspartate antagonists protect against sound-induced seizures in DBA/2 mice. Eur J Pharmacol 166:201, 1989

86. Roth JE, Zhang G, Murray TF, Franklin PH: Dextrorotatory opioids and phencyclidine exert anticonvulsant action in prepiriform cortex. Eur J Pharmacol 215:293, 1992

87. Rothman SM, Olney JW: Excitotoxicity and the NMDA receptor. Trends Neurosci 10:299, 1987

88. Choi DW, Koh J-Q, Peters S: Pharmacology of glutamate neurotoxicity in cortical cell culture: attenuation by NMDA antagonists. J Neurosci 8:185, 1988

89. Goldberg NP, Viseskul V, Choi DW: Phencyclidine receptor ligands attenuate cortical neuronal injury after N-methyl-D-aspartate exposure or hypoxia. J Pharmacol Exp Ther 245:1081, 1988

90. Olney JW, Price MT, Fuller TA et al: The anti-excitotoxic effects of certain anesthetics, analgesics and sedative-hypnotics. Neurosci Lett 68:29, 1986

91. Weiss J, Goldberg MP, Choi DW: Ketamine protects cultured neocortical neurons from hypoxic injury. Brain Res 380:186, 1986

92. Monyer H, Goldberg MP, Choi DW: Glucose deprivation neuronal injury in cortical culture. Brain Res 483:347, 1989

93. Lucas JH, Wolf A: In vitro studies of multiple impact injury to mammalian CNS neurons: prevention of perikaryal damage and death by ketamine. Brain Res 543:181, 1991

94. Choi DW: Ketamine reduces NMDA receptor mediated neurotoxicity in cortical cultures. In Domino EF (ed): Status of Ketamine in Anesthesiology. p. 549. NPP Books, Ann Arbor, 1990

95. Didier M, Heaulme M, Gonalons N et al: 35mM K$^+$-stimulated ^{45}Ca^{++} uptake in cerebellar granule cell cultures mainly results from NMDA receptor activation. Eur J Pharmacol 244:57, 1993

96. Bliss TVP, Lomo T: Long-lasting potentiation of synaptic transmission in the dentate area of the anaesthetized rabbit following stimulation of the perforant path. J Physiol (Lond) 232:331, 1973

97. Stringer JL, Guyenet PG: Elimination of long-term potentiation in the hippocampus by phencyclidine and ketamine. Brain Res 258:159, 1983

98. Tocco G, Maren S, Shors TJ et al: Long-term potentiation is associated with increased [^{3}H]AMPA binding in rat hippocampus. Brain Res 573:228, 1992

99. Alessandri B, Bättig K, Welzl H: Effects of ketamine on tunnel maze and water maze performance in the rat. Behav Neural Biol 52:194, 1989

100. Jones KW, Bauerle LM, DeNoble VJ: Differential effects of σ and phencyclidine receptor ligands on learning. Eur J Pharmacol 179:97, 1990

101. Lalond R, Joyal CC: Effects of ketamine and l-glutamic acid diethyl ester on concept learning in rats. Pharmacol Biochem Behav 39:828, 1991

102. Contreras PC, Monahan JB, Lanthorn TH et al: Phencyclidine: physiological actions, interactions with excitatory amino acids and endogenous ligands. Mol Neurobiol 1:191, 1987

103. McCarron MM: Phencyclidine intoxication. In Clouet DH (ed): Phencyclidine: An Update. NIDA Research Monograph 64. p. 209. United States Government Printing Office, Washington, DC, 1986

104. Siegel RK: Phencyclidine and ketamine intoxication: a study of four populations of recreational users. In Petersen RC, Stillman RC (eds): Phencyclidine (PCP) Abuse: An Appraisal. NIDA Research Monograph 21. p. 119. United States Government Printing Office, Washington, DC, 1978

105. Holtzman SG: Phencyclidine-like discriminative effects of opioids in the rat. J Pharmacol Exp Ther 214:614, 1980

106. Young AM, Herling S, Wenger GD, Woods JH: Comparison of discriminative and reinforcing effects of ketamine and related compounds in the rhesus monkey. In Harris LS (ed): Problems of Drug Dependence, 1980. NIDA Research Monograph 34. p. 173. United States Government Printing Office, Washington, DC, 1981

107. Brady KT, Balste RL: Discriminative stimulus properties of ketamine stereoisomers in phencyclidine-trained rats. Pharmacol Biochem Behav 17:291, 1982

108. Johnson KM, Snell LD: Effects of phencyclidine (PCP)-like drugs on turning behavior, ^{3}H-dopamine uptake and ^{3}H-PCP binding. Pharmacol Biochem Behav 22:731, 1985

109. Kuhar MJ, Boja JW, Cone EJ: Phencyclidine binding to striatal cocaine receptors. Neuropharmacology 29:293, 1990

110. Koek W, Colpaert FC, Woods JH, Kamenka J-M: The phencyclidine (PCP) analog N-[1-(2-benzo(B)-thiophenyl)cyclohexyl] piperidine shares cocaine-like but not other characteristic behavioral effects with PCP, ketamine and MK-801. J Pharmacol Exp Ther 250:1019, 1989

111. Martin DC, Introna RP, Aronstam RS: Inhibition of neuronal 5-HT uptake by ketamine, but not halothane, involve disruption of substrate recognition by the transporter. Neurosci Lett 112:99, 1990

112. Schwartz DA, Horwitz LD: Effects of ketamine on left ventricular performance. J Pharmacol Exp Ther 194:410, 1975

113. Ivankovich AD, Miletich DJ, Reimann C et al: Cardiovascular effects of centrally administered ketamine in goats. Anesth Analg 53:924, 1974

114. Cook DJ, Carton EG, Housmans PR: Mechanism of the positive inotropic effect of ketamine in isolated ferret ventricular papillary muscle. Anesthesiology 74:880, 1991

115. Lundy P, Gverzdys S, Frew R: Ketamine: evidence of tissue specific inhibition of neuronal and extraneuronal catecholamine uptake processes. Can J Physiol Pharmacol 63:298, 1985

116. Lundy PM, Lockwood PA, Thompson G, Frew R: Differential effect of ketamine isomers on neuronal and extraneuronal catecholamine uptake mechanisms. Anesthesiology 64:359, 1986

117. Endou M, Hattori Y, Nakaya H et al: Electrophysiologic mechanisms responsible for inotropic responses to ketamine in guinea pig and rat myocardium. Anesthesiology 76:409, 1992

118. Ogawa A, Uemura M, Kataoka Y et al: Effects of ketamine on cardiovascular responses mediated by N-methyl-D-aspartate receptor in the rat nucleus tractus soltarius. Anesthesiology 78:163, 1993

119. Johnson KM, Snell LD: Involvement of dopaminergic, cholinergic and glutamatergic mechanisms in the actions of phencyclidine-like drugs. In Clouet DH (ed): Phencyclidine: An Update. NIDA Research Monograph 64. p. 52. United States Government Printing Office, 1986

120. Church J, Lodge D: N-Methyl-D-aspartate (NMDA) antagonism is central to the actions of ketamine and other phencyclidine receptor ligands. In Domino EF (ed): Status of Ketamine in Anesthesiology. p. 501. NPP Books, Ann Arbor, 1990

121. Wood JD, Hertz L: Ketamine-induced changes in the GABA system of mouse brain. Neuropharmacology 19:805, 1980

122. Lodge D, Anis NA: Effects of ketamine and three

other anaesthetics on spinal reflexes and inhibitions in the cat. Br J Anaesth 56:1143, 1984

123. Drejir J, Honore T: Phencyclidine analogues inhibit NMDA-stimulated [^{3}H]GABA release from cultured cortex neurons. Eur J Pharmacol 143:287, 1987

124. Little HJ, Atkinson HD: Ketamine potentiates the responses of the rat superior cervical ganglion to GABA. Eur J Pharmacol 98:53, 1984

125. Maayani S, Weinstein H, Ben-Zui N et al: Psychotomimetics as anticholinergic agents: I. 1-Cyclohexylpiperidine derivatives: anticholinesterase activity and antagonist activity to acetylcholine. Biochem Pharmacol 23:1263, 1974

126. Aronstum RS, Narayanan L, Wenger DA: Ketamine inhibition of ligand binding to cholinergic receptors and ion channels. Eur J Pharmacol 78:367, 1982

127. Murray TF, Cheney DL: The effect of phencyclidine on the turnover rate of acetylcholine in various regions of rat brain. J Pharmacol Exp Ther 217:733, 1981

128. Ngai SH, Cheney DL, Finck AD: Acetylcholine concentrations and turnover in rat brain structures during anesthesia with halothane, enflurane and ketamine. Anesthesiology 48:4, 1978

129. Wachtel RE: Ketamine decreases the open time of single-channel currents activated by acetylcholine. Anesthesiology 68:563, 1988

130. Lodge D, Johnston GAR: Effect of ketamine on amino acid-evoked release of acetylcholine from rat cerebral cortex in vitro. Neurosci Lett 56:371, 1985

131. Azzaro AJ, Smith DJ: The inhibitory action of ketamine HCl on [^{3}H]5-hydroxytryptamine accumulation by rat brain synaptosomal-rich fractions: comparison with [^{3}H]catecholamine and [^{3}H]γ-aminobutyric acid uptake. Neuropharmacology 16:349, 1977

132. Mason ST, King RAJ, Banks P, Angel A: Brain noradrenaline and anaesthesia: behavioral and electrophysiological evidence. Neuroscience 10:177, 1983

133. Bartschat DK, Blaustein MP: Phencyclidine in low doses selectively blocks a presynaptic voltage-regulated potassium channel in rat brain. Proc Natl Acad Sci U S A 83:189, 1986

134. Rothman S: Noncompetitive N-methyl-D-aspartate antagonists affect multiple ionic currents. J Pharmacol Exp Ther 246:137, 1988

135. Erecinska M, Nelson D, Silver IA: Interactions of benzotropine, atropine and ketamine with veratridine-activated sodium channels: effects on membrane depolarization, K$^+$-efflux and neurotransmitter amino acid release. Br J Pharmacol 94:871, 1988

136. Allaoua H, Chicheportiche R: Anaesthetic properties of phencyclidine (PCP) and analogues may be related to their interaction with NA$^+$ channels. Eur J Pharmacol 163:327, 1989

Chapter 17

Pharmacokinetics of Ketamine

Evan D. Kharasch

The dissociative anesthetic ketamine has been administered by intravenous, intramuscular, rectal, oral, epidural, and intrathecal routes. The pharmacokinetics of ketamine have been studied extensively and are perhaps better understood than those of many other anesthetic agents.

INTRAVENOUS BOLUS ADMINISTRATION

Administered intravenously, ketamine has a rapid onset and relatively short duration of hypnotic effect, followed by prolonged analgesia. A typical concentration versus time profile for an intravenous ketamine bolus is shown in Figure 17-1. The plasma disappearance curve is biphasic, with an initial rapid distribution phase lasting up to 45 minutes and a longer elimination phase lasting several hours. Typical plasma concentrations during surgical anesthesia are 1 to 3 μg/ml. The principal ketamine metabolite, norketamine, appears in the blood within 2 minutes and possesses significant pharmacologic activity. Most investigators report norketamine concentrations that approximate or exceed those of the parent drug after the initial peak of formation.[1-6] A secondary metabolite, 5,6-dehydronorketamine, a "pseudometabolite" reflecting the formation of 5-hydroxynorketamine

(see subsequent discussion), also is found in significant concentrations in the blood following intravenous ketamine. Another secondary norketamine metabolite, 6-hydroxynorketamine, is quantitatively more important than is 5-hydroxynorketamine based on urinary metabolite recovery data.[7,8] However, there is no information on 6-hydroxynorketamine plasma concentration after ketamine administration.

There is considerable evidence that norketamine, the primary metabolite of ketamine, is pharmacologically active and contributes significantly to the clinical effects observed after parent drug administration. Norketamine produces a spectrum of pharmacologic effects similar to those of ketamine; however, it is 1/10 to 1/3 less potent on a molar basis.[9-12] In contrast, the hydroxylated metabolites of norketamine have relatively little pharmacologic activity.[12]

Most investigators have characterized ketamine pharmacokinetics according to a two compartment open model that consists of a highly perfused central compartment and a less well-perfused peripheral compartment. Distribution (intercompartmental clearance) occurs from the central to the peripheral compartment, and elimination is presumed to occur from the central compartment.[1,4,13-16] In this model, the central compart-

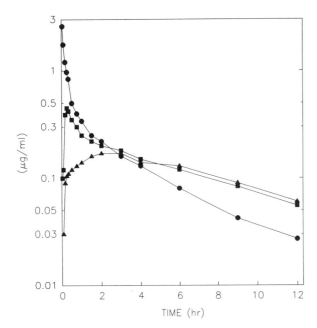

Fig. 17-1 Pharmacokinetics of intravenous ketamine. Mean serum concentrations of ketamine (●), norketamine (■), and 5,6-dehydronorketamine (▲) are shown following intravenous injection of 2.5 mg/kg of racemic ketamine to five patients. 5,6-Dehydronorketamine is a pseudometabolite, an artifact of the assay method used in this investigation, which reflects the concentration of 5-hydroxynorketamine from which it is derived. (Modified from Wieber et al.,[1] with permission.)

ment includes the brain, as a result of the high lipid solubility of ketamine.[1,10,17] One group of investigators has used a three compartment open model to describe intravenous ketamine pharmacokinetics.[2,3] For this alternative model, the brain is placed in a rapidly equilibrating peripheral compartment. Animal experiments directly measuring tissue ketamine concentrations have substantiated these pharmacokinetic models.[18,19] After intravenous administration, ketamine concentrations in the plasma, brain, heart, and kidney peak within 1 minute; those in the muscle, liver, gut, and skin rise more slowly, achieving a peak in 10 to 20 minutes. Redistribution of ketamine into fat occurs after a substantial time delay.

The pharmacokinetic parameters for intravenous ketamine disposition in humans are provided in Table 17-1. These parameters and the pharmacokinetic behavior of ketamine are independent of the dose administered. Volumes of distribution, clearance, and half-lives have been shown to be similar over a 30-fold dose range, from 0.125 to 3.7 mg/kg.[1,13,15]

INTRAVENOUS INFUSION

More recent investigations have focused on the use of ketamine infusions, either alone or in combination with other intravenous agents, for prolonged

Table 17-1 Ketamine Pharmacokinetics[a]

Dose (mg/kg)	Compartments	Last Time Point Assayed (hr)	$t_{1/2\pi}$(min)	$t_{1/2\alpha}$(min)	$t_{1/2\beta}$(min)	CL (ml/kg/min)	V_c (L/kg)	V_β (L/kg)	V_{ss} (L/kg)	Reference
2.5 IV bolus	2	12		11 ± 4	151 ± 59	17.1 ± 8.9[b]	0.9 ± 0.1[b]	3.1 ± 1.1[b]	3.0 ± 0.7[b]	1
0.125 IV bolus	2	7		16 ± 1	178 ± 41	16.3 ± 2.9		4.2 ± 0.4	2.1 ± 0.7	13
0.25 IV bolus	2	7		18 ± 3	182 ± 22	19.1 ± 2.5		5.1 ± 0.7	3.1 ± 0.9	13
2.0 IV bolus	2	6		8 ± 6	176 ± 57	17.8 ± 8.5[b]	0.7 ± 0.3[b]	6.2 ± 2.6[b]	2.6 ± 0.5[b]	4
3.7 IV infusion	2	8		13 ± 9	132 ± 32	16.1 ± 4.6	1.0 ± 0.4	2.9 ± 0.5		15
2.0 IV bolus	3	24	0.5 ± 0.2	9 ± 4	158 ± 36	20.8 ± 8.8	0.05 ± 0.05	4.3 ± 1.6	2.3 ± 1.1	2
2.2 IV bolus	3	24	0.5 ± 0.3	8 ± 6	135 ± 27	14.2 ± 5.3	0.06 ± 0.05		1.8 ± 0.7	3

Abbreviations: CL, clearance; $t_{1/2\alpha}$, ; $t_{1/2\beta}$, ; $t_{1/2\pi}$, ; V_β, ; V_c, initial volume of distribution; V_{ss}, steady-state volume of distribution.

[a] All values are mean ± standard deviation.

[b] Recalculated from the original data by the present author, assuming a patient weight of 70 kg.

surgical anesthesia or sedation.[20–26] The apparent kinetic behavior of ketamine, used in infusions with midazolam, fentanyl, or droperidol, did not differ significantly from that when it was given as a bolus.[22–24] The one major difference was the elevated and sustained plasma concentrations of norketamine, which probably contributed to the observed pharmacologic effects. Ketamine infusions may be titrated to specific targeted end points, such as a predetermined plasma concentration, with predictable results. Schüttler et al.[26] devised a microprocessor-controlled infusion pump that predictably achieves target ketamine blood concentrations preset by an anesthesiologist by turning a single dial.

INTRAMUSCULAR ADMINISTRATION

Intramuscular ketamine, conveniently used for induction of anesthesia in patients without venous access, is rapidly absorbed into the central circulation (Fig. 17-2).[27] Ketamine administered intra-

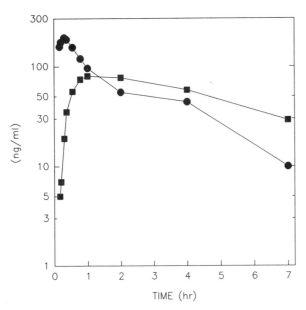

Fig. 17-2 Mean plasma ketamine (●) and norketamine (■) concentrations following intramuscular ketamine administration (0.5 mg/kg) to six healthy volunteers. (Modified from Grant et al.,[28] with permission.)

muscularly is almost completely absorbed, with a systemic bioavailability exceeding 90 percent in both humans and dogs.[28,29] Following a typical intramuscular induction dose of 6 mg/kg in adults, mean peak plasma concentrations of 1.7 μg/ml were achieved within 15 to 30 minutes.[30] These peak plasma concentrations were equivalent to those seen after 2 mg/kg of intravenous ketamine. In adults following a subhypnotic intramuscular dose of 0.5 mg/kg, mean peak plasma ketamine concentrations of 0.24 μg/ml were reached after an average of 22 minutes, with a lag time of 1 minute before the appearance of ketamine in the plasma.[28] Analgesia occurred within 15 minutes, the first time point examined after injection.

Intramuscular administration in adults significantly prolongs the duration of ketamine effects compared with intravenous injection. In operations lasting 1 to 2 hours, during which anesthesia was maintained with halothane and nitrous oxide, adults induced with intravenous ketamine awoke immediately after surgery, but those induced with intramuscular ketamine did not regain consciousness for an additional hour (3 hours after induction).[30]

In children, intramuscular ketamine is more rapidly absorbed and eliminated than in adults.[30] Peak plasma ketamine concentrations occur 5 to 15 minutes after intramuscular injection in children, compared with 15 to 30 minutes in adults. The volumes of distribution are similar, but the half-life and mean residence time are shorter in children. The plasma clearance is greater in children compared with that in adults. Awakening after identical doses of intramuscular ketamine (mg/kg) is more rapid in children than in adults.

RECTAL ADMINISTRATION

Rectal administration of ketamine for induction of anesthesia in children has been described repeatedly,[31–36] with two detailed pharmacokinetic investigations reported.[33,34] Typical induction doses are 10 to 15 mg/kg. Rectal ketamine is rapidly absorbed, with unconsciousness achieved within 6 to 15 minutes. The bioavailability, however, is low because of poor absorption and extensive first-pass metabolism, thereby necessitating the use of larger doses than those used intravenously or intramuscularly.

Idvall et al.[33] induced anesthesia with rectal ketamine in solution (average dose, 9 mg/kg) 1 hour after premedication with rectal atropine and diazepam. Loss of consciousness and the ability to tolerate venous cannulation were achieved after 7 to 15 minutes and were associated with mean plasma ketamine concentrations of 0.2 μg/ml. Peak ketamine plasma concentrations of 0.7 μg/ml were reached 40 minutes after rectal induction (Fig. 17-3). The elimination half-life was 109 minutes, similar to that observed after intravenous administration. In another investigation, Pedraz et al.[34] administered ketamine (10 mg/kg) as a rectal suppository in lipophilic stearine. Compared with the aqueous solution dosing form, ketamine in lipid suppositories had a slower release, and plasma concentrations were diminished but prolonged. The apparent rate of ketamine absorption was similar to that after ketamine rectal solution, with peak plasma concentrations occurring after 45 minutes. However, no

child lost consciousness, and the mean peak plasma ketamine concentration was only 0.16 μg/ml. Plasma concentrations were sustained, however, and postoperative analgesia was excellent, consistent with a terminal half-life (190 minutes) that was significantly longer than that observed after ketamine rectal solution. The differences in peak plasma concentrations and apparent ketamine half-life can be attributed to the use of lipid suppositories rather than a ketamine solution.

In both investigations, the plasma concentrations of the primary metabolite norketamine exceeded those of the parent ketamine at all times after rectal administration (Fig. 17-3). This suggests extensive hepatic first-pass metabolism following absorption into the rectal venous plexus and transport to the liver by the portal circulation. Norketamine undoubtedly contributed to the pharmacologic effects of the parent drug. Plasma ketamine concentrations alone were subtherapeutic (0.2 μg/ml) at the time the children fell asleep, but plasma concentrations of the equally effective metabolite were 0.4 μg/ml.[33] The extensive first-pass hepatic metabolism probably accounts for the relatively low bioavailability of rectal ketamine, estimated by Idvall et al.[33] to be similar to that following oral administration, between 11 and 25 percent.

ORAL ADMINISTRATION

After oral administration, ketamine absorption is incomplete and delayed, plasma concentrations are lower compared with parenteral administration, and the drug undergoes significant first-pass metabolism.[28] In adults receiving 0.5 mg/kg, a mean peak ketamine concentration of only 0.045 μg/ml was reached after an average of 30 minutes with an absorption lag time of 8 minutes compared with a peak of 0.24 μg/ml reached after 22 minutes following the same dose administered intramuscularly (Fig. 17-4). The oral bioavailability was only 16 percent,[28] which is exactly that predicted from a ketamine extraction ratio of 0.85, calculated from the intravenous clearance of ketamine and an estimate of hepatic blood flow. Plasma norketamine concentrations, normally less than those of ketamine for the 2 hours after parenteral administration, were substantially higher than ketamine con-

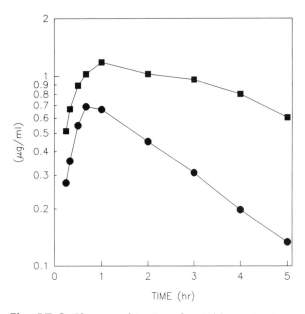

Fig. 17-3 Pharmacokinetics of rectal ketamine in children. Plasma concentrations of ketamine (●) and norketamine (■) are shown after rectal administration of ketamine (mean dose, 9 mg/kg) to eight children (mean age, 8 years). (Modified from Idvall et al.,[33] with permission.)

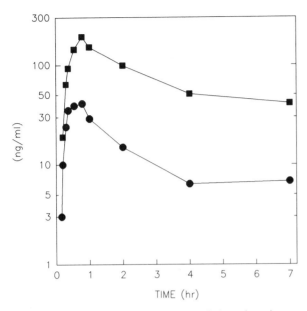

Fig. 17-4 Mean plasma ketamine (●) and norketamine (■) concentrations following administration of ketamine 0.5 mg/kg orally to six healthy volunteers. (Modified from Grant et al.,[28] with permission.)

centrations at all times after oral administration. Norketamine's contribution to ketamine analgesia was apparent because the plasma concentrations of ketamine (10 to 50 ng/ml) were far below the threshold for analgesia (150 ng/ml). These results indicate a substantial hepatic first-pass metabolism of ketamine prior to reaching the systemic circulation.

The data of Grant et al.[28] indicate an intrinsic hepatic clearance, as approximated from the oral clearance, of approximately 7 L/min. A similar finding was reported by Pedraz et al.,[37] who projected an unbound intrinsic hepatic clearance of 5.2 L/min. The high intrinsic clearance reflects the high rate of hepatic metabolism.

EPIDURAL ADMINISTRATION

The analgesic efficacy of neuraxial ketamine is controversial. Epidural ketamine (4 mg) administered postoperatively following lower abdominal, perineal, or lower extremity procedures, produced analgesia within 5 to 10 minutes, which was maximal within 15 to 30 minutes with a mean duration of 4

hours.[38] In contrast, two randomized investigations comparing epidural ketamine with epidural morphine found that 4 to 10 mg of ketamine was unable to relieve pain following gynecologic or lower extremity surgery.[39,40] Larger doses, however, have been efficacious in some studies. Following cholecystectomy, pain scores were reduced by both 10 mg and 30 mg of epidural ketamine, with a greater decrease produced by the higher dose.[41] In the study by Ravat et al.,[39] 30 mg of epidural ketamine provided analgesia in a setting in which 10 mg was inadequate. A comparison of 30 mg administered intramuscularly with 30 mg administered epidurally found a similar reduction of pain scores, although a longer duration was found in the patients who received epidural ketamine.[41]

The pharmacokinetics of epidural ketamine have been investigated in humans and dogs. In two groups of patients with normal hepatic and renal function, the disposition of 5 mg/kg of epidural ketamine was compared with that of 2 mg/kg administered as an intravenous bolus (Fig. 17-5).[4]

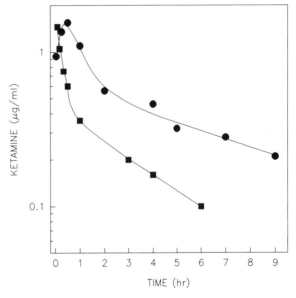

Fig. 17-5 Comparative pharmacokinetics of epidural and intravenous ketamine in humans. Plasma ketamine concentrations are shown following epidural (5 mg/kg, ●) and intravenous (2 mg/kg, ■) administration. (Modified from Pedraz et al.,[4] with permission.)

Epidural ketamine underwent rapid systemic absorption, reaching a maximum plasma concentration of 1.6 μg/ml 20 minutes after administration, which was above the threshold for analgesia. The rate of uptake following epidural administration was greater than that observed following intramuscular injection.[28] The systemic bioavailability was 77 percent of the dose, slightly less than that attained after intramuscular administration but substantially greater than that after oral administration. The apparent terminal plasma half-life of ketamine was significantly longer after epidural compared with intravenous administration, suggesting a rate-limiting slow release from the epidural space.[4]

A comparison of epidural and intravenous ketamine administration showed that peak plasma concentrations reached after epidural injection were similar to those attained after intravenous dosing (Fig. 17-5). The rapid systemic appearance of epidural ketamine suggested that the reported efficacy of high dose epidural ketamine (30 mg) may result from the significant plasma concentrations and systemic pharmacologic effects.[39] Thus, there appears to be no pharmacokinetic or therapeutic advantage to the epidural administration of ketamine compared with intravenous administration.

In dogs, epidural ketamine was rapidly absorbed across the dura into the cerebrospinal fluid (CSF).[42] Cervical CSF ketamine concentrations were maximal 30 minutes after epidural injection. CSF ketamine concentrations exceeded plasma concentrations at all times after 3 mg/kg of epidural ketamine was administered. Systemic absorption of epidural ketamine is also rapid, with the time to peak plasma concentrations similar to that reported for peak CSF concentrations. Because of facile systemic ketamine uptake, plasma concentrations were never less than one-half the CSF concentrations. The small plasma-CSF concentration difference for ketamine, a highly lipid-soluble drug, is in contrast to that observed following epidural administration of more water-soluble drugs, such as morphine. Following epidural administration, plasma morphine concentrations are approximately 20-fold less than are CSF morphine concentrations.[43]

The pharmacokinetics of ketamine administered intrathecally[44] or for intravenous regional anesthesia, both rare forms of administration, have not been studied. However, it is apparent that the plasma concentrations of ketamine following intravenous regional anesthesia are high, as evidenced by the loss of consciousness or psychotomimetic side effects experienced after tourniquet release.[45,46]

DISTRIBUTION AND PLASMA PROTEIN BINDING

The values reported for the initial volume of distribution (V_c) vary widely as a result of differences in blood sampling intervals and the compartmental models chosen for analysis. Nevertheless, the initial volume of distribution exceeds that of the intravascular space. The total apparent volume of distribution (V_{ss}) is large, indicating extensive tissue distribution, similar to that observed with other lipid-soluble intravenous anesthetics, such as barbiturates. The apparent volume during the elimination phase (V_β) overestimates V_{ss} because ketamine is rapidly cleared from the central compartment with a relatively short half-life.[47]

Ketamine is not highly bound to plasma proteins.[1,48,49] Dayton et al.[49] extensively studied ketamine binding to human plasma proteins. Ketamine binding in normal subjects averaged 27 percent but was as high as 47 percent in one patient. Ketamine was bound to both human serum albumin and α_1 acid glycoprotein. Although ketamine's affinity for α_1 acid glycoprotein is reported to be higher than for human serum albumin, the total binding at normal protein concentrations in the plasma is greater for albumin than for α_1 acid glycoprotein. The binding is dependent on the protein concentration, but it is independent of the concentration of ketamine. Ketamine's protein binding is pH dependent, with lower binding to albumin occurring at a lower pH. Pregnancy does not alter maternal ketamine plasma protein binding, but binding in the fetal plasma is substantially less (10 percent) than that in the maternal plasma (35 percent). There is no difference in the binding of racemic ketamine or ketamine enantiomers to α_1 acid glycoprotein. Norketamine, at 10-fold greater concentrations, does not displace ketamine from human serum albumin or from α_1 acid glycoprotein. In dogs, the protein binding of norketamine (60 percent) is similar to that of ketamine (54 percent).

The high extraction ratio and intrinsic hepatic clearance of ketamine, coupled with the relatively high free fraction of ketamine, implies that changes in plasma protein binding will have negligible effects on ketamine clearance.[50,51] Displacement of ketamine from plasma proteins will also have insignificant effects on the clearance.

CLEARANCE AND METABOLISM

Ketamine is cleared from the body almost exclusively by hepatic biotransformation with subsequent renal excretion of primary and secondary metabolites. Less than 3 percent of the dose is eliminated as the unchanged drug.[1] More than 90 percent of an intravenous dose is recovered in the urine, with less than 3 percent recovered in the feces.[52] Because ketamine is almost completely metabolized in the liver, systemic clearance (CL_S) is equivalent to total hepatic clearance (CL_H). The total hepatic clearance is the product of hepatic blood flow and the hepatic extraction ratio (ER), which describes the ability of the liver to extract a drug from blood perfusing the liver, represented as a fraction between 0 and 1.[53] The maximal ability of the liver to remove a drug in the absence of any limitations imposed by blood flow is the intrinsic hepatic clearance (CL_I), which reflects the capacity of hepatic biotransformation enzymes. From the "well-stirred" model relationship between CL_S, CL_H, and CL_I, for a hepatically cleared drug,

$$CL_S = CL_H = Q \cdot ER = Q \left[\frac{CL_I}{Q + CL_I} \right]$$

it is apparent that the hepatic clearance of the drug can be influenced by hepatic blood flow and intrinsic hepatic clearance.

Ketamine is a high-extraction drug with a high systemic clearance and a high intrinsic hepatic clearance. The systemic clearance in humans (16 to 20 ml/kg/min, Table 17-1) approaches that of the hepatic blood flow, with a hepatic extraction ratio of approximately 0.8. The intrinsic clearance, calculated from these clinical data and the foregoing equation is also high, roughly 6 to 8 L/min. Compounds with an extraction ratio exceeding 0.7 are considered high-extraction drugs. This mathematic relationship predicts that, for high-extraction drugs, hepatic clearance predominantly reflects hepatic blood flow, with a lesser dependence on intrinsic clearance. Consequently, systemic ketamine clearance will be sensitive to changes in hepatic blood flow but relatively less influenced by changes in hepatic metabolism. However, changes in hepatic metabolism can affect ketamine clearance and the bioavailability of ketamine following oral or rectal administration.[53]

METABOLISM

Ketamine is rapidly and extensively metabolized shortly after administration. As mentioned, more than 97 percent of an intravenous dose is metabolized prior to excretion.[1] The major biotransformation products are norketamine ("metabolite I" in early publications) and several hydroxylated norketamine metabolites (Fig. 17-6). Several early investigators of ketamine metabolism reported the formation of 5,6-dehydronorketamine, initially identified as "metabolite II."[1,9,54,55] Norketamine and 5,6-dehydronorketamine were considered by most investigators for several years to be the primary metabolites of ketamine. It is now well appreciated that 5,6-dehydronorketamine is not formed in the liver enzymatically but, rather, is an artifact of the plasma extraction and gas chromatography assay used originally to measure ketamine and its metabolites. Metabolite II is thus a "pseudometabolite," derived from the nonenzymatic dehydration of hydroxynorketamine metabolites, specifically, 5-hydroxynorketamine.[7,8] Whereas some investigators suspected initially that 5,6-dehydronorketamine could arise from either 5- or 6-hydroxynorketamine, it has since been shown conclusively that 6-hydroxynorketamine does not decompose to 5,6-dehydronorketamine.[7] Although it is a pseudometabolite, the quantitation of 5,6-de-

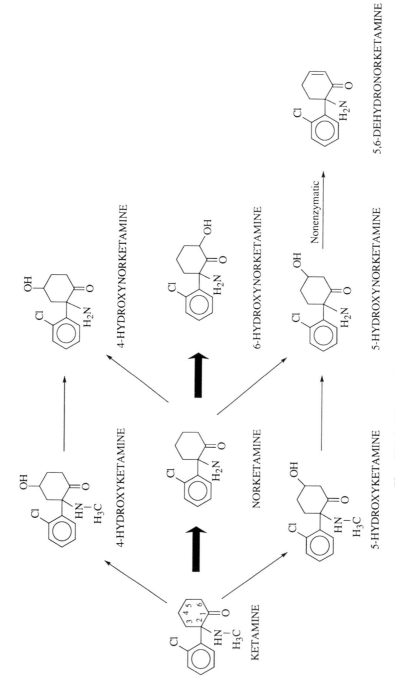

Fig. 17-6 Biotransformation of ketamine in humans.

hydronorketamine in the plasma is still used as an indirect measure of 5-hydroxynorketamine metabolite formation.[3,4,14,42,56,57] In humans, the cumulative excretion of norketamine and 5,6-dehydronorketamine is 2 percent and 16 percent, respectively, of an administered ketamine dose.[1] The remaining 80 percent is thought to be glucuronic acid conjugates of hydroxynorketamine metabolites.[1,9] The apparent terminal half-lives of norketamine and 5,6-dehydronorketamine are approximately 4 and 7 hours, respectively, compared with 2 to 3 hours for ketamine.[1]

Ketamine is metabolized by cytochrome P-450, primarily in the liver, although extrahepatic metabolism, specifically in the lung, has been reported.[58] There is no evidence for ketamine metabolism in the brain.[17] Hepatic microsomal ketamine metabolism in vitro has been studied extensively.[59] The major pathways of ketamine metabolism are shown in Figure 17-6.[8] N-demethylation to norketamine is the major pathway of biotransformation. Norketamine undergoes further metabolism, with hydroxylation at positions 4, 5, and 6 on the cyclohexanone ring, forming 4-, 5-, and 6-hydroxynorketamine. These are subsequently conjugated to form water-soluble glucuronides, which are renally excreted. Human and rodent hepatic microsomes preferentially hydroxylate norketamine at the 6 position. Thus, 6-hydroxynorketamine is the major hydroxylated ketamine metabolite formed.[7,8] Ketamine itself can be hydroxylated on the cyclohexanone ring, forming 4-, 5-, and 6-hydroxyketamine. Human hepatic microsomes selectively hydroxylate at the 4 position; rat hepatic microsomes form predominantly 5-hydroxyketamine.[7,8] Hydroxylation of the parent compound is, however, a quantitatively insignificant pathway of metabolism. Ketamine is not metabolized on the aromatic ring, and phenolic metabolites are not formed. Hydroxylation on the cyclohexanone ring introduces a second chiral center (see discussion on stereochemistry later) in the molecule. Both isomers of 5-hydroxynorketamine are formed by rodent and human hepatic microsomes.[7,8] In contrast, hydroxylation of norketamine in the 6 position is stereoselective. The (Z)-6-hydroxynorketamine (the cis-diastereomer) is formed ex-

clusively, with no formation of the (E)- or trans-diastereomer).

Human hepatic ketamine metabolism has been studied in vitro.[60–62] There are at least two isoforms of cytochrome P-450 that are capable of catalyzing ketamine N-demethylation, although the activity of only one predominates at therapeutic ketamine concentrations.[61] The identity of these P-450 isoforms is not yet known.

SPEED OF ONSET

Following intravenous administration, the onset of anesthesia (hypnosis) occurs within 1 minute. A rapid penetration into the brain accounts for the swift speed of onset. Ketamine concentrations in the brain peak within 1 minute after intravenous injection and decline rapidly in parallel with the concentration in the plasma.[12,17,18] The drug's accessibility to the central nervous system is a result of its high lipid solubility. Ketamine is a tertiary amine with a pK_a of 7.5, so that nearly one-half of the drug exists in the more lipid soluble un-ionized form at physiologic pH.[10] Furthermore, ketamine has an extremely high organic solvent/buffer partition coefficient, conferring a lipid solubility 5 to 10 times greater than that of thiopental.[10] Ketamine preferentially accumulates in brain tissue, at concentrations 2 to 6 times those in the plasma or surrounding medium.[10,11,17,18,63] Ketamine's enhancement of cerebral blood flow may augment the rapid brain entry already afforded by the high lipid solubility of the drug.[17]

Norketamine appears in the brain within 1 minute after ketamine injection.[17] This metabolite is only slightly less lipid soluble than is ketamine, and with a pK_a of 6.6, an even greater fraction than ketamine exists in the lipid-soluble un-ionized form.[10] Like ketamine, norketamine accumulates in the brain, reaching concentrations exceeding those in the plasma.[10,11,17] Following intravenous ketamine administration, norketamine concentrations in the brain continue to rise for several minutes while ketamine concentrations in the plasma decline.[10,12] Although norketamine is pharmacologically active, cerebral norketamine penetration probably contributes minimally to hypnosis after intravenous ketamine because norketamine concentrations in the brain after intravenous ketamine are substantially less than those required to cause hypnosis.[10,12] Norketamine may however contribute to the onset of clinical effects after enteral ketamine administration as a result of significant first-pass metabolism.

Less information is available regarding the speed of onset following routes of administration other than intravenous. In adults, a subhypnotic ke-

tamine dose of 0.5 mg/kg increased pain thresholds within 15 minutes of intramuscular injection.[28] In children, 5 mg/kg of intramuscular ketamine produced nystagmus within 2 to 4 minutes of injection and unconsciousness within 5 minutes.[64] Also in children, rectal ketamine (5 to 10 mg/kg) produced unconsciousness in 7 to 15 minutes.[33,35] The onset following oral ketamine is dose dependent. Doses of 3 or 6 mg/kg in children produced sedation within 11 to 12 minutes and maxi-

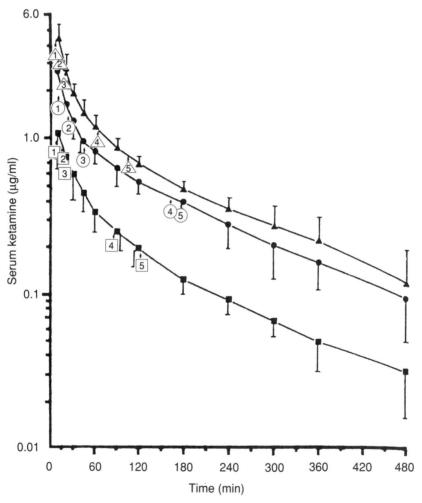

Fig. 17-7 Venous serum concentrations of ketamine (mean ± standard deviation) after infusion of racemic ketamine (●), S(+) ketamine (■), or R(−) ketamine (▲). The arrows indicate the time of awakening, for example, opened eyes (1); ability to follow simple command, for example, squeezed hand (2); orientation to person, place, and time (3); and return to predrug scores for Treiger (4) and symbol-digit (5) tests. (From White et al.,[15] with permission.)

mal sedation in 20 minutes.[65] A lower oral dose (0.5 mg/kg) in adults produced analgesia after 30 minutes.[28]

DURATION OF ACTION

The duration of ketamine anesthesia will be determined by the brain's concentrations of ketamine and norketamine, as reflected by plasma concentrations, and the time course of these concentration changes (Fig. 17-7). Table 17-2 summarizes plasma ketamine concentration thresholds for surgical anesthesia, awakening, return of psychomotor function, and analgesia. The termination of pharmacologic effects is influenced both by ketamine redistribution and biotransformation.

Termination of hypnosis following an intravenous bolus occurs at relatively high concentrations (0.6 to 1.1 μg/ml), during the initial phase of the plasma concentration-time curve. The primary mechanism is rapid redistribution (intercompartmental clearance) from the brain to peripheral tissues. There is also a contribution of metabolic

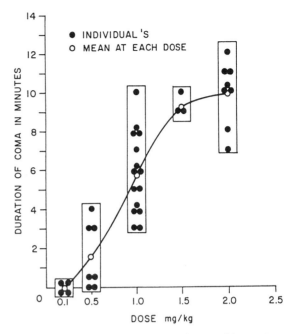

Fig. 17-8 Effects of increasing doses of ketamine on duration of hypnosis. (From Domino et al.,[83] with permission.)

Table 17-2 Therapeutic Plasma Ketamine Concentrations in Adults[a]

| Clinical Effect | Dose | Racemic Ketamine | | S(+) Ketamine | | R(−) Ketamine | | Reference |
		Ketamine	Norketamine	Ketamine	Norketamine	Ketamine	Norketamine	
Surgical anesthesia (with 65 percent nitrous oxide, during abdominal surgery)	IV infusion	2.2	0.4–1.1					73
Surgical anesthesia (with 70 percent nitrous oxide, during superficial surgery)	IV infusion	1.1	0.4					21
Awakening	IV infusion	0.6	~0.7					73
	IV bolus	0.7–1.1	~0.2					54
	IV bolus	0.9	0.6	0.5	0.15	1.7	0.5	5
Return of psychomotor scores to baseline	IV infusion	0.4	ND	0.2	ND	1.0	ND	15
Analgesia	IV bolus	0.1–0.2	ND					13
	IM	0.15	0.055					28
	PO	0.04	0.16					28

Abbreviations: ND, not determined.

[a] All concentrations are in micrograms per milliliter.

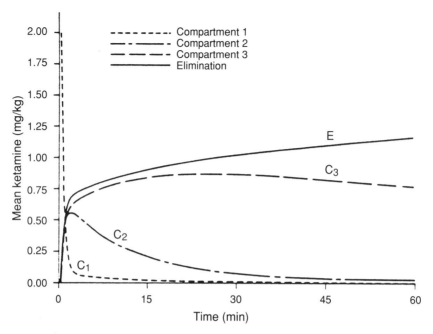

Fig. 17-9 Estimated amounts of ketamine in each compartment of a three compartment open model. Note rapid reduction of ketamine concentration in compartment 1. Compartment 2 levels peak within 2 minutes and decline over 30 or more minutes. In contrast, compartment 3 accumulates ketamine with rapid elimination of approximately one-half the dose in the first 30 minutes. (From Domino et al.,[2] with permission.)

clearance to the termination of hypnosis,[1,2,18,21] although the precise magnitude of this contribution is not known. The duration of hypnosis following typical ketamine induction doses is shown in Figure 17-8. Figure 17-9 shows the computer-predicted ketamine concentration in compartment 2, thought to include the brain, which declines coincident with emergence from anesthesia.[2] Like other lipid-soluble drugs whose pharmacologic effect is terminated by redistribution, most of the ketamine dose is still present in the body when patients awaken.

Termination of analgesia following an intravenous bolus occurs at much lower plasma ketamine concentrations, during the shallow portion of the plasma disappearance curve. Termination results predominantly from hepatic metabolism during this elimination phase. The predominant role of metabolic clearance in the termination of analgesia at lower plasma ketamine concentrations and at later times after injection is also apparent from Figure 17-9.

KETAMINE ENANTIOMERS

Ketamine contains an asymmetric carbon atom and is thus a chiral compound. It is used clinically as a racemate, the equal mixture of optically active enantiomers; however, the S(+) and R(−) enantiomers differ in their pharmacokinetic and pharmacodynamic properties. The analgesic and hypnotic potency of S(+) ketamine is approximately four times greater than that of the R(−) isomer, which is only a partial agonist.[15,66,67] In contrast, psychic emergence reactions and agitated behavior are far less common with S(+) ketamine than with its R(−) antipode or with the racemate.[5,15]

Recent improvements in synthetic and chromatographic techniques now afford a better understanding of ketamine enantiomer pharmacokinetics (Table 17-3). White et al.[15] first described the kinetic behavior of ketamine enantiomers in humans. When the enantiomers were administered individually, the plasma clearance of S(+) ketamine was 22 percent greater than that of the

Table 17-3 Pharmacokinetics of Ketamine Enantiomers[a]

Design	Dose	Assay	$t_{1/2\alpha}$(min)	$t_{1/2\beta}$(min)	CL(ml/kg/min)	V_{ss}	V_c	V_β	Reference
Three-way crossover ketamine infusion (n=5)	3.7 mg/kg RS	Nonselective	13 ± 9	132 ± 32	16.1 ± 4.6		1.0 ± 0.4	2.9 ± 0.5	15
	1.9 mg/kg S(+)		23 ± 15	158 ± 45	21.3 ± 1.6		1.6 ± 0.7	4.7 ± 1.1	
	5.7 mg/kg R(−)		12 ± 9	155 ± 42	17.4 ± 2.5		0.9 ± 0.7	3.9 ± 1.3	
Two-way crossover ketamine infusion (n=10)	0.2 μg/kg/min RS	Nonselective		76 ± 18	15.7 ± 1.5		0.27 ± 0.07		68
	0.1 μg/kg/min S(+)			74 ± 19	18.5 ± 1.1		0.35 ± 0.10		
Parallel groups ketamine bolus	2.0 mg/kg RS (n=24)	S(+) selective		149 ± 48	19.1 ± 7.2	3.3 ± 1.3			16
		R(−) selective		155 ± 57	16.5 ± 4.8	3.0 ± 1.2			
	1.0 mg/kg S(+) (n=10)	S(+) selective		143 ± 76	16.4 ± 5.7	2.8 ± 1.6			

Abbreviations: CL, clearance; $t_{1/2\alpha}$, distribution half-life; $t_{1/2\beta}$, elimination half-life; V_β, elimination phase volume of distribution; V_C, initial volume of distribution; V_{ss}, steady-state volume of distribution.
[a] All values are mean ± standard deviation.

R(−) enantiomer, although this difference was not statistically significant. Similarly, anesthetic recovery from racemic ketamine was significantly slower than recovery from either of the individual enantiomers. Geisslinger et al.[16] recently showed, using a stereoselective assay, that when the racemate was administered, the clearance of S(+) ketamine was significantly greater (15 percent) than that of R(−) ketamine. Schüttler et al.[68] compared the disposition of S(+) ketamine with that of the racemate in normal volunteers and found a greater clearance of the single enantiomer compared with the racemate.

The apparent mechanism for differences in ketamine enantiomer clearance was explained by Kharasch and Labroo.[61] They studied human hepatic microsomal ketamine N-demethylation and found that the rate of S(+) ketamine demethylation was greater than that of either R(−) ketamine or the racemate. In addition, an interaction was observed whereby R(−) ketamine inhibited the demethylation of the more rapidly metabolized S(+) enantiomer.

Stereoselective differences in ketamine enantiomer pharmacokinetics and metabolism were first observed in rodents.[69,70] Preferential accumulation in the brain of S(+) norketamine compared with racemic and R(−) norketamine was observed in rats and mice. Differences in the pharmacologic effects of norketamine enantiomers[71] may contribute to those of the parent compounds. Rodent livers, like human livers, demethylated ketamine enantiomers at different rates.

HEPATIC AND RENAL DISEASE

As a high-extraction drug, the clearance of ketamine should be relatively insensitive to changes in intrinsic hepatic clearance,[53] which for ketamine, is roughly equivalent to hepatic metabolism. This has also been observed clinically. No significant differences were found in the infusion rate required for anesthesia[72] or in the metabolism of ketamine in patients with hepatic insufficiency compared with those with normal hepatic function.[73] Thus, ketamine dosing need not be altered in patients with moderate hepatocellular disease.

Because unchanged ketamine undergoes negligible urinary excretion, renal insufficiency a priori would not be expected to influence the elimination of ketamine or its metabolism. Patients with acute renal failure who received ketamine infusions for 3 days had steady-state plasma ketamine and norketamine concentrations that were not different from those of patients with normal renal function.[57] However, 5,6-dehydronorketamine plasma concentrations (representing 5-hydroxynorketamine) were significantly greater in renal failure. This most likely represents diminished renal excretion of this metabolite and its water-soluble glucuronide rather than increased hepatic formation. Because hydroxynorketamine metabolites possess minimal pharmacologic activity,[12,19] there is no apparent need to alter the dose of ketamine in patients with impaired renal function. In contrast, in rabbits with experimentally induced renal impairment, the metabolism of ketamine to norketamine and 5-hydroxynorketamine was impaired, and plasma concentrations of both ketamine and 5,6-dehydronorketamine (but not norketamine) were elevated compared with those in rabbits with normal renal function.[56] These animal data suggest that doses used for long-term infusions should be evaluated periodically and readjusted if necessary. The discrepancy between animal and human data for renal failure effects on intravenous ketamine disposition has not yet been resolved.

DRUG INTERACTIONS

Although ketamine is a high-extraction drug, alterations in hepatic microsomal enzyme activity can influence ketamine disposition and the duration of effect in humans and animals. The induction of hepatic P-450 activity can increase the metabolism and excretion of ketamine. Enzyme induction by chronic phenobarbital treatment in rats increased ketamine N-demethylation in vitro, diminished brain and plasma ketamine concentrations in vivo, and shortened the duration of the pharmacologic effect.[10,18] In phenobarbital-induced patients who received ketamine infusions for 3 days, steady-state plasma ketamine concentrations were one-third those in controls who received the same dose.[57] Chronic treatment with phenobarbital or diazepam reduced the elimination half-life of ketamine and increased its metabolism, as evidenced by higher plasma hydroxynorketamine concentrations.[14] Ketamine may also induce its own metabolism[18] and the metabolism of other drugs.[74,75] The clinical significance of chronic ketamine induction of drug metabolism in humans, if any, is not known. For example, sequential pharmacokinetics in pediatric patients undergoing frequent ketamine anesthesia for radiologic procedures has not been examined.

Inhibition of hepatic enzyme activity alters ketamine disposition and the duration of effect; this is seen most commonly after concomitant administration of drugs that compete for or otherwise inhibit the activity of hepatic cytochrome P-450.[10] The most studied interaction is that between ketamine and benzodiazepines, which are used today almost ubiquitously to ameliorate the psychomimetic side effects of ketamine.[76–79] Pediatric patients pretreated with intramuscular diazepam (0.15 mg/kg) 30 minutes before induction with intramuscular ketamine (10 mg/kg) had a longer duration of hypnosis and prolonged ketamine half-life compared with untreated controls.[80] Similarly, ketamine metabolism was diminished and the plasma half-life was prolonged compared with controls in adults given rectal diazepam 1 hour before anesthesia with intravenous ketamine (2 mg/kg for induction and 2 to 3 mg/min by infusion).[14] Compared with untreated controls, patients pretreated with diazepam (0.3 mg/kg) 10 minutes before induction with ketamine (2.2 mg/kg IV) showed higher plasma ketamine concentrations for the 30 minutes following induction and a slightly diminished ketamine clearance.[3] Thus, there is a significant metabolic interaction between diazepam and ketamine. More recent investigations have examined the combination of midazolam and ketamine.[78,79] The half-life of ketamine in patients receiving a midazolam-ketamine infusion was significantly shorter than the half-life in those receiving a diazepam-ketamine infusion,[79] suggesting that midazolam may have a smaller effect on the metabolism and disposition of ketamine.

Other classes of anesthetics have also been shown to interact kinetically with ketamine. Halothane, which noncompetitively inhibited ketamine N-demethylation in vitro, increased the half-lifes of ketamine in the brain and plasma in vivo and prolonged the pharmacologic effect.[19] Ketamine metabolism was also inhibited by etomidate in vitro, but etomidate had no effect on ketamine disposition in vivo.[81,82]

PEDIATRIC PHARMACOKINETICS

Unfortunately, there is little information regarding the pharmacokinetics of intravenous ketamine in children. One study found that intramuscular ketamine was more rapidly absorbed, exhibited earlier peaks in plasma concentration, was eliminated faster, and produced faster recovery in children compared with adults.[30] Oral ketamine kinetics in children were described earlier in this chapter.

REFERENCES

1. Wieber J, Gugler R, Hengstmann JH, Dengler HJ: Pharmacokinetics of ketamine in man. Anaesthesist 24:260, 1975
2. Domino EF, Zsigmond EK, Domino LE et al: Plasma levels of ketamine and two of its metabolites in surgical patients using a gas chromatographic mass fragmentographic assay. Anesth Analg 61:87, 1982
3. Domino EF, Domino SE, Smith RE et al: Ketamine kinetics in unmedicated and diazepam-premedicated subjects. Clin Pharmacol Ther 36:645, 1984
4. Pedraz JL, Lanao JM, Calvo MB et al: Pharmacokinetic and clinical evaluation of ketamine administered by i.v. and epidural routes. Int J Clin Pharmacol Ther Toxicol 25:77, 1987
5. White PF, Ham J, Way WL, Trevor AJ: Pharmacology of ketamine isomers in surgical patients. Anesthesiology 52:231, 1980
6. Geisslinger G, Menzel-Soglowek S, Kamp H-D, Brune K: Stereoselective high-performance liquid chromatographic determination of the enantiomers of ketamine and norketamine in plasma. J Chromatogr 568:165, 1991
7. Woolf TF, Adams JD: Biotransformation of ketamine, (Z)-6-hydroxyketamine, and (E)-6-hydroxyketamine by rat, rabbit, and human liver microsomal preparations. Xenobiotica 17:839, 1987
8. Adams JD Jr, Baillie TA, Trevor AJ, Castagnoli N Jr: Studies on the biotransformation of ketamine. 1. Identification of metabolites produced in vitro from rat liver microsomal preparations. Biomed Mass Spectrom 8:527, 1981
9. Chang T, Glazko AJ: Biotransformation and disposition of ketamine. Int Anesthesiol Clin 12:157, 1974
10. Cohen ML, Trevor AJ: On the cerebral accumulation of ketamine and the relationship between metabolism of the drug and its pharmacological effects. J Pharmacol Exp Ther 189:351, 1974
11. White PF, Johnston RR, Pudwill CR: Interaction of ketamine and halothane in rats. Anesthesiology 42:179, 1975
12. Leung LY, Baillie TA: Comparative pharmacology in the rat of ketamine and its two principal metabolites, norketamine and (Z)-6-hydroxynorketamine. J Med Chem 29:2396, 1986
13. Clements JA, Nimmo WS: Pharmacokinetics and analgesic effect of ketamine in man. Br J Anaesth 53:27, 1981
14. Idvall J, Aronsen KF, Stenberg P, Paalzow L: Pharmacodynamic and pharmacokinetic interactions between ketamine and diazepam. Eur J Clin Pharmacol 24:337, 1983
15. White PF, Schüttler J, Shafer A et al: Comparative pharmacology of the ketamine isomers. Br J Anaesth 57:197, 1985
16. Geisslinger G, Hering W, Thomann P et al: Pharmacokinetics and pharmacodynamics of ketamine enantiomers using a stereoselective analytical method. Br J Anaesth 70:666, 1993
17. Cohen ML, Chan S-L, Way WL, Trevor AJ: Distribution in the brain and metabolism of ketamine in the rat after intravenous administration. Anesthesiology 39:370, 1973
18. Marietta MP, White PF, Pudwill CR et al: Biodisposition of ketamine in the rat: self-induction of metabolism. J Pharmacol Exp Ther 196:536, 1976
19. White PF, Marietta MP, Pudwill CR et al: Effects of halothane anesthesia on the biodisposition of ketamine in rats. J Pharmacol Exp Ther 196:545, 1976
20. White PF: Use of continuous infusion versus intermittent bolus administration of fentanyl or ketamine during outpatient anesthesia. Anesthesiology 59:294, 1983
21. White PF, Dworsky WA, Horai Y, Trevor AJ: Comparison of continuous infusion fentanyl or ketamine versus thiopental—determining the mean effective serum concentrations for outpatient surgery. Anesthesiology 59:564, 1983
22. Kawamata M, Ujike Y, Miyabe M et al: Continuous infusion of ketamine and midazolam for prolonged sedation in the intensive care unit. Masui 40:1793, 1991
23. Matsuki A, Ishihara H, Kotani N et al: A clinical study on total intravenous anesthesia with droperidol, fentanyl and ketamine—2. Pharmacokinetics following the end of continuous ketamine infusion. Masui 40:61, 1991
24. Kudo T, Kudo M, Ishihara H et al: Clinical study on total intravenous anesthesia with droperidol, fentanyl and ketamine—3. Pharmacokinetics during prolonged continuous ketamine infusion. Masui 40:179, 1991
25. Mayer M, Ochmann O, Doenicke A et al: The effect of propofol-ketamine anesthesia on hemodynamics and analgesia in comparison with propofol-fentanyl. Anaesthesist 39:609, 1990
26. Schüttler J, Schüttler M, Kloos S et al: Optimierte dosierungsstrategien fur die totale intravenose

anaesthesie mit propofol und ketamin. Anaesthesist 40:199, 1991

27. Wyant GM: Intramuscular ketalar (CI-581) in paediatric anaesthesia. Can J Anaesth 18:72, 1971

28. Grant IS, Nimmo WS, Clements JA: Pharmacokinetics and analgesic effects of i.m. and oral ketamine. Br J Anaesth 53:805, 1981

29. Loscher W, Ganter M, Fassbender CP: Correlation between drug and metabolite concentrations in plasma and anesthetic action of ketamine in swine. Am J Vet Res 51:391, 1990

30. Grant IS, Nimmo WS, McNichol LR, Clements JA: Ketamine disposition in children and adults. Br J Anaesth 55:1107, 1983

31. Saint-Maurice C, Laguenie G, Couturier C, Goutail-Flaud F: Rectal ketamine in paediatric anaesthesia. Br J Anaesth 51:573, 1979

32. Cetina J: Schonende narkoseeinleitung bei kindern durch orale oder rektale ketamin-dehydrobenzperidol-applikation. Anaesthesist 31:277, 1982

33. Idvall J, Holasek J, Stenberg P: Rectal ketamine for induction of anaesthesia in children. Anaesthesia 38:60, 1983

34. Pedraz JL, Calvo MB, Lanao JM et al: Phamacokinetics of rectal ketamine in children. Br J Anaesth 63:671, 1989

35. Holm-Knudsen R, Sjogren P, Laub M: Midazolam und ketamin zur rektalen prämedikation und narkoseeinleitung bei kindern. Anaesthesist 39:255, 1990

36. Jantzen JP, Diehl P: Die rektale medikamentenverabreichung. Grundlagen und anwendung in der anaesthesie. Anaesthesist 40:251, 1991

37. Pedraz JL, Lanao JM, Dominguez-Gil A: Interspecies pharmacokinetics of ketamine. p. 285. In Domino EF (ed): Status of Ketamine in Anesthesiology. NPP Books, Ann Arbor, 1990

38. Islas JA, Astorga J, Laredo M: Epidural ketamine for control of postoperative pain. Anesth Analg 64:1161, 1985

39. Ravat F, Dorne R, Baechle JP et al: Epidural ketamine or morphine for postoperative analgesia. Anesthesiology 66:819, 1987

40. Kawana Y, Sato H, Shimada H et al: Epidural ketamine for postoperative pain relief after gynecologic operations: a double-blind study and comparison with epidural morphine. Anesth Analg 66:735, 1987

41. Naguib M, Adu-Gyamfi Y, Absood GH et al: Epidural ketamine for postoperative analgesia. Can J Anaesth 33:16, 1986

42. Pedraz JL, Calvo MB, Gascon AR et al: Pharmaco-

kinetics and distribution of ketamine after extradural administration to dogs. Br J Anaesth 67:310, 1991

43. Durant PAC, Yaksh TL: Distribution in cerebrospinal fluid, blood, and lymph of epidurally injected morphine and inulin in dogs. Anesth Analg 65:583, 1986

44. Bion JF: Intrathecal ketamine for war surgery. A preliminary study under field conditions. Anaesthesia 39:1023, 1984

45. Amiot JF, Bouju P, Palacci JH, Balliner E: Intravenous regional anaesthesia with ketamine. Anaesthesia 40:899, 1985

46. Durrani Z, Winnie AP, Zsigmond EK, Burnett ML: Ketamine for intravenous regional anesthesia. Anesth Analg 68:328, 1989

47. Gibaldi M, Perrier D: Pharmacokinetics. Marcel Dekker, New York, 1982

48. Kaka JS, Hayton WL: Pharmacokinetics of ketamine and two metabolites in dog. J Pharmacokinet Biopharm 8:193, 1980

49. Dayton PG, Stiller RL, Cook DR, Perel JM: The binding of ketamine to plasma proteins: emphasis on human plasma. Eur J Clin Pharmacol 24:825, 1983

50. Wilkinson GR: Clearance approaches in pharmacology. Pharmacol Rev 39:1, 1987

51. Wood M: Plasma drug binding: implications for anesthesiologists. Anesth Analg 65:786, 1986

52. Chang T, Savory A, Albin M et al: Metabolic disposition of tritium-labelled ketamine in normal human subjects. Clin Res 18:597, 1970

53. Wilkinson GR, Shand DG: A physiologic approach to hepatic drug clearance. Clin Pharmacol Ther 18:377, 1975

54. Little B, Chang T, Chucot L et al: Study of ketamine as an obstetric anesthetic agent. Am J Obstet Gynecol 113:247, 1972

55. Chang T, Glazko AJ: A gas chromatographic assay for ketamine in human plasma. Anesthesiology 36:401, 1972

56. Pedraz JL, Lanao JM, Dominguez-Gil A: Kinetics of ketamine and its metabolites in rabbits with normal and impaired renal function. Eur J Drug Metab Pharmacokinet 10:33, 1985

57. Koppel C, Arndt I, Ibe K: Effects of enzyme induction, renal and cardiac function on ketamine plasma kinetics in patients with ketamine long-term analgosedation. Eur J Drug Metab Pharmacokinet 15:259, 1990

58. Pedraz JL, Lanao JM, Hdez JM, Dominguez-Gil A: The biotransformation kinetics of ketamine "in vitro" in rabbit liver and lung microsome fractions. Eur J Drug Metab Pharmacokinet 11:9, 1986

59. Trevor AJ: Biotransformation of ketamine. p. 93. In Domino EF (ed): Status of Ketamine in Anesthesiology. NPP Books, Ann Arbor, 1990

60. Trevor AJ, Woolf TF, Baillie TA et al: Stereoselective metabolism of ketamine enantiomers. p. 279. In Kamenka JM, Domino EF, Geneste P (ed): Phencyclidine and Related Arylcyclohexylamines: Present and Future Applications. NPP Books, Ann Arbor, 1983

61. Kharasch ED, Labroo R: Metabolism of ketamine stereoisomers by human liver microsomes. Anesthesiology 77:1201, 1992

62. Kharasch ED, Herrmann S, Labroo R: Ketamine as a probe for medetomidine stereoisomer inhibition of human liver drug metabolism. Anesthesiology 77:1208, 1992

63. Gole DJ, French J, Houser J, Domino EF: Plasma ketamine: relation to brain concentrations and the hippocampal electroencephalogram. p. 297. In Domino EF (ed): Status of Ketamine in Anesthesiology. NPP Books, Ann Arbor, 1990

64. Bennett JA, Bullimore JA: The use of ketamine hydrochloride anaesthesia for radiotherapy in young children. Br J Anaesth 45:197, 1973

65. Gutstein HB, Johnson KL, Heard MB, Gregory GA: Oral ketamine preanesthetic medication in children. Anesthesiology 76:28, 1992

66. Schüttler J, Stanski DR, White PF et al: Pharmacodynamic modeling of the EEG effects of ketamine and its enantiomers in man. J Pharmacokinet Biopharm 15:241, 1987

67. Klepstad P, Maurset A, Moberg ER, Oye I: Evidence of a role for NMDA receptors in pain perception. Eur J Pharmacol 187:513, 1990

68. Schüttler J, Kloos S, Ihmsen H, Pelzer E: Pharmacokinetic/-dynamic properties of S(+)-ketamine vs. racemic ketamine: a randomized double-blind study in volunteers. Anesthesiology 77:A330, 1993

69. Ryder S, Way WL, Trevor AJ: Comparative pharmacology of the optical isomers of ketamine in mice. Eur J Pharmacol 49:15, 1978

70. Marietta MP, Way WL, Castagnoli N, Trevor AJ: On the pharmacology of the ketamine enantiomorphs in rats. J Pharmacol Exp Ther 202:157, 1977

71. Hong SC, Davisson JN: Stereochemical studies of demethylated ketamine enantiomers. J Pharm Sci 71:912, 1982

72. Schaps D, Hauenschild E: Anwendung von ketamin bei lebergeschädigten patienten. Anaesthesist 26:172, 1977

73. Idvall J, Ahlgren I, Aronsen KF, Stenberg P: Ketamine infusions: pharmacokinetics and clinical effects. Br J Anaesth 51:1167, 1979

74. Marietta MP, Vore ME, Way WL, Trevor AJ: Characterization of ketamine induction of hepatic microsomal drug metabolism. Biochem Pharmacol 26:2451, 1977

75. Kammerer RC, Schmitz DA, Hwa JJ, Cho AK: Induction of phencyclidine metabolism by phencyclidine, ketamine, ethanol, phenobarbital and isosafrole. Biochem Pharmacol 33:599, 1984

76. Coppel DL, Bovill JG, Dundee JW: The taming of ketamine. Anaesthesia 28:293, 1973

77. Dundee JW, Lilburn JK: Ketamine-lorazepam. Attenuation of psychic sequelae of ketamine by lorazepam. Anaesthesia 33:312, 1978

78. Cartwright PD, Pingel SM: Midazolam and diazepam in ketamine anaesthesia. Anaesthesia 39:439, 1984

79. Toft P, Romer U: Comparison of midazolam and diazepam to supplement total intravenous anaesthesia with ketamine for endoscopy. Can J Anaesth 34:466, 1987

80. Lo JN, Cumming, JF: Interaction between sedative premedicants and ketamine in man and in isolated perfused rat livers. Anesthesiology 43:307, 1975

81. Horai Y, White PF, Trevor AJ: Effect of etomidate on rabbit liver microsomal drug metabolism in vitro. Drug Metab Dispos 13:364, 1985

82. Atiba JO, Horai Y, White PF et al: Effect of etomidate on hepatic drug metabolism in humans. Anesthesiology 68:920, 1988

83. Domino EF, Chodoff P, Corssen G: Pharmacologic effects of CI-581, a new dissociative anesthetic, in man. Clin Pharmacol Ther 6:279, 1965

Chapter 18

Clinical Pharmacology and Applications of Ketamine

Noor Gajraj and Paul F. White

Ketamine was synthesized in the 1960s and its pharmacology was reported in detail by Domino et al.[1] in 1965. Although approved for general clinical use in 1970, the clinical usefulness of ketamine has been limited because of its cardiovascular-stimulating properties and high incidence of psychomimetic emergence reactions. However, supplementation with other drugs, such as the benzodiazepines, has reduced the incidence of these side effects, and ketamine remains a valuable drug for use in selected situations (Tables 18-1 and 18-2). The clinical pharmacology and therapeutic uses of ketamine were initially reviewed in 1982[2] and updated in 1989.[3]

CLINICAL PHARMACOLOGY

Optical Isomers of Ketamine

The commercially available ketamine solutions contain equal amounts of two isomers, S(+) and R(−) ketamine (Fig. 18-1). In animal studies, the S(+) isomer was shown to have a higher therapeutic index, produce more profound sedation and analgesia, and cause less excitatory activity than the R(−) isomer.[4,5]

In a randomized double-blind clinical study, the S(+) isomer of ketamine produced more effective anesthesia than did either the racemic mixture or the R(−) isomer.[6] Quantification of verbal responses in the postanesthetic period suggested that R(−) ketamine was associated with more agitation and psychic emergence reactions than was the racemic compound or S(+) ketamine. A study in healthy young volunteers indicated that S(+) ketamine was three to five times more potent in terms of its anesthetic effects.[7] However, both isomers produced similar degrees of cardiovascular stimulation and psychomimetic activity. The pharmacokinetic variables for the ketamine isomers did not differ from those for the racemic mixture. Pharmacodynamic modeling of the electroencephalographic (EEG) effects of ketamine and its enantomers revealed that R(−) ketamine was less effective than racemic or S(+) ketamine in causing EEG slowing (Fig. 18-2).[8] These data suggest that the R(−) isomer may function as a partial agonist (or an agonist-antagonist) with respect to its effect on the central nervous system (CNS).

Given the minor qualitative differences between the ketamine isomers with regard to their side effects, the American pharmaceutical industry has been reluctant to pursue further studies with S(+) ketamine. However, S(+) ketamine is currently be-

Table 18-1 Clinical Uses of Ketamine in the Practice of Anesthesiology

Induction of anesthesia in high risk patients
  Shock or cardiovascular instability
  Severe dehydration
  Bronchospasm
  Severe anemia
  One-lung anesthesia

Obstetric patients
  Induction of general anesthesia
    Severe hypovolemia
    Acute hemorrhage
    Acute bronchospasm
  Low dose for analgesia
    To supplement regional anesthetic techniques
  At the time of delivery or during the postpartum period

Adjunct to local and regional anesthetic techniques
  For sedation and analgesia during performance of nerve block procedures
  To supplement an inadequate block

Outpatient surgery
  For brief diagnostic and therapeutic procedures
  To supplement local and regional block techniques

Uses outside the operating room
  In burn units (e.g., débridement, dressing changes)
  In emergency rooms (e.g., closed reductions)
  In intensive care units (e.g., sedation, painful procedures)
  In recovery rooms (e.g., postoperative sedation and analgesia)

Table 18-2 Contraindications to Use of Ketamine

Cardiovascular disease
  Poorly controlled hypertension
  Intracranial, thoracic, or abdominal aneurysms
  Unstable angina or recent myocardial infarction
  Right or left heart failure[a]

Central nervous system disorders
  Cerebral trauma
  Intracerebral mass or hemorrhage

Open globe injury to eye or increased intraocular pressure[a]

Thyrotoxic states[a]

Otolaryngologic procedures involving pharynx, larynx, or trachea[a]

Psychiatric disorders (e.g., schizophrenia or history of adverse reactions to ketamine or one of its congeners[a])

[a] Indicates a relative contraindication to the use of ketamine.

ing developed for clinical use in Europe. It is possible that a structural analog of S(+) ketamine could prove to be a clinically useful anesthetic.

Effects of Ketamine on Central Nervous System

Ketamine produces a "dissociated" anesthetic state that has been described as a functional and electrophysiologic dissociation between the thalamo-

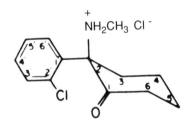

S, (+) - Ketamine hydrochloride   R,(-) - Ketamine hydrochloride

Fig. 18-1 Structural configuration of the two optical isomers of ketamine. The commercial formulation consists of the two isomers. (From White et al.,[2] with permission.)

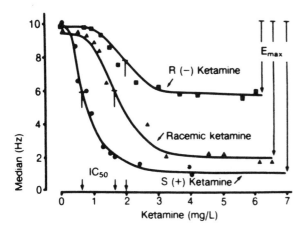

Fig. 18-2 Relationship between the changes in the electroencephalographic median frequency and serum ketamine concentrations in a volunteer receiving racemic ketamine, *S(+)*, and *R(−)* ketamine on separate occasions. (From Schuttler et al.,[8] with permission.)

neocortical and limbic systems. Early EEG studies reported that ketamine depressed thalamocortical pathways and concomitantly activated the limbic system. Subsequent studies demonstrated that ketamine produced excitatory activity in both the thalamus and limbic systems; however, there was no clinical evidence that this seizure-like activity spread to cortical areas. In fact, ketamine has been used successfully to treat status epilepticus.[9]

The EEG changes produced by racemic ketamine (and the S(+) isomer) can be classified into three sequential phases (Fig. 18-3).[8] The unique clinical anesthetic state, which is produced by ketamine and its isomers, has been characterized as a state of catalepsy, in which the eyes often remain open with a slow nystagmic gaze, while corneal and light reflexes remain intact. Reduced glucose use in the somatosensory and auditory systems suggests that a selective sensory deprivation occurs during ketamine-induced anesthesia.[10] Anesthesia is considered adequate when there is no purposeful response to noxious stimuli. However, varying degrees of hypertonus and occasional spontaneous movements, seemingly unrelated to painful stimuli, may be noted when surgical anesthesia is adequate.

Clinical observations suggest that ketamine's analgesia may outlast its anesthesia; thus, this analgesic effect may occur even at subanesthetic doses. There is evidence in animals to suggest that ketamine's analgesic action is mediated in part through interactions with the opioid receptor system.[11,12] Yet, the analgesic effects of subanesthetic doses of ketamine remain highly controversial. In volunteer studies, investigators suggested that it was possible to provide effective analgesia without producing undesirable side effects by using a ketamine infusion.[13] However, Owen et al.[14] reported that a ketamine infusion was ineffective in providing postoperative analgesia. More recently, in a double-blind clinical study, the effects of low-dose intramuscular ketamine (1 mg/kg) were compared with meperidine (1 mg/kg) in the treatment of pain after thoracic surgery.[15] Ketamine was as effective as meperidine in providing postoperative analgesia without producing respiratory depression.

Ketamine is a potent N-methyl-D-aspartate (NMDA) antagonist that has been demonstrated in vitro to reduce neuronal death associated with hypoxia or neurotransmitter toxicity.[16] However, in vivo, variable effects on rodent outcome following

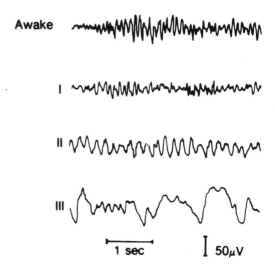

Fig. 18-3 Progressive changes in the electroencephalogram produced by ketamine. Phases I to III were seen with racemic ketamine and its S(+) isomer. With R(−) ketamine, the maximal EEG effect was phase II. (From Schuttler et al.,[8] with permission.)

cerebral ischemia have been reported.[17–19] Ketamine was also found in rats to improve the neurologic severity score and decrease the cerebral infarct volume following head injury.[20] The value of ketamine in these situations in humans remains to be established.

Postanesthesia Emergence Reactions

The psychotomimetic activity produced by ketamine can be disturbing to physicians and nurses and may upset other patients in the recovery room. Typically, the psychic sensations during emergence from ketamine anesthesia are described as alterations in mood state and body image, extracorporeal (out-of-body) experiences, floating sensations, vivid dreams or illusions, "weird trips," and occasional frank delirium.[6] The loss of skin and musculoskeletal sensations decreases the patient's ability to feel gravity, thereby producing a sensation of body detachment or floating in space. The vivid dreams and visual illusions disappear on wakening, although recurrent illusions (flashbacks) have been reported several weeks after ketamine administration in adults and children.

The reported incidence of psychic disturbances following ketamine vary from less than 5 to more than 30 percent. Factors associated with a higher incidence of emergence reactions include: age (older than 16 years of age), sex (females more than males), subjects who frequently dream during sleep, large doses of ketamine (more than 2 mg/kg IV), rapid intravenous administration (more than 40 mg/min), and a history of personality problems. Compared with thiopental, ketamine was found to be associated with a significantly greater incidence of psychological abnormalities in the immediate postoperative period.[21] The ketamine induced changes were short-lived (less than 24 hours), and no differences were found between the two groups with regard to long-term changes in personality.

Despite many statements in the literature to the contrary, neither covering the eyes during the operative and postoperative periods nor allowing patients to emerge in a quiet area alters the incidence of emergence reactions. In fact, it is important to discuss the common side effects of ketamine (e.g., dreaming, floating sensations, dizziness, and blurred vision) with the patient, both before and after the operation. Adverse reactions to ketamine can be minimized by informing the patient in advance of the likelihood of "vivid visual imagery" during the anesthetic experience.

Several premedicants and adjunctive agents have been evaluated in preventing emergence reactions caused by ketamine. Recently, the effect of music on emergence phenomena was investigated.[22] Although the incidence of emergence phenomena was not reduced, the effects tended to be more pleasant and acceptable to those to whom music was played. Atropine premedication before ketamine administration may increase the incidence of unpleasant dreams. Although droperidol was first reported to reduce the incidence of adverse emergence reactions when used as a premedicant, others found that it could increase the incidence of vivid dreams. Furthermore, patients receiving droperidol tend to be significantly less responsive and more disoriented during the recovery period. Several investigators reported a decrease in emergence reactions when ketamine was used with thiobarbiturates or other general anesthetics. Concomitant use of nitrous oxide significantly decreased the ketamine dose required for surgical anesthesia, resulting in a decreased incidence of emergence reactions, and shortened the recovery-room stay.

Benzodiazepines appear to be the most effective drugs for attenuating the psychic actions of ketamine during the emergence period. Diazepam (0.15 to 0.3 mg/kg IV) was reported to decrease significantly the incidence of dreams and to eliminate postoperative illusions when administered before induction with ketamine. Others have reported diazepam to be equally effective in attenuating emergence sequelae, whether administered at the start or the end of the procedure. Although diazepam is highly effective in preventing vivid emergence reactions and delirium following ketamine, a high incidence of floating sensations, dizziness, and dreaming can occur even in the presence of diazepam.

Of the currently available benzodiazepines, lorazepam (2 to 5 mg PO or IV) is reported to be the most effective in preventing unpleasant dreams and emergence sequelae after ketamine. The enhanced effectiveness of lorazepam may be related to its ability to produce more effective and longer lasting amnesia than does diazepam. Flunitrazepam (0.03 mg/kg IV) also attenuates emergence sequelae. Freuchen et al.[23] found that a combination of flunitrazepam and ketamine for induction, followed by a ketamine infusion and nitrous oxide for maintenance anesthesia, compared favorably with an inhalational anesthetic technique. Similarly, diazepam-ketamine-nitrous oxide-induced anesthesia was associated with fewer adverse sequelae than was a droperidol-fentanyl-nitrous oxide combination.[24]

The water-soluble benzodiazepine, midazolam, also prevents unpleasant dreaming and emergence sequelae when used as an adjunct to ketamine for inducing general anesthesia.[25] The midazolam-ketamine combination was associated with fewer postoperative side effects and a shorter recovery period than either midazolam or ketamine alone. Cartwright and Pingel[26] reported that midazolam was more effective than was diazepam in preventing unpleasant dreams when used as an adjuvant to ketamine-induced anesthesia.

Cardiovascular Effects

Ketamine produces a dose-related rise in the rate-pressure product (often in excess of 100 percent), with a transient rise in the cardiac index, but without significantly altering the stroke index.[27]

Traber et al.[28] suggested that the sympathomimetic effects of ketamine might be mediated within the CNS because ganglionic blockade and thoracic epidural block were capable of ablating its cardiostimulatory properties. In fact, when ketamine is injected directly into the cerebral circulation, an immediate increase in blood pressure, heart rate, and cardiac output is produced, and these effects can be markedly attenuated by prior administration of pentobarbital.[29] Based on these and other studies, it is believed that ketamine produces its sympathomimetic actions primarily by direct stimulation of the CNS.

In the absence of autonomic control, ketamine has direct myocardial depressant properties.[30–33] However, its effects on cardiac rhythm are controversial. There is evidence to suggest that ketamine has the ability to sensitize the myocardium to catecholamines and thereby enhance the arrhythmogenicity of epinephrine. Cabbabe and Behbahani[34]

reported two cases of serious arrhythmias in patients undergoing plastic surgery who received 0.5 mg/kg IV ketamine for sedation during infiltration of lidocaine solutions that contained epinephrine. However, there is also evidence for a dose-related antiarrhythmic effect.

Ketamine may have both inhibitory and excitatory effects on the peripheral sympathetic nervous system. Juang et al.[35] demonstrated that ketamine depressed smooth muscle contraction in response to preganglionic stimulation while it produced a transiently increased contraction in response to postganglionic stimulation, suggesting that ketamine has an effect at the level of the sympathetic ganglia. The effects of ketamine on postganglionic adrenergic neurons include inhibition of intraneuronal uptake of catecholamines (i.e., a cocaine-like effect) and a dose-dependent inhibition of extraneuronal norepinephrine uptake. Ketamine directly dilates vascular smooth muscle while causing sympathetically mediated vasoconstriction. The net effect is that systemic vascular resistance is not significantly altered by ketamine. Even though ketamine increases coronary blood flow, it may be insufficient to meet the increased metabolic demand of the myocardium.

Ketamine markedly elevates pulmonary artery pressure and right ventricular stroke work secondary to increased pulmonary vascular resistance. Thus, ketamine is probably contraindicated in patients with minimal right ventricular reserve. In patients without cardiopulmonary disease, ketamine produced a 40 percent increase in pulmonary vascular resistance, a secondary increase in right heart work, and a transient 20 percent increase in the intrapulmonary shunt.[36] However, in children with increased pulmonary vascular resistance and right-to-left shunts, ketamine did not worsen the shunt when used for induction of anesthesia.

The use of ketamine and thiopental as part of a balanced anesthetic technique decreases the degree of cardiac stimulation produced by ketamine.[25] Others showed that ketamine-induced cardiovascular stimulation and the concomitant rise in plasma free norepinephrine levels may be significantly decreased by premedication with diazepam (0.2 to 0.5 mg/kg IV).[37,38] Although lorazepam is more effective than diazepam in preventing emergence reactions, it is unable to block the cardiovascular stimulation produced by ketamine. Of the newer benzodiazepines, flunitrazepam and midazolam appear to be the most effective in attenuating the cardiostimulatory properties of ketamine. Nevertheless, the clinical significance of ketamine-induced cardiovascular stimulation in patients without hypertension, coronary artery disease, or cerebral vascular disease is yet to be established.

Ketamine produces an increase in cerebrospinal fluid (CSF) pressure that appears to be related to an increase in cerebral blood flow. Although the increase in cerebral blood flow produced by ketamine can be effectively blunted by prior administration of either thiopental or diazepam, ketamine should probably be avoided in patients with abnormal CSF flow dynamics or intracranial pathologic conditions. Case reports describe ketamine-induced apnea secondary to medullary compression, resulting from increased intracranial pressure.

Pulmonary Effects

Clinically useful doses of ketamine produce only mild respiratory depression. However in patients spontaneously breathing room air, ketamine (2 mg/kg IV) given as a rapid bolus injection produced significant reductions in PaO_2 lasting from 5 to 10 minutes.[39] In contrast, patients premedicated with diazepam (10 to 15 mg IM) who received ketamine (2 mg/kg IV over 60 seconds) while spontaneously breathing room air showed no significant change in either PaO_2 or $C(a-v)O_2$.[40] Furthermore, when an infusion of ketamine (1 mg/kg IV) was administered during vaginal deliveries, no significant changes were noted in either maternal or infant arterial blood gas values.[41] The respiratory response to CO_2 challenge is maintained during ketamine anesthesia.[42] Thus, ketamine only produces significant respiratory depression in those situations in which it is given as a rapid intravenous infusion or large bolus injection. In fact, a recent study reported that low doses of ketamine were capable of producing mild ventilatory stimulation.[43]

Lumb et al.[44] found a consistently lower shunt fractions and higher PaO_2 values when a continuous infusion of ketamine was compared with halothane during one-lung anesthesia in dogs. Mankikian et al.[45] studied the ventilatory pattern and chest wall mechanics during ketamine anesthesia. They reported maintenance of functional residual capacity, minute ventilation, and tidal volume, with an increase in the intercostal muscle contribution to tidal volume relative to the diaphragmatic component. Functional residual capacity is also preserved in young children during ketamine anesthesia.[46]

.In early clinical studies, an increase in pulmonary compliance and a decrease in airway resistance and bronchospasm were noted following administration of ketamine to patients with reactive airway disease. In vitro bronchial smooth muscle studies demonstrated that ketamine produces muscle relaxation, antagonism of the spasmogenic effects of carbachol and histamine, and a potentiation of the antispasmodic effects of epinephrine. Moreover, although propranolol blocked the relaxant effect of epinephrine, it did not alter ketamine's effects. These data suggest that in vitro ketamine acts at sites other than β receptors. Ketamine was found to be as effective as halothane or enflurane in preventing experimentally induced bronchospasm in dogs. The ability of ketamine to antagonize antigen-induced bronchospasm might be related to its vagolytic and direct smooth muscle relaxant properties. However, in vivo, ketamine's bronchodilatory properties appear to be dependent on its sympathomimetic actions because the protective effect against antigen-induced bronchospasm is decreased in the presence of β adrenergic blockade.

Salivary and tracheobronchial mucus gland secretions are increased by ketamine, necessitating prophylactic administration of an antisialogogue. Despite alleged retention of the protective pharyngeal and laryngeal reflexes, tracheal soiling and aspiration has been reported following induction of anesthesia with ketamine. The physician should not assume that the use of ketamine obviates the need for careful airway management.

Miscellaneous Pharmacologic Effects

Ketamine frequently produces an increase in skeletal muscle tone and occasionally muscle spasms, although it has been used safely in patients with myopathies and malignant hyperthermia. In the rat phrenic nerve-hemidiaphragm preparation, ketamine was shown to increase indirectly evoked twitch tension, but it produced no effect on directly stimulated skeletal muscle. However, a more recent study reported that ketamine produces neuromuscular effects by a direct postsynaptic action, initially potentiating and then blocking the twitch response elicited by direct muscle stimulation.[47] These data suggest that ketamine may interfere with calcium binding or its fluxes and thereby contribute to the initial potentiation and subsequent depression of twitch tension. These actions might explain ketamine's enhancement of the neuromuscular actions of succinylcholine, tubocurarine, and pancuronium.

The reduction in blood loss that has been reported when ketamine is used as an induction agent for first trimester abortions may be related to its ability to increase both uterine tone and the intensity of uterine contractions. In parturients, ketamine was reported to have variable effects on uterine tone and contractility. Oats et al.[48] found that ketamine was able to induce contractions equal to those after ergonovine when it was administered during the first trimester of pregnancy, but exerted no effect in the third trimester. Although ketamine had no effect on basal uterine tone in the parturient, Marx et al.[49] reported that ketamine produced dose-related changes in uterine activity in the term pregnant uterus. Analgesic doses of ketamine (0.2 to 0.4 mg/kg IV) produced no significant effects; larger induction doses (more than 1 mg/kg IV) produced increases in the intensity of uterine contractions.

Ketamine has reportedly been used safely in a patient with acute intermittent porphyria. Nevertheless, it can increase ALA synthetase activity in animals and, therefore, should be used with caution in patients with porphyria.

Ketamine has also been used in the treatment of persistent penile erection during general anesthesia.[50] Given intravenously, 20 to 30 mg is reported to produce detumescence within 1 to 2 minutes without unwanted side effects.

Ketamine produces only a mild elevation in blood glucose (12 percent) compared with that produced by halothane (55 percent) or thiopental (72 percent). Serum free fatty acid levels are decreased by ketamine (13 percent) in contrast to halothane and thiopental, which produce 59 percent and 34 percent increases, respectively. Thyroxine levels are not altered by ketamine; however, triiodothyronine levels are reduced. Therefore, the dose-dependent hypothermia produced by ketamine in rats at ambient temperatures may be the result of decreased heat production and increased heat loss secondary to cutaneous vasodilation.

Initial studies indicated that ketamine increased plasma renin activity, an effect that was attenuated by prior treatment with antihypertensive agents.[2] However, more recent studies found no change in renin activity during ketamine anesthesia, even though the pressor response to angiotension I and II was accentuated compared with that produced under halothane-induced anesthesia. In addition, ketamine produces an activation of the pituitary-adrenal axis, with adrenal-mediated release of catecholamines and corticosteroids. During deep ketamine-induced anesthesia, inhibition of this pituitary activation was reported, although intense and prolonged stimulation was noted on emergence.

Badrinath et al.[51] studied the effects of ketamine (with atracurium) on intraocular pressure. They found that intraocular pressure decreased significantly after anesthetic induction. Following intubation, intraocular pressure returned to the preinduction control level. Ketamine's effects were similar to those of thiopental and etomidate.

Atkinson et al.[52] showed that intramuscular ketamine irreversibly inhibits the aggregation of platelets in baboons. However, Heller et al.[53] found no significant hemostatic changes in humans undergoing ketamine-midazolam-induced anesthesia.

PRACTICAL APPLICATIONS

Use of Ketamine in Cardiothoracic Anesthesia

The cardiostimulatory properties of ketamine can produce serious sequelae in patients with cardiac disease. Although labetalol (1 mg/kg IV) is effective in attenuating the ketamine-induced rise in heart rate and blood pressure, benzodiazepines are also used for this purpose.[2] When a ketamine infusion was administered in combination with high-dose diazepam and nitrous oxide for cardiac anesthesia, adequate anesthetic conditions were produced with minimal effect on the cardiorespiratory system. There was excellent anterograde amnesia, satisfactory analgesia, and no postoperative emergence reactions. Diazepam (0.3 to 0.5 mg/kg IV) effectively prevents the increase in the rate-pressure product following administration of ketamine. As mentioned earlier, ketamine-induced cardiovascular stimulation and the concomitant rise in plasma norepinephrine levels can be significantly decreased by premedication with diazepam. Flunitrazepam and midazolam also effectively attenuate the cardiostimulatory response produced by ketamine.

In a study comparing a morphine-diazepam-nitrous oxide combination with ketamine-nitrous oxide-induced anesthesia for coronary bypass surgery, Reeves et al.[54] found that, although the overall number of changes in this rate-pressure product were similar, the mean maximal increases in systolic blood pressure and rate-pressure product were significantly higher in the ketamine group. The incidence of changes in the rate-pressure product might have been less if diazepam had also been incorporated as part of the ketamine regime. Nevertheless, these investigators found no significant difference between the two treatment groups with respect to perioperative morbidity and mortality rates.

In a controlled study of the circulatory responses during induction and maintenance of anesthesia in patients undergoing heart valve replacement, Dhadphale et al.[55] found no significant differences between the diazepam-ketamine-nitrous oxide and morphine-nitrous oxide techniques. These investigators believed that high-dose diazepam (0.5 mg/kg IV) combined with ketamine (1 to 2 mg/kg for induction and 15 to 30 μg/kg/min for maintenance) was a satisfactory alternative to morphine-nitrous oxide-induced anesthesia for patients with coronary artery disease and for those undergoing heart valve replacement. A potential advantage of the diazepam-ketamine technique is that the nitrous oxide concentration is not critical, and therefore, 100 percent oxygen can be used. As with any "balanced" anesthetic technique, there may be re-call of intraoperative events during cardiac surgery with diazepam-ketamine-induced anesthesia. Apart from its intrinsic anesthetic properties, ketamine produces minimal, if any, anterograde amnesia. The adjunctive use of either lorazepam or midazolam would be expected to decrease the possibility of intraoperative recall when ketamine is used without nitrous oxide.

High-dose opioid techniques (e.g., fentanyl 50 to 150 μg/kg or sufentanil 5 to 15 μg/kg) are popular for anesthetic induction of hemodynamically unstable patients undergoing cardiac surgery. In a comparison of ketamine and sufentanil for the induction of patients with severe cardiomyopathy undergoing cardiac transplantation, Gutzke et al.[56] reported that ketamine maintained a stable cardiac index and heart rate at the expense of increased wall tension. In patients undergoing elective coronary bypass surgery, fentanyl (50 μg/kg) effectively obtunded the sympathomimetic actions of ketamine (1.5 mg/kg).[57] In contrast to the commonly used sedative hypnotics (thiopental and etomidate), the use of ketamine to supplement fentanyl-induced anesthesia was not associated with significant hemodynamic changes. Furthermore, when ketamine or fentanyl were administered as intravenous adjuncts during thoracic surgery, ketamine was associated with more prolonged postoperative analgesia than was fentanyl.[58]

Many cardiac anesthesiologists consider ketamine the drug of choice for inducing and maintaining anesthesia in patients with cardiac tamponade or constrictive pericarditis because ketamine maintains sympathetic nervous system activity, even though ketamine may further increase the pulmonary vascular resistance. In these patients, the hemodynamic response to ketamine varies considerably, especially if the pulmonary capillary wedge pressure exceeds 15 mmHg. Further studies are needed in these surgical populations.

Extensive experience with the use of ketamine for pediatric cardiac catherizations would suggest that it provides adequate sedative-hypnotic conditions with fewer catheter associated arrhythmias than do the volatile anesthetics. Compared with propofol, the mean systolic blood pressure is better maintained, although the recovery time is longer.[59]

Yet, clinical evidence suggests that ketamine can sensitize the myocardium to circulating catecholamines. Nevertheless, a combination of midazolam and low-dose ketamine has been used successfully for sedation and analgesia during electrical cardioversions. Interestingly, when ketamine is used for adult cardiac catherization, it can produce significant decreases in blood pressure.

Use of Ketamine in Critically Ill Patients

Ketamine has been used in critically ill patients in whom a period of hypotension or apnea could be life threatening. Park et al.[60] described the use of a ketamine infusion as a sedative, inotrope, and bronchodilator in a critically ill patient. Also Sharma[61] reported the use of intravenous ketamine in two patients with acute severe asthma who did not respond to conventional therapy. An infusion of ketamine at a rate of 0.15 mg/kg/min was used in each case to prevent a recurrence of bronchospasm. When ketamine was used in critically ill patients, it was reported to provide good surgical anesthesia with a greater margin of safety than "conventional" anesthesia. However, it is difficult to draw meaningful conclusions from anecdotal clinical reports.

The use of ketamine during major surgical procedures in elderly patients has been reported to be associated with hemodynamic stability and a rapid emergence, with a low incidence of unpleasant dreams. Stefansson et al.[62] reported that using ketamine as the sole anesthetic for hip fracture surgery in the geriatric patient resulted in a survival rate that did not differ significantly from other common anesthetic techniques, including epidural and volatile anesthetics. Furthermore, Pedersen et al.[63] reported that ketamine, in contrast to thiopental, did not decrease the cardiac output when used for the induction of anesthesia in critically ill patients. The so-called "slow-dose" ketamine technique, which consists of a benzodiazepine (e.g., diazepam 2 to 5 mg IV) followed by an infusion of ketamine (2 to 4 mg/min) can also be extremely useful in aged and high risk patients.[64]

Ketamine is regarded by some as advantageous for patients in hemorrhagic shock; others dispute its usefulness in this situation. In contrast to the marked pressor response following ketamine administration to normovolemic subjects, induction with ketamine in patients who are hypovolemic secondary to acute hemorrhage causes no significant change or even a slight decrease in blood pressure. Rather than clarifying the cardiovascular and metabolic actions of ketamine, animal studies have produced conflicting results.

In experimental hemorrhagic and septic shock, ketamine significantly increases both systolic and diastolic blood pressure. Compared with hypovolemic barbiturate anesthetized rats, hypovolemic rats anesthetized with ketamine had significantly greater perfusion to their vital organs. Using a dog model, ketamine was found to be more effective than either thiopental or diazepam in maintaining renal blood flow.[65] Furthermore, a higher survival rate was reported in hypotensive rats anesthetized with ketamine compared with halothane. In contrast to the volatile anesthetics, Longnecker et al.[66] demonstrated that ketamine diminished the arteriolar response to hemorrhage, and therefore, tissue hypoxia did not occur. On the other hand, Weiskopf et al.[67] found that ketamine produced a greater base deficit and larger increases in arterial lactate concentration than did the volatile agents. These investigators reported that, in spite of its ability to increase catecholamine levels, the use of ketamine was associated with cardiovascular depression and metabolic acidosis.[68]

Critically ill patients occasionally respond to ketamine with an unexpected drop in blood pressure, which may result from the inability of the sympathomimetic actions of ketamine to counterbalance its direct myocardial depressant and vasodilatory effects. A diminished catecholamine response to ketamine following prolonged stress could result in a maldistribution of systemic blood flow. Waxman et al.[69] observed occasional decreases in cardiac and pulmonary performance when ketamine was used to induce anesthesia in critically ill and acutely traumatized patients.

Use of Ketamine in Patients With Pulmonary Disease

As a result of its salutary effects on airway resistance, ketamine may be the agent of choice for the rapid induction of anesthesia in patients with reactive airway disease. Furthermore, ketamine is an alternative to the volatile agents for maintenance of anesthesia in patients who are receiving parenteral bronchodilators. However, concurrent administration of ketamine and aminophylline may decrease the seizure threshold.[70]

Ketamine is an excellent alternative to the volatile agents for one-lung anesthesia in patients with pre-existing pulmonary disease and abnormal preoperative blood gas values. When one-lung anesthesia was used during thoracic surgery, patients with impaired pulmonary function had improved oxygenation and decreased pulmonary shunt fractions when a diazepam-ketamine infusion-muscle relaxant anesthetic technique was used as an alternative to conventional inhalation techniques. The difference appeared to be a result of ketamine's ability to preserve the hypoxic vasoconstrictor reflex. Ketamine would also be advantageous in clinical situations where a high inspired oxygen concentration is required to maintain adequate tissue oxygenation (e.g., severe anemia and cerebrovascular insufficiency).

Use of Ketamine for Obstetric Anesthesia and Analgesia

Early studies using ketamine anesthesia for routine vaginal deliveries reported an unacceptably high incidence of maternal complications and depressed infants with low Apgar scores. These problems were shown to be dose related. When lower doses of ketamine (0.2 to 0.5 mg/kg IV) were used, neonates were not depressed, and complications were minimal with high patient acceptance. Nevertheless, even when subanesthetic doses of ketamine are used to produce obstetric analgesia, a majority of these patients will experience a dream-like state.

Ketamine given in combination with nitrous oxide for obstetric anesthesia produces virtually no recall of pain during delivery, and although dreaming occurs in many patients, a majority of the dreams are pleasant with excellent patient acceptance. The use of larger doses of ketamine (more than 1.5 mg/kg IV) for inducing anesthesia in unpremedicated parturients produces good surgical anesthesia; however, recovery from anesthesia is often unpleasant. In a large obstetric series comparing low-dose ketamine (0.5 mg/kg IV) with methoxyflurane (0.25 to 10 percent), ketamine produced a more rapid onset of action and was the superior analgesic; patient acceptance was similar for the two groups. The use of droperidol as an adjunct to ketamine prolonged the recovery period without decreasing the incidence of adverse emergence reactions.

Compared with thiopental for induction of anesthesia prior to cesarean section, ketamine provided rapid induction and greater analgesia and amnesia, with a similar incidence of unpleasant emergence reactions. However, the incidence of undesirable psychotomimetic reactions was low following both induction agents. Using ketamine as the sole anesthetic for cesarean section in Third World countries has been reported to result in lower fetal mortality rates than with other general anesthetic techniques.

In comparison with thiopental, ketamine is advantageous for hypovolemic patients (e.g., abruptio placentae and placenta previa) and for patients with acute bronchospasm. Some investigators suggest that ketamine may be a useful analgesic for managing the hemodynamically unstable preeclamptic patient because of its anticonvulsant properties; however, it should be used with caution in this situation because its cardiostimulatory properties could precipitate a hypertensive crisis.

There have been no clinical reports regarding fetal acid base changes following ketamine anesthesia; however, animal studies indicate that ketamine increases uterine blood flow without adversely affecting fetal cardiovascular or acid base status. Using a chronic sheep preparation with induced fetal acidosis, Pickering et al.[71] found better preservation of blood pressure and cerebral blood flow following administration of ketamine compared with thiopental. Arterial blood gas evaluations in mothers and infants receiving ketamine-induced analgesia for vaginal delivery showed no significant differences compared with those who received regional anesthesia. In a comparative study of ketamine and thiopental for rapid intravenous induction prior to cesarean section, ketamine treated patients showed higher maternal umbilical artery and vein pH and base excess values.[72]

Neonatal arterial blood pressure has been reported to be less depressed after maternal ketamine anesthesia compared with a similar group receiving thiopental. Neonatal neurobehavioral scores following vaginal delivery with ketamine, 0.7 mg/kg IV, and 50 percent nitrous oxide; thiopental, 4 mg/kg IV, and 50 percent nitrous oxide; or 2 percent chloroprocaine epidural anesthesia revealed the greatest percentage of high scores in the epidural group, intermediate values following ketamine-nitrous oxide, and the lowest scores after thiopental-nitrous oxide.

The reduced blood loss that has been reported when ketamine was used as an induction agent for first trimester abortions may be related to its ability to increase both uterine tone and the intensity of uterine contractions. However, a study comparing ketamine-midazolam with methohexital found no difference in blood loss.[73] In parturients, ketamine has been reported to have variable effects on uterine tone and contractility. Ketamine can induce contractions equal to ergonovine when administered during the first trimester of pregnancy, and it produces dose-related changes in uterine activity in the full-term pregnant uterus. So called "analgesic" doses of ketamine (0.2 to 0.4 mg/kg IV) increase the intensity of uterine contractions. Similarly, ketamine increases both basal uterine tone and the intensity of contractions in the nonpregnant uterus.

Pediatric Anesthesia

Ketamine has been used by the oral route to premedicate pediatric patients. In a recent study, 6 mg/kg of ketamine mixed with 0.2 ml/kg of cola-flavored drink was well accepted.[74] Predictable sedation occurred within 20 to 25 minutes without significant side effects. Intramuscular ketamine (4 to 8 mg/kg) was also proved to be extremely useful for induction of anesthesia prior to administering an inhalational agent and for diagnostic and minor surgical procedures not requiring intravenous cannulae or endotracheal intubation.

Ketamine has been used successfully for oral surgical procedures and diagnostic muscle biopsies lasting from 5 to 30 minutes (doses, 1 to 3 mg/kg IM or 0.5 to 1.0 mg/kg IV). However, the side effects that have been reported include cardiovascular stimulation, partial airway obstruction, and minor postanesthetic complications, including un-

pleasant dreams. Diazepam (5 to 10 mg PO) combined with ketamine (3 mg/kg IM) can provide excellent sedation with few side effects for children requiring oral surgical procedures lasting 45 to 60 minutes.[75]

In children undergoing minor otolaryngologic procedures, ketamine (2 mg/kg IV) compared favorably with thiopental (4 mg/kg).[76] Although the operating conditions were similar, thiopental produced more cardiorespiratory depression and a greater need for postoperative analgesics; ketamine was associated with a higher incidence of restlessness and a somewhat more prolonged recovery period. Ketamine (10 mg/kg IM) has also been used for bronchoscopy in children without significant complications. However, ketamine stimulated the production of copious amounts of upper airway secretions, necessitating concomitant use of an antisialagogue. Furthermore, anecdotal reports indicate that ketamine may produce "hyper-reactive" airway reflexes, especially when the upper respiratory tract is inflamed (e.g., in burned patients).

Finally, rectal ketamine (7.5 to 15 mg/kg) has been used successfully as an induction agent in pediatric anesthesia. Compared with rectal methohexital (25 mg/kg), the use of ketamine (15 mg/kg per rectum) for induction was associated with a higher incidence of airway complications during the perioperative period.[77] Although there is a high degree of acceptance of ketamine in children undergoing repeated anesthesia for radiotherapy anesthesia, tolerance to its CNS effects may develop.

Anesthesia for Burned Patients

Ketamine has also been used extensively in burn units for dressing changes and skin grafting procedures in children and adults. Intramuscular ketamine (2 to 6 mg/kg) produces excellent surgical conditions for eschar excision. The relatively rapid recovery from ketamine caused minimal delays in resuming nutritional intake. Rare emergence reactions (mild excitement and/or illusions) were noted in these unpremedicated burned patients. In premedicated patients, even lower doses of ketamine (1 to 2 mg/kg IM) can produce good operating conditions, amnesia, and satisfactory analgesia with a rapid recovery and resumption of normal activities. However, tolerance to ketamine appeared to develop in all patients receiving more than two exposures, and the dose requirement increased progressively in patients receiving repeated doses of ketamine.

Use of Ketamine for Sedation and Analgesia

During the performance of a painful nerve block, the ideal adjunctive drug would provide analgesia, sedation, and amnesia without cardiorespiratory depression. In comparing the clinical effectiveness and acceptability of diazepam, droperidol-fentanyl, and ketamine for sedation and analgesia prior to intercostal nerve blocks, ketamine was reported to produce more optimal conditions during the block procedure and higher patient acceptance.[78] Furthermore, the use of a diazepam (0.15 mg/kg)-ketamine (0.5 mg/kg) combination was not associated with increased side effects or a greater need for postoperative care than found in an unpremedicated group undergoing similar nerve block procedures. More importantly, patient acceptance was significantly higher in the diazepam-ketamine group. Low-dose ketamine combined with a benzodiazepine has become increasingly popular during the injection of local anesthetics for outpatient cosmetic procedures. Patients are reported to be more comfortable and cooperative with this drug combination.[79]

In a randomized double-blind study, midazolam was compared with diazepam for sedation when administered as an adjuvant to ketamine during local anesthesia.[80] Midazolam (0.05 to 0.15 mg/kg IV) was found to produce a spectrum of CNS activity that was similar to that of diazepam (0.1 to 0.3 mg/kg IV). However, the slope of midazolam's dose-response curve for sedation appeared to be steeper (i.e., a narrower therapeutic dosage range). In a comparative evaluation, midazolam (0.1 mg/kg IV) was found to produce more profound sedation and amnesia than diazepam (0.2 mg/kg IV). Midazolam was associated with significantly less pain on injection and a lower incidence of postoperative venoirritation. Although recovery characteristics were similar for the two benzodiazepines when used as adjuvants to ketamine, overall patient acceptance was higher with midazolam than diazepam.

Ketamine infusions (1 to 1.5 mg/min) have been used during the early postoperative period for sedation and analgesia. In achieving adequate postoperative analgesia with ketamine, profound sedation also is produced. When used to sedate patients requiring postoperative ventilatory support, ketamine was reported to decrease agitation and the analgesic requirements.[81]

Outpatient Anesthesia

It appears that ketamine can be used for induction and maintenance for outpatient anesthesia if the minimal effective dose of ketamine (0.5 to 1.0 mg/kg for induction followed by continuous infusion of 15 to 30 μg/kg/min) is administered in combination with nitrous oxide and thiopental (1 to 3 mg/kg) or midazolam (0.7 to 0.15 mg/kg). To provide for a more rapid recovery following brief outpatient procedures, a combination of propofol (1 to 3 mg/kg IV) for induction followed by a continuous infusion of ketamine (3 to 6 mg/min) and nitrous oxide (70 percent in oxygen) is recommended. The use of a continuous infusion of ketamine significantly decreases the drug dosage requirement, improves intraoperative conditions, and decreases recovery time compared with the traditional intermittent bolus technique.[82] Although ketamine and nitrous oxide produced superior intraoperative conditions compared with a fentanyl-nitrous oxide combination, recovery times were more prolonged, and side effects were more frequent with the ketamine-based technique.[83]

Use of Ketamine Infusions

The titration of intravenous anesthetics like ketamine using small incremental bolus doses has been performed by anesthesiologists for many years. Continuous infusion is a logical extension of this method of titration; it minimizes the fluctuations in blood and brain ketamine concentrations that follow bolus injections.[82] To achieve a therapeutic blood level more rapidly, it is necessary to administer a "loading" dose. To maintain a desired drug concentration, it is necessary to infuse the drug continuously. Although infusions are usually administered on an empiric basis, a knowledge of pharmacokinetic principles may allow the anesthesiologist to predict more accurately the dosage requirements. Pharmacokinetic data for ketamine can be used to calculate the loading dose and the initial maintenance infusion rate (MIR).

Two simple equations can be used to estimate the loading dose and MIR for ketamine as follows:

$$\text{Loading dose } (\mu g/kg) = Cp\ (\mu g/ml) \times V\ (ml/kg)$$

and

$$MIR\ (\mu g/kg/min) = Cp\ (\mu g/ml) \times CL\ (ml/kg/min)$$

where Cp = plasma drug concentration, V = volume of distribution, and CL = clearance of drug.

The range of ketamine population pharmacokinetic values are:

$$Cp = 0.25 \text{ to } 2.5\ \mu g/ml,$$
$$V = 0.6 \text{ to } 3.0\ ml/kg, \text{ and}$$
$$CL = 15 \text{ to } 20\ ml/kg/min.$$

The loading dose can be administered as either a bolus or as a rapid "priming" infusion. Because side effects appear to be more severe with rapid fluctuations in plasma drug concentrations, a loading infusion may be preferred to a loading bolus. The required plasma drug concentration will depend on the desired pharmacologic effect (e.g., sedation and hypnosis), the presence of other centrally active drugs, the type of operation, and the individual's sensitivity to the drug (e.g., age, level of anxiety, and drug history). The influence of premedication, adjunctive drugs, nitrous oxide, and type of operation on the maintenance requirement for ketamine is shown in Table 18-3.

Which clinical signs are most useful in deciding whether to increase or decrease the MIR of ketamine? Although the most sensitive clinical signs of depth of anesthesia appear to be changes in muscle tone and ventilatory pattern, the physician must rely on evidence of autonomic hyperactivity (e.g., sweating, lacrimation, tachycardia, hypertension, and pupillary dilatation) if the patient has received muscle relaxants. Although the blood pressure response to surgical stimulation may be a

Table 18-3 Use of Ketamine Infusion as Part of a Balanced Anesthetic Technique for Major Abdominal Surgery, Cardiac Surgery, and Gynecologic Surgery

Investigator	Premedication	Adjunct	Induction (mg/kg)	Induction Ketamine (mg/kg)	Nitrous Oxide (%)	Maintenance Ketamine (µg/kg/min)
Major abdominal surgery						
Hatano et al.[96] (1979)	Diazepam	Diazepam	0.2–0.3	1.3–2.0	66	10–15
Houlton and Downing[97] (1978)	Omnopon (papaveretum)	Flunitrazepam	0.3	—	—	33
Idvall et al.[98] (1979)	Atropine/meperidine, droperidol/fentanyl	—	—	2.0	50	41
Cardiac surgery						
Hatano et al.[99] (1976)	Diazepam		0.5–0.5	1.0	50	12
Jackson et al.[38] (1978)	Morphine		0.4	2.0	—	90
Dhadphale et al.[55] (1979)	Morphine		0.4	2.0	50	17
Gynecologic surgery						
El-Naggar et al.[101] (1977)	Diazepam	Diazepam	0.2	0.5–1.0	66	17–34
Liburn et al.[102] (1978)	Lorazepam		—	1.0	—	66–83
Barclay et al.[103] (1980)	Papaveretum, atropine	Flunitrazepam, atropine	0.3	—	40–60	16–81
Freuchen et al.[23] (1981)	Flunitrazepam	Flunitrazepam	0.3	1.0	60	18

Table 18-4 Using Ketamine as a Sedative, Analgesic, or Anesthetic During the Perioperative Period

Premedication
    A benzodiazepine administered either orally (e.g., diazepam, 15–30 mg or lorazepam, 2–5 mg) 60–90 minutes before surgery or IV (e.g., midazolam 0.05–0.1 mg/kg) immediately prior to induction as an adjunct to ketamine.
    If preoperative sedation is contraindicated, a benzodiazepine can be administered IV prior to termination of surgery. An antisialagogue (e.g., glycopyrrolate, 0.005 mg/kg IV) can decrease secretions if administered 10 minutes before induction.

Induction of anesthesia
    Ketamine, 0.5–1.5 mg/kg IV, or 4–6 mg/kg IM. Lower doses of ketamine are use if thiopental (1–2 mg/kg IV) midazolam (0.075–0.15 mg/kg), or propofol (0.75–1.5 mg/kg IV) is used as an adjunct in place of the premedicant or if the patient is elderly or critically ill.

Maintenance of anesthesia
    Ketamine 15–45 μ/kg/min (1–3 mg/min) by continuous IV infusion with supplemental nitrous oxide, 50–70% in oxygen.
    If ketamine is infused in combination with nitrous oxide, 70%, following a barbiturate or propofol induction, a higher initial maintenance infusion rate will be required (e.g., 30–90 μg/kg/min).

Sedation and analgesia
    Ketamine, 0.2–0.8 mg/kg IV (over 2–3 minutes) or 2–4 mg/kg IM, followed by continuous ketamine infusion (5–20 μg/kg/min) with or without supplemental oxygen.

useful guide in judging the depth of anesthesia with volatile anesthetics, it is a less reliable index when intravenous anesthetics are used. Table 18-4 summarizes an approach to using a ketamine infusion as part of a "balanced" anesthetic technique and for sedation and analgesia during local and regional anesthesia.

Epidural Ketamine

Theoretically, the administration of ketamine by the epidural or intrathecal route should be able to produce analgesia without sympathetic blockade or respiratory depression.[84,85] Epidural ketamine was reported to be effective in producing postoperative analgesia. In an uncontrolled study of 50 patients, Islas et al.[86] claimed potent analgesia from 4 mg of epidural ketamine. Naquib et al.[87] reported using up to 30 mg of epidural ketamine in patients who underwent cholecystectomy, with 54 percent of patients receiving 30 mg having adequate analgesia for up to 24 hours. In a more recent study, ketamine was compared with bupivacaine for caudal analgesia in 50 children undergoing inguinal herniotomy.[88] Caudal administration of ketamine 0.5 mg/kg produced postoperative analgesia comparable to that associated with caudal injection of 0.25 percent bupivacaine, 1 ml/kg. However, in two studies comparing epidural ketamine with epidural morphine, morphine was the more potent and longer acting analgesic.[89,90]

Use of Ketamine in Patients With Uncommon Diseases

Although ketamine can increase skeletal muscle tone and occasionally produce muscle spasms, it was used safely in patients with a variety of myopathies and in those with a history compatible with malignant hyperthermia.[91] Even though ketamine increases ALA synthetase activity in animals, it was used successfully to anesthetize patients with acute intermittent porphyria and hereditary coproporphyria.[92,93] A diazepam and ketamine combination was used successfully to provide anesthesia for a patient with malignant carcinoid syndrome and associated tricuspid valvular disease.[94] Ketamine was also used for a patient with Shy-Drager syndrome.[95]

SUMMARY

Ketamine is a safe, rapid-acting, parenteral anesthetic and analgesic agent. Ketamine alone increases blood pressure and heart rate and produces profuse salivation, lacrimation, sweating, skeletal muscle hypertonus, involuntary purposeless movements, and agitation or even transient delirium during emergence. The use of a continuous infusion technique allows the anesthesiologist to titrate the drug more closely and, thereby, reduce the amount of drug required. Benzodiazepines are highly effective in preventing the marked cardiovascular responses and unpleasant emergence reactions associated with ketamine anesthesia. A combination of ketamine and midazolam (a benzodiazepine with a pharmacokinetic profile similar to that of ketamine) was useful for rapid induction of anesthesia and can also be used for maintenance of anesthesia and sedation during total intravenous anesthesia.

Numerous clinical studies have appeared in the literature over the last 15 years using ketamine infusion techniques (Table 18-3). Clinical applications for ketamine in anesthesia include a role in total intravenous anesthesia for major surgery, in the management of acute trauma, and in ambulatory surgery. Ketamine is widely used for sedation and analgesia during procedures under local anesthesia. In addition, ketamine can be used in intensive care units and emergency rooms for providing acute pain relief during brief procedures or painful manipulations. Although it is apparent that ketamine does not possess all the physicochemical and pharmacologic properties of an ideal intravenous anesthetic,[2] its diverse pharmacologic properties may provide important insights in the continuing search for an intravenous drug that will be closer to the ideal.

REFERENCES

1. Domino EF, Chodoff P, Corssen G: Pharmacologic effects of CI-581, a new dissociative anesthetic in man. Clin Pharmacol Ther 6:279, 1965
2. White PF, Way WL, Trevor AJ: Ketamine—its pharmacology and therapeutic uses. Anesthesiology 56:119, 1982
3. Reich DL, Silvay G: Ketamine: an update on the first twenty-five years of clinical experience. Can J Anaesth 36:186, 1989
4. Marietta MP, Way WL, Castagnoli N et al: On the pharmacology of the ketamine enantiomorhs in the rat. J Pharmacol Exp Ther 202:157, 1977
5. Ryder S, Way WL, Trevor AJ: Comparative pharmacology of the optical isomers of ketamine in mice. Eur J Pharmacol 49:15, 1978
6. White PF, Ham J, Way WL et al: Pharmacology of ketamine isomers in surgical patients. Anesthesiology 52:231, 1980
7. White PF, Schuttler J, Shaffer A et al: Comparative pharmacology of ketamine isomers. Studies in volunteers. Br J Anaesth 57:197, 1985
8. Schuttler J, Stanski DR, White PF et al: Pharmacodynamic modelling of the EEG effects of ketamine and its enantomers in man. J Pharmacokinet Biopharm 15:241, 1987
9. Sybert JW, Kyff JV: Ketamine treatment of status epilepticus. Anesthesiology 58:203, 1983
10. Crosby G, Crane AM, Sokoloff L: Local changes in cerebral glucose utilization during ketamine anesthesia. Anesthesiology 56:437, 1982
11. Smith DJ, Pekoe GM, Martin LL, Coalgate B: The interaction of ketamine with the opiate receptor. Life Sci 26:789, 1980
12. Finck AD, Ngai SH: A possible mechanism of ketamine-induced analgesia. Anesthesiology 56:291, 1982
13. Clements JA, Nimmo WS, Grant IS: Bioavailability, pharmacokinetics, and analgesic activity of ketamine in humans. J Pharm Sci 71:539, 1982
14. Owen H, Reekie RM, Clements JA et al: Analgesia from morphine and ketamine—a comparison of infusions of morphine and ketamine for postoperative analgesia. Anaesthesia 42:1051, 1987
15. Dich-Nielsen JO, Svendsen LB, Berthelsen P: Intramuscular low-dose ketamine versus pethidine for postoperative pain treatment after thoracic surgery. Acta Anaesthesiol Scand 36:583, 1992
16. Rothman SM, Thurston JH, Hauhart RE et al: Ketamine protects hippocampal neurons from anoxia in vitro. Neuroscience 21:673, 1987
17. Church J, Zeman S, Lodge D: The neuroprotective action of ketamine and MK-801 after transient cerebral ischemia in rats. Anesthesiology 69:702, 1988
18. Warner DS, Ridenour TR, Todd MM et al: Ketamine does not reduce infarct volume in rats undergoing focal cerebral ischemia. Anesthesiology 73:A727, 1990
19. Hoffman WE, Pelligrino DA, Werner C et al: Ketamine decreases plasma catecholamines and improves outcome from incomplete cerebral ischemia in rats. Anesthesiology 76:755, 1992
20. Shapira Y, Artru AA, Lam AM: Protective effect of ketamine following closed cranial impact in rats. Anesthesiology 75:A203, 1991
21. Moretti RJ, Hassan SZ, Goodman LI et al: Comparison of ketamine and thiopental in healthy volunteers: effects on mental status, mood, and personality. Anesth Analg 63:1087, 1984
22. Kumar A, Bajaj A, Sarkar P, Grover VK: The effect of music on ketamine induced emergence phenomena. Anaesthesia 47:438, 1992
23. Freuchen I, Ostergaard J, Mikkelsen BO: Anaesthe-

sia with flunitrazepam and ketamine. Br J Anaesth 53:827, 1981

24. Klausen N-O, Wiberg-Jorgensen F, Chraemmer-Jorgensen B: Psychotomimetic reactions after low dose ketamine infusion—comparison with neuroleptanaesthesia. Br J Anaesth 55:297, 1983

25. White PF: Comparative evaluation of intravenous agents for rapid sequence induction—thiopental, ketamine, and midazolam. Anesthesiology 57:279, 1982

26. Cartwright PD, Pingel SM: Midazolam and diazepam in ketamine anesthesia. Anaesthesia 39:439, 1984

27. Tweed WA, Minuck MS, Mymin D: Circulatory responses to ketamine anesthesia. Anesthesiology 37:613, 1972

28. Traber DL, Wilson RD, Priano LL et al: Blockade of the hypertensive response to ketamine. Anesth Analg 49:420, 1970

29. Ivankovich AD, Miletich DJ, Reimann C et al: Cardiovascular effects of centrally administered ketamine in goats. Anesth Analg 53:924, 1974

30. Schwartz DA, Horwitz LD: Effects of ketamine on left ventricular performance. J Pharmacol Exp Ther 194:410, 1975

31. Stowe DF, Bosnjak ZJ, Kampine JP: Comparison of etomidate, ketamine, midazolam, propofol and thiopental on function and metabolism of isolated hearts. Anesth Analg 74:547, 1992

32. Pagel PS, Kampine JP, Schmeling WT et al: Ketamine depresses myocardial contractility as evaluated by the preload recruitable stroke work relationship in chronically instrumented dogs with autonomic system blockade. Anesthesiology 76:564, 1992

33. Pagel PS, Schemeling WT, Kampine JP et al: Alteration of canine left ventricular diastolic function by intravenous anesthetics in vivo. Ketamine versus propofol. Anesthesiology 76:419, 1992

34. Cabbabe EB, Behbahani PM: Cardiovascular reactions associated with the use of ketamine and epinephrine in plastic surgery. Ann Plast Surg 15:50, 1985

35. Juang MS, Konemura K, Morioka T et al: Ketamine acts on the peripheral sympathetic nervous system of guinea pigs. Anesth Analg 59:45, 1980

36. Gooding JM, Dimick AR, Tavakoli M: A physiologic analysis of cardiopulmonary responses to ketamine anesthesia in non-cardiac patients. Anesth Analg 56:813, 1977

37. Zsigmond EK, Korthary SP, Martinez OA et al: Diazepam for the prevention of the rise in plasma catecholamines caused by ketamine. Clin Pharmacol Ther 15:223, 1974

38. Jackson APF, Dhadphale PR, Callaghan ML: Haemodynamic studies during induction of anaesthesia for open-heart surgery using diazepam and ketamine. Br J Anaesth 50:375, 1978

39. Zsigmond EK, Matsuki A, Kothary SP et al: Arterial hypoxemia caused by intravenous ketamine. Anesth Analg 55:311, 1976

40. Rust M, Landauer B, Kolb E: Stellenwert von ketamin in der notfallsituation. Anaesthesist 27:205, 1978

41. Maduska AL, Hajghassemali M: Arterial blood gases in mothers and infants during ketamine anesthesia for surgical delivery. Anesth Analg 57:121, 1978

42. Soliman MG, Brinale GF, Kuster G: Response to hypercapnia under ketamine anaesthesia. Can J Anaesth 22:486, 1975

43. Morel DR, Forster A, Gemperie M: Noninvasive evaluation of breathing pattern and thoraco-abdominal motion following the infusion of ketamine or droperidol in humans. Anesthesiology 65:392, 1986

44. Lumb PD, Silvay G, Weinreich AI et al: A comparison of the effects of continuous ketamine infusion and halothane on oxygenation during one-lung anesthesia in dogs. Can J Anaesth 26:394, 1979

45. Mankikian B, Cantineau JP, Sartene R et al: Ventilatory pattern and chest wall mechanics during ketamine anesthesia in humans. Anesthesiology 65:492, 1986

46. Shulman D, Beardsmore CS, Aronson HB, Godfrey S: The effect of ketamine on the functional residual capacity in young children. Anesthesiology 62:551, 1985

47. Marwaha J: Some mechanisms underlying actions of ketamine on electromechanical coupling in skeletal muscle. J Neurosci Res 5:43, 1980

48. Oats JN, Vasey OP, Waldren BA: Effects of ketamine on the pregnant uterus. Br J Anaesth 51:1163, 1979

49. Marx GF, Hwang HS, Candra P: Postpartum uterine pressures with different doses of ketamine. Anesthesiology 50:163, 1979

50. Hutchinson WF: Persistent erection and general anaesthesia. Anaesthesia 45:794, 1990

51. Badrinath SK, Vazeery A, McCarthy RJ, Ivankovich AD: The effect of different methods of inducing anesthesia on intraocular pressure. Anesthesiology 65:431, 1986

52. Atkinson PM, Taylor DI, Chetty N: Inhibition of

platelet aggregation by ketamine hydrochloride. Thromb Res 40:227, 1985

53. Heller W, Fuhrer G, Kuhner M et al: Haemostaseologische untersuchungen unter der anwendung von midazolam/ketamin. Anaesthesist 35:419, 1986

54. Reeves JG, Lell WA, McCraken LE et al: Comparison of morphine and ketamine. Anesthetic techniques for coronary surgery: a randomized study. South Med J 71:33, 1978

55. Dhadphale PR, Jackson APF, Alseri S: Comparison of anesthesia with diazepam and ketamine vs. morphine in patients undergoing heart-valve replacement. Anesthesiology 51:200, 1979

56. Gutzke GE, Shah K, Glisson SN et al: Sufentanil or ketamine: induction in cardiomyopathy patients. Anesthesiology 67:64, 1987

57. Newsome LR, Moldenhauer CC, Hug CC et al: Hemodynamic interactions of moderate doses of fentanyl with etomidate and ketamine. Anesth Analg 64:260, 1985

58. Benumof JL, Canada ED, Scanlon TS: Intravenous anesthesia and postoperative analgesia. Anesth Analg 60:240, 1981

59. Lebovic S, Reich DL, Steinberg LG et al: Comparison of propofol versus ketamine for anesthesia in pediatric undergoing cardiac catheterization. Anesth Analg 74:490, 1992

60. Park GR, Manara AR, Mendel L et al: Ketamine infusion—its use as a sedative, inotrope, and bronchodilator in a critically ill patient. Anaesthesia 42:980, 1987

61. Sharma VJ: Use of ketamine in acute severe asthma. Acta Anaesthesiol Scand 36:106, 1992

62. Stefansson T, Wickstom I, Haljamae H: Hemodynamic and metabolic effects of ketamine anesthesia in the geriatric patient. Acta Anaesthesiol Scand 26:371, 1982

63. Pedersen T, Engback J, Klausen NO et al: Effects of low-dose ketamine and thiopentone on cardiac performance and myocardial oxygen balance in high risk patients. Acta Anaesthesiol Scand 26:235, 1982

64. Sher MH: Slow dose ketamine—a new technique. Anaesth Intensive Care 8:359, 1980

65. Priano LL: Alterations of renal hemodynamics by thiopental, diazepam and ketamine in conscious dogs. Anesth Analg 61:853, 1982

66. Longnecker DE, Ross DC, Silver IA: Anesthetic influence on arteriolar diameters and tissue oxygen tension in hemorrhaged rats. Anesthesiology 57:177, 1982

67. Weiskopf RB, Townsley MI, Riordan KK et al: Comparison of cardiopulmonary responses to graded hemorrhage during enflurane, halothane, isoflurane and ketamine anesthesia. Anesth Analg 60:481, 1981

68. Bogetz MS, Weiskopf RB, Roizen MF: Ketamine increases catecholamines but causes cardiovascular depression and acidosis in hypovolemic swine. Anesthesiology 57:29, 1982

69. Waxman K, Shoemaker WC, Lippmann M: Cardiovascular effects of anesthetic induction with ketamine. Anesth Analg 59:355, 1980

70. Hirshman CA, Krieger W, Littlejohn G et al: Ketamine aminophylline induced decrease in seizure threshold. Anesthesiology 56:464, 1982

71. Pickering BG, Palahniuk RJ, Cote J et al: Cerebral vascular responses to ketamine and thiopentone during foetal acidosis. Can J Anaesth 29:463, 1982

72. Dich-Nielsen J, Holasek J: Ketamine as induction agent for cesarean section. Acta Anaesthesiol Scand 26:139, 1982

73. Coad NR, Mills PJ, Verma R, Ramasubramanian R: Evaluation of blood loss during suction termination of pregnancy: ketamine compared with methohexitone. Acta Anaesthesiol Scand 30:253, 1986

74. Gutstein HB, Johnson KL, Heard MB et al: Oral ketamine preanesthetic medication in children. Anesthesiology 76:28, 1992

75. Duperon DF, Jedrychowski JR: Preliminary report on the use of ketamine in pediatric dentistry. Pediatr Dentist 5:75, 1983

76. Saarnivaara L: Comparison of thiopentone, althesin and ketamine in anesthesia for otolaryngological surgery in children. Br J Anaesth 49:363, 1977

77. Jantzen JP, Tzanova I, Klein AM et al: A clinical evaluation of methohexitone and ketamine for anorectal induction of anesthesia in children. Anasthesiol Intensivmed Notfallmed Schmerzther 28:56, 1987

78. Thompson GE, Moore DC: Ketamine, diazepam, and Innovar: a computerized comparative study. Anesth Analg 50:458, 1971

79. White PF: Use of ketamine for sedation and analgesia during injection of local anaesthetics. Ann Plast Surg 15:53, 1985

80. White PF, Vasconez LE, Mathes S et al: Comparison of midazolam and diazepam for sedation during plastic surgery. Plast Reconstr Surg 81:703, 1988

81. Joachimsson PO, Hedstrand U, Ekland A: Low dose ketamine infusion for analgesia during postoperative ventilator treatment. Acta Anaesthesiol Scand 30:697, 1986

82. White PF: Use of continuous infusions versus inter-

mittent bolus administration of fentanyl or ketamine during outpatient anesthesia. Anesthesiology 59:294, 1983

83. White PF, Dworsky WA, Horai Y et al: Comparison of continuous infusion fentanyl or ketamine versus thiopentone—determining the mean effective serum concentrations for outpatient surgery. Anesthesiology 59:564, 1983

84. Havalda HS, Borison RL, Diamond BI: Ketamine anesthesia and analgesia: neurochemical differentiation. Anesthesiology 53:S57, 1980

85. Tung S, Yaksh TL: Analgesic effect of intrathecal ketamine in the rat. Reg Anesth 6:91, 1981

86. Islas JA, Astorga J, Loredo M: Epidural ketamine for control of postoperative pain. Anesth Analg 64:1161, 1985

87. Naquib M, Adu-Gyamfi Y, Absood GM et al: Epidural ketamine for postoperative analgesia. Can J Anaesth 33:16, 1986

88. Naquib M, Sharif AM, Seraj M et al: Ketamine for caudal analgesia in children: comparison with caudal bupivacaine. Br J Anaesth 67:559, 1991

89. Ravat F, Dorne R, Baechle JP et al: Epidural ketamine or morphine for postoperative analgesia. Anesthesiology 66:819, 1987

90. Kawana Y, Sato H, Shimada H: Epidural ketamine for postoperative pain relief after gynecologic operations. Anesth Analg 66:735, 1987

91. Lees DE, Kim YD, MacNamara TE: The safety of ketamine in pediatric neuromuscular disease. Anesth Rev 9:17, 1982

92. Bancroft GH, Lauria JI: Ketamine induction for caesarian section in a patient with acute intermittent porphyria and achondroplastic dwarfism. Anesthesiology 53:143, 1983

93. Capouet V, Dernovoi B, Azagra JS: Induction of anesthesia with ketamine during an acute crisis of hereditary coproporphyria. Can J Anaesth 34:388, 1987

94. Eisenkraft JB, Dimich I, Miller R: Ketamine-diazepam anesthesia in a patient with carcinoid syndrome. Anaesthesia 36:881, 1981

95. Saarnivaara L, Kautto U-M, Teravainen H: Ketamine anesthesia for a patient with the Shy-Drager syndrome. Acta Anaesthesiol Scand 27:123, 1983

96. Hatano S, Nishiwada M, Matsumura M: Ketamine-diazepam anesthesia for abdominal surgery. Anaesthesist 27:172, 1978

97. Houlton PJC, Downing JW: General anaesthesia with intravenous flunitrazepam, continuous ketamine infusion and muscle relaxant. Afr Med J 54:1048, 1978

98. Idvall J, Ahlgren I, Aronsen KF et al: Ketamine infusions: Pharmacokinetics and clinical effects. Br J Anaesth 51:1167, 1979

99. Hatano S, Keane DM, Boggs RE et al: Diazepam-ketamine anaesthesia for open heart surgery—a micro-mini drip administration technique. Can Anaesth Soc J 23:648, 1976

100. Reves JG, Lell WA, McCracken LE et al: Comparison of morphine and ketamine. Anesthetic techniques for coronary surgery: a randomized study. South Med J 71:33, 1978

101. El-Naggar M, Letcher J, Middleton E et al: Administration of ketamine or Innovar by the microdrip method—a double blind study. Anesth Analg 56:279, 1977

102. Lilburn JK, Dundee JW, Moore J: Ketamine infusions—observations on technique dosage and cardiovascular effects. Anaesthesia 33:315, 1978

103. Barclay A, Houlton PC, Downing JW: Total intravenous anesthesia—a technique using flunitrazepam, ketamine, muscle relaxants and controlled ventilation of the lung. Anaesthesia 35:287, 1980

Chapter 19

Basic Pharmacology of Neuromuscular Blockers

Eugene M. Silinsky

The skeletal neuromuscular junction is designed to produce the expeditious generation of a muscle twitch in response to an electrical impulse in the motor neuron. The rapidity of this biologic event is so striking that, for many years, it was believed that neuromuscular transmission took place by direct transfer of electrical activity from nerve to muscle without any intervening neurotransmitter substance. Indeed, it was only with the advent of the intracellular recording microelectrode that the idea of direct electrical neuromuscular transmission was ultimately refuted.[1,2]

We now know that the speed of neuromuscular transmission is caused by the inherent swiftness of each of the stages that intervenes between the initiation signal in the nerve ending and the activation of receptors on the muscle. Each participating stage occurs through rapid physicochemical processes rather than by the slower catalytic cascades associated with the synthesis of second messenger substances.[3] A nerve action potential opens voltage-gated ion channels, permitting the entry of intracellular Ca^{++}, which stimulates presynaptic release of the preformed neurotransmitter acetylcholine (ACh), which in turn, activates nicotinic receptors in the postjunctional membrane. The nicotinic receptors are members of a superfamily of receptors that incorporate an ion channel as part of their structure; thus, activation of nicotinic receptors can produce channel opening in the submillisecond time scale.[4–6]

This chapter provides an overview of the biophysical aspects of neuromuscular transmission and a brief description of the electrophysiologic methods that provide the basis for this understanding. The postjunctional nicotinic receptor-ion channel complex will be described, along with the biophysical characteristics of different categories of blocking drugs; included in this discussion will be the electrophysiologic properties of single ACh receptors and their associated ion channels. The chapter concludes with a consideration of twitch tension measurements used to evaluate neuromuscular block during surgical procedures.

OVERVIEW OF PROCESSES UNDERLYING SKELETAL NEUROMUSCULAR TRANSMISSION

Generally Accepted Scheme

Neuromuscular transmission can be conveniently divided into prejunctional events associated with the release of ACh and postjunctional events associated with the action of ACh on receptors in the skeletal muscle membrane (Figs. 19-1 and 19-2).

Prejunctional Events

Molecules of ACh are synthesized and then stored in vesicles (together with adenosine triphosphate [ATP], to be discussed later) in the presynaptic terminals. The initiating event for evoked neuromuscular transmission is the normal wave of depolarization associated with the nerve action potential, which propagates near the nerve ending (Fig. 19-2). The depolarization associated with the upstroke of the action potential opens voltage-sensitive Ca^{++} channels. Ca^{++} flows into the cell down an electrochemical gradient. Once in the cytoplasm, Ca^{++} reduces an electrostatic energy barrier between the negatively charged synaptic vesicles and the nerve terminal membranes, bringing these membranes together and distorting them. The synaptic vesicles fuse with the nerve terminal membrane, and ACh is secreted by exocytosis into the synaptic cleft. The process of ACh release also occurs randomly and spontaneously in the absence of an action potential; the action potential accelerates the release process into synchronous discharges of about 100 to 200 ACh-containing vesicles.

Postjunctional Events

After a brief diffusion time in the narrow 40 to 50-nm synaptic cleft, ACh combines with the recognition site on the nicotinic receptor-ion channel complex. This interaction with the receptor gates (opens) a nonselective channel through which Na^+ and other cations flow down an electrochemical gradient. The entry of Na^+ through the ACh-gated channel depolarizes the membrane from its resting state. This postjunctional depolarization produced in response to ACh is termed the end plate potential (EPP) (Figs. 19-2 and 19-3). The EPP is generally so large that a suprathreshold muscle action potential is generated by voltage-sensitive Na^+ channels. This action potential then causes muscle contraction by the mechanisms underlying excitation-contraction coupling. The action of ACh is terminated by acetylcholinesterase (AChE), and the choline released from this process is retrieved by the nerve ending for resynthesis of ACh.

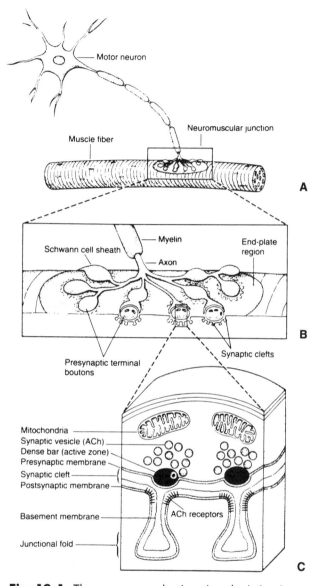

Fig. 19-1 The neuromuscular junction depicting in progressively enlarged views the terminal end of an individual presynaptic bouton. **(A)** Shows the terminals of the motorneurons innervating the skeletal muscle fiber. **(B)** Represents an enlargement of the terminal and of the presynaptic boutons (swellings) or varicosities arranged adjacent to the muscle end plate. **(C)** Depicts an individual presynaptic bouton separated from the muscle end plate membrane by the synaptic cleft. The end plate is represented as a specialized region of the muscle membrane in which high densities of ACh receptors are localized. ACh, acetylcholine. (Modified from Kandel and Schwartz,[65] with permission.)

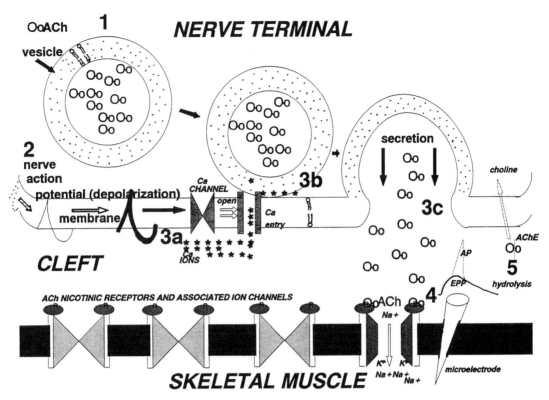

Fig. 19-2 Summary of the mechanisms involved in neuromuscular transmission at a single site. The prejunctional events associated with evoked ACh release are numbered *1–3c* and the postjunctional events associated with the action of ACh on its nicotinic receptor and the hydrolysis of ACh are numbered *4* and *5*, respectively. Presynaptically, * represent Ca^{++} ions, which enter the cytoplasm by voltage-gated Ca^{++} channels. Other channel types (e.g., tetrodotoxin-sensitive Na^+ channel and a variety of voltage- and Ca^{++}-gated K^+ channels) are not shown. Postjunctionally, *R* = is the recognition site for ACh on the nicotinic ACh receptor, *EPP* = is the end plate potential, and *AP* = is the action potential generated in the muscle when the EPP has reached threshold. ACh, acetylcholine; AChE, acetylcholinesterase. (For further details of specific vesicular and nerve terminal proteins, see refs. 67–71.)

Basic Electrophysiologic Method

When a glass pipette microelectrode is inserted into the interior of a skeletal muscle fiber, a recording device (e.g., a cathode ray oscilloscope) registers a downward deflection of −70 to −90 mV (negative inside), which represents the resting potential of the muscle cell (Fig. 19-3, Vm). If the pipette is inserted at the innervated region of the skeletal muscle, then small deflections, termed miniature EPPs (MEPPs) are observed in association with the random spontaneous release of ACh from the nerve terminal. The quantal theory of synaptic transmission states that the MEPP represents the basic "coin" or quantum of transmitter secretion.[2] The nerve impulse harmonizes these discrete quantal units into the synchronous release of many quanta (normally 100 to 200) detected electrophysiologically as the EPP. The EPP thus represents integral multiples of the MEPP. MEPPs and EPPs are decreased in size by postjunctional ACh receptor blockers, such as curare alkaloids, and increased by anticholinesterases, which decrease the hydrolysis of ACh.

For ACh to be released in packets that are approximately the same size, it was necessary to postulate a packaging mechanism that maintained the uniformity of the secretory product. The observa-

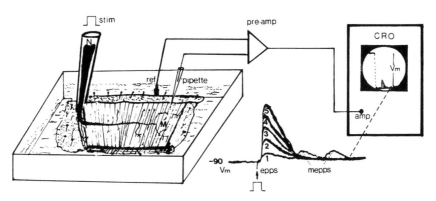

Fig. 19-3 Electrophysiologic method for studying neuromuscular transmission. A glass pipette micro-electrode records the potential as referenced to an indifferent ground electrode (*ref*). The signal is fed into a preamplifier with high input impedance (*pre-amp*) and then into the plug-in amplifier (*amp*) of a cathode ray oscilloscope (*CRO*). When skeletal muscle is impaled with the microelectrode, the resting potential of the muscle is registered (V_m = −70 to −90 mV). See text for further details of the spontaneous events recorded at the end plate region of skeletal muscle in the absence of nerve stimulation (*mepps*) and the evoked potentials (*epps*) recorded when the motor nerve (*N*) is stimulated (_⌐⌐_stim). The many epps represent superimposed sweeps from a storage oscilloscope. Physiologic solutions contained low Ca^{++} (0.1 mM). This experiment was done on a frog cutaneous pectoris nerve-muscle junction. Each *mepp* was approximately 1 mV in amplitude with a 1 to 2 ms in rise time. epp, end plate potential, mepp, miniature epp.

tion of synaptic vesicles and the finding that they contained high concentrations of ACh provided such a mechanism.[2,3] In accordance with the vesicle hypothesis, the MEPP is thought to correspond to the all-or-none release of the ACh contents of one synaptic vesicle (see ref. 3 for further discussion).

MEPP frequency is dependent on intracellular Ca^{++} concentrations. Neurally evoked responses (EPPs), however, are intimately related to extracellular Ca^{++} because nerve stimulation causes voltage-sensitive Ca^{++} channels to open; Ca^{++} then enters the nerve ending and promotes ACh release. As the extracellular Ca^{++} concentration is raised, more Ca^{++} can enter the nerve ending through the open Ca^{++} channels, and the EPP becomes larger until, at 2 mM Ca^{++}, some 100 to 200 quanta are released, producing a muscle action potential.

Changes in EPPs and MEPPs are used to determine sites of neuromuscular blocking drug action.[2,3,7] For example, if drug X blocks neuromuscular transmission but the MEPPs remain constant in amplitude, then it is almost certain that drug X does not influence the action of ACh on the receptor; drug X must work presynaptically. However, if the MEPPs are decreased in size, then it is

highly probable that the drug acts at the postsynaptic nicotinic receptor-ion channel complex. It is theoretically possible for a drug to decrease MEPP amplitude by reducing the number of ACh molecules per vesicle. However, this generally requires repetitive high frequency stimulation to deplete the available stores of preformed ACh vesicles. Confirmation of the locus of drug action may be made by ACh iontophoresis, whereby ACh is locally applied from a micropipette by brief pulses of electric current. The response of the skeletal muscle to iontophoretically applied ACh is decreased if the inhibitory drug acts on the ACh receptor.

A quantitative assessment of presynaptic drug effects is made from the ratio of the average amplitude of the EPP to the average amplitude of the MEPP. The EPP/MEPP ratio reflects the mean number of ACh packets released by a nerve impulse and is referred to as the "mean quantal content." If drug X decreases the mean quantal content without a change in spontaneous MEPP frequency, then an inhibitory effect of the agent on Ca^{++} entry into nerve endings is likely. This inhibition could occur directly by an effect on Ca^{++} channels or, indirectly, as a consequence of decreases in

Na$^+$ currents or increases in K$^+$ currents. Newer recording methods can usually distinguish between effects of drugs on Na$^+$, K$^+$, or Ca^{++} currents in motor nerve endings.[8–11] In some instances, the frequency of spontaneous MEPPs is decreased when a drug inhibits transmitter release (e.g., adenosine, discussed later).

PREJUNCTIONAL PHYSIOLOGY AND PHARMACOLOGY

Drugs Acting to Impair Synthesis and Storage

ACh synthesis proceeds normally only when choline can be recaptured into the nerve ending, acetylated to ACh, and then packaged into synaptic vesicles. The uptake of choline by the nerve ending takes place through a saturable, high affinity carrier (K$_m$, 1 to 5 μM), which is dependent on Na$^+$ and ATP. The hemicholinium analogs, and especially hemicholinium 3, are competitive inhibitors of this choline transport mechanism.[12,13] When the neuromuscular junction is blocked by hemicholinium 3, which requires repetitive nerve stimulation to deplete the available stores of ACh, MEPPs become extremely small as a result of the decrease in the number of ACh molecules in a quantum.

Vesamicol (AH5183), produces the same apparent electrophysiologic dysfunction as does hemicholinium 3, namely, a presynaptic reduction in MEPP amplitude after repetitive nerve stimulation.[14] However, vesamicol blocks ACh synthesis at a later stage than do the hemicholiniums; it prevents the transport of ACh from the nerve terminal cytoplasm across the vesicle membrane.

Drugs That Block Conduction of Action Potential Into the Nerve Terminals by Effects on Na$^+$ and K$^+$ Channels

Tetrodotoxin is the active ingredient found in fugu (puffer fish), from which a delicacy served in fashionable restaurants in Japan is prepared.[15–17] The dish must be prepared by specially licensed chefs because tetrodotoxin, found mainly in specific internal organs of the fish, can produce severe poisoning by blocking Na$^+$ channels in neurons and thus prevent the initiation and propagation of the action potential. Tetrodotoxin-sensitive Na$^+$ channels also generate action potentials in muscle cells (see below).

Drugs and Conditions in Which Ca^{++} Entry and Thus Evoked ACh Release Is Impaired

Mg^{++} and all other impermeant polyvalent cations (e.g., Co^{++}, Mn^{++}, Cd^{++}, and La^{+++}) compete with Ca^{++} for entry through the Ca^{++} channel and decrease neurally evoked ACh release. The effects of these ions are reflected electrophysiologically as a decrease in EPP amplitude with little to no change in the amplitude or frequency of MEPPs. Aminoglycoside antibiotics (e.g., streptomycin, kanamycin, neomycin, and gentamicin) also block stimulated ACh release,[18,19] as a consequence of Ca^{++} channel blockade (Redman RS, Silinsky EM: unpublished observations). There is also a postsynaptic blocking action of these and other antibiotics, but only at higher concentrations.

Based on conventional methods for distinguishing between Ca^{++} channel subtypes (i.e., toxins, venoms, and dihydropyridine derivatives for differentiating N, L, T, and P subtypes), it is impossible to generalize as to the specific subset of Ca^{++} channels that mediate ACh release from vertebrate nerve endings.[11] In clinically relevant concentrations, verapamil blocks Ca^{++} channels in mammalian motor nerve endings.[9,20]

Very recently, we have obtained additional information as to specific vesicular, cytoplasmic, and nerve terminal membrane proteins that constitute a fusion machine for neurotransmitter release.[67–71] Briefly, the vesicular protein, synaptotagmin, a calcium-binding protein, is linked via cytoplasmic proteins to a plasma membrane protein (syntaxin); syntaxin in turn is linked to voltage-sensitive calcium channels (N-type). Several of the cytoplasmic proteins important to the secretory apparatus, abbreviated as SNAPS (with various flavors indicated by Greek letters or numbers) form the targets for various toxins and venoms (see below). Other proteins such as the vesicular protein VAMP (synatobrevin) and the plasma membrane protein neurexin also bind toxins and venoms. Finally, small GTP-binding proteins and synapsins associated with the vesicles are important respectively for vesicle docking and for attachment of vesicles to the cytoskeleton.

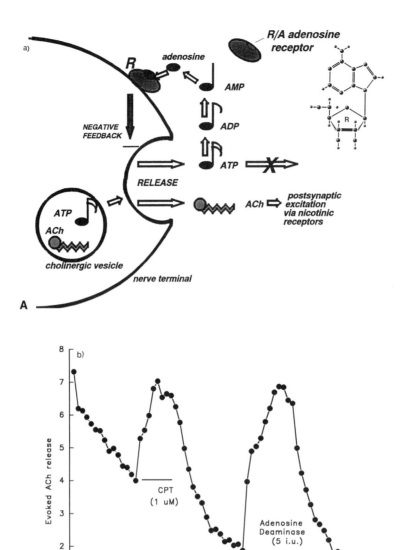

Fig. 19-4 A model for the action of adenosine in mediating prejunctional neuromuscular depression **(A)** and the evidence for such a model **(B)**. **(A)** Note the corelease of ATP with ACh, the hydrolysis of ATP to adenosine, and the binding of adenosine to its receptors (Rs) on the motor nerve ending. **(B)** Shows that presynaptic neuromuscular depression produced by continuous prejunctional stimulation of frog motor nerve at 1 stimulus per 10 seconds is fully reversed by an antagonist of A_1 adenosine receptors (CPT) or by adenosine deaminase, which degrades adenosine.[28,29] Evoked ACh release is shown in arbitrary units and reflects the EPP amplitude in millivolts in a solution containing blockers of K^+ channels, tetraethylammonium (250 μM) and 3,4-diaminopyridine (100 μM). The solution also contained tubocurarine (5 mg/L), 0.9 mM Ca^{++}, and 10 mM Mg^{++}. The K^+ channel blockers increase ACh release by prolonging the action potential in the nerve ending and also allow for measurements of Ca^{++} currents, which were not altered by the action of endogenous adenosine during this experiment. Similar results were observed in absence of K^+ channel blockers. A similar mechanism is likely to occur at mouse motor nerve.[29] ACh, acetylcholine; ATP, adenosine triphosphate; CPT, cyclopentyltheophylline; EPP, end plate potential; R, receptor.

Drugs That Affect ACh Release Mechanism

Botulinum toxin (type A), produced by the bacterium *Clostridium botulinum*,[21] is one of the most potent toxins known (several hundred grams could poison the entire population of the world). This toxin binds to a nerve terminal ganglioside, is internalized by endocytosis, and then acts at the internal face of the membrane to inhibit ACh release. Botulinum toxin appears to obstruct Ca^{++} from initiating the exocytosis process inside the nerve ending by reducing the apparent affinity of Ca^{++} to promote exocytosis.[22] Thus a higher level of intracellular Ca^{++} is necessary to produce a given level of ACh secretion. Type A botulinum toxin binds to a specific cytoplasmic protein in the fusion machine SNAP-25.[71] Other fractions of this toxin bind to VAMP syntoxin and to other SNAP proteins.[67–71] The electrophysiologic manifestation in botulism is a reduction in MEPP frequency and in stimulated ACh release.

Black widow spider venom blocks ACh release by a different mechanism. The active ingredient, α-latrotoxin,[23] causes a tremendous barrage of MEPPs associated with the appearance of a considerable number of exocytotic vesicles. Indeed, morphologic studies on muscles poisoned by α-latrotoxin provide some of the clearest evidence for the vesicle hypothesis. In poisoned patients, the enormous release of ACh induced by the toxin causes asynchronous muscle twitches, leading to painful muscle rigidity. If allowed to persist, the population of ACh-containing vesicles in the nerve ending is severely depleted. The underlying mechanism of this effect of α-latrotoxin has not been fully elucidated, but it may be related to a cation ionophore action or to an effect on phosphoinositide turnover.[24] Furthermore, α-latrotoxin binds specifically to the plasma membrane protein neurexin, which is linked to the calcium-binding vesicular protein synaptotagmin.[67–71]

Adenosine is a unique inhibitor of evoked ACh release because it is an endogenous physiologic modulator of presynaptic function. Adenosine acts extracellularly at specific presynaptic adenosine receptors located on cholinergic neuron terminals (Fig. 19-4).[25] The adenosine is derived from ATP, which is packaged and released together with ACh

in synaptic vesicles.[26] On release, ATP is hydrolyzed to adenosine, which binds to prejunctional receptors to inhibit the release of ACh. Adenosine is responsible for all or most of the neuromuscular depression that ensues with repetitive nerve stimulation at physiologic levels of ACh release.[27–29] Adenosine decreases both evoked ACh release and MEPP frequency.[30] The mechanism is probably a reduction in the ability of intracellular Ca^{++} to promote ACh release,[11,31,32] although small effects on Ca^{++} currents have also been observed in some species.[33] 8-Cyclopentyltheophylline (1 μM), a selective blocker of adenosine receptors, antagonizes neuromuscular depression as does adenosine deaminase, which degrades adenosine to the inactive inosine (Fig. 19-4).

Nicotinic receptors are also present on motor nerve endings.[34,35] These presynaptic nicotinic receptors appear to maintain ACh stores in a readily releasable state. ACh released into the synaptic cleft tonically mobilizes ACh stores by positive feedback on presynaptic nicotinic receptors.[34] Nondepolarizing neuromuscular blocking drugs, used clinically primarily to block postsynaptic nicotinic receptors, may also produce presynaptic impairment of ACh release by preventing mobilization of ACh (discussed subsequently in Assessing Types of Neuromuscular Block From Patterns of Twitch Tension Measurements). Conversely, depolarizing neuromuscular blocking drugs may act on presynaptic nicotinic receptors to enhance ACh release. Stimulation of ACh release by presynaptic receptor activation is thought to underlie the mechanism of succinycholine-induced muscle fasciculations.[36] Similarly, small ("defasciculating") doses of nondepolarizing blockers prevent succinylcholine-induced fasciculation by blocking these presynaptic receptors.

POSTJUNCTIONAL PHYSIOLOGY AND PHARMACOLOGY

Drugs that block postsynaptic receptors of the neuromuscular junction revolutionized anesthesiology when they were introduced in 1942.[37] Prior to the availability of drugs that selectively blocked neuromuscular transmission, large doses of general anesthetic were used to produce a nonspecific membrane depressant effect at the postsynaptic membrane. Neuromuscular blockers selectively reduce muscle tone during surgery and thus allow the use of lower and safer doses of general anesthetics.

Acetylcholine Receptor-Ion Channel Complex

The nicotinic ACh receptor (AChR) is probably the best defined of all neurotransmitter receptors currently known. The characterization of this receptor was facilitated by the discovery of its great abundance in the organs of the Torpedo ray and the electric eel, *Electrophorus electricus*.[38] The electric organs of these species contain some 1,000 times more AChRs than do mammalian skeletal muscle, enabling investigators to identify, purify, and subsequently, isolate the receptor.[39] More recently, the cloning and sequencing of the complementary DNA and genes encoding the subunits of the receptor were accomplished. The nicotinic receptor of the electric organ and neuromuscular junction is now known to exist in a pentameric complex consisting of subunits designated as α, β, γ, or δ, with a stoichiometry of two α and one each of the other subunits (i.e., α_2, β, γ, δ). These five subunits are arranged in a petal-like fashion around a central cavity that is thought to represent the ion channel (Fig. 19-5).[6,40,41] Models constructed from sequencing data proposed that four or five spanning regions traverse the membrane (M1 to M4) with one

possessing the amino terminus located on the extracellular surface. Site-directed mutagenesis and photolabelling the channel with channel blockers suggest that the M2 segment represents the ion transport system of the receptor-channel complex. Only the α subunits appear to possess the recognition sites for ACh and other agonists and competitive antagonists. The binding site of both α subunits must be occupied by an agonist for receptor activation and subsequent channel opening. Therefore, two molecules of ACh are needed to activate the receptor.

A major breakthrough was made in 1963 when Chang and Lee[43] discovered that the venom from the banded krait, *Bungarus multicinctus*, contained a toxin, α-bungarotoxin, that bound avidly to the nicotinic receptor of the electric organ and mammalian neuromuscular junction. Subsequently, the α-toxin from cobra venom also showed similar high affinity binding to the receptor. By radioactively labeling these toxins, it became possible to develop chromatographic columns with which to isolate and purify the receptor. Physicochemical studies of the purified receptor revealed that the toxins are bound to the two α subunits of the AChR in a virtually irreversible manner.[44]

The autonomic and central nervous systems also contain nicotinic receptors. It has been known since the early 1900s that autonomic ganglia possessed receptors that were activated and blocked by

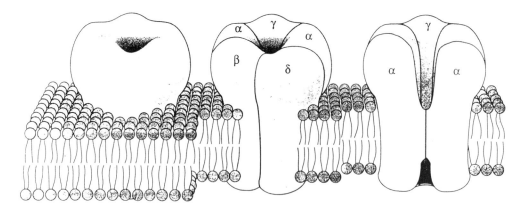

Fig. 19-5 Schematic representation of the arrangement of the nicotinic ACh receptor-channel complex within the muscle membrane. The receptor, together with the channel, is composed of two α and one each of β, γ (or ε), and δ subunits. The binding sites for ACh are located on α subunits. When two molecules of ACh bind to the two α subunits, the channel opens to allow flow of ions across the muscle membrane (From Kandel and Schwartz,[65] with permission.)

nicotine and that they were related to, but different from, the neuromuscular nicotinic receptors. More recently, nicotinic receptors were also found in various areas of the brain. Because no high density sources of the neuronal nicotinic receptors have been found (as in the case of the electric organs for muscle nicotinic receptors), their properties are not as well defined as in the case of the neuromuscular junction. However, it is now clear that the neuronal nicotinic receptor has subunits different from those of muscle, seven of which have been cloned and designated as $\alpha_2–\alpha_8$ subunits.[41,45] Because the α subunit represents the binding sites for ACh and its antagonists, these findings of different α subunits offer an explanation for the differences in activities of various neuromuscular blocking agents at the neuromuscular junction and autonomic ganglia, as will be discussed later. The neuronal nicotinic receptors are generally not blocked by α-bungarotoxin, which as discussed earlier, produces a near-irreversible block of the muscle receptor in extremely low concentrations, but are blocked by neuronal (κ) bungarotoxin.[42] Thus far, the neuronal receptor appears to be a tetramer or pentamer, but it consists only of the α and β subunits in an $\alpha_2\beta_3$ arrangement.

Types of Postjunctional Block

Nondepolarizing Block

Nondepolarizing blockers are competitive antagonists of ACh at the recognition sites of the nicotinic receptor. They are generally large bulky molecules possessing two ACh-like moieties as part of a more elaborate ring structure (see Fig. 19-11A and later discussion). They bind to the recognition site on the nicotinic receptor but do not have the favorable steric structure to promote opening of the ion channel. In contrast, nicotinic receptor agonists (e.g., ACh) are generally smaller molecules (see Fig. 19-11B).

Depolarizing Block

As a prelude to discussing depolarizing block, it is necessary to review first the types of ionic channels that populate the membranes of the skeletal muscle fiber.[1,2,4,5,17] Both chemically gated ion channels (the ACh receptor-ion channel complex) and electrically gated channels (Na^+ and K^+ channels) span the plasma membrane of skeletal muscle (Fig. 19-6). Synaptic communication occurs when ACh activates the ACh receptor, opening the relatively nonselective receptor-cation channel to admit Na^+ and allow K^+ to exit.[17] The influx of Na^+ begins to depolarize the membrane toward an equilibrium potential (between -15 and 0 mV), which is midway between the Na^+ and K^+ equilibrium potentials. ACh-induced depolarization, in turn, rapidly activates the voltage-sensitive membrane sodium channel. Sodium entry through the electrically gated sodium channel is responsible for the upstroke of the muscle action potential. The sodium channels activate within milliseconds and then inactivate. This inactivation process and the activation of depolarization-gated K^+ channels, which develops more slowly, restores the membrane potential to its polarized resting level. In addition to activation by motor nerve stimulation, the muscle can be stimulated directly. Stimulation of the muscle membrane itself activates the voltage-sensitive muscle membrane sodium channels, eliciting a muscle action potential.

The normal activation sequence of the nicotinic ACh receptor goes awry when excessive agonist (depolarizing agent) is present. High concentrations of agonist may desensitize the nicotinic receptor[46] or block by depolarization prior to desensitization.[46,47] Indeed, ACh, the normal neuromuscular transmitter, is also a neuromuscular blocker. A high concentration of a depolarizing agent, such as ACh or succinylcholine, first depolarizes the muscle fibers at the end plate, causing trains of action potentials and muscle fasciculations (Fig. 19-7). After this phase of uncoordinated muscle contraction, muscle twitches in response to nerve stimulation are rapidly abolished. The muscle remains depolarized and is now refractory to any form of stimulus. Neither nerve nor muscle stimulus produces a response (Fig. 19-7). Transmission is thus blocked by depolarization, termed *phase I block*. If the depolarizing drug remains in contact with the neuromuscular junction for a prolonged period, the muscle membrane potential returns to its resting undepolarized value, despite the continued presence of the depolarizing drug. It appears that the end plate has become less sensitive to the agonist over time. This phase of block is termed *desensitization block* or *phase II block*.

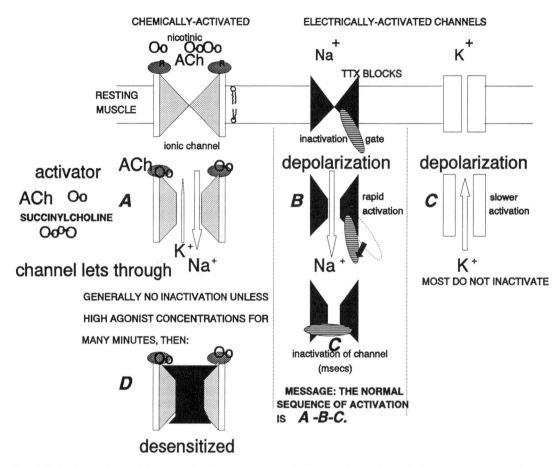

Fig. 19-6 Overview of the chemically activated and electrically activated channels that populate the muscle fiber membrane. The chemically activated channel (*left*) is part of the nicotinic ACh receptor, which when gated by ACh (or its analogs, such as succinylcholine), depolarizes the membrane by the entry of Na^+ through its nonselective cation pore (*A*). This depolarization rapidly (in milliseconds) activates the TTX-sensitive Na^+ channel (*B*), further depolarizes the membrane, and normally generates an action potential. The membrane potential is restored by inactivation of the Na^+ channel and by the slower activation of K^+ channels (*C*). The normal sequence of activation by neurally released ACh is thus A to B to C. If enough exogenous depolarizing drug is applied, a desensitized receptor (*D*) may result. ACh, acetylcholine; TTX, tetrodotoxin.

Phase I block is characterized by a depolarized but electrically inexcitable muscle in and around the end plate region, thereby blocking synaptic communication. After first initiating a series of action potentials through the electrically activated Na^+ channel, the persistent depolarization produced through the chemically activated nicotinic cation channel causes the inactivation of the electrically activated Na^+ channel. The zone of chemically depolarized but electrically inactivated muscle membrane at and around the end plate prevents effective communication between the nerve and

muscle. The exogenous agonist present on ACh receptors also prevents endogenous ACh released from presynaptic nerve terminals from reaching the receptor. In the continued presence of the depolarizing drug, the membrane potential may return to its resting level. This produces phase II block.

Phase II block is characterized by a muscle membrane that has repolarized and thus regained its normal direct electrical excitability, that is, voltage-gated Na^+ channel function is restored. The repolarization is probably caused by the conversion of

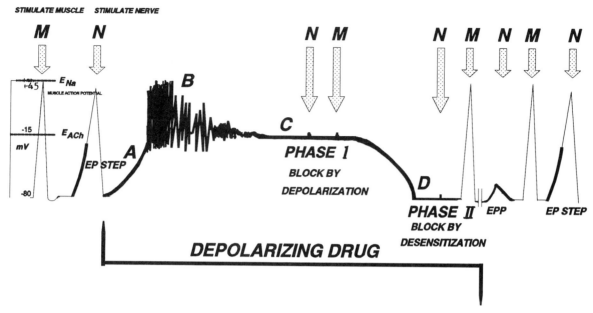

Fig. 19-7 The effect of a depolarizing blocking drug on the action potentials evoked by direct muscle stimulation (M) and by the release of ACh from nerve endings (N). With a microelectrode in the end plate, direct muscle stimulation elicits an action potential (M) as the Na^+ channel activated by the depolarizing stimulus drives the membrane potential to E_{Na}. Stimulation of the motor nerve (N) releases ACh, which acts on the nicotinic receptors to drive the membrane potential to the equilibrium potential for the action of ACh = E_{ACh}. Because ACh activates a relatively nonselective cation channel, E_{ACh} is midway between the K^+ and Na^+ equilibrium potential (between -15 and 0 mV). Before E_{ACh} is reached, however, the entry of Na^+ through the nicotinic receptor-channel has depolarized the membrane potential to threshold for excitation of an action potential.

Application of a depolarizing agent (applied between the arrows) first depolarizes the muscle fibers at the end plate (A) and produces trains of action potentials and muscle fasciculations (B). After this uncoordinated electrical and mechanical activity has subsided, the muscle remains depolarized and refractory to any form of stimulus, a state known as phase I block (C). If the drug is allowed to remain in the muscle bath for a prolonged period, the membrane potential returns to its resting undepolarized state, despite the continued presence of the drug (D). It appears that the end plate has become less sensitive to the drug over time. This phase of block is called desensitization block or phase II block. During phase II block, the muscle membrane potential repolarizes and regains excitability to direct muscle stimulation (M), but synaptic communication (N) is still blocked. Finally, withdrawal of the drug allows neuromuscular transmission to return slowly to normal. ACh, acetylcholine.

nicotinic receptors into a desensitized conformation that is inactive and thus cannot conduct Na^+ ions to maintain the membrane in a depolarized state (Fig. 19-7). Muscle stimulation can directly produce an action potential, but synaptic communication is still blocked. Nerve stimulation does not produce a muscle action potential. Because some investigators observed an improvement with anticholinesterase drugs during phase II block, it was suggested that the agonist achieved a competitive-like nature, rather than that the receptor was desensitized. However, such an explanation is not

required to explain the effects of anticholinesterases.[47]

Channel Block

The preceding discussion of phase I and II blocks was somewhat idealized. In reality, depolarization during phase I block is never complete because nicotinic agonists may also plug ACh receptor-ion channels during depolarization, producing open channel block.[47] The agonist thus opposes its own depolarizing action by occluding the entry of Na^+ through the nicotinic receptor channel.

Current understanding of open channel block derives from the ability to measure the membrane currents, which generate the MEPPs and EPPs, caused by ions passing through the open nicotinic receptor-ion channel. The technique for measuring these end plate currents is called voltage clamp.[48] In voltage clamp, two electrodes are used, and the membrane potential is specifically prevented from changing ("clamped") by what is essentially a high gain negative feedback device (Fig. 19-8). As before, one electrode records the membrane potential. A second electrode is used to pass

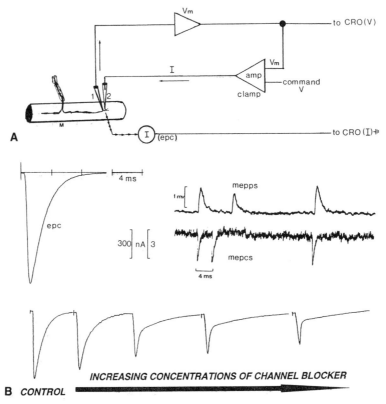

Fig. 19-8 Diagram representing the two electrode voltage clamp for studying (a) epcs and mepcs and (b) the effects of open channel blockers. **(A)** The typical circuit is shown. The end plate is impaled with a recording electrode (1) that carries an electrical signal (V_m) to the voltage clamp amplifier. Another input supplies the amplifier with the command signal (*command V*), which is under the control of the experimenter. A second electrode (2) is also inserted into the muscle for the purpose of passing current to prevent the membrane potential from changing (i.e., voltage clamping the membrane). After ACh release from motor neuron terminals, electrode 2 injects a current identical to that generated by ACh to produce the muscle depolarization into the muscle. This current delivered by the electrode can be measured and recorded and reflects the magnitude and time course of the ACh-induced current. If this current is evoked by nerve stimulation it is referred to as the end plate current (EPC), and if it occurs spontaneously, as the miniature EPC (MEPC).

The effect of the open channel blocker, isobutylmethylxanthine, on the EPC in frog muscle is shown in (b). Note the progressive reduction in amplitude and conversion into a biphasic decay of the EPC on exposure of the muscle to progressive increases in drug concentration. The early phase of the decay occurs because the channel blocking effect of the drug curtails the rise of the EPC. The slower decay is caused by the flickering of the channel between the open and blocked states. Flickering reduces the time the channel is in the conducting state and, thus, decreases the amplitude of the current, but the drug prevents the channel from closing and thus prolongs the duration of the EPC beyond that of the control. ACh, acetylcholine. (From Silinsky and Vogel,[66] with permission.)

current into the membrane, the amount of which is determined by the difference between Vm and the command voltage. For example, suppose the muscle membrane is commanded to remain at the resting potential. ACh is released and attempts to depolarize the membrane but cannot because the clamping electrode is passing current to prevent the membrane potential from changing. The clamping current reflects the magnitude and time course of the ACh-induced current. Spontaneously occurring currents are called miniature end plate currents (MEPC), and currents evoked by nerve stimulation are called end plate currents (EPC), analogous to the MEPPs and EPPs described previously. Clamping membrane voltage also eliminates the effects of drugs and neurotransmitters on voltage-gated channels, thereby permitting isolated study of the chemically gated nicotinic receptor-ion channel.

Voltage clamp has been used to assess the mechanism of channel block. Open channel block in which the blocker prevents the channel from closing alters the normal EPC and its associated monophasic decay by reducing the peak amplitude and converting monophasic decay to biphasic decay (Fig. 19-8).[47] The early rapid phase of decay occurs because the channel blocking effect of the drug curtails the rise of the EPC. The slower decay is the result of flickering of the channel between open and blocked states; the drug plugging the channel prevents the channel from closing and thus prolongs the EPC duration beyond normal. Nicotinic agonists, such as ACh, succinylcholine, and decamethonium, all produce open channel block.[49] The first demonstration of channel block was with charged molecules, such as local anesthetics, which produce block that is voltage dependent because hyperpolarizing the membrane drives the positively charged drug into the channel.[47] Uncharged drugs can also produce channel block. In addition, curare, at very polarized membrane potentials (-90 mV and more), produces channel block in addition to acting as a competitive antagonist at the ACh recognition site on the nicotinic receptor.

Single Ion Channels

Interactions between drugs and receptors can now be studied at the level of individual receptors. The method used to observe a single ion channel in a patch of membrane, the patch clamp, in essence, electrophysiologically purifies a single functioning receptor (Fig. 19-9A). When a blunt-snouted microelectrode is filled with ACh, attached to a voltage clamp amplifier, pressed cautiously against the innervated region of a skeletal muscle fiber, and a high resistance seal achieved, the rectangular pulses of current indicating the opening and closing of individual nicotinic receptor ion channels may be recorded. The development and use of this technique resulted in the Nobel Prize for Physiology and Medicine for Sakmann and Neher[50,51] in 1992.

The currently accepted kinetic scheme for nicotinic receptor activation is depicted in Figure 19-9B. Two ACh molecules bind to the receptor to form an inactive bound state (ACh_2R), which then isomerizes into the active state (ACh_2R^*), and the ion channel is opened. The *binding* of any drug to the receptor is described by K_d, the equilibrium dissociation constant, which is the ratio of the backward and forward rate constants for receptor drug binding. The *efficacy* of any drug represents the ability of the drug, once bound to the receptor, to produce channel opening. This is represented by an isomerization constant for drug efficacy, the ratio of the opening and closing rate constants for receptor activation (β/α). The ability to observe single channel events thus changed the notion of efficacy, traditionally an abstract concept, to a concrete physicochemical concept.

Single Channel Agonists

In a traditional dose-response curve for ACh concentration versus membrane depolarization, the response increases as the concentration of ACh is raised because more AChRs are active. Increasing the agonist concentration increases the frequency and the time in which the channel is opened, thus permitting a net increase in ion flow across the muscle membrane (Fig. 19-10A).[52]

How then do weaker agonists, such as partial agonists (agonists that cannot produce a maximum biologic effect even with all receptors occupied and which antagonize the action of full agonists), behave at the level of single channels? There are several possibilities shown in Fig. 19-10B. First, the partial agonist could produce the same frequency pattern of opening and closing as is shown for the

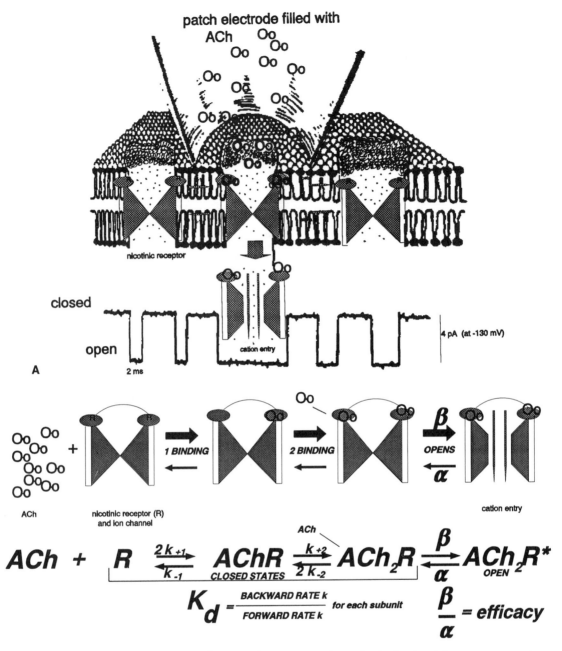

Fig. 19-9 The patch clamp technique for recording currents through single nicotinic receptors and their associated ion channels and the kinetic scheme that describes the ACh-receptor interaction is shown. **(A)** A patch electrode containing ACh is pressed against the skeletal muscle fiber. In the receptor under the patch, the binding of two ACh molecules causes channel opening, cation entry, and downward rectangular single channel currents, which reflect the abrupt opening and closing of the ion channel. The calibration is 4 pA at a holding potential of -130 mV. **(B)** Illustrates the kinetic model. Rate constants for forward and backward reactions are shown. Note that there are three closed states (R, AChR, and ACh$_2$R) and one open state (ACh$_2$R*). The equilibrium dissociation constant, K$_d$ in reciprocal molar units, refers to the binding of ACh. In an ideal case with one ACh molecule bound K$_d$ = k_{-1}/k_{+1}. Because two ACh molecules are required to activate the receptor, K$_d$/2 = k_{-1}/k_{+1}. It is possible to simplify the scheme by assuming that the affinity for each of two ACh binding sites is the same, but this may not be strictly true.[53] The ability of the bound drug to generate the ACh$_2$R* state is the efficacy of the drug and reflects the ratio of β to α (this ratio is an isomerization constant). The units of rate constants may be found in reference 53. For further details, see text. ACh, acetylcholine.

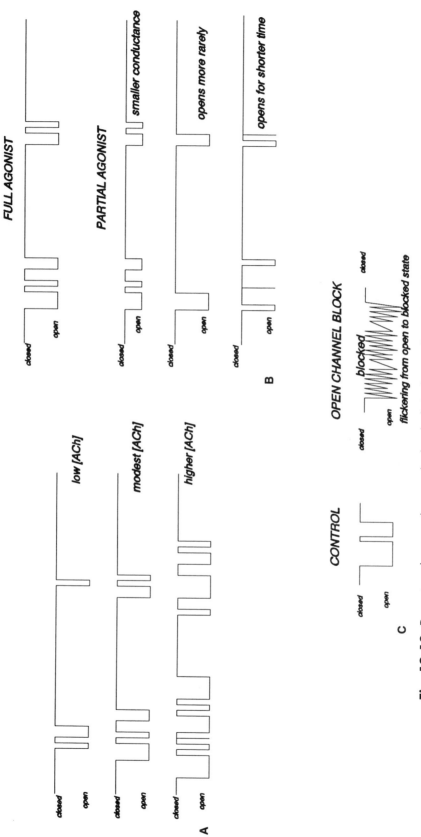

Fig. 19-10 Receptor pharmacology at the level of single ion channels. (**A**) A single channel evaluation of dose-response curves for ACh. (**B**) Drug efficacy for agonists. (**C**) The action of antagonists that block open channels. Nondepolarizing blockers shift the dose-response curve to appear as if lower concentrations of agonist are present. ACh, acetylcholine.

full agonist, but the channel might not open as far (i.e., it has a smaller conductance). This does not happen at nicotinic receptors. Second, the partial agonist could cause channel openings to occur less frequently, thus reflecting a reduced β for the weaker agonist. Third, the weak agonist could cause each opening to occur for a shorter period, which would indicate that it has a faster rate constant of channel closure, α, than the stronger agonists.

It appears that both the second and third mechanisms contribute to the different efficacies of agonists at nicotinic receptors. For example, carbamylcholine is a weaker agonist than ACh because it has a reduced β and an increased α compared with ACh. Thus, the isomerization constant β/α, which reflects drug efficacy, is lower for carbamycholine.[53] Because a reduction in this isomerization constant reflects a reduction in the relative amount of ACh_2R^* relative to ACh_2R, the amount of time the weaker agonist spends conducting ions in the active (ACh_2R^*) state is less than that for the stronger agonist. For a true partial agonist β/α must be less than 1. The situation is even more complex, however, because many drugs produce channel block and desensitization. Thus, the differences in maximal effects that occur with different agonists in equilibrium dose-response curves may reflect, not only differences in the rate constants of channel opening and closing, but also differences in the ability of drugs to block channels and to desensitize the receptors.

Nicotinic ACh receptors at the adult neuromuscular junction are largely localized to the innervated region of skeletal muscle. In fetal muscles or in adult muscles after denervation or immobilization, however, AChRs are present along the entire surface of the muscle as a result of the increased synthesis of extrajunctional receptors.[1] These new extrajunctional receptors have a smaller single channel conductance and longer open times than do those situated at junctional regions.[6,50] Because these extrajunctional receptors are kinetically different and proliferate beyond the region of muscle innervation, agents that activate ACh receptors (e.g., succinylcholine) can produce profound changes in the serum levels of ions that move through AChR-gated channels (e.g., succinylcholine-induced hyperkalemia).

Single Channel Antagonists

Competitive (Nondepolarizing) Blockers

Nondepolarizing blockers produce a powerful equilibrium block and are the most widely used clinically of all the neuromuscular blocking agents. These drugs, however, are rather uninteresting at the single channel level because they make the current record appear as if a lower agonist concentration is present. Competitive inhibitors represent the most extreme of partial agonists, with β so much smaller than α that the β/α ratio is equivalent to zero. The receptor is thus never persuaded to enter the conducting conformation, and the effects of agonists are antagonized by the presence of the drug on the receptor.

Open Channel Block

Open channel block in which the blocker prevents the channel from closing at the level of the single channel is shown in Fig. 19-10C. The channel flickers back and forth from the open to blocked state, and the channel opening time is prolonged. Biophysicists have an experimental interest in this form of block in that it may play a part in the level of steady depolarization achieved during phase I block.[47,49] However, open channel blockers are highly ineffective blockers at equilibrium and, therefore, of little clinical relevance. Indeed, at low agonist concentrations, open channel blockers do not even reduce the equilibrium effect of the agonist.

Structure-Activity Relationships for Specific Neuromuscular Blockers

Nondepolarizing Blockers

Tubocurarine

Tubocurarine, the prototype drug, was the first to be introduced into use in general anesthesia.[37] Curare is a generic term used for a number of poisonous substances isolated from plants found in the Amazon rain forests (species Strychnos and Chondodendron). This drug is still used by the Amazon River Indians to coat the tips of darts, which are blown at appetizing prey (death of the animals results from paralysis of the skeletal muscles of respiration). The name tubocurarine was derived from the packaging of this agent; the Amazonian

Indians originally kept curare in bamboo tubes. Tubocurarine contains two nitrogen atoms positively charged at physiologic pH, one quaternary and the other a protonated tertiary amine (Fig. 19-11A). Nondepolarizing blockers are bulky molecules compared with ACh and depolarizing drugs, such as succinylcholine and decamethonium (Fig. 19-11B). In addition to blocking the nicotinic neuromuscular junction receptor, tubocurarine also blocks the nicotinic receptor in ganglia of the sympathetic nervous system (albeit at higher doses). The resulting vasodilatation can produce hypotension. Vasodilatation may also result from the release of histamine from mast cells. Histamine release is also a common property of benzylquinolinium neuromuscular blocking drugs; the order of potency for releasing histamine is tubocurarine > metocurine > atracurium > mivacurium > doxacurium.[54]

Metocurine

Metocurine is a semisynthetic derivative of tubocurarine prepared by adding three methyl groups to tubocurarine, one to quaternize the tertiary nitrogen and two others to O-methylate the two phenolic groups. It was originally misnamed dimethyltubocurarine when it was believed that tubocurarine had two quaternary nitrogens (and, thus, the only substrate for the methylation reactions were thought to be the two phenolic hydroxyl groups). Metocurine is two to three times more potent than tubocurarine.[9,55]

Pancuronium

Pancuronium is a synthetic derivative that represents rational drug design based on the chemistry and pharmacology of the neuromuscular junction, incorporating the following features.[55] First, quaternary nitrogen atoms were chosen in preference to other charged atoms, such as sulfur (S^+) because they have the greatest blocking potency. Second, two quaternary nitrogens were combined because bisquaternary structures have higher potencies than drugs with only a single cationic moiety. Third, the steroid nucleus (the -curonium suffix signifies the steroidal structure) was selected to form the rigid backbone of the molecule because it allowed the two positively charged nitrogen groups to be constrained at the distance (1.11 nm) that was

optimal for neuromuscular blockade and yet produced minimal effects on autonomic ganglia. The girth of this molecule and the bulky substituents on the nitrogen atoms favor nondepolarizing blockade. Fourth, ACh was included as part of the molecule to increase the affinity of the drug for the receptor and to allow for biotransformation in a manner similar to ACh hydrolysis. The resultant drug, pancuronium (Fig. 19-11A), is 5 to 10 times more potent than tubocurarine, does not release histamine, and produces minimal ganglionic blockade. Pancuronium does, however, antagonize cholinergic muscarinic receptors in the heart, blocking the vagal tone on the heart and thus producing tachycardia.[56]

Vecuronium

Vecuronium is another steroidal neuromuscular blocker that is similar in potency to pancuronium.[56] It is a structural analog of pancuronium but is missing a methyl group on one of the nitrogen atoms, thus making it monoquaternary (Fig. 19-11A). Vecuronium has no effect on ganglionic nicotinic receptors and therefore is relatively devoid of cardiovascular side effects.

Pipecuronium

Pipecuronium is a steroidal pancuronium analog that possesses high potency, long duration, and minimal cardiovascular effects.

Rocuronium

Closely related to pancuronium is the compound rocuronium. Based on suggestions that the desacetoxy analogs of pancuronium might produce extremely rapid neuromuscular block,[57] extensive clinical investigations of this agent were undertaken. Rocuronium is about threefold more rapid in onset but of similar duration to mivacurium. Cardiovascular effects are minimal. Results from recent clinical trials suggest that this drug might replace vecuronium as the drug of choice when rapid intubation and moderate duration of neuromuscular block is desired.[56]

Atracurium

Atracurium was the first of a series of benzylisoquinolinium derivatives and represents a different structural motif from the steroidal agents discussed

Tubocurarine

Pancuronium

Pipecuronium

Vecuronium

Atracurium

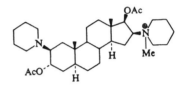

Mivacurium

A **Doxacurium**

Fig. 19-11 Structural formulae for the **(A)** nondepolarizing blocking drugs (tubocurarine, pancuronium, pipecuronium, vecuronium, atracurium, doxacurium, and mivacurium). (*Figure continues.*)

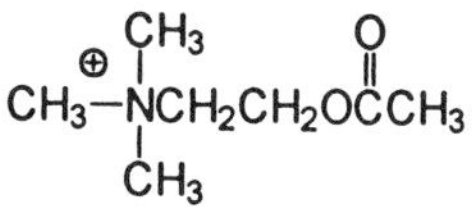

CH₃—⊕NCH₂CH₂OCCH₃
(Acetylcholine structure)

CH₃COCH₂CH₂N⊕—CH₃
(Acetylcholine structure)

Acetylcholine 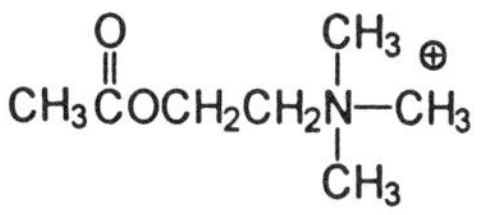　　　　　　**Acetylcholine**

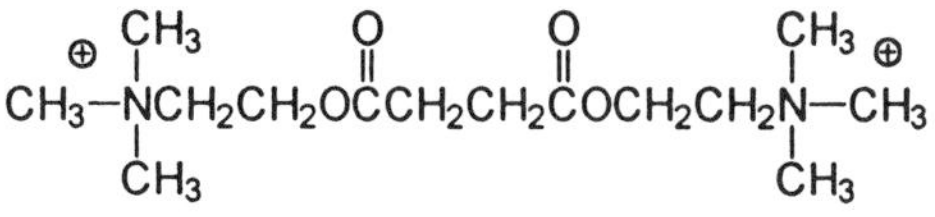

CH₃—⊕NCH₂CH₂OCCH₂CH₂COCH₂CH₂N⊕—CH₃
(Succinylcholine structure)

Succinylcholine

CH₃—⊕NCH₂CH₂CH₂CH₂CH₂CH₂CH₂CH₂CH₂N⊕—CH₃
(Decamethonium structure)

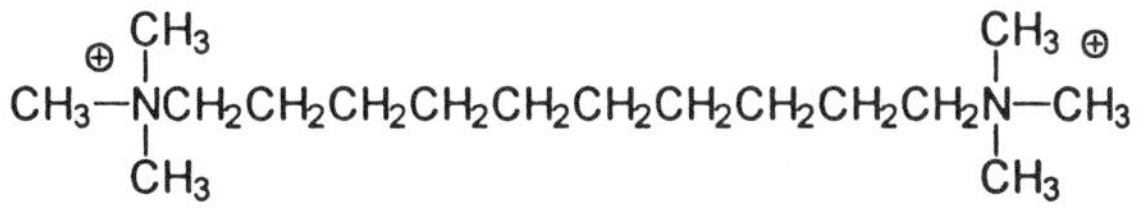

B　　　**Decamethonium**

Fig. 19-11 (*Continued*). **(B)** Acetylcholine and the depolarizing blocking drugs (succinylcholine and decamethonium). For the nondepolarizing agents, there are really two broad categories currently in use, the steroidal agents (pancuronium is the prototype of this class) and the benzylisoquinolinium agents (atracurium is the prototype of this class). Vecuronium is a pancuronium analog with one less N-methyl group. Vecuronium is thus monoquaternary rather than bisquanternary. Pipecuronium is similar to pancuronium and vecuronium, except that the substituent six-membered rings attached to either end of the steroid nucleus each possess two nitrogen moieties (one quaternary and one tertiary per substituent). The benzylisoquinolinium drugs, atracurium and mivacurium, have two ACh-like moieties attached end to end by benzylquinoline groups. For mivacurium, the double bonded oxygen is on the "correct" side of the molecule with respect to the quaternary nitrogen head (like ACh) to provide a more favorable substrate for ChE. In contrast to the short acting benzylisoquinolinium agents, doxacurium has a long duration because of a reduced alkyl chain length. The carboxylic groups are separated by only two carbon atoms in doxacurium in contrast to six carbons in mivacurium. This pushes the carboxylic oxygens close together and minimizes hydrolysis. For details on the depolarizing blockers, see text. ACh, acetylcholine.

earlier.[58,59] Drugs that possess this structure are identifiable by the *-curium* suffix. The middle section of the molecule has two ACh-like moieties escorted on each side by ring structures (Fig. 19-11A). Atracurium does not produce vagal or ganglionic block. It is only one-third as potent as pancuronium.

Doxacurium

Doxacurium is a benzylisoquinolinium derivative with a long duration of action. The potential for hypotension with this agent is less than with other isoquinolinium drugs.[60] Doxacurium is the most potent of the neuromuscular blockers currently available. It is also the slowest in onset of the nondepolarizing blockers (see Ch. 20).

Mivacurium

Mivacurium is a benzylisoquinolinium compound with a short duration of action (Fig. 19-11A). It is similar structurally to atracurium but was modified to permit rapid hydrolysis by pseudocholinesterases.[54] Bolus administration showed that the onset was similar to that of atracurium, but the duration of block was intermediate between that produced by atracurium and the depolarizing blocker succinylcholine.

Depolarizing Blockers

Depolarizing blockers are all nicotinic receptor agonists. Two agents will be considered, succinylcholine and decamethonium. The block is generally phase I, unless excessive amounts of drug are administered, in which case the block proceeds to phase II. Other agents, such as nicotine and carbamylcholine, are also in this category.[46]

Succinylcholine

Succinylcholine is equivalent to two ACh molecules connected end to end (Fig. 19-11B). It is therefore hydrolyzed by AChE in two steps, first to succinylmonocholine and then to succinic acid.

ACh activates ganglionic nicotinic receptors and muscarinic receptors on the effector organs innervated by the autonomic nervous system and nicotinic receptors at the neuromuscular junction. Therefore, it is not surprising that succinylcholine, because of its resemblance to ACh, also activates ganglionic nicotinic and muscarinic receptors. Succinylcholine may thus stimulate muscarinic receptors in the heart to produce bradycardia. It may also stimulate nicotinic receptors of the vagal ganglia and sympathetic ganglia to produce slowing or speeding, respectively, of the heart rate. Succinylcholine thus produces complex and variable cardiovascular effects.

Succinylcholine may also induce malignant hyperthermia, a condition in which massive skeletal muscle contracture is associated with a hypermetabolic state and an elevation in body temperature. The Ca^{++}-release mechanism from the sarcoplasmic reticulum is hypersensitive in patients with malignant hyperthermia.[61]

Decamethonium

Decamethonium (C-10) is a bisquaternary drug that structurally resembles succinylcholine (Fig. 19-11B). Its use was prevalent in the past because of the mistaken notion that it spared the muscles of respiration. This drug may also produce presynaptic blocking activity.[47]

Acetylcholinesterase and Its Inhibitors

Reversible anticholinesterases are competitive antagonists of AChE, the enzyme that hydrolyzes ACh into choline and acetic acid. The normal synaptic position of AChE is in the basal lamina external to the cell membrane in close proximity to the nicotinic receptor-ion channel complex. Because of the efficiency of the enzyme and its proximity to the nicotinic receptors, much of the ACh that is released is degraded before it reaches and reacts with the receptors. Under normal conditions, the local concentration of ACh in the vicinity of the end plate is high only long enough to produce one muscle action potential. On treating a muscle with an AChE agent, a maximal stimulus to the motor nerve produces a larger than normal muscle contraction because some of the muscle fibers twitch repetitively. This occurs because AChE inhibitors block ACh hydrolysis, which raises the ACh concentration in the synaptic cleft to a higher level for a longer period. There is thus an increase in the number of times ACh can bind to its receptors as it slowly diffuses out of the synaptic cleft, with diffusion being slowed by repetitive binding of ACh to receptors.[1] Transmitter action is thus intensified.

When neuromuscular transmission is impaired by a mechanism other than excessive receptor activation (and subsequent depolarization), anticholinesterases improve transmission. Clinical use is thus made of drugs that competitively inhibit cholinesterases. The inhibitors of AChE, such as neostigmine and the longer acting pyridostigmine and ambenonium, increase synaptic ACh concentrations sufficiently to reverse the muscle paralysis produced by the nondepolarizing blockers.

ASSESSING TYPE OF NEUROMUSCULAR BLOCK FROM PATTERNS OF TWITCH TENSION MEASUREMENTS

Safety Factor for Neuromuscular Transmission

The ultimate effect of the local depolarization by ACh released from the nerve ending is to produce a twitch of the entire muscle fiber. It is from twitch tension measurements that the degree and type of neuromuscular block are assessed. The data gleaned from such measurements are less precise than are those from electrophysiologic measurements because neuromuscular transmission operates with an enormous safety factor. Either transmitter release or the number of functional ACh receptors may be substantially decreased without altering the twitch of the muscle. If a nondepolarizing blocker decreases the number of active receptors by about 80 percent, the twitch response to nerve stimulation remains unchanged. However, if ACh release is decreased by even a small amount in the presence of 80 percent receptor blockade, the twitch will then be diminished. Thus, a nerve-muscle junction in which 80 percent of the receptors are blocked, although allowing twitches to occur, is said to have a low safety factor because now any additional impairment of synaptic transmission will subsequently block the neurally evoked muscle twitch in that fiber.

When the motor nerve is stimulated at low frequencies (i.e., one stimulus per 5 to 10 seconds), ACh release (reflected as the EPP) is well maintained (Fig. 19-12, upper trace). However, when

the nerve is stimulated repetitively at the higher frequencies (i.e., 25 Hz), ACh release per impulse declines (depression). Then, if allowed to recover briefly, it rebounds to higher levels than the original control level. This rebound phenomenon is termed post-tetanic potentiation (Fig. 19-12, lower trace). Depression was traditionally attributed to a depletion of the immediately available vesicular store of ACh.[3] Although this is certainly true after exhaustive stimulation, the more likely mechanism of normal depression is the release of endogenous adenosine, which acts as a negative feedback modulator of ACh release (see Prejunctional Physiology and Pharmacology). Post-tetanic potentiation is caused by an increased availability of ACh or an increased probability of ACh release because of Ca^{++} or Ca^{++}-dependent phosphorylation that occurs after the cessation of repetitive nerve stimulation.[2,3,62] Depression and post-tetanic potentiation occur normally at unblocked neuromuscular junctions. However, because of the high safety factor for neuromuscular transmission, depression and post-tetanic potentiation are not normally reflected in changes in the twitch response of the muscle

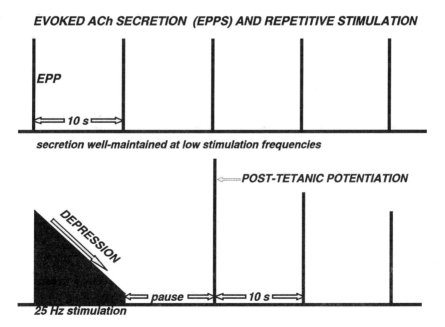

Fig. 19-12 Effects of repetitive stimulation on evoked ACh release recorded electrophysiologically as EPPs. The EPPs were sketched on a slow time scale and thus appear as spikes in this figure. For further details, see text. ACh, acetylcholine; EPP, end plate potential.

fiber. Only when the safety factor for neuromuscular transmission is markedly reduced can they be observed in the twitch response.

Assessment of Blockade From Twitch Tension Measurements

The degree of neuromuscular blockade is typically monitored by stimulating the ulnar nerve and measuring the contractile force of the thumb generated as a consequence of contraction of the adductor pollicis muscle.[63] This method monitors the summated contraction of many muscle fibers simultaneously; a decrease in the twitch thus reflects the loss of the ability of individual fibers to contract. When normal muscle receives four consecutive stimuli at 2 Hz, the so-called train of four, muscle twitch is well maintained (Fig. 19-13A). High frequency tetanic stimulation at 25 Hz also produces a well maintained tetanus, which is larger than that produced by a single stimulus as a result of the summated events in the muscle contractile machinery. There is no reflection of the presynaptic processes of depression and post-tetanic potentiation, even though they are likely to be occurring.

In the presence of nondepolarizing blockers, the presynaptic processes of depression and post-tetanic potentiation are evident in the twitch tension measurements. When a train-of-four stimulus is applied in the presence of a nondepolarizing blocker, the absolute size of the first twitch response in the muscle mass is reduced from normal to approximately 20 percent of normal as a result of the complete elimination of the twitch in 80 to 90 percent of the muscle fibers (Fig. 19-13B). Furthermore, there is a decrement in the twitch tension of the unblocked fibers during the train of four. Tetanic high frequency stimulation (25 Hz) also reveals depression during the tetanus. After a post-tetanic pause, post-tetanic potentiation is observed. The reasons for these observations are twofold. First, the 20 percent of the fibers that are not blocked have a low safety factor. They respond to the first stimulus with a twitch, but the presynaptic depression that ensues with repetitive stimulation causes individual fibers of low safety factor to be reduced below threshold for action potential generation. Thus, the loss of twitches in individual fibers as a result of presynaptic depression produces

the fade seen in the train of four. The other important consideration is that blockade of presynaptic nicotinic receptors occurs with nondepolarizing blockers,[34,35] exacerbating the neuromuscular depression that occurs normally. When ACh release rebounds after post-tetanic stimulation, even fibers that were blocked at the time of the first stimulus may be recruited into the twitch tension pattern, and the overall measured twitch is thus increased.

In depolarizing block (phase I, Fig. 19-13C), the absolute size of the twitch is reduced as a result of blockade of 80 percent of the muscle fibers by muscle membrane depolarization. The unblocked fibers produce patterns that appear normal but have a reduced amplitude. No depression or post-tetanic potentiation is observed in the twitch tension measurements, possibly because depolarizing drugs do not block presynaptic nicotinic receptors. The unblocked fibers also might have a high safety factor; they may be depolarized enough to be boosted closer to threshold but not enough for Na^+ channel inactivation to occur. If depolarizing block proceeds to phase II, then generally the train of four exhibits a decrement in amplitude,[47] and tetanic contractions are no longer well maintained. It is also possible that presynaptic block occurs during phase II.

DRUG INTERACTIONS AT NEUROMUSCULAR JUNCTION

ACh released from nerve endings acts on skeletal muscle to initiate a complex chain of events that ultimately leads to muscle contraction. There are many processes along this chain at which various drugs may interact (e.g., nerve terminal, postsynaptic receptor, ACh-gated ion channel, membrane lipid, and contractile machinery). If two drugs block at the same site, then their effects are generally less than additive. When two blockers act at different sites along the chain, then the effects of these blockers are greater than additive and are termed synergistic.

Knowledge of these interactions may be helpful in the judicious selection of combinations of nondepolarizing blockers. For example, two nondepolarizing blockers may be used synergistically if one of the two has a pronounced presynaptic blocking

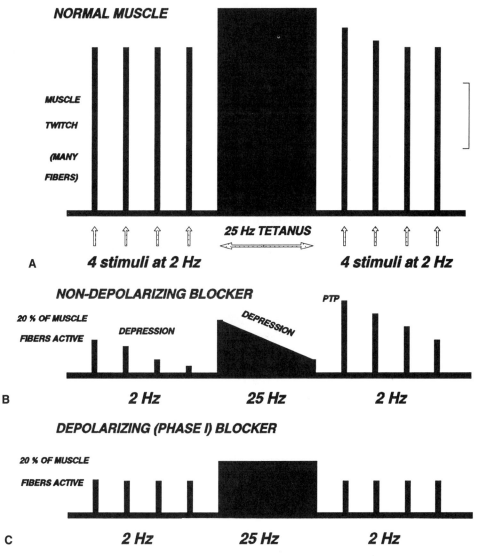

Fig. 19-13 Patterns of twitch tension measurements seen in the absence of neuromuscular blockade (**A**), during nondepolarizing block (**B**) and during depolarizing block (**C**). Such records are generally made by measuring the twitch of the adductor pollicis muscle in response to ulnar nerve stimulation. Note that it is only with nondepolarizing block (or with phase II block, not depicted) that the patterns of twitch tension measurements reflect the presynaptic phenomena seen electrophysiologically (see Fig. 19-12). (**B** and **C**) The level of blocker was chosen to eliminate the twitch in 80 percent of muscle fibers. The train of four is applied at the beginning of each trace (four stimuli at 2 Hz), with the ratio of the amplitude of the first to the fourth twitch used to quantify neuromuscular block. For further details, see text.

effect. Tubocurarine and metocurine were reported to have a more pronounced presynaptic effect than pancuronium, which acts largely postjunctionally.[64] The combination of pancuronium and tubocurarine (or metocurine) thus synergistically increases neuromuscular blockade and can be used clinically in this manner. In general, benzylisoquinolinium compounds and steroidal nondepolarizing blockers exhibit synergistic effects when used in combination. General anesthetics (which produce membrane stabilizing effects) also act synergistically with the nondepolarizing blockers.

In contrast to the beneficial effects of synergism, multiplicative effects of synergism may be disadvantageous when drugs used for other purposes incidentally interfere with neuromuscular transmission. For example, intraperitoneal lavage with antibiotics that block presynaptic Ca^{++} channels (kanamycin or streptomycin) may cause profound neuromuscular block following even modest doses of nondepolarizing blockers as a result of synergy. Similarly, profound neuromuscular block may ensue with nondepolarizing blockers in patients treated with magnesium salts. Mg^{++} multiplies the postsynaptic blocking action of the nondepolarizing drug by blocking Ca^{++} entry. This unwanted synergism makes it difficult to reverse muscle relaxation with anticholinesterases if the patient has been treated with agents that block presynaptically.

REFERENCES

1. Kuffler SW, Nichols JG, Martin AR: From Neuron to Brain. Sinauer Associates, Sunderland, MA, 1984
2. Katz B: The Release of Neural Transmitter Substances. Sherrington Press, London, 1969
3. Silinsky EM: The biophysical pharmacology of calcium-dependent acetylcholine release. Pharmacol Rev 37:81, 1985
4. Gage PW: Generation of end-plate potentials. Physiol Rev 56:177, 1976
5. Peper K, Bradley RJ, Dreyer F: The acetylcholine receptor at the neuromuscular junction. Physiol Rev 62:1271, 1982
6. Konno T, Busch C, von Kitzing E et al: Rings of anionic amino acids as structural determinants of ion selectivity in the acetylcholine receptor channel. Proc R Soc Lond [Biol] 244:69, 1991
7. Silinsky EM: Electrophysiological methods for studying acetylcholine Secretion. p. 255. In Poisner A, Trifaro J (eds): In Vitro Methods for Studying Secretion. Elsevier Science Publishing, Amsterdam, 1987
8. Brigant JL, Mallart A: Presynaptic currents in mouse motor endings. J Physiol (Lond) 333:619, 1982
9. Anderson AJ, Harvey AL: ω-Conotoxin does not block the verapamil-sensitive calcium channels at mouse motor nerve terminals. Neurosci Lett 82:177, 1987
10. Penner R, Dreyer F: Two different presynaptic calcium currents in mouse motor nerve terminals. Pflugers Arch 406:190, 1986
11. Silinsky EM, Solsona CS: Calcium currents at motor nerve endings: absence of effects of adenosine receptor agonists in the frog. J Physiol (Lond) 457:315, 1992
12. Potter LT: Synthesis, storage and release of [^{14}C] acetylcholine in isolated rat diaphragm muscles. J Physiol (Lond) 206:145, 1970
13. Elmqvist D, Quastel DMJ: Presynaptic action of hemicholinium at the neuromuscular junction. J Physiol (Lond) 177:463, 1965
14. Marshall IG, Parsons SM: The vesicular acetylcholine transport system. Trends Neurosci 10:174, 1987
15. Chicago Tribune: Potentially lethal fish on seven New York menus. Friday April 7, 1989, section 1, p. 16
16. Narahashi T, Moore JW, Scott WR: Tetrodotoxin blockage of sodium conductance increase in lobster giant axons. J Gen Physiol 47:965, 1992
17. Hille B: Ionic Channels of Excitable Membranes. Sinauer Associates, Sunderland, MA, 1992
18. Singh YN, Marshall IG, Harvey AL: Depression of transmitter release and postjunctional sensitivity during neuromuscular block produced by antibiotics. Br J Anaesth 51:1027, 1979
19. Gilman AG, Rall TW, Nies AS, Taylor P: Goodman and Gilman's The Pharmacological Basis of Therapeutics. Pergamon Press, Elmsford, NY, 1990
20. Swash M, Ingram DA: Adverse effect of verapamil in myasthenia gravis. Muscle Nerve 15:396, 1992
21. Simpson LL: Molecular pharmacology of botulinum toxin and tetanus toxin. Annu Rev Pharmacol Toxicol 26:427, 1986
22. Cull-Candy SG, Lundh H, Thesleff S: Effects of botulinum toxin on neuromuscular transmission in the rat. J Physiol (Lond) 260:177, 1976
23. Finkelstein A, Rubin LL, Tzeng MC: Black widow spider venom: effect of purified toxin on lipid bilayer membranes. Science 193:1009, 1976
24. Vincentini LM, Meldolesi J: Alpha-latrotoxin of black widow spider venom binds to a specific receptor

coupled to phosphoinositide breakdown in PC12 cells. Biochem Biophys Res Commun 121:538, 1984

25. Silinsky EM: Evidence for specific adenosine receptors at cholinergic nerve endings. Br J Pharmacol 71:191, 1980

26. Silinsky EM: On the association between transmitter secretion and the release of adenine nucleotides from mammalian motor nerve terminals. J Physiol (Lond) 247:145, 1975

27. Ribeiro JA, Sebastiao AM: On the role, inactivation, and origin of endogenous adenosine at the frog neuromuscular junction. J Physiol (Lond) 384:571, 1987

28. Redman RS, Silinsky EM: A selective adenosine antagonist (8-cyclopentyl-1,3-dipropylxanthine) eliminates neuromuscular depression and the action of exogenous adenosine by an effect of A_1 receptors. Mol Pharmacol 44:835, 1993

29. Redman RS, Silinsky EM: ATP released together with acetylcholine as the mediator of neuromuscular depression at frog motor nerve endings. J Physiol (in press, 1994)

30. Ginsborg BL, Hirst GDS: The effect of adenosine on the release of the transmitter from the phrenic nerve of the rat. J Physiol (Lond) 224:629, 1972

31. Silinsky EM: On the calcium receptor that mediates depolarization-secretion coupling at cholinergic motor nerve terminals. Br J Pharmacol 73:413, 1981

32. Silinsky EM: On the mechanism by which adenosine receptor activation inhibits the release of acetylcholine from motor nerve endings. J Physiol (Lond) 346:243, 1984

33. Hamilton BR, Smith DO: Autoreceptor-mediated purinergic and cholinergic inhibition of motor nerve terminal calcium currents in the rat. J Physiol (Lond) 432:327, 1991

34. Bowman WC, Prior C, Marshall IG: Presynaptic receptors in the neuromuscular junction. Ann N Y Acad Sci 604:69, 1990

35. Bowman WC, Marshall IG, Gibb AJ: Is there feedback control of transmitter release at the neuromuscular junction? Semin Anesthesiol 3:275, 1984

36. Riker WF: Prejunctional effects of neuromuscular blocking and facilitatory drugs. p. 59. In Katz R (ed): Muscle Relaxants. Excerpta Medica, Amsterdam, 1975

37. Griffith HR, Johnson GE: The use of curare in general anesthesia. Anesthesiology 3:418, 1942

38. Cohen JB, Changeux J-P: The cholinergic receptor protein in its membrane environment. Annu Rev Pharmacol 15:83, 1975

39. Potter LT: Acetylcholine receptors in vertebrate skeletal muscles and electric tissues. p. 295. In Rang HP (ed): Drug Receptors. University Park Press, Baltimore, 1973

40. Changeux J-P, Giraudat J, Dennis M: The nicotinic acetylcholine receptor: molecular architecture of a ligand-regulated ion channel. Trends Pharmacol Sci 8:459, 1987

41. Taylor P, Brown JH: Acetylcholine. p. 203. In Siegel G, Agranoff B, Albers RW, Molinoff P (eds): Basic Neurochemistry. 4th Ed. Raven Press, New York 1989

42. Sargent P: The diversity of neuronal nicotinic receptors. Ann Rev Neurosci 16:403, 1993

43. Chang CC, Lee CY: Isolation of neurotoxins from the venom of *Bungarus multicinctus* and their modes of neuromuscular blocking action. Arch Int Pharmacodyn Ther 144:241, 1963

44. Smith CUM: Ligand-gated channels. p. 203. In: Elements of Molecular Neurobiology. Wiley, Chichester, 1989

45. Colquhoun D, Ogden DC, Mathie A: Nicotinic acetylcholine receptors or nerve and muscle: functional aspects. Trends Pharmacol Sci 8:465, 1987

46. Zaimis E, Head S: Depolarizing neuromuscular blocking drugs. p. 365. In Zaimis E (ed): Neuromuscular Junction: Handbook of Experimental Pharmacology. Springer-Verlag, New York, 1976

47. Lingle CJ, Steinbach JH: Neuromuscular blocking agents. Int Anesthesiol Clin 26:288, 1988

48. Silinsky EM: Intracellular recording methods. p. 29. In Stamford JA (ed): Monitoring Neuronal Activity: A Practical Approach. Oxford University Press, London, 1992

49. Marshall CG, Ogden DC, Colquhoun D: The actions of suxamethonium (succinyldicholine) as an agonist and channel blocker at the nicotinic receptors of frog muscle. J Physiol (Lond) 428:155, 1990

50. Sakmann B, Neher E: Single-Channel Recording. Plenum, New York, 1983

51. Sakmann B: Elementary steps in synaptic transmission revealed by currents through single ion channels. Science 256:503, 1992

52. Palotta B: Single ion channel's view of classical receptor theory. FASEB J 5:2035, 1991

53. Colquhoun D, Ogden DC, Cachelin AB: Mode of action of agonists on nicotinic receptors. p. 255. In Ritchie JM, Keynes RD, Bolis L (eds): Ion Channels in Neural Membranes. Alan R. Liss, New York, 1986

54. Savarese JJ, Hassan HA, Basta SJ et al: The clinical pharmacology of mivacurium chloride (BW B1090U). Anesthesiology 68:723, 1988

55. Bowman WC, Rand MJ: Textbook of Pharmacology. Blackwell Scientific Publications, London 1980

56. Bowman WC, Rodger IW, Houston J et al: Structure: action relationships among some desacetoxy analogues of pancuronium and vecuronium in the anesthetized cat. Anesthesiology 69:57, 1988

57. Mirakhur RK: Newer neuromuscular blocking drugs. An overview of their clinical pharmacology and therapeutic use. Drugs 44:192, 1992

58. Lennon RL, Olson RA, Gronert GA: Atracurium or vecuronium for rapid sequence endotracheal intubation. Anesthesiology 64:510, 1986

59. Hughes R, Chapple DJ: The pharmacology of atracurium: a new competitive neuromuscular blocking agent. Br J Anaesth 53:31, 1981

60. Reich DL: Transient systemic arterial hypotension and cutaneous flushing in response to doxacurium chloride. Anesthesiology 71:783, 1989

61. MacLennan DH: The genetic basis of malignant hyperthermia. Trends Pharmacol Sci 13:330, 1992

62. Parnas H, Dudel J, Parnas I: Neurotransmitter release and its facilitation in crayfish. VII. Another voltage dependent process besides Ca entry controls the time course of phasic release. Pflugers Arch 406:121, 1986

63. Dripps RD, Eckenhoff JE, Vandam LD: Introduction to Anesthesia. WB Saunders, Philadelphia, 1988

64. Lebowitz PW, Ramsey FM, Savarese JJ et al: Combination of pancuronium and metocurine: neuromuscular and hemodynamic advantages over pancuronium alone. Anesth Analg 60:12, 1981

65. Kandel WER, Schwartz JH: Principles of Neural Science. 3rd Ed. Appleton & Lange, Norwalk, CT, 1993

66. Silinsky EM, Vogel SM: Independent regulation of channel closure and block of open channels by methylxanthines at acetylcholine receptors in the frog. J Physiol (Lond) 390:33, 1987

67. Jahn R, Südhoff TC: Synaptic vesicle traffic: rush hour in the nerve terminal. J Neurochem 61:12, 1993

68. Bennett MK, Scheller RH: The molecular machinery for secretion is conserved from yeast to neurons. Proc Natl Acad Sci USA 90:2559, 1993

69. DeBello WM, Betz H, Augustine GJ: Synaptotagmin and neurotransmitter release. Cell 74:947, 1993

70. Barinaga M: Secrets of secretion revealed. Science 260:487, 1993

71. Huttner WB: Snappy exocytoxins. Science 365:104, 1993

Chapter 20

Pharmacokinetics of Neuromuscular Blockers

Colin A. Shanks

Neuromuscular blockade is quantified as the evoked muscular responses to motor nerve stimulation, usually the ulnar nerve. This chapter discusses neuromuscular blocking agents (NMBAs) in terms of their onset and duration, as they affect the twitch responses of the adductor pollicis muscle, (Table 20-1) although it is recognized that not all muscle groups are the same.[1] The graded twitch response is the basis of most pharmacologic studies, quantified between 0 and 100 percent effect (twitch depression) for a given nerve-muscle group. The dose-response relationship is usually expressed as an ED_{95}, the mean effective dose producing 95 percent depression of the single twitch response in a single individual.

ROUTES OF ADMINISTRATION

The NMBAs are almost exclusively administered intravenously, although intramuscular and subcutaneous routes can both produce therapeutic effects given sufficient dosage. The dose used to facilitate endotracheal intubation in the anesthetized patient ("intubating dose") is normally 1.5 to 2 times the ED_{95}. Subsequent maintenance bolus doses may be one-quarter to one-half this amount, usually administered when recovery to 75 percent twitch depression occurs. For continuous effect,

NMBAs may be administered as an infusion, adjusted to maintain the desired intensity of paralysis. Both the bolus dose and the infusion rate can be predicted from the pharmacokinetic parameters and the desired plasma concentration, if known, where the desired concentration might be that associated with 95 percent twitch depression (EC_{95}).

Most pharmacokinetic studies which use a predetermined dosage regimen use the equations of Mitenko and Ogilvie[2]:

$$\text{Loading dose} = C_p * V_d \qquad (1)$$

$$\text{Infusion rate} = C_p * CL \qquad (2)$$

where C_p refers to the desired plasma concentration, V_d is the volume of distribution, CL is the total clearance, and the loading dose is administered as a bolus. The goal of these equations is to rapidly achieve a desired plasma concentration without overshoot, and then to maintain that concentration. Using the initial volume of distribution (V_1) for V_d will result in insufficient plasma concentrations. The area-based or terminal-phase volume of distribution (V_{area} or V_β) usually gives adequate results. Alternatively, using the steady-state volume of distribution (V_{ss}), bolus doses close to those used clinically are predicted.[3] While use of Equa-

419

Table 20-1 Modified Classification of the NMBAs, Based on the Average Time-Course of Paralysis Induced by a Clinically Useful Bolus Dose.

Intervals From Injection to Percent Twitch Depression

Class	Useful Duration, (minutes to 75% twitch depression)	Minimal Effect (minutes to 5% twitch depression)
Ultrashort	5–8	10–15
Short	15–20	25–35
Intermediate	20–30	40–60
Long-acting	45–60	90–180

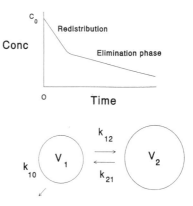

Fig. 20-1 A traditional two-compartment model. Above, the concentration-time curve for the central compartment, V_1. Below, depiction of the model, its volumes and rate constants. For details see text.

tion 1 with either V_β or V_{ss} gives initial plasma concentrations in excess of those desired, effective concentrations in the biophase are rapidly achieved, resulting in prompt onset of paralysis.

DISTRIBUTION AND PLASMA PROTEIN BINDING

Pharmacokinetic Models

The majority of studies report the pharmacokinetics of the NMBAs with values for V_{ss}, or V_{area} or V_β, the elimination clearance (CL), and the elimination half-life ($t_{1/2}\beta$). These are based on either "model-independent" or compartmental models that characterize plasma concentration-time data. There may also be an additional compartment to characterize the pharmacodynamic effect of the NMBA, the effect compartment. This compartment does not participate directly in the pharmacokinetic model. A classical two-compartment model is depicted in Figure 20-1, with drug being administered into, and eliminated from, the central compartment, V_1. With a bolus dose the central volume is instantaneously full at time zero; initially drug is lost from the central compartment through both intercompartmental clearance to the peripheral compartment V_2 and elimination clearance (the distribution phase). Pseudoequilibrium is reached when drug concentrations in V_1 and V_2 are equal. Once pseudoequilibrium has been

reached, drug continues to be cleared by systemic elimination and is simultaneously being returned by redistribution from the peripheral compartment to the central compartment (the elimination phase). The elimination clearance can be calculated from the product of V_1 and the rate constant, k_{10}. Similarly, intercompartmental clearance can be calculated as the product of V_1 and the rate constant, k_{12}. The V_{ss} is the sum of V_1 and V_2. The V_β is obtained by dividing the dose by the product of the elimination rate constant and the area under the concentration-time curve; this is usually a little larger than V_{ss}. The volume of the central compartment can be obtained by backextrapolation of the concentration-time curve to time zero; division of the intercept concentration, C_{zero} (in units of mass per volume), by the dose (mass) gives the volume. This implies an assumption of instantaneous mixing throughout V_1 at time zero. While useful as a simplification, observation of a dye-dilution cardiac output curve shows the assumption to be invalid (Fig. 20-2). Dye is seen to arrive at the arterial sampling site after a time lag; the initial peak is followed by one or more recirculatory peaks. Modelling these oscillations is complex.[4] Although elaborate, such models permit insights into the effects of rate of drug administration, which is an important consideration for NMBAs producing a dose- and time-related release of histamine.[5]

Concentration versus Dose Rate

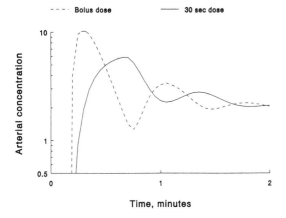

Fig. 20-2 Arterial concentrations with a seven-compartment model,[4] showing its ability to depict concentrations during the first 2 minutes after a dose. The initial peak after a 1-second dose duration is almost double that for a 30-second dose.

Distribution Pharmacokinetics of NMBAs

The NMBAs have one or more positively charged quaternary ammonium groups, which remain ionized irrespective of pH. This reduces their ability to cross lipid membranes and would predict distribution, which is restricted to the extracellular fluid, to little more than 20 percent of the ideal body weight. Table 20-2 gives the mean values reported for the distribution volumes of the NMBAs in adult patients (excluding where possible those series with less than seven subjects). Where possible, V_{ss} is reported in preference to V_β.

Distribution to the periphery produces a rapid fall in plasma drug concentrations following bolus administration (Fig. 20-1). If this occurs through a range of concentrations associated with recovery from paralysis, then return of motor power will be more rapid than would be predicted from the elimination half-life alone (derived from the slope of the elimination phase, Fig. 20-1). This concept is important clinically, as in spontaneous recovery from vecuronium-induced paralysis.

The studies reported in Table 20-2 involved surgical patients, in which plasma samples were sel-

Table 20-2 Steady-State Volumes of Distribution of the NMBAs, Citing Studies With More Than Seven Adult Patients[a]

	Volume of Distribution (L/kg)	Number of Subjects	Reference
Short			
Mivacurium	0.1	8	6
	0.1–0.3(β)	9	7
Intermediate			
Atracurium	0.15(β)	19	8
	0.16(β)	12	9
	0.18(β)	10	10
	0.15	10	11
	0.14	15	12
	0.12	16	12
	0.12	10	12
	0.14	10	13
	0.11	8	13
Rocuronium	0.27	10	14
	0.21	10	15
Vecuronium	0.25	14	16
	0.46	13	17
	0.18	10	18
	0.20	10	19
	0.20	10	20
	0.48	7	21
	0.41	10	14
Long			
Alcuronium	0.32	19	22
	0.27	12	23
Doxacurium	0.15	8	24
	0.22	9	25
Metocurine	0.35	9	26
	0.51(β)	14	27
Pancuronium	0.28(β)	18	28
	0.20	18	29
	0.30	16	30
	0.18	11	31
Pipecuronium	0.31	20	29
	0.31	10	32
	0.35	8	33
Tubocurarine	0.52	20	34
	0.30	14	35
	0.42(β)	9	36
	0.60(β)	12	37
	0.30	8	38

[a] Volumes reported as Vβ are marked as β; all others are V_{ss}.

dom obtained for more than 6 hours. Animal studies, using longer sampling times, indicate considerable distribution to cartilaginous tissues.[39] With an insufficiently long sampling period NMBA binding to such sites would appear as elimination instead of distribution. Sampling for 96 hours markedly increases the distribution volume and half-life for tubocurarine.[36]

Plasma Protein Binding

Table 20-3 shows plasma protein binding data for the NMBAs. Binding data vary, depending on the experimental technique used: using equilibrium dialysis, most NMBAs are 20 to 50 percent protein bound. Binding to this low extent makes it unlikely that small differences in the degree of binding will have a major influence on free drug concentration at the site of action. A technique based on the inhibitory effect on human plasma butyrylcholinesterase reports 77 to 91 percent binding.[49] Other workers, using ultrafiltration or electrophoretic techniques, have found NMBA-plasma protein binding in the range of 70 to 80 percent.[41] For the NMBAs, binding is chiefly to albumin and gamma globulin.[50,51]

Table 20-3 Plasma Protein Binding of the NMBAs

	Binding (%)	Technique	Reference
Intermediate			
Atracurium	37	—	40
Vecuronium	30	UC	41
Long			
Alcuronium	40	ED	42
Metocurine	42	ED	43
	35	ED	44
Pancuronium	13	ED	45
	20	ED	39
	29	ED	41
	72	UF	46
Tubocurarine	51	ED	44
	51	ED	47
	56	UC	41
	50	ED	48

Abbreviations: ED, equilibrium dialysis; UC, ultraCentrifuge; UF, ultraFiltration.

CLEARANCE AND BIOTRANSFORMATION

Elimination clearance is a time-dependent volume from which all drug appears to have been removed. It is the chief determinant of the duration of paralysis in prolonged NMBA administration. When NMBAs are to be infused, the terminal infusion rate can be calculated as the product of the desired plasma concentration and the elimination clearance (Eq. 2). Table 20-4 shows the mean values for NMBA elimination clearance and half-lives.

NMBA clearance associated with blood loss can be calculated from known pharmacokinetic parameters. With moderate blood loss, this is almost negligible.[52,53] For example, calculating from data with vecuronium[19] in Table 20.5, 95 percent paralysis is associated with a plasma concentration of 0.34 μg/ml. Losses totalling three liters of plasma would then result in removal of 1 mg of vecuronium for the whole procedure. Only with massive blood loss, as in liver transplantation, is NMBA clearance likely to be affected with hemorrhage.

Urinary Excretion

Renal excretion of the NMBAs appears to be predominantly related to glomerular filtration, since the permanently charged quaternary ammonium groups preclude tubular reabsorption. Pharmacokinetic studies of the long-acting NMBAs typically collect 40 to 70 percent of the dose in urine in the first 24 hours.[52,58-62] Recovery percentages tend to rise in the presence of hepatobiliary dysfunction.[63] Some of the remaining dose appears in the bile, but much remains unaccounted for.

Metabolic Clearance

The steroidal NMBAs are desacetylated, undergoing hydrolysis at the 3- and 17- positions; both 3-desacetylpancuronium and 3-desacetylvecuronium have been detected in plasma. The presence of 3-desacetylvecuronium confounds the pharmacokinetic parameters derived for vecuronium when the metabolite is not distinguished from the parent compound during analysis of plasma.[20] The presence of 17-hydroxyvecuronium has been suggested as a cause for apparent resistance to vecuronium.[64] Animal studies suggest that 3-desacetylpancuro-

Table 20-4 Elimination Clearance and Half-Life of NMBAs

	Clearance (ml/kg¹/min¹)	Half-Life (min)	Number of Subjects	Reference
Short				
Mivacurium	70.4	18	8	6
	53–59	2.1–2.3	9	7
Intermediate				
Atracurium	5.1	20	19	8
	5.5	20	12	9
	6.1	21	10	10
	5.9	20	10	11
	6.7[a]	19	15	12
	5.3[b]	20	16	12
	5.6[c]	19	10	12
	6.6	20	10	13
	5.0	20	8	13
Rocuronium	4.0	131	10	14
	2.9	71	10	15
Vecuronium	4.3	58	14	16
	3.8	113	13	17
	4.5	58	10	18
	3.2	84	10	19
	5.0	55	10	20
	4.0	116	7	21
Long				
Alcuronium	1.3	200	19	22
	1.3	199	12	23
Doxacurium	2.2	86	8	24
	2.7	99	9	25
Metocurine	1.1	240	9	26
	1.1	345	7	27
Pancuronium	1.8	107	18	28
	1.5	115	18	29
	2.1	94	16	30
	0.8	169	11	31
Pipecuronium	2.4	137	20	29
	2.5	154	10	32
	3.0	111	8	33
Tubocurarine	1.81	275	20	34
	2.25	119	14	35
	1.8	166	9	36
	2.7	172	12	37
	3.0	89	8	38

[a] Patients receiving isoflurane.
[b] Patients receiving halothane.
[c] Patients receiving midazolam.

Table 20-5 Pharmacodynamics of the NMBAs for Pharmacokinetic-Pharmacodynamic Models

	EC$_{50}$, mg/min	Gamma (γ)	k$_{eo}$/min	No of Subjects	Reference
Intermediate					
Atracurium	0.65	4.3	0.10	19	8
	0.45	6.1	0.07	8	13
	0.31	5.6	0.09	10	13
	0.38	5.4	0.09	8	54
	0.65	4.3	0.10	5	55
Vecuronium	0.20	5.5	0.10	10	19
	0.11	—	0.11	7	21
	0.09	5.8	0.17	5	56
Long					
Alcuronium	0.50	5.4	0.24	12	23
Metocurine	0.26	—	—	6	57
Pancuronium	0.21	5.5	0.48	10	31
	0.15	—	0.15	5	21
	0.11	4.8	0.17	7	56
Pipecuronium	0.06	—	—	10	32
Tubocurarine	0.61	4.5	0.16	10	57
	0.60	—	0.15	14	35
	0.53	—	0.10	7	38
	0.45	—	—	6	57

Sigmoid E$_{max}$ equation: Fractional Effect $= \dfrac{\text{Concentration}^{\gamma}}{\text{EC50}^{\gamma} + \text{Concentration}^{\gamma}}$

nium and 3-desacetylvecuronium are pharmacologically active at clinically relevant concentrations.[65,66]

The clearance of atracurium occurs in both central and peripheral compartments. There are two mechanisms of atracurium clearance—metabolism by tissue carboxylases and spontaneous degradation by Hofmann elimination.[67] Systemic atracurium clearance is composed of organ-dependent and non-organ-dependent pathways. An in vitro metabolic rate constant for atracurium elimination (degradation) can be determined from blood drawn prior to drug administration. Assuming this rate to be the value for nonorgan elimination from all compartments, then organ elimination of atracurium from the central compartment can be calculated by subtraction from the total elimination rate. Organ clearance of atracurium has been confirmed in intensive care unit patients.[68] Hemofiltration clears both atracurium and laudanosine, but does not alter the plasma clearance values.

Atracurium is a mixture of ten isomers, which can be separated into three geometrical isomer groups: cis-cis, cis-trans, and trans-trans, of which the cis-cis and cis-trans are the most important.[69] For the cis-trans group the apparent elimination half-life and clearance are 18 minutes and 9 ml/kg/min, respectively, but this is the average rate of decomposition of a mixture of isomers, each with its own properties.

The main breakdown products of atracurium are the tertiary amine, laudanosine, and a monoquaternary acrylate, both resulting from Hofmann degradation (see Fig. 21-12).[67] Laudanosine does not possess neuromuscular blocking activity. One of the rare investigations that incorporates metabolite pharmacokinetics with those of a parent drug has been reported for atracurium and laudanosine.[70] Plasma laudanosine concentrations peak within 2 minutes after atracurium administration and remain near peak concentrations for several minutes.[71] Laudanosine readily penetrates into the brain, causes central nervous system stimulation, increases the MAC for volatile anesthetics at clinically relevant concentrations, and causes convulsions at high concentrations.[72] Nevertheless, although of great initial concern, CNS activation by laudanosine is probably of little clinical significance.

Ester hydrolysis, catalyzed by nonspecific tissue esterases, is a quantitatively less significant atracurium breakdown pathway.[71] Plasma pseudocholinesterase does not participate significantly in atracurium ester hydrolysis, as evidenced by unaltered atracurium kinetics in patients with pseudocholinesterase abnormalities.

Mivacurium is metabolized by plasma cholinesterase, at approximately 88 percent of the rate for succinylcholine (Fig. 20-3).[73] Plasma cholinesterase activity does not correlate with the duration of blockade, suggesting additional routes of elimination.[73] Like atracurium, mivacurium is a mixture of isomers. The cis-trans (36 percent) and trans-trans (57 percent) isomers are equipotent and are rapidly hydrolyzed by plasma cholinesterase (clinical $t_{1/2}$ 2 minutes for both), while the cis-cis isomer (6 percent of the total) is one-tenth as potent and hydrolyzed more slowly (clinical $t_{1/2}$ 55 minutes).[7]

In contrast to atracurium and mivacurium, the benzylisoquinoline doxacurium is relatively resistant to metabolic breakdown. Only about 5 percent of doxacurium is metabolized by plasma cholinesterase.[74]

There is a direct relationship between duration of action of succinylcholine and cholinesterase activity.[75,76] Studies of succinylcholine pharmacokinetics in humans are not based on assays of succinylcholine plasma concentrations. Rather, pharmacokinetic parameters are based on a bioassay: twitch depression combined with the assumption of a one-compartment model.[77]

SPEED OF ONSET

Paralysis following intravenous injection of a NMBA does not occur instantaneously, even with high initial plasma concentrations. It may take several minutes to produce full paralysis of all mus-

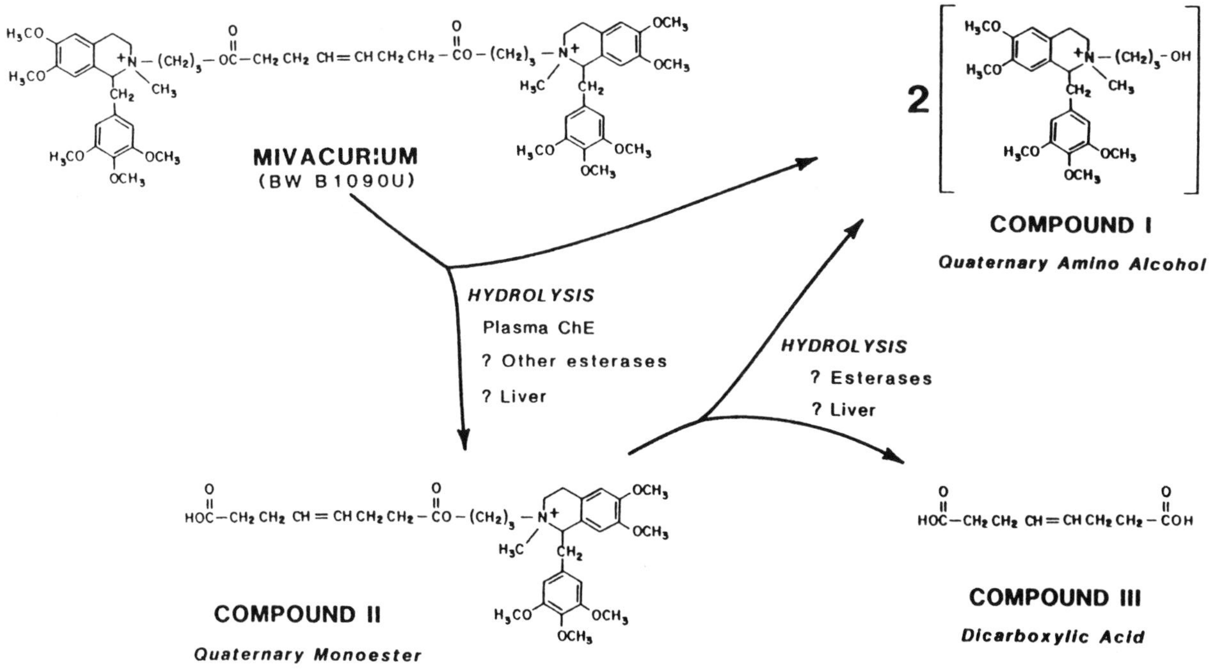

Fig. 20-3 Breakdown pathway of mivacurium. (From Savarese et al.,[73] with permission.)

cles, and even then the pattern of onset differs among the various muscle groups. Paralysis occurs when a critical concentration is reached at the site of action, and its timing depends on many factors: kinetics at the neuromuscular junction, tissue blood flow, dose, and the concentration-effect relationship.[78] Models of onset based on two venous samples taken in the first 10 minutes are likely to be unrealistic, regardless of the number of samples taken subsequently. Arterial blood sampling is necessary to model drug arrival at the neuromuscular junction. A new model, based on arterial blood sampling every 10 seconds in the first 2 minutes, found different pharmacokinetic parameters compared with previous studies using fewer, venous samples.[79] Most different was the estimate for the effect compartment rate constant, k_{eo}.

A major factor influencing the speed of onset of NMBAs is drug-receptor kinetics at the neuromuscular junction. Recent investigations have demonstrated a reciprocal relationship between the speed of onset of block and drug potency. A study with structurally related analogs of pancuronium and vecuronium showed that fast onset and brief duration were produced only with compounds of relatively low potency (see Fig. 21-7).[80] Similar results were obtained with equipotent doses of the structurally unrelated NMBAs gallamine, tubocurarine, and pancuronium. There was an inverse log linear relationship between the onset time to 50 percent single twitch depression in seconds, and drug potency expressed as the ED_{95}.[81] Rapid onset with highly potent drugs, which by definition have a high affinity for the receptor, can only be achieved at the expense of prolonged effect. Conversely, for brief duration, low receptor affinity and thus low potency is necessary.[80] The faster onset of less potent NMBAs has been explained as follows[81]: A critical number of NMBA molecules must block the receptors, and this critical number will be carried in a larger volume of blood if the drug is more potent. The larger volume of blood containing the more potent agent will reach the neuromuscular junction more slowly, therefore increasing the onset time. Onset and offset times of NMBAs were measured directly by local application to the motor endplate via iontophoresis.[82] The time constants for onset of block (gallamine < tubocurarine <

atracurium < doxacurium) were directly related to drug potency, with the most potent NMBA having the longest time constant. The initial appearance of a potent NMBA is likely to be associated with considerable drug-receptor binding of these first molecules, resulting in slow increase in drug concentrations, and reduced rate of drug onset. As the low-potency drug is present in large numbers of molecules, the free concentrations is minimally affected by such binding. This effect can be modelled as a change in distribution volume at the biophase.[83,84]

Tissue perfusion also has an effect on the speed of onset of NMBAs. The interval between injection of succinylcholine and 95 percent depression of twitch height is proportional to the circulation time.[85] For pancuronium, this time interval is related both to the arm-arm circulation time and to the dose.[86] The onset of vecuronium-induced blockade is influenced by the cardiac output.[87] The onset and intensity of paralysis produced by gallamine are related directly to muscle blood flow.[88] Succinylcholine and the nondepolarizing NMBAs all show more rapid onset of blockade at the diaphragm than that of the adductor pollicis, despite the greater sensitivity of the latter.[89–91] Perhaps the diaphragm, owing to its proximity to the aorta, receives a greater blood supply than the adductor pollicis. Alternatively, ultrastructural differences in the neuromuscular junction at the two muscles may affect NMBA access and thus speed of onset.[91]

Pharmacokinetic-Pharmacodynamic Models

Complex relationships between NMBA dose, concentration at the site of action, and pharmacologic effect can be examined, both for individual subjects and for patient groups. Simultaneous measurements of plasma NMBA concentrations and twitch response permit concomitant characterization of pharmacokinetics and pharmacodynamics, and the building of pharmacokinetic-pharmacodynamic models.

The first kinetic-dynamic model applied to NMBAs was developed by Sheiner et al.[92] for tubocurarine. The sigmoid E_{max} relationship [Eq. 3] assumes that a sigmoid curve characterizes the relationship between NMBA concentration in the effect compartment (biophase) and NMBA effect (percent paralysis).

$$\text{Fractional Effect} = \frac{E_{max} \cdot C^\gamma}{EC_{50}^\gamma + C^\gamma} \quad (3)$$

The sigmoidal relationship is characterized by the unitary maximal response (E_{max}), the drug concentration producing 50 percent of the maximal response (EC_{50}), the drug concentration (C), and a slope, or exponent (γ), relating the change in response to the change in drug concentration. When an effect compartment is included, another parameter is required to characterize in the model (k_{eo}). This rate constant describes drug removal from the effect compartment, characterizing the temporal aspects of equilibrium between plasma drug concentration and response. Table 20-5 provides the pharmacodynamic parameters for certain NMBAs. The usefulness of this model is that rapidity of NMBA onset can be described by the two parameters EC_{50} and k_{eo}. The kinetic-dynamic model may not, however, be static; time-dependent increases in sensitivity to tubocurarine suggest that certain model parameters may change during anesthesia.[93]

GERIATRICS

Table 20-6 provides NMBA pharmacokinetic parameters reported for the elderly. Age-related changes in NMBA pharmacokinetics are most likely to produce differences in onset, due to slower cardiovascular delivery of drug to the neuromuscular junction, and more prolonged recovery when organ clearance is the rate-limiting step. There does not appear to be any age-related change in sensitivity of the neuromuscular junction to NMBAs; the EC_{50}'s for metocurine,[57] atracurium,[94] vecuronium,[56] and pipecuronium[32] do not differ between the elderly and young patients (Table 20-5).

OBSTETRICS

NMBAs follow the usual time-course and intensity in pregnant patients as in other adults; the pharmacokinetics of vecuronium and pancuronium[100] are in good agreement with those in Tables 20-2 and 20-4. Magnesium treatment of preeclampsia produces muscle relaxation and reduces dose requirements for the nondepolarizing

Table 20-6 Pharmacokinetics of the NMBAs in Elderly Patients

	Steady-State Distribution Volume (l/kg)	Elimination Clearance (ml/kg/min)	Elimination Half-Life (min)	Reference
Intermediate				
Atracurium	0.15	5.4	23[a]	11
	0.19[a]	6.5	22[a]	94
Rocuronium	0.62[a]	3.4	137	95
Vecuronium	0.44	2.6[a]	125[a]	96
	0.18[a]	3.7[a]	58	56
Long				
Alcuronium	0.29	1.2[a]	191[a]	97
Doxacurium	0.22[a]	2.5	96	24
	0.30	2.4	118	98
Metocurine	0.28[a]	0.4[a]	530[a]	57
Pancuronium	0.32	1.2	204	28
	0.22	1.2	151	56
	0.25	0.8	168	99
Pipecuronium	0.39	2.4	181	32
Tubocurarine	0.22[a]	1.2[a]	151[a]	57

[a] Differed from values obtained for a control group of younger patients.

NMBAs; however, dose-response studies for this important drug interaction seem not to be available. NMBAs administered to the mother are transferred to the fetus, with the placenta functioning as an incomplete barrier. This means that prolonged exposure, as in an intensive care unit case requiring weeks of continued NMBAs, would result in comparable paralysis of the fetus.

A major concern in obstetric anesthesia is the amount of NMBA in the fetal blood at the time of delivery. This is usually reported as the ratio between concentrations in the umbilical venous blood and those in the maternal venous blood (UV/MV). These samples are collected at delivery, usually 3 to 20 minutes after the time of NMBA administration. The UV/MV ratio typically is in the range of 0.1 to 0.4.[100-104] With the usual clinical doses, significant effects on the neonate are unlikely. With

use of atracurium the UV/MV ratio for laudanosine averages 0.19.[104]

PEDIATRICS

The pharmacokinetic parameters shown in Table 20-7 indicate that the pharmacokinetics of several NMBAs differ in pediatric patients compared with adults, although not uniformly. The dose-response relationships for infants and children may not be the same as, or even parallel to those in adults. The pharmacodynamic parameters for adults (Table 20-5) may also not apply to children. For example, infants and children are more sensitive to tubocurarine.[38] Infants are more sensitive than children to vecuronium, but also have a larger distribution volume[109]; however, these opposing factors result in similar dose requirements for the two age groups.

Table 20-7 Pharmacokinetics of the NMBAs in Pediatric Patients

	Steady-State Volume (l/kg)	Elimination Clearance (ml/kg/min)	Elimination Half-Life (min)	Reference
Intermediate				
Atracurium	0.17	9.1	14	105[a]
	0.14	5.1	19	105
	0.21[b]	7.9[b]	20	106[a]
	0.13	6.8[b]	17	106
Rocuronium	0.30[b]	13.5	56[b]	107[c]
	0.22	11.4	38	107
Vecuronium	0.32[b]	2.8[b]	123	108
	0.13	4.8	28	109
	0.36[b]	5.6	65	110
	0.20	5.9	41	110
Long				
Pancuronium	0.20	1.7	103	108
Pipecuronium	0.19	1.3[b]	125[b]	111[a]
	0.17	2.1	59	111
Tubocurarine	0.51	1.1[b]	311[b]	112[c]
	0.47	1.0[b]	306[b]	112[a]
	0.34	1.5	171	112
	0.74[b]	3.7	174[b]	38[c]
	0.52	3.3	130	38
	0.41	4.0	90	38

[a] Infants.

[b] Differed from control adults.

[c] Neonates.

SPECIFIC DISEASE STATES

Hepatic and Renal Disease

Most NMBAs are excreted in urine and bile. In patients with renal or hepatic dysfunction, decreased clearance is likely to be associated with an increased duration of effect when large or repeated doses are administered, due to delayed removal of drug from the effect site. In both renal and hepatic failure, sensitivity of the neuromuscular junction to NMBAs appears unaltered. Thus observed alterations in the time course of paralysis are entirely a function of altered pharmacokinetics.

NMBA pharmacokinetic parameters in patients with renal disease are provided in Table 20-8. In general, the effects of renal failure are more pronounced with NMBAs of long duration, whereas the kinetics of shorter-acting NMBAs such as atracurium and vecuronium are minimally affected if at all. Resistance to pancuronium has been reported in patients with chronic renal failure, which is probably related to an increase in the volume of distribution.

Pharmacokinetic parameters are NMBAs in patients with hepatic or biliary disease are provided in Table 20-9. In patients with cirrhosis, there is an initial "resistance" to a bolus dose of pancuronium.[63] This is because the volume of distribution is increased and plasma concentrations will be lower for any given dose. However, with continued administration, pancuronium clearance becomes increasingly important in terminating the drug's effect, and decreased hepatic clearance results in increased "sensitivity" to pancuronium.

Atracurium

Liver failure makes little difference to atracurium kinetics[122,127] or dynamics,[128] even when acute hepatic failure is combined with acute renal failure.[123] Clearance of the atracurium metabolite laudanosine is reduced in patients with hepatic cirrhosis.[122]

Vecuronium

The liver exerts a major influence on the disposition of vecuronium, which is extensively deacetylated in the liver prior to excretion.[17] Unlike pancuronium,[63] the V_{ss} of vecuronium is unchanged in hepatic disease, and there is no initial "resistance" to drug effect.[16] Vecuronium may have an altered duration of effect in patients with liver dysfunc-

Table 20-8 Pharmacokinetics of the NMBAs in Patients With Renal Failure

	Steady State Distribution Volume (l/kg)	Elimination Clearance, (ml/kg/min)	Elimination Half-Life (min)	Reference
Intermediate				
Atracurium	0.14	5.8	20	113
	0.22(β)	6.7	24	10
	0.17	6.3	18	114
Rocuronium	0.26	3.0	97[a]	15
Vecuronium	0.47	2.6	149	17
	0.24	2.5	97	115
	0.24	3.1[a]	83[a]	116
Long				
Doxacurium	0.27	1.2[a]	221	25
Metocurine	0.35(β)	0.4	684	58
Pancuronium	0.21	0	1,050	117
	0.24[a]	0.3[a]	489[a]	118
	0.26	0.9[a]	238[a]	119
Pipecuronium	0.44[a]	1.6[a]	263[a]	120
Tubocurarine	0.25	1.5	330	121

[a] Differed from control patients with normal renal function.

Table 20-9 Pharmacokinetics of the NMBAs in Patients With Hepatic or Biliary Disease

	Steady-State Distribution Volume (l/kg)	Elimination Clearance (ml/kg/min)	Elimination Half-Life (min)	Reference
Intermediate				
Atracurium	0.28[a]	8.0[a]	25	122
	0.21(β)[a]	6.5[a]	20	123[b]
Rocuronium	0.32[a]	3.0	173	124
Vecuronium	0.25	2.7	84	16
	0.22	4.3[a]	51[a]	18
	0.21	2.4	98[a]	125
	0.20	4.5	49	20
Long				
Doxacurium	0.29	2.3	115	25
Pancuronium	0.35[a]	1.5[a]	208[a]	63
	0.43[a]	1.5	224[a]	60
	0.31	1.1[a]	270[a]	126
Pipecuronium	0.30	1.3[a]	99[a]	33

[a] Differs significantly from control patients without hepatic or biliary disease.

[b] Acute, combined with renal failure.

tion, cirrhosis, or cholestasis. In patients with cirrhosis, prolongation of effect[16] was related to reduced clearance and greater elimination half-life.[16] In contrast, patients with alcoholic liver disease showed no change in vecuronium pharmacokinetics or duration of neuromuscular block.[18] Human liver biopsies show that more than one-half the dose of vecuronium remains in the liver at 30 minutes. These results suggest prolonged redistribution could occur, as the low hepatic extraction of vecuronium in man accounts for only 18 percent to 35 percent of its total clearance.[129] Renal failure was reported initially not to alter the kinetics of vecuronium,[17] but its clearance has been found by others to be reduced.[116]

Long-Acting NMBAs

Most long-acting NMBAs are eliminated mainly by the kidney, with lesser removal by the liver. In patients with renal failure, there is reduced clearance and prolongation of the elimination half-life. Reduced clearance seldom affects the response to the initial dose of NMBA, but is likely to prolong the paralysis with additional doses.

Prolonged Use, Intensive Care Unit

In a national survey on the use of NMBAs by anesthesiologists in intensive care units, 52 percent of respondents listed vecuronium as their primary NMBA.[130] Pancuronium (28 percent), metocurine (5 percent) and atracurium (3 percent) were also used. The most frequently cited justification for the use of vecuronium was the absence of hemodynamic side effects. In more than one-half the intensive care units, dosage was monitored by clinical observation alone, without twitch monitoring. Pancuronium and alcuronium are most popular for intensive care unit use in Britain.

Prolonged use of neuromuscular blocking agents to facilitate mechanical ventilation can be followed by disuse atrophy, myopathies, and weakness of skeletal muscles.[131,132] Large doses over a prolonged period may produce drug accumulation in undesirable sites; for example, tubocurarine is known to enter the CSF.[133]

In general, NMBA metabolite pharmacokinetics are of little importance during intraoperative NMBA administration. However, metabolite kinetics are important during long-term NMBA use.

Avoidance of atracurium has been suggested for patients in renal failure who require prolonged relaxation due to concerns over accumulation of laudanosine, and possible CNS toxicity. However it seems unlikely that toxic levels of laudanosine would ever be reached.[134] Pharmacokinetics of atracurium itself are unaffected by combined renal and hepatic failure.[123] Case reports have implicated sustained use of vecuronium in intensive care unit patients in the development of prolonged neuromuscular blockade. A recent study of vecuronium found an association between persistent paralysis and high plasma concentrations of the active metabolite 3-desacetyl vecuronium, low pH, high plasma magnesium, female sex, and renal failure.[135] Prolonged neuromuscular block could particularly occur if the active metabolite is inadequately excreted due to insufficient renal function. Isobolograms indicate that 3-desacetyl vecuronium acts additively with vecuronium.[136] Studies of vecuronium disposition in rodents indicate that both parent drug and vecuronium metabolites are excreted into the bile and a fraction of drug excreted undergoes enterohepatic cycling, with intestinal reabsorption.[137] Further studies are required to determine whether enterohepatic cycling contributes to prolonged neuromuscular blockade by vecuronium in man.

Morbid Obesity

Limited data are available regarding the pharmacokinetics of NMBAs in obesity. Table 20-10 provides pharmacokinetic parameters for atracurium and vecuronium in patients with morbid obesity.[138,139] The clearance and V_{ss} of both atracurium and vecuronium, calculated per kilogram of actual body weight, are diminished in morbidly obese patients compared with normal weight controls. However, when normalized to ideal body weight, these values are not different from those normalized values in normal weight patients. Vecuronium, administered as a bolus dose based on actual body weight, showed prolonged effect compared to controls, and recovery time was linearly related to percent ideal body weight.[140] In contrast, the duration of effect of atracurium, administered as a bolus dose based on actual body weight, was not prolonged.[140] Plasma vecuronium concentrations producing equivalent neuromuscular blockade were not different in obese patients compared to controls, suggesting no effect of obesity on NMBA pharmacodynamics.[139]

Thermal Injury

Patients with thermal injury are resistant to the nondepolarizing NMBAs. Increases in plasma protein binding partially accounted for the altered requirement, unbound V_c and clearance were significantly increased whereas $t_{1/2}$, V_{ss} and intrinsic clearance were unchanged. Thus pharmacokinetic changes are minimally responsible for resistance in burn patients.[59] There is a marked increase in the number of acetylcholine receptors in response to 45 to 55 percent burns,[141] and the neuromuscular receptors are up-regulated.[141] Thus pharmacodynamic effects predominate in resistance to NMBAs in burns.

Table 20-10 Pharmacokinetics of the NMBAs in Patients With Morbid Obesity[a]

	Steady State Distribution Volume (l/kg)	Elimination Clearance (ml/kg/min)	Elimination Half-Life (min)	Reference
Intermediate				
Atracurium	0.07^b (0.14)	3.5^b (7.3)	20	138
Vecuronium	0.47^b (0.79)	2.8^b (4.7)	119	139

[a] Values in parentheses are normalized to ideal body weight. Unlike the values based on actual body weight, these do not differ significantly from control.

[b] Differed from control patients with normal body weight.

Table 20-11 Pharmacokinetics of the NMBAs in Patients Whose Surgery Involves Cardiopulmonary Bypass

	Steady State Distribution Volume (l/kg)	Elimination Clearance (ml/kg/min)	Elimination Half-Life (min)	Reference
Long				
Alcuronium	0.33	0.8[a]	532[a]	142
Metocurine	0.35	1.3[a]	264	26
Pancuronium	0.31	1.0[b]	296[b]	61
Pipecuronium	0.35	1.8	161	61
Tubocurarine	0.42	0.6[a]	633[a]	142

[a] Differed from control.
[b] Reduced with use of dopamine.

Cardiopulmonary Bypass

Pharmacokinetic parameters of NMBAs during cardiopulmonary bypass (CPB) are shown in Table 20-11. Physiologic changes associated with alterations in bloodflow, temperature, and acid-base balance are among the factors which make alterations to both pharmacokinetics and pharmacodynamics unpredictable.

REFERENCES

1. Donati F, Bevan DR: Not all muscles are the same. Br J Anaesth 68:239, 1992
2. Mitenko PA, Ogilvie RI: Rapidly achieved plasma concentration plateaus, with observations on theophylline kinetics. Clin Pharmacol Ther 13:329, 1972
3. Shanks CA: Pharmacokinetics of the nondepolarizing neuromuscular relaxants applied to calculation of bolus and infusion dosage regimens. Anesthesiology 64:72, 1986
4. Henthorn TK, Avram MJ, Krecjie TC et al: Minimal compartmental model of circulatory mixing of indocyanine green. Am J Physiol 31:H903, 1992
5. Scott RP, Savarese JJ, Basta SJ et al: Atracurium: clinical strategies for preventing histamine release and attenuating the haemodynamic response. Br J Anaes 57:550, 1985
6. Cook DR, Freeman JA, Lai AA et al: Pharmacokinetics of mivacurium in normal patients and in those with hepatic or renal failure. Br J Anaesth 69:580, 1992
7. Lien CA, Schmith VD, Wargin WA et al: Pharmaco-
kinetics and pharmacodynamics of mivacurium stereoisomers during a two-step infusion. Anesthesiology 77:A910, 1992
8. Weatherley BC, Williams SG, Neill EA: Pharmacokinetics pharmacodynamics and dose-response relationships of atracurium administered i.v. Br J Anaesth 55(suppl 1):39S, 1983
9. Ward S, Neill EAM, Weatherley BC et al: Pharmacokinetics of atracurium besylate in healthy patients (after a single i.v. bolus dose). Br J Anaesth 55:113, 1983
10. Fahey MR, Rupp SM, Fisher DM et al: The pharmacokinetics and pharmacodynamics of atracurium in patients with and without renal failure. Anesthesiology 61:699, 1984
11. Kent AP, Parker CJR, Hunter JM: Pharmacokinetics of atracurium and laudanosine in the elderly. Br J Anaesth 63:661, 1989
12. Parker CJR, Hunter JM, Snowden SL: Effects of age, sex and anaesthetic technique on the pharmacokinetics of atracurium. Br J Anaesth 69:439, 1992
13. Donati F, Gill SS, Bevan DR et al: Pharmacokinetics and pharmacodynamics of atracurium with and without previous suxamethonium administration. Br J Anaesth 66:557, 1991
14. Wierda JM, Kleef UW, Lambalk LM et al: The pharmacodynamics and pharmacokinetics of ORG 9426, a new non-depolarizing neuromuscular blocking agent, in patients anaesthetized with nitrous oxide, halothane and fentanyl. Can J Anaesth 38:430, 1991
15. Szenohdradszky J, Fisher DM, Segredo V et al: Pharmacokinetics of rocuronium bromide in patients with normal renal function or patients undergoing cadaver renal transplantation. Anesthesiology 77:899, 1992

16. Lebrault C, Berger JL, d'Hollander AA et al: Pharmacokinetics and pharmacodynamics of vecuronium (ORG NC45) in patients with cirrhosis. Anesthesiology 62:601, 1985

17. Bencini A, Scaf AHJ, Sohn YJ et al: Disposition and urinary excretion of vecuronium in anesthetized patients with normal renal function or renal failure. Anesth Analg 65:245, 1986

18. Arden JR, Lynam DP, Castagnoli KP et al: Vecuronium in alcoholic liver disease: a pharmacokinetic and pharmacodynamic analysis. Anesthesiology 68:771, 1988

19. Shanks CA, Avram MJ, Fragen RJ: Pharmacokinetics and pharmacodynamics of vecuronium administered by bolus and infusion during halothane or balanced anesthesia. Clin Pharmacol Ther 42:459, 1987

20. Castagnoli KP, Caldwell JE, Canfell PC et al: Does the independent measurement of 3-desacetylvecuronium influence the pharmacokinetics of vecuronium? Anesthesiology 69:A479, 1988

21. Sohn YJ, Bencini AF, Scaf AH et al: Comparative pharmacokinetics and dynamics of vecuronium and pancuronium in anesthetized patients. Anesth Analg 65:233, 1986

22. Walker JS, Triggs EJ, Shanks CA: Clinical pharmacokinetics of alcuronium chloride in man. Eur J Clin Pharm 17:449, 1980

23. Walker JS, Shanks CA, Brown KF: Alcuronium kinetics and plasma concentration-effect relationship. Clin Ther Pharmacol 33:510, 1983

24. Dresner DL, Basta SJ, Ali HH et al: Pharmacokinetics and pharmacodynamics of doxacurium in young and elderly patients during isoflurane anesthesia. Anesth Analg 71:498, 1990

25. Cook DR, Freeman JA, Lai AA et al: Pharmacokinetics and pharmacodynamics of doxacurium in normal patients and in those with hepatic or renal failure. Anesth Analg 72:145, 1991

26. Avram MJ, Shanks CA, Henthorn TK et al: Metocurine kinetics in patients undergoing operations requiring cardiopulmonary bypass. Clin Pharmacol Ther 42:576, 1987

27. Matteo RS, Brotherton WP, Nishitateno K et al: Pharmacodynamics and pharmacokinetics of metocurine in humans: comparison to d-tubocurarine. Anesthesiology 57:183, 1982

28. Duvaldestin P, Saada J, Berger JL et al: Pharmacokinetics, pharmacodynamics and dose-response relationships of pancuronium in control and elderly patients. Anesthesiology 56:36, 1982

29. Caldwell JE, Castagnoli KP, Canfell PC et al: Pipecuronium and pancuronium: comparison of pharmacokinetics and duration of action. Br J Anaesth 61:693, 1988

30. Somogyi AA, Shanks CA, Triggs EJ: Combined i.v. bolus and infusion of pancuronium bromide. Br J Anaesth 50:575, 1978

31. Evans MA, Shanks CA, Brown KF et al: Pharmacokinetic and pharmacodynamic modelling with pancuronium. Eur J Clin Pharmacol 26:243, 1984

32. Ornstein E, Matteo RS, Schwartz AE et al: Pharmacokinetics and pharmacodynamics of pipecuronium bromide (Arduan) in elderly surgical patients. Anesth Analg 74:841, 1992

33. d'Honneur G, Khalil M, Dominique C et al: Pharmacokinetics and pharmacodynamics of pipecuronium in patients with cirrhosis. Anesth Analg 77:1203, 1993

34. Shanks CA, Ramzan MI, Triggs EJ: Studies in man with a constant-rate infusion of tubocurarine. Anaesth Intensive Care 7:209, 1979

35. Stanski DR, Ham J, Miller RD et al: Pharmacokinetics and pharmacodynamics of d-tubocurarine during nitrous oxide-narcotic and halothane anesthesia in man. Anesthesiology 51:235, 1979

36. Matteo RS, Nashitateno K, Pua EK et al: Pharmacokinetics of d-tubocurarine in man: Effect of an osmotic diuretic on urinary excretion. Anesthesiology 52:335, 1980

37. Ramzan MI, Shanks CA, Triggs EJ: Pharmacokinetics of tubocurarine administered by combined i.v. bolus and infusion. Br J Anaesth 52:893, 1980

38. Fisher DM, O'Keefe C, Stanski DR et al: Pharmacokinetics and pharmacodynamics of d-tubocurarine in infants, children and adults. Anesthesiology 57:203, 1982

39. Waser PG: Localization of ^{14}C-pancuronium by histo- and wholebody-autoradiography in normal and pregnant mice. Naunyn-Schmiedberg's Arch Pharmacol 279:399, 1973

40. Hunter JM: Resistance to non-depolarizing neuromuscular blocking agents. Br J Anaesth 67:511, 1991

41. Duvaldestin P, Henzel D: Binding of tubocurarine, fazadinium, pancuronium, and ORG NC 45 to serum proteins in normal man and in patients with cirrhosis. Br J Anaesth 54:513, 1982

42. Raaflaub VJ, Frey P: Zur pharmacokinetik von diallyl-nor-toxiferin beim menschen. Arzneim-Forsch 22:73, 1972

43. Olsen GD, Chan EM, Riker WK: Binding of d-tubocurarine di(methyl- ^{14}C) ether iodide and other amines to cartilage, chondroitin sulfate and human

plasma proteins. J Pharmacol Exp Ther 195:242, 1975

44. Meijer DKF, Weitering JG, Vermeer GA et al: Comparative pharmacokinetics of d-tubocurarine and metocurine in man. Anesthesiology 51:402, 1979

45. Wood M, Stone WJ, Wood AJ: Plasma binding of pancuronium: effects of age, sex, and disease. Anesth Analg 62:29, 1983

46. Thompson JM: Pancuronium binding by plasma proteins. Anaesthesia 31:219, 1976

47. Leibel WS, Martyn JA, Szyfelbein SK et al: Elevated plasma binding cannot account for the burn-related d-tubocurarine hyposensitivity. Anesthesiology 54:378, 1981

48. Walker JS, Shanks CA, Brown KF: Determinants of d-tubocurarine plasma protein binding in health and disease. Anesth Analg 62:870, 1983

49. Foldes FF, Deery A: Protein binding of atracurium and other short-acting neuromuscular blocking agents and their interaction with human cholinesterases. Br J Anaesth 55(Suppl 1):31S, 1983

50. Ghoneim MM, Pandya H: Binding of tubocurarine to specific serum protein fractions. Br J Anaesth 47:853, 1975

51. Skivington MA: Protein binding of three tritiated muscle relaxants. Br J Anaesth 44:1030, 1972

52. Shanks CA, Avram MJ, Ronai AK et al: The pharmacokinetics of d-tubocurarine with surgery involving salvaged autologous blood. Anesthesiology 62:161, 1985

53. Ramzan IM, Shanks CA, Triggs EJ: Relationship between gallamine plasma concentration and neuromuscular paralysis in surgical patients. J Clin Pharm 23:243, 1983

54. Donati F, Varin F, Ducharme J et al: Pharmacokinetics and pharmacodynamics of atracurium obtained with arterial and venous blood samples. Clin Pharmacol Ther 49:515, 1991

55. Weatherley BC, Williams SG, Neill EAM: Pharmacokinetics, pharmacodynamics and dose-response relationships of atracurium administered i.v. Br J Anaesth 55:395, 1983

56. Rupp SM, Castagnoli KP, Fisher DM et al: Pancuronium and vecuronium pharmacokinetics and pharmacodynamics in young and elderly adults. Anesthesiology 67:45, 1987

57. Matteo RS, Backus WW, McDaniel DD et al: Pharmacokinetics and pharmacodynamics of d-tubocurarine and metocurine in the elderly. Anesth Analg 64:23, 1985

58. Brotherton WP, Matteo RS: Pharmacokinetics and pharmacodynamics of metocurine in humans with

and without renal failure. Anesthesiology 55:273, 1981

59. Martyn JAJ, Matteo RS, Greenblatt DJ et al: Pharmacokinetics of d-tubocurarine in patients with thermal injury. Anesth Analg 61:241, 1982

60. Westra P, Vermeer GA, de Lange AR et al: Hepatic and renal disposition of pancuronium and gallamine in patients with extrahepatic cholestasis. Br J Anaesth 53:331, 1981

61. Wierda JM, Karliczek GF, Vandenbrom RH et al: Pharmacokinetics and cardiovascular dynamics of pipecuronium bromide during coronary artery surgery. Can J Anaesth 37:183, 1990

62. Wierda JM, Szenohradszky J, De Wit AP et al: The pharmacokinetics, urinary and biliary excretion of pipecuronium bromide. Eur J Anaesthesiol 8:451, 1991

63. Duvaldestin P, Agoston S, Henzel D et al: Pancuronium pharmacokinetics in patients with liver cirrhosis. Br J Anaesth 50:1131, 1978

64. Cozanitis DA: Probable resistance to vecuronium involving the 17-hydroxy metabolite. Br J Anaesth 69:110, 1992

65. Miller RD, Agoston S, Booij LH et al: The comparative potency and pharmacokinetics of pancuronium and its metabolites in anesthetized man. J Pharmacol Exp Ther 207:539, 1978

66. Segredo V, Shin YS, Sharma ML et al: Pharmacokinetics, neuromuscular effects, and biodisposition of 3-desacetylvecuronium (Org 7268) in cats. Anesthesiology 74:1052, 1991

67. Stenlake JB, Hughes R: In vitro degradation of atracurium in human plasma. Br J Anaes 59:806, 1987

68. Shearer ES, O'Sullivan EP, Hunter JM. Clearance of atracurium and laudanosine in the urine and by continuous venovenous haemofiltration. Br J Anaesth 67:569, 1991

69. Tsui D, Graham GG, Torda TA. The pharmacokinetics of atracurium isomers in vitro and in humans. Anesthesiology 67:722, 1987

70. Nigrovic V, Banoub M: Pharmacokinetic modelling of a parent drug and its metabolite. Atracurium and laudanosine. Clin Pharmacokinet 22:396, 1992

71. Nigrovic V, Fox JL: Atracurium decay and the formation of laudanosine in humans. Anesthesiology 74:446, 1991

72. Shi W-Z, Fahey MR, Fisher DM et al: Laudanosine (a metabolite of atracurium) increases the minimum alveolar concentration of halothane in rabbits. Anesthesiology 63:584, 1985

73. Savarese JJ, Ali HH, Basta SJ et al: The clinical neuromusular pharmacology of mivacurium chlo-

ride (BW B1090U): a short-acting nondepolarizing ester neuromuscular blocking drug. Anesthesiology 67:723, 1988

74. Basta SJ, Savarese JJ, Ali HH et al: Clinical pharmacology of doxacurium chloride. A new long-acting nondepolarizing muscle relaxant. Anesthesiology 69:478, 1988

75. Ritter DM, Rettke SR, Ilstrup DM et al: Effect of plasma cholinesterase activity on the duration of action of succinylcholine in patients with genotypically normal enzyme. Anesth Analg 67:1123, 1988

76. Perez-Guillermo F, Martinez-Pretel CM, Tarin-Royo F et al: Prolonged suxamethonium-induced neuromuscular blockade associated with organophosphate poisoning. Br J Anaes 61:233, 1988

77. Cook DR, Wingard LB: Pharmacokinetics of succinylcholine in infants, children and adults. Clin Pharmacol Ther 20:493, 1976

78. Donati F: Onset of action of relaxants. Can J Anaesth 35:552, 1988

79. Ducharme J, Varin F, Theoret Y et al: Influence of blood sampling schedule on vecuronium kinetic (PK) and dynamic (PD) parameters. Anesthesiology 75:A803, 1991

80. Bowman WC, Rodger IW, Houston J et al: Structure:action relationships among some desacetoxy analogues of pancuronium and vecuronium in the anesthetized cat. Anesthesiology 69:57, 1988

81. Kopman AF: Pancuronium, gallamine, and d-tubocurarine compared: is speed of onset inversely related to drug potency? Anesthesiology 70:915, 1989

82. Law Min JC, Bekavac I, Glavinovic MI et al: Iontophoretic study of speed of action of various muscle relaxants. Anesthesiology 75:A811, 1991

83. Bartkowski RR, Epstein RH: The influence of receptor binding on the onset of neuromuscular blockade. Anesthesiology 76:A916, 1992

84. Hull CJ: Review lecture. 4th International Neuromuscular Meeting, Montreal, 1992

85. Harrison GA, Junius F: The effect of circulation time on the neuromuscular action of suxamethonium. Anaesth Intensive Care 1:33, 1972

86. Harrison GA: The relationship between the arm-arm circulation time and the neuromuscular action of pancuronium. Anaesth Intensive Care 2:91, 1974

87. Iwasaki H, Igarashi M, Yamakagi M et al: Influence of cardiac output on the onset of neuromuscular blockade after vecuronium. Anesthesiology 77:A945, 1992

88. Goat VA, Yeung ML, Blakeney C et al: The effect of blood flow upon the activity of gallamine triethiodide. Br J Anaesth 48:69, 1976

89. Donati F, Antzaka C, Bevan DR: Potency of pancuronium at the diaphragm and the adductor pollicis muscle in humans. Anesthesiology 65:1, 1986

90. Chauvin M, Lebrault C, Duvaldestin P: The neuromuscular blocking effect of vecuronium on the human diaphragm. Anesth Analg 66:117, 1987

91. Pansard J-L, Cauvin M, Lebrault C et al: Effect of intubating dose of succinylcholine and atracurium on the diaphragm and the adductor pollicis muscle in humans. Anesthesiology 67:326, 1987

92. Sheiner LB, Stanski DR, Vozeh S et al: Simultaneous modeling of pharmacokinetics and pharmacodynamics: Application to d-tubocurarine. Clin Pharmacol Ther 25:358, 1979

93. Stanski DR, Ham J, Miller RD et al: Time-dependent increase in sensitivity to d-tubocurarine during enflurane anesthesia in man. Anesthesiology 52:483, 1980

94. Kitts JB, Fisher DM, Canfell PC et al: Pharmacokinetics and pharmacodynamics of atracurium in the elderly. Anesthesiology 72:272, 1990

95. Matteo RS, Ornstein E, Schwartz AE et al: Pharmacokinetics and pharmacodynamics of ORG 9426 in elderly surgical patients. Anesth Analg 77:1193, 1993

96. Lien CA, Matteo RS, Ornstein E et al: Distribution, elimination, and action of vecuronium in the elderly. Anesth Analg 73:39, 1991

97. Stephens ID, Ho PC, Holloway AM et al: Pharmacokinetics of alcuronium in elderly patients undergoing total hip replacement or aortic reconstructive surgery. Br J Anaesth 56:465, 1984

98. Lepage JY, Malinovsky JM, Debord P et al: Pharmacokinetics of doxacurium in elderly patients. Anesthesiology 77:A911, 1992

99. McLeod K, Hull CJ, Watson MJ: Effects of ageing on the pharmacokinetics of pancuronium. Br J Anaesth 51:435, 1979

100. Dailey PA, Fisher DM, Shnider SM et al: Pharmacokinetics, placental transfer and neonatal effects of vecuronium and pancuronium administered during cesarean section. Anesthesiology 60:569, 1984

101. Duvaldestin P, Demetriou M, Henzel D et al: The placental transfer of pancuronium and its pharmacokinetics during caesarian section. Acta Anaesth Scand 22:327, 1978

102. Booth PN, Watson MJ, MacLeod K: Pancuronium and the placental barrier. Anaesthesia 32:320, 1977

103. Demetriou M, Depoix JP, Diakite B et al: Placental transfer of ORG NC 45 in women undergoing Caesarean section. Br J Anaesth 54:643, 1982

104. Shearer ES, Fahy LT, O'Sullivan EP et al: Transpla-

cental distribution of atracurium, laudanosine and monoquaternary alcohol during elective caesarean section. Br J Anaesth 66:551, 1991

105. Brandom BW, Stiller RL, Cook DR et al: Pharmacokinetics of atracurium in anaesthetized infants and children. Br J Anaesth 58:1210, 1986

106. Fisher DM, Canfell PC, Spellman MJ et al: Pharmacokinetics and pharmacodynamics of atracurium in infants and children. Anesthesiology 73:33, 1990

107. O'Kelly B, Fiset P, Meistelman C et al: Pharmacokinetics of rocuronium in pediatric patients during halothane anesthesia. Anesthesiology 77:A907, 1992

108. Meistelman C, Agoston S, Kersten UW et al: Pharmacokinetics and pharmacodynamics of vecuronium and pancuronium in anesthetized children. Anesth Analg 65:1319, 1986

109. Steinbereithner K, Fitzal S, Schwarz S: Pharmacokinetics and pharmacodynamics of vecuronium in children. Can Anesthesiol 32:5, 1984

110. Fisher DM, Castagnoli K, Miller RD: Vecuronium kinetics and dynamics in anesthetized infants and children. Clin Pharmacol Ther 37:402, 1985

111. Tassonyi E, Pittet J-F, Schopfer C et al: Pharmacokinetics of pipecurium in infants, children and adults. Anesthesiology 75:A777, 1991

112. Matteo RS, Lieberman IG, Salanitre Et et al: Distribution, elimination, and action of d-tubocurarine in neonates, infants, children, and adults. Anesth Analg 63:799, 1984

113. Ward S, Boheimer N, Weatherley BC et al: Pharmacokinetics of atracurium and its metabolites in patients with normal renal function, and in patients with renal failure. Br J Anaesth 59:697, 1987

114. deBros F, Lai A, Scott R et al: Pharmacokinetics and pharmacodynamics of atracurium under isoflurane anesthesia in normal and anephric patients. Anesth Analg 64:207, 1985

115. Fahey MR, Morris RB, Miller RD et al: Pharmacokinetics of ORG NC45 (norcuron) in patients with and without renal failure. Br J Anaesth 53:1049, 1991

116. Lynam DP, Cronnelly R, Castagnoli PC et al: The pharmacodynamics and pharmacokinetics of vecuronium in patients anesthetized with isoflurane with normal renal function or with renal failure. Anesthesiology 69:227, 1988

117. Buzello W, Agoston S: Pharmacokinetics of pancuronium in patients with normal and impaired renal function. Anaesthesist 27:291, 1987

118. McLeod K, Watson MJ, Rawlins MD: Pharmacokinetics of pancuronium in patients with normal and impaired renal function. Br J Anaesth 48:341, 1976

119. Somogyi AA, Shanks CA, Triggs EJ: The effect of renal failure on the disposition and neuromuscular blocking action of pancuronium bromide. Eur J Clin Pharmacol 12:23, 1977

120. Caldwell JE, Canfell PC, Castagnoli KP et al: The influence of renal failure on the pharmacokinetics and duration of action of pipecuronium bromide in patients anesthetized with halothane and nitrous oxide. Anesthesiology 70:7, 1989

121. Miller RD, Matteo RS, Benet LZ et al: The pharmacokinetics of d-tubocurarine in man with and without renal failure. J Pharmacol Exp Ther 202:1, 1977

122. Parker CJ, Hunter JM: Pharmacokinetics of atracurium and laudanosine in patients with hepatic cirrhosis. Br J Anaesth 62:177, 1989

123. Ward S, Neill EA: Pharmacokinetics of atracurium in acute hepatic failure (with acute renal failure). Br J Anaesth 55:1169, 1983

124. Magorian T, Wood P, Caldwell JE et al: Pharmacokinetics, onset, and duration of action of rocuronium in humans: normal vs hepatic dysfunction. Anesthesiology 75:A1069, 1991

125. Lebrault C, Duvaldestin P, Henzel D et al: Pharmacokinetics and pharmacodynamics of vecuronium in patients with cholestasis. Br J Anaesth 58:983, 1986

126. Somogyi AA, Shanks CA, Triggs EJ: Disposition kinetics of pancuronium bromide in patients with total biliary obstruction. Br J Anaesth 49:1103, 1977

127. Cook DR, Brandom BW, Stiller RL et al: Pharmacokinetics of atracurium in normal and liver failure patients. Anesthesiology 61:A433, 1984

128. Simpson DA, Green DW: Use of atracurium during major abdominal surgery in infants with hepatic dysfunction from biliary atresia. Br J Anaes 58:1214, 1986

129. Goldfarb G, Ganeau P, Ang ET et al: Hepatic extraction and clearance of vecuronium in humans. Anesthesiology 69:A480, 1988

130. Klessig HT, Geiger HJ, Murray MJ et al: A national survey on the practice of anesthesiologist intensivists in the use of muscle relaxants. Crit Care Med 20:1341, 1992

131. Buck ML, Reed MD: Use of nondepolarizing neuromuscular blocking agents in mechanicaly ventilated patients. Clin Pharm 10:32, 1991

132. Douglass JA, Tuxen DV, Horne M et al: Myopathy in severe asthma. Am Rev Resp Dis 145:517, 1992

133. Matteo RS, Pua EK, Khambatta HJ et al: Cerebrospinal fluid levels of d-tubocurarine in man. Anesthesiology 46:396, 1977

134. Parker CJ, Jones JE, Hunter JM. Disposition of infusions of atracurium and its metabolite, laudanosine, in patients in renal and respiratory failure in an ITU. Br J Anaesth 61:531, 1988

135. Segredo V, Caldwell JE, Matthay MA et al: Persistent paralysis in critically ill patients after long-term administration of vecuronium. N Engl J Med 327:524, 1992

136. Khuenl-Brady K, Mair P, Koller J et al: Antagonism of vecuronium by one of its metabolites in vitro. Anesthesiology 75:A800, 1991

137. Waser PG, Wiederkehr H, Chang Sin-Ren A, Kaiser-Schonenberger E: Distribution and kinetics of ^{14}C-vecuronium in rats and mice. Br J Anaesth 59:1044, 1987

138. Varin F, Ducharme J, Theoret Y et al: Influence of extreme obesity on the body disposition and neuromuscular blocking effect of atracurium. Clin Pharmacol Ther 48:18, 1990

139. Schwartz AE, Matteo RS, Ornstein E et al: Pharmacokinetics and pharmacodynamics of vecuronium in the obese surgical patient. Anesth Analg 74:515, 1992

140. Weinstein JA, Matteo RS, Ornstein E et al: Pharmacodynamics of vecuronium and atracurium in the obese surgical patient. Anesth Analg 67:1149, 1988

141. Kim C, Martyn JAJ, Fluke N: Burn injury to rat causes denervation-like responses in the gastrocnemius muscle. J Appl Physiol 65:1745, 1988

142. Walker JS, Brown KF, Shanks CA: Alcuronium kinetics in patients undergoing cardiopulmonary bypass surgery. Br J Clin Pharmacol 15:237, 1983

143. Wierda JMKH, van der Starre PIA, Scaf AHJ et al: Pharmacokinetics of pancuronium in patients undergoing coronary artery surgery with and without low dose dopamine. Clin Pharmacokin 19:491, 1990

144. Walker JS, Shanks CA, Brown KF: Altered d-tubocurarine disposition during cardiopulmonary bypass surgery. Clin Pharmacol Ther 35:686, 1984

Chapter 21

Clinical Pharmacology and Applications of Neuromuscular Blockers

Cynthia A. Lien, John J. Savarese, and
Aaron F. Kopman

The history of anesthesia may be logically divided into periods before and after the introduction of muscle relaxants into clinical practice. In the era prior to curare, "anesthesia was more an art possessed by a privileged few than a science that could be taught to many."[1] The anesthesiologist was frequently forced to choose between the respiratory, cardiovascular, and metabolic effects of deep general anesthesia and providing the surgeon with adequate operating conditions. The introduction of curare in 1942[2] and succinylcholine in 1952,[3] for all practical purposes, eliminated the concept of inoperability as a result of advanced age and general patient debility. It is doubtful if the progress we have seen in cardiac, transplant, and neurosurgery during the last 40 years would have been possible without the advent of neuromuscular blocking agents.[4] These advances are, in effect, a reflection of the wide therapeutic index that muscle relaxants display.

This wide margin of safety is, however, not without limits. A fundamental concept that must be kept in mind when discussing dosing of nondepolarizing relaxants is that absolute overdosage is possible. The depth of neuromuscular block can be so great that pharmacologic antagonism is not possible. Anticholinesterases do not have an unlimited capacity to antagonize curare-like drugs. It has long been known that the time to return of single twitch to control following neostigmine antagonism of tubocurarine is a function of the depth of pre-existing neuromuscular block.[5–8] If the concentration of neuromuscular blocking drug at the myoneural junction is high enough, the extent of recovery that can be induced is finite.[9] Several concepts follow from this. If these drugs are to be administered on a rational basis, the clinician must have (1) some means of determining the extent of neuromuscular block; (2) a familiarity with the potency, pharmacokinetics, side effects, and expected duration of action of individual neuromuscular blockers; and (3) an understanding of the indications for relaxant administration and the needs, both real and imagined, of the operating surgeon.

CLINICAL USE OF MUSCLE RELAXANTS IN ANESTHESIA

Intraoperative Monitoring of Neuromuscular Function

Because neuromuscular blocking agents produce their effects by interrupting synaptic transmission, their pharmacologic actions are best assessed by indirect stimulation of a suitable muscle. The muscle-nerve group that is most widely used clinically is the ulnar nerve-adductor pollicis nerve muscle unit. Thumb adduction as a result of ulnar nerve stimulation has been the most extensively studied because this nerve-muscle unit is readily accessible. The thumb is easily attached to a force transducer, and when stimulating electrodes are applied at the wrist, the muscle is relatively immune to direct stimulation. From the vast literature that has centered on the effects of muscle relaxants on the adductor pollicis, it might be supposed that this muscle is representative of other muscle groups in the body, such as the diaphragm and adductors of the vocal cords, which are important to the anesthesiologist. This is not, however, the case. Both of the latter muscles are more resistant to the effects of neuromuscular blocking agents and have more rapid onset and offset profiles than does the adductor pollicis.[10–13]

In actual clinical practice, however, it is not necessary to measure directly the degree of paralysis of specific muscle groups of particular interest. Their degree of paresis can be inferred from an assessment of the response of the adductor pollicis and a knowledge of their relative sensitivities to the effects of muscle relaxants. The occurrence of coughing or "bucking," when there is no response to peripheral nerve stimulation at the wrist, is not a failure of monitoring, but rather, it reflects the different responses of the diaphragm and adductor pollicis to neuromuscular blocking drugs.

Peripheral Nerve Stimulation

A discussion of such topics as the characteristics of an ideal nerve stimulator, the relative merits of mechanical versus electromyographic (EMG) recording techniques, and current requirements for supramaximal stimulation are beyond the scope of this chapter. Several excellent general reviews of this topic are available.[14–18]

Stimulus Patterns

Traditionally, the extent of neuromuscular block was evaluated by quantifying the force of a single muscle twitch evoked by indirect supramaximal stimulation. Following the administration of a depolarizing muscle relaxant, the twitch height is relatively independent of the rate of stimulation. In a partially paralyzed individual, the evoked response to stimulation at 1.0 and 0.1 Hz will be essentially the same. In contrast, neuromuscular block that is induced with a nondepolarizing agent shows marked fade on repetitive stimulation. Under stable levels of competitive neuromuscular block, there will be some degree of diminished response after the rate of stimulation exceeds 0.10 to 0.15 Hz.[19]

In 1970, Ali et al.[20] first suggested that the train-of-four (TOF) fade ratio might be a useful measure of neuromuscular block in humans. They reported that, when four stimuli were delivered at 0.5-second intervals, there was a progressive fade of successive twitch responses in curarized subjects, with the magnitude of fade appearing to depend on the extent of curarization. The height of the fourth response divided by the height of the first was defined as the TOF ratio. Because this parameter did not require a control measurement, it was eminently suitable for common clinical situations. If TOFs are separated by 15 to 20 seconds, the first response to TOF stimulation is not different in magnitude to single twitches delivered at 0.15 Hz. As neuromuscular block deepens, the fourth then the third, second, and first twitch disappear, in that order (Fig. 21-1).[21] Counting the number of twitches in the train, therefore, permits a subjective assessment of the magnitude of competitive block. As a general rule, the first, second, third, and fourth responses of the adductor pollicis become palpable when the twitch height first returns to 5, 15, 25, and 35 percent of control, respectively.[22]

During intense neuromuscular block, it may be impossible to evoke any muscle response, regardless of the stimulus sequence used. Under these conditions, it is impossible to tell if the plasma level of blocker is just sufficient to produce 100 percent twitch depression or if it is greatly in excess of the required amount. However, another characteristic of competitive neuromuscular block with nondepolarizing muscle relaxants, the phenomenon of post-tetanic facilitation (PTF), offers a mechanism by which moderate "overdosage" can be quantified. During partial nondepolarizing block, tetanic nerve stimulation is normally followed by a transient increase in twitch height.[23] The degree and duration of PTF depend on the magnitude of neuromuscular blockade, and this facilitation usually disappears within 30 seconds of the end of tetanic

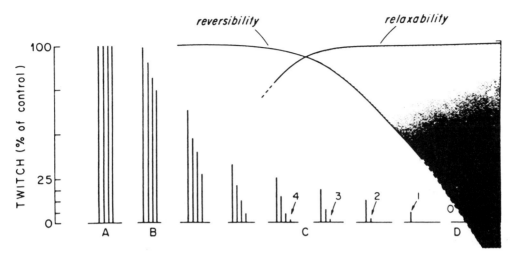

Fig. 21-1 Monitoring of train-of-four response to stimulation. Increasing depth of neuromuscular block versus height of T_1 as a percent of control. **A:** Baseline response to stimulation. **B:** A 25 percent fade in the train of four with onset of neuromuscular block. **C:** With increasing depth of neuromuscular block, loss of the fourth response to stimulation. **D:** 100 percent neuromuscular block. No response to train-of-four stimulation. As shown, with increasing depth of neuromuscular block, pharmacologic antagonism becomes more difficult. (From Lee,[273] with permission.)

stimulation. If the plasma concentration of the neuromuscular blocker is not too high, it is often possible, using PTF, to elicit a response at a time when TOF stimulation still evokes no twitch. This level of paralysis may be quantified by using a standardized stimulus pattern consisting of 50-Hz tetanus of 5-second duration, a 3-second pause, and then single stimuli given at 1 Hz for 26 to 20 seconds. The number of twitches that can be detected is known as the post-tetanic count (PTC).[24] The fewer the number of post-tetanic responses seen, the deeper is the block. During recovery, after the PTC approaches a value of 10, the first response to TOF stimulation generally returns.[25] The PTC has been correlated with the ability to cough or buck on tracheal stimulation under light general anesthesia. A PTC of three or less is necessary to prevent strong coughing on carinal stimulation, and a value of zero is required to ensure that no detectable response ensues.[26]

Indications for Neuromuscular Relaxants

Situations arise in which periods of intense neuromuscular block (PTC less than three) are indicated. Examples of such circumstances might include la-

ser microsurgery of the larynx, manipulation of displaced fractures, tracheal suction in a patient with raised intracranial pressure, or an open eye injury. In addition, there are times when the anesthesiologist may intentionally administer an "overdose" of relaxant to achieve a rapid onset of action. An example of the latter practice might be to facilitate rapid sequence tracheal intubation.

However, the majority of surgical operations do not require this depth of neuromuscular block. Good operating conditions for most abdominal procedures, for example, can be achieved with TOF counts of one or two, and frequently, three. It should be remembered that neuromuscular blockers are not anesthetic agents but they are adjuvants to general anesthetics to be used with discretion. Amnesia, analgesia, and reflex suppression, in addition to relaxation, are all required components of the anesthetic state. Patient movement (especially when the TOF count is less than three) should be viewed as a sign of light anesthesia, not as an indication for the administration of more relaxant. Likewise, poor "surgical relaxation" is not always improved by giving additional muscle relaxant. Adequate relaxation for an intra-abdominal procedure can be achieved with one or two responses to

TOF stimulation with an opioid-based anesthetic, and with three responses to TOF stimulation with a volatile agent-based anesthetic.

Tracheal Intubation

Facilitation of tracheal intubation is perhaps the most common indication for the administration of neuromuscular blockers. Optimal intubating conditions require relaxation of the masseter muscle and adductor muscles of the larynx. If coughing or bucking is to be avoided, complete diaphragmatic paralysis is also probably necessary.[26] Inasmuch as the latter two muscle groups are less sensitive to the neuromuscular effects of muscle relaxants than are the adductors of the thumb, by common usage an "intubating dose" of a relaxant has come to mean a dose twice the ED_{95}, or twice the dose causing 95 percent neuromuscular block, as measured at the adductor pollicis. Despite this decreased sensitivity, the onset of neuromuscular blockade occurs earlier at the diaphragm[27] and larynx[10] than at the thumb. This is perhaps a function of better perfusion of airway and respiratory muscles.

Satisfactory intubating conditions may also be obtained without relaxant administration, providing that adequate depth of anesthesia is provided. In patients premedicated with 1 mg midazolam who had Mallampati class I airways, vocal cord exposure, cord position during laryngoscopy, and patient response to intubation were not different in patients induced with alfentanil (40 to 60 μg/kg IV) and propofol (2 mg/kg IV) compared with those induced with thiamylal (4 mg/kg IV) and succinylcholine (1 mg/kg IV).[28]

Routine Tracheal Intubation

Succinylcholine remains unrivaled for its rapid onset of effect and short duration of action, and it is the most commonly used muscle relaxant for routine tracheal intubation. However, some anesthesiologists have changed from succinylcholine to a nondepolarizing muscle relaxant of short or intermediate duration of action because of the side effects of succinylcholine. Following a dose of twice the ED_{95} of any nondepolarizing muscle relaxant, satisfactory intubating conditions can be anticipated in 2.5 to 3.0 minutes. In the majority of elec-

tive cases, the 60- to 90-second prolongation of the intubation time interval associated with these drugs, compared with that of succinylcholine, is not of consequence to clinicians using nondepolarizing relaxants for routine intubation.

Rapid Sequence Induction

When tracheal intubation must be performed rapidly to prevent pulmonary aspiration of gastric contents, succinylcholine remains, at present, the most reliable relaxant available. When precurarization is avoided, doses of succinylcholine of 1 to 1.5 mg/kg produce complete neuromuscular block in less than 90 seconds, and laryngoscopy may be attempted within 60 seconds of induction. However, clinical trials with rocuronium, a new steroidal agent of low potency and intermediate duration, offer a promising alternative. At a dose of 1.5 to 1.75 times the ED_{95} (0.6 mg/kg), rocuronium produces complete twitch depression of the adductor pollicis in 75 to 150 seconds and good to excellent intubating conditions at 60 and 90 seconds.[29–32] A recent report suggests that rocuronium (0.6 mg/kg) may be used successfully as a substitute for succinylcholine as part of a "crash-induction" sequence.[33]

Until rocuronium becomes available, if succinylcholine is deemed to be contraindicated, alternate nondepolarizing agents and induction techniques must be used. As larger multiples of the ED_{95} are administered (two to four times the ED_{95}), onset times get progressively shorter. For example, vecuronium (0.1 mg/kg) produces total twitch depression in 60 to 360 seconds, and the duration of clinical effect (time to recovery of 25 percent single twitch height) is about 45 minutes.[34] As this dose is increased to 0.2, 0.3, and 0.4 mg/kg, the average (and range) onset times decrease to 120 (100 to 140), 88 (60 to 120), and 78 (60 to 100) seconds, respectively; but the clinical duration gradually increases to more than 2 hours.[35] The "point of diminishing returns" appears once the initial bolus exceeds six to eight times the ED_{95}. Increasing the dose beyond this point yields little improvement in the onset time, and the duration of effect becomes progressively longer and less predictable.

In 1985, a technique was suggested for improving the onset time of currently available nondepolarizing relaxants without prolonging the duration of effect.[36,37] The "priming principle," as it was called, is based on the concept that, because a large proportion of acetylcholine receptors must be occupied by a nondepolarizing blocking agent before twitch depression is detectable, the onset is really a two-step process.[38] The first step consists of drug binding to "spare" receptors (no effect observed). This step takes a finite amount of time. Step two represents the actual development of overt neuromuscular block. It follows that the onset time would be reduced if a small "priming" dose completes step one before the administration of a larger subsequent "paralyzing" dose.

Rather extravagant initial claims for this technique led to a veritable avalanche of articles attempting to define the optimal priming sequence. Unfortunately, the possible permutations in protocol were almost limitless. Variations in anesthetic technique, choice of the priming drug, size of the priming dose, duration of the priming interval, size of the paralyzing dose, choice of the monitoring technique, and definition of "satisfactory conditions for intubation" made interpretation of the literature on this subject difficult. There is general agreement that the priming dose should not exceed 20 percent of the drug's ED_{95}. However, recent evidence suggests that doses of this magnitude depress EMG activity of the muscles of swallowing by more than 50 percent.[39] Such partially paralyzed patients are at increased risk for aspiration of pharyngeal contents. Because individual variability in response to neuromuscular blocking drugs is so great, some experts believe that the maximum priming dose should be limited to 10 percent of the ED_{95}, not 10 percent of the "intubating dose."[40]

Priming appears to work. However, the extent to which priming shortens the time to intubation is still unclear. Decreases in onset time of more than 30 seconds should not be expected, and the benefits of priming are clearest when the intubating dose is modest. Not all investigators agree that priming offers any clinical benefit. Jones,[41] in a recent editorial, noted that, although priming does hasten the onset of paralysis, it produces intubating conditions less uniformly than those provided with succinylcholine. He concluded that the potential problems associated with the technique out-

weigh its advantages and, hence, it has no useful role in clinical anesthesia. Although this judgment may be unduly harsh, the early enthusiasm that greeted the description of the technique has largely waned.

Interactions With Potent Inhalation Anesthetics

The addition of even small amounts of a potent volatile anesthetic markedly reduces muscle relaxant requirements.[42] Enflurane and isoflurane at end-tidal concentrations of 1.4 and 1.0 percent, respectively, may decrease vecuronium infusion requirements by as much as 65 percent compared with a balanced nitrous oxide-opioid anesthetic.[43] In one study of tubocurarine potentiation by enflurane, plasma levels of the blocker were kept constant at approximately 0.2 μg/ml. At end-tidal concentrations of 2.2, 1.35, and 0.5 percent enflurane induced twitch heights were depressed by 92, 42, and 9 percent, respectively.[44] Although most investigators have not found reductions of this magnitude, decreases of 30 to 40 percent are commonly reported.[45] The mechanism of this interaction is still controversial, but recent evidence suggests an effect on the acetylcholine receptor channel.[46] Although general anesthetics have important interactions with neuromuscular blocking agents, an important part of their ability to produce muscular relaxation cannot be quantified with a peripheral nerve stimulator. These agents have actions in the central nervous system, such as depression of reflex pathways at the spinal level, which also contribute to relaxation in the clinical setting.

Potentiation of neuromuscular block by volatile agents may provide additional safety for patients. After the administration of volatile agents is withdrawn at the end of a case, neuromuscular function should theoretically start to recover even in the absence of a fall in the plasma level of the blocking drug. This makes perfect sense in theory, but there is little experimental data to substantiate this effect. There is evidence, however, that the anticholinesterases are less effective antagonists of neuromuscular blockade in the presence of inhalation anesthetics.[47] If volatile agents are discontinued 15 minutes in advance of the attempted reversal, they do not render pharmacologic antagonism of residual neuromuscular block more difficult.[48]

Rational Dosing of Muscle Relaxants in Anesthesia

As noted earlier, anticholinesterases have a "ceiling" regarding the extent of block that can be antagonized completely. When reversal of neuromuscular block greater than this ceiling (twitch height less than 30 percent of control) is attempted, the peak effect of the antagonist is followed by a plateau phase that represents the balance between diminishing anticholinesterase activity and spontaneous recovery of neuromuscular block. The latter becomes the major determinant of recovery at profound levels of neuromuscular block (twitch height less than 10 percent).[49]

It follows, therefore, that antagonism of residual neuromuscular block is most efficacious when the TOF count has been allowed to return to three or four palpable responses before antagonism is attempted. Long-, intermediate-, and short-acting relaxants, consequently, require different dosing strategies if these conditions are to be obtained at the termination of surgery.

Agents of Long Duration

Doxacurium is a typical example of this drug class. Following a doxacurium dose of 50 to 80 μg/kg (1.6 to 2.7 times the ED$_{95}$), the single twitch 5 to 25 percent recovery time averaged 25 to 34 minutes.[50] This indicates that, after some evoked response to TOF stimulation becomes evident, antagonism may be attempted with a reasonable certainty of success in 30 to 45 minutes, providing no additional relaxant is given. Hence it is prudent, when using drugs of this duration, to anticipate the need for surgical relaxation so that "top-up" doses may be avoided just prior to the end of surgery. Giving an intermediate- or short-acting blocker as the last incremental dose is not a satisfactory alternate maneuver because the duration of these latter drugs is markedly extended by the prior administration of a longer-acting blocker.[51,52]

Using careful monitoring and proper timing, traditional long-acting agents may be used successfully even for cases of moderate duration. However, even with special expertise in the use of mus-

cle relaxants, undetected residual neuromuscular block in the recovery room is more common following the administration of long-acting agents.[53] Thus, some experts in the clinical use of relaxants suggest that long-acting relaxants are best reserved for situations in which tracheal extubation is not anticipated at the end of surgery and a rapid full return of neuromuscular function is not required.

Agents of Intermediate Duration

In contrast, profound atracurium or vecuronium induced neuromuscular block may be allowed to persist until almost the end of surgery with the expectation that reliable antagonism can still be achieved in a reasonable amount of time. Following the termination of a continuous atracurium or vecuronium infusion at 95 percent twitch depression, the recovery time to a T_1 of 25 percent is only about 12.5 minutes.[54] After the TOF count reaches four palpable responses, satisfactory antagonism may be achieved within 2 to 5 minutes with edrophonium 0.75 mg/kg.[22] Even if antagonism is attempted at 90 percent T_1 depression (TOF count equals one), TOF ratios more than 0.70 are readily achieved if 20 minutes are allowed to elapse after reversal.[55]

Agents of Short Duration

Mivacurium allows even more flexibility as the end of surgery approaches. The time for 95 percent recovery of twitch height, after some evoked response to TOF stimulation can be felt (T_1, 5 to 95 percent), averages about 14 minutes, with a 5 to 25 percent recovery interval of about 4 minutes. The time from T_1 equals 95 percent to a TOF ratio more than 0.70 averages 3.5 minutes.[56] This has several implications. If some evoked response to TOF stimulation is maintained at all times, then rapid antagonism can be achieved within 5 minutes. A knowledge of this recovery pattern is helpful in deciding whether antagonism will be required at all. The amount of time from a TOF count of one to a TOF count of three approximates one-quarter of the interval from T_1 of 5 percent to a TOF ratio of 70 percent. This interval is best measured at the beginning of the case, during recovery from the initial intubating dose of relaxant. If the time required for the TOF count to increase from one to three is less than 5 minutes, it can be safely assumed that, after some response to TOF stimulation is elicited, adequate spontaneous recovery is less than 20 minutes away.

SIDE EFFECTS OF MUSCLE RELAXANTS

Cardiovascular

Neuromuscular blocking agents, in large part because they are designed to interact with acetylcholine receptors, tend to cause cardiovascular side effects. These side effects can occur by several mechanisms (Table 21-1). In general, cardiovascular effects occur either because a muscle relaxant interferes with autonomic function or it causes histamine release. The clinical nature of each of these two mechanisms is different. Histamine release can

Table 21-1 Causes of Cardiovascular Side Effects

Autonomic stimulation through
Ganglionic blockade
Binding to muscarinic receptors
Vagolysis
Sympathomimetic activity
Histamine release

be attenuated with slower administration of the drug (Fig. 21-2) and is less with repeated doses of the same or a smaller amount of drug. In contrast, cardiovascular effects secondary to autonomic effects of the muscle relaxants are not attenuated with slower administration of the drug and are undiminished following repeated administration of

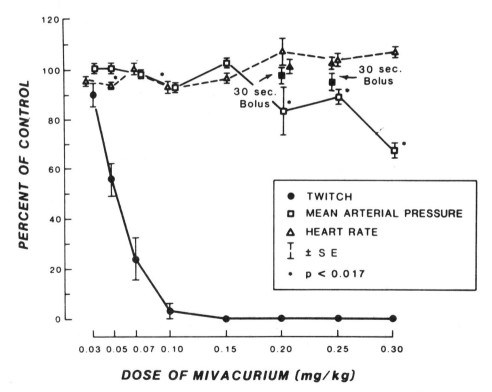

Fig. 21-2 Maximal changes in heart rate, △, and mean arterial pressure, □, following bolus doses of various sizes of mivacurium, a benzylisoquinolinium. The decrease in mean arterial pressure with doses of 0.2 mg/kg or more of mivacurium are secondary to histamine release and are minimized by administration of the drug over 30 seconds, ■. (From Savarese et al.,[62] with permission.)

the drug. Generally, muscle relaxants of different structures cause side effects through different mechanisms. For example, nondepolarizing muscle relaxants with a steroidal nucleus tend to be vagolytic; nondepolarizing muscle relaxants that are benzylisoquinoliniums tend to cause histamine release. With a continuously improving knowledge of structure-activity relationships, nondepolarizing muscle relaxants may be developed that are free of cardiovascular side effects.

The majority of muscle relaxants do, however, still possess cardiovascular side effects (Table 21-2). Nevertheless these side effects may be used to clinical advantage. All muscle relaxants if given in sufficient quantities will cause cardiovascular side effects; however, many of these adverse side effects occur outside the clinical dose range or at the upper end of this range. The distinction between doses required for neuromuscular blocking action and those required to cause cardiovascular side effects are defined in terms of the drug's "margin of safety." This is usually described in terms of the ED_{50} for cardiac vagal blockade, ganglionic blockade, or histamine release in cats divided by the dose required for 95 percent neuromuscular block in humans. This ratio indicates the multiples of the dose required for 95 percent neuromuscular block that need to be administered to cause a given cardiovascular side effect.

The dose of muscle relaxant required to cause cardiovascular side effects varies from 0.6 times the ED_{95} to greater than 100 times the ED_{95} (Table 21-3). The margin of safety for muscle relaxant administration in terms of cardiovascular side effects improved with the development of the two new long-acting muscle relaxants, pipecuronium and doxacurium, and intermediate-acting and the short-acting muscle relaxants.

The vagolytic side effects of muscle relaxants are the result of block of the muscarinic receptors at the sinoatrial node. Pancuronium is weakly vagolytic; therefore, with large doses, as may be used to facilitate intubation (Table 21-4), a moderate increase in heart rate may be observed.

Changing the $2,16\beta$ piperadino substitutions of pancuronium to $2,16\beta$ piperazino substitutions with quaternizations of the distal nitrogens yields pipecuronium (Fig. 21-3). In addition to increasing

Table 21-2 Cardiovascular Side Effects Caused by Muscle Relaxants

Muscle Relaxant	Cardiovascular Side Effect
Depolarizing	
Succinylcholine	Stimulates autonomic ganglia
	Stimulates cardiac muscarinic receptors
	Histamine release
Nondepolarizing	
Drugs of long duration	
Doxacurium	None
Pipecuronium	None
Pancuronium	Vagolytic, sympathomimetic
Tubocurarine	Histamine release
Gallamine	Vagolytic
Metocurine	Histamine release
Drugs of intermediate duration	
Vecuronium	None
Atracurium	Histamine release
Rocuronium	Vagolytic
Drugs of short duration	
Mivacurium	Histamine release

Table 21-3 Margins of Safety for Muscle Relaxants

Muscle Relaxant	Margin of Safety[a]		
	Ganglion Block	Vagal Block	Histamine Release
Benzylisoquinolines			
Mivacurium	>100	>100	3
Atracurium	36	9	3
Doxacurium	>100	>100	>4
Tubocurarine	3	0.6	1
Metocurine	19	3	2
Steroids			
Rocuronium	>100	5	High
Vecuronium	89	41	High
Pipecuronium	>100	25	High
Pancuronium	329	3	High

[a] $\dfrac{ED_{50} \text{ effect (mg/kg)}}{ED_{95} \text{ neuromuscular block (mg/kg)}}$

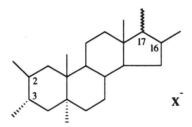

Number/Name	Positions and configurations of substitutions				
of compound	2	3	16	17	X
Pancuronium	—N⁺(CH₃)⟨piperidine⟩	—OCCH₃ (O)	—N⁺(CH₃)⟨piperidine⟩	—OCCH₃ (O)	2Br
Vecuronium	—N⟨piperidine⟩	—OCCH₃ (O)	—N⁺(CH₃)⟨piperidine⟩	—OCCH₃ (O)	Br
Pipecuronium	—N⟨piperazine⟩N⁺(CH₃)₂	—OCCH₃ (O)	—N⟨piperazine⟩N⁺(CH₃)₂	—OCCH₃ (O)	2Br
Rocuronium	—N⟨morpholine⟩O	—OH	—N⁺(CH₂CH=CH₂)⟨piperidine⟩	—OCCH₃ (O)	Br

Fig. 21-3 Chemical structure of steroidal muscle relaxants. (Adapted from Ducharme and Donati,[274] with permission.)

Table 21-4 Doses of Muscle Relaxants That Produce Cardiovascular Side Effects

Muscle Relaxant	Cardiovascular Side Effect	Dose at Which Side Effect Is Likely to Occur (mg/kg)
Doxacurium	None	>0.10
Pipecuronium	None	>0.20
Pancuronium	Vagolytic	0.1–0.15
Tubocurarine	Histamine release	0.5–0.6
Vecuronium	None	>1.0
Atracurium	Histamine release	0.60
Rocuronium	Vagolytic	0.6–0.9
Mivacurium	Histamine release	0.25

the potency of the compound by a factor of approximately 1.5, this structural change decreases the compound's vagolytic activity approximately 10-fold. Therefore, in the clinical dose range of pipecuronium, it is free of cardiovascular side effects (Table 21-4).[57]

In developing rocuronium, structural changes were deliberately made to lower its potency as a neuromuscular blocking agent (Fig. 21-3). In so doing, the onset of block is faster. However, the margin of cardiovascular safety is lower. The dose ratio of vagolytic to neuromuscular blocking potency is 5 compared with 50 for vecuronium, which is free of cardiovascular side effects. Indeed, the margin of safety with rocuronium approaches that of pancuronium, and dose related increases in heart rate do occur (Table 21-5).[58] This means that,

Table 21-5 Dose Related Increases in Heart Rate for Rocuronium

Rocuronium (μg/kg)	Heart Rate (% basal heart rate 5 minutes after administration)
120	100 ± 8
200	107 ± 8
300	107 ± 5
500	108 ± 6
600	115 ± 11
680	126 ± 30

(Data from Mellinghoff et al.[58])

at doses recommended for intubation, tachycardia may occur.

Benzylisoquinolinium compounds tend to cause some histamine release. In large measure, this is caused by the presence of a tertiary amine.[59] Bisquaternary structures cause less histamine release.[60,61] Clinically, histamine release manifests as a transient increase in the heart rate and a transient decrease in blood pressure, both occurring approximately 2 minutes after the administration of muscle relaxant, and facial erythema. Clinical experience has demonstrated that these clinical manifestations can be minimized or even eliminated with slower administration of a given dose, administration of a smaller dose, or by pretreatment with both H_1 and H_2 blocking agents.[62–66]

The benzylisoquinoline muscle relaxants, metocurine, atracurium, and mivacurium, cause histamine release when given in doses two to three times the ED_{95}.[62,64] Mivacurium has been studied in doses up to four times the ED_{95}.[62] Rapid administration of 0.20 mg/kg of mivacurium causes decreases in blood pressure and increases in heart rate secondary to histamine release.[62] In otherwise healthy patients, these hemodynamic changes are short-lived, resolving spontaneously within 5 minutes. Histamine release associated with mivacurium doses of 0.20 mg/kg or more can be attenuated by slow administration of the muscle relaxant to keep patients hemodynamically stable.[62] The new long-acting benzylisoquinolinium, doxacurium, causes neither histamine release nor cardiovascular side effects at doses up to and including 0.08 mg/kg (three times the ED_{95}).[50,67]

Prolonged Neuromuscular Block

Vecuronium

Vecuronium is eliminated primarily by the liver, with approximately 50 percent of a dose found unchanged in the bile.[68] The kidney plays a minor role in vecuronium's elimination, with less than 25 percent of a dose excreted in the urine. Despite the minor role of renal elimination, vecuronium's duration of block is longer and its plasma clearance is decreased in patients with renal failure.[69] Waser et al.[70] found that, in rodents, renal excretion of vecuronium increased after administration of the drug; after 5 minutes, the density of ^{14}C-vecuronium in the kidney was similar to that in the liver. After 60 minutes, renal elimination was found to be prominent. Repeated doses of vecuronium in patients with renal failure have a significantly more prolonged effect than they do in patients with normal renal function (Fig. 21-4).[71] There have been reports of excessively prolonged recovery from vecuronium induced neuromuscular block in patients with renal failure in intensive care units.[72-74] Why this occurs, when the drug does not depend on the kidney to any great extent for its metabolism and elimination, is not intuitively obvious. However, because of the variable dose requirements and the prolonged recovery of muscle strength after discontinuation of an infusion in patients with renal failure, it has been recommended that the drug be administered as repeated boluses rather than as an infusion in patients in the intensive care unit.[72]

Vecuronium is metabolized in the liver. During its metabolism, the acetoxy substituents at the 3 and/or 17 positions of the steroid nucleus are re-moved to produce 3-desacetyl, 17-desacetyl, and 3,17-desacetyl vecuronium. The 3-desacetylvecuronium metabolite is 50 to 70 percent as potent as vecuronium in terms of its neuromuscular blocking potential.[75,76] The reported cases of prolonged paralysis were associated with renal failure and elevated plasma concentrations of 3-desacetylvecuronium, which has been reported to cause 90 percent depression of muscle strength at a concentration of 165 mg/ml.[75] However, 3-desacetylvecuronium is cleared primarily through the liver.[76] This was confirmed in a recent study[77] that did not demonstrate elevated plasma concentrations of 3-desacetylvecuronium in cats with ligated renal pedicles following a single intravenous dose of 3-desacetylvecuronium. The cats with hepatic failure, in this same study, did have significantly decreased clearance of the drug. Therefore, a ready explanation for prolonged paralysis and elevated plasma concentrations of 3-desacetylvecuronium in patients with renal failure who receive long-term infusions of vecuronium in intensive care units is not available.

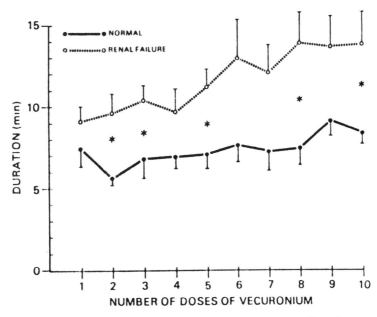

Fig. 21-4 Duration of action (minutes) after multiple doses of 0.01 mg/kg of vecuronium. Significant differences (* = $P < 0.05$) are seen between the responses of otherwise healthy patients and those with renal disease. In patients with renal disease, there is an increase of approximately 50 percent in the duration of effect with 8 to 10 repeated doses. (From Bevan et al.,[71] with permission.)

Mivacurium

Mivacurium's short duration of action is dependent on hydrolysis by plasma cholinesterase.[56,78] Therefore, in patients with decreased levels of cholinesterase activity or abnormal plasma cholinesterase levels, this muscle relaxant becomes a longer acting drug. In vitro, the half-life of mivacurium was found to increase as plasma cholinesterase activity decreased.[78] In vivo, the clearance of the two potent isomers of mivacurium, the cis-trans and the trans-trans isomers, was found to decrease with decreased levels of plasma cholinesterase levels in patients who had normal plasma cholinesterase activity (Lien C: unpublished results). Phenotypically normal patients have a recovery following mivacurium (0.2 mg/kg) that is inversely correlated with their plasma cholinesterase activity. With higher levels of plasma cholinesterase activity, patients recovered more quickly from mivacurium induced neuromuscular block.[79] The rate of infusion of mivacurium required to maintain a stable degree of neuromuscular block was also related to plasma cholinesterase activity.[54] In four patients homozygous for the atypical plasma cholinesterase gene, mivacurium (0.03 mg/kg) was shown to cause 100 percent neuromuscular block in 3 to 4.6 minutes. This block was markedly prolonged, with the first twitch in the TOF reappearing in 62 minutes.[80] Although further studies are needed to define more completely the dose-response relationship of mivacurium in patients homozygous for this atypical gene, these preliminary results indicate that mivacurium is both a long-acting muscle relaxant and the most potent of the nondepolarizing muscle relaxants in these patients.

Not surprisingly, therefore, there have been several case reports of prolonged neuromuscular block in patients homozygous for atypical plasma cholinesterase.[81–83] The four patients described in these case reports ranged in age from 3 months to 31 years and were homozygous for atypical plasma cholinesterase. They received 0.12 to 0.2 mg/kg of mivacurium, and all experienced markedly prolonged neuromuscular block. The postoperative management of each patient varied from sedating the patient and waiting for spontaneous recovery from neuromuscular block to antagonizing with neostigmine and/or edrophonium at varying levels of neuromuscular block. Both spontaneous recovery and pharmacologically induced recovery from deep levels of neuromuscular block proceed slowly in these patients. Because mivacurium is a nondepolarizing muscle relaxant, pharmacologic antagonism is possible. However, mivacurium is a long-acting muscle relaxant in this patient population, and antagonism should not be attempted until a significant degree of spontaneous recovery has occurred (two to three twitches in the TOF), as with other long-acting muscle relaxants.

Because of mivacurium's rather unique means of metabolism, another potential means of hastening the recovery from neuromuscular block in patients homozygous for atypical plasma cholinesterase exists. Purified human cholinesterase was given to patients with pseudocholinesterase deficiency who received succinylcholine to speed recovery from neuromuscular block, with some success.[84,85] Either purified enzyme or whole blood possessing cholinesterase activity may be used to hasten the recovery from mivacurium induced neuromuscular block in patients homozygous for atypical pseudocholinesterase. Butyrylcholinesterase was given to cats that received mivacurium; it was shown to speed the recovery from deep neuromuscular block.[86]

An unexpectedly prolonged duration of action of mivacurium was reported in a patient with end-stage renal disease.[87] In this patient, no responses were present to a TOF stimulus 45 minutes after the administration of 0.17 mg/kg of mivacurium. Similarly, in a study of mivacurium infusions in anephric patients,[88] the time to 5 percent recovery following a 0.15 mg/kg dose of mivacurium was approximately 1.5 times longer than in patients with normal renal function, and the infusion rate of mivacurium required to maintain 95 percent muscle relaxation was approximately 60 percent of that required in patients with normal renal function. There are two possible explanations for the increase in mivacurium's duration of action in patients with renal failure. First, patients with renal failure may have decreased levels of plasma cholinesterase activity.[89] In the cited reports,[87,88] the patients with renal failure had decreased cholinesterase activity. This decreased level of activity is most likely secondary to uremia rather than hemodialysis, because the latter does appear to affect cholinesterase activity consistently.[90,91] In patients with end-stage renal disease undergoing renal transplantation, there were no significant differences in mivacurium's (0.15 mg/kg) pharmacokinetics compared with those in patients with normal renal function.[92] Although both patients with renal disease and control patients had comparable levels of cholinesterase activity, the duration of action was modestly but not significantly prolonged. The second possible explanation for the increased mivacurium duration of effect in renal failure is renal elimination. The kidney is a secondary pathway of elimination for mivacurium, with approximately 7 percent of a dose being eliminated unchanged in the urine.[92] Therefore, decreased renal elimination may account in some part for the longer mivacurium duration of action in patients with renal failure. It may be especially important in terms of the pharmacokinetics of the cis-cis isomer of mivacurium, which has a clearance that is approximately 12 times slower than that of the more potent cis-trans and trans-trans isomers (Lien C: unpublished results), for which renal elimination is, most likely, less prominent.

Succinylcholine

Succinylcholine, like mivacurium, is metabolized by plasma cholinesterase. Substantial reductions in plasma cholinesterase activity must be present before even moderate delays in recovery time from succinylcholine become apparent.[93] However, clinically significant prolongations in recovery have been reported in pregnancy,[94] hepatic disease,[95] cancer,[96] and following plasmapheresis. Because it is uncommon, even in overt hepatic failure, for cholinesterase activity to fall by much more than 75 percent, the overall prolongation that is seen under these circumstances is at most a two- to threefold increase in the duration of action.

Prior or concomitant anticholinesterase therapy will also prolong succinylcholine's duration of action. Such interactions have been reported after organophosphate insecticides, echothiophate eye drops, and such cytotoxic drugs as cyclophosphamide. Prolonged activity was also reported following neostigmine and pyridostigmine administration.[97]

Although plasma cholinesterase activity is essential for the metabolism of succinylcholine and mivacurium, the normal physiologic function of cholinesterase is unknown. There are now at least four known allelic genes for plasma cholinesterase (i.e., the normal, dibucaine-resistant, fluoride-resistant, and silent genes). These can combine to form 10 genotypes. A detailed account of these various genotypes is beyond the scope of this discussion, but patients possessing at least one atypical gene probably account for about 4 percent of the general population.[98] In these individuals, the duration of succinylcholine is prolonged by perhaps 50 percent. However, patients homozygous for either the silent or the dibucaine-resistant gene exhibit prolonged neuromuscular block with succinylcholine. Following administration of 1 mg/kg of succinylcholine, 2.5 to 3.5 hours may be required for recovery of these individuals.[84]

Increases in Intracranial Pressure

The use of succinylcholine is generally accepted to be associated with increases in intracranial pressure.[99,100] It is currently believed that afferent muscle spindle input to the central nervous system follows succinylcholine induced depolarization of the neuromuscular junction. The sudden afferent input results in increased cerebral blood flow, an increase in cerebral blood volume, and ultimately, an increase in intracranial pressure.[101] This increase may be blunted by prior precurarization.[102] Although this is the prevailing opinion, others point out that much of the increase in intracranial pressure seen after succinylcholine may be caused by laryngoscopic stimulation under light anesthesia. Increases in ICP are of theoretic concern, but there are no reports of patients herniating after receiving succinylcholine.

Increases in Intraocular Pressure

Soon after its introduction into clinical practice, succinylcholine was found to produce a significant rise in intraocular pressure such that loss of the vitreous humor was a distinct possibility if the drug was administered in the presence of an open eye injury.[103] This observation was confirmed by many authors.[104,105] It was suggested that pretreatment with small doses of competitive neuromuscular blocking drugs would diminish this increase.[106] However, this protective effect is not reliable.[107] Although some clinicians, despite theoretic objections, continue to use succinylcholine in the presence of an open globe,[108] this is a minority position.

Postoperative Myalgia

Moderate to severe myalgia on the day after surgery is the most common side effect associated with succinylcholine administration. This discomfort was described as similar to the aches and pains that follow strenuous exercise in a normally sedentary individual. A recent meta-analysis of 45 published articles revealed a reported incidence of succinylcholine induced myalgia that ranged from 5 to 83 percent. Forty-one of the 45 studies found the incidence to be at least 30 percent, and in 22 studies, the overall incidence exceeded 50 percent.[109] Atracurium, tubocurarine, gallamine, pancuronium, diazepam, and lidocaine all significantly decreased the frequency of myalgias by about 30 percent.

Malignant Hyperthermia

The clinical picture of malignant hyperthermia (MH) was first described in 1966,[110] and almost from the outset, succinylcholine was recognized as a potent triggering agent for MH.[111] It is also generally agreed that masseter muscle rigidity (MMR) may be an early sign of impending MH.[112] However, a transient, moderate increase in masseter muscle tone after succinylcholine administration is probably a normal response to this drug.[113] The acute management of MMR has thus become a controversial topic. Some authors suggest that an isolated episode of MMR is not sufficient grounds for terminating anesthesia.[114] Other experts disagree strongly with this position.[115] Susceptibility to MH is a relatively rare condition, but MMR is not. Because of the quandary that this creates, some anesthesiologists now try to reserve the use of succinylcholine, especially in children, for situations that require extremely rapid control of the airway.[116]

Hyperkalemia

In normal individuals, succinylcholine administration may result in small increases (less than 0.5 mEq/L) in serum potassium concentration.[117] However, acute life-threatening hyperkalemia may follow succinylcholine administration in patients with burns,[118] massive trauma,[119] upper and lower motor neuron lesions,[120] disuse atrophy,[121] and numerous other disease states.[122] The common denominator in all these conditions is probably a proliferation of extrajunctional receptors throughout the muscle membrane. In these patients, potassium efflux is no longer limited to the end plate region, and large amounts of potassium may be released when these cholinoceptors are activated.[123]

DOSE-EFFECT RELATIONSHIPS

Neuromuscular block is dose dependent with respect to the onset, depth of block, and duration of effect, but not necessarily with respect to the speed of recovery. Neuromuscular blocking drugs that are not actively metabolized and depend on processes of distribution, redistribution, and organ-based elimination (liver and kidney) to facilitate recovery from neuromuscular block demonstrate a dose-dependent increase in the time for spontaneous recovery. This slowing of recovery is related both to increasing single-bolus doses and to the total cumulative dose. Pancuronium, doxacurium, tubocurarine, vecuronium, and rocuronium are examples of such drugs. In the case of rocuronium, the increase in recovery time is manifested as a lengthening of the 25 to 75 percent recovery index, which increases from about 13 to 17 minutes at a dose of two times the ED$_{95}$[124,125] to a recovery that is 35 to 55 percent longer with a dose of three times the ED$_{95}$.[126]

In contrast, neuromuscular blockers, such as mivacurium and atracurium, which are actively degraded or metabolized in the plasma, either by Hofmann elimination or by cholinesterase-catalyzed hydrolysis, have constant slopes of recovery which appear to be independent of the dose. This occurs because recovery from block with these compounds does not depend on redistribution or on organ-based elimination. Mivacurium, for example, has a 25 to 75 percent recovery index of about 6.5 minutes following doses from one (0.07 to 0.08 mg/kg) to four times (0.30 mg/kg) the ED$_{95}$.[56]

Onset of Block

The onset of neuromuscular block is usually defined as the time from the completion of drug injection to the maximum depression of the twitch response of the adductor pollicis. It should be noted that the speed of twitch suppression following the administration of nondepolarizing muscle relaxants is a function of the stimulus frequency. At faster stimulus rates (e.g., 1.0 Hz), the twitch is suppressed more quickly than at slower rates, such as 0.1 Hz. This is an important relationship with much clinical relevance, particularly with respect to the timing of tracheal intubation. In general, clinical relaxation corresponds well with depression of adductor pollicis twitch at the stimulus rate of 0.1 Hz.

In clinical practice, the twitch response of the adductor pollicis, when elicited at 0.1 Hz, is visibly weakened at 70 percent or more blockade, and tracheal intubation can be performed under good conditions when 90 to 95 percent or more block is present. For this reason, the onset to 90 percent block is a frequently measured indicator of the timing of tracheal intubation. This degree of block of the adductor pollicis is easily observed during clinical monitoring and signals that tracheal intubation can be initiated. In fact, the clinician should not wait for complete abolition of the twitch response for two important reasons: First, complete abolition of the response may take as much as 1 minute longer than 90 percent suppression, thus unnecessarily delaying the maneuver of intubation. Second, the onset of block in the muscles of the airway, such as the larynx, jaw, and diaphragm, occurs about 1 minute earlier than in the thumb; therefore, the timing of the onset of about 90 percent twitch suppression in the thumb corresponds with the onset of complete blockade in the muscles of the airway (discussed later).[10]

When the onset is measured at the time from the injection of the relaxant to maximum twitch suppression, there is an obvious dose-response relationship with all relaxants; increased doses results in shorter onset times. For example, with mivacurium, the onset of the ED$_{95}$ is 4.2 minutes, whereas the onset at two, three, and four times the ED$_{95}$ is 3.3, 2.5, and 1.9 minutes, respectively.[56] Similarly, with vecuronium, the onset at the ED$_{95}$ is about 5.7 minutes,[10] whereas the onset at two, four, and eight times the ED$_{95}$ averages 2.5, 2, and 1.5 minutes.[34,35,127,128]

Muscles of Airway

The dose-response curves of various muscles, such as the thumb, jaw, larynx, and diaphragm, are similar, with perhaps only the diaphragm showing about a 50 percent rightward shift of the curve. In contrast to this pharmacodynamic similarity, there is an important and clinically relevant kinetic difference in the evolution of blockade in the airway muscles (larynx, jaw, and diaphragm) compared with that of the adductor pollicis.[10–13,129–134]

The airway muscles are central structures with a better blood supply than the peripheral thumb musculature. For this reason, relaxant delivery to the airway muscles is likely faster and more efficient, resulting in faster onset (Fig. 21-5). For the same reason, drug removal (clearance) from these sites is more efficient, resulting in earlier recovery of the airway musculature than of the thumb.

This difference is important in clinical practice for two reasons. First, traditional monitoring of block development in the thumb delays clinical estimates of patient readiness for tracheal intubation by about 1 minute. Second, estimation of a normal recovery from block in the thumb is a safety measure as far as the airway muscles are concerned

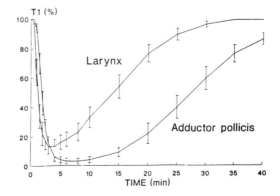

VECURONIUM, 0.07 mg/kg

Fig. 21-5 Onset of neuromuscular block in the larynx and the adductor pollicis following a dose of vecuronium 0.07 mg/kg (mean ± SE of the mean). (From Donati,[10] with permission.)

because the return of normal function in the thumb always *follows* the recovery in the jaw, larynx, and diaphragm. As a reminder, however, after TOF response is detected, without fade, patients may still be clinically weak, although able to breathe adequately, as long as their airway is secured with an endotracheal tube.

This description indicates two important changes in clinical practice. First, clinicians have hitherto been advised to proceed with tracheal intubation when the twitch response in the thumb is abolished. Because the responses of the airway muscles are abolished 1 minute earlier, intubation should be performed at this time (which corresponds to about 70 to 90 percent depression of the thumb response). At this point, the response of the thumb is visibly weakened. Another good indicator of readiness for intubation is abolition of the twitch in the orbicularis oculi. This muscle shows a time course of block development and recovery similar to that of the larynx (Fig. 21-6). Second, clinicians should be reassured that evidence derived from monitoring of evoked responses in the thumb, sug-

gesting that the thumb has recovered to a state of clinically adequate function, indicates that the airway musculature has already recovered to a similar level of function.

Potency, Clearance, and Onset of Block

In a series of steroidal relaxants studied in the cat, Bowman et al.[135] observed that the speed of onset of block was inversely related to the potency (Fig. 21-7); the less potent compounds have the fastest onset and the most potent substances, the slowest onset.

Kopman[136] studied the onset of equipotent doses of gallamine, tubocurarine, and pancuronium in patients (Fig. 21-8) and found that the least potent drug (gallamine) had the fastest onset, whereas the most potent (pancuronium) had the slowest onset.

The accelerated onset of relaxants of low potency compared with that of relaxants of high potency is explained by a process of "buffered diffusion," in which there are a greater number of relaxant molecules available for binding to a fixed

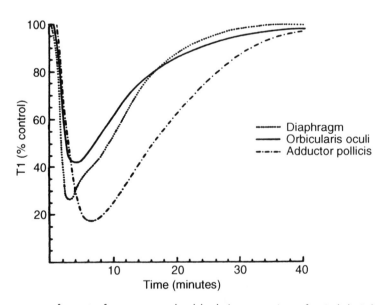

Fig. 21-6 Time course of onset of neuromuscular block (suppression of twitch height, T_1), as a function of time, simultaneously in the diaphragm, orbicularis oculi, and adductor pollicis following a dose of 0.04 mg/kg of vecuronium. The onset of neuromuscular block in the larynx is more closely represented by the twitch response of the orbicularis oculi than by that of the adductor pollicis. (From Donati et al.,[275] with permission.)

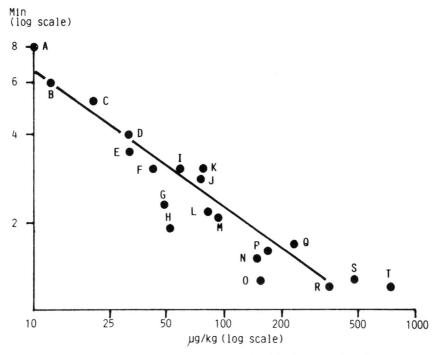

Fig. 21-7 Minutes to onset of 50 percent neuromuscular block versus log dose of compounds *A* through *T*. All compounds have steroidal structures. The onset of neuromuscular block is inversely related to potency. Compound *A* is pipecuronium, *C* is pancuronium, and *D* is vecuronium. (From Bowman et al.,[135] with permission.)

population of receptors during the first few minutes following injection. Drugs of lower potency have weaker binding constants, diffuse away from receptors, and are cleared from the tissue phase more readily by the circulation, thus limiting the duration of neuromuscular block. For drugs that are not metabolized, this process of clearance from the vicinity of junctional receptors is largely a distribution-redistribution phenomenon, depending ultimately on renal and hepatic function. The process can become "overloaded" or "saturated" in proportion to the bulk quantity or the total dose of the drug injected, leading to "cumulation" or an increasing length of block following a supplemental dosage, and a slower rate of spontaneous recovery, reflected in longer 25 to 75 percent or 5 to 95 percent twitch recovery indices.

For drugs that undergo metabolism or degradation in the plasma (e.g., atracurium [Hofmann elimination] and mivacurium [cholinesterase-cata-

lyzed hydrolysis]), the process of clearance from junctional receptors depends largely on two processes: diffusion away from the neuromuscular junction and destruction of the drug in the plasma. It has little to do with organ function. The more rapid the clearance is, the shorter the duration of action and the faster the recovery from block are. For drugs with a rapid clearance, the injection of larger doses will provide a greater number of molecules for binding to receptors, thereby accelerating the onset. The rapid plasma clearance limits the duration of effect of first bolus doses and keeps the duration of action and speed of recovery from supplemental doses relatively constant. Injection of larger doses of potent drugs constitutes a reasonable clinical strategy to speed the time to tracheal intubation. Two disadvantages, however, of injecting larger numbers of relaxant molecules are a longer duration of blocking effect and/or an increased incidence and intensity of side effects.

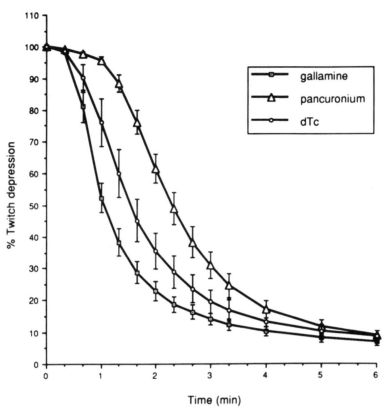

Fig. 21-8 Time course of onset with equipotent doses of gallamine (2.4 mg/kg), pancuronium (0.07 mg/kg), and tubocurarine (*dTc*) (0.45 mg/kg). (From Kopman,[136] with permission.)

CLINICAL PHARMACOLOGY OF INDIVIDUAL DRUGS

Depolarizing Muscle Relaxants

Succinylcholine

Background

Four decades after its introduction into the practice of anesthesia,[3,137,138] succinylcholine remains in widespread use. Its continued popularity is a function of its unique capacity to produce rapid onset of profound relaxation with a short duration of effect.

Mechanism of Neuromuscular Block

Succinylcholine is the only currently available depolarizing relaxant. The drug consists of two acetylcholine molecules joined together (see Fig. 19-11) and mimics the effects of acetylcholine at the postjunctional receptor, thereby triggering end plate depolarization. Both agonists attach to the receptor only briefly (less than 1 ms), and in this regard, there is little difference in the action of acetylcholine and succinylcholine. However, acetylcholine is broken down so rapidly by true acetylcholinesterase at the neuromuscular junction that the synaptic cleft is cleared of transmitter prior to the arrival of the next nerve impulse. In contrast, succinylcholine is not a substrate for this enzyme, and it is cleared from the neuromuscular junction only when plasma levels of the drug begin to decline. As a consequence, succinylcholine molecules are free to combine repetitively with receptors and, hence, depolarize the end plate continuously. This leads to the formation of a zone in the muscle membrane surrounding each end plate of sodium channels, which are fixed in an inactivated state, and prevents the propagation of nerve impulses to normal muscle membranes. The inactivated perijunctional zone blocks all such transmission.

Another characteristic of succinylcholine induced paralysis is that the nature of the block changes with time. Initially, the block is characterized by a diminished response to indirect muscle stimulation, but any evoked response is well sustained. Tetanic or TOF fade on repetitive stimulation is not prominent. This initial or "phase I" block is gradually superseded by a "phase II" block, which is characterized by fade with repeated stimulation and the development of post-tetanic potentiation. Phase II block is usually defined as a TOF ratio less than 0.50.[139,140] The time and dose of succinylcholine necessary for its development varies widely, but after the cumulative dose approaches 7 mg/kg, significant TOF fade is usually present.[141]

Metabolism and Pharmacokinetics

Succinylcholine is hydrolyzed by plasma cholinesterase (butyrylcholinesterase) to succinylmonocholine and choline. The monocholine has weak neuromuscular blocking properties, with a potency of 5 to 10 percent that of succinylcholine.[142] Succinylmonocholine is then broken down to choline and succinic acid at a rate approximately 3 to 4 percent of the parent compound[143]

Because of difficulties in assay techniques and the changing nature of succinylcholine induced neuromuscular blockade, a typical pharmacokinetic profile for succinylcholine is not available. However, approximate values for succinylcholine clearance may be estimated by comparison with those of mivacurium, a short-acting nondepolarizing muscle relaxant. The hydrolytic rate of mivacurium in vitro is 70 percent that of succinylcholine.[78] The recovery index (the time for 25 to 75 percent recovery of twitch height) of succinylcholine is one-half that of mivacurium.[144] Although mivacurium is a mixture of stereoisomers with somewhat different rates of hydrolysis, the overall clearance of the drug in normal individuals approximates 70 ml/kg/min, and the elimination half-life is 2 minutes.[92,145,146] It is probable, therefore, that the clearance of succinylcholine in individuals with

normal butyrylcholinesterase activity exceeds 100 ml/kg/min and that the drug has an elimination half-life of less than 2 minutes.

Potency

In the presence of inhalation anesthetics, succinylcholine has an ED_{95} between 0.20 and 0.30 mg/kg.[147,148] In the absence of potent volatile agents and nitrous oxide, as much as 0.50 to 0.60 mg/kg is necessary to produce 95 percent twitch suppression of the adductor pollicis.[149] This latter figure is the more clinically relevant value because the most common indication for succinylcholine administration is to facilitate tracheal intubation immediately following an intravenous anesthesia induction sequence. There is, however, great interpatient variability in sensitivity to the drug. Even in a relatively small group (n = 15), a single bolus of 0.3 mg/kg may produce responses ranging from 4 to 90 percent single twitch depression.[150] In addition, similar to other muscle relaxants, all muscles do not show identical sensitivity to the effects of succinylcholine. Although the masseter muscle and adductor pollicis require similar doses of succinylcholine to produce comparable effects,[151] the diaphragm has an ED_{95} that is 1.8 times that of the muscles of the hand. To eliminate the fasciculations caused by succinylcholine, a small (one-tenth of the ED_{95}) dose of nondepolarizing muscle relaxant can be administered 2 to 3 minutes prior to the succinylcholine. This defasciculation or precurarization will decrease the potency of succinylcholine by 30 to 50 percent.[149,152] For all these reasons, the standard intubating dose of succinylcholine is generally quoted to be 1.0 to 1.5 mg/kg.

Onset and Recovery

Even following the administration of subparalyzing doses of succinylcholine, the peak effect is evident within 75 to 90 seconds. At doses of 1.0 mg/kg or greater, complete twitch suppression is usually present in about 60 seconds,[153,154] although this may be delayed in the presence of a prolonged circulation time or pretreatment with a nondepolarizing blocker.[155,156] In genotypically normal individuals, this dose of succinylcholine produces apnea lasting on average 6 minutes with 90 percent recovery of twitch height occurring in about 10 minutes. A 60 percent reduction in butyrylcholinesterase activity from normal levels is associated with only modest increases in the total duration of action.[93]

This onset-offset profile is unmatched by any other muscle relaxant. Succinylcholine has therefore been classified as the only available "ultrashort-acting relaxant."[157] Despite its unique characteristics, anesthesiologists have long sought to replace it with a nondepolarizing blocker of similar duration[158] because of the potential complications associated with its use.

Long-Acting Muscle Relaxants

Pancuronium

Background

Hewitt and Savage conceived the idea of incorporating acetylcholine-like moieties into a steroidal ring system. The first compound, pancuronium (see Fig. 19-11), developed in 1964, revolutionized neuromuscular blocking drugs at the time. Pancuronium was the first synthetic substance that improved on naturally occurring materials, such as tubocurarine. Not only is pancuronium six times more potent than tubocurarine, it also has fewer cardiovascular side effects, does not cause histamine release, and provides a minor route of metabolism. Whereas all older nondepolarizing blockers introduced into clinical practice are not metabolized, pancuronium has a minor route of metabolism through hydrolysis of its acetoxy groups.

Dosage and Duration of Effect

The ED_{95} for blockade of the adductor pollicis single twitch under nitrous oxide anesthesia is about 0.07 mg/kg. The dosage for intubation, 0.08 to 0.12 mg/kg, allows laryngoscopy and intubation within 2 to 3 minutes following intravenous induction of anesthesia. Recovery to 25 percent of control twitch height following intubating doses (the "clinical duration of effect") requires 1.5 to 2.0 hours. Supplemental doses of 0.01 to 0.02 mg/kg normally require 30 to 60 minutes for return of twitch to 25 percent of control.

Metabolism and Elimination

Pancuronium is eliminated primarily by the kidneys, with minor elimination by the liver. A small amount of metabolism (10 to 15 percent of an injected dose) occurs in the liver by deacetylation at the 3 position. Because the elimination half-life and clinical duration of action are prolonged in renal or hepatic failure, pancuronium should be used with considerable caution in patients with these conditions.

Cardiovascular and Autonomic Effects

The principal cardiovascular side effect of pancuronium, an increase in heart rate of 10 to 25 percent, is the result of partial vagolytic activity. This effect resides in the acetylcholine-like substitution on the A-ring of the molecule. Vagolysis is often used to advantage to counteract the sinus bradycardia induced by opioid-based anesthetic techniques. Pancuronium also has a stimulating effect on the sympathetic nervous system, which results from augmented catecholamine release from adrenergic nerve terminals, and from the inhibition of reuptake of these neurotransmitters from these terminals. This property may contribute to elevated blood pressures in lightly anesthetized patients or to an increased incidence of ventricular dysrhythmias in susceptible patients.

Tubocurarine ("Curare")

Background

The prototypic benzylisoquinolinium neuromuscular blocking drug in anesthesia, tubocurarine (Fig. 21-9), was first administered to a patient under cyclopropane anesthesia in 1942 by Griffith and Johnson in Montreal. Its introduction at once revolutionized clinical practice and initiated a search for improved compounds. The main side effect (prominent histamine release) is significant enough, however, that clinicians have always been taught to administer curare cautiously and in divided doses.

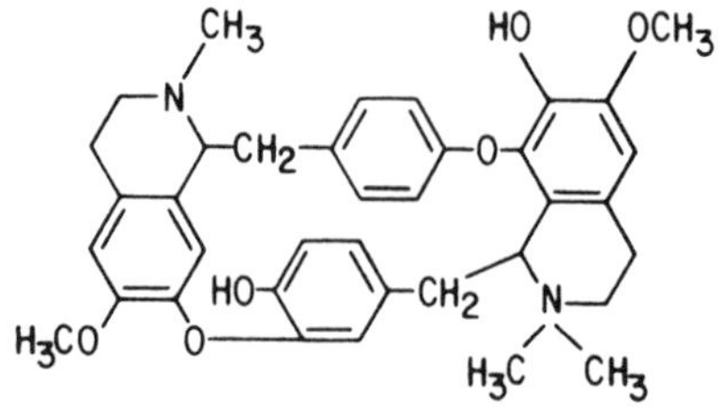

Fig. 21-9 Chemical structure of tubocurarine.

Dosage and Duration of Effect

The ED_{95} of tubocurarine under nitrous oxide-narcotic anesthesia is 0.5 mg/kg. The intubating dose is usually quoted as 0.6 mg/kg. The clinical duration of action of this dose is about 80 minutes. Larger doses are not given as a single bolus for two reasons: Histamine release becomes too severe, and large doses of tubocurarine can cause ganglionic blockade. Because of this, tubocurarine has never been popular for tracheal intubation. Supplemental doses of 0.10 to 0.15 mg/kg provide additional clinical relaxation lasting 30 to 45 minutes.

Metabolism and Elimination

There is little or no metabolism of tubocurarine. The principle route of elimination is the kidney. The liver is a secondary pathway. The elimination half-life and the clinical duration of effect are extended by renal or hepatic disease and in elderly patients. Therefore, the drug is rarely used with these patients.

Cardiovascular and Autonomic Effects

A decrease in blood pressure together with facial flushing is likely when doses greater than 0.3 mg/kg are given as a rapid intravenous bolus. The mechanism for this is histamine release. The prominence of this side effect is related both to the size of the dose and to the speed of administration. Although blockade of autonomic ganglia can easily be demonstrated in animals, this side effect does not occur in clinical practice most likely because it occurs at doses exceeding those used clinically. There is normally little effect on the heart rate because the dose affecting the autonomic nervous system is greater than that usually administered to patients. Both sympathetic and parasympathetic ganglia are blocked simultaneously. This is another reason why the heart rate is little affected by curare. When an increase in heart rate does occur following tubocurarine injection, there is also usually a decrease in blood pressure and facial flushing, all manifestations of the syndrome of histamine release. The popularity of tubocurarine persisted throughout the 1970s largely because, in contrast with pancuronium and gallamine, the heart rate usually remains stable following its administration.

Metocurine

Background

Formerly called "dimethyltubocurarine," metocurine (Fig. 21-10) is actually the trimethyl derivative of tubocurarine. When first given to patients in 1948 by V. K. Stoelting, metocurine's greater potency and relative lack of side effects compared with those of tubocurarine were noted. Metocurine is used less frequently today since the introduction of the more potent pancuronium and the long-acting drugs, doxacurium and pipecuronium, which are free of cardiovascular effects.

Dosage and Duration of Effect

The ED_{95} of metocurine in patients receiving nitrous oxide anesthesia is 0.28 mg/kg. Doses of 0.3 or 0.4 mg/kg are recommended for tracheal intubation. The clinical duration of effect of the larger dose is 90 to 100 minutes. Supplemental doses of 0.05 to 0.1 mg/kg provide additional relaxation lasting 30 to 60 minutes.

Metabolism and Elimination

Metocurine is not metabolized. The molecule is excreted unchanged almost exclusively in the urine, and clearance approximates the glomerular filtration rate. There is probably no biliary elimination of any importance. Because clearance is markedly reduced in renal failure and in elderly patients, metocurine is not recommended for use in these patients.

Cardiovascular and Autonomic Effects

Metocurine has greater safety ratios for ganglionic blockade and histamine release than does tubocurarine. It does not block the vagus. For these reasons, cardiovascular responses in humans are

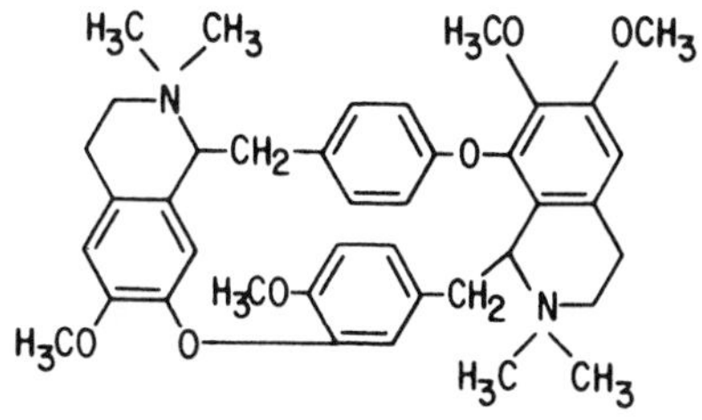

Fig. 21-10 Chemical structure of metocurine.

normally stable following metocurine administration. The only cardiovascular effect, a fall in blood pressure together with facial flushing, occurs only when large bolus doses result in histamine release. This becomes prominent at about 1.5 times the ED_{95} of metocurine (0.4 mg/kg), whereas it is obvious at about 0.8 times the ED_{95} (also 0.4 mg/kg) of tubocurarine.

Doxacurium

Background

Doxacurium chloride (see Fig. 19-11) is a bisbenzylisoquinolinium diester, which is a long-acting nondepolarizing muscle relaxant. It was introduced into clinical practice as an alternative to metocurine, tubocurarine, and pancuronium. With an ED_{95} of 0.025 mg/kg,[50] it is the most potent of the nondepolarizing muscle relaxants (Table 21-6). Doxacurium is a potent neuromuscular blocker requiring the use of small doses, and the doses that cause cardiovascular side effects are large, resulting in a high margin of safety (Table 21-3). Doxacurium is relatively free of cardiovascular side effects.[159–161]

Potency and Onset of Action

Because potency is inversely related to onset (Figs. 21-7 and 21-8),[135,136] the onset of neuromuscular block with the markedly potent doxacurium is slower than with all other nondepolarizing neuro-

Table 21-6 Potency of Nondepolarizing Muscle Relaxants

Drug	Potency[a] (mg/kg)
Gallamine	2.8
Rocuronium	0.40
Metocurine	0.28
Atracurium	0.23
Mivacurium	0.08
Pancuronium	0.07
Vecuronium	0.05
Pipecuronium	0.04
Doxacurium	0.025

[a] ED_{95} in humans.

muscular blocking agents. A dose of 0.05 mg/kg (twice the ED_{95}) and a dose of 0.08 mg/kg cause 90 percent inhibition of twitch response in 5.4 and 3.5 minutes, respectively.[162] A dose of 0.025 mg/kg (ED_{95}) has a mean time to maximal block of 9 minutes.[160] Increasing the dose from 0.05 to 0.06 mg/kg does not significantly shorten the onset time. With a dose two to three times the ED_{95}, patients can be intubated, generally with good to excellent intubating conditions, in 3 to 5 minutes. With a dose of 0.05 mg/kg intubating conditions at 5 minutes are better than at 4 minutes, and with a dose of 0.08 mg/kg, intubating conditions at 4 minutes are better than those at 3 minutes. At each dose, however, more than one-half of patients can be intubated with good to excellent conditions at the shorter time.[162]

To accelerate intubation by 30 seconds, the clinician can prime or pretreat with a fraction of the intubating dose (0.005 mg/kg of doxacurium) 4 minutes prior to administering the full intubating dose. An alternative to this would be to intubate patients with succinylcholine and then maintain neuromuscular block with doxacurium.

Dosage and Duration of Effect

Doxacurium is a long-acting blocking agent. A dose of 0.05 mg/kg (twice the ED_{95}) has a clinical duration (time from injection to return to 25 percent of baseline muscle strength) of 85 minutes.[162] Increasing the dose to 0.08 mg/kg essentially doubles the duration of effect, with patients returning to 25 percent of their baseline muscle strength in approximately 160 minutes.[50,162]

Similar to all other long-acting nondepolarizing muscle relaxants, pharmacologic antagonism of residual doxacurium neuromuscular block may be difficult. The time required for full antagonism depends on the depth of neuromuscular block at the time of the administration of the antagonist. Patients with greater than 90 percent neuromuscular block at the time of administration of 0.06 mg/kg of neostigmine may require up to 28 minutes to recovery of 95 percent of the single twitch height.[50] Adequate recovery of the TOF response to stimulation can take more than 35 minutes when neostigmine is administered at 90 percent neuromuscular block.[163,164]

Metabolism and Elimination

There is essentially no hepatic metabolism of doxacurium, accounting in part for its long duration of action. Although it is a benzylisoquinolinium diester, doxacurium is eliminated unchanged primarily in the urine and, to a lesser extent, in the bile.

The clearance of doxacurium is similar to that of other long-acting nondepolarizing muscle relaxants (2.7 ml/kg/min).[165] The elimination half-life is 100 minutes. Not surprisingly, the clearance is decreased in patients with renal failure, and the elimination half-life is prolonged. As a result, the clinical duration of action is doubled in these patients. These kinetic and dynamic data indicate that dosing intervals should be lengthened in patients with renal failure, and the drug should be used with extreme caution in these patients.

Because renal blood flow and glomerular filtration decrease with aging, the clinician would expect the pharmacokinetics of doxacurium to be altered in elderly patients. Dresner et al.[159] found that the clearance, elimination half-life, and time to 25 percent recovery of muscle strength were not significantly different in elderly patients compared with a group of young adults. Interpatient variability in the duration of effect was, however, markedly increased in elderly patients. The authors attributed the lack of altered pharmacokinetics and pharmacodynamics in elderly patients to the presence of secondary routes of elimination; hepatic elimination and hydrolysis by plasma cholinesterase.

Cardiovascular and Autonomic Effects

Although doxacurium is a benzylisoquinolinium, it does not cause histamine release in clinically used doses. It offers some clinical advantage over certain older longer acting muscle relaxants in that its use is free of cardiovascular side effects.[159–161]

Pipecuronium

Background

Pipecuronium (see Fig. 19-11) is a long-acting nondepolarizing muscle relaxant, introduced into clinical practice as a nonvagolytic alternative to pancuronium. Structurally, it is similar to pancuronium (see Fig. 19-11).

Potency and Onset of Action

The structural changes made to decrease the vagolytic potential of pipecuronium also increased its potency. In humans, pipecuronium (ED_{95} of 35 to 45 μg/kg) is about 1.5 times as potent as pancuronium, which has an ED_{95} of 70 μg/kg.[166,167]

The onset of neuromuscular block with pipecuronium is similar to that of pancuronium. Larijani et al.[168] reported that pipecuronium (70 to 100 μg/kg) produced 90 percent suppression of twitch height in 2 to 3 minutes and 100 percent neuromuscular block in 3 to 4 minutes. Intubating conditions 3 minutes after a dose of 70 μg/kg were good ("slight diaphragmatic movement") to excellent ("complete relaxation"). To speed the onset of neuromuscular block, the clinician can prime with one-tenth of the intubating dose of muscle relaxant 2 to 4 minutes prior to the administration of the full intubating dose.

Dosage and Duration of Effect

Although Larijani et al.[168] were unable to demonstrate a significant dose-effect relationship for the onset of neuromuscular block with the doses studied (70, 85, and 100 μg/kg), the clinical duration of effect (time from administration to 25 percent recovery) increased significantly from 70 minutes with 70 μg/kg to 98 and 95 minutes with 85 and 100 μg/kg, respectively.

Similar to any long-acting nondepolarizing muscle relaxant, the pharmacologic antagonism of residual pipecuronium induced neuromuscular block should be undertaken with care. The ease of antagonism varies with the depth of neuromuscular block at the time of antagonism. Although the majority of patients in Larijani et al.'s study[168] could have their blockade readily antagonized with neostigmine, 10 patients who had a T_4/T_1 ratio of 0 at the time of neostigmine administration required more than 10 minutes or a second dose of neostigmine for full antagonism. The clearance of pipecuronium and elimination half-life are 2.4 ml/kg/min and 137 minutes, respectively,[169] and these are similar to the clearance and elimination half-life of pancuronium. The long duration of pipecuronium's effect reflects its pharmacokinetics.

Metabolism and Elimination

Pipecuronium is cleared primarily (70 to 80 percent) by renal elimination and, to a lesser extent, by the liver.[169–171] It undergoes little or no metabolism. The pharmacokinetics and pharmacodynamics of pipecuronium are significantly altered in the presence of renal failure.[169,171] Although Caldwell et al.[169] were unable to demonstrate a significantly prolonged recovery from pipecuronium induced neuromuscular block in patients with renal disease, they did find that there was a marked degree of interpatient variability in terms of recovery in these patients. Recovery may be more prolonged with repeated doses of pipecuronium. The pharmacokinetics and pharmacodynamics of pipecuronium appear to not be affected by advanced age.[172]

Cardiovascular and Autonomic Effects

Modification of the 2,16-β-piperidino substitutions of pancuronium to 2,16-β-piperazino substitutions, by moving the nitrogen atom to the distal (4 position) aspect of the compound, lessened its acetylcholine-like nature. As a result, pipecuronium is approximately 10 times less vagolytic than is pancuronium and its margin of safety for vagolysis (ED_{50} vagolysis in the cat/ED_{95} neuromuscular block) was increased from 2.9 for pancuronium to 25 (Table 21-3). As with other steroidal relaxants, the ganglion-blocking potency of pipecuronium is low, and histamine release does not occur. Within the clinical dose range, pipecuronium is free of vagolytic side effects. Patients undergoing coronary artery bypass grafting remained hemodynamically stable when given doses up to three times the ED_{95} of pipecuronium.[57] Decreases in heart rate and mean arterial pressure were noted during this study of hemodynamic effects and occurred to a large extent prior to the administration of muscle relaxant. They were most likely secondary to the vagal effects of the anesthetic.

Intermediate-Acting Muscle Relaxants

In 1975, an editorial in *Anesthesiology* suggested a need for nondepolarizing blockers with a duration of action intermediate between succinylcholine and the relaxants then available.[158] Older longer acting agents, such as curare, may be associated with un-suspected residual postoperative neuromuscular blockade.[173] When used to produce profound blockade (single twitch depression to 10 percent of control), longer acting agents, such as pancuronium, may be more difficult to antagonize than shorter acting agents, such as vecuronium and atracurium, under certain conditions.[55] Some subjective measurements of residual neuromuscular blockade, such as diplopia or weakness, were more common immediately postoperatively in patients receiving pancuronium than in those receiving atracurium.[174] These issues have received increasing attention with the growth in ambulatory surgery.

Vecuronium

Background

Vecuronium (see Fig. 19-11) is a steroidal muscle relaxant that differs in structure from pancuronium only in the nature of its 2β-nitrogen atom, which is tertiary rather than quaternary. This seemingly minor structural alteration results in a molecule with pharmacokinetic and pharmacodynamic properties that are different from those of its parent compound. As a monoquaternary analog, it is more lipophilic than is pancuronium, which modifies distribution within the body and probably accounts for a greater rate of hepatic uptake. Demethylation also reduced the acetylcholine-like properties associated with the A ring of the pancuronium molecule.

Potency

Vecuronium has a potency slightly greater than pancuronium. Its ED_{50} and ED_{95} average 0.027 and 0.045 mg/kg, respectively, under balanced anesthesia.[12,175–178] Isoflurane and enflurane may reduce these dose requirements by more than 50 percent.[43]

Onset

The onset of action of vecuronium is not substantially different from that of other drugs with similar potency, such as pancuronium or pipecuronium. Following a subparalyzing dose, the peak effect occurs in about 6 to 7 minutes. An intubating dose of 0.1 mg/kg will produce total twitch depression in about 3 minutes.[34] This time can be decreased to less than 90 seconds if doses of 0.3 to 0.4 mg/kg are administered.[35]

Metabolism and Elimination

Vecuronium depends on both the kidney and liver for its elimination. It is deactylated in the liver to various alcohol metabolites. The 3-hydroxy metabolite has approximately 50 to 60 percent of the potency of vecuronium (in cats). As previously discussed, this metabolite may be associated with prolonged neuromuscular blockade (lasting days) when vecuronium is administered for extended periods in an intensive care setting.[74]

It has been estimated that more than 40 percent of administered vecuronium is excreted in the bile in 24 hours, and liver biopsies indicate that the liver may contain more than 50 percent of the intravenous dose within 30 minutes after injection.[179] Not surprisingly, hepatic cirrhosis is associated with a 40 percent increase in the elimination half-life of vecuronium and 100 percent increase in most of the measured indices of recovery.[180]

Renal elimination of vecuronium appears less important. Initial reports comparing normal patients and those with renal failure indicated that these groups did not differ in the duration of effect or rate of recovery from vecuronium.[181] Nonetheless, significant amounts of the drug may be eliminated by the kidney. Thirty percent of the parent compound and its 3-hydroxy derivative can be recovered in the urine within 24 hours.[68] More recent information suggests that renal failure impairs the elimination of vecuronium. In patients without renal function, the clearance is reduced 40 percent, and the elimination half-life is increased by almost 60 percent, with a resulting 80 percent prolongation in clinical effect.[69]

Pharmacokinetics, Dose, and Duration of Action

Vecuronium has a plasma clearance of 4 to 5.5 ml/ kg/min. This is two to three times the rate reported with long-acting agents, such as pancuronium or pipecuronium.[182] The elimination half-life of vecuronium ranges from a low of 50 to 75 minutes to more than 2 hours (Table 21-7). Despite the fact that the elimination half-life of vecuronium may approach that of longer acting blockers and is at least three times that of atracurium, the drug is an agent of intermediate duration.

Recovery from modest doses of vecuronium can be rapid. Following a dose of 0.043 mg/kg (91 percent block), 90 percent twitch recovery may be present within 20 minutes, and even at three times this dose, similar degrees of recovery require only 1 hour.[188,189] Following doses of 0.1 mg/kg, the time for recovery of twitch height from 25 to 75 percent averages about 10 minutes, and the time from 25 percent recovery of twitch height to restoration of a TOF ratio more than 0.75 approximates 36 minutes.[190] Volatile anesthetics, however, will slow these rates of recovery significantly. An end-tidal isoflurane concentration is 0.7 to 0.9 percent will slow vecuronium (0.1 mg/kg) TOF recovery to 75 percent to 123 minutes.[7,48] Repeated or large doses of vecuronium result in even slower recovery. After the total dose of drug reaches 0.3 mg/kg, these slower recovery times may become clinically impor-

Table 21-7 Pharmacokinetics of Vecuronium

$T_{1/2}\pi$ (min)	$T_{1/2}\alpha$ (min)	$T_{1/2}\beta$ (min)	V_1 (ml/kg)	V_{ss} (ml/kg)	CL (ml/kg/min)	Ref.
—	7.5	53	—	199	5.3	69
2	15	70	52	244	5.2	183
2.2	13	71	50	270	5.2	184
1.4	13.3	108	76	413	4.6	185
1.3	10	118	48	690	4.1	186
—	15	133	83	933	5.4	187

Abbreviations: CL, clearance; $T_{1/2}\alpha$, distribution half-life; $T_{1/2}\beta$, elimination half-life; $T_{1/2}\pi$, rapid distribution half-life; V_1, volume of the central compartment; V_{ss}, steady state volume of distribution.

tant. For example, the recovery index (recovery from 25 to 75 percent twitch height) increases from 10 to 20 minutes with large doses.[191]

The dose-dependent nature of the vecuronium recovery has a pharmacokinetic basis.[192] With small doses of drug (twice the ED_{95}), rapid return of neuromuscular function takes place because of redistribution. Vecuronium has a large total volume of distribution relative to the volume of the central compartment; hence, redistribution continues to play an important role in recovery even after many multiples of the ED_{95} have been administered. Eventually, however, peripheral storage sites become saturated, and drug elimination becomes the dominant recovery mechanism.

As noted previously, hepatic and, to a lesser extent, renal failure are associated with a prolongation of the duration of effect of vecuronium. Any condition that alters the elimination of vecuronium is likely to have a similar effect. For example, delayed recovery from vecuronium has been associated with morbid obesity[193] and extremes of age.[194–196]

Cardiovascular and Autonomic Effects

In 1979, vecuronium was selected for study from a series of pancuronium analogs because it was most likely to produce neuromuscular block without concomitant cardiovascular side effects.[197] Vecuronium exhibited negligible ganglionic blocking activity and a wide safety margin between neuromuscular and vagal blocking doses in animals.[198] In addition, even in large doses, vecuronium is not associated with significant increases in plasma histamine concentration.[199,200] As a consequence, vecuronium was the first clinically available nondepolarizing neuromuscular blocker that is essentially devoid of cardiovascular side effects in humans when given in amounts up to eight times the ED_{95}. Doses of 0.3 to 0.4 mg/kg produce no significant alterations in heart rate, blood pressure, systemic vascular resistance, or cardiac output.[201]

Rocuronium

Background

Rocuronium is the 2-morpholino, 3-desacetyl, 16-allyl-pyrrolidino analog of vecuronium. It is another steroidal nondepolarizing neuromuscular blocking drug, classified as having an intermediate duration of effect (Fig. 21-11). It is the first nondepolarizing muscle relaxant with a fast onset of action.

Potency and Onset

Rocuronium is approximately one-seventh as potent as vecuronium, with an ED_{95} that averages 0.35 mg/kg. Reported figures for this value range from 0.27 to 0.43 mg/kg.[202–207] The drug, therefore, has a low potency, which has major implications in regard to its rate of onset of action.

In 1988, Bowman et al.,[135] after studying a series of desacetoxy analogs of vecuronium (in cats), reported that fast onset, coupled with brief duration, may be produced only with compounds of relatively low potency. The importance of potency as a determinant of speed of action was also confirmed

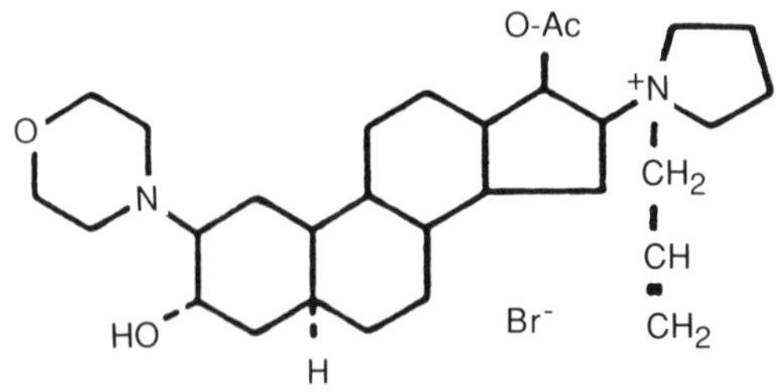

Fig. 21-11 Chemical structure of rocuronium.

in humans.[136] Inasmuch as rocuronium is a drug of relatively low potency, it should have a relatively rapid onset of action. This is indeed the case.

Uniformly excellent intubating conditions were reported 60 seconds after a bolus of 1.0 mg/kg (3 times the ED_{95}), at which time T_1 averages only 12 percent of control. Even at lower doses, extremely short onset times were described. Following a dose of 0.6 mg/kg, 80 percent block may occur in less than 1 minute with complete twitch suppression evident in 90 seconds. Although the onset times following this dose vary (range, 75 to 150 seconds), there is general agreement that rocuronium 0.6 mg/kg produces good to excellent intubating conditions at 60 to 90 seconds.[29]

Recovery from small doses of rocuronium (0.45 mg/kg) can be rapid with a clinical duration (bolus to 25 percent recovery of twitch height) of 21 minutes and a recovery index of only 9 minutes.[208] The clinical duration of the effect of rocuronium following 0.6 mg/kg under balanced anesthesia is between 30 and 40 minutes, with a recovery index of 13 to 17 minutes.[124,209] As the total dose of rocuronium increases, recovery slows. The recovery index following an initial bolus of 0.9 mg/kg is 35 to 55 percent greater than after a dose of 0.6 mg/kg.[126] Similarly, following a 2-hour infusion of rocuronium at rates sufficient to produce 95 percent twitch suppression (10 μg/kg/min under balanced anesthesia), the time to 90 percent recovery of T_1 after termination of the infusion is 46 minutes. Comparable levels of twitch depression under isoflurane anesthesia require infusions of only 6 μg/kg/min, but 90 percent recovery time after stopping the infusion is even more prolonged (75 minutes), with a recovery index in excess of 1 hour.[210]

Metabolism and Elimination

The pharmacokinetic profile of rocuronium is essentially the same as that of vecuronium. In normal adults, the elimination half-life was reported between 56 and 97 minutes, with a plasma clearance of 2.9 to 5.8 ml/kg/min.[211–213] Similar to vecuronium, more than 50 percent of the drug is eliminated in the bile in the first 6 hours, the majority within 1 hour of administration. Renal elimination is of secondary importance, with about 30 percent

excreted in the first 24 hours. In contrast to vecuronium, measurable amounts of metabolites seem to be absent.[214]

In the cat, although rocuronium appears to be mainly excreted by the liver,[215] renal disease also appears to impair elimination. In patients with renal dysfunction sufficient to require dialysis, plasma clearance is reduced by one-third compared with normal controls, and 90 percent recovery times recorded following a dose of 0.6 mg/kg during isoflurane anesthesia increased from 70 to 100 minutes. However, in patients undergoing renal transplantation, drug clearance was not found to differ from that in controls.[213] Hence, the suitability of rocuronium in patients with renal failure is still unsettled.

Similar to vecuronium, recovery is delayed in older patients.[212,216] The prolongation in the duration of action is secondary to a decreased plasma clearance of rocuronium.

Cardiovascular and Autonomic Effects

In animal studies, the cardiovascular effects of rocuronium are slight. It blocks bradycardia produced by vagal stimulation only in doses greater than those necessary to produce neuromuscular block. This is, however, only one-tenth the margin of safety seen with vecuronium. Ganglionic block is seen only in doses several times those producing vagal block.[217] Most investigations of rocuronium's effects in humans focused on the drug's neuromuscular effects. Changes in heart rate and blood pressure appear to be minimal.[218] There is, however, some evidence that doses as small as 0.6 mg/kg may produce at least transient tachycardia in humans.[58]

Atracurium

Background

Atracurium (see Fig. 19-11) belongs to the benzylisoquinolinium class of neuromuscular blockers and is a bis-quaternary nitrogen compound. It is an intermediate-acting neuromuscular blocking agent that was developed in a search for a short-acting neuromuscular blocking agent capable of rapid biodegradation by a purely chemical pathway.[219] When incubated in an aqueous buffer solution at 37°C and pH 7.3 to 7.4, atracurium has an in vitro half life between 60 and 80 minutes. This nonenzymatic degradation is mediated by the clinical process known as the Hofmann reaction. The atracurium molecule is also subject to ester hydrolysis, and when incubated in plasma at physiologic pH and temperature, the in vitro half-life is reduced by 50 to 65 percent compared with that when incubated in buffer alone.[220,221] Postulated breakdown pathways and products are illustrated in Figure 21-12. The extent to which Hofmann elimination versus ester hydrolysis contribute to the breakdown of atracurium in humans has been the subject of much debate.[222,223] Current evidence suggests that both processes are important, with ester hydrolysis probably playing a somewhat more dominant role in humans.

Potency, Onset, and Duration of Effect

Atracurium is approximately one-fifth as potent as vecuronium. Reported ED_{95} values range from 0.20 to 0.34 mg/kg,[224–228] but the generally accepted figure is 0.25 mg/kg, with an ED_{50} of about 0.13 mg/kg.

Atracurium has an onset time of the same order of magnitude as vecuronium and pancuronium. Following a bolus of 0.6 mg/kg (2.4 times the ED_{95}), the time to 100 percent twitch depression averages 130 seconds compared with 70 seconds for succinylcholine.[153] When equipotent doses (1.3 times the ED_{95}) of atracurium and vecuronium are compared, the onset times to 95 percent block are identical, 161 versus 168 seconds, respectively.[229] These onset times, however, should be read with a certain degree of skepticism because values from respected investigators can disagree widely.[230]

Atracurium, 0.3 mg/kg (1.2 times the ED_{95}), has a clinical duration of approximately 25 minutes, and single twitch returns to 95 percent of control in 45 to 50 minutes.[231] Increasing the dose to 0.5 mg/kg results in a clinical duration of 40 to 45 minutes, and 90 to 95 percent return of T_1 occurs in 60 to 65 minutes.[144,232] The 25 to 75 percent and 5 to 95 percent recovery intervals are essentially independent of the dose or duration of atracurium administration and are constant at 11 to 14 and 25 to 30 minutes, respectively.[54,233]

Atracurium has also been used for longer surgical procedures. To maintain neuromuscular block in a narrow range (TOF count, one to three), incremental injections are needed approximately every 8 to 10 minutes. Atracurium has also been administered by continuous infusion. After steady state conditions are achieved, adjustments to the rate of infusion should be infrequent. Under balanced an-

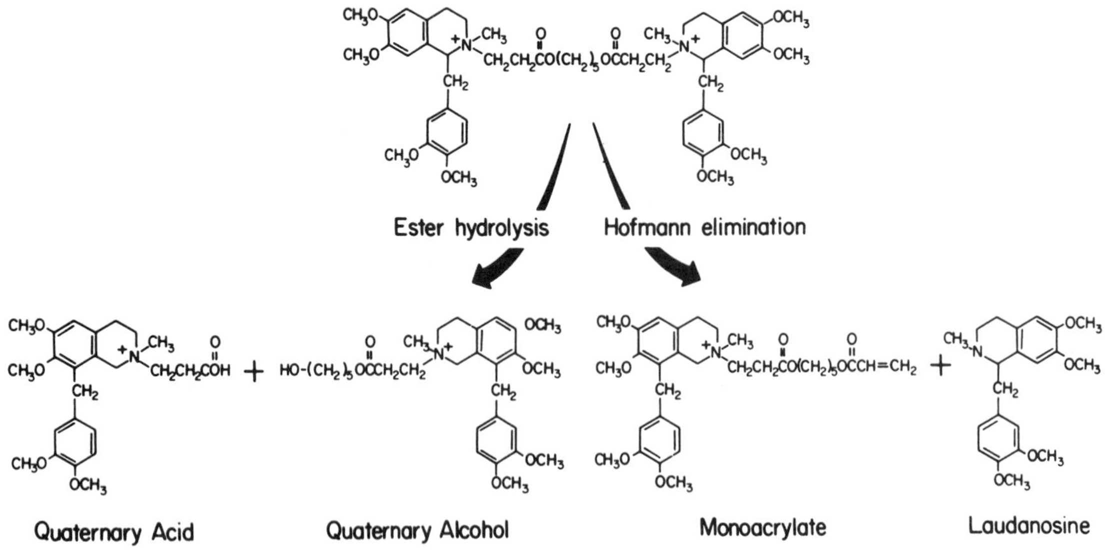

Fig. 21-12 Breakdown pathways of atracurium. The compound undergoes both Hofmann elimination and ester hydrolysis. (From Miller and Savarese,[276] with permission.)

esthesia, infusion rates of 6 μg/kg/min usually result in 90 to 95 percent twitch depression.[234–236] However, several caveats need to be noted. Similar to all relaxants, individual sensitivity varies widely. Therefore, even in a relatively small patient population, infusion requirements vary considerably, with rates ranging from 2.5 to 10 μg/kg/min. In addition, when administered with potent inhalation anesthetics, these requirements may be reduced by 30 to 50 percent.

Pharmacokinetics

In normal adults, atracurium has a clearance of 5 to 6 ml/kg/min and a small total volume of distribution (Table 21-8). The elimination half-life of 20 minutes is little different from the value determined for plasma or whole blood in vitro.[243] Although it has been suggested that organ-based elimination (primarily liver) may account for one-half of the elimination of atracurium,[244] there is little direct evidence to support this position. Because the elimination of atracurium is essentially independent of organ function, the pharmacokinetic profile and clinical duration are unmodified in patients with hepatic[245,246] or renal disease.[247,248] Likewise, effects of atracurium are not altered in obesity or in elderly patients.[249–251] At the extremes of age, the ED$_{95}$ and duration of action of atracurium are not different in infants, children, or adolescents,[252] although children do require somewhat higher infusion rates than adults.[253,254]

Cardiovascular and Autonomic Effects

In experimental animals, atracurium has a wide margin of safety between the neuromuscular blocking dose and the dose that causes autonomic side effects.[255] This is also true in humans. When administered in doses of 0.4 mg/kg or less, changes in heart rate and blood pressure from control average 5 percent or less.[256] However, changes in vital signs may accompany doses of atracurium equal to or greater than 0.5 mg/kg, and these alterations are the result of histamine release.[64]

At 2.5 times the ED$_{95}$ (0.6 mg/kg), the mean blood pressure has been reported to fall by 20 percent, with an 8 percent increase in heart rate. At doses of 0.8 to 0.9 mg/kg, decreases in the mean arterial blood pressure average 25 percent, and the heart rate increases by 10 to 15 percent if the administration is rapid (5 to 30 seconds).[257] If the dose is increased still further (1.5 mg/kg, six times the ED$_{95}$), average mean arterial pressure decreases of 35 to 40 percent are seen.[258] These effects are most prominent at 2 minutes after administration, and generally, they start to return toward baseline by 5 minutes postbolus. Histamine release may be avoided (in doses of atracurium up to 0.8 mg/kg) if the drug is given slowly over 75 seconds or longer. The hemodynamic consequences of histamine release, but not the histamine liberation itself, may be almost totally blunted if H$_1$ and H$_2$ receptor blocker prophylaxis is given 15 to 30 minutes prior to atracurium administration.[258,259]

Table 21-8 Pharmacokinetics of Atracurium

T$_{1/2\alpha}$ (min)	T$_{1/2\beta}$ (min)	V$_1$ (ml/kg)	V$_{ss}$ (ml/kg)	CL (ml/kg/min)	Ref.
2.1	19.9	49	157	5.5	237
3.6	20.1	80	141	5.8	238
3.3	16.9	50	142	5.9	239
3.4	20.6	60	182	6.1	240
2.1	19.9	49	157	5.5	241
2.0	20.4	41	145	5.0	242

Abbreviations: CL, clearance; T$_{1/2\alpha}$, distribution half-life; T$_{1/2\beta}$, elimination half-life; V$_1$, volume of the central compartment; V$_{ss}$, steady state volume of distribution.

Potential Toxicity

Laudanosine is one of the major products of atracurium metabolism. This compound is a known central nervous system stimulant. Following a large dose of atracurium (3.5 mg/kg) in dogs under halothane anesthesia, electroencephalographic evidence of cerebral arousal has been observed. This cerebral stimulation, which is not accompanied by significant increases in cerebral blood flow or oxygen consumption, is presumed to be secondary to laudanosine.[260] Laudanosine at plasma concentrations of 0.5 to 0.9 μg/ml was also found to increase the minimum alveolar concentration in rabbits by 20 to 30 percent.[261] However, at similar laudanosine levels, no increased incidence of seizure activity was detected using a typical antibiotic induced epilepsy model in rabbits.[262] After the continuous infusion of laudanosine to conscious dogs, plasma concentrations in the order of 1.2 μg/ml did not cause behavioral disturbances. In anesthetized dogs, laudanosine plasma concentrations of more than 6 μg/ml caused hypotension and bradycardia, laudanosine concentrations larger than 10 μg/ml induced epileptic electroencephalographic spiking, and plasma concentrations more than 17 μg/ml produced prolonged seizures.[263] However, in unanesthetized rabbits, purposeless uncoordinated whole body movements began at laudanosine plasma concentrations of 5 μg/ml.[264] These data notwithstanding there is no information available as to the central nervous system effects of different laudanosine plasma levels in humans.

In contrast to the short elimination half-life of atracurium, laudanosine has an elimination half-life in normal individuals of 197 minutes.[237] In renal failure or severe hepatic disease, this value rises to 234 and 560 minutes, respectively. Concern has therefore been expressed about the possibility of significant elevations of plasma laudanosine concentrations (and potential toxicity) in patients with reduced renal and hepatic function. In a study of eight patients scheduled for renal transplantation, a single bolus of atracurium 0.5 mg/kg produced higher peak laudanosine levels than in a group of normal controls. However, in the renal failure group, the highest recorded value was less than 0.8 μg/ml, and average values 20 minutes after injection were only 0.2 μg/ml. Hence, plasma concentrations are probably not high enough to cause overt toxicity.[265]

A study of laudanosine plasma concentrations in six patients receiving prolonged atracurium infusions (2 to 6 days) did in fact reveal elevated concentrations of laudanosine. The maximum concentrations ranged from 1.9 to 5.1 μg/ml, with an indication of a plateau after 2 to 3 days.[266] Of interest, the patient with the highest concentration had no evidence of renal or hepatic disease. Despite incomplete neuromuscular blockade, there was no evidence of seizure activity in any patient. In two individuals, electroencephalograms performed on days 5 and 6 showed no evidence of cerebral excitation. Another study of 14 patients in the intensive care unit who were receiving atracurium infusions for 11 to 47 hours showed similar results. Seven of the patients had normal renal function, and seven were in acute renal failure. In the patients with normal renal function, the plasma laudanosine concentration reached a plateau of approximately 1.2 μg/ml within 10 hours. In patients with renal failure, there was greater variation in the plasma laudanosine concentration; the highest value recorded was 4.3 μg/ml.[267] In summary, even with long-term infusions of atracurium in patients with renal failure, there are no data substantiating any causally related adverse patient outcome.

51W89

Background

This new benzylisoquinolinium compound (Fig. 21-13) is the R-cis, R'-cis stereoisomer of atracurium. It was identified following the evaluation of six of the isomers of atracurium for possible shorter duration of effect or decreased side effects. 51W89 is about three times as potent as atracurium in humans, does not release histamine, and is degraded by Hofmann elimination.

Dose and Duration of Effect

The ED_{95} of 51W89 in patients receiving nitrous oxide-opioid anesthesia is 0.05 mg/kg. 51W89 has an intermediate duration of action similar to that of atracurium; at twice the ED_{95}, the clinical duration of action is about 45 minutes. At four times the

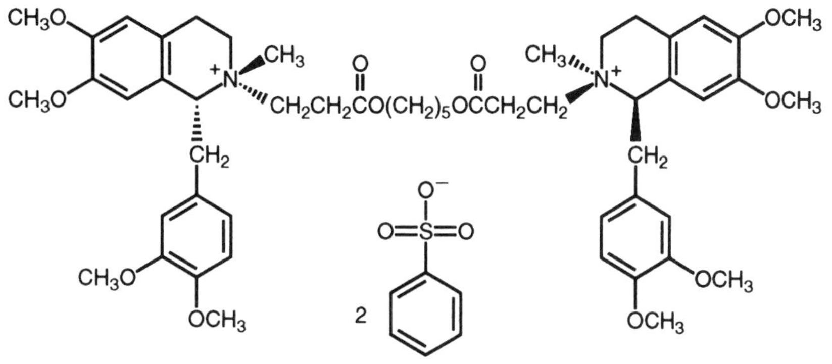

Fig. 21-13 Chemical structure of 51W89.

ED_{95}, the clinical duration is about 65 minutes. Tracheal intubation may be carried out at 150 seconds following a dose of twice the ED_{95} and at 120 or 90 seconds following doses of three or four times the ED_{95} (0.15 or 0.2 mg/kg). A supplemental dose of 0.01 to 0.015 mg/kg yields additional relaxation lasting 10 to 20 minutes.

Supplemental doses of 51W89 show a constant duration of effect and constant rate of spontaneous recovery regardless of the duration of administration. The 5 to 95 percent recovery interval for the adductor pollicis twitch is about 30 to 35 minutes, and the 25 to 75 percent recovery index is about 12 to 13 minutes. 51W89 can be given by continuous infusion to maintain a stable degree of neuromuscular block. Infusion rates of 1 to 2 $\mu g/kg/min$ are typical.

Metabolism and Elimination

Because the drug is new, the data in this area are preliminary. Hofmann elimination is the likely principal route of degradation, with a half-life in vitro and in vivo of about 20 to 25 minutes. Other minor pathways, such as enzymatic hydrolysis of the ester groups, are possible, although less likely than in the case of atracurium.

Cardiovascular and Autonomic Effects

The principal advantage of 51W89 versus atracurium is lack of histamine release. In patients receiving nitrous oxide-opioid-barbiturate anesthesia, variations in heart rate and arterial pressure measured through a radial arterial catheter were less than 5 percent following doses from one to eight times the ED_{95} (0.05 to 0.4 mg/kg).

Short-Acting Muscle Relaxants

Mivacurium

Background

Mivacurium (see Fig. 19-11), a benzylisoquinolinium diester, is a short-acting nondepolarizing muscle relaxant. It is currently the only nondepolarizing muscle relaxant with a short duration of action.

Potency and Duration of Effect

With an ED_{95} of 0.08 mg/kg mivacurium is approximately three times more potent than atracurium. Administration of three times the ED_{95} dose (0.25 mg/kg) causes 100 percent neuromuscular block in approximately 2 to 3 minutes. Twenty minutes is required for 25 percent recovery and 30 minutes for recovery to 95 percent of twitch height (Fig. 21-14).[56]

Interestingly, recovery from mivacurium induced neuromuscular block is apparently unaffected by either the size of an intravenous bolus dose or the duration of an infusion.[56] The slope of recovery curves is constant, following any number of doses (Fig. 21-15). Recovery indices of 25 to 75 percent or 5 to 95 percent are not different for any of several different doses (Table 21-9).

These findings suggest that mivacurium can be used in an infusion, providing reliable recovery even after prolonged administration. To maintain

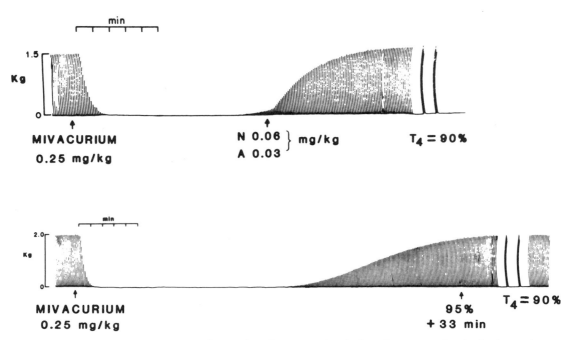

Fig. 21-14 Spontaneous recovery (bottom) and neostigmine induced recovery (top) of mivacurium (0.25 mg/kg) induced neuromuscular block. The 5 to 95 percent recovery interval is 14 minutes during spontaneous recovery, and the time from mivacurium administration to 95 percent recovery is 33 minutes. (From Savarese et al.,[56] with permission.)

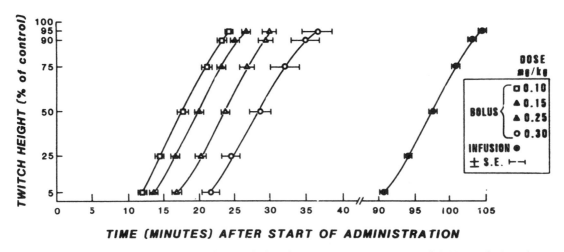

Fig. 21-15 Spontaneous recovery following bolus doses (0.10, 0.15, 0.25, and 0.30 mg/kg) and infusions of mivacurium. The 5 to 95 percent recovery index is 13 to 14 minutes in all cases, indicating that, under nitrous-opioid anesthesia, recovery is not related to muscle relaxant dose. From the infusion data (n = 38), it also appears to be unrelated to the duration of administration. (From Savarese et al.,[56] with permission.)

Table 21-9 Spontaneous Recovery From Mivacurium Induced Neuromuscular Block

Dose (mg/kg)	Recovery Index (min ± SE)	
	25–75%	5–95%
0.15	6.6 ± 0.6	13.6 ± 0.9
0.20	6.9 ± 0.4	14.7 ± 0.8
0.25	6.6 ± 0.5	13.8 ± 0.7
0.30	7.2 ± 1.2	14.5 ± 2.3
Infusion (35–324 min)	6.5 ± 0.3	14.4 ± 0.6

Abbreviations: SE, standard error.
(Adapted from Savarese et al.,[56] with permission.)

90 to 99 percent neuromuscular block, infusion rates of 5 to 15 μg/kg/min are necessary. Recovery after a mivacurium infusion occurs in approximately 50 percent of the time required for recovery from atracurium or vecuronium infusions (Table 21-10).

In spite of the rapid recovery from mivacurium induced neuromuscular block, there are times when the clinician may want to shorten the time required for recovery further. Because mivacurium is a nondepolarizing relaxant, and in spite of its metabolism by plasma cholinesterase (discussed later), pharmacologic antagonism with anticholinesterases is possible. Although there is theoretic concern that the metabolism of mivacurium may be inhibited by administration of an anticholinesterase, clinical recovery is shortened by anticholinesterases.[56] As is the case with neuromuscular block

Table 21-10 Spontaneous Recovery Following Mivacurium, Atracurium, or Vecuronium Infusions[a]

Muscle Relaxant	Recovery Indices (min)	
	25–75%	5–95%
Mivacurium	6.4	13.6
Atracurium	10.9	26.6
Vecuronium	13.8	32.0

[a] Duration of infusions 58–122 min.
(Adapted from Ali et al.,[54] with permission.)

induced with other nondepolarizing neuromuscular blockers, neostigmine will not effectively antagonize profound (100 percent) mivacurium induced neuromuscular block.[86] Recovery from 95 percent neuromuscular block, however, is shortened to approximately 7 minutes by the administration of neostigmine.[268] Cook et al.[269] demonstrated the in vitro inhibition of mivacurium metabolism by neostigmine but not edrophonium, suggesting that edrophonium is a better antagonist of mivacurium than is neostigmine. A small but statistically significant decrease in the amount of time required for recovery to TOF of 70 percent from approximately 90 percent neuromuscular block, from 11.2 to 8.2 minutes, was observed with 0.75 mg/kg of edrophonium.[270] Further studies are needed to determine the effect of cholinesterase inhibition on the in vivo pharmacokinetics of mivacurium.

Mivacurium actually consists of a mixture of three geometric noninterconvertible stereoisomers: a cis-trans, a trans-trans, and a cis-cis isomer, which differ in terms of their potency and pharmacokinetics. The least potent isomer, the cis-cis isomer, comprises 4 to 8 percent of mivacurium; the trans-trans and cis-trans isomers, each being approximately 13 times more potent than the cis-cis isomer, comprise 52 to 62 percent and 30 to 45 percent of mivacurium, respectively.[271]

The more potent cis-trans and trans-trans isomers of mivacurium have half-lives of 1.8 and 1.9 minutes, respectively, and clearances of 92 and 53 ml/min/kg, respectively.[145] The brief duration of mivacurium effect is caused in part by the pharmacokinetics of the more potent isomers.

The rapid clearance and short elimination half-life of mivacurium are the result of extensive metabolism by plasma cholinesterase. The rate of hydrolysis of mivacurium is 70 to 88 percent that of succinylcholine.[56,78] Mivacurium and its metabolites have been identified in the urine, indicating that the kidney is a likely secondary route of elimination.

Theoretically, the lack of overall dependence on the kidney and the liver for elimination and metabolism suggests that mivacurium pharmacokinetics should be unaffected by hepatic or renal failure or by advanced age. However, plasma cholinesterase is synthesized by the liver, and cholinesterase plasma concentration is affected by uremia. Thus, mivacurium pharmacodynamics and, in the case of hepatic failure, mivacurium pharmacokinetics are altered in end-organ failure. Cook et al.,[92] in a study of the pharmacokinetics and pharmacodynamics of mivacurium in patients with hepatic failure, found that the 25 to 75 percent recovery index was approximately three times longer in patients with hepatic failure compared with that in patients with normal hepatic function (15.7 versus 5.5 minutes, respectively). This prolongation of effect was apparently the result of decreased clearance (33.3 versus 70.4 ml/min/kg in patients with hepatic failure and normal hepatic function, respectively) and an increase in mean residence time (4.2 versus 1.5 minutes, respectively). The altered pharmacokinetics were likely secondary to the significantly decreased dibucaine numbers and plasma cholinesterase activity found in patients with hepatic failure.

Uremia, rather than hemodialysis, is also associated with decreased levels of plasma cholinesterase activity;[90,91] this may be responsible for the prolonged duration of action of mivacurium in patients with renal failure. These patients may take significantly longer to recover from mivacurium induced neuromuscular block and require significantly less drug to maintain paralysis.[87,88] Another potential reason for prolonged neuromuscular block in this group of patients is that they are unable to eliminate any drug through renal routes. Further kinetic studies need to be done with a stereospecific assay to elucidate fully the pharmacokinetics of mivacurium in this patient population.

Preliminary results indicate that the pharmacodynamics of mivacurium are not significantly altered by advanced age. In elderly patients, there is a tendency toward a slight (but not significant) prolongation of the duration of mivacurium (0.1 mg/kg) block in patients under isoflurane anesthesia.[272] However the pharmacokinetics of mivacurium in elderly patients are unknown.

Cardiovascular and Autonomic Effects

Because mivacurium is a benzylisoquinolinium, it causes histamine release in large doses and with rapid administration. This histamine release can be attenuated by either administration of smaller doses or slower administration of the drug (Fig. 21-2).

SUMMARY

The choice of muscle relaxant and dosing regimen depends on the needs of the individual patient. These needs are, in part at least, dictated by underlying disease processes, patient age, and the nature of the surgical procedure. Through the rational use of muscle relaxants, the anesthesiologist can optimize patient care by ensuring both adequate relaxation for the surgical procedure and complete recovery of muscle strength at the completion of surgery if the patient is to be extubated.

REFERENCES

1. Foldes F: Life before and after curare. p. 5. In Bowman WC, Denissen PAF, Feldman S (eds): Neuromuscular Blocking Agents: Past, Present, and Future. Excerpta Medica, Princeton, 1990
2. Griffith HR, Johnson GE: The use of curare in general anesthesia. Anesthesiology 3:412, 1942
3. Foldes GG, McNall PG, Borrego-Hinojosa JM: Succinylcholine: a new approach to muscular relaxation in anesthesiology. N Engl J Med 247:596, 1952
4. Foldes FF: The impact of neuromuscular blocking agents on the development of anaesthesia and surgery. In Agoston S, Bowman WC (eds): Muscle Relaxants: Monographs in Anaesthesiology 2nd Ed. Vol. 19. Elsevier, New York, 1990
5. Baraka A: Irreversible curarization. Anaesthesiol Intensive Care 5:244, 1977
6. Caldwell JE, Robertson EN, Baird WLM: Antagonism of profound neuromuscular blockade induced by vecuronium or atracurium: comparison of neostigmine with edrophonium. Br J Anaesth 58:1285, 1986
7. Magorian T, Lynam DP, Caldwell JE et al: Can early administration of neostigmine, in single or repeated doses, alter the course of neuromuscular recovery from a vecuronium-induced neuromuscular blockade? Anesthesiology 73:410, 1990
8. Donati F, Lahoud J, McCready D et al: Neostigmine, pyridostigmine, and edrophonium as antagonists of deep pancuronium blockade. Can J Anaesth 34:589, 1987
9. Kalow W: The distribution, destruction, and elimination of muscle relaxants. Anesthesiology 20:505, 1959

10. Donati F, Plaud B, Meistelman D: Vecuronium neuromuscular blockade at the adductor muscles of the larynx and at the adductor pollicis. Anesthesiology 74:833, 1991

11. Meistelman C, Plaud B, Donati F: Rocuronium (ORG 9426) neuromuscular blockade at the adductor muscles of the larynx and adductor pollicis in humans. Can J Anaesth 39:665, 1992

12. Lebrault C, Chauvin M, Guirmand F et al: Relative potency of vecuronium on the diaphragm and the adductor pollicis. Br J Anaesth 63:389, 1989

13. Laycock JRD, Donati F, Smith CE et al: Potency of atracurium and vecuronium at the diaphragm and the adductor pollicis muscle. Br J Anaesth 61:286, 1988

14. Beemer GH, Reeves JH, Bjorksten AR: Accurate monitoring of neuromuscular blockade using a peripheral nerve stimulator—a review. Anaesthesiol Intensive Care 18:490, 1990

15. Hudes E, Lee KC: Clinical use of peripheral nerve stimulators in anaesthesia. Can J Anaesth 34:525, 1987

16. Viby-Mogensen J: Clinical assessment of neuromuscular transmission. Br J Anaesth 54:209, 1982

17. Ali HH, Savarese JJ: Monitoring of neuromuscular function. Anesthesiology 45:216, 1976

18. Ali HH: Monitoring of neuromuscular function and clinical interaction. p. 447. In Norman J (ed): Clinics in Anesthesiology. Vol. 3. WB Saunders, Philadelphia, 1985

19. Ali HH, Savarese JJ: Stimulus frequency and dose response to d-tubocurarine in man. Anesthesiology 52:36, 1980

20. Ali HH, Utting JE, Gray TC: Stimulus frequency in the detection of neuromuscular block in man. Br J Anaesth 42:967, 1970

21. Lee CM: Train-of-four quantitation of competitive neuromuscular block. Anesth Analg 54:649, 1975

22. Kopman AF: Tactile evaluation of train-of-four count as an indicator of reliability of antagonism from vecuronium or atracurium-induced neuromuscular blockade. Anesthesiology 75:588, 1991

23. Gissen AJ, Katz RL: Twitch, tetanus, and post tetanic potentiation as indices of neuromuscular block in man. Anesthesiology 30:481, 1969

24. Viby-Mogensen J, Howardy-Hansen P, Chraemmer-Jorgensen B et al: Postetanic count (PTC): a new method of evaluating an intense nondepolarizing block. Anesthesiology 55:458, 1981

25. Bonu AK, Viby-Mogensen J, Fernando PUE et al: Relationship of post-tetanic count and train-of-four response during intense neuromuscular blockade

caused by atracurium. Br J Anaesth 59:1089, 1987

26. Fernando PUE, Viby-Mogensen J, Bonus AK et al: Relationship between posttetanic count and response to carinal stimulation during vecuronium-induced neuromuscular blockade. Acta Anaesthesiol Scand 31:593, 1987

27. Chauvin M, Lebrault C, Duvaldestin P: The neuromuscular blocking effect of vecuronium on the human diaphragm. Anesth Analg 66:117, 1987

28. Scheller MS, Zornow MH, Saidman LJ: Tracheal intubation without the use of muscle relaxants: a technique using propofol and varying doses of alfentanil. Anesth Analg 75:788, 1992

29. Vandenbrom RHG, Wierda JMKH, Huizinga ACT et al: Intubation conditions and time-course of action of ORG 9426. Anesthesiology 75:A788, 1991

30. Dubois M, Shearrow T, Tran D et al: ORG 9426 used for endotracheal intubation: a comparison with succinylcholine. Anesthesiology 75:A1066, 1991

31. Puhringer FK, Khuenl-Brady KS, Koller J et al: Evaluation of the endotracheal intubating conditions of rocuronium (ORG 9426) and succinylcholine in outpatient surgery. Anesth Analg 75:37, 1992

32. Cooper R, Mirakhur RK, Clarke RSJ et al: Comparison of intubating conditions after administration of ORG 9426 (rocuronium) and suxamethonium. Br J Anaesth 69:269, 1992

33. Tryba M, Zorn A, Thole H et al: Crash-induction with ORG 9426 vs succinylcholine: a randomized double blind study. Anesthesiology 77:A962, 1992

34. Tullock WC, Duana P, Cook DR et al: Neuromuscular and cardiovascular effects of high-dose vecuronium. Anesth Analg 70:86, 1990

35. Ginsberg B, Glass PS, Quill T et al: Onset and duration of neuromuscular blockade following high-dose vecuronium administration. Anesthesiology 71:201, 1989

36. Schwartz S, Ilias W, Lachner F et al: Rapid tracheal intubation with vecuronium: the priming principle. Anesthesiology 62:388, 1985

37. Mehta MP, Choi WW, Gergis SD et al: Facilitation of rapid endotracheal intubation with divided doses of nondepolarizing neuromuscular blocking drugs. Anesthesiology 62:392, 1985

38. Waud BE, Waud DR: The margin of safety of neuromuscular transmission in the muscle of the diaphragm. Anesthesiology 37:417, 1972

39. D'Honneur G, Gall O, Gerard A et al: Priming doses of atracurium and vecuronium depress swallowing in humans. Anesthesiology 77:1070, 1992

40. Donati F: The priming saga: where do we stand now? Can J Anaesth 35:1, 1988

41. Jones RM: The priming principle: how does it work and should we be using it? Br J Anaesth 63:1, 1989

42. Maizner J: Awareness, muscle relaxants, and balanced anesthesia. Can J Anaesth 26:386, 1979

43. Cannon JW, Fahey MR, Castagnoli KP et al: Continuous infusion of vecuronium: the effect of anesthetic agents. Anesthesiology 67:503, 1987

44. Gencarelli PJ, Miller RD, Eger EI et al: Decreasing enflurane concentrations and d-tubocurarine neuromuscular blockade. Anesthesiology 56:192, 1982

45. Weber S, Brandom BW, Bowers DM et al: Mivacurium chloride (BW B1090U)-induced neuromuscular blockade during N_2O-isoflurane and N_2O-narcotic anesthesia in adult surgical patients. Anesth Analg 67:495, 1988

46. Brett RS, Dilger JP, Yland KF: Isoflurane causes "flickering" of the acetylcholine receptor channel: observations using the patch clamp. Anesthesiology 69:161, 1988

47. Gill SS, Bevan DR, Donati FF: Edrophonium antagonism of atracurium during enflurane anaesthesia. Br J Anaesth 64:300, 1990

48. Baurain MJ, d'Hollander AA, Melot C et al: Effects of residual concentrations of isoflurane on the reversal of vecuronium-induced neuromuscular blockade. Anesthesiology 74:474, 1991

49. Beemer GH, Bjorksten AR, Dawson PJ et al: Determinants of the reversal time of competitive neuromuscular block by anticholinesterases. Br J Anaesth 66:469, 1991

50. Basta SJ, Savarese JJ, Ali HH et al: Clinical pharmacology of doxacurium chloride. Anesthesiology 69:478, 1988

51. Brandom BW, Meretoja OA, Taivainen et al: Accelerated onset and delayed recovery of neuromuscular block induced by mivacurium preceded by pancuronium in children. Anesth Analg 76:998, 1993

52. Kay B, Chesnut RJ, Sum Ping JST et al: Economy in the use of muscle relaxants. Anaesthesia 42:277, 1987

53. Bevan DR, Smith CE, Donati F: Postoperative neuromuscular blockade: A comparison between atracurium, vecuronium, and pancuronium. Anesthesiology 69:272, 1988

54. Ali HH, Savarese JJ, Embree PB et al: Clinical pharmacology of mivacurium chloride (BW1090U) infusion: comparison with vecuronium and atracurium. Br J Anaesth 61:541, 1988

55. Kopman AF: Recovery times following edrophonium and neostigmine reversal of pancuronium, atracurium, and vecuronium steady-state infusions. Anesthesiology 65:572, 1986

56. Savarese JJ, Ali HH, Basta SJ et al: The clinical neuromuscular pharmacology of mivacurium chloride (BW B10909U). Anesthesiology 68:723, 1988

57. Tassonyi E, Neidhart P, Pittet J et al: Cardiovascular effects of pipecuronium and pancuronium in patients undergoing coronary artery bypass grafting. Anesthesiology 69:793, 1988

58. Mellinghoff H, Diefenbach CL, Buzello W: Neuromuscular and cardiovascular properties of ORG 9426. Anesthesiology 75:A807, 1991

59. Paton WDM: Histamine release by compounds of single chemical structure. Pharmacol Rev 9:269, 1957

60. Hughes R, Chapple DJ: Effects of non-depolarizing neuromuscular blocking agents on peripheral autonomic mechanisms in cats. Br J Anaesth 48:59, 1976

61. Hughes R, Chapple DJ: Cardiovascular and neuromuscular effects of dimethyltubocurarine in anaesthetized cats and rhesus monkeys. Br J Anaesth 48:847, 1976

62. Savarese JJ, Ali HH, Basta SJ et al: The cardiovascular effects of mivacurium chloride (BW B1090U) in patients receiving nitrous oxide-opioid-barbiturate anesthesia. Anesthesiology 70:386, 1989

63. Scott RPF, Savarese JJ, Ali HH et al: Atracurium: clinical strategies for preventing histamine release and attenuating the hemodynamic response. Anesthesiology 61:A287, 1984

64. Basta SJ, Savarese JJ, Ali HH et al: Histamine-releasing properties of atracurium, dimethyltubocurarine, and tubocurarine. Br J Anaesth 55:1055, 1983

65. Choi WW, Mehta MP, Murray DJ et al: Neuromuscular and cardiovascular effects of mivacurium chloride in surgical patients receiving nitrous oxide-narcotic or nitrous oxide-isoflurane anaesthesia. Can J Anaesth 36:641, 1989

66. From RP, Pearson KS, Choi WW et al: Neuromuscular and cardiovascular effects of mivacurium chloride (BW B1090U) during nitrous oxide-fentanyl-thiopentane and, nitrous oxide-halothane anaesthesia. Br J Anaesth 64:193, 1990

67. Stoops CM, Curtis CA, Kovach DA et al: Hemodynamic effects of doxacurium chloride in patients receiving oxygen sufentanil anesthesia for coronary artery bypass grafting or valve replacement. Anesthesiology 69:356, 1988

68. Upton RA, Nguyen TL, Miller RD et al: Renal and biliary elimination of vecuronium (ORG NC 45) and pancuronium in rats. Anesth Analg 61:313, 1982

69. Lynam DP, Cronnelly R, Castagnoli KP et al: The pharmacokinetics and pharmacodynamics of vecuronium in patients anesthetized with isoflurane with normal renal function or with renal failure. Anesthesiology 69:227, 1988

70. Waser PG, Wiederkehr H, Sin-Ren AC et al: Distribution and kinetics of vecuronium in rats and mice. Br J Anaesth 59:1044, 1987

71. Bevan DR, Donati F, Gyasi H et al: Vecuronium in renal failure. Can J Anaesth 31:491, 1984

72. Smith CL, Hunter JM, Jones RS: Vecuronium infusions in patients with renal failure in an ITU. Anaesthesia 42:387, 1987

73. Segredo V, Matthay MA, Sharma ML et al: Prolonged neuromuscular blockade after long-term administration of vecuronium in two critically ill patients. Anesthesiology 72:566, 1990

74. Segredo V, Caldwell JE, Matthay MA et al: Persistent paralysis in critically ill patients after long-term administration of vecuronium. N Engl J Med 327:524, 1992

75. Marshall IG, Gibb AJ, Durant NN: Neuromuscular and vagal blocking actions of pancuronium bromide, its metabolites, and vecuronium bromide (ORG NC45) and its potential metabolites in the anaesthetized cat. Br J Anaesth 55:703, 1983

76. Bencini AF, Houwertjes MC, Agoston S: Effects of hepatic uptake of vecuronium bromide and its putative metabolites on their neuromuscular blocking actions in the cat. Br J Anaesth 57:789, 1985

77. Segredo V, Shin Y-S, Sharma ML et al: Pharmacokinetics, neuromuscular effects, and biodisposition of 3-desacetylvecuronium (ORG 7268) in cats. Anesthesiology 74:1052, 1991

78. Cook DR, Stiller RL, Weakly JN et al: *In vitro* metabolism of mivacurium chloride (BW B1090U) and succinylcholine. Anesth Analg 68:452, 1989

79. Ostergaard D, Jensen FS, Jensen E et al: Influence of plasma cholinesterase activity on recovery from mivacurium-induced neuromuscular blockade in phenotypically normal patients. Acta Anaesthesiol Scand 36:702, 1992

80. Ostergaard D, Jensen E, Jensen FS et al: The duration of action of mivacurium-induced neuromuscular block in patients homozygous for the atypical plasma cholinesterase gene. Anesthesiology 75:A774, 1991

81. Petersen RS, Bailey PL, Kalameghan R et al: Prolonged neuromuscular block after mivacurium. Anesth Analg 76:194, 1993

82. Goudsouzian NG, d'Hollander AA, Viby-Mogensen J: Prolonged neuromuscular block from mivacu-

83. Maddineni VR, Mirakhur RK: Prolonged neuromuscular block following mivacurium. Anesthesiology 78:1181, 1993

84. Viby-Mogensen J: Succinylcholine neuromuscular blockade in subjects homozygous for atypical plasma cholinesterase. Anesthesiology 55:429, 1981

85. Scholler KL, Goedde HW, Benkman H-G: The use of serum cholinesterase in succinylcholine apnoea. Can J Anaesth 24:396, 1977

86. Bownes PB, Hartman GS, Chisolm D et al: Antagonism of mivacurium blockade by purified human butyryl cholinesterase in cats. Anesthesiology 77:A909, 1992

87. Mangar D, Kirchoff GT, Rose PT et al: Prolonged neuromuscular block after mivacurium in a patient with end-stage renal disease. Anesth Analg 76:866, 1993

88. Phillips BJ, Hunter JM: Use of mivacurium chloride by constant infusion in the anephric patient. Br J Anaesth 68:492, 1992

89. Robertson GS: Serum cholinesterase deficiency. 1: Disease and inheritance. Br J Anaesth 38:355, 1966

90. Thomas JL, Holmes JH: Effect of hemodialysis on plasma cholinesterase. Anesth Analg 49:323, 1970

91. Ryan DW: Preoperative serum cholinesterase concentration in chronic renal failure. Clinical experience of suxamethonium in 81 patients undergoing renal transplant. Br J Anaesth 49:945, 1977

92. Cook DR, Freeman JA, Lai AA et al: Pharmacokinetics of mivacurium in normal patients and in those with hepatic or renal failure. Br J Anaesth 69:580, 1992

93. Viby-Mogensen J: Correlation of succinylcholine duration of action with plasma cholinesterase activity in subjects with the genotypically normal enzyme. Anesthesiology 53:517, 1980

94. Wildsmith JAW: Serum cholinesterase, pregnancy, and suxamethonium. Anaesthesia 27:90, 1972

95. Viby-Mogensen J, Hanel HK: Prolonged apnoea after suxamethonium. An analysis of the first 225 cases reported to the Danish Cholinesterase Research Unit. Acta Anaesthesiol Scand 22:371, 1978

96. Kaniaris P, Fassoulaki A, Liarmakopoulou K et al: Serum cholinesterase levels in patients with cancer. Anesth Analg 58:82, 1979

97. Sunew KY, Hicks RG: Effects of neostigmine and pyridostigmine on duration of succinylcholine action and pseudocholinesterase activity. Anesthesiology 49:188, 1978

98. Lubin AH, Garry PJ, Owen GM: Sex and popula-

tion differences in the incidence of plasma cholinesterase varient. Science 173:161, 1971

99. Cottrell JE, Hartung J, Griffin JP: Intracranial and hemodynamic changes after succinylcholine administration in cats. Anesth Analg 62:1006, 1983

100. McLeskey CH, Cullen BF, Kennedy RD et al: Control of cerebral perfusion pressure during induction of anesthesia in high-risk neurosurgical patients. Anesth Analg 53:985, 1974

101. Lanier WL, Milde JH, Michenfelder JD: Cerebral stimulation following succinylcholine in dogs. Anesthesiology 64:551, 1986

102. Minton MD, Grosslight K, Stirt JA et al: Increases in intracranial pressure with succinylcholine: Prevention with prior non-depolarizing blockade. Anesthesiology 65:165, 1986

103. Dillon JB, Sabaeala P, Taylor DB et al: Action of succinylcholine on extraocular muscles and intraocular pressure. Anesthesiology 18:44, 1957

104. Pandey K, Badola RP, Kumr S: Time course of intraocular hypertension produced by suxamethonium. Br J Anaesth 44:191, 1972

105. Lavery GG, McGailliard JN, Mirakhur RK et al: The effects of atracurium on intraocular pressure during steady state and rapid sequence induction: a comparison with succinylcholine. Can J Anaesth 33:437, 1986

106. Miller RD, Way WL, Hickey RF: Inhibition of succinylcholine induced increased intraocular pressure by non-depolarizing muscle relaxants Anesthesiology 29:123, 1968

107. Myers EF, Krupin T, Johnson M et al: Failure of nondepolarizing blockers to inhibit succinylcholine induced increased intraocular pressure, a controlled study. Anesthesiology 48:149, 1978

108. Libonati MM, Leahy JJ, Ellison N: The use of succinylcholine in open eye surgery. Anesthesiology 62:637, 1985

109. Pace NL: Prevention of succinylcholine myalgias: a meta-analysis. Anesth Analg 70:477, 1990

110. Gordon RA: Malignant hyperpyrexia during general anesthesia. Can J Anaesth 13:415, 1966

111. Hall LW, Woolf N, Bradley JWP et al: Unusual reaction to suxamethonium chloride. BMJ 2:1305, 1966

112. Donlon JV, Newfield P, Streter F et al: Implications of masseter spasm after succinylcholine. Anesthesiology 49:298, 1978

113. Van Der Spek AFL, Fang WB, Aston-Miller JA et al: Increased masticatory muscle stiffness during limb muscle flaccidity associated with succinylcholine administration. Anesthesiology 69:11, 1988

114. Gronert GA: Management of patients in whom trismus occurs following succinylcholine (letter). Anesthesiology 68:653, 1988

115. Rosenberg H: Trismus is not trivial. Anesthesiology 67:453, 1987

116. Fisher DM: Should succinylcholine continue to be used routinely in pediatric anesthesia? p. 394. In Rupp SM (ed): Problems in Anesthesia. Vol. 3. JB Lippincott, Philadelphia, 1989

117. Weintraub HD, Heisterkamp DV, Cooperman LH: Changes in plasma potassium concentration after depolarizing blockers in anaesthetized man. Br J Anaesth 41:1048, 1969

118. Martyn J, Goldhill DR, Goudsouzian NG: Clinical pharmacology of muscle relaxants in patients with burns. J Clin Pharmacol 26:680, 1986

119. Mazze RI, Escue HM, Houston JB: Hyperkalemia and cardiovascular collapse following administration of succinylcholine to the traumatized patient. Anesthesiology 31:540, 1969

120. Smith RB: Hyperkalemia following succinylcholine administration in neurological disorders. Can J Anaesth 18:199, 1971

121. Fung DL, White DA, Jones BR et al: The onset of disuse-related potassium efflux to succinylcholine. Anesthesiology 75:650, 1991

122. Gronert GA, Theye RA: Pathophysiology of hyperkalemia induced by succinylcholine. Anesthesiology 43:89, 1975

123. Martyn JAJ, White DA, Gronert GA et al: Up-and-down regulation of skeletal muscle acetylcholine receptors. Anesthesiology 76:822, 1992

124. Wierda JMKH, De Wit APM, Kuizenga K et al: Clinical observations on the neuromuscular blocking action of ORG 9426, a new steroidal non-depolarizing agent. Br J Anaesth 64:521, 1990

125. Rolly G, Debrock M, De May JC: Intubating conditions and time course of action of rocuronium bromide. Anesthesiology 77:A963, 1992

126. Cooper RA, Mirakhur RK, Maddineni VR: Neuromuscular effects of rocuronium bromide (ORG 9426) during fentanyl and halothane anaesthesia. Anaesthesia 48:103, 1993

127. Kaufman JA, Dubois MY, Chen YJ et al: Pharmacodynamic effects of vecuronium: a dose-response study. J Clin Anesth 1:434, 1989

128. Kerr WJ, Baird WLM: Clinical studies on ORG NC45: comparison with pancuronium. Br J Anaesth 54:1159, 1982

129. Cantineau JP, Parte F, Horns JB et al: Neuromuscular blocking effect of ORG 9426 on human diaphragm. Anesthesiology 75:A785, 1991

130. Donati F: Onset of action of relaxants. Can J Anaesth 35:S52, 1988

131. Donati F, Antzaka C, Bevan DR: Potency of pancuronium at the diaphragm and the adductor pollicis muscles in humans. Anesthesiology 65:1, 1986

132. Pansard JL, Chauvin M, Lebrault C et al: Effect of an intubating dose of succinylcholine or atracurium on the diaphragm and the adductor pollicis muscle in humans. Anesthesiology 67:326, 1987

133. Plaud B, Legueau F, Debaene B et al: Mivacurium neuromuscular blockade at the adductor muscles of the larynx and adductor pollicis in man. Anesthesiology 77:A908, 1992

134. Plaud B, Meistleman C, Donati F: Organon 9426 neuromuscular blockade at the adductor muscles of the larynx and adductor pollicis in man. Anesthesiology 75:A784, 1991

135. Bowman WC, Rodger IW, Houston J et al: Structure:action relationships among some desacetoxy analogues of pancuronium and vecuronium in the anesthetized cat. Anesthesiology 69:57, 1988

136. Kopman AF: Gallamine, pancuronium and d-tubocurarine compared: is onset time related to drug potency? Anesthesiology 70:915, 1989

137. Brucke H, Ginzel KH, Klupp H et al: Bis-cholinester von dicarbonsäuren als muskelrelaxantien in der narkose. Wien Klin Wochenschr 63:464, 1951

138. Browne JG, Collier HOJ, Somers GF: Succinylcholine (succinoxylcholine): muscle relaxant of short duration. Lancet 1:1225, 1952

139. Lee C, Katz RL: Dose relationships of phase II, tachyphylaxis, and train-of-four fade in suxamethonium induced neuromuscular block in man. Br J Anaesth 47:841, 1975

140. Ramsey FM, Lebowitz PW, Savarese JJ et al: The clinical characteristics of long term succinylcholine neuromuscular blockade during balanced anesthesia. Anesth Analg 59:110, 1980

141. Hilgenberg JC, Stoelting RK: Characteristics of succinylcholine-induced phase II neuromuscular block during enflurane, halothane, and fentanyl anesthesia. Anesth Analg 60:192, 1981

142. Foldes FF, McNall PG, Birch JH: The neuromuscular activity of succinylmonocholine in man. BMJ 1:967, 1954

143. Litwiller RW: Succinylcholine hydrolysis: a review. Anesthesiology 29:1014, 1969

144. Caldwell JE, Heir T, Kitts JB et al: Comparison of the neuromuscular block induced by mivacurium, suxamethonium, or atracurium during nitrous oxide-fentanyl anaesthesia. Br J Anaesth 63:393, 1989

145. Lien CA, Schmith VD, Wargin WA et al: Pharmacokinetics and pharmacodynamics of mivacurium stereoisomers during a two-step infusion. Anesthesiology 77:A910, 1992

146. Head-Rapson AG, Devlin JC, Lovell GG Et al: Pharmacokinetics of the isomers of mivacurium chloride in the healthy adult. Br J Anaesth 70:487P, 1993

147. Smith CE, Donati F, Bevan DR: Potency of succinylcholine at the diaphragm and at the adductor pollicis muscle. Anesth Analg 67:625, 1988

148. Smith CE, Donati F, Bevan DR: Dose-response curves for succinylcholine: single vs cumulative techniques. Anesthesiology 69:338, 1988

149. Szalados JE, Donati F, Bevan DR: Effect of d-tubocurarine pretreatment on succinylcholine twitch augmentation and neuromuscular blockade. Anesth Analg 71:55, 1990

150. Chestnut RJ, Healy TEJ, Harper NJN et al: Suxamethonium—the relation between dose and response. Anaesthesia 44:14, 1989

151. Smith CE, Donati F, Bevan DR: Effects of succinylcholine at the masseter and adductor pollicis muscles in adults. Anesth Analg 69:158, 1989

152. Eisenkraft JB, Mingus ML, Herlich A et al: A defasciculating dose of d-tubocurarine causes resistance to succinylcholine. Can J Anaesth 37:538, 1990

153. Scott RPF, Goat VA: Atracurium: its speed of onset. A comparison with suxamethonium. Br J Anaesth 54:909, 1982

154. Blackburn CL, Morgan M: Comparison of speed of onset of fazadinium, pancuronium, d-tubocurarine, and suxamethonium. Br J Anaesth 50:361, 1978

155. Harrison GA, Junius F: Effect of circulation time on the neuromuscular action of suxamethonium. Anaesthesiol Intensive Care 1:33, 1972

156. Manchikanti L, Grow JB, Colliver JA et al: Atracurium pretreatment for succinylcholine-induced fasciculations and postoperative myalgia. Anesth Analg 64:1010, 1985

157. Fragen RJ, Shanks CA: Is there an ideal outpatient muscle relaxant? p. 69. In Wetchler BV (ed): Problems in Anesthesia—Outpatient Anesthesia. JB Lippincott, Philadelphia, 1988

158. Savarese JJ, Kitz R: Does clinical anesthesia need new neuromuscular blocking agents? Anesthesiology 42:236, 1975

159. Dresner DL, Basta SJ, Ali HH et al: Pharmacokinetics and pharmacodynamics of doxacurium in young and elderly patients during isoflurane anesthesia. Anesth Analg 71:498, 1990

160. Murray DJ, Mehta MP, Choi WW et al: The neuromuscular blocking and cardiovascular effects of doxacurium chloride in patients receiving nitrous

oxide narcotic anesthesia. Anesthesiology 69:472, 1988

161. Emmot RS, Bracey BJ, Goldhill DR et al: Cardiovascular effects of doxacurium, pancuronium, and vecuronium in anaesthetized patients presenting for coronary artery bypass surgery. Br J Anaesth 65:480, 1990

162. Lennon R, Hosking MP, Houck PC et al: Doxacurium chloride for neuromuscular blockade before tracheal intubation and surgery during nitrous oxide-oxygen-narcotic-enflurane anesthesia. Anesth Analg 68:255, 1989

163. Lien CA, Matteo RS, Ornstein E et al: Neostigmine antagonism of doxacurium or pancuronium blockade under isoflurane. Anesthesiology 77:A959, 1992

164. Stinson LW, Lennon RL: Comparison of doxacurium, pancuronium, and pipecuronium train-of-four recovery after pharmacological antagonism. Anesthesiology 77:A928, 1992

165. Cook DR, Freeman JA, Lai AA et al: Pharmacokinetics and pharmacodynamics of doxacurium in normal patients and in those with hepatic or renal failure. Anesth Analg 72:145, 1991

166. Boros M, Szenohradsky J, Marosi G et al: Comparative clinical study of pipecuronium bromide and pancuronium bromide. Drug Res 30:389, 1980

167. Wierda JMKH, Richardson FJ, Agoston S: Dose-response relation and time course of action of pipecuronium bromide in humans anesthetized and nitrous oxide and isoflurane, halothane, or droperidol and fentanyl. Anesth Analg 68:208, 1989

168. Larijani GE, Bartkowski RR, Azad SS et al: Clinical pharmacology of pipecuronium bromide. Anesth Analg 68:734, 1989

169. Caldwell JE, Canfell PC, Castagnoli KP et al: The influence of renal failure on the pharmacokinetics and duration of action of pipecuronium bromide in patients anesthetized with halothane and nitrous oxide. Anesthesiology 70:7, 1989

170. Vereczkey L, Szporny L: Disposition of pipecuronium bromide in rats. Drug Res 30:364, 1980

171. Khuenl-Brady KS, Sharma M, Chung K et al: Pharmacokinetics and disposition of pipecuronium bromide in dogs with and without ligated renal pedicles. Anesthesiology 71:919, 1989

172. Ornstein E, Matteo RS, Schwartz AE et al: Pharmacokinetics and pharmacodynamics of pipecuronium bromide (Arduan) in elderly surgical patients. Anesth Analg 74:841, 1992

173. Viby-Mogensen J, Jørgensen BC, Ørding H: Residual curarization in the recovery room. Anesthesiology 50:539, 1979

174. Hutton P, Burchett KR, Madden AP: Comparison of recovery after neuromuscular blockade by atracurium or pancuronium. Br J Anaesth 60:36, 1988

175. Gibson FM, Mirakhur RK, Clarke RSJ et al: Comparison of cumulative and single bolus dose technique for determining the potency of vecuronium. Br J Anaesth 57:1060, 1985

176. O'Hara DA, Fragen RJ, Shanks CA: The effects of age on the dose response curve of vecuronium in adults. Anesthesiology 63:542, 1985

177. Ørding H, Skovgaard LT, Engbaek J et al: Dose response curves for vecuronium during halothane and neurolept anesthesia: single bolus vs cumulative method. Acta Anaesthesiol Scand 29:121, 1985

178. Engbaek J, Ørding H, Pedersen T et al: Dose response relationships and neuromuscular blocking effects of vecuronium and pancuronium during ketamine anesthesia. Br J Anaesth 56:953, 1984

179. Bencini AF, Scaf AHJ, Sohn YJ et al: Hepatobiliary disposition of vecuronium bromide in man. Br J Anaesth 58:988, 1985

180. Lebrault C, Berger JL, D'Hollander AA et al: Pharmacokinetics and pharmacodynamics of vecuronium (ORG NC45) in patients with cirrhosis. Anesthesiology 62:601, 1985

181. Fahey MR, Morris RB, Miller RD et al: Pharmacokinetics or ORG 45 (Norcuron) in patients with and without renal failure. Br J Anaesth 53:1049, 1981

182. Caldwell JE, Castagnoli KP, Canfell PC et al: Pipecuronium and pancuronium: comparison of pharmacokinetics and duration of action. Br J Anaesth 61:693, 1988

183. Rupp SM, Castagnoli KP, Fisher DM et al: Pancuronium and vecuronium pharmacokinetics and pharmacodynamics in young and elderly adults. Anesthesiology 67:45, 1987

184. Cronnelly R, Fisher DM, Miller RD et al: Pharmacokinetics and pharmacodynamics of vecuronium (NC 45) and pancuronium in anesthetized humans. Anesthesiology 58:405, 1983

185. Bencini AF, Scaf AHJ, Sohn YJ et al: Disposition and urinary excretion of vecuronium bromide in anesthetized patients with normal renal function or renal failure. Anesth Analg 65:245, 1986

186. Sohn YJ, Bencini AF, Scaf AHJ et al: Comparative pharmacokinetics and dynamics of vecuronium and pancuronium in anesthetized patients. Anesth Analg 65:233, 1986

187. Schwartz AE, Matteo RS, Ornstein E et al: Pharmacokinetics and pharmacodynamics of vecuronium in

the obese surgical patients. Anesth Analg 74:515, 1992

188. Robertson EN, Booij LHDJ, Fragen RJ et al: Clinical comparison of atracurium and vecuronium (ORG NC 45). Br J Anaesth 55:125, 1983

189. Agoston S, Salt P, Newton D et al: The neuromuscular blocking action of ORG NC 45, a new pancuronium derivative, in anaesthetized patients. Br J Anaesth 52:53S, 1980

190. Erkola O, Karhunen U, Sandelin-Hellqvist E: Spontaneous recovery of residual neuromuscular blockade after atracurium or vecuronium during isoflurane anaesthesia. Acta Anaesthesiol Scand 33:290, 1989

191. Buzello W, Noldge G: Repetitive administration of pancuronium and vecuronium (ORG NC 45, Norcuron) in patients undergoing long lasting operations. Br J Anaesth 54:1151, 1982

192. Fisher DM, Rosen JI: Pharmacokinetic explanation for increasing recovery time following larger or repeated doses of nondepolarizing muscle relaxants. Anesthesiology 65:286, 1986

193. Weinstein JA, Matteo RS, Ornstein E et al: Pharmacodynamics of vecuronium and atracurium in the obese surgical patient. Anesth Analg 67:1149, 1988

194. d'Hollander A, Massaux F, Nelelstein M et al: Age dependent dose response relationships or ORG NC 45 in anesthetized patients. Br J Anaesth 54:653, 1982

195. Meretoja OA: Is vecuronium a long-acting neuromuscular blocking agent in infants and neonates? Br J Anaesth 62:184, 1989

196. Lien CA, Matteo RS, Ornstein E et al: Distribution, elimination and action of vecuronium in the elderly. Anesth Analg 73:39, 1991

197. Durant NN, Marshall IG, Savage DS et al: The neuromuscular and autonomic blocking activities of pancuronium. ORG NC 45, and other pancuronium analogs in the cat. J Pharm Pharmacol 31:831, 1979

198. Marshall IG, Agoston S, Booij LHDJ et al: Pharmacology of ORG NC 45 compared with other nondepolarizing neuromuscular blocking drugs. Br J Anaesth 52:11S, 1980

199. Goudsouzian NG, Young ET, Moss J et al: Histamine release during administration of atracurium or vecuronium in children. Br J Anaesth 58:1229, 1986

200. Cannon JE, Fahey MR, Moss J et al: Large doses of vecuronium and plasma histamine concentrations. Can J Anaesth 35:350, 1988

201. Morris RB, Cahalan MK, Miller RD et al: The cardiovascular effects of vecuronium (ORG NC 45) and pancuronium in patients undergoing coronary artery bypass surgery. Anesthesiology 58:438, 1983

202. Tullock WC, Wilks DH, Brandom BW et al: ORG 9426: single-dose response, onset, and duration with halothane anesthesia. Anesthesiology 73:A877, 1990

203. Quill TJ, Begin M, Glass PSA et al: Clinical responses to ORG 9426 during isoflurane anesthesia. Anesth Analg 72:203, 1991

204. Oris B, Vandermeersch E, Van Aken H et al: Dose-response relationship of ORG 9426 during halothane, isoflurane, enflurane, and intravenous anesthesia. Anesthesiology 75:A1063, 1991

205. Lambalk LM, De Wit APM, Wierda JMKH et al: Dose-response relationship and time course of action of ORG 9426. Anaesthesia 46:907, 1991

206. Cooper RA, Mirakhur RK, Elliot P: Estimation of the potency of ORG 9426 using two different modes of peripheral stimulation. Can J Anaesth 39:139, 1992

207. Booij LHD, Knape HTA: The neuromuscular blocking effect of ORG 9426. Anaesthesia 46:341, 1991

208. Tullock WC, Wilks DH, Brandom BW et al: ORG 9426: onset, intubating conditions, and clinical duration. Anesthesiology 75:A789, 1991

209. Foldes F, Nagashima H, Nguyen HD et al: The neuromuscular effects of ORG 9426 in patients receiving balanced anesthesia. Anesthesiology 75:191, 1991

210. Shanks CA, Fragen RJ, Ling D: Continuous intravenous infusion of rocuronium (ORG 9426) in patients receiving balanced, enflurane, or isoflurane anesthesia. Anesthesiology 78:649, 1993

211. Cooper R, Maddineni VR, Mirakhur RK et al: Pharmacokinetics of rocuronium (ORG 9426) in patients with and without impaired renal function. Br J Anaesth 70:482P, 1993

212. Matteo RS, Ornstein E, Schwartz AE et al: Pharmacokinetics and pharmacodynamics of ORG 9426 in elderly surgical patients. Anesthesiology 75:A1065, 1991

213. Szenohradszky J, Fisher DM, Segredo V et al: Pharmacokinetics of rocuronium bromide (ORG 9426) in patients with normal renal function or patients undergoing cadaver renal transplantation. Anesthesiology 77:899, 1992

214. Wierda JMKH, Kleef UW, Lambalk LM et al: The pharmacodynamics and pharmacokinetics of ORG 9426, a new non-depolarizing neuromuscular block-

ing agent, in patients anaesthetized with nitrous oxide, halothane, and fentanyl. Can J Anesth 38:430, 1991

215. Khuenl-Brady K, Castagnoli KP, Canfell PC et al: The neuromuscular blocking effects and pharmacokinetics of ORG 9426 and ORG 9616 in the cat. Anesthesiology 72:669, 1990

216. Bevan DR, Fiset P, Balendran P et al: Pharmacodynamic behavior of rocuronium in the elderly. Can J Anaesth 40:127, 1993

217. Muir AW, Houston J, Green KL et al: Effects of a new neuromuscular blocking agent (ORG 9426) in anaesthetized cats and pigs and in isolated nerve-muscle preparations. Br J Anaesth 63:400, 1989

218. Foldes FF, Nagashima H, Nguyen H et al: The clinical pharmacology of ORG 9426. In Bowman WC, Denissen PAF, Feldman S (eds): Neuromuscular Blocking Agents: Past, Present and Future. Excerpta Medica, Princeton, 1990

219. Stenlake JB, Waigh RD, Urwin J et al: Atracurium: conception and inception. Br J Anaesth 55:3S, 1983

220. Merrett RA, Thompson CW, Webb FW: In vitro degradation of atracurium in human plasma. Br J Anaesth 55:61, 1983

221. Stiller RL, Cook DR, Chakrovorti S: In vitro degradation of atracurium in human plasma. Br J Anaesth 57:1085, 1985

222. Cook DR, Stiller R, Ingram M: In vitro degradation of atracurium. Anesth Analg 65:543, 1986

223. Nigrovic V, Pandya JB, Auen M et al: Inactivation of atracurium in human and rat plasma. Anesth Analg 64:1047, 1985

224. Basta SJ, Ali HH, Savarese JJ et al: Clinical pharmacology of atracurium besylate (BW33A): a new non-depolarizing muscle relaxant. Anesth Analg 61:723, 1982

225. Gibson FM, Mirakhur RK, Lavery GG et al: Potency of atracurium: a comparison of single bolus and cumulative dose techniques. Anesthesiology 62:657, 1985

226. Ramsey FM, White PA, Stullken EH et al: Clinical use of atracurium during N_2O/O_2, fentanyl, and N_2O/O_2 enflurane regimens. Anesthesiology 61:328, 1984

227. Sokoll MD, Gergis SD, Mehta M et al: Safety and efficacy of atracurium (BW33A) in surgical patients receiving balanced or isoflurane anesthesia. Anesthesiology 58:450, 1983

228. Meretoja OA, Wirtavuori K: Two-dose technique to create an individual dose-response curve for atracurium. Anesthesiology 70:732, 1989

229. Gramstad L, Lilleaasen P, Minaas B: Onset time and

230. duration of action of atracurium, ORG NC 45, and pancuronium. Br J Anaesth 54:827, 1982

230. Mirakhur RK, Lavery GG, Clarke RSJ et al: Atracurium in clinical anaesthesia: effect of dosage on onset, duration, and conditions for tracheal intubation. Anaesthesia 40:801, 1985

231. Katz RL, Stirt J, Murray A et al: Neuromuscular effects of atracurium in man. Anesth Analg 61:730, 1982

232. Ornstein E, Matteo RS, Schwartz AE et al: The effect of phenytoin on the magnitude and duration of neuromuscular block following atracurium and vecuronium. Anesthesiology 67:191, 1987

233. Scott RPF, Savarese JJ, Basta SJ et al: Clinical pharmacology of atracurium given in high dose. Br J Anaesth 58:834, 1986

234. Haraldsted VY, Nielsen JW, Madsen JV et al: Maintenance of constant 95% neuromuscular blockade by adjustable infusion rates of pancuronium and atracurium. Br J Anaesth 60:491, 1988

235. d'Hollander AA, Luyckx C, Barvais L et al: Clinical evaluation of atracurium besylate requirements for a stable muscle relaxation during surgery. Lack of age related effects. Anesthesiology 59:237, 1983

236. Gramstad L, Lilleaasen P: Neuromuscular blocking effects of atracurium, vecuronium, and pancuronium during bolus and infusion administration. Br J Anaesth 57:1052, 1985

237. Ward S, Weatherley BC: Pharmacokinetics of atracurium and its metabolites. Br J Anaesth 58:6S, 1986

238. Ward S, Boheimer N, Weatherley BC et al: Pharmacokinetics of atracurium and its metabolites in patients with normal renal function, and in patients in renal failure. Br J Anaesth 59:697, 1987

239. de Bros FM, Lai A, Scott R et al: Pharmacokinetics and pharmacodynamics of atracurium during isoflurane anesthesia in normal and anephric patients. Anesth Analg 65:743, 1986

240. Fahey MR, Rupp SM, Fisher DM et al: The pharmacokinetics and pharmacodynamics of atracurium in patients with and without renal failure. Anesthesiology 61:699, 1984

241. Ward S, Neil EAM, Weatherley BC et al: Pharmacokinetics of atracurium besylate in healthy patients (after a single IV bolus dose). Br J Anaesth 55:113, 1983

242. Donati F, Gill SS, Bevan DR et al: Pharmacokinetics and pharmacodynamics of atracurium with and without previous suxamethonium administration. Br J Anaesth 66:557, 1991

243. Tsui D, Graham GG, Torda TA: The pharmacokinetics of atracurium isomers in vitro and in humans. Anesthesiology 67:722, 1987

244. Fisher DM, Canfell PC, Fahey MR et al: Elimination of atracurium in humans: contribution of Hofmann elimination and ester hydrolysis vs organ-based elimination. Anesthesiology 65:6, 1986

245. Parker CJR, Hunter JM: Pharmacokinetics of atracurium and laudanosine in patients with hepatic cirrhosis. Br J Anaesth 62:177, 1989

246. Ward S, Neill EAM: Pharmacokinetics of atracurium in acute hepatic failure (with acute renal failure). Br J Anaesth 55:1169, 1983

247. Mongin-Long D, Chabrol B, Baude C et al: Atracurium in patients with renal failure. Br J Anaesth 58:44S, 1986

248. Hunter JM, Jones RS, Utting JE: Use of atracurium in patients with no renal function. Br J Anaesth 54:1251, 1982

249. Kitts JB, Fisher DM, Canfell PC et al: Pharmacokinetics and pharmacodynamics of atracurium in the elderly. Anesthesiology 72:272, 1990

250. Bell PF, Mirakhur RK, Clarke RSJ: Dose-response studies of atracurium, vecuronium and pancuronium in the elderly. Anaesthesia 44:925, 1989

251. Kent AP, Parker CJR, Hunter JM: Pharmacokinetics of atracurium and laudanosine in the elderly. Br J Anaesth 63:661, 1989

252. Goudsouzian N, Liu LMP, Gionfriddo M et al: Neuromuscular effects of atracurium in infants and children. Anesthesiology 62:75, 1985

253. Goudsouzian NG, Martyn J, Rudd GD et al: Continuous infusion of atracurium in children. Anesthesiology 64:171, 1986

254. Brandom BW, Cook DR, Woelfel SK et al: Atracurium infusion requirements in children during halothane, isoflurane, and narcotic anesthesia. Anesth Analg 64:471, 1985

255. Sutherland GA, Squire IB, Gibb AJ et al: Neuromuscular blocking and autonomic effects of vecuronium and atracurium in the anaesthetized cat. Br J Anaesth 55:1119, 1983

256. Stirt JA, Murray AL, Katz RL et al: Atracurium during halothane anesthesia in humans. Anesth Analg 62:207, 1983

257. Hughes R, Payne JP: Clinical assessment of atracurium using single twitch and tetanic responses of the adductor pollicis muscles. Br J Anaesth 55:47S, 1983

258. Hosking MP, Lennon RL, Gronert GA: Combined H1 and H2 receptor blockade attenuates the cardiovascular effects of high dose atracurium for rapid sequence endotracheal intubation. Anesth Analg 67:1089, 1988

259. Scott RPF, Savarese JJ, Basta SJ: Atracurium; clinical strategies for preventing histamine release and attenuating the haemodynamic response. Br J Anaesth 57:550, 1985

260. Lanier WL, Milde JH, Michenfelder JD: The cerebral effects of pancuronium and atracurium in halothane anesthetized dogs. Anesthesiology 63:589, 1985

261. Shi W, Fahey MR, Fisher DM et al: Laudanosine (a metabolite of atracurium) increases the MAC of halothane in rabbits. Anesthesiology 63:584, 1985

262. Tateishi A, Zornow MH, Scheller MS et al: Electroencephalographic effects of laudanosine in an animal model of epilepsy. Br J Anaesth 62:548, 1989

263. Chapple DJ, Miller AA, Ward JB et al: Cardiovascular and neurological effects of laudanosine. Br J Anaesth 59:218, 1987

264. Shi WZ, Fahey MR, Fisher DM et al: Modification of central nervous system effects of laudanosine by inhalation anesthetics. Br J Anaesth 63:598, 1989

265. Fahey MR, Rupp SM, Canfell C et al: Effect of renal failure on laudanosine excretion in man. Br J Anaesth 57:1049, 1985

266. Yate PM, Flynn PJ, Arnold RW et al: Clinical experience and plasma laudanosine concentrations during infusion of atracurium in the ICU. Br J Anaesth 59:211, 1987

267. Parker CJR, Jones JE, Hunter JM: Disposition of infusions of atracurium and its metabolite laudanosine, in patients in renal and respiratory failure. Br J Anaesth 61:531, 1988

268. Curran MJ, Shaff L, Savarese JJ et al: Comparison of spontaneous recovery and neostigmine-accelerated recovery from mivacurium neuromuscular blockade. Anesthesiology 69:A528, 1988

269. Cook DR, Chakravorti S, Brandom BW et al: Effects of neostigmine, edrophonium, and succinylcholine on the *in vitro* metabolism of mivacurium: clinical correlates. Anesthesiology 77:A948, 1992

270. Goldhill DR, Whitehead JP, Emmot RS et al: Neuromuscular and clinical effects of mivacurium chloride in healthy adult patients during nitrous oxide-enflurane anaesthesia. Br J Anaesth 67:289, 1991

271. Maehr RB, Belmont MR, Wray DL et al: Autonomic and neuromuscular effects of mivacurium and its isomers in cats. Anesthesiology 75:A772, 1991

272. Basta SJ, Dresner DL, Shaff LP et al: Neuromuscular effects and pharmacokinetics of mivacurium in elderly patients under isoflurane anesthesia. Anesth Analg 68:S1, 1989

273. Lee C, Katz RL: Neuromuscular pharmacology: a clinical update and commentary. Br J Anaesth 52:173, 1980

274. Ducharme J, Donati F: Pharmacokinetics and pharmacodynamics of steroidal muscle relaxants. Anesthesiology Clin North Am 11:283, 1993

275. Donati F, Meistleman C, Plaud D: Vecuronium neuromuscular blockade at the diaphragm, the obicularis oculi and adductor pollicis muscles. Anesthesiology 73:870, 1990

276. Miller RD, Savarese JJ: Pharmacology of muscle relaxants and their antagonists. p. 394. In Miller RD (ed): Anesthesia. 3rd Ed. Churchill Livingstone, New York, 1990

Chapter 22

Clinical Pharmacology of Reversal of Neuromuscular Blockade

David R. Bevan

It is now more than 50 years since the introduction of neuromuscular blocking drugs (NMBDs) into clinical anesthetic practice.[1] Initially, in North America, they were used in small doses to supplement the muscle relaxation provided by inhalational agents, such as cyclopropane. At the end of surgery, recovery from paralysis was allowed to occur spontaneously, and reversal agents were seldom employed. However, when tubocurarine was introduced in England much larger doses were used,[2] and this, together with the realization that the use of curare seemed to be associated with increased anesthetic mortality rates,[3] encouraged the routine use of neostigmine to restore neuromuscular activity.

In the last 20 years, anesthetic practice has changed. Other anticholinesterase reversal agents, pyridostigmine and edrophonium, have been introduced as alternatives to neostigmine. Nevertheless, residual neuromuscular blockade remains a cause of postoperative morbidity and mortality. The introduction of nondepolarizing NMBDs with a more rapid rate of spontaneous recovery, such as atracurium and vecuronium, and more recently mivacurium, has again questioned the place of routine reversal of neuromuscular block. The widespread use of neuromuscular monitoring during anesthesia has heightened this awareness.

This chapter reviews the current status of reversal of neuromuscular blockade during anesthesia, describes the pharmacology of the commonly used reversal agents, discusses factors that may modify their effectiveness, summarizes problems that they may cause, and suggests a therapeutic regimen to ensure the return of adequate neuromuscular function. The aim of reversal is to restore effective neuromuscular activity, particularly with regard to the restoration of pulmonary ventilation and airway protection.

RESIDUAL NEUROMUSCULAR BLOCKADE

In 1979, Viby-Mogensen et al.[4] in Denmark demonstrated that 30 of 72 patients who had received NMBDs during anesthesia without monitoring of neuromuscular activity but with reversal using anticholinesterase demonstrated a train-of-four (TOF) ratio of less than 0.7 when examined in the recovery room after anesthesia. Since then, there have been several similar reports from centers around the world (Table 22-1). Characteristically, residual neuromuscular blockade can be identified in 20 to 50 percent of adult patients after the use of long-acting NMBDs, such as tubocurarine (d-tubo-curarine), pancuronium, gallamine, or alcuro-

Table 22-1 Incidence of Residual Neuromuscular Blockade After Anesthesia

Reference	Origin	NMBD	TOF <0.7	
			No.	%
Viby-Morgensen et al.[4] (1979)	Copenhagen, Denmark	TC/P/G	30/72	42
Lennmarken et al.[5] (1984)	Linköping, Sweden	P	12/48	25
Beemer and Rozental[6] (1986)	Melbourne, Australia	TC/P/G/Al	21/100	21
Andersen et al.[7] (1988)	Arhus, Denmark	P	6/30	20
		A	0/30	0
Bevan et al.[8] (1988)	Montreal, Canada	P	17/47	36
		A	2/46	4
		V	5/57	9
Brull et al.[9] (1991)	New Haven, CT	P	14/29	48
		V	2/24	8
Howardy-Hansen et al.[10] (1989)	Copenhagen, Denmark	G	5/10	50
		A	0/9	0
Jensen et al.[11] (1990)	Denmark	P	62/159	39
		A	3/171	2
		V	6/158	4

Abbreviations: A, atracurium; Al, alcuronium; TC, tubocurarine; G, gallamine; NMBD, neuromuscular blocking drug; TOF, train of four; V, vecuronium.

nium.[5–12] The weakness occurs despite the use of reversal agents and intraoperative neuromuscular monitoring. The incidence is much reduced when the intermediate-acting NMBDs, atracurium and vecuronium, are used.[8,11] In the only study performed in children, residual neuromuscular blockade was not seen after the use of pancuronium, vecuronium, or atracurium.[12]

The recognition of small degrees of neuromuscular weakness is difficult despite the use of several clinical tests, measurement of ventilatory variables, and neuromuscular monitoring. It may be impossible to obtain patient cooperation in the postanesthetic state, particularly for respiratory testing. Consequently, correlations have been established between neuromuscular monitoring and ventilatory function in conscious volunteers and with crude tests of muscle weakness, such as the head lift and hand grip, in awake volunteers and in patients after anesthesia.

Neuromuscular Monitoring

Usually, because of easy accessibility, neuromuscular monitoring during anesthesia is achieved by stimulating the ulnar nerve and observing or recording the response of the adductor pollicis or small muscles of the hand. Other nerve-muscle groups, such as the lateral popliteal-foot extensors and facial nerve-orbicularis oculis, have also been used, but their responses may not be equivalent to ulnar nerve-adductor pollicis monitoring. When small doses of d-tubocurarine were given to awake volunteers with simultaneous neuromuscular and ventilatory measurement, it was shown that statistically significant reductions in maximum inspiratory force were found only when the TOF was less than 0.7, although there was no reduction in vital capacity (Fig. 22-1).[13] Thus, a TOF of greater than 0.7 has become accepted as the "gold standard" toward which to aim in assessing the adequacy of recovery. However, it should be realized that even lesser degrees of block may be associated with minor symptoms of heavy eyelids, blurred vision, and difficulty in swallowing.[14,15] Also, TOF values of 0.5 have been suggested as adequate indices of recovery from atracurium and vecuronium because of their more rapid rate of recovery.[16]

Unfortunately, small degrees of neuromuscular

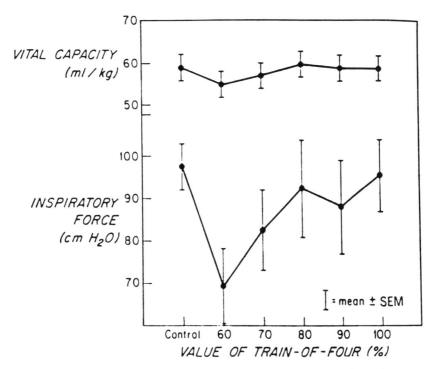

Fig. 22-1 Train-of-four ratio, inspiratory force, and vital capacity in awake volunteers given tubo-curarine. (From Ali et al.,[13] with permission.)

block are difficult to detect clinically either by tactile or visual inspection of the response to TOF stimulation. Experienced observers can correctly identify TOF fade clinically only when the average TOF ratio is less than 0.44.[17] Greater sensitivity is possible with double burst stimulation. Double burst stimulation consists of two short (60 ms) bursts of 50 Hz tetanic stimulation, separated by 75 ms, with a response of two short muscle contractions. Although the extent of double burst stimulation and TOF fade are similar, small degrees of neuromuscular block (equivalent to TOF of 0.6) can be detected with double burst stimulation but not with manual TOF monitoring (Fig. 22-2).[18] Tetanic stimulation with tactile evaluation of the response is no more sensitive than TOF monitoring.[19] The only means of detecting small degrees of fade is by recording the response by electromyography, accelerography, or mechanography.

Clinical testing of more profound block is sensitive and reproducible. Another variation of TOF monitoring, the TOF count, can also identify neuromuscular block. Using the TOF count, the fourth twitch becomes palpable when the ratio of T_1 to control (T_1/T_c) recovers to about 35 percent.[20] The TOF count can be used to predict the ease with which neuromuscular blockade can be reversed.

Clinical Tests

The most sensitive clinical test of residual neuromuscular blockade is the ability to maintain head lift for 5 seconds, but this is less sensitive than neuromuscular monitoring recorded by a force-displacement transducer. Of 26 patients who exhibited TOF less than 0.7 in the postanesthetic care unit, clinical weakness was detected in only nine patients (head lift in seven, hand grip in six, tongue protrusion in four, and eye opening in two). How-

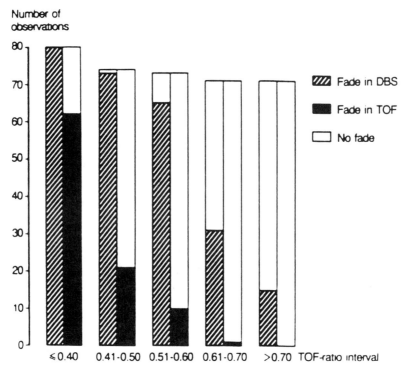

Fig. 22-2 Ability to detect responses to train-of-four and double burst stimulation during recovery from neuromuscular block. (From Drenck et al.,[18] with permission.)

ever, to ensure that no patient exhibited weakness, a TOF of 0.9 was required.[8] Head lift could not be sustained by any patient when the TOF was 0.5, by only 50 percent of patients at a TOF of 0.6, but by all patients at a TOF more than 0.8.[21]

Measurement of Ventilation

Measurement of ventilation is an inadequate monitor of neuromuscular blockade. Vital capacity and minute volume are maintained despite extensive neuromuscular block as long as airway patency is maintained. In contrast, measurement of maximum inspiratory force is a more sensitive monitor.[13] In awake volunteers given tubocurarine, Pavlin et al.[22] demonstrated that when the maximum inspiratory pressure (MIP) was reduced to -25 cmH$_2$O, none could swallow, maintain a patent airway, or lift their heads, although vital capacity was reduced by only 60 percent and the PaCO$_2$ remained normal. Head lift and leg raising required MIPs, of -55 and -50 cmH$_2$O, respectively.

Thus, in the absence of recording of neuromuscular activity, the ability of patients to maintain 5-second head lift is usually compatible with adequate ventilatory function.

REVERSAL AGENTS

Anticholinesterase Pharmacology

The anticholinesterases, neostigmine, edrophonium, and pyridostigmine, are the usual agents utilized to reverse nondepolarizing neuromuscular blockade. Experiments with 4-aminopyridine, which increases acetylcholine (ACh) release, have been limited because this drug acts slowly and because it crosses the blood-brain barrier to cause excitement.[23] Similarly, germine acetate, which has been used in the treatment of myasthenic syndrome, has not been introduced into clinical practice, although it has been shown to improve neuromuscular conduction after depolarizing and nondepolarizing NMBDs.[24]

Mechanism of Action

Neostigmine, edrophonium, and pyridostigmine inhibit acetylcholinesterase (AChE), which lies in the synaptic cleft. Inhibition of AChE leads to an increase in the number and lifetime of ACh molecules that compete with the NMBD for the Ach receptor at the neuromuscular junction, thereby increasing the number of end plate currents that reach threshold and generate muscle action potentials. Anti-ChEs increase the size and duration of muscle action potentials. The increase in size occurs predominately because inhibition of AChE allows a greater number of ACh molecules to reach the postsynaptic membrane. The ACh molecules are present at the junction for a longer time, allowing repeated binding at the receptor and prolonging the duration of the muscle action potential.[25–27]

Edrophonium, neostigmine, and pyridostigmine differ in their mechanisms of inhibition of AChE. Edrophonium contains a quaternary nitrogen group that interacts reversibly with the anionic site on AChE to inhibit, in a competitive and reversible fashion, the binding of endogenous ACh released presynaptically.[28] Neostigmine and pyridostigmine, in addition to containing a quaternary nitrogen group that interacts with the anionic site on AChE, also contain a carbamoyl group that binds to the ester site on AChE. Neostigmine and pyridiostigmine are hydrolyzed by AChE, which is itself carbamoylated in the hydrolysis reaction. The carbamoylated AChE is inactive, thereby incapable of terminating the action of released ACh. Carbamoylated AChE then slowly hydrolyzes to restore the active enzyme. Neostigmine and pyridostigmine are inactivated enzymatically by AChE; termination of the effect of edrophonium depends on plasma clearance. These different mechanisms of action, however, appear to have little impact on the clinical effect of AChE inhibitors. In particular, they do not appear responsible for the faster time course of the edrophonium effect.

AChE inhibitors have several other actions, unrelated to inhibition of postsynaptic AChE and ACh accumulation that may contribute to the reversal of NMBDs. The anticholinesterase activity may produce presynaptic and postsynaptic effects. When given in the absence of NMBDs, antiChEs generate action potentials in the nerve terminal that may be seen clinically as fasciculations.[29] The nerve action potentials spread antidromically and then orthodromically; therefore, the generation of an action potential in one nerve terminal results in the contraction of all muscle cells supplied by that nerve. When the contractions occur after stimulation of the nerve, repetitive stimulation will result in a greater than normal twitch response.

The return of TOF fade following pancuronium, for the same degree of return of T_1, is slower following reversal with neostigmine than after edrophonium, suggesting that these two drugs may act by different mechanisms.[30] Also, neostigmine and edrophonium increase muscle action potential amplitude and duration even after AChE activity has been completely inhibited by methanesulfonyl fluoride, an irreversible inhibitor.[31] Furthermore antiChEs, at high doses, interact with the ACh receptor and decrease the mean channel opening time.[32]

When reversal of an intense block of the phrenic nerve-diaphragm preparation is attempted in vitro, the anticholinesterases demonstrate a ceiling effect.[33] In addition, reversal may be affected by autonomic effects; atropine[34] and adrenaline[35] augment the anticurare effect of neostigmine.

Administration of large doses of antiChEs in the absence of NMBDs may cause neuromuscular blockade. This has been termed neostigmine block. Increasing fade in response to tetanic stimulation has been described when neostigmine,[36] but not edrophonium,[37] was given to reverse neuromuscular blockade. Surprisingly, this effect is antagonised by small doses of nondepolarizing NMBDs. Neostigmine block appears to be of little clinical importance and should not be interpreted as a contraindication to the reversal of neuromuscular blockade.

Pharmacodynamics

The potency of anticholinesterases has been determined by administering the reversal agents during recovery from NMBDs and producing dose-response curves. The ED_{50} and ED_{80} for T_1 obtained 10 minutes after administering the agents at 10 percent spontaneous recovery from bolus doses of several relaxants demonstrate that neostigmine is 10 to 20 times more potent than edrophonium (Table 22-2).[38,39] Approximately twice as much anticholinesterase is required to reverse the effects of the intermediate compared with the long-acting drugs. However, d-tubocurarine requires more anticholinesterase than pancuronium, and vecuronium requires more than atracurium. For TOF recovery, the potency ratio for edrophonium and neostigmine is different from that for recovery of T_1. When reversal is attempted at 10 percent T_1 spontaneous recovery, the dose of edrophonium required to achieve TOF ratio of 0.5 is 25 times greater for edrophonium than for neostigmine when reversing either pancuronium or vecuronium.[40] When reversal is attempted at more intense 99 percent block, the dose-response curves are shifted to the right (Fig. 22-3).[41] More anticholinesterase is required to achieve the same effect. For neostigmine, the curves for reversal of 90 and 99 percent block are parallel; for edrophonium, the curve for reversal of 99 percent block is flatter, indicating that the potency ratio for edrophonium and neostigmine is greater for more intense block.

The onset of action of edrophonium is more rapid than that of neostigmine which, in turn, is more rapid than that of pyridostigmine. When administered during the course of a continuous infusion of relaxant, the peak effect of edrophonium is achieved in 1 to 2 minutes and that of neostigmine is 7 to 11 minutes.[42] Pyridostigmine may take up to 16 minutes to achieve its maximum effect.[38] Similar onset times are seen following spontaneous recovery from bolus doses of pancuronium.[43] The reason for the differences is not known but may

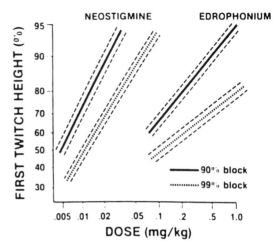

Fig. 22-3 Dose-response curves for T_1 following reversal of atracurium at 90 and 99 percent neuromuscular block with edrophonium or neostigmine. (From Donati et al.,[41] with permission.)

not be simply a reflection of the different binding rates of anticholinesterase to the enzyme. The slow onset of pyridostigmine makes it unsuitable for routine use for reversal of neuromuscular block.

Pharmacokinetics

The anticholinesterases are ionized, water soluble compounds excreted primarily in the urine. Their plasma clearances are greater than the glomerular filtration rate because they are normally secreted into the tubular lumen by an active process.[47] Consequently, their excretion is impaired more than that of the NMBDs in patients with renal failure (Table 22-3).

Table 22-2 Doses of Neostigmine or Edrophonium[a] Required for 50 and 80 percent Recovery of First Twitch Height 10 Minutes After Injection of Reversal Agent at 10 percent T_1 Twitch Height

	d-Tubocurarine	Pancuronium	Atracurium	Vecuronium
Neostigmine				
ED_{50}	17 ± 1.2	13 ± 1.5	10 ± 1	10 ± 1
ED_{80}	45 ± 3.4	45 ± 5.5	22 ± 2	24 ± 2
Edrophonium				
ED_{50}	270 ± 27	170 ± 24	110 ± 30	180 ± 50
ED_{80}	880 ± 93	680 ± 102	440 ± 110	460 ± 13

[a] In micrograms per kilogram.
(Data from Donati et al.[40,41])

Table 22-3 Mean Pharmacokinetic Variables[a] of the Anticholinesterases Neostigmine, Edrophonium, and Pyridostigmine in Normal Subjects and Patients with Renal Failure

Drug	Patients	$T_{1/2\beta}$ (min)	V_{SS}(L/kg)	CL(ml/kg/min)
Neostigmine	N	77 ± 47	0.7 ± 0.2	9.2 ± 2.6
	RF	181 ± 54	1.6 ± 0.2	7.8 ± 2.6
Edrophonium	N	110 ± 34	1.1 ± 0.2	9.6 ± 2.7
	RF	206 ± 62	0.7 ± 0.1	2.7 ± 1.4
Pyridostigmine	N	112 ± 12	1.1 ± 0.3	8.6 ± 1.7
	RF	379 ± 16	1.0 ± 0.1	2.1 ± 0.6

Abbreviations: CL, clearance; N, normal subjects; R, renal failure; $T_{1/2\beta}$, elimination half-life; V_{SS}, steady-state volume of distribution.

[a] Mean ± standard deviation.

(Data from Cronnelly et al.,[44] Morris et al.[45,46])

The duration of action is similar for all the anticholinesterases and reflects their similar pharmacokinetic profiles (Table 22-3).

Complications

The cholinergic activity of the anticholinesterases leads to vagal stimulation with bradycardia and other escape bradyarrhythmias, such as ventricular escape and asystole. The time course of the cardiac effects is similar to their neuromuscular effect, that is, rapid for edrophonium, slower for neostigmine, and slowest for pyridostigmine. These effects can be attenuated or prevented by the administration of the anticholinergics, atropine or glycopyrrolate. Atropine has a more rapid onset of action than does glycopyrrolate, and it alone passes the blood-brain barrier.[48] When given simultaneously the time course of the anticholinergic drug should match that of the anticholinesterase. Thus, atropine is an appropriate choice with edrophonium, in doses of 0.6 mg of atropine for 25 mg of edrophonium.[38,49] Glycopyrrolate has a time course similar to that of neostigmine in doses one-quarter those of neostigmine. If atropine is used with neostigmine it should be given in approximately one-half the dose of neostigmine (i.e., 40 μg/kg neostigmine requires 20 μg/kg atropine or 10 μg/kg glycopyrrolate.[38] Equivalent doses of edrophonium require only one-half the dose of anticholingeric to prevent the cardiac effects. Pyridostigmine appears to require similar anticholinergic doses as neostigmine.[38] However, the anticholinergic dose is variable; therefore, bradycardia requiring further treatment may still occur.

Anticholinergic drugs have been used in the treatment of asthma, and anticholinesterases may cause bronchospasm. However, the combination of anticholinergic-anticholinesterase at the end of surgery does not appear to provoke bronchoconstriction.

Anticholinesterases increase salivation and stimulate peristalsis, which is not blocked by anticholinergics. Despite reports of increased bowel anastomotic leakage after the use of anticholinesterases,[50,51] the hazard of avoiding reversal of neuromuscular block is likely to be even greater. The combination of atropine-neostigmine reduces gastroesophageal sphincter tone[52] and may increase the risk of regurgitation. In day-care patients, reversal with neostigmine has been suggested as a cause of postoperative vomiting.[53]

FACTORS AFFECTING REVERSAL
Dose of Reversal Agent

Dose-response curves constructed in the reversal of 90 and 99 percent block demonstrated that the greater the dose of reversal agent, the greater the extent of recovery. Furthermore, greater recovery was achieved with the intermediate- than with the long-acting NMBDs, following the same dose of anticholinesterase.[38–41] The small differences described among the long-acting[38,54,55] and intermediate-acting drugs[39] are clinically unimportant. The ceiling effect[33] demonstrated in vitro does not seem to occur for the doses used in clinical practice. Thus, the time to achieve a given degree of reversal is inversely proportional to the dose of reversal agent. However, when spontaneous recovery is almost complete, large doses are unnecessary and may induce greater cardiovascular effects.

Differences may exist in reversal of neuromuscular blockade produced by intermittent bolus compared with infusions of NMBDs. For example, the same dose of reversal agent was less effective after continuous infusions of atracurium, vecuronium, or pancuronium than during recovery from bolus injections. Furthermore, following pancuronium, atracurium, and vecuronium infusions, neostigmine (0.05 mg/kg) produced more rapid and complete recovery than did edrophonium (0.75 mg/kg).[56] When given by prolonged infusion, the recovery from vecuronium is slower than after bolus injections.[57] This occurs presumably because recovery becomes dependent on NMBD elimination rather than redistribution, and the differences between vecuronium and pancuronium tend to disappear because of their similar elimination half-lives.[58]

Priming With Anticholinesterases

Attempts have been made to accelerate the action of the reversal agents by administering them in divided doses. Naguib and Abdulatif[59] demonstrated that a TOF of 0.75 is achieved more rapidly when the initial dose (15 to 25 percent of the total) is given at the 10 percent T_1 recovery followed 3 minutes later by the remaining 75 to 85 percent of the dose ("priming"), compared with recovery when the entire dose is administered together. However, the clinical importance of such observations is small.[60]

Intensity of Neuromuscular Block

The time to reach any specific end point (e.g., TOF of 0.7, T_1 of 95 percent) is inversely dependent on the degree of recovery when any fixed dose of reversal agent is administered. Similar observations have been made after d-tubocurarine,[61] pancuronium,[62] atracurium,[63] vecuronium,[63] doxacurium,[64] or mivacurium[65] administered either by bolus or infusion.[56] Although the recovery time for the short-acting agent, mivacurium, is more rapid than for the intermediate-acting drugs, which is

less than for the long-acting agents, the general pattern relating recovery time to block intensity is similar (Fig. 22-4). The place of reversal agents in accelerating recovery from mivacurium block has not been evaluated adequately. However, the concern that the administration of anticholinesterases would impair recovery, because they also may modify the action of plasma cholinesterase that is responsible for the rapid spontaneous recovery from mivacurium, has not been substantiated.[65]

For all agents, the reversal time is considerably prolonged when spontaneous recovery at the time of reversal is less than 10 percent T_1. Thus, it has been recommended that administration of reversal agents not be attempted until at least this level of spontaneous recovery has been achieved. If reversal agents are given earlier, their effect is less predictable and overall, recovery is seldom quicker than by waiting.[55]

One means of combating the slower recovery following a fixed dose of reversal agent is to relate its dose to the intensity of block (i.e., the dose response of reversal agents is shifted to the right in the presence of profound block.[41] However, edrophonium and pyridostigmine are more af-

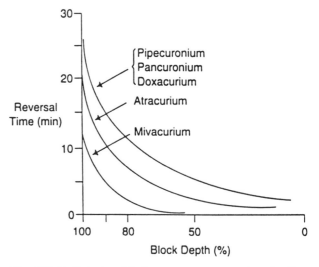

Fig. 22-4 Relationship between recovery time (to T_1 95 percent) and block intensity at the time of reversal (after neostigmine 50 to 60 μg/kg) with short- intermediate-, and long-acting NMBDs. (From Savarese,[66] with permission.)

fected in the presence of profound block than is neostigmine.[67] Therefore, deeper blocks should only be reversed with neostigmine.

Inhalational Anesthetic Agents

Although several drugs have been shown to interact with NMBDs, few have been demonstrated to affect reversal. However, when reversal of pancuronium was attempted in the presence of enflurane,[68] or vecuronium in the presence of enflurane[69] or isoflurane, reversal was impaired. However, if the administration of the anesthetic vapor ceases at the same time as reversal, the impairment is reduced, if not eliminated.[70] Thus, in practice, inhalational agents are unlikely to be responsible for inadequate reversal of neuromuscular blockade.

Age

Reversal of neuromuscular blockade occurs more rapidly in infants and children than in adults. When neostigmine or edrophonium were given after bolus doses of pancuronium[71] or vecuronium[72] at 90 percent T_1 block in children, reversal occurred more rapidly than after similar doses in adults (Fig. 22-5). Similarly, when dose-response curves for neostigmine were determined during continuous infusion of d-tubocurarine sufficient to maintain 90 percent T_1 block, the dose required to produce 50 percent reversal was 13.1 μg/kg in infants, 15.5 μg/kg in children, and 22.9 μg/kg in adults.[73] Thus, reversal of nondepolarizing block in children should be at least as rapid as in adults. Indeed, in one study designed to detect postoperative residual neuromuscular blockade in children, the authors were unable to detect residual block in any of 98 children after pancuronium, vecuronium, or atracurium.[12] This is in stark contrast to several studies performed in adults. Consequently, reluctance to use NMBDs in children because of the fear of persistent block is misplaced.

Spontaneous recovery from neuromuscular block achieved with most non-depolarizing NMBDs occurs more slowly in the elderly, perhaps as a consequence of age-related changes in hepatic metabolism and/or glomerular filtration. This has been shown for pancuronium[74] and metocurine[75] but not for atracurium.[76] Nevertheless, impair-

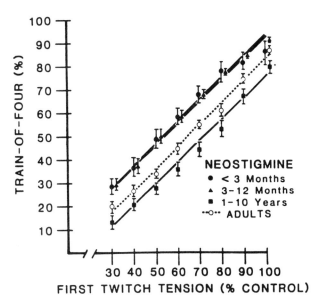

Fig. 22-5 Recovery of T_1 in pediatric and adult patients after reversal of pancuronium at 10 percent T_1 with neostigmine 0.36 or 0.71 mg/kg. (From Meakin et al.,[71] with permission.)

ment of reversal in the elderly patient has not been demonstrated. In addition, the duration of action and antagonism elicited by neostigmine and edrophonium are prolonged in elderly patients, matching the prolongation of NMBD action.[75]

Reversal of Phase II Succinylcholine Block

In many respects, the characteristics of the neuromuscular block produced by prolonged administration of succinylcholine resemble nondepolarizing block. In particular, there is a gradual decrease in the TOF ratio; a phase II block is defined as TOF less than 0.5. Also, the block can be reversed rapidly with edrophonium or neostigmine.[77,78] However, caution should be exercised before assuming that a neuromuscular block that is associated with TOF fade is reversible with anticholinesterases. For example, on recovery from the prolonged block following administration of succinylcholine to patients with atypical plasma cholinesterase, there is considerable TOF fade. Administration of either edrophonium or neostigmine at this time does not lead to recovery.[79] It

Table 22-4 Recommended Doses of Neostigmine or Edrophonium According to Response to Train-of-Four Stimulation

TOF Visible Twitches	Fade	Agent	Dose (mg/kg)
None	Postpone reversal until some evoked response		
≤2	++++	Neostigmine	0.07
3–4	+++	Neostigmine	0.04
4	++	Edrophonium	0.5
4	+/−	Edrophonium	0.25

Abbreviations: TOF, train of four.

is preferable, in this situation, to continue pulmonary ventilation until adequate spontaneous recovery has occurred.

REVERSAL REGIMEN

From the preceding discussion, it is clear that reversal regimens should be based on those factors that modify neuromuscular block. In particular, the choice of NMBD, intensity of the block, and dose of the reversal agent should attempt to achieve adequate recovery of neuromuscular block promptly after surgery. Reversal agents should always be given after administration of NMBDs during anesthesia because small but clinically important residual block may be undetected despite careful monitoring. The only exception may be after mivacurium, although current experience is limited. Intense blocks require neostigmine to achieve recovery. Otherwise, the rapid recovery and reduced cholinergic effects following reversal with edrophonium make it attractive when some return of neuromuscular activity is established. One suggested regimen is provided (Table 22-4), based on TOF monitoring of the ulnar nerve and adductor pollicis. The aim has been to achieve TOF of more than 0.7 within 10 minutes. Recovery from neuromuscular block must be confirmed by clinical testing when the patient has recovered from anesthesia.

In conclusion, residual neuromuscular blockade remains a serious complication of the use of NMBDs during anesthesia. The incidence of postoperative weakness may be reduced by the appropriate use of NMBDs and their reversal agents. Although precise clinical testing is difficult, the avoidance of long-acting relaxants, the use of neuromuscular monitoring, and administration of the appropriate reversal agent in the proper dose should result in fewer complications.

REFERENCES

1. Griffith HG, Johnson GE: The use of curare in general anesthesia. Anesthesiology 3:418, 1943
2. Gray TC, Halton J: A milestone in anaesthesia (d-tubocurarine chloride)? Proc R Soc Med 39:400, 1946
3. Beecher HK, Todd DP: A study of the deaths associated with anesthesia and surgery. Ann Surg 140:2, 1954
4. Viby-Mogensen J, Jørgensen BC, Ørding H: Residual curarization in the recovery room. Anesthesiology 50:539, 1979
5. Lennmarken C, Löfström JB: Partial curarization in the postoperative period. Acta Anaesthesiol Scand 28:260, 1984
6. Beemer GH, Rozental P: Postoperative neuromuscular function. Anaesth Intensive Care 14:41, 1986
7. Andersen BN, Madsen JV, Schurizek BA, Juhl B: Residual curarisation: a comparative study of atracurium and pancuronium. Acta Anaesthesiol Scand 32:79, 1988
8. Bevan DR, Smith CE, Donati F: Postoperative neuromuscular blockade: a comparison between atracurium, vecuronium, and pancuronium. Anesthesiology 69:272, 1988
9. Brull SJ, Ehrenwerth J, Connelly NR, Silverman DG: Assessment of residual curarization using low-current stimulation. Can J Anaesth 38:164, 1991
10. Howardy-Hansen P, Rasmussen JA, Jensen BN: Residual curarization in the recovery room: atracurium

versus gallamine. Acta Anaesthesiol Scand 33:167, 1989

11. Jensen E, Engbaek J, Andersen BN et al: The frequency of residual neuromuscular blockade following atracurium (A), vecuronium (V) and pancuronium (P). A multicenter randomized study. Anesthesiology 73:A914, 1990

12. Baxter MRN, Bevan JC, Samuel J et al: Post-operative neuromuscular function in pediatric day-care patients. Anesth Analg 72:504, 1991

13. Ali HH, Wilson RS, Savarese JJ, Kitz RJ: The effect of tubocurarine on indirectly elicited train-of-four muscle response and respiratory measurements in humans. Br J Anaesth 47:570, 1975

14. Howardy-Hansen P, Jørgensen BC, Ørding H, Viby-Mogensen J; Pretreatment with non-depolarizing muscle relaxants: the influence on neuromuscular transmission and pulmonary function. Acta Anaesthesiol Scand 24:419, 1980

15. Engbaek J, Howardy-Hansen P, Ørding J, Viby-Mogensen J: Precurarization with vecuronium and pancuronium in awake, healthy volunteers: the influence on neuromuscular transmission and pulmonary function. Acta Anaesthesiol Scand 29:117, 1985

16. Jones RM, Pearce AC, Williams JP: Recovery characteristics following antagonism of atracurium with neostigmine or edrophonium. Br J Anaesth 56:453, 1984

17. Saddler JM, Bevan JC, Donati F, Bevan DR, Pinto SR: Comparison of double-burst and train-of-four stimulation to assess neuromuscular blockade in children. Anesthesiology 73:401, 1990

18. Drenck NE, Ueda N, Olsen NV et al: Manual evaluation of residual curarization using double burst stimulation: a comparison with train-of-four. Anesthesiology 70:578, 1989

19. Dupuis JY, Martin R, Tessonnier JM, Tétrault JP: Clinical assessment of the muscular response to tetanic nerve stimulation. Can J Anaesth 37:397, 1990

20. Kopman AF: Tactile evaluation of train-of-four count as an indicator of reliability of antagonism of vecuronium- or atracurium-induced neuromuscular blockade. Anesthesiology 75:588, 1991

21. Engbaek J, Østergaard D, Viby-Mogensen J, Skovgaard LT: Clinical recovery and train-of-four ratio measured mechanically and electromyographically following atracurium. Anesthesiology 71:391, 1989

22. Pavlin EG, Holle RH, Schoene RB: Recovery of airway protection compared with ventilation in humans after paralysis with curare. Anesthesiology 70:381, 1989

23. Agoston S, Langreter D, Newton DEF: Pharmacol-

ogy and possible clinical applications of 4-aminopyridine. Semin Anesth 4:81, 1985

24. Higashi H, Yonemura K, Slimoji K: Antagonism of neuromuscular blocks by germine monoacetate. Anesthesiology 38:145, 1973

25. Fiekers JF: Interactions of edrophonium, physostigmine and methanesulfonyl fluoride with the snake end-plate acetylcholine receptor-channel complex. J Pharmacol Exp Ther 234:539, 1985

26. Kordas M, Brzin M, Majcen Z: A comparison of the effect of cholinesterase inhibitors on end-plate current and on cholinesterase activity in frog muscle. Neuropharmacology 14:791, 1975

27. Bowman WC: Pharmacology of Neuromuscular Function. 2nd Ed. Wright, London, 1990

28. Taylor P: In Goodman GA, Rall TW, Nies AS, Taylor P (eds): Goodman and Gilman's The Pharmacological Basis of Therapeutics. 8th Ed. Pergamon Press, New York, 1990

29. Blaber LC, Bowman WC: Studies on the repetitive discharges evoked in motor nerve and skeletal muscle after injection of anti-cholinesterase drugs. Br J Pharmacol 20:326, 1963

30. Donati F, Ferguson A, Bevan DR: Twitch depression and train-of-four ratio after antagonism of pancuronium with edrophonium, neostigmine, or pyridostigmine. Anesth Analg 62:314, 1983

31. Akaike A, Ikeda SR, Brookes N et al: The nature of the interactions of pyridostigmine with the nicotinic acetylcholine receptor-ionic channel complex II. Patch clamp studies. Mol Pharmacol 25:102, 1984

32. Wachtel RE: Comparison of anticholinesterases and their effects on acetylcholine-activated ion channels. Anesthesiology 72:496, 1990

33. Bartkowski RR: Incomplete reversal o pancuronium neuromuscular blockade by neostigmine, pyridostigmine, and edrophonium. Anesth Analg 66:594, 1987

34. Alves-do-Prado W, Corrado AP, Prado WA: Reversal by atropine of tetanic fade induced in cats by antinicotinic and anticholinesterase agents. Anesth Analg 66:492, 1987

35. Drury PJ, Birmingham AT, Healy TEJ: Interaction of adrenaline with neostigmine and tubocurarine at the skeletal neuromuscular junction. Br J Anaesth 59:784, 1987

36. Payne JP, Hughes R, Al Azawi S: Neuromuscular blockade by neostigmine in anaesthetized man. Br J Anaesth 52:69, 1980

37. Astley BA, Katz RL, Payne JP: Electrical and mechanical responses after neuromuscular blockade with vecuronium, and subsequent antagonism with

neostigmine or edrophonium. Br J Anaesth 59:983, 1987

38. Cronnelly R, Morris RB, Miller RD: Edrophonium: duration of action and atropine requirement in humans during halothane anesthesia. Anesthesiology 57:261, 1982

39. Gencarelli PJ, Miller RD: Antagonism of ORG NC45 (vecuronium) and pancuronium neuromuscular blockade by neostigmine. Br J Anaesth 54:53, 1982

40. Donati F, McCarroll SM, Antzaka C et al: Dose-response curves for edrophonium, neostigmine, and pyridostigmine after pancuronium and d-tubocurarine. Anesthesiology 66:471, 1987

41. Donati F, Smith CE, Bevan DR: Dose-response relationships for edrophonium and neostigmine as antagonists of moderate and profound atracurium blockade. Anesth Analg 68:13, 1989

42. Miller RD, Van Nyhuis LS, Eger EI II et al: Comparative times to peak effect and durations of action of neostigmine and pyridostigmine. Anesthesiology 41:27, 1974

43. Ferguson A, Egerszegi P, Bevan DR: Neostigmine, pyridostigmine, and edrophonium as antagonists of pancuronium. Anesthesiology 53:390, 1980

44. Cronnelly R, Stanski DR, Miller RD, Sheiner LB: Pyridostigmine kinetics with and without renal function. Clin Pharmacol Ther 28:78, 1980

45. Morris RB, Cronnelly R, Miller RD et al: Pharmacokinetics of edrophonium in anephric and renal transplant patients. Br J Anaesth 53:1311, 1981

46. Morris RB, Cronnelly R, Miller RD et al: Pharmacokinetics of edrophonium and neostigmine when antagonizing d-tubocurarine neuromuscular blockade in man. Anesthesiology 54:399, 1981

47. Rennick BR: Renal tubule transport of organic cations. Am J Physiol 19:F83, 1981

48. Mirakhur RK, Dundee JW: Glycopyrrolate: pharmacology and clinical use. Anaesthesia 38:1195, 1983

49. Urquhart ML, Ramsey RM, Royster RL et al: Heart rate and rhythm following an edrophonium/atropine mixture for antagonism of neuromuscular blockade during fentanyl/N_2O/O_2 anesthesia. Anesthesiology 67:561, 1987

50. Aitkenhead AR: Anaesthesia and bowel surgery. Br J Anaesth 56:95, 1984

51. Child CS: Prevention of neostigmine-induced colonic activity. A comparison of atropine and glycopyrronium. Anaesthesia 39:1083, 1984

52. Turner DAB, Smith G: Evaluation of the combined effects of atropine and neostigmine on the lower oesophageal sphincter. Br J Anaesth 57:956, 1985.

53. King MJ, Milazkiewicz R, Carli F, Deacock AR: Influence of neostigmine on postoperative vomiting. Br J Anaesth 61:403, 1988

54. Engbæk J, Østergaard D, Skovgaard LT, Viby-Mogensen J: Reversal of intense neuromuscular blockade following infusion of atracurium. Anesthesiology 72:803, 1990

55. Caldwell JE, Robertson EN, Baird WLM: Antagonism of profound neuromuscular blockade induced by vecuronium or atracurium: comparison of neostigmine with edrophonium. Br J Anaesth 58:1285, 1986

56. Kopman AF: Recovery times following edrophonium and neostigmine reversal of pancuronium, atracurium, and vecuronium steady-state infusions. Anesthesiology 65:572, 1986

57. Noeldge G, Hinsken H, Buzello W: Comparison between the continuous infusion of vecuronium and the intermittent administration of pancuronium and vecuronium. Br J Anesth 56:473, 1984

58. Sohn YJ, Bencini AF, Scaf AHJ et al: Comparative pharmacokinetics and dynamics of vecuronium and pancuronium in anesthetized patients. Anesth Analg 65:233, 1986

59. Naguib M, Abdulatif M: Priming with anticholinesterases—the effect of different combinations of anticholinesterases and different priming intervals. Can J Anaesth 35:47, 1988

60. Donati F, Smith CE, Wiesel S, Bevan DR: "Priming" with neostigmine: failure to accelerate reversal of single twitch and train-of-four responses. Can J Anaesth 36:30, 1989

61. Katz RL: Neuromuscular effects of d-tubocurarine, edrophonium and neostigmine in man. Anesthesiology 28:327, 1967

62. Katz RL: Clinical neuromuscular pharmacology of pancuronium. Anesthesiology 34:550, 1972

63. Rupp SM, McChristian JW, Miller RD et al: Neostigmine and edrophonium antagonism of varying intensity neuromuscular blockade induced by atracurium, pancuronium, or vecuronium. Anesthesiology 64:711, 1986

64. Basta SJ, Savarese JJ, Ali HH et al: Clinical pharmacology of doxacurium chloride. A new long-acting nondepolarizing muscle relaxant. Anesthesiology 69:478, 1988

65. Curran MJ, Shaff L, Ali HH, Risner M: Comparison of spontaneous recovery and neostigmine accelerated recovery from mivacurium neuromuscular blockage. Anesthesiology 69:A528, 1988

66. Savarese JJ: Reversal of non-depolarizing blocks: more controversial than ever? Anesth Analg, suppl: 77, 1993

67. Donati F, Lahoud J, McCready D, Bevan DR: Neostigmine, pyridostigmine and edrophonium as antagonists of deep pancuronium blockade. Can J Anaesth 34:589, 1987

68. Delisle S, Bevan DR: Impaired neostigmine and antagonism of pancuronium during enflurance anaesthesia in man. Br J Anaesth 54:441, 1982

69. Dernovoi B, Agoston S, Barvais L et al: Neostigmine antagonism of vecuronium paralysis during fentanyl, halothane. Anesthesiology 66:698, 1987

70. Gill SS, Bevan DR, Donati F: Edrophonium antagonism of atracurium during enflurance anaesthesia. Br J Anaesth 64:300, 1990

71. Meakin G, Sweet PT, Bevan JC, Bevan DR: Neostigmine and edrophonium as antagonists of pancuronium in infants and children. Anesthesiology 59:316, 1983

72. Debaene B, Meistelman C, d'Hollander A: Recovery from vecuronium neuromuscular blockade following neostigmine administration in infants, children, and adults during halothane anesthesia. Anesthesiology 71:840, 1989

73. Fisher DM, Cronnelly R, Miller RD, Sharma M: The neuromuscular pharmacology of neostigmine in infants and children. Anesthesiology 59:220, 1983

74. Marsh RHK, Chmielewski AT, Goat VA: Recovery from pancuronium. A comparison between old and young patients. Anesthesia 35:1193, 1980

75. Young WL, Matteo RS, Ornstein E: Duration of action of neostigmine and pyridostigmine in the elderly. Anesth Analg 67:775, 1988

76. d'Hollander AA, Luyckx C, Barvais L, de Ville A: Clinical evaluation of atracurium besylate requirement for a stable muscle relaxation during surgery: lack of age-related effects. Anesthesiology 59:237, 1983

77. Lee C: Train-of-four fade and edrophonium antagonism of neuro-muscular block by succinylcholine in man. Anesth Analg 55:663, 1976

78. Futter ME, Donati F, Sadikot AS, Bevan DR: Neostigmine antagonism of succinylcholine phase II block: a comparison with pancuronium. Can J Anaesth 30:575, 1983

79. Bevan DR, Donati F: Succinylcholine apnoea: attempted reversal with anticholinesterases. Can J Anaesth 30:536, 1983

Chapter 23

Basic Pharmacology of Inhalational Anesthetic Agents

James P. Dilger

Inhalational general anesthetics have been in clinical use since 1846. An important relationship between anesthetic structure and activity was described before 1900. The first synthetic inhalational anesthetic with relatively high potency was available in 1956. Inhalational anesthetics are extremely effective, relatively safe, and used in operating rooms throughout the world. However, despite a long and successful clinical history, the basic mechanisms underlying the mode of action of general anesthetics are still unknown.

In one respect, this is not surprising. General anesthetics produce a variety of effects on the central nervous system (CNS), for example, unconsciousness, sleep, analgesia, and amnesia, and our understanding of these processes is primitive. Our ignorance regarding anesthetics, however, goes beyond our inability to define cognitive states. Even if we could identify the relevant structures in the brain, we still would not be certain whether anesthetics produce their effects by binding to specific sites within that structure or by producing a nonspecific disturbance in that region of the CNS. Realistically, we simply do not know what these drugs do.

This is not for lack of concentrated efforts to solve the problem. The question has stimulated research, both experimental and theoretical, by both

physicians and scientists of many disciplines. These include anesthesiologists, pharmacologists, neuroscientists, physicists, physical chemists, biochemists, and behavioral scientists. Moreover, whenever a new experimental tool is introduced, it soon becomes employed to study the action of anesthetics or the phenomenon of anesthesia.

All this means that a textbook chapter about basic mechanisms of anesthesia may contain diverse information derived from a wide variety of sources but will provide few definitive answers or "take home messages." An all-inclusive review would be overwhelming and confusing. Although this might provide an accurate description of our present level of understanding, it would not be useful. It is difficult to predict which portions of the available data are truly relevant to anesthesia and anesthetic mechanisms. Rather than attempting to summarize and critique many results, this chapter will concentrate on the current hypotheses and experimental methods. It is hoped that this will provide the reader with sufficient background to approach newly published studies critically. At the end of each section are questions designed to stimulate further thinking about anesthetic mechanisms and to be used in evaluating new research and hypotheses.

This chapter begins with a discussion of how the

potency of inhalational anesthetics is measured. Then, the structure and chemical properties of anesthetics and the known correlations between structure and potency are discussed. This is followed by sections on the effects of general anesthetics on physiologic structures of increasing complexity: lipid and protein molecules, the nervous system, experimental animals, and humans.

MEASURING POTENCY

Inhalational general anesthetics differ from many other pharmacologic agents in several ways; for example, their route of administration (as a mixture with air supplied into the lungs), their speed of onset and recovery (minutes), and their effects on the body (functioning of the CNS). It is not surprising that a unique method of assessing the "dose-response" relationship of inhalational anesthetics had to be devised. The clinical observation that the "depth" of anesthesia quickly responds to changes in the amount of anesthetic in the inspired gas implies that there is a rapid equilibration of anesthetic in the lungs with anesthetic in the brain. At equilibrium, the partial pressure (percentage of 1 atm) of anesthetic in the inspired or expired gas is equal to the partial pressure or "dose" of anesthetic in the brain.

The "response" end of the dose-response relationship is more difficult to quantify. Patients cannot inform the anesthesiologist about their states of consciousness, and thus far, there exists no unambiguous method of quantifying the depth of anesthesia. Fortunately, there are practical methods for determining whether a patient is adequately anesthetized for surgery. Unfortunately, these methods do not provide a direct measure of the level of unconsciousness or even analgesia; therefore, they must be used cautiously by investigators of anesthetic mechanisms.

The currently available methods for determining the depth of anesthesia involve the ability of a patient (or experimental animal) to move. This movement may be spontaneous (awakening or righting reflex) or evoked in response to a painful stimulus (surgical incision in humans or animals or electric current or tail clamp for a mouse). Depth of anesthesia measured in this way is a discrete or "all-or-none" measurement; the subject either moves or remains still. Measurements are performed on a population of subjects. The results are compiled as the number of subjects exhibiting the movement at each anesthetic dose. The dose at which only one-half of the population moves is the effective dose, ED_{50}.

The most widely used index of anesthetic depth in humans and other mammals is the minimum alveolar concentration (MAC).[1,2] For humans, MAC 1.0 is defined as the amount of an inhalational anesthetic needed to prevent movement in response to surgical skin incision of 50 percent of a population of unparalyzed patients.[2] Thus, MAC 1.0 is an ED_{50}. For other animals, surgical incision or another noxious stimulus may be used to assess anesthesia. The type of stimulus appears to be unimportant as long as its intensity is supramaximal.[3] The muscular response is defined as a "gross purposeful muscular movement,"[3] that is, a movement suggesting that the subject is experiencing nociception.

A rigorous determination of MAC requires allowing sufficient time for equilibration of the anesthetic gas between the alveoli and the brain. In most studies, a 15-minute equilibration time was considered to be sufficient.[4] The amount of anesthetic in the brain can be measured in vivo with a magnetic resonance technique sensitive to fluorine. These measurements show that the time constant for the elimination of halothane from the brain is on the order of 35 minutes.[5] However, MAC is usually determined by making small adjustments to the inspired anesthetic concentration; thus, the effective time for equilibration is much shorter than 35 minutes.

A variety of physiologic variables have been tested for effects on MAC.[4] Some have significant effects; many others do not. Ultimately, these factors may provide clues about the mechanism of action of anesthetics, but at present, they are of more use to the clinician than the basic scientist.

From a mechanistic standpoint, it is important to determine the reliability of MAC as a standard measure of anesthetic potency. In particular, can results obtained from nonhuman species of animals be extrapolated to humans? Species variation in the MAC (or ED_{50}) of halothane is shown in

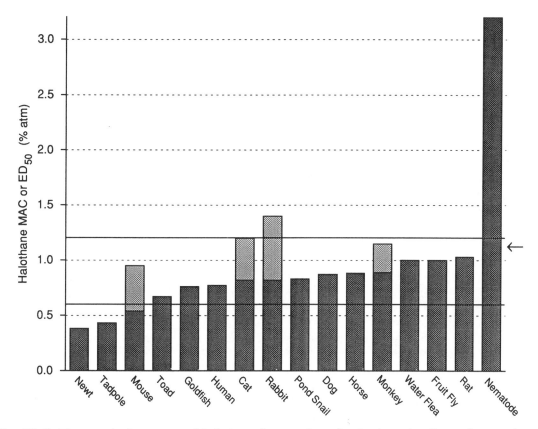

Fig. 23-1 The anesthetic potency of halothane for a variety of animal species. Two values each are given for the mouse, cat, rabbit, and monkey because there is substantial disparity in published values. The two solid horizontal lines are at 0.6 and 1.2 percent halothane. The arrow indicates the ED_{50} of the halothane-sensitive *unc*-79 mutant of the nematode. (*References:* newt,[122] tadpole[123] (converted from 0.223 mM to percent atmospheric pressure at 25°C using a water/gas partition coefficient of 1.2[124]), mouse,[22,125] toad,[126] goldfish,[33] human,[127] cat,[128,129] rabbit,[130,131] pond snail,[132] dog,[133] horse,[134] monkey,[135,136] water flea,[117] fruit fly,[116] rat,[125] and nematode.[115])

Figure 23-1. Most of the values of halothane MAC for these 16 animals, which includes mammals, amphibians, fish, and arthropods, fall within a factor of two: 0.6 to 1.2 percent atm. Two of the values outside this range, the lower value for mouse and the higher value for rabbit, might be attributed to experimental uncertainties, because MAC values for mouse and rabbit obtained by other investigators do fall within the range. The MAC values for the newt and the tadpole, however, differ from the MAC value for the wild-type strain of nematode by almost a factor of 10.

Naturally, the experimental conditions (stimulus, response, temperature, and dose measurement) used to determine MAC must be appropriate for the physiology of the animal being studied. In this light, the overall uniformity of MAC for different animals is impressive. (With the current level of understanding of anesthetic mechansims, factors of two are usually too small to worry about.) In addition, a pattern similar to that in Figure 23-1 is seen when the MAC of other anesthetics is compared for different animals. In a study of seven anesthetics, the MAC for both rats and dogs was between 1.2 and 2.0 times higher than the MAC for humans.[6]

There is an intrinsic limitation to MAC as a measure of depth of anesthesia; it provides only a single point on the dose-response curve (a plot of depth of anesthesia versus anesthetic concentration).[7-11] The dose-response curves for two anesthetics may not be parallel. This means that even though 1 MAC of halothane and 1 MAC of diethylether (ether) each achieve the same result, the effect of 1.5 MAC of halothane is not necessarily the same as the effect of 1.5 MAC of ether. Also, a mixture of 0.5 MAC of halothane and 0.5 MAC of ether does not necessarily add up to make 1 MAC of anesthetic. If any measure successfully replaces MAC as the standard for determining depth of anesthesia, it should be a graded response, one that can be quantified at all concentrations of anesthetic.[7] This requirement excludes measures similar to MAC, such as MAC awake.[12] The most likely place to look for a graded response is in the electrical[13-15] or metabolic activity of the brain itself.

What does MAC tell us about anesthesia? It is possible that MAC reflects a certain level of consciousness within the CNS. Another possibility is that MAC is an index for analgesia, that is, the absence of nociception. Alternatively, it might mean that MAC is consistently measuring something else, perhaps a critical link between the perception of pain and muscle movement. The answer is not yet known, but the question will be posed repeatedly as our understanding of the brain improves.[16]

Question: What criteria must an index of depth of anesthesia meet?
What sort of measurement might meet these criteria?

STRUCTURE AND POTENCY

The molecular structures of volatile and gaseous anesthetics used in humans are shown in Figures 23-2 and 23-3. Six of these agents are halogenated ethers (Fig. 23-2), with fluorine being the most common substitution for the hydrogens of ether. Halogenated ethers are less flammable and, with the exception of desflurane, less volatile (have a lower vapor pressure) than ether itself. Figure 23-3 shows the structures of anesthetic agents not related to ether. These include an inert gas, xenon; three obsolete anesthetics, chloroform, cyclopro-

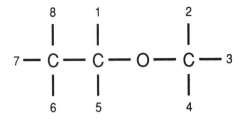

	MW	1	2	3	4	5	6	7	8
Diethyl ether	74	H	H	CH_3	H	H	H	H	H
Fluroxene	126	H	H	$=CH_2$		H	F	F	F
Methoxyflurane	165	F	H	H	H	F	Cl	H	Cl
Desflurane	168	H	F	H	F	F	F	F	F
Isoflurane	184	H	F	H	F	Cl	F	F	F
Enflurane	184	F	F	H	F	F	Cl	H	F
Sevoflurane	200	H	H	F	H	CF_3	F	F	F

Fig. 23-2 The structure of ether-based volatile anesthetics. The chart indicates the molecular weight of each anesthetic (in Daltons) and the atoms or chemical groups attached to each of the eight available carbon bonds.

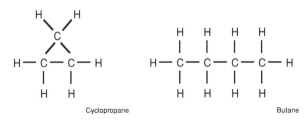

Fig. 23-3 The structure of other inhalational agents that are known to induce general anesthesia in humans.

pane, and butane; and two familiar agents, nitrous oxide and halothane. Observation of these molecules reveals that there are no chemical groups shared by all anesthetics. This becomes even more evident if we consider other molecules (not all of them volatile) that act as general anesthetics in experimental animals but have not been used in humans, for example, alkanes (C_nH_{2n+2}, where n = 1 to 10), perfluoro alkanes ($C_n F_{2n+2}$; where n = 1 or 2), alcohols ($C_nH_{2n+1} OH$, where n = 2 to 13), benzyl alcohol, diols ($C_nH_{2n}(OH)_2$, where n = 5 to 12),[17] acetone, sulfur hexafluoride, hydrogen, nitrogen, argon, krypton, and thiomethoxyflurane. All these general anesthetics are relatively small molecules (with molecular weights less than 200 Daltons), but they do vary considerably in size (molar volumes range between 28 and 240 ml) or shape (spheric to hot dog-shaped).

The only chemical features that general anesthetics seem to share are that they are small and either nonpolar or only moderately polar. Both of these features can be related to anesthetic potency; the more potent anesthetics are larger and less po-

lar. The importance of polarity was discovered in 1899, independently by Hans Horst Meyer,[18] a pharmacologist, and Charles Ernst Overton,[19,20] an anesthesiologist. They found that the potency of general anesthetics is strongly correlated with the drug's solubility in olive oil, a nonpolar solvent. This relationship has become known as the Meyer-Overton correlation. Figure 23-4 shows the correlation for 13 inhalational anesthetics used in humans. The MAC of the anesthetic is plotted against the partition coefficient between oil and gas. Both axes are displayed with logarithmic scales so the correlation extends over a range of 1,000 in both partition coefficient and anesthetic potency. The line is the best fit regression line and has a slope of −1.0. When the correlation is extended to include anesthetics not used in humans, the range would be about five orders of magnitude, and the slope would still be −1.0.

To appreciate fully the meaning of the Meyer-Overton correlation, it is necessary to clarify the concept of partition coefficient. The partition coefficient is the (dimensionless) ratio of the concentra-

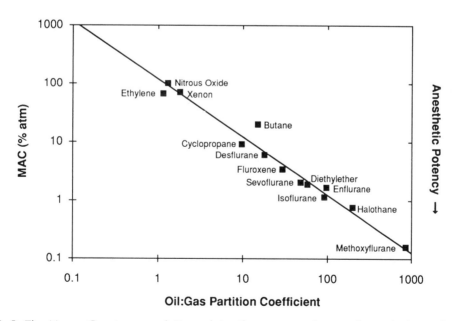

Fig. 23-4 The Meyer-Overton correlation relates the potency of general anesthetics to their oil gas partition coefficient. Here, the MAC of the anesthetic (the reciprocal of potency) is plotted against the oil gas partition coefficient on a log-log scale. The most potent inhalational agent administered to humans, methoxyflurane, has the highest oil gas partition coefficient.[124,137] MAC, minimum alveolar concentration.

tion of a substance in one solvent to the concentration in a second solvent at equilibrium. In Figure 23-4, the first solvent is oil, and the second is air. Because we generally express concentrations in moles per liter of a liquid solvent and as a partial pressure of a gaseous solvent, a conversion factor (the molar volume of anesthetic vapor at standard temperature and pressure) is needed to arrive at a dimensionless value for partition coefficient. To convert a partial pressure, p, to a concentration in oil, c_{oil}, the following formula is used:

$$c_{oil}(mM) = \frac{1000}{22.4} * p(atm) * PC_{oil/gas}$$

where $PC_{oil/gas}$ is the oil/gas partition coefficient. For example, $PC_{oil/gas} = 197$; so, halothane vapor at 0.008 atm is in equilibrium with 70 mM halothane in oil. The partition coefficient between oil and water, $PC_{oil/water}$, can also be measured. The partition coefficient between water and gas can be calculated from the other two numbers

$$PC_{water/gas} = \frac{PC_{oil/gas}}{PC_{oil/water}}.$$

Table 23-1 lists each of these partition coefficients for the anesthetics in Figure 23-4.

Figure 23-5 is a schematic illustration of the equilibration of 1 MAC of both nitrous oxide and halothane between air, water, and oil. To achieve anesthesia, the partial pressure of nitrous oxide must be more than 100 times higher than that of halothane. At that partial pressure, however, both nitrous oxide and halothane equilibrate at a concentration of 60 to 70 mM in oil. This is the message of the Meyer-Overton correlation. At equipotent partial pressures, all inhalational anesthetics will reach a concentration of about 70 mM at a site with chemical properties resembling oil. If all anesthetics produce anesthesia by the same mechanism, then the site at which they act must have a chemical environment similar to oil.

The oil for Meyer and Overton was olive oil. The partitioning of anesthetics into other solvents has been measured in the following: hexadecane,[21] octanol,[6,21] lipid bilayers,[22] benzene,[6] and lipids.[6] In general, amphiphilic solvents (molecules, such as octanol or lecithin [phosphatidylcholine], that have both polar and nonpolar functional groups) produce a stronger Meyer-Overton correlation than do nonpolar solvents. If the Meyer-Overton corre-

Table 23-1 Anesthetic and Chemical Properties of Inhalational Anesthetics

	MAC		Partition Coefficients		
Anesthetic	% atm	mM	Water/Gas	Oil/Gas	Oil/Water
Methoxyflurane	0.16	0.30	4.2	850	200
Halothane	0.77	0.22	0.63	200	310
Isoflurane	1.15	0.28	0.54	91	170
Enflurane	1.68	0.58	0.78	97	120
Diethyl ether	1.9	9.3	11	57	5.2
Sevoflurane	2.0	1.4	1.5	48	32
Fluroxene	3.4	1.1	0.71	29	41
Desflurane	6.0	2.7	1	18	18
Cyclopropane	9.2	0.83	0.20	9.7	48
Butane	20	0.17	0.019	15	790
Ethylene	67	2.5	0.085	1.1	13
Xenon	71	2.4	0.075	1.8	24
Nitrous oxide	101	18	0.39	1.3	3.3

Abbreviations: MAC, minimum alveolar concentration.
(Data from Firestone et al.[124] and Wrigley and Jones.[137])

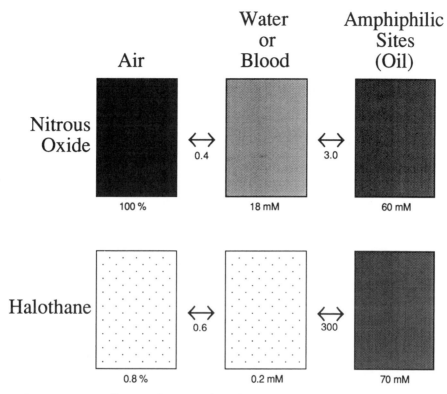

Fig. 23-5 The partition coefficient of an anesthetic between two compartments is the ratio of the equilibrium concentration of the drug in each compartment. The equilibrium concentrations of 1 MAC of nitrous oxide and halothane are given below each compartment. Inhalational anesthetics are administered in the gas phase, equilibrate with blood, and then with unknown binding sites in the brain. The Meyer-Overton correlation suggests that these binding sites are in an amphiphilic chemical environment.

lation teaches us something about the site of anesthetic action, then it indicates that this site is in an amphiphilic (not simply hydrophobic) environment.

Other studies used the Meyer-Overton correlation to obtain more information about the site of anesthetic action. A theoretic analysis of the types and strengths of intermolecular forces that might underlie the Meyer-Overton correlation suggests that the anesthetic site is relatively hydrophilic and might possess a formal charge.[23] The ability of anesthetics to form hydrogen bonds is also relevant.[24] An anesthetic that can accept a hydrogen bond is less potent than one that cannot. The ability of an anesthetic to donate a hydrogen bond does not affect its potency (Fig. 23-6).

Molecular size is important in determining anesthetic potency in two respects. In general, "bigger

is better," but a molecule can also be too big to be an anesthetic. There is a cutoff in anesthetic potency at a certain point in a homologous series of compounds.[25–27] The potency of alcohols increases through C_{13}, but C_{14} is not an anesthetic. There is a cutoff in the potency of alkanes between C_6 and C_{10} and in the potency of perfluoroalkanes at C_3. Size is clearly relevant to anesthetic potency, but size alone cannot explain why the cutoff occurs at different chain lengths for different homologous series.

What does the Meyer-Overton correlation tell us about the site of anesthetic action? Two answers to this question could be defended: (1) nothing whatsoever or (2) many generalities but no specifics. The advocate of the first answer would say that a correlation does not imply a mechanistic association. The relationship between potency and oil sol-

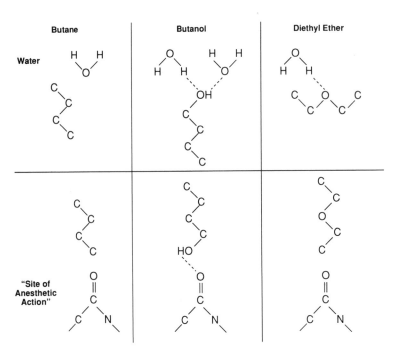

Fig. 23-6 The hydrogen bonding capacity of anesthetics is a secondary factor in determining anesthetic potency. The three anesthetics, butane, butanol, and diethyl ether all have four carbon atoms and are approximately the same size but have different hydrogen-bonding capacities. Butane cannot form hydrogen bonds, diethyl ether can accept a hydrogen bond, and butanol can accept and donate hydrogen bonds. The anesthetic binding site can accept hydrogen bonds. Of the three anesthetics, butane is the most potent ($ED_{50} \approx 0.2$ mM) because it can partition between water and the anesthetic site without breaking hydrogen bonds. Both butanol and diethyl ether must break a hydrogen acceptor bond to reach the anesthetic site. Butanol must also break a hydrogen-donor bond, but it regains the lost energy by forming a hydrogen-donor bond at the anesthetic site. Thus, butanol and diethyl ether have about the same anesthetic potency ($ED_{50} \approx 10$ mM). The "site of anesthetic action" is modeled as an amide linkage in a protein, one of several possible hydrogen-bond acceptor groups found in biological molecules.

ubility might be an epiphenomenon or a side effect and have nothing to do with anesthesia. Also, the correlation would have no meaning at all if different anesthetics acted by different mechanisms. General anesthetics do exhibit agent-specific effects on patients, so why should we assume that there is a unitary mechanism of action?

The more popular response to the question is choice 2. (For one thing, it is easier to construct and test models that assume a unitary mechanism for anesthetics.) The supporter of this answer would say that the Meyer-Overton correlation tells us that the site of anesthetic action is amphiphilic and can accommodate molecules no larger than about 200 Daltons. However, there are many areas in the CNS that fit this description. Both lipid and protein

molecules are amphiphilic. The Meyer-Overton correlation does not provide us with any hints that lead us directly to the anesthetic site. Most investigators would probably agree that we have learned all that can be learned from this correlation; now we must turn to other experimental and theoretic tools. The rest of this chapter is about these newer approaches, but first, there are a few more things to discuss about the anesthetics themselves.

Table 23-1 lists MAC values in terms of aqueous (or blood) concentrations and partial pressures. When the potency of anesthetics is expressed in this way, the order of potencies appears to change. Ether is more potent than cyclopropane when partial pressures are compared (1.9 versus 9.2 percent), but ether is less potent than cyclopropane when aqueous concentrations are compared (9.3 versus 0.83 mM). There is no contradiction here; we just need to consider how the drugs equilibrate among all three phases. Ether partitions more favorably from air into water than does cyclopropane ($PC_{water/gas}$ = 11 versus 0.2), but it partitions less favorably from water into oil ($PC_{oil/water}$ = 5.2 versus 48). The net result is that ether has a larger oil/gas partition coefficient than cyclopropane (57 versus 9.7). The Meyer-Overton correlation is equally well presented in terms of the aqueous concentration of anesthetic versus the oil/water partition coefficient (then, nonvolatile anesthetics also can be included).

A partition coefficient is an equilibrium property, not a kinetic property. The oil/gas partition coefficient can be expressed as the ratio of two kinetic properties, the rate of the gas to oil transition to the rate of the oil to gas transition. It is reasonable to assume that the gas to oil transition rate is about the same for all anesthetics and is limited only by diffusion. This means that more potent anesthetics have a slower oil to gas transition rate. This is only one of many factors that determine the rates at which inhalational anesthetics enter and leave the CNS.[28-30]

MAC decreases at lower temperatures.[31-34] Several factors may contribute to this temperature dependence as follows: (1) oil/gas partition coefficients usually increase as the temperature is lowered, (2) normal physical and neuronal activities of many animals, especially homeotherms, decrease at lower temperature, and (3) a genuine change in efficacy of the anesthetic. No study of temperature dependence is complete unless the roles of all three factors are considered.

One difficulty in the study of general anesthetics is that there are no known drugs that specifically antagonize or reverse the effects of anesthesia. However, reversal of general anesthesia can be achieved by high pressure.[35] Anesthetized tadpoles will "wake up" and resume swimming when the hydrostatic pressure is increased above 100 atm. Just as with the effects of temperature on anesthetic potency, caution must be used in interpreting high pressure experiments. The effect of pressure could arise either from the displacement of anesthetic molecules from their site of action or

from activation of some mechanism that tends to counter the effects of anesthetics.

Although anesthesiologists often refer to halothane, isoflurane, and enflurane as "potent agents," this is true only in comparison with nitrous oxide. Drugs with effective concentrations in the millimolar range are not considered potent by pharmacologists. Intravenous anesthetics like etomidate and fentanyl (ED_{50} = 4.0 and 0.06 μM) are much more potent than inhalational anesthetics.

Question: If a unitary mechanism for anesthesia by inhalational anesthetics is found, will it also apply to intravenous anesthetics?

EFFECTS ON BIOLOGIC MOLECULES

Much of the debate about anesthetic mechanisms centers around the question "are lipids or proteins the primary targets of general anesthetics?"[36-39] The word "primary" is crucial. In the fluid mosaic model of the cell membrane, proteins play a more active role than do lipids in electrical and chemical signaling within the CNS. Lipids literally play a supporting role. A reasonable hypothesis is that, during anesthesia, some critical membrane protein (or proteins) malfunctions. However, this could be caused by either a direct effect of anesthetics on the protein or an effect of anesthetics on the lipids surrounding the protein that modifies the behavior of the protein.

Modern cell physiology challenges this dichotomy between the roles of lipids and proteins. There are lipids that are active participants in membrane signaling.[40] There are cytoskeletal structural proteins that help maintain the shape and organization of the membrane.[41] Finally, there are intracellular enzymes that modulate the processing of information in the cell membrane.[42]

These developments have begun to change our way of thinking about anesthetics, but most of what can be read about anesthetic mechanisms is written from the perspective that the interaction of anesthetics with lipids implies a nonspecific and indirect mode of action, whereas the interaction of anesthetics with proteins implies a specific and direct mode of action. Even if it is not entirely accurate, this provides a convenient formalism for organizing hypotheses and experimental results (Table 23-2). In the future, this formalism can easily accommodate changes in what is considered specific and nonspecific.

Saturation of the binding of anesthetics in the brain has been the subject of recent studies. If anesthetics bind to a limited number of specific sites on proteins, it should be possible to saturate those sites completely with a high enough concentration of anesthetic. If anesthetics bind nonspecifically in the lipid membrane, saturation is not expected. The experiments require many controls to distinguish between saturable and nonsaturable binding. The results are mixed. Although some studies have found evidence for saturable binding of halothane in the brain,[43,44] others have not.[45] One study suggests that even a lipid bilayer system can exhibit saturable binding at clinical levels of halothane.[46] It appears that this line of experimentation will not provide a quick settlement of the protein versus lipid controversy.

A second lead that has been followed is stereoselectivity. The argument here is that a protein binding site might be able to distinguish two optical isomers of an anesthetic,[47] whereas a lipid binding site should not. A recent study measuring anesthetic sleep time in mice showed that the potencies of two stereoisomers of isoflurane were significantly different.[48] The two isoflurane isomers also have different potencies for activating and inhibit-ing ionic currents in neurons.[49] Additional evidence, especially determinations of MAC, must be presented before stereoselectivity can become the "acid test" for direct actions of inhalational anesthetics on proteins.

Another potential distinction between specific and nonspecific sites of action concerns the additive effects of two anesthetics. If two anesthetics act at specific sites, they may compete for those sites and show evidence of either synergism or antagonism. The same argument holds for two anesthetics acting at different sites, but if the target sites are nonspecific and nonsaturable, the combined effect of those two anesthetics should be additive. As mentioned earlier, MAC is not a graded scale of anesthetic potency; therefore, it is not appropriate to equate 0.5 MAC of one anesthetic with 0.5 MAC of another. Nevertheless, investigators have tested the additivity of anesthetics using MAC. Much,[50] but not all,[51] of the evidence favors the idea that the potency of a mixture of anesthetics is additive. Progress cannot be made in this area until a graded scale of anesthetic potency is found.

Cell membranes contain many amphiphilic sites at which anesthetics may bind (Fig. 23-7). Anesthetics may interact with just the lipids (at the center of the bilayer, near the surface, or selectively with lipids near proteins), with just the proteins (at binding sites in contact with the extracellular or intracellular solutions, within the membrane, between protein subunits, or at sites accessible only in certain conformations of the protein), or at the in-

Table 23-2 Comparison of Lipids and Proteins in Their Possible Interactions With Anesthetics

	Lipids	Proteins
Link to proteins	Indirect	Direct
Binding site	Diffuse and nonspecific	Well defined and specific or diffuse and nonspecific
Binding curve	Linear	Saturable
Drug specificity	None	Possible
Combined effect of two drugs	Additive	Additive, synergistic, or antagonistic
Drug concentration	Drug molecules per lipid	Fraction of occupied sites
Nonanesthetics	Critical concentration not reached or bilayer unaffected by drug	Site has low affinity for drug, or drug is bound but not efficacious
Stereoselectivity	Unlikely	Possible
Genetic control	Yes	Yes

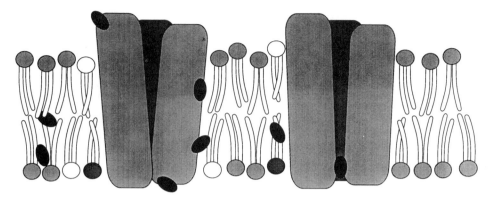

Fig. 23-7 Some possible sites of action of general anesthetics in a cell membrane. Shown are several types of lipid molecules, distinguished by different shading of the head groups; some lipids (boundary lipids) are preferentially located near the protein. Three subunits of a protein are drawn, and the two protein molecules are in different conformational states. The black ellipses represent anesthetic molecules. It is important to remember that the components of membranes are in constant thermal motion; this drawing represents a snapshot taken with an extremely short exposure time. (Modified from Franks and Lieb,[38] with permission.)

terface between lipids and proteins.[52] The next two sections deal with attempts to distinguish between lipid and protein sites of action for anesthetics.

Question: Does it really matter whether anesthetics bind to lipids or proteins?
How do we distinguish between specific and nonspecific binding?

Lipids

Considerable research has been directed toward determining the effects of anesthetics on lipids and lipid bilayers. The results have been disappointing, especially because 1 MAC of anesthetic exerts little effect on the properties of lipids.[53–56] This does not mean that all lipid-based hypotheses of anesthetic action are incorrect; it is possible that there are lipids or mixtures of lipids that are particularly sensitive to anesthetics that have not yet been identified, or perhaps, we have not been clever enough to measure the relevant property of the lipid bilayer. At any rate, the concepts and techniques that have been applied to the study of "simple" lipid systems are now being applied to complex systems containing proteins. Besides, we cannot afford to dismiss the lipid theories before we have a clear viable alternative. Protein theories have their own set of problems.

The effect of anesthetics on a lipid bilayer may be looked on as follows. Assume that, at MAC, the concentration of anesthetic in a cell membrane is 70 mM and that anesthetic molecules are distributed uniformly throughout the lipid bilayer. For a 50-Å thick membrane, this amounts to about one anesthetic molecule per 2,000 Å^2 or one anesthetic molecule for each 60 lipid molecules (a pair of lipid molecules occupies about 70 Å^2 in cross-sectional area). Anesthetic molecules would comprise only 1.5 percent of the total number of molecules in the membrane[53] or less than 0.5 percent of the total volume.[54] It would appear that the anesthetic is merely a minor contaminant in the membrane. Are the assumptions reasonable? Might anesthetics partition into a lipid bilayer more strongly than into bulk oil? Probably, this does not occur; some lipid/gas partition coefficients have been measured and they are actually somewhat smaller than oil/gas partition coefficients.[6,22,57] Do anesthetics partition uniformly throughout the bilayer? We do not know the answer to this question. If anesthetics partitioned preferably into a 5 Å thick layer within the lipid head groups[58] (where they are more likely to accept a hydrogen bond), there would be one anesthetic molecule for each 12 lipid molecules.

Lipid-based hypotheses of anesthetic action postulate that some physical or chemical property of the lipid bilayer is modified by anesthetics. Changes in the dimensions (thickness,[59] area per lipid molecule, volume,[60] or curvature[61]) of the bilayer on adsorption of anesthetics would alter the physical environment sensed by proteins. If anesthetics increase the fluidity of the membrane,[62,63] the rates at which proteins undergo conformational changes might increase.[64] The adsorption of anesthetics has been postulated to increase the ionic permeability of lipid bilayers.[65] If this occurred in the membrane of a synaptic vesicle, the proton gradient across the vesicle would be reduced, resulting in a decreased concentration of neurotransmitter in the vesicle. Anesthetics have also been considered to change the dielectic properties[66,67] of membranes and the temperature at which lipid phase transitions take place.[68,69]

Membrane fluidity deserves particular mention because it is often considered as a possible anesthetic mechanism.[70,71] Fluidity in a two-molecule thick nonisotropic structure (a lipid bilayer) differs from the fluidity of a bulk liquid phase.[72] The spectroscopic techniques used to determine membrane fluidity (nuclear magnetic resonance, electron spin resonance, and fluorescence depolarization) measure the mobility of a "probe" molecule at some position(s) within the membrane. These methods provide information about different types and time scales of movements.[73] What these measurements mean for lipid-protein interactions is not well understood, but recent studies have attempted to clarify[74] and extend[63] the definitions of fluidity.

Question: If a new effect of anesthetics on lipids is being considered as a mechanism for anesthetic action, ask...

What anesthetic concentrations are needed to produce the effect?

Does the effect require special conditions (e.g., lipid composition) and are these found in cell membranes?

How large is the effect of 1 MAC of anesthetic compared with the effect of a change in temperature of 1°C?

Proteins

There has been considerable reluctance to set aside the notion of the lipid bilayer as the primary target for general anesthetics. Although the lipid bilayer hypothesis still has its proponents, the view that proteins play a major role in anesthesic action has gained considerable favor. Proteins do offer several advantages over lipids as targets for anesthetics. Anesthetics may interact with lipid molecules in a limited number of ways, whereas macromolecules like proteins offer more opportunities for interactions. Many proteins are designed to undergo structural changes in response to the binding of small substrates; therefore, the binding of a single anesthetic molecule to a protein might produce an appreciable effect.

Direct evidence for the binding of general anesthetics to proteins comes from studies of a water soluble protein, luciferase. This enzyme, found in the lanterns of fireflies, binds to a substrate, luciferin, and produces light. General anesthetics bind to the luciferin binding site on luciferase and inhibit the light-emitting reaction.[75] This action of anesthetics meets all the requirements for competitive inhibition; the same interaction that underlies the inhibition of acetylcholine receptor channels by tubocurarine. Surprisingly, the general anesthetics bind to luciferase at concentrations that are essentially the same as their ED_{50} for anesthesia.

The molecular picture that arises from these results is that the luciferase molecule has an amphiphilic pocket that can accommodate small molecules. Two molecules of relatively small anesthetics (halothane) or one molecule of larger anesthetics (decanol) can fit into the pocket. Luciferin itself has about the same molecular volume as decanol. The amphiphilic pocket of luciferase has several properties in common with the unknown site of general anesthesia (correlation with oil/water partition coefficients,[75] cutoff at long chain length alcohols,[76] and hydrogen bonding[24]), but it does not exhibit pressure reversal.[77]

Because luciferase is water soluble, there is no question that anesthetics interact directly with this protein. Unfortunately, luciferase is not found in the CNS; therefore, it is not an ideal model system for the study of general anesthesia. The luciferin story serves to direct serious attention toward proteins as the primary targets of anesthetics. Another factor that contributes to the current interest in proteins is the development of experimental tools for studying proteins, especially those found in excitable cells.[78] These tools are now extremely powerful. This is particularly true for ion channel proteins. The structure of ion channels can be determined and modified at the level of single amino acids. The electrical behavior of normal and modified ion channels can then be examined using methods sensitive enough to detect the activity of a single channel. These methods may eventually reveal how a single anesthetic molecule interacts with a single protein.

Ion channel proteins are pores that control the flow of ions across membranes.[79] The proteins are made up of several subunits that align within the membrane to form an aqueous pore, the pathway for ions. The pores have gates that are opened and closed in response to a stimulus (the membrane potential, the binding of an extracellular ligand, or the effect of an intracellular messenger). The stim-

ulus and channel gating are separate molecular processes. The stimulus (e.g., binding of the ligand) does not really open the channel, but it promotes conditions energetically more favorable for the channel to open. Gating of the channel is a conformational change that probably involves movement of all of the protein subunits.

Open channels are usually selective for one particular ion (Na^+, K^+, Ca^{++}, or Cl^-). Ions flow through open channels by passive electrochemical diffusion; the driving force is a combination of the difference in ion concentration across the membrane and the membrane potential. When ion channels are studied with the patch clamp or single channel recording technique,[80,81] gating of the channel is detected as rectangular steps of current (Fig. 23-8a). These "microscopic" currents are sev-

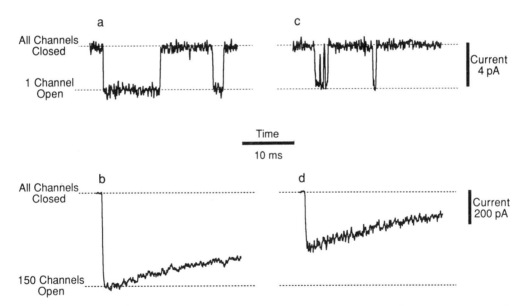

Fig. 23-8 Microscopic (single channel) and macroscopic (multiple channel) currents measured in patch clamp experiments. (ACh receptor channels at −100 mV are activated by 200 nM ACh [a and c] or 100 μM ACh [b and d]). (Unpublished data from the author's laboratory.) (a) Two single channel events. Steps in the current level correspond to the opening (downward steps) and closing (upward steps) of a single ion channel in a small patch of membrane. Single channel currents generally have a uniform current amplitude but a wide distribution of open durations. (b) A macroscopic current composed of currents from an ensemble of 150 channels. Single channel steps are too small to be resolved. The current was activated by rapid perfusion of the ligand (ACh). The current decay is the result of receptor desensitization. (c) Single channel events recorded while the patch was exposed to 2 percent isoflurane. The current amplitudes are essentially the same as in a, but the open durations are shorter and occur in bursts.[89] Isoflurane causes the channel to spend much less time in the open conformation. (d) A macroscopic current from the same patch as b during exposure to 2 percent isoflurane. The macroscopic current is smaller because each of the 150 channels has a smaller probability of being open. The number of active channels and the microscopic currents are not changed by isoflurane. ACh, acetylcholine.

eral picoamperes (pA) (1 pA = 10^{-12} Amperes) in amplitude and several milliseconds in duration. There may be several hundred copies of one type of channel gating simultaneously in a cell. The individual currents superimpose to form a larger smoother "macroscopic" current (Fig. 23-8b).

Three factors determine the amplitude of the macroscopic current (I): the number of active channels (N), the amplitude of the microscopic current (i), and the probability of any one channel being open (p). The macroscopic current is the product of the three factors.

$$I = N \times i \times p$$

If a drug affects the macroscopic current, it changes at least one of these factors. Single channel recording can help to determine which factors have been changed by the drug (Fig. 23-8c and d). Using this information, we can construct testable models to describe the action of the drug on the ion channel protein.

There are three major classes of ion channels, distinguished by the stimulus that gates the channel. The structure and function of each class will be considered separately. In addition, a few of the reported effects of inhalational anesthetics on channels will be reviewed to suggest what might happen to neurons containing these channels when an anesthetic is present. Finally, the possible relationship of the effects to the structure of the channel will be examined. This is somewhat speculative because, within each class of channels, a variety of subtypes have been found; the subtypes often exhibit different responses to drugs. (The question of whether these effects are relevant to general anesthesia is deferred [see Effects on the Central Nervous System].)

Voltage-gated ion channels are usually selectively permeable to one particular ion and are named after that ion (Table 23-3). They are responsible for setting the resting potential of the cell and for propagating action potentials along nerve axons. In addition, Ca^{++} channels at nerve terminals play a role in synaptic transmission. Ca^{++} influx through these channels triggers the fusion of synaptic vesicles with the presynaptic membrane, resulting in the release of neurotransmitter molecules into the synapse.

Voltage-gated channels possess a "molecular voltmeter" that senses the electrical potential across the cell membrane (Fig. 23-9). A change in potential opens (activates) the channel. For many voltage-gated channels, the activation gate is closed at resting membrane potentials (around −75 mV) and open at depolarized potential (greater than −50 mV). The inward rectifier K^+ channel has the opposite voltage dependence. Some voltage-gated channels have a second gate, which is called the inactivation gate. In Na^+ channels, the inactivation gate is open at resting potentials and closes when the membrane potential is depolarized for pro-

Table 23-3   Roles of Some Voltage-Gated Ion Channels in Neurons

Channel	Ion	Role
Sodium	Na^+	Action potential depolarization
Delayed rectifier	K^+	Action potential repolarization
A-current	K^+	Depolarization during repetitive action potentials
Inward rectifier	K^+	Sustained depolarization
Ca^{++}-activated K^{+a}	K^+	Spike frequency adaptation
? Potassium[b]	K^+	Resting potential
? Chloride[b]	Cl^-	Resting potential
Calcium	Ca^{++}	Action potential depolarization and fusion of synaptic vesicles with nerve terminal membrane

[a] This channel is gated by intracellular calcium and voltage.

[b] Little is known about the channels underlying the resting membrane potential.

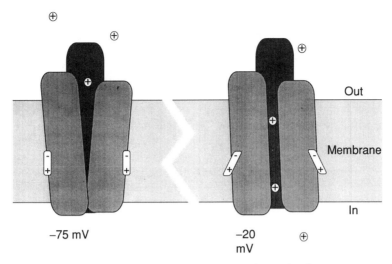

Fig. 23-9 Voltage-gated ion channel (e.g., the axonal Na^+ channel). The activation gate of the channel is closed at the -75 mV resting potential of the cell (left) and open at a depolarized potential of -20 mV (right). The voltage sensor of the channel is represented as a charged mobile portion of the channel protein. In this gating scheme, movement of the sensor causes the subunits of the protein to move relative to each other and form a patent pathway for ions.

longed periods. Closing of the inactivation gate helps terminate the action potential. Voltage-gated channels may have binding sites for drugs that modify the behavior of the channel. L-type Ca^{++} channels have a high affinity site for dihydropyridines (Ca^{++} channel blockers like nifedipine); Ca^{++} currents may either increase or decrease in the presence of dihydropyridines.

Anesthetics may interact with voltage-gated channels at any of the functional parts of the channel protein. One of the effects of halothane on axonal Na^+ channels is to change the voltage sensitivity of gating so that a larger depolarization than normal is required to activate the channel.[82] This increases the time needed to initiate an action potential in the neuron. An action potential may even fail to fire in response to a low level of stimulation. The portion of the Na^+ channel protein that functions as the voltage sensor has not been identified; therefore, it is difficult to localize the site of this action of halothane.

Halothane does not affect the gating of Ca^{++} channels in sensory neurons, but it does reduce macroscopic currents.[83] If the action of halothane is to reduce the microscopic current through each Ca^{++} channel, then the binding site for halothane

might be near the pore of the channel. Alternatively, halothane might decrease the number of functional Ca^{++} channels. Because halothane also decreases the number of dihydropyridine binding sites,[84] this site is a candidate for the target of halothane on Ca^{++} channels. It is also possible that halothane binds to the protein at a site distant from both the channel pore and the dihydropyridine binding site and affects these sites allosterically, that is, by causing a conformational change in the protein that distorts many parts of the protein.

The hyperpolarization of the resting membrane potential of neurons produced by halothane has been attributed to the opening of K^+ channels.[85,86] It is easy to understand why this would inhibit the firing of action potentials in the cell. However, there is no information about the location or nature of halothane's effect because little is known about the K^+ channels that are responsible for maintaining the resting membrane potential.

Ligand-gated ion channels are generally found in the postsynaptic membranes of neurons. They are named after the neurotransmitter that activates them (Table 23-4). Excitatory synapses contain channels permeant to Na^+ and Ca^{++}; when these channels are opened, the postsynaptic neuron is

Table 23-4 Roles of Some Ligand-Gated Ion Channels in Neurons

Channel	Transmitter	Ion	Role
Nicotinic	ACh	Na^+	Excitatory synaptic transmission
Glutamate	Glutamate[c]	Na^+, Ca^{++}	Excitatory synaptic transmission
GABA$_A$ receptor	GABA	Cl^-	Inhibitory synaptic transmission
Glycine	Glycine	Cl^-	Inhibitory synaptic transmission
Anesthetic-activated[a]	?	K^+	Cell hyperpolarization?
Anesthetic-activated[b]	GABA?	Cl^-	Cell hyperpolarization?

Abbreviations: ACh, acetylcholine; GABA, γ-aminobutyric acid.

[a] Found in certain neurons in pond snail, *Lymnaea stagnalis.*[87]

[b] Found in rat hippocampal neurons.[88]

[c] Different subtypes are activated by different agonists: N-methyl-D-aspartate, kainate, and quisqualate.

depolarized. Inhibitory synapses contain channels permeant to Cl^-; when these channels are opened, the postsynaptic neuron is hyperpolarized.

Ligand-gated channels have one or more ligand binding sites (Fig. 23-10). When no ligand is bound, the channel is closed. Ligand binding promotes the conformational change that opens the gate of the channel. Competitive antagonists compete with agonists at this binding site to prevent or attenuate the agonist from initiating the process of channel opening. Glutamate receptor channels have a binding site for glycine and glutamate; both ligands are required for channel opening. Other drug binding sites have been identified on some ligand-gated channels. The γ-aminobutyric acid-A

(GABA$_A$) receptor has binding sites for benzodiazepines, steroids, and barbiturates (see Chs. 10 and 13). Prolonged exposure to ligands causes ligand-gated channels to close again or desensitize. Desensitization of ligand-gated channels is analogous to inactivation of voltage-gated channels; it involves a separate gating mechanism. Desensitization also results in an increased affinity of the receptor for the ligand.

The structure of ligand-gated channels suggests several possible sites for anesthetic action. Anesthetics increase the apparent affinity of the muscle acetylcholine (ACh) receptor for ACh[87] (much less is known about the neuronal ACh receptor). This may have two opposing consequences, that is, in-

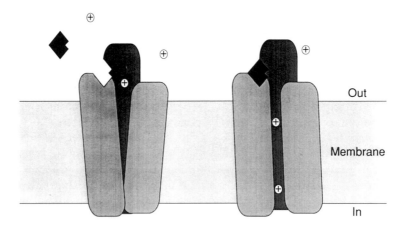

Fig. 23-10 Ligand-gated ion channel (e.g., glutamate receptor channel at an excitatory synapse). Binding of a ligand molecule induces a conformational change in the channel protein from closed (left) to open (right).

creased activation of the channel and increased desensitization of the channel. It is not known which effect is more important in vivo. The gating of different ligand-gated channels is affected by anesthetics in different ways. Inhalational anesthetics increase the open time of GABA$_A$ receptor channels[88] but decrease the open time of ACh[89] and glutamate receptor channels.[90] Curiously, these effects both result in less excitability in the CNS, that is, an increase in inhibitory synaptic transmission through GABA$_A$ receptors and a decrease in excitatory synaptic transmission through glutamate receptors.

The one instance for which the effect of an anesthetic can clearly be associated with a specific binding site on an ion channel is the action of a local anesthetic on the muscle-ACh receptor channel. QX222 (N^1-trimethylaminomethyl)-2'-6'-xylidine), a derivative of lidocaine, binds within the pore of the ion channel and blocks the flow of ions through the pore. This mechanism of action for QX222 had been suspected,[91] but it was demonstrated conclusively by site-directed mutagenesis.[92] Mutations of the normal ACh receptor were made by changing the DNA code for the amino acid sequences of the channel subunits. Messenger RNA for this new code was injected into a frog oocyte, and the oocyte expressed the mutated channels in its membrane. When mutations were made in the region of the protein that forms the pore, the blocking action of QX222 was specifically modified.[93] Site-directed mutagenesis will be an important tool for studying the actions of other drugs on proteins.

The last two entries in Table 23-4 are recently discovered currents that have the unexpected property of being activated by general anesthetics.

Their classification as ligand-gated channels is speculative at this point. The first anesthetic-activated current was found in a neuron in the pond snail *Lymnaea stagnalis*.[94] Exposure of this neuron to inhalational anesthetics opens a K$^+$ selective channel, which hyperpolarizes the cell and suppresses its spontaneous firing activity. The properties of this current are different from other known K$^+$ currents, and the endogenous activator of this current is unknown.

The second anesthetic-activated current is a Cl$^-$ selective channel found in rat hippocampal neurons.[95] The current is inhibited by drugs that block the GABA$_A$ receptor channel, which suggests that inhalational anesthetics may enhance GABA-mediated synaptic transmission, much like the barbiturates and steroids. Thus, activation of this Cl$^-$ current might suppress CNS activity in two ways: (1) by hyperpolarizing the cell and (2) by increasing transmission through inhibitory synapses.

The third class of ion channels are indirectly gated by ligands. At least three membrane proteins are linked to form the signaling system: a receptor that binds the ligand, a guanosine triphosphate-binding protein (G protein), and an ion channel (Fig. 23-11). In some cases, the system is even more complex and also involves intracellular messengers. Because of the intermediate steps, channel activation generally occurs more slowly in synapses using G protein-coupled receptors than in synapses with ligand-gated channels.

The biochemical pathways used by the receptors, G proteins, and ion channels are still being mapped out.[96] Receptors that bind specific ligands may be coupled to more than one type of ion channel (Table 23-5), and a given ion channel may be

Table 23-5 Modulatory Roles of Some G-Protein-Coupled Receptors in Neurons

Receptor	Transmitter	Associated Channels	Presynaptic Role	Postsynaptic Role
Muscarinic	ACh	Ca^{++}, K$^+$	Depression	Both
Catecholamine	Dopamine	Ca^{++}, K$^+$	Depression	Depression
GABA$_B$	GABA	Ca^{++}, K$^+$	Depression	Depression
5-HT$_{1,2}$	Serotonin	K$^+$	Sensitization	
Opioid	Opioids	Ca^{++}, K$^+$	Depression	Depression
Purine	Adenosine	Ca^{++}, K$^+$	Depression	Depression

Abbreviations: ACh, acetylcholine; GABA, γ-aminobutyric acid; 5-HT, serotonin.

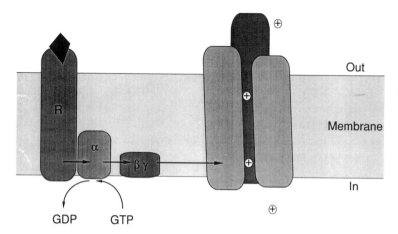

Fig. 23-11 G protein-coupled receptor (e.g., muscarinic acetylcholine receptor). Binding of a ligand molecule to the receptor (*R*) activates the G protein (subunits α, β, and γ). Intracellular GTP replaces GDP on the α subunit. The βγ complex dissociates from α and interacts with a K^+ channel protein, causing it to open. GDP, guanosine diphosphate; GTP, guanosine triphosphate.

associated with more than one G protein. Because of the complex nature of these systems, there are potentially many sites at which drugs like general anesthetics may act to disrupt normal signaling. Investigations into the effects of anesthetics on G protein-coupled receptors have just begun.[97]

Question: If a protein is relevant to general anesthesia, will the effects of anesthetics on this protein necessarily...

be consistent with the Meyer-Overton correlation?

be reversed by high pressure?

show a cutoff at some point in a homologous series of compounds?

EFFECTS ON THE CENTRAL NERVOUS SYSTEM

It is a big jump from ion channels to the CNS. First of all, each neuron has its own collection of ion channels that are localized in specific areas of the cell (Fig. 23-12). The soma contains the K^+ and Cl^- channels that set the resting potential, dendrites contain ligand-gated channels and G-protein-coupled receptors and ion channels, the soma and axon hillock (the connection between the soma and the axon) contain Na^+ or Ca^{++} channels that initi-

ate action potentials, the axon contains Na^+ and K^+ channels to propagate action potentials, and the nerve terminal contains Ca^{++} channels to promote neurotransmitter release. Then, consider the connections each cell makes with its neighbors and how these connections integrate excitatory and inhibitory inputs (Fig. 23-13). Finally, when we multiply this by 10^{11} or 10^{12}, the number of neurons in the human brain, it is not surprising why it is so difficult to determine how nonspecific drugs like general anesthetics act.

Attempts at understanding the effects of general

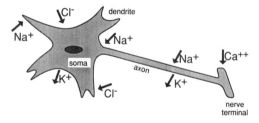

Fig. 23-12 Ion channels in a neuron. Every neuron has its own complement of ion channels that allow the cell to maintain its resting potential, respond to both excitatory and inhibitory synaptic input, generate and propagate action potentials, and regulate intracellular Ca^{++} levels.

normal   with anesthetic

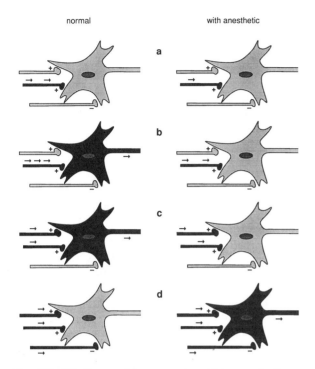

Fig. 23-13 Some of the ways in which anesthetics may interfere with synaptic integration in the central nervous system. A neuron with two excitatory (+) and one inhibitory (−) synaptic inputs. Arrows denote action potentials. Depolarized cells are drawn darker than nondepolarized cells. Normal synaptic events are depicted in the left panels, possible scenarios in the presence of anesthetic are depicted in the right panels. (*a*) Low frequency input from excitatory synapse does not depolarize neuron. Anesthetic reduces input from excitatory synapses but has no effect on the neuron. (*b*) High frequency input from excitatory synapse depolarizes neuron. Anesthetic reduces input from excitatory synapse and prevents depolarization of the neuron. (*c*) Simultaneous input from two excitatory synapses depolarizes neuron. Anesthetic disrupts timing of excitatory inputs and prevents depolarization of the neuron. (*d*) Input from inhibitory synapse opposes input from excitatory synapses and prevents depolarization of neuron. Anesthetic delays the arrival of inhibitory input so the neuron depolarizes. (Modified from Urban,[138] with permission.)

anesthetics on the CNS have centered around three unitary hypotheses: (1) anesthetics depress conduction of action potentials through axons, (2) anesthetics depress excitatory synaptic transmission, and (3) anesthetics potentiate inhibitory syn-aptic transmission.[98] All three hypotheses assume that anesthesia results from (or is accompanied by) a decrease in the level of electrical activity of the CNS. This assumption is not usually questioned[99] and, therefore, will not be raised during the following discussion. (However, it will be raised again at the end of this section.)

Many investigators point out that axonal conduction is relatively insensitive to inhalational anesthetics and consider it unlikely that a reduction in axonal transmission is relevant to general anesthesia. The history of this view goes back to 1905.[98] This view appears to be supported by voltage-clamp measurements of Na^+ currents in axons, 18 MAC of halothane is needed to reduce the current by one-half,[82] and 2 MAC of halothane has only a small effect.[100] However, it may be too early to dismiss axonal conduction as a factor in the action of general anesthetics. First, the rate of stimulation may amplify seemingly small effects of clinical concentrations of anesthetics.[101] Second, most experiments have been done with large myelinated axons. A significant slowing of the action potential is seen in small unmyelinated axons in the hippocampus exposed to 1 to 2 MAC of isoflurane.[102] These axons may have a higher sensitivity to anesthetics as a result of either a lower margin of safety for action potential propagation (caused by a lower density of channels) or differences between Na^+ channels in the peripheral and central nervous systems.[103]

By most accounts, clinical concentrations of inhalational anesthetics depress excitatory synaptic transmission. This is apparent at the level of single channel currents,[89,90] voltage-clamped synaptic currents,[104] excitatory postsynaptic potentials,[105] and somatosensory-evoked potentials.[106] In measurements of single channel and voltage-clamped currents, it is clear that the anesthetics are acting on a component of the postsynaptic cell. However, measurements of postsynaptic potentials activated by direct application of neurotransmitter suggest that the suppression of excitatory postsynaptic potentials by inhalational anesthetics may have a presynaptic origin.[105]

Although there is much evidence for barbiturate anesthetics potentiating inhibitory synaptic transmission,[107] the issue of whether inhalational anesthetics act similarly is controversial. The hypothesis is supported by single channel measurements on GABA$_A$ receptors[88,95] and inhibitory postsynaptic currents in hippocampal neurons.[108,109] Inhalational anesthetics depress[110] inhibitory postsynaptic potentials in some systems, but they have no effect on these potentials in other systems.[111] Similarly, inhalational anesthetics may augment or depress GABA$_A$ receptor channel currents, depending on whether or not there is desensitization.[112]

Some argue that, because none of the three unitary hypotheses of anesthetic action is consistently supported by experimental evidence, "there may be as many mechanisms [of anesthetic action] as there are anesthetics."[98] A nonunitary hypothesis is supported by observations that two similar anesthetics, enflurane and isoflurane, have different effects on the membrane potential and conductance of hippocampal neurons.[86] Hippocampal synaptic responses are also affected differently by different inhalational anesthetics.[113]

Is it time to abandon the notion of a unitary hypothesis of anesthetic action? Perhaps not. Our understanding of normal neuronal signaling is still primitive. We have not yet identified all classes and subclasses of ion channels that participate in this process. The channel species studied in one type of experiment, such as single channel recording, may have significantly different properties from those studied in a brain slice preparation. The kinetics of channel activation, inactivation, and desensitization are known for only a few channel subtypes. The "wiring diagram" of even small areas of the CNS is incomplete. The time course of neurotransmitter release, diffusion, and recycling at synapses is largely unknown. In short, it is premature to interpret disparate results as evidence for multiple mechanisms of inhalational anesthetic action.

Question: Why do general anesthetics exist? Is it just an accident of nature or might there be an endogenous pain control system in the CNS similar to opioid receptors?

Might the site of general anesthetic action undergo an increase in electrical activity during anesthesia, even though the CNS as a whole is less active?

EFFECTS ON EXPERIMENTAL ANIMALS AND HUMANS

Genetic variability in the sensitivity of animals to anesthetics provides another tool for studying the mechanisms of anesthetic action. Selective breeding of mice,[114] nematodes (round worms),[115] fruit flies,[116] and water fleas[117] produced mutant species that are either less or more sensitive to inhalational anesthetics. The nematode and fruit fly mutants that have been studied appear to have altered sensitivity to only some inhalational anesthetics.[116,118]

The ultimate goal of these experiments is to map the genetic locus of mutations that govern an animal's sensitivity to anesthetics. This should direct us to the physical location of anesthetic targets (lipid or protein) in the CNS. Mutants may have either a different number of these targets or targets with abnormal properties. Each animal model has its own niche in studies of anesthetic sensitivity. Nematodes have a simple and well understood CNS consisting of 302 neurons. The CNS of fruit flies, consisting of tens of thousands of neurons, may contain synaptic connections not found in simpler animals but essential to higher animals.

There are a limited number of ways in which anesthetic mechanisms can be studied in humans subjects. This is unfortunate because, even though worms and insects can teach us something, what we really want to know is what happens to humans when we are anesthetized. Some human research appeared recently.[119] The research was prompted by the controversial issue of awareness during anesthesia.[120,121] It will be interesting to determine whether a series of well designed experiments can provide insights into the mechanisms of consciousness and anesthesia.

Question: The unanesthetized behavior of some anesthetic-sensitive mutants is different from normal. Does this detract from their usefulness as model systems?

REFERENCES

1. Merkel G, Eger EI II: A comparative study of halothane and halopropane anesthesia. Including method for determining equipotency. Anesthesiology 24:346, 1963

2. Saidman LJ, Eger EI II: Effect of nitrous oxide and narcotic premedication on the alveolar concentration of halothane required for anesthesia. Anesthesiology 25:302, 1964

3. Eger EI II, Saidman LJ, Brandstater B: Minimum alveolar anesthetic concentration: a standard of anesthetic potency. Anesthesiology 26:756, 1965

4. Quasha AL, Eger EI II, Tinker JH: Determination and applications of MAC. Anesthesiology 53:315, 1980

5. Litt L, González-Méndez R, James TL et al: An in vivo study of halothane uptake and elimination in the rat brain with fluorine nuclear magnetic resonance spectroscopy. Anesthesiology 67:161, 1987

6. Taheri S, Halsey MJ, Liu J et al: What solvent best represents the site of action of inhaled anesthetics in humans, rats, and dogs? Anesth Analg 72:627, 1991

7. Waud BE, Waud DR: On dose-response curves and anesthetics. Anesthesiology 33:1, 1970

8. Eger EI: MAC and dose-response curves. Anesthesiology 34:202, 1971

9. Shim CY, Anderson NB: Minimal alveolar concentration (MAC) and dose-response curves in anesthesia. Anesthesiology 36:146, 1972

10. Kissin I, Morgan PL, Smith LR: Anesthetic potencies of isoflurane, halothane, and diethyl ether for various end points of anesthesia. Anesthesiology 58:88, 1983

11. Deady JE, Koblin DD, Eger EI II et al; Anesthetic potencies and the unitary theory of narcosis. Anesth Analg 60:380, 1981

12. Stoelting RK, Longnecker DR, Eger EI II: Minimum alveolar concentrations in man on awakening from methoxyflurane, halothane, ether and fluroxene anesthesia: MAC awake. Anesthesiology 33:5, 1970

13. Schwilden H, Stoeckel H: Quantitative EEG analysis during anaesthesia with isoflurane in nitrous oxide at 1.3 and 1.5 MAC. Br J Anaesth 59:738, 1987

14. Stanksi DR: Pharmacodynamic modeling of anesthesic EEG drug effects. Annu Rev Pharmacol Toxicol 32:423, 1992

15. Drummond JC, Brann CA, Perkins DE, Wolfe DE: A comparison of median frequency, spectral edge frequency, a frequency band power ratio, total power, and dominance shift in the determination of depth of anesthesia. Acta Anaesthesiol Scand 35:693, 1991

16. Llinas RR, Pare D: Of dreaming and wakefulness. Neuroscience 44:521, 1991

17. Moss GWJ, Curry S, Franks NP, Lieb WR: Mapping the polarity profiles of general anesthetic target sites using normal-alkane-(alpha, omega)-diols. Biochemistry 30:10551, 1991

18. Meyer HH: Theorie der alkoholnarkose. Arch Exp Pathol Pharmakol 42:109, 1899

19. Overton CE: Studien Uber die Narkose, zugleich ein Beitrag zur allgemeinen Pharmakologie. Fischer G, Jena, 1901

20. Overton CE: Studies of Narcosis. Lipnick RL (ed). Routledge, Chapman and Hall, New York, 1991

21. Franks NP, Lieb WR: Where do general anaesthetics act? Nature 274:339, 1978

22. Smith RA, Porter EG, Miller KW: The solubility of anesthetic gases in lipid bilayers. Biochim Biophys Acta 645:327, 1981

23. Katz Y, Simon SA: Physical parameters of the anesthetic site. Biochim Biophys Acta 471:1, 1977

24. Abraham MH, Lieb WR, Franks NP: Role of hydrogen bonding in general anesthesia. J Pharm Sci 80:719, 1991

25. Meyer KH, Hemmi H: Beiträge zur theorie der narkose. Biochem Z 277:39, 1935

26. Pringle MJ, Brown KB, Miller KW: Can the lipid theories of anesthesia account for the cutoff in anesthetic potency in homologous series of alcohols? Mol Pharmacol 19:49, 1981

27. Alifimoff JK, Firestone LL, Miller KW: Anaesthetic potencies of primary alkanols: implications for the molecular dimensions of the anaesthetic site. J Pharmacol 96:9, 1989

28. Eger EI II: Anesthetic Uptake and Action. Williams & Wilkins, Baltimore, 1974

29. Lockhart SH, Cohen Y, Yasuda N et al: Cerebral uptake and elimination of desflurane, isoflurane and halothane from rabbit brain: an *in vivo* NMR study. Anesthesiology 74:575, 1991

30. Yasuda N, Lockhart SH, Eger EI II et al: Comparison of kinetics of sevoflurane and isoflurane in humans. Anesth Analg 72:316, 1991

31. Eger EI II, Saidman LJ, Brandstater B: Temperature dependence of halothane and cyclopropane anesthesia in dogs: correlation with some theories of anesthetic action. Anesthesiology 26:764, 1965

32. Regan MJ, Eger EI II: Effect of hypothermia in dogs on anesthetizing and apneic doses of inhalational agents. Determination of the anesthetic index (apnea/MAC). Anesthesiology 28:689, 1967

33. Cherkin A, Catchpool JF: Temperature dependence of anesthesia in goldfish. Science 144:1460, 1964

34. McKenzie JD, Calow P, Clyde J et al: Effects of temperature on the anesthetic potency of halothane,

enflurane and ethanol in *Daphnia magna* (Cladocera, Crustacea). Comp Biochem Physiol 101C:15, 1992

35. Johnson FH, Flagler EA: Hydrostatic pressure reversal of narcosis in tadpoles. Science 112:92, 1951

36. Richards CD: In search of the mechanisms of anaesthesia. Trends Neurosci 3:9, 1980

37. Miller KW: Are lipids or proteins the target of general anaesthetic action? Trends Neurosci 9:49, 1986

38. Franks NP, Lieb WR: What is the molecular nature of general anaesthetic target sites? Trends Pharmacol Sci 8:169, 1987

39. Franks NP, Lieb WR: Mechanisms of general anesthesia. Environ Health Perspect 87:199, 1990

40. Berridge MJ: Inositol trisphosphate and diacylglycerol: two interacting second messengers. Annu Rev Biochem 56:159, 1987

41. Steinert PM, Roop DR: Molecular and cellular biology of intermediate filaments. Annu Rev Biochem 57:593, 1988

42. Schramm M, Selinger Z: Message transmission: receptor controlled adenylate cyclase system. Science 225:1350, 1984

43. Evers AS, Berkowitz BA, d'Avignon DA: Correlation between the anaesthetic effect of halothane and saturable binding in brain. Nature 341:766, 1989

44. El-Maghrabi EA, Eckenhoff RG, Shuman H: Saturable binding of halothane to rat brain synaptosomes. Proc Natl Acad Sci U S A 89:4329, 1992

45. Lockhart SH, Cohen Y, Yasuda N et al: Absence of abundant binding sites for anesthetics in rabbit brain—an *in vivo* NMR study. Anesthesiology 73:455, 1990

46. Yoshida T, Okabayashi H, Kamaya H, Ueda I: Saturable and unsaturable binding of a volatile anesthetic enflurane with model lipid vesicle membranes. Biochim Biophys Acta 979:287, 1989

47. Calvey TN: Chirality in anaesthesia. Anaesthesia 47:93, 1992

48. Harris B, Moody E, Skolnick P: Isoflurane anesthesia is stereoselective. Eur J Pharmacol 217:215, 1992

49. Franks NP, Lieb WR: Stereospecific effects of inhalational general anesthetic optical isomers on nerve ion channels. Science 254:427, 1991

50. Murray DJ, Mehta MP, Forbes RB: The additive contribution of nitrous oxide to isoflurane MAC in infants and children. Anesthesiology 75:186, 1991

51. Cole DJ, Kalichman MW, Shapiro HM, Drummond JC: The nonlinear potency of sub-MAC concentrations of nitrous oxide in decreasing the anesthetic requirement of enflurane, halothane, and isoflurane in rats. Anesthesiology 73:93, 1990

52. Fraser DM, Louro SRW, Horvath LI et al: A study of the effect of general anesthetics on lipid protein interactions in acetylcholine receptor enriched membranes from *Torpedo nobiliana* using nitroxide spin-labels. Biochemistry 29:2664, 1990

53. Franks NP, Lieb WR: The structure of lipid bilayers and the effects of general anesthetics. An x-ray and neutron diffraction study. J Mol Biol 133:469, 1979

54. Franks NP, Lieb WR: Is membrane expansion relevant to anaesthesia? Nature 292:248, 1981

55. King GI, Jacobs RE, White SH: Hexane dissolved in dioleoyl-lecithin bilayers has a partial volume of approximately zero. Biochemistry 24:4637, 1985

56. Akeson MA, Deamer DW: Steady-state catecholamine distribution in chromaffin granule preparations: a test of the pump-leak hypothesis of general anesthesia. Biochemistry 28:5120, 1989

57. Simon SA, McIntosh TJ, Bennett PB, Shrivastav BB: Interaction of halothane with lipid bilayers. Mol Pharmacol 16:163, 1979

58. Craig NC, Bryant GJ, Levin IW: Effects of halothane on dipalmitoyl-phosphatidylcholine liposomes. A Raman spectroscopic study. Biochemistry 26:2449, 1987

59. Haydon DA, Hendry BM, Levinson SR, Requena J: The molecular mechanism of anesthesia. Nature 268:356, 1977

60. Miller KW, Paton WDM, Smith RA: The pressure reversal of general anesthesia and the critical volume hypothesis. Mol Pharmacol 9:131, 1973

61. Gruner S, Shyamsunder E: Is the mechanism of general anesthesia related to lipid membrane spontaneous curvature? Ann N Y Acad Sci 625:685, 1991

62. Metcalfe JC, Seeman P, Burgen ASV: The proton relaxation of benzyl alcohol in erythrocyte membranes. Mol Pharmacol 4:87, 1968

63. Ueda I, Hirakawa M, Arakawa K, Kamaya H: Do anesthetics fluidize membranes? Anesthesiology 64:67, 1986

64. Lee AG, Michelangeli F, East JM: Tests for the importance of fluidity for the function of membrane proteins. Biochem Soc Trans 17:962, 1989

65. Bangham AD, Mason WT: Anaesthetics may act by collapsing pH gradients. Anesthesiology 53:135, 1980

66. Gage PW, McBurney RN, Schneider GT: Effects of some aliphatic alcohols on the conductance change caused by a quantum of acetylcholine at the toad endplate. J Physiol (Lond) 244:409, 1975

67. Enders A: The influence of general, volatile anesthetics on the dynamic properties of model membranes. Biochim Biophys Acta 1029:43, 1990

68. Trudell J: A unitary theory of anesthesia based on lateral phase separations in nerve membranes. Anesthesiology 46:5, 1977

69. Suezaki Y, Tamura K, Takasaki M et al: A statistical mechanical analysis of the effect of long-chain alcohols and high pressure upon the phase transition temperature of lipid bilayer membranes. Biochim. Biophys Acta 1066:225, 1991

70. Gage PW, Hamill O: General anesthetics: synaptic depression consistent with increased membrane fluidity. Neurosci Lett 1:61, 1975

71. Lechleiter J, Wells M, Gruener R: Halothane-induced changes in acetylcholine receptor channel kinetics are attenuated by cholesterol. Biochim Biophys Acta 856:640, 1986

72. Gennis RB: Biomembranes. Molecular Structure and Function. Springer-Verlag, New York, 1989

73. Trudell JR: Role of membrane fluidity in anesthetic action: p. 1. In Aloia RC, Curtain CC, Gordon LM (eds): Drug and Anesthetic Effects on Membrane Structure and Function. Wiley-Liss, New York, 1991

74. Bloom M, Mouritsen OG: The evolution of membranes. Can J Chem 66:707, 1988

75. Franks NP, Lieb WR: Do general anaesthetics act by competitive binding to specific receptors? Nature 310:599, 1984

76. Franks NP, Lieb WR: Mapping of general anaesthetic target sites provides a molecular basis for cutoff effects. Nature 316:349, 1985

77. Moss GWJ, Lieb WR, Franks NP: Anesthetic inhibition of firefly luciferase, a protein model for general anesthesia, does not exhibit pressure reversal. Biophys J 60:1309, 1991

78. Richards CD, Martin K, Gregory S et al: Degenerate perturbations of protein structure as the mechanism of anaesthetic action. Nature 276:775, 1978

79. Hille B: Ionic Channels of Excitable Membranes. 2nd Ed. Sinauer Associates, Sunderland, MA, 1992

80. Neher E: Ion channels for communication between and within cells. Science 256:498, 1992

81. Sakmann B: Elementary steps in synaptic transmission revealed by currents through single ion channels. Science 256:503, 1992

82. Haydon DA, Urban BW: The effects of some inhalation anaesthetics on the sodium current of the squid giant axon. J Physiol (Lond) 341:429, 1983

83. Takenoshita M, Steinbach JH: Halothane blocks low-voltage-activated calcium current in rat sensory neurons. J Neurosci 11:1404, 1991

84. Drenger B, Heitmiller ES, Quigg M, Blanck TJJ: Depression of calcium channel blocker binding to rat brain membranes by halothane. Anesth Analg 74:758, 1992

85. Nicoll RA, Madison DV: General anesthetics hyperpolarize neurons in the vertebrate central nervous system. Science 217:1055, 1982

86. MacIver MB, Kendig JJ: Anesthetic effects on resting membrane potential are voltage-dependent and agent-specific. Anesthesiology 74:83, 1991

87. Miller KW, Braswell LM, Firestone LL et al: General anesthetics act both specifically and nonspecifically on acetylcholine receptors. p. 125. In Roth SH, Miller KW (eds): Molecular and Cellular Mechanisms of Anesthetics. Plenum, New York, 1986

88. Yeh JZ, Quandt FN, Tanguy J et al: General anesthetic action of γ-aminobutyric acid-activated channels. Ann N Y Acad Sci 625:155, 1991

89. Dilger JP, Brett RS, Lesko LA: Effects of isoflurane on acetylcholine receptor channels. 1. Single-channel currents. Mol Pharmacol 41:127, 1992

90. Yang J, Zorumski CF: Effects of isoflurane on N-methyl-D-aspartate gated ion channels in cultured rat hippocampal neurons. Ann N Y Acad Sci 625:287, 1991

91. Neher E, Steinbach JH: Local anaesthetics transiently block currents through single acetylcholine-receptor channels. J Physiol (Lond) 277:153, 1978

92. Kunkel TA, Roberts JD, Zakour RA: Rapid and efficient site-specific mutagenesis without phenotypic selection. Methods Enzymol 154:367, 1987

93. Charnet P, Labarca C, Leonard RJ et al: An open-channel blocker interacts with adjacent turns of α-helices in the nicotinic acetylcholine receptor. Neuron 2:87, 1990

94. Franks NP, Lieb WR: Volatile general anesthetics activate a novel neuronal K+ current. Nature 333:662, 1988

95. Yang J, Isenberg KE, Zorumski CF: Volatile anesthetics gate a chloride current in postnatal rat hippocampal neurons. FASEB J 6:914, 1992

96. Neer EJ, Clapham DE: Roles of G protein subunits in transmembrane signalling. Nature 333:129, 1988

97. Maze M: Transmembrane signalling and the Holy Grail of anesthesia. Anesthesiology 72:959, 1990

98. Richards CD: Actions of general anaesthetics on synaptic transmission in the CNS. Br J Anaesth 55:201, 1983

99. Winters WD: A review of the continuum of drug-induced states of excitation and depression. Prog Drug Res 26:225, 1982

100. Haydon DA, Simon AJB: Excitation of the squid giant axon by general anaesthetics. J Physiol (Lond) 402:375, 1988

101. Strichartz G: Use-dependent conduction block produced by volatile central anesthetic agent. Acta Anaesthesiol Scand 24:402, 1980

102. Berg-Johnsen J, Langmoen IA: Mechanisms concerned in the direct effect of isoflurane on rat hippocampal and human neocortical neurons. Brain Res 507:28, 1990

103. Haydon DA, Hendry BM: Nerve impulse blockage in squid axons by n-alkanes: the effect of axon diameter. J Physiol (Lond) 333:393, 182

104. Gage PW, Hamill OP: Effects of anesthetics on ion channels in synapses. p. 1. In Porter R (ed): International Review of Physiology. University Park Press, Baltimore, 1981

105. Berg-Johnsen J, Langmoen IA: The effect of isoflurane on excitatory synaptic transmission in the rat hippocampus. Acta Anaesthesiol Scand 36:350, 1992

106. Shimoji K, Fujioka H, Fukazawa T et al: Anesthetics and excitatory/inhibitory responses of midbrain reticular neurons. Anesthesiology 61:151, 1984

107. Olsen RW, Sapp DM, Bureau MH et al: Allosteric actions of central nervous system depressants including anesthetics on subtypes of the inhibitory γ-aminobutyric acid$_A$ receptor-chloride channel complex. Ann N Y Acad Sci 615:145, 1991

108. Gage PW, Robertson B: Prolongation of inhibitory postsynaptic currents by pentobarbitone, halothane and ketamine in CA1 pyramid cells in rat hippocampus. Br J Pharmacol 85:675, 1985

109. Mody I, Tanelian DL, MacIver MB: Halothane enhances tonic neuronal inhibition by elevating intracellular calcium. Brain Res 538:319, 1991

110. Fujiwara N, Higashi H, Nishi S et al: Changes in spontaneous firing patterns of rat hippocampal neurons induced by volatile anesthetics. J Physiol (Lond) 402:155, 1988

111. McGivern J, Scholfield CN: General anaesthetics and field currents in unclamped, unmyelinated axons of rat olfactory cortex. Br J Pharmacol 101:217, 1990

112. Nakahiro M, Yeh JZ, Brunner E, Narahashi T: General anesthetics modulate GABA receptor channel complex in rat dorsal root ganglion neurons. FASEB J 3:1850, 1989

113. MacIver MB, Roth SH: Inhalational anaesthetics exhibit pathway-specific differential actions on hippocampal synaptic responses in vitro. Br J Anaesth 60:680, 1988

114. Koblin DD, Doug DE, Deady JE et al: Selective breeding alters murine resistance to nitrous oxide without alteration in synaptic membrane composition. Anesthesiology 62:401, 1980

115. Sedensky MM, Meneely PM: Genetic analysis of halothane sensitivity in *Caenorhabditis elegans*. Science 236:952, 1987

116. Krishnan KS, Nash HA: A genetic study of the anesthetic response—mutants of *Drosophila melanogaster* altered in sensitivity to halothane. Proc Natl Acad Sci U S A 87:8632, 1990

117. McKenzie JD, Calow P, Nimmo WS: Effects of inhalational general anaesthetics on intact *Daphnia magna* (Cladocera, Crustacea). Comp Biochem Physiol 101C:9, 1992

118. Morgan PG, Sedensky M, Meneely PM: Multiple sites of action of volatile anesthetics in *Caenorhabditis elegans*. Proc Natl Acad Sci U S A 87:2965, 1990

119. Dwyer R, Bennett HL, Eger EI, Peterson N: Isoflurane anesthesia prevents unconscious learning. Anesth Analg 75:107, 1992

120. Jessop J, Jones JG: Conscious awareness during general anaesthesia—what are we attempting to monitor? Br J Anaesth 66:635, 1991

121. Ghoneim MM, Block RI: Learning and consciousness during general anesthesia. Anesthesiology 76:279, 1992

122. Smith RA: Investigations into the mechanism of anaesthesia: the relationship between anaesthesia and pressure, thesis. Oxford University, Oxford, 1974

123. Kita Y, Bennett LJ, Miller KW: The partial molar volumes of anesthetics in lipid bilayers. Biochim Biophys Acta 647:130, 1981

124. Firestone LL, Miller JC, Miller KM: Tables of physical and pharmacological properties of anesthetics. p. 267. In Roth SH, Miller KW (eds): Molecular and Cellular Mechanisms of Anesthetics. Plenum, New York, 1986

125. Mazze RI, Rice SA, Baden JM: Halothane, isoflurane, and enflurane MAC in pregnant and nonpregnant female and male mice and rats. Anesthesiology 62:339, 1985

126. Shim CY, Andersen NB: The effect of oxygen on minimal anesthetic requirements in the toad. Anesthesiology 34:333, 1971

127. Saidman LJ, Eger EE II, Munson ES et al: Minimum alveolar concentrations of methoxyflurane, halothane, ether and cyclopropane in man: correlation with theories of anesthesia. Anesthesiology 28:994, 1967

128. Brown BR, Crout JR: A comparative study of the effects of five general anesthetics on myocardial

contractility: I. Isomeric conditions. Anesthesiology 34:236, 1971

129. Drummond JC, Todd MM, Shapiro HM: Minimal alveolar concentrations for halothane, enflurane, and isoflurane in the cat. J Am Vet Med Assoc 182:1099, 1983

130. Davis NL, Nunnally RL, Malinin TI: Determination of the minimum alveolar concentration (MAC) of halothane in the white New Zealand rabbit. Br J Anaesth 47:341, 1975

131. Drummond JC: MAC halothane, enflurane, and isoflurane in the New Zealand white rabbit and a test for the validity of MAC determination. Anesthesiology 62:336, 1985

132. Cruickshank SGH, Girdlestone D, Winlow W: The effects of halothane on the withdrawal response of *Lynmaea*. J Physiol (Lond) 367:8P, 1985

133. Eger EI II, Brandstater B, Saidman LJ et al: Equipotent alveolar concentration of methoxyflurane, halothane, diethylether, fluroxene, cyclopropane, xenon and nitrous oxide in the dog. Anesthesiology 26:771, 1965

134. Steffey EP, Howland D Jr, Giri S et al: Enflurane, halothane, and isoflurane potency in horses. Am J Vet Res 38:1037, 1977

135. Steffey EP, Gillespie Jr, Berry JD et al: Anesthetic potency (MAC) of nitrous oxide in the dog, cat and stump-tail monkey. J Appl Physiol 36:530, 1974

136. Tinker JH, Sharbrough FW, Michenfelder JD: Anterior shift of the dominant EEG rhythm during anesthesia in the Java monkey: correlation with anesthetic potency. Anesthesiology 46:252, 1977

137. Wrigley SR, Jones RM: Inhalational agents—an update. Eur J Anaesthesiol 9:185, 1992

138. Urban BW: The anaesthetic site of action—an overview. Anasthesiol Intensivmed Notfallmed Schmerzther 27:68, 1992

Chapter 24

Pharmacokinetics of Inhalational Anesthetics

Jerrold Lerman

For more than 150 years inhalational anesthetics have been the cornerstone of general anesthesia. Their success has been predicated on an understanding of the factors that control the partial pressure of anesthetic within the brain. A knowledge of these factors should provide for fine control of the speed of induction of and emergence from anesthesia, precise control of the depth of anesthesia, and minimal adverse physiologic effects.

WASH-IN OF ANESTHETICS INTO THE LUNG

General Principles

The increase in the ratio of the anesthetic fraction or partial pressure in the alveoli (F_A) to that in the inspired (F_I) fresh gas is known as the *wash-in* of the anesthetic. The relationship between F_A/F_I and time during this wash-in period is described by the differential equation:

$$dF_A/dF_I = -t/\tau \qquad (1)$$

where t is time and τ is the time constant. The units of τ are time and thus the ratio dF_A/dF_I is dimensionless. To solve this differential equation, the ratio, F_A/F_I, must be defined at the extremes of time:

at t = 0, F_A/F_I is zero whereas as t $\Rightarrow \infty$, $F_A/F_I \Rightarrow 1.0$. Equation 1 is then integrated to yield the following solution:

$$F_A/F_I = 1 - e^{-t/\tau} \qquad (2)$$

The time constant, τ, for the wash-in of anesthetic is defined as the ratio of the capacity of the reservoir (V) into which the anesthetic is being delivered to the flow rate of anesthetic (Q) into the reservoir as follows:

$$\tau = V \cdot Q^{-1} \qquad (3)$$

Using equations 2 and 3, we can now estimate the time to equilibration of alveolar and inspired anesthetic partial pressures in the lung, assuming the uptake of anesthetic from the lungs is negligible. For a lung with a function residual capacity of 2 liters and an alveolar ventilation of 4 l/min, as in the case of an adult, τ is 2/4 or 0.5 minutes. When t equals 1τ, the ratio t/τ becomes 1 and $F_A/F_I = 1 - e^{-1}$ or 0.63. The values for F_A/F_I for larger multiples of τ are shown in Table 24-1. Based on these values, it takes approximately 2 minutes to fully equilibrate the partial pressure of anesthetic in the alveoli with that in the inspired gas in the adult lung.

Table 24-1 Values for F_A/F_I

Number of Time Constants (τ)	Extent of Equilibration of Anesthetic Partial Pressure in the Reservoir With the Inspired Pressure
1	0.63
2	0.86
3	0.95
4	0.98

Determinants of the Wash-In

The rate of rise of alveolar to inspired anesthetic partial pressures (wash-in) depends on a balance of the rate of delivery of anesthetic to and removal (or uptake) from the lungs. The wash-in of inhalational anesthetics depends upon six factors (Table 24-2)[1]: the first three factors determine the rate of delivery of inhalational anesthetics to the alveoli; the second three determine its rate of removal from the alveoli.

Ventilation

The fraction of the minute ventilation that determines the delivery of anesthetics to the lungs is that fraction involved in gas exchange, (i.e., alveolar ventilation). Alveolar ventilation comprises approximately two-thirds of the minute ventilation, which in the case of the adult is approximately 4 L/min (60 ml/kg). Throughout this chapter, ventilation will refer exclusively to alveolar ventilation.

Alveolar ventilation directly affects the wash-in of inhalational anesthetics in the lungs; changes in ventilation lead to parallel changes in the rate of rise of alveolar to inspired anesthetic partial pressure (Fig. 24-1). This effect of ventilation on the wash-in of inhalational anesthetics may be explained in terms of its effect on the τ defined in

Table 24-2 Factors Responsible for the Wash-In of Inhalational Anesthetics[1]

Inspired concentration
Alveolar ventilation
Functional residual capacity
Cardiac output
Solubility
Alveolar to venous partial pressure gradient

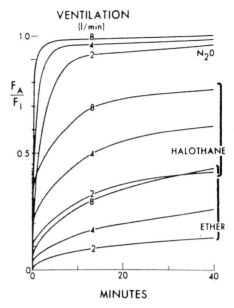

Fig. 24-1 Effect of alveolar ventilation on the rate of rise of alveolar (F_A) to inspired (F_I) anesthetic partial pressure at a constant cardiac output. The effect of ventilation on F_A/F_I increased with increasing solubility in blood. (From Eger,[1] with permission.)

Equation 3. As the alveolar ventilation, Q, increases, τ decreases and the time to equilibration of anesthetic partial pressures also decreases. Hence, an increase in alveolar ventilation increases the rate of rise of alveolar to inspired anesthetic partial pressures. The converse also holds true; that is, as alveolar ventilation decreases, τ increases and thus, the time to equilibration of anesthetic partial pressure increases.

Functional Residual Capacity

The time constant, t, depends on the ratio of volume of the reservoir, FRC (V), to alveolar ventilation (Q), as described by Equation 3. Changes in FRC lead to parallel changes in τ during the wash-in of inhalational anesthetics into the lungs, provided alveolar ventilation remains constant. In clinical situations, such as obesity and restrictive lung defects where the FRC is reduced, the wash-in of anesthetic into the lungs will be more rapid than in the presence of a normal FRC.

Inspired Concentration

The inspired concentration of an inhalational anesthetic is the driving force of anesthetic into the lungs, blood, and tissues. The greater the inspired concentration, the greater the driving force and thus, the more rapid the increase in alveolar to inspired anesthetic partial pressures. However, with most inhalational anesthetics administered in concentrations between 3 and 5 percent, the effect of the inspired concentration on wash-in is relatively small.

Uptake of Anesthetic from the Lung

The increase of alveolar to inspired anesthetic partial pressures is the net result of the delivery of anesthetic to and removal from the lungs. If delivery to the lung is unopposed (zero uptake), then the increase in alveolar to inspired partial pressure progresses rapidly, as in the case of nitrous oxide and desflurane (Fig. 24-2).[2] However, the rate of rise of F_A/F_I slows after the first few minutes because of the uptake of anesthetic from the alveoli.

Uptake of anesthetic from the alveoli is the product of three factors: cardiac output, blood/gas partition coefficient, and the alveolar to venous partial pressure gradient. If any one or more of these factors decreases, uptake of anesthetic from the alveoli decreases in parallel. As a consequence, the partial pressure of anesthetic remaining in the alveoli increases more rapidly until it equilibrates with the inspired partial pressure.

Solubility

Inhalational anesthetics partition into two physiologic compartments in body fluids and tissues: an aqueous phase and a protein/lipid phase. This is analogous to the distribution of oxygen and carbon dioxide in blood between the aqueous phase and hemoglobin. The fraction of anesthetic that is dissolved in the aqueous phase determines the partial pressure of the anesthetic. As in the case of oxygen, inhalational anesthetics move from phases of high partial pressure to phases of low partial pressure and not along concentration gradients between fluids and tissues within the body. The remainder of the anesthetic is located in the protein and lipid phases of liquids and tissues. The sites on proteins

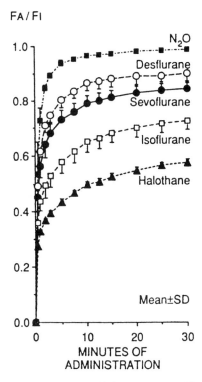

Fig. 24-2 Increase in F_A/F_I for nitrous oxide, desflurane, sevoflurane, isoflurane, and halothane in adults over time. The wash-in of anesthetics increases as the solubility of the anesthetics in blood decreases. (From Yasuda et al.,[2] with permission.)

and lipids that attract inhalational anesthetics are unknown. However, we do know that the interaction of anesthetics with liquids and tissues is reversible and that the anesthetic molecule that is recovered appears to be unchanged in its physical and chemical properties.

The solubility of an anesthetic is defined as the ratio of the concentrations of anesthetic in two phases when the partial pressure of the anesthetic in the two phases has equilibrated. For example, a blood/gas partition coefficient of 0.5 indicates an anesthetic concentration in the blood phase that is one-half that in the gas phase. Similarly, a brain/blood partition coefficient of 2.0 indicates an anesthetic concentration in the brain that is twice that in the blood. Thus, solubility reflects the relative solubility of an anesthetic in one phase compared with its solubility in a second phase.

The rate of increase of alveolar to inspired anesthetic partial pressures is inversely related to the solubility of inhalational anesthetics in blood. That is, the wash-in of anesthetics that are less soluble in blood is very rapid whereas the wash-in of more soluble anesthetics is slower. Because soluble anesthetics are taken up by blood more readily than are less soluble anesthetics, the partial pressure of the more soluble anesthetics in the alveoli increases more slowly compared with the less soluble anesthetics. This is illustrated by the relative rate of increase of alveolar to inspired partial pressures for five inhalational anesthetics (Fig. 24-2). Here, the order of the wash-in of anesthetics from fastest to slowest (nitrous oxide to methoxyflurane) varies inversely with their solubilities in blood: nitrous oxide > desflurane > sevoflurane > isoflurane > enflurane > halothane > methoxyflurane (Table 24-3).[2] Thus, the alveolar partial pressure of less soluble anesthetics equilibrates more rapidly with the inspired partial pressure than does the pressure of the more soluble anesthetics. The same holds true for the tissue partial pressure of anesthetics.

After a stepwise increase in the inspired concentration during the wash-in, the end-tidal concentration of less soluble anesthetics equilibrates very rapidly with the new inspired concentration (Fig. 24-2).[2] The wash-out of less soluble anesthetics is also rapid.[2] Therefore, anesthetists should be able to control the depth of anesthesia more rapidly and effectively with the newer, less soluble inhalational anesthetics than they could with the older, more soluble anesthetics.

Cardiac Output

Uptake of inhalational anesthetics from the lung involves movement of the anesthetic across the alveolar capillary membrane and then its removal by the blood traversing the pulmonary capillaries. Because the alveolar–capillary membrane offers no resistance to the movement of inhalational anesthetics, it does not merit further discussion. Removal of anesthetic from the lung depends then, on the pulmonary blood flow or cardiac output and the alveolar to venous partial pressure gradient. The greater the pulmonary blood flow, the greater the uptake of anesthetic by blood which in turn increases the delivery of anesthetic to tissues. However, the greater uptake of anesthetic from the alveoli actually slows the rate of rise of F_A/F_I. Because the partial pressure difference between the alveoli or blood and tissues determines the rate of rise of anesthetic partial pressure in the tissues, the slower rate of rise of alveolar partial pressure slows the distribution of anesthetic into fluids and tissues. Thus, an increased cardiac output actually slows the rate of rise of both alveolar to inspired anesthetic partial pressures and tissue anesthetic partial pressures (Fig. 24-3). Conversely, as cardiac output decreases, so too does the uptake of anesthetic from the lung. This speeds the increase in alveolar to inspired anesthetic partial pressures. With the blood flow to vital organs such as brain and heart preserved in a low cardiac output state, these organs become vulnerable to depression by the rapidly increasing alveolar and blood anesthetic partial pressures. Thus, in the presence of a low cardiac

Table 24-3   Partition Coefficients for Blood and Tissues in Adults

Inhalational Anesthetic	Blood/Gas	Brain/Blood	Liver/Blood	Kidney/Blood	Muscle/Blood	Fat/Blood
Nitrous oxide	0.47	1.1	0.8	—	1.2	2.3
Desflurane	0.42	1.3	1.3	0.94	2.0	27
Sevoflurane	0.69	1.7	1.8	1.15	3.1	48
Isoflurane	1.4	1.6	1.75	1.05	2.9	45
Enflurane	1.8	1.4	2.1	—	1.7	36
Halothane	2.4	1.9	2.1	1.2	3.4	51
Methoxyflurane	15	1.4	2.0	0.9	1.6	61

(Data from references 1, 18, 25, 29, 95–97.)

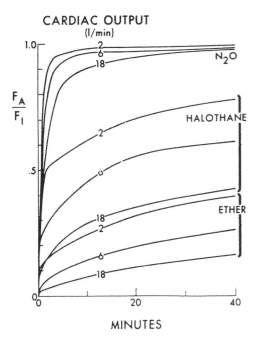

Fig. 24-3 Effect of cardiac output on the rate of rise of alveolar (F_A) to inspired (F_I) anesthetic partial pressure at a constant alveolar ventilation. The effect of cardiac output on F_A/F_I increased with increasing solubility in blood. (From Eger,[1] with permission.)

output state, the inspired anesthetic partial pressure must be carefully adjusted to prevent excessive depression of the vital organs.

Alveolar to Venous Partial Pressure Gradient

The alveolar to venous partial pressure gradient is the driving force for movement of inhalational anesthetics from the alveolus to venous blood. As the anesthetic partial pressure in tissues approaches that in blood, so too does the partial pressure of anesthetic in the blood returning to the lungs. The net effect is a decrease in the alveolar to venous anesthetic partial pressure gradient and therefore a decrease in the uptake of anesthetic from the lung. As this gradient approaches zero (i.e., the anesthetic partial pressures in the tissues, blood and alveoli approach partial pressure equilibrium), uptake of anesthetic from the lungs also approaches zero.

Specific Conditions

Ventilation

Changes in Ventilation

The effect of ventilation on the rate of increase of alveolar to inspired anesthetic partial pressure affects more soluble inhalational anesthetics to a greater extent than it does less soluble anesthetics (Fig. 24-1). We can explain this differential effect of ventilation as follows: the rate of increase of alveolar to inspired anesthetic partial pressures of less soluble anesthetics is rapid because there is little uptake of anesthetic from the alveoli. In the case of the less soluble anesthetics, the alveolar to inspired anesthetic partial pressures equilibrate rapidly. In contrast, the rate of increase of alveolar to inspired anesthetic partial pressures for more soluble anesthetics is slow. This slow wash-in may be attributed to the rapid removal of anesthetics from the alveoli because of their large solubilities in blood and tissues. If the delivery of the soluble anesthetic were increased, the balance of the delivery to and uptake from the alveoli would favor an increased delivery and thus, an increase in the rate of wash-in of anesthetic. Ether, an example of a soluble anesthetic, depends on an adequate alveolar ventilation for a rapid increase in F_A/F_I. At 4 L/min alveolar ventilation, the rate of increase of alveolar to inspired methoxyflurane partial pressures (F_A/F_I) is indicated by the middle curve for methoxyflurane in Figure 24-1. At 20 minutes, F_A/F_I is 0.2. If ventilation were doubled to 8 L/min, then the wash-in would follow the uppermost curve and the F_A/F_I at 20 minutes would also double to 0.4. Conversely, if alveolar ventilation were halved to 2 L/min, the wash-in would follow the lowermost curve and the F_A/F_I at 20 minutes would also be halved to 0.1. Hence, the rate of wash-in of soluble anesthetics parallels changes in alveolar ventilation.

In contrast, the rate of increase of F_A/F_I for less soluble anesthetics is affected to only a small extent by changes in alveolar ventilation. Because the uptake of less soluble anesthetics from the alveoli is small, F_A/F_I rapidly approaches at least 90 percent within the first few minutes of ventilation. This is depicted for nitrous oxide in Figure 24-1. After 20 minutes of ventilation at a rate of 4 L/min, F_A/F_I for nitrous oxide reaches 0.95. If the alveolar ventilation were doubled to 8 L/min, F_A/F_I increases minimally, to 0.98 (3 percent increase). In contrast, if alveolar ventilation were halved to 2 L/min, F_A/F_I decreases minimally to 0.90 (5 percent decrease). Thus, changes in alveolar ventilation minimally affect the rate of rise of alveolar to inspired anesthetic partial pressure of less soluble anesthetics. Alveolar ventilation directly affects the rate of rise of alveolar to inspired anesthetic partial pressures of more soluble anesthetics to a greater extent than that of less soluble anesthetics.

Hyperventilation

Based on the above discussion, increases in ventilation (or hyperventilation) should speed the rate of rise of tissue to blood anesthetic partial pressures. Ventilation increases the delivery of anesthetic to the alveoli, which in turn increases the rate of rise of blood anesthetic partial pressure and thus the tissue anesthetic partial pressure. At the same time, however, increases in alveolar ventilation decrease the arterial carbon dioxide tension which decreases cerebral blood flow. Because the delivery of anesthetic to the brain depends on the cerebral blood flow, hyperventilation may increase the time constant for anesthetic partial pressure equilibration in the brain. Thus, hyperventilation confers two opposing effects: it increases the delivery of anesthetic to the alveoli through increased partial pressure on the one hand, but decreases the delivery of anesthetic to the brain by decreasing cerebral blood flow on the other hand.

The effect of hyperventilation on the rate of increase of anesthetic partial pressure in the brain depends on the blood solubility of the anesthetic (Fig. 24-4).[3] In the case of the more soluble anesthetics, hyperventilation increases the rate of rise of alveolar to inspired anesthetic partial pressures. This effect is of greater physiologic importance than the decrease in cerebral blood flow. As a result, hyperventilation with a soluble anesthetic speeds the net rate of rise of anesthetic partial pressure in the brain. In contrast, hyperventilation contributes in only a small way to the rate of rise of alveolar anesthetic partial pressure of the less soluble anesthetics. Hyperventilation minimally in-

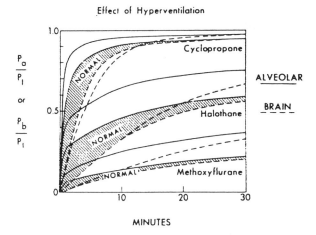

Fig. 24-4 Wash-in of three inhalational anesthetics: cyclopropane (less soluble), methoxyflurane (very soluble), and halothane (intermediate solubility). The *solid curves* denote the alveolar anesthetic partial pressure and the *dashed curves* the brain anesthetic partial pressure. Two conditions are delineated: normocapnia denoted by the curves joined by the diagonals, and hypocapnia induced by hyperventilation. Compared with the normocapnic state, hyperventilation speeds the rise of alveolar anesthetic partial pressure for all three anesthetics, although the effect is greatest with the most soluble and least with the least soluble anesthetic. In contrast, hyperventilation delays the rise of brain anesthetic partial pressure most with the least soluble and least with the most soluble anesthetic. The effect on halothane is intermediate. (Adapted from Munson and Bowers,[3] with permission.)

creases the rate of rise of alveolar to inspired anesthetic partial pressures. However, the decrease in carbon dioxide tension decreases cerebral blood flow. The net effect of hyperventilation with a less soluble anesthetic (i.e., desflurane or sevoflurane) is a slowing of the rate of rise of the brain anesthetic partial pressure during the first 15 minutes of anesthesia. After this initial period, however, the effect of hyperventilation on the delivery of anesthetic prevails and the rate of rise of the brain anesthetic partial pressure increases more rapidly than it does with normocapnic ventilation.

For anesthetics of intermediate solubility such as halothane, the effects of hyperventilation are offsetting: the increased delivery of anesthetic to the alveoli and therefore the increased rate of rise of alveolar to inspired anesthetic partial pressures is offset by the decrease in cerebral blood flow during the first 10 minutes of anesthesia (Fig. 24-4). After the first 10 minutes of anesthesia however, the rate of rise of brain anesthetic partial pressure exceeds that during normal ventilation.

These effects of hyperventilation on the rate of rise of brain anesthetic partial pressure are important not only during the first 15 minutes of anesthesia but also whenever the inspired partial pressure of anesthetic is changed during the anesthetic. The net effect of hyperventilation on the rate of rise of brain anesthetic partial pressure depends on both the solubility of the anesthetic and the time after the change in alveolar ventilation.

Modes of Ventilation: Spontaneous versus Controlled Ventilation

Two feedback mechanisms exist in response to inhalational anesthesia: respiratory and cardiovascular. The respiratory feedback mechanism is a negative feedback loop in which spontaneous ventilation decreases as the depth of anesthesia increases. This limits the depth of anesthesia by attenuating the delivery of anesthetic to the lungs. Although the delivery of anesthetic to the lungs subsides, anesthetic already present in tissues is redistributed from organs in which it is present at a high partial pressure (such as the brain) to others in which its partial pressure is low (such as muscle). When the partial pressure of anesthetic in the brain has decreased to a threshold level, respiration resumes. This feedback loop is a protective mechanism that helps to prevent an anesthetic overdose.

The second feedback mechanism is a positive feedback loop in which cardiac output decreases as the depth of anesthesia increases. As cardiac output decreases, the quantity of anesthetic that is taken up from the alveoli decreases and thus, the rate of rise of alveolar to inspired anesthetic partial pressures increases further. This increase in alveolar partial pressure is reflected in an increase in the partial pressure of anesthetic in blood and a greater driving force for anesthetic delivery to vital organs. The increase in anesthetic partial pressure in tissues further depresses organ function such as cardiac output with a further increase in anesthetic partial pressure in the alveoli, blood and tissues.

This downward spiral continues until there is an intervention that reverses the downward spiral or a cardiac arrest ensues.

The significance of these two feedback loops on the pharmacokinetics of inhalational anesthetics has been investigated in adult dogs.[4] During spontaneous ventilation in the presence of between 0.3 and 4 percent inspired halothane, the F_A/F_I increased to ≈ 0.65 where it plateaued for up to 50 minutes (Fig. 24-5A). All of the dogs survived. During controlled ventilation however, the F_A/F_I plateaued only in those dogs who were given up to 1.5 percent inspired halothane. The F_A/F_I increased relentlessly until it reached ≈ 1.0 in those dogs given 4 percent and 6 percent and within 1 hour most of those dogs experienced cardiovascular collapse (Fig. 24-5B). Thus, spontaneous ventilation remains an effective negative feedback control mechanism for preventing an anesthetic overdose of inhalational anesthetic. In contrast, controlled ventilation exposes a positive feedback mechanism that may result in a relentless downward spiral of cardiovascular depression unless the anesthetic partial pressure is attenuated. These data in dogs should also hold true for humans.

The Concentration Effect

When an inhalational anesthetic is administered in a small concentration (1 percent), uptake of half of this anesthetic results in a concentration of 0.5 percent. If however, the anesthetic is administered in an 80 percent concentration, uptake of one-half of the anesthetic results in a contracted gas volume. The net concentration is 90 percent, rather than 50 percent of the original concentration (Fig. 24-6). The concentration effect results from two factors: a concentrating effect and an increase in inspired ventilation. Uptake of 50 percent of a small concentration of anesthetic does not change the alveolar gas volume whereas uptake of a large concentration of anesthetic concentrates the residual anesthetic. As a result of the contraction of the alveolar gas volume when the anesthetic is administered in large concentrations, the void is filled with additional inspired gas. This gas augments the concentration of the anesthetic such that the final concentration in the alveoli is greater than 70 percent.

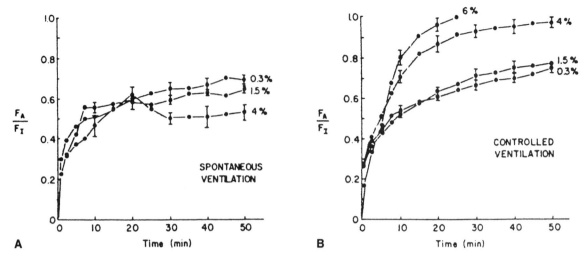

Fig. 24-5 Effect of mode of ventilation on the rate of rise of alveolar (F_A) to inspired (F_I) anesthetic partial pressure. In **A** the negative feedback effect of spontaneous ventilation limited the rate of rise of F_A/F_I. All dogs survived. **(B)** The positive feedback effect of controlled ventilation resulted in death in those dogs anesthetized with both 4 percent and 6 percent halothane. (From Gibbons et al.,[4] with permission.)

Second Gas Effect

When two anesthetics are administered, one in a large concentration and the second in a small concentration, the concentration effect of the first anesthetic increases the concentration of the second anesthetic (Fig. 24-6). This effect is produced by the same two mechanisms that explained the concentration effect above, as demonstrated in dogs.[5]

Induction of Anesthesia

It is commonly believed that the rapid rise of alveolar to inspired partial pressures of less soluble anesthetics induces anesthesia more rapidly than the more soluble anesthetics. However, this is a misconception that merits correction.

The speed of induction of anesthesia depends upon several factors including:

1. Solubility of the anesthetic
2. Rate of increase of the inspired concentration
3. Maximum inspired concentration
4. Airway reflex responses

The wash-in of less soluble anesthetics into the alveoli is rapid. F_A/F_I values for the less soluble anesthetics desflurane and sevoflurane vary from 20 to 40 percent greater than corresponding F_A/F_I values for halothane at comparable times and using a similar induction technique. This modest increase in the F_A/F_I ratio, however, is more than offset by the difference in the minimum alveolar concentration (MAC) values of these anesthetics. For example, the MAC values of desflurane and sevoflurane are approximately 800 percent and 500 percent greater than that of halothane, respectively.[6-8] Thus, at comparable inspired concentrations, the rate of induction of anesthesia with less soluble anesthetics will actually lag behind that of the more soluble anesthetics. To ensure equipotent anesthetic partial pressures during induction of anesthesia, the incremental increases in the inspired concentration and the maximum inspired concentration of less soluble anesthetics must compensate for these differences in solubility and MAC values. The maximum inspired concentration that the vaporizer must deliver to provide for a comparable induction of anesthesia with less soluble anesthetics

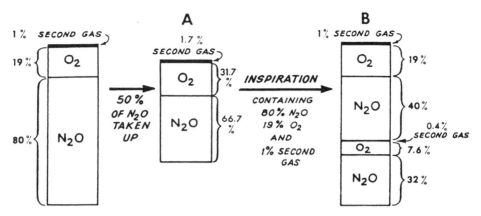

Fig. 24-6 The concentration effect and the second gas effect. The concentration effect depends on the rapid uptake of anesthetic that is present in a large concentration. This decreases the gas volume (concentrating the residual gases) **(A)** and draws fresh gas into the alveoli **(B)**. The second gas effect is evidenced by the increase in concentration of the second gas under A and B. (From Stoelting and Eger[5], with permission.)

depends on several factors, including age-related MAC values, F_A/F_I values during the wash-in, and physicochemical properties of the anesthetic. Induction of anesthesia will not, however, be similar if the anesthetic triggers airway reflex responses.

Overpressure Technique

In order to achieve the desired partial pressure in the brain rapidly, the inspired anesthetic partial pressure is usually adjusted to a value that is several-fold greater than the desired partial pressure. In this way, the partial pressure of anesthetic in the brain will very rapidly approach that needed to facilitate surgery.

The maximum inspired concentration of an anesthetic that can be delivered by a vaporizer is crucial to the success of the ovepressure technique. In the case of halothane, the maximum inspired concentration delivered by the vaporizer is 5 percent. Thus, within the first few minutes of induction of anesthesia, the maximum anesthetic partial pressure that can be achieved within the brain is the product of F_A/F_I (0.3) and the inspired concentration (5 percent) or 1.5 MAC halothane. This is equivalent to twice the MAC of halothane. By delivering a 5 percent inspired concentration of halothane, the partial pressure of halothane in the

brain will rapidly achieve an adequate anesthetic depth.

The maximum inspired concentration of sevoflurane that can be delivered by commercial vaporizers in Japan, where sevoflurane is in clinical use, is also 5 percent. With a MAC between 2.5 and 3.3 percent for infants and children,[9] the maximum inspired concentration of sevoflurane that can be delivered is barely twice the MAC for this age group. To provide for a rapid induction of anesthesia with this anesthetic, at least one major pediatric institution has arranged two sevoflurane vaporizers in series to deliver 7 to 10 percent inspired sevoflurane, equivalent to two to three times MAC. If sevoflurane is to find a meaningful role in pediatric anesthesia, vaporizers will have to deliver an inspired concentration of sevoflurane of 8 percent. This will provide induction of anesthesia with sevoflurane as rapid as that with halothane.

Vital Capacity Inductions

The traditional technique used for induction of anesthesia by inhalation is a stepwise increase in the inspired concentration of the anesthetic every few breaths. This technique is considered by many to be rapid, free from airway reflex responses, and acceptable to patients. However, despite these beliefs, an inhalational induction of anesthesia using this technique is not rapid. More recently, an alternate technique has been developed for rapid induction of anesthesia by inhalation. This involves priming the anesthetic circuit with the maximum concentration of anesthetic that the vaporizer can deliver and having the patient perform one or more vital capacity breaths.[10,11] Both halothane and sevoflurane have been used in this regard with success in comparison to the traditional inhalational induction technique.

Cardiac Output

The effect of changes in cardiac output on the rate of rise of alveolar to inspired anesthetic partial pressure is similar to that of ventilation: soluble anesthetics are affected to a greater extent than less soluble anesthetics. Soluble anesthetics are removed from the alveoli in greater quantities per unit blood flow through the lungs than are less soluble anesthetics. Therefore, in the presence of an increased cardiac output, the rate of rise of alveolar to inspired partial pressures of soluble anesthetics is slower than that of less soluble anesthetics (Fig. 24-3). This is reflected in parallel changes in the partial pressure of more soluble anesthetics in tissues since the anesthetic partial pressure in the blood equilibrates with that in the alveoli. In contrast, the rate of rise of alveolar to inspired partial pressures of the less soluble anesthetics depends less on the speed of delivery of anesthetic to or removal from the alveoli. Accordingly, changes in blood flow through the lungs have much less impact on the rate of rise of less soluble anesthetics than on the more soluble anesthetics. Cardiac output, like alveolar ventilation, affects the rate of rise of alveolar to inspired partial pressures of more soluble anesthetics to a greater extent than the less soluble anesthetics.

Shunts

Two types of blood shunts exist in the heart and lungs: left-to-right and right-to-left. Left-to-right shunts (where blood is recirculated through the lungs) do not usually affect the wash-in of inhalational anesthetics, provided cardiac output and its distribution remain unchanged. In contrast, right-

to-left shunts (where venous blood bypasses the lungs and mixes with arterial blood) exert a significant effect on the wash-in of inhalational anesthetics. The magnitude of this effect depends on the solubility of the anesthetic: right-to-left shunts affect less soluble anesthetics (i.e., nitrous oxide, desflurane and sevoflurane) to a greater extent than they affect the more soluble anesthetics (i.e., halothane and methoxyflurane) (Fig. 24-7).[1,12,13] In this model,[12] the rate of rise of the blood anesthetic partial pressure in the pulmonary veins is slower with a less soluble anesthetic than with a more soluble anesthetic in the presence of a right-to-left shunt. These effects are independent of the anatomic level of right-to-left shunts: intrapulmonary (as in the case of an endobronchial intubation) or intracardiac. The importance of right-to-left

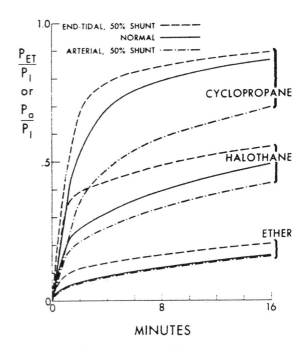

Fig. 24-7 Effect of right-to-left shunts on the wash-in of three inhalational anesthetics. From the solid (normal) curves and the dot-dashed (pulmonary venous anesthetic pressures with a 50% right-to-left shunt) it is apparent that the shunt does not affect the wash-in of a soluble anesthetic (ether) but dramatically affects the wash-in of the less soluble anesthetic, cyclopropane. The effects of halothane are intermediate. (From Eger,[1] with permission.)

shunts has recently received increased attention with the introduction into clinical practice of the less soluble inhalational anesthetics, desflurane and sevoflurane.

The effect of a right-to-left shunt on the wash-in of inhalational anesthetics is illustrated in a simplified model of the lungs in which each lung is represented by one alveolus and is perfused by one pulmonary artery (Fig. 24-8).[14] When the tracheal tube is positioned at the mid-trachea level (Fig. 24-8A), ventilation is divided equally between both lungs, thereby yielding equal anesthetic partial pressures in both pulmonary veins. However, when the tip of the tube is advanced into one bronchus (Fig. 24-8B), all of the ventilation is delivered to one lung, that is, ventilation to the intubated lung is doubled whereas ventilation to the second lung is zero. Under these conditions, normocapnia is maintained. The partial pressure of a more soluble anesthetic in the combined pulmonary venous

drainage of the lungs is approximately the same as under normal conditions because the increased ventilation to the intubated lung speeds the rise of alveolar to inspired anesthetic partial pressure such that it compensates for the presence of the shunt. However, when a less soluble anesthetic is administered in the presence of a right-to-left shunt (Fig. 24-8C) the increased ventilation to the intubated lung minimally affects the rate of rise of alveolar to inspired anesthetic partial pressures in that lung, since changes in ventilation do not appreciably affect the wash-in of less soluble anesthetics. In this case, the anesthetic partial pressure in the combined pulmonary venous drainage lags behind that which would occur in the absence of a right-to-left shunt (Fig. 24-8A).

In the presence of right-to-left shunts, the gradient between end-tidal concentrations of less soluble anesthetics and the anesthetic partial pressure in blood is greater than for more soluble anesthetics,

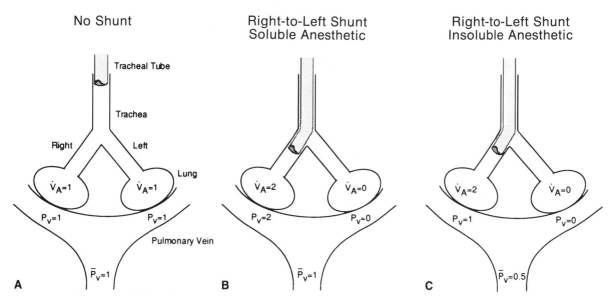

Fig. 24-8 Right-to-left shunts affect the rate of rise of the partial pressure of less soluble anesthetics in the pulmonary vein. In **(A)**, the normal situation without a shunt, ventilation is equal in both lungs and normocapnia is maintained. In **(B)**, a soluble anesthetic is administered in the presence of a right-to-left shunt from an endobronchial intubation. Normocapnia is maintained and hypoxic pulmonary vasoconstriction is negligible. Here, the increase in ventilation to the intubated lung offsets the effect of the shunt. In **(C)**, a right-to-left shunt in the presence of a less soluble anesthetic limits the increase in anesthetic partial pressure in the pulmonary vein. Since an increase in alveolar ventilation does not affect the wash-in of a less soluble anesthetic substantially, the shunted blood has a dramatic effect to slow the rate of rise of anesthetic partial pressure in the pulmonary vein. (From Lerman,[14] with permission.)

as with the end-tidal-to-arterial carbon dioxide partial pressure differences in children with cyanotic heart disease.[15] As desflurane and sevoflurane are introduced into clinical practice, this issue becomes increasingly important for patients with right-to-left shunts.

Others

Temperature

The solubility of inhalational anesthetics in blood and tissues is inversely related to the temperature (i.e., as the temperature decreases, the solubility increases). The effect of temperature on the solubility of inhalational anesthetics has been reported for isoflurane, enflurane, halothane, and methoxyflurane.[16-18] Solubility increases 4 to 5 percent for each degree centigrade decrease in temperature.

Temperature has a predictable effect on the pharmacokinetics of inhalational anesthetics. As the temperature decreases and solubility increases, the wash-in of inhalational anesthetics is delayed. This would be expected to significantly affect the pharmacokinetics of inhalational anesthetics administered during cardiopulmonary bypass when the patient temperature is decreased.

WASH-IN OF ANESTHETICS INTO TISSUES

The uptake of anesthetic by the body is the sum of the uptake by each of the tissues in the body. The uptake of anesthetics by tissues determines the uptake of anesthetic from the lung and the alveolar to venous partial pressure gradient. Early in the anesthetic, the uptake of anesthetic by tissues is great and the partial pressure of anesthetic in the venous return is low. As the partial pressure of anesthetic in tissues approaches the partial pressure in the alveoli, the venous partial pressure increases and the uptake of anesthetic from the alveoli subsides.

We can estimate the uptake of anesthetic by grouping tissues according to the time to anesthetic partial pressure equilibration in the tissue, based on the relative solubility of the inhalational anesthetics in those tissues and the perfusion to the tissues.

Four tissue groups have been defined: vessel-rich group, muscle group, fat, and vessel-poor

groups.[1] The vessel-rich group is comprised of five organs: brain, heart, kidney, splanchnic (liver), and endocrine glands.

The time constant for equilibration of anesthetic partial pressure in a tissue is defined as the ratio of the capacity of the organ and the blood flow to the organ as in equation 3. The capacity of the tissue reservoir for anesthesia is the product of the volume of the tissue (or organ) and the solubility of the anesthetic in that tissue (tissue/blood partition coefficient). Thus, the time constant for organs is the ratio of this capacity to the blood flow to the organ:

$$\tau = (V \cdot \lambda_{t/b}) \cdot Q^{-1} \qquad (4)$$

where $\lambda_{t/b}$ is the tissue/blood partition coefficient for the anesthetic. Since the volume of and blood flow to most organs is constant, changes in the time constant for an organ is determined by differences in the $\lambda_{t/b}$. For example, we can estimate the time to equilibration of anesthetic partial pressures in tissues such as the brain by determining the time constant for the brain. The time constant (τ) for the brain is described by the following ratio:

$$\tau = \frac{\text{Volume of the brain (ml)} \times \text{Brain/blood solubility}}{\text{Brain blood flow (ml/min)}} \qquad (5)$$

If the blood flow to the brain is approximately 50 ml/min/100 gm of brain and the brain/blood solubility for a particular inhalational anesthtic is 2.0, then the time constant is:

$$\tau = \frac{100 \text{ ml} \times 2}{50 \text{ ml/min}} = 4 \text{ min} \qquad (6)$$

assuming the density of the brain tissue is 1 gm/ml. Thus, the time to 98 percent equilibration of anesthetic partial pressures (that is, four time constants) is 16 minutes. If the brain/blood solubility of a second anesthetic were one-half that of the first (i.e., 1.0), then the time to 98 percent equilibration would be reduced to only 8 minutes. Hence, the time to equilibration of anesthetic partial pressure within the brain with this second anesthetic would be approximately one-half that with the first anesthetic.

The rate of rise of anesthetic partial pressure in tissues and organs follows a pattern that is determined by the delivery of anesthetic to these organs. That is, organs that are perfused with a greater fraction of the cardiac output equilibrate anesthetic partial pressure with that in the alveoli more rapidly than organs with a smaller fraction of the cardiac output. Based on equations 4 to 6, we can predict the time constants for groups of organs with similar perfusion as shown in Table 24-4. The order of equilibration of tissue halothane partial pressure is from first to last as follows: vessel-rich group, muscle, vessel-poor group, and fat.

Uptake of anesthetic by the vessel-rich group is denoted by the initial flattening of the wash-in curve for inhalational anesthetics. Without uptake by the vessel-rich group, the increase in F_A/F_I would continue with the same rapid increase as it does in the first minutes of the wash-in. Thus, the effect of uptake of anesthetic by the vessel-rich group is to slow the rate of rise of alveolar to inspired anesthetic partial pressures. Thereafter, uptake of anesthetic from the alveoli occurs by the remaining tissues in the body.

The wash-in of inhalational anesthetics into the vessel-rich group is usually complete within the first 15 to 20 minutes of anesthesia. In adults, these organs comprise 10 percent of the body weight but receive 75 percent of the cardiac output. Accordingly, the time constant for this group is small and anesthetic partial pressure equilibrates rapidly in these organs (Table 24-4). For example, one time constant or 66 percent equilibration of halothane partial pressure in the vessel-rich organs is 3.3 minutes and the time to 98 percent equilibration is 13 minutes. The magnitude of the range in the time constants for different tissues is determined by the tissue/blood solubility; the greater the solubility, the greater the time constant and vice versa (Table 24-4).

After equilibration of the anesthetic partial pressure in the vessel-rich group, F_A/F_I should increase rapidly. However, the rate of increase of F_A/F_I is slower than expected because of the uptake of anesthetic by the tissue group with the second smallest time constant, the muscle group. Substantial uptake by this group begins approximately 20 minutes after induction of anesthesia and continues for approximately 200 minutes.[1] The time constant for anesthetic in the muscle group is greater than that in the vessel-rich group by approximately 10- to 30-fold (Table 24-4). This may be attributed to a relatively smaller perfusion per unit muscle mass and a greater solubility of anesthetics in the muscle tissues. The time to equilibration of the anesthetic partial pressure in muscle is approximately 2 to 6 hours depending on the particular anesthetic (Table 24-4).

After equilibration of the anesthetic partial pressure in the muscle group, uptake continues by the vessel-poor group and fat as reflected by the large time constants for these tissue groups (Table 24-4). Fat represents 20 percent of the body weight but receives only 6 percent of the cardiac output in the healthy adult. Although the perfusion of fat per

Table 24-4   Tissue Group Characteristics[a]

	Vessel-Rich Group (VRG)	Muscle Group (MG)	Fat Group (FG)	Vessel-Poor Group (VPG)
Body mass (%)	9	50	19	22
Volumes (L)	6	33	14.5	12.5
Cardiac output (% of total)	75	18.1	5.4	1.5
Time constant (τ) (min) for N_2O	1.3	30	100	160
Time constant (τ) (min) for halothane	3.3	106	2,720	390

[a]Data (from Eger[1]) are based on a 70-kg adult.

unit volume is only 10 to 20 percent less than that of muscle, the solubility of anesthetics in fat is 10 to 30 times greater than that in muscle (Table 24-3). On the basis of Equation 5, the time constant for fat is 10 to 30 times that in muscle or 1.5 to 40 hours depending on the anesthetic. With time constants of this duration, uptake of anesthetic by fat usually contributes minimally to the total tissue uptake.

Several investigators have modeled the wash-in of anesthetic in the body using a multi-exponential model as follows[19]:

$$\sum_{i=1}^{n} \frac{A_i}{\lambda_i} (1 - e^{-\lambda_i t}) \qquad (7)$$

A_i is the compartmental coefficient (accounting for tissue characteristics), λ_i is the tissue/blood solubility and t is time. The time constants for individual compartments were calculated as:

$$\tau = 1/\lambda_i \qquad (8)$$

Carpenter et al.[19] measured the wash-in of four inhalational anesthetics isoflurane, enflurane, halothane and methoxyflurane simultaneously in healthy adults. Surprisingly, they were able to predict only a two or three compartment model of uptake and distribution of inhalational anesthetics with this model. They attributed their failure to identify the four tissue compartments to the brief period (120 minutes) of wash-in measured.

In contrast to the limited period of wash-in, Carpenter et al. also measured the wash-out of the same four inhalational anesthetics for an extended period, 5 to 9 days[1] in the same study. On the basis of their wash-out data, they predicted a five-compartment model of uptake and distribution of anesthetics within the body.[19] These five compartments corresponded to: lungs, vessel-rich group, muscle group, a fourth group, and fat. Furthermore, their estimates of the time constants for four of the tissue groups were similar to those published previously (Table 24-4). The fourth tissue group was explained by an inter-tissue group such as fat tissue near a highly perfused tissue (i.e., omental, pericardial, perirenal, or subcutaneous fat). Further refinement of this model and additional human data are required before the pharmacokinetics of inhalational anesthetics are fully understood.

The effects of two other variables, duration of anesthesia and age of the patients, on the time constants of the tissue compartments were determined using a similar model. Duration of anesthesia between 30 and 120 minutes had little effect on time constants.[20] Elimination of volatile anesthetics in the elderly was delayed compared to young adults.[21] This difference in elimination was attributed to a decrease in tissue perfusion and increase in the fat/lean body weight ratio in the elderly compared to young adults. Similar modeling of the pharmacokinetics of inhalational anesthetics in infants and children remains to be completed.

Kinetics in Infants and Children

Although it is generally accepted that the rates of rise of alveolar to inspired anesthetic partial pressures in neonates and young infants are more rapid than that in adults, there is little evidence to support this notion. Salanitre and Rackow[22] first demonstrated that the rate of rise of alveolar to inspired partial pressures of halothane is more rapid in young children (1 to 3 years of age) than it is in adults (Fig. 24-9). In two separate studies, investigators reported a more rapid increase in F_A/F_I of nitrous oxide in neonates compared with that in adults.[22,23] However, these observations have not been verified with other inhalational anesthetics in neonates and infants. Gallagher and Black[24] reported the rate of rise of F_A/F_I in infants and children up to 2 years of age, but they grouped neonates and young infants together with older infants and children. Recent observations have suggested that the pharmacokinetics of inhalational anesthetics in neonates requires further investigation (see Elimination below).

Table 24-5 Factors Responsible for the Rapid Wash-In of Inhalational Anesthetics in Infants

Greater alveolar ventilation to functional residual capacity ratio
Greater fraction of the cardiac output distributed to the vessel rich group
Lower blood/gas solubility
Lower tissue/blood solubility

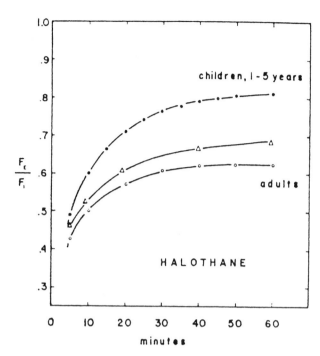

Fig. 24-9 Rate of rise of alveolar to inspired partial pressures of halothane in children and adults. The wash-in of halothane in children (*upper curve*) exceeds that in adults (*two lower curves*). (From Salanitre and Rackow,[22] with permission.)

The more rapid rate of rise of anesthetic partial pressures in children compared with adults has been attributed to four differences between these two age groups: alveolar ventilation to FRC ratio, cardiac output, tissue/blood solubility, and blood/gas solubility (Table 24-5).

Alveolar Ventilation to FRC Ratio

The ratio of alveolar ventilation to FRC has already been identified as an important determinant of the rate of rise of alveolar to inspired anesthetic partial pressure. The greater the ratio, the more rapid the wash-in of inhalational anesthetic (Fig. 24-1). In neonates, this ratio is approximately 5 : 1 compared with only 1.5 : 1 in adults. The greater ratio in neonates is attributable to the threefold greater metabolic rate in neonates compared with adults. Additionally, previous studies have demonstrated that changes in alveolar ventilation (as well as cardiac output) affect more soluble anesthetics to a greater extent than less soluble anesthetics (Figs. 24-1 and

24-3). Halothane is the most commonly used inhalational anesthetic in pediatric anesthesia and the greater alveolar ventilation to FRC ratio in neonates will speed the wash-in of this soluble anesthetic.

Cardiac Output

In adults, increases in cardiac output slow the rate of rise of alveolar to inspired anesthetic partial pressures (Fig. 24-3).[1] Paradoxically, the greater cardiac index in neonates actually speeds the rise of alveolar to inspired anesthetic partial pressures. This has been attributed to the preferential distribution of the cardiac output to the vessel-rich group of tissues in neonates. The vessel-rich group of tissues receives a greater proportion of the cardiac output in neonates because it comprises 18 percent of the body weight in neonates compared with only 8 percent in adults. As a result of the increased blood flow, the partial pressure of anesthetic in the vessel-rich group equilibrates with that in the alveoli more rapidly in neonates than it does in adults. Since the uptake of anesthetic by tissues other than those of the vessel-rich group in neonates is small, the rapid equilibration of anesthetic partial pressures in the vessel-rich group will lead to a greater partial pressure of anesthetic in the venous blood returning to the lungs. Uptake of anesthetic from the lung then rapidly diminishes. The net effect of the greater cardiac output in neonates is to speed equilibration of anesthetic partial pressure in the vessel-rich group.

Solubility

The solubility of inhalational anesthetics in blood varies with age.[25] The blood solubilities of the inhalational anesthetics halothane, isoflurane, enflurane and methoxyflurane are 18 percent less in neonates and the elderly than they are in young adults (Fig. 24-10). In contrast, the solubilities of the less soluble anesthetic sevoflurane in preterm and full-term neonates are not significantly different from those in adults.[26] The effect of gestational age on the solubility of desflurane in blood has not been determined, although based on the data for sevoflurane, the effect is probably small and clinically insignificant.

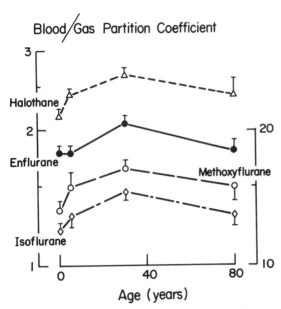

Fig. 24-10 Effect of age on the solubility of inhalational anesthetics in blood. Solubility is 18 percent less in neonates than in adults for all four inhalational anesthetics. (From Lerman et al.,[25] with permission.)

The precise site of binding of inhalational anesthetics to the constituents in blood is poorly understood. Using multiple regression analysis, we attempted to identify the blood constituent(s), protein and/or lipid, that determined the blood/gas partition coefficients of isoflurane, enflurane, halothane and methoxyflurane.[25] We found that the blood/gas partition coefficients of isoflurane and enflurane correlated directly with the serum albumin and triglyceride concentrations, that of halothane correlated directly with the serum cholesterol, albumin, triglyceride and globulin concentrations, and that of methoxyflurane correlated directly with the serum cholesterol, albumin, and globulin concentrations.[25] These data were consistent with previous studies.[27] Binding of inhalational anesthetics to α_1-acid glycoprotein does not appear to be significant.[28]

The solubilites of the inhalational anesthetics, halothane, isoflurane, enflurane and methoxyflurane in the tissues of the vessel-rich group in neonates are approximately one-half those in adults (Fig. 24-11).[29] The decreased tissue solubilities are attributable to two differences in the composition of tissues between neonates and adults: (1)

greater water content and (2) decreased protein and lipid concentrations in neonates. The decreased tissue solubility of inhalational anesthetics decreases the time for partial pressure equilibration of anesthetics in these tissues and therefore the time constant. Although the partial pressures of inhaled anesthetics in tissues cannot easily be measured in vivo, they may be estimated by the anesthetic partial pressure in the exhaled or alveolar gases. Thus, the decrease in the solubility of inhalational anesthetics in tissues speeds the rate of rise of alveolar to inspired anesthetic partial pressures in neonates compared with that in adults.

The solubilities of the inhalational anesthetics isoflurane, enflurane, halothane and mexthoxyflurane in muscle increase in a semilogarithmic fashion with age between neonates and the elderly (Fig. 24-12).[29] The decrease in the solubility of anesthetics in the muscle of neonates may be attributed to the small protein content of muscle in the first few months of life whereas the increased solu-

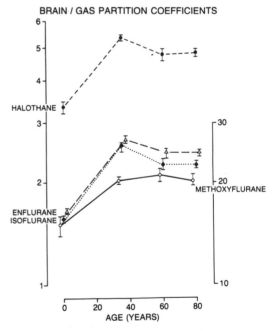

Fig. 24-11 Effect of age on the solubility of isoflurane, enflurane, halothane, and methoxyflurane in human brain. The solubilities of all anesthetics in neonatal brain are less than those in adults. (From Lerman et al.,[29] with permission.)

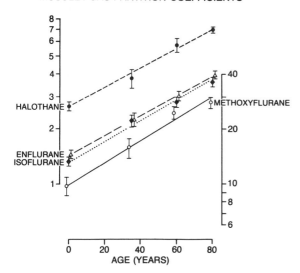

MUSCLE / GAS PARTITION COEFFICIENTS

Fig. 24-12 The solubility of inhalational anesthetics in muscle increases with age. This semilogarithmic relationship is attributed to smaller protein content in neonates and larger protein and fat content in the elderly. (From Lerman et al.,[29] with permission.)

bility in the elderly reflects the increased protein and fat content of muscle in this age group. The importance of the decreased solubility of inhalational anesthetics in muscle in neonates is reflected in the more rapid equilibration of inhalational anesthetic partial pressure in muscle during the uptake of anesthetic by muscle, between 20 and 200 minutes after introduction of the inhalational anesthetic. Thus, the low solubility of inhalational anesthetics in muscle in neonates speeds the wash-in and contributes to the striking difference in the wash-in of inhalational anesthetics between neonates and adults.

The net effect of the various differences between neonates and adults is to speed the equilibration of anesthetic partial pressures in alveoli and tissues and thereby speed the rate of rise of alveolar to inspired anesthetic partial pressures in infants and children compared with adults. This has been shown to hold true for the more soluble anesthetics halothane, enflurane, and isoflurane. However, the factors responsible for the more rapid wash-in of soluble anesthetics in infants and children may

not confer similar effects for the less soluble anesthetics, desflurane and sevoflurane. Hence, age-related differences in the speed of wash-in of these less soluble anesthetics may be attenuated compared with the published data for the more soluble anesthetics. This hypothesis awaits verification.

ELIMINATION

General Principles

The wash-out of inhalational anesthetics follows an exponential decay (the inverse of the wash-in curve). The rapidity of wash-out varies, in part, with blood/gas solubility (Fig. 24-2, Table 24-3). However, the elimination of inhalational anesthetics depends on other factors as well, including duration of anesthetic exposure and metabolism.

After 30 to 40 minutes of anesthesia, the anesthetic partial pressure in the vessel-rich group of tissues has equilibrated with that in the alveoli whereas the anesthetic partial pressure in the muscle lags behind that in the vessel-rich group and that in fat is even less than that in the muscle group. At the conclusion of anesthesia, the inhalational anesthetic moves along the partial pressure gradient from the vessel-rich tissues into blood and then into the alveoli. However, the anesthetic partial pressure gradient between tissues outside the vessel-rich group and blood may vary considerably. For example, the anesthetic partial pressure in muscle will be less than that in the vessel-rich tissues. After a brief anesthetic (i.e., 30 minutes), the anesthetic partial pressure in muscle will be very small, and the release of anesthetic from the vessel-rich group will increase the anesthetic partial pressure in blood and maintain the uptake by muscle. In contrast, after 3 or 4 hours the partial pressure of anesthetic in muscle will be similar to that in the vessel-rich group and alveoli. Here, the anesthetic will be released by both the vessel-rich group and muscle. Similar considerations also hold true for fat except that the time constant for partial pressure equilibration would be significantly greater.

The effect of the duration of anesthesia on the rate of wash-out of anesthetic depends in part on the solubility of the anesthetic.[30] The greater the solubility of the anesthetic, the greater the effect of duration of anesthesia on the wash-out. For anesthetics with low solubilities (such as nitrous oxide, desflurane, and sevoflurane), the wash-out is rapid and the duration of anesthesia has little effect on the wash-out. On the other hand, for anesthetics that are very soluble (such as methoxyflurane), the rate of wash-out varies inversely with the duration of anesthesia: that is, the longer the duration, the slower the wash-out.[30]

Percutaneous loss of inhalational anesthetics result in small losses relative to expired losses and metabolism. These losses depend on the blood solubility of the anesthetic. Quantitatively, percutaneous losses of inhalational anesthetics do not affect their pharmacokinetics.[31,32]

Metabolism

Metabolism is an important mechanism for the elimination of some inhalational anesthetics. Metabolism occurs in patients of all ages. Metabolism of inhalational anesthetics depends primarily on the cytochrome P-450 enzyme systems located in the endoplasmic reticulum of hepatocytes. Two of the metabolic pathways followed are the oxidative and reductive pathways. Of the oxidative pathways, dehalogenation and O-dealkylation have been described for inhalational anesthetics. Dehalogenation is the result of hydroxylation of the halogenated carbon that decomposes to a carboxylic acid and inorganic halogens. The presence of two halogens on the terminal carbon provides optimal conditions for dehalogenation, whereas the presence of three halogens dramatically reduces the probability of dehalogenation. O-dealkylation is the result of hydroxylation of an alkyl group adjacent to the oxygen of the ether bond. The intermediate compound rapidly decomposes to an alcohol and an aldehyde. The aldehyde may be oxidized by aldehyde oxidase to carboxylic acid or reduced by alcohol dehydrogenase to an alcohol. The reductive pathway has only been demonstrated for halothane.[33-36]

The extent of metabolism of inhalational anesthetics ranges from 50 percent for methoxyflurane to 0.02 percent for desflurane (Table 24-6). With the exception of halothane and methoxyflurane, the metabolism of inhalational anesthetics accounts for the elimination of less than 3 percent of the

Table 24-5   Extent of Metabolism of Inhalational Anesthetics

Anesthetic	Metabolism (%)[a]
Methoxyflurane	50
Halothane	15–20
Sevoflurane	3.3
Enflurane	2.4
Isoflurane	0.2
Desflurane	0.02

[a]Estimated extent of metabolism based on both animal and human studies.

total anesthetic administered. Insofar as halothane and methoxyflurane are concerned, their rates of metabolism significantly affect the pharmacokinetics. The wash-out of halothane in adults is similar to that of enflurane, despite a 100 percent difference in the blood solubility between these anesthetics.[19] The similar rates of washout of these two anesthetics may be attributed to the offsetting effects of the greater metabolism of halothane and the lesser solubility of enflurane.

Methoxyflurane is metabolized to a greater extent (50 percent) than any other inhalational anesthetic (Table 24-6). This ether anesthetic is oxygenated either at the methyl carbon or at the dichloroethyl carbon with the release of large quantities of inorganic fluoride, dichloroacetic acid and possibly methoxydifluoroacetic acid.[37-39] Defluorination of methoxyflurane occurs in the presence of cytochrome P-450, glutathione-s-transferase and possibly a nonenzymatic pathway that requires B12 and glutathione.[40-43] Metabolism of methoxyflurane is increased after pretreatment with phenobarbital,[44] phenytoin,[45] ethanol,[46,47] diazepam,[48] and isoniazid.[49,50]

Halothane is extensively metabolized oxidatively and reductively through the cytochrome P-450 mixed function oxidase system.[51-54] The products of the oxidative pathway are inorganic bromide, chloride, and trifluoroacetic acid, whereas the products of the reductive pathway are inorganic bromide and fluoride. An alternate reductive pathway requires an electron donor (usually the cytochrome P-450 enzyme system) and an anaerobic milieu. This pathway results in several volatile halogenated compounds (1,1-difluoro-2-chloro-ethylene, 1,1,1-trifluoro-2-chloroethane and 1,1-difluoro-2-bromo-2-chloroethylene) and inorganic fluoride is also released.[36,55] Peak inorganic fluoride concentrations remain low (less than 15 μm) even after 19.5 MAC · h halothane in adults.[56] Metabolism of halothane is increased after administration of phenobarbital,[57] isoniazid,[58] and prolonged exposure to subanesthetic concentrations of halothane.[59] The role of metabolism in the elimination of halothane is important, particularly in adults, as evidenced by wash-out comparable to enflurane, an anesthetic with one-half the solubility of halothane.[19]

The rate of metabolism of sevoflurane in vivo (3.3 percent) approximates that of enflurane. Sevoflurane is metabolized by cytochrome P-450 II E1 through oxidation of the α-carbon rather than the trifluoromethyl carbons.[60] The profile of inorganic fluoride after sevoflurane anesthesia in adults without hepatic enzyme induction is similar to that of enflurane. Maximum fluoride concentrations reach 25 to 35 μm within 1 or 2 hours of discontinuation of the anesthetic but decrease to less than 5 μm by several hours.[61,62] The rapid decrease in serum inorganic fluoride after discontinuation of the anesthetic is attributed to the rapid wash-out of sevoflurane (Table 24-3) and minimal metabolism of sevoflurane. Plasma inorganic fluoride concentrations are approximately 20 percent greater after prolonged exposure (13.4 ± 0.9 h) and in mildly obese patients.[63,64] Organic fluoride in the form of hexafluoroisopropanol is the route of elimination of most of the fluoride. This organic metabolite is rapidly conjugated and eliminated in the urine.[65] Defluorination of sevoflurane is increased after pretreatment with phenobarbital,[66] phenytoin,[45] ethanol,[47] and isoniazid.[49,50] The importance of metabolism in the elimination of this anesthetic remains to be clarified.[19]

Enflurane is metabolized to only a small extent (Table 24-6). Enflurane is metabolized via oxidative dehalogenation at the chlorofluoromethyl carbon on enflurane by cyctochrome P-450 II E1 isozyme.[60] The resultant inorganic fluoride yields serum concentrations that are considered subtoxic.

Isoflurane is metabolized to only a small extent (Table 24-6), approximately one-tenth that of enflurane. Metabolism occurs via oxidation of the α-carbon yielding trifluororacetic acid, inorganic fluoride and several intermediate compounds. The maximum serum concentration of inorganic fluoride after isoflurane is less than 5 μm,[67,68] although plasma fluoride concentrations in excess of 50 μm have been reported after prolonged administration of isoflurane (19.2 MAC · h).[56] Enzyme induction increases metabolism of isoflurane, although metabolism does not contribute significantly to the elimination of this anesthetic.

Desflurane is the least metabolized of the inhalational anesthetics (Table 24-6). The reduced metabolism is attributed to the substitution of fluorine for chlorine on the α-carbon, thereby decreasing the affinity of this substrate for the cytochrome enzymes. Inorganic fluoride after desflurane is <3 μm even after prolonged exposure.[69–71] Metabolism does not contribute substantially to the termination of the action or elimination of this anesthetic.

Infants and Children

The wash-out of inhalational anesthetics in neonates and infants has been incompletely studied. Recently, we reported the wash-out ratios for desflurane and sevoflurane at 2 and 5 minutes after discontinuation of anesthesia in six age groups of neonates, infants, and children.[9,72] During the wash-out period, ventilation was controlled to maintain an end-tidal PCO_2 of 35 to 45 mmHg. For both anesthetics, the ratio, F_A/F_{AO}, was 20 to 50 percent greater in neonates at 2 and 5 minutes after discontinuation of anesthesia than it was for older infants. (F_A, the alveolar fraction during washout. F_{AO}, the alveolar fraction at the time of discontinuation of anesthesia.) Consistent with these prolonged wash-out data were longer times to extubation and recovery of neonates compared with the older infants.[9,72] These observations were surprising in view of our previous understanding of the effect of age on the wash-in and wash-out of inhalational anesthetics in the pediatric age range.[22–24] The pharmacokinetics of inhalational anesthetics in neonates and older infants requires further investigation.

Age significantly affects the rate of metabolism of inhalational anesthetics. The metabolism of inhalational anesthetics in neonates and infants is less than that in adults. This has been attributed to reduced activity of hepatic microsomal enzymes,[73] reduced fat stores, and more rapid exhalation of the anesthetics.[22] For example, the plasma profile of inorganic fluoride after methoxyflurane anesthesia in children is diminished compared with that in adults.[74] This includes both the maximum plasma concentration of inorganic fluoride as well as the area under the curve. Similar data holds true for sevoflurane.[9] In contrast to the substantially increased plasma fluoride concentrations reported after prolonged exposure to isoflurane in adults, peak plasma fluoride concentrations after up to 440 MAC · h isoflurane in children were less than 30 μm.[75] Indeed, in contrast to adults, fluoride-induced nephrotoxicity has never been reported in children. Decreased metabolism of methoxyflurane in children compared with adults has been attributed to several factors, including reduced activity of the hepatic microsomal enzymes, reduced fat stores, increased uptake of inorganic fluoride by bone, and more rapid wash-out.[74] The impact of the reduced metabolism of inhalational anesthetics in neonates and infants should be most apparent for those anesthetics that undergo extensive metabolism, i.e., methoxyflurane and halothane. Accordingly, the rates of elimination of these anesthetics in younger patients should lag behind that of enflurane. Decreased metabolism in infants will likely have less impact on the elimination of the newer less soluble anesthetics than on the more soluble ones.

Recovery

Recovery from anesthesia depends on the wash-out of anesthetic partial pressure from the brain. The rate of wash-out of anesthetic from the brain should be rapid because the brain/blood solubility of inhalational anesthetics is modest (Table 24-3) and the brain receives a large fraction of the cardiac output.

Recovery of motor function in rats parallels the wash-out of inhalational anesthetics: desflurane > sevoflurane > isoflurane > halothane.[76] Although similar studies in infants and children are not available, it is reasonable to expect that the order of wash-out of inhalational anesthetics in children will be similar to that in adults.

CIRCUITS
Wash-in

The rate of wash-in of anesthetic into the anesthetic circuit is determined by the fresh gas flow and the volume within the anesthetic circuit. With Mapleson D and F (i.e., Bain and Ayre's t piece circuits), the volume of the circuit is small and the wash-in of anesthetic is determined by the fresh gas flow. With these circuits, the wash-in of anesthetic is fast even under low fresh gas flow conditions (0.5 to 2.0 L/minute). However, under low fresh gas flow conditions, rebreathing may occur. In this case, the inspired anesthetic partial pressure will reflect a mixture of the anesthetic partial pressures in the fresh gas and that in the exhaled gas.

In most circumstances, the volume of the circuit is small relative to the fresh gas flow and does not delay the onset of delivery of inhalational anesthesia to the patient. In the case of the adult circle circuit, however, this may not hold true. These circuits consist of a large reservoir bag, carbon dioxide canister and large bore corrugated tubing with gas volumes approaching 7 L. Under conditions of low flow (0.5 L/min), the gas volume of the circuit is 14-fold greater than the fresh gas flow, giving a time constant for this circuit of 14 minutes. Accordingly, the time to 98 percent equilibration of anesthetic concentration is this circuit would be 56 minutes! This illustrates the difficulty in effecting rapid changes in anesthetic partial pressures with a low fresh gas flow in this type of circuit. Increasing the fresh gas flow to 3.5 liters/minute will decrease the time to 98 percent equilibration of anesthetic partial pressures by 5 fold, to 8 minutes. With these circuits, large fresh gas flows are required when a rapid increase or decrease in anesthetic partial pressure is required.

The kinetics of inhalational anesthetics in cardiopulmonary bypass circuits is incompletely understood. In a model of one such circuit, Nussmeier et al.[77] determined the wash-in of isoflurane, enflurane and halothane and the factors that affect the wash-in. They found that in a circuit with a hematocrit of 27 percent maintained at 24 to 26°C, the wash-in of the 3 inhalational anesthetics was similar. The solubility of anesthetics in the diluted blood prime was similar to that reported for whole blood. They attributed this to offsetting effects of hemodilution and hypothermia.[78,79] Increasing the gas inflow to the oxygenator fourfold only slightly affected the wash-in and wash-out whereas increasing the pump flow 60 percent had no effect. The kinetics of inhalational anesthetics in a blood-primed bypass circuit at modest hypothermia are rapid and similar for isoflurane, enflurane, and halothane.

Fiscal restraint and concerns over local and atmospheric pollution have led to a reduction in fresh gas flows during anesthesia. Economic pressures to control anesthetic costs have motivated anesthetists to decrease fresh gas flows, particularly when using the newer anesthetics, desflurane and sevoflurane, and to monitor adequacy of ventilation and anesthetic gas concentrations. In contrast, minimal savings will be recognized by decreasing the fresh gas flow during halothane anesthesia as these costs are approximately $0.50 per hour at a 6-liter fresh gas flow rate. Isoflurane and enflurane are intermediate in cost between halothane and desflurane.

Local pollution is easily managed by the use of scavenging systems in the operating theater; however, these waste gases are then emitted into the atmosphere. Most reports suggest that polyfluorinated ether anesthetics are ozone neutral, neither aggressively destroying the ozone layer in the stratosphere nor remaining in the atmosphere for extended periods (half-life 5 y).[80,81] In contrast, nitrous oxide produces free radicals and resides in the stratosphere for up to 150 years.

Anesthetic Loss to Circuitry and Carbon Dioxide Absorbers

Inhalational anesthetics may be removed from the fresh gas flow at several sites in the delivery circuit including the gas tubing, carbon dioxide absorber, and bag. All inhalational anesthetics are soluble in the plastic and rubber components of the circuit. This poses a serious problem for methoxyflurane and halothane use, as both are soluble in polyethylene, rubber, and polyvinyl chloride.[82–86] However, for desflurane and sevoflurane this is not an issue. Isoflurane and enflurane are intermediate and are not significantly affected.

Uptake of anesthetic in the carbon dioxide absorber is a potentially serious problem. Delivery of the inhalational anesthetics through a carbon dioxide absorber with dry soda lime or baralyme may substantially decrease the inspired partial pressure of anesthetic. Several inhalational anesthetics, including halothane[87–89] and sevoflurane, are adsorbed by and degraded in dry carbon dioxide absorbers. At high temperatures, halothane is degraded to 2-bromochloroethylene, although the concentration of this degradation product is less than 3 percent of its lethal concentration. Insofar as halothane is concerned, neither its disappearance nor its degradation in soda lime have been clinical problems. Isoflurane, enflurane and desflurane are absorbed and degraded to small extents in the presence of soda lime.[88,89]

Sevoflurane is both absorbed and degraded in part, by alkaline hydrolysis in the presence of both soda lime and baralyme.[89–91] Factors that affect the disappearance of sevoflurane in carbon dioxide cannisters include the water content and temperature of the absorbent and the type of absorbent. Fresh dry soda lime absorbs more sevoflurane than moist soda lime. Furthermore, as the temperature of soda lime increases, so too does the rate of disappearance of sevoflurane. We found that sevoflurane disappeared more rapidly when it was incubated with baralyme than with soda lime.[90] Absorption of sevoflurane by soda lime might delay the wash-in of sevoflurane.[91] However, recent data suggests that absorption of sevoflurane by soda lime is not likely to be clinically significant even in low flow systems.[92] Further studies are warranted to establish the possible clinical implications of in vitro disappearance of sevoflurane.

Closed Circuit or Low Flow Anesthesia

Closed circuit anesthesia is based on the principle that the anesthetic requirements can be predicted by the wash-in of inhalational anesthetics and that based on the uptake, no more and no less anesthetic need be administered. If this technique is to be safe for patients it requires: (1) a measure of the oxygen partial pressure within the circuit, particularly in the presence of nitrous oxide, and (2) a measure of the partial pressure of anesthetic being delivered. Today, both of these monitors are available and should allow the safe use of this type of circuitry.

Empirical formulas were developed to predict the anesthetic requirements of patients during closed circuit anaesthesia. The uptake of anesthetic during the first minute of anesthesia could be predicted from the modified uptake equation:

$$U_1 = \lambda \cdot Q \cdot A/BP$$

where U_1 is the uptake in the first minute, λ is the blood/gas solubility of the anesthetic, Q is the cardiac output and A is the alveolar partial pressure corrected for barometric pressure. The A/BP is abbreviated from $(A - v)/BP$ where v is the anesthetic partial pressure in the venous blood, which is zero at the commencement of anesthesia. Severinghaus[94] then suggested that the uptake at any time U_t may be expressed as follows:

$$U_t = U_1 \cdot t^{-1/2}$$

Although these formulae provided an estimate of the amount of liquid anesthetic that was required each minute in the circuit, the interindividual variability in the dose required was substantial. Factors that contributed to this variability included body mass and surface area, anesthetic requirements, and pathophysiologic conditions. With the widespread availability of anesthetic agent monitoring, precise control of the end-tidal concentration of anesthetic is possible for each patient with each breath. This addition to our monitoring armamentarium has simplified closed circuit anesthesia and the level of safety attendant with its use.

REFERENCES

1. Eger EI II: Anesthetic Uptake and Action. Williams & Wilkins, Baltimore, 1974
2. Yasuda N, Lockhart SH, Eger EI II et al: Comparison of kinetics of sevoflurane and isoflurane in humans. Anesth Analg 72:316, 1991
3. Munson ES, Bowers DL: The effects of hyperventilation on the rate of cerebral anesthetic equilibration. Anesthesiology 28:377, 1967
4. Gibbons RT, Steffey EP, Eger EI II: The effect of spontaneous versus controlled ventilation on the rate of rise of alveolar halothane concentration in dogs. Anesth Analg 56:32, 1977
5. Stoelting RK, Eger EI II: An additional explanation for the second gas effect: A concentrating effect. Anesthesiology 30:273, 1969
6. Rampil IJ, Lockhart SH, Zwass MS et al: Clinical characteristics of desflurane in surgical patients: minimum alveolar concentration. Anesthesiology 74:429, 1991
7. Katoh T, Ikeda K: The minimum alveolar concentration (MAC) of sevoflurane in humans. Anesthesiology 66:301, 1987
8. Gregory GA, Eger EI II, Munson ES: The relationship between age and halothane requirement in man. Anesthesiology 30:488, 1969
9. Lerman J, Sikich N, Kleinman S, Yentis S: The pharmacology of sevoflurane in infants and children. Anesthesiology 80:814, 1994
10. Wilton NCT, Thomas VL: Single breath induction of anaesthesia, using a vital capacity breath of halothane, nitrous oxide and oxygen. Anaesthesia 41:472, 1986
11. Yurino M, Kimura H: Vital capacity rapid inhalation induction technique: comparison sevoflurane and halothane. Can J Anaesth 40:440, 1993
12. Stoelting RF, Longnecker DF: The effect of right-to-left shunt on the rate of increase of arterial anesthetic concentration. Anesthesiology 36:352, 1972
13. Tanner GE, Angers DG, Barash PG et al: Effect of left-to-right, mixed left-to-right, and right-to-left shunts on inhalational anesthetic induction in children: a computer model. Anesth Analg 64:101, 1985
14. Lerman J: Pharmacology of inhalational anaesthetics in infants and children. Pediatric Anaesthesia 2:191, 1992
15. Burrows FA: Physiologic dead space, venous admixture, and the arterial to end-tidal carbon dioxide difference in infants and children undergoing cardiac surgery. Anesthesiology 70:219, 1989
16. Weathersby PK, Homer LD: Solubility of inert gases in biological fluids and tissues: a review. Undersea Biomed Res 7:277, 1980
17. Steward A, Allott PR, Cowles AL, Mapleson WW: Solubility coefficients for inhaled anaesthetics for water, oil and biological media. Br J Anaesth 45:282, 1973
18. Eger RR, Eger EI II: Effect of temperature and age on the solubility of enflurane, halothane, isoflurane, and methoxyflurane in human blood. Anesth Analg 64:640, 1985
19. Carpenter RL, Eger EI II, Johnson JH et al: Pharmacokinetics of inhaled anesthetics in humans: measurements during and after the simultaneous administration of enflurane, halothane, isoflurane, methoxyflurane, and nitrous oxide. Anesth Analg 65:575, 1986

20. Carpenter RL, Eger EI II, Johnson BH et al: Does the duration of anesthetic administration affect the pharmacokinetics or metabolism of inhaled anesthetics in humans? Anesth Analg 66:1, 1987

21. Strum D, Eger EI II, Unadkat JD et al: Age affects the pharmacokinetics of inhaled anesthetics in humans. Anesth Analg 73:310, 1991

22. Salanitre E, Rackow H: The pulmonary exchange of nitrous oxide and halothane in infants and children. Anesthesiology 30:388, 1969

23. Steward DJ, Creighton RE: The uptake and excretion of nitrous oxide in the newborn. Can Anaesth Soc J 25:215, 1978

24. Gallagher TM, Black GW: Uptake of volatile anaesthetics in children. Anaesthesia 40:1073, 1985

25. Lerman J, Willis MM, Gregory GA, Eger EI II: Age and the solubility of volatile anesthetics in blood. Anesthesiology 61:139, 1984

26. Malviya S, Lerman J: The blood/gas solubilities of sevoflurane, isoflurane, halothane, and serum constituent concentrations in neonates and adults. Anesthesiology 72:79, 1990

27. Pang YC, Reid PE, Brooks DE: Solubility and distribution of halothane in human blood. Br J Anaesth 52:851, 1980

28. Sinclair L, Strong HA, Lerman J: Effects of AAGP, local anesthetics and pH on the partition coefficients of halothane, enflurane and sevoflurane in blood and buffered saline, (abstracted). Can J Anaesth 35:S99, 1988

29. Lerman J, Schmitt-Bantel BI, Willis MM et al: Effect of age on the solubility of volatile anesthetics in human tissues. Anesthesiology 65:307, 1986

30. Stoelting RK, Eger EI II: The effects of ventilation and anesthetic solubility on recovery from anesthesia: an in vivo and analog analysis before and after equilibration. Anesthesiology 39:290, 1969

31. Fassoulaki A, Lockhart SH, Freire BA et al: Percutaneous loss of desflurane, isoflurane and halothane in humans. Anesthesiology 74:479, 1991

32. Lockhart SH, Yasuda N, Peterson N et al: Comparison of percutaneous losses of sevoflurane and isoflurane in humans. Anesth Analg 72:212, 1991

33. Van Dyke RA, Baker MT, Jansson I, Schenkman J: Reductive metabolism of halothane purified by cytochrome P-450. Biochem Pharmacol 37:2357, 1988

34, Van Dyke RA, Gandolfi AJ: Anaerobic release of fluoride from halothane. Relationship to the binding of halothane metabolites to hepatic cellular constituents. Drug Metab Dispos 4:40, 1976

35. Maiorino RM, Sipes IG, Gandolfi AJ et al: Factors affecting the formation of chlorotrifluorethane and chlorodifluoroethylene from halothane. Anesthesiology 53:383, 1981

36. Ahr HJ, King LJ, Nastainczk W et al: The mechanism of reductive dehalogenation of halothane by liver cytochrome P-450. Biochem Pharmacol 31:383, 1982

37. Holaday DA, Rudofsky S, Treuhaft PS: Metabolic degradation of methoxyflurane in man. Anesthesiology 33:579, 1970

38. Van Dyke RA, Wood CL: Metabolism of methoxyflurane: release of inorganic fluoride in human and rat hepatic microsomes. Anesthesiology 39:613, 1973

39. Yoshimura N, Holaday DA, Fiserova-Bergerova V: Metabolism of methoxyflurane in man. Anesthesiology 44:372, 1976

40. Madelian V, Warren WA: Defluorination of methoxyflurane by a glutathione-dependent enzyme. Res Commun Chem Pathol Pharmacol 16:385, 1977

41. Warren W, Madelian V: Defluorination of methoxyflurane by glutathione and coenzyme B12. Res Commun Chem Pathol Pharmacol 35:515, 1982

42. Wang S-L, Rice SA, Serra MT, Gross B: Purification and identification of rat cytosolic enzymes responsible for defluorination of methoxyflurane and fluoroacetate. Drug Metab Dispos 14:392, 1986

43. Rice SA, Wang S-L: Defluorination by hepatic glutathione S-transferases? Toxicologist 7:217, 1987

44. Mazze RI, Hitt BA, Cousins MJ: Effect of enzyme induction with phenobarbital on the in vivo and in vitro defluorination of isoflurane and methoxyflurane. J Pharmacol Exp Ther 190:523, 1974

45. Caughey GH, Rice SA, Kosek JC et al: Effect of phenytoin (DPH) treatment on methoxyflurane metabolism in rats. J Pharmacol Exp Ther 210:180, 1979

46. Van Dyke RA: Enflurane, isoflurane, and methoxyflurane metabolism in rat hepatic microsomes from ethanol-treated animals. Anesthesiology 58:22, 1983

47. Rice SA, Dooley JR, Mazze RI: Metabolism by rat hepatic microsomes of fluorinated ether anesthetics following ethanol consumption. Anesthesiology 58:237, 1983

48. Biermann JS, Rice SA, Gallagher EJ, West JA: Effect of diazepam treatment on hepatic microsomal anesthetic defluorinase activity. Arch Int Pharmacol Ther 283:181, 1986

49. Rice SA, Talcott RE: Effects of isoniazid treatment on selected hepatic mixed function oxidases. Drug Metab Dispos 7:260, 1979

50. Rice SA, Sbordone L, Mazze RI: Metabolism by rat hepatic microsomes of fluorinated ether anesthetics

following isoniazid administration. Anesthesiology 53:489, 1980

51. Van Dyke RA, Chenoweth MB, Van Poznak A: Metabolism of volatile anesthetics. I. Conversion in vivo of several anesthetics to $^{14}CO_2$ and chloride. Biochem Pharmacol 13:1239, 1964

52. Stier A: Trifluoroacetic acid as a metabolite of halothane. Biochem Pharmacol 12:544, 1964

53. Stier A, Alter H, Hessler O, Rehder K: Urinary excretion of bromide in halothane anesthesia. Anesth Analg 43:723, 1964

54. Greunke LD, Konopka K, Koop DR, Waskell LA: Characterization of halothane oxidation by hepatic microsomes and purified cytochrome P-450 using a gas chromatographic mass spectrometric assay. J Pharmacol Exp Ther 246:454, 1988

55. Sharp JH, Trudell JR, Cohen EN: Volatile metabolites and decomposition products of halothane in man. Anesthesiology 50:2, 1979

56. Murray JM, Trinick TR: Plasma fluoride concentrations during and after prolonged anesthesia: a comparison of halothane and isoflurane. Anesth Analg 74:236, 1992

57. de Groot H, Harnisch U, Noll T: Suicidal activation of microsomal cytochrome P-450 by halothane under hypoxic conditions. Biochem Biophys Res Commun 107:885, 1982

58. Rice SA, Maze M, Smith CM et al: Halothane hepatotoxicity in Fischer 344 rats pretreated with isoniazid. Toxicol Appl Pharmacol 87:411, 1987

59. Duvaldestin P, Mazze RI, Nivoche Y et al: Occupational exposure to halothane results in enzyme induction in anesthetists. Anesthesiology 54:57, 1981

60. Kharasch ED, Thummel K: Human liver volatile anesthetic defluorination: role of cytochrome P450IIE1, abstracted. Anesthesiology 75:A350, 1991

61. Shiraishi Y, Ikeda K: Uptake and biotransformation of sevoflurane in humans: a comparative study of sevoflurane with halothane, enflurane, and isoflurane. J Clin Anesth 2:381, 1990

62. Frink EJ, Hantous H, Malan P et al: Plasma inorganic fluoride with sevoflurane anesthesia: correlation with indices of hepatic and renal function. Anesth Analg 74:231, 1992

63. Kobayashi Y, Ochiai R, Takeda J et al: Serum and urinary inorganic fluoride concentrations after prolonged inhalation of sevoflurane in humans. Anesth Analg 74:753, 1992

64. Higuchi H, Satoh T, Arimura S et al: Serum inorganic fluoride levels in mildly obese patients during and after sevoflurane anesthesia. Anesth Analg 77:1018, 1993

65. Kikuchi H, Morio M, Fujii K et al: Clinical evaluation and metabolism of sevoflurane in patients. Hiroshima J Med Sci 36:93, 1987

66. Cook TL, Beppu WJ, Hitt BA et al: Renal effects and metabolism of sevoflurane in Fischer 344 rats. An in vivo and in vitro comparison with methoxyflurane. Anesthesiology 43:70, 1975

67. Mazze RI, Cousins MJ, Barr GA: Renal effects and metabolism of isoflurane in man. Anesthesiology 40:536, 1974

68. Holaday DA, Fiserova-Bergerova V, Latto IP et al: Resistance of isoflurane to biotransformation in man. Anesthesiology 54:383, 1981

69. Jones RM, Koblin DD, Cashman JN et al: Biotransformation and hepato-renal function in volunteers after exposure to desflurane (I-653). Br J Anaesth 64:482, 1990

70. Zaleski L, Abello D, Gold MI: Desflurane versus isoflurane in patients with chronic hepatic and renal disease. Anesth Analg 76:353, 1993

71. Sutton TS, Koblin DD, Gruenke LD et al: Fluoride metabolites after prolonged exposure of volunteers and patients to desflurane. Anesth Analg 73:180, 1991

72. Taylor RH, Lerman J: Induction and recovery characteristics for desflurane in children. Can J Anaesth 39:6, 1992

73. Aranda JV, MacLeod SM, Renton KW, Eade NR: Hepatic microsomal drug oxidation and electron transport in newborn infants. J Pediatr 85:534, 1974

74. Stoelting RK, Peterson C: Methoxyflurane anesthesia in pediatric patients: evaluation of anesthetic metabolism and renal function. Anesthesiology 42:26, 1975

75. Arnold JH, Truog RD, Rice SA: Prolonged administration of isoflurane to pediatric patients during mechanical ventilation. Anesth Analg 76:520, 1993

76. Eger EI II, Johnson BH: Rates of awakening from anesthesia with I-653, halothane, isoflurane and sevoflurane: a test of the effect of anesthetic concentration and duration in rats. Anesth Analg 66:977, 1987

77. Nussmeier NA, Moskowitz GJ, Weiskopf RB et al: In vitro anesthetic washin and washout via bubbler oxygenators: influence of anesthetic solubility and rates of carrier gas inflow and pump blood flow. Anesth Analg 67:982, 1988

78. Lerman J, Gregory GA, Eger EI II: Hematocrit and the solubility of volatile anesthetics in blood. Anesth Analg 63:911, 1984

79. Lerman J, Gregory GA, Eger EI II: Effects of anaes-

thesia and surgery on the solubility of volatile anaesthetics in blood. Can J Anaesth 34:14, 1987

80. Brown AC, Canosa-Mas CE, Parr AD et al: Troposphere lifetimes of halogenated anaesthetics. Nature 341:635, 1989

81. Logan M, Farmer JG: Anaesthesia and the ozone layer (editorial). Br J Anaesth 63:645, 1989

82. Eger EI II, Larson CP Jr, Severinghaus JW: The solubility of halothane in rubber, soda lime and various plastics. Anesthesiology 23:356, 1962

83. Titel JH, Lowe HJ, Elam JO, Grosholz JR: Quantitative closed-circuit halothane anesthesia. Anesth Analg 47:560, 1968

84. Tang AG, Yasuda N, Eger EI II: Anesthetic plastic solubility. Anesthesiology 69:A297, 1988

85. Munson ES, Eger EI II: Methoxyflurane solubility in plastics. Anesthesiology 26:828, 1965

86. Eger EI II, Brandstater B: Solubility of methoxyflurane in rubber. Anesthesiology 24:679, 1963

87. Grodin WK, Epstein MAF, Epstein RA: Mechanisms of halothane adsorption by dry soda-lime. Br J Anaesth 54:516, 1982

88. Eger EI II, Strum DP: The absorption and degradation of isoflurane and I-653 by dry soda lime at various temperatures. Anesth Analg 66:1312, 1987

89. Strum DP, Eger EI II: The degradation, absorption, and solubility of volatile anesthetics in soda lime depend on water content. Anesth Analg 78:340, 1994

90. Wong DT, Lerman J: Factors affecting the rate of disappearance of sevoflurane in Baralyme. Can J Anaesth 4:366, 1992

91. Hanaki C, Fuju K, Mario M, Tashima T: Decomposition of sevoflurane by soda lime. Hiroshima J Med Sci 36:61, 1987

92. Liu J, Laster MJ, Eger EI II, Taheri S: Absorption and degradation of sevoflurane and isoflurane in a conventional anesthetic circuit. Anesth Analg 72:785, 1991

93. Severinghaus JW: The rate of uptake of nitrous oxide in man. J Clin Invest 33:1183, 1954

94. Yasuda N, Targ AG, Eger EI II: Solubility of I-653, sevoflurane, isoflurane, and halothane in human tissues. Anesth Analg 69:370, 1989

95. Strum DP, Eger EI II: Partition coefficients for sevoflurane in human blood, saline, and olive oil. Anesth Analg 66:654, 1987

96. Eger EI II: Partition coefficients of I-653 in human blood, saline and olive oil. Anesth Analg 66:971, 1987

Chapter 25

Clinical Pharmacology and Applications of Inhalational Anesthetic Agents

R. Joseph Isner and Burnell R. Brown, Jr.

Inhalational anesthetics are a most important group of drugs for the anesthesiologist. These agents have advantages of providing a route of administration and elimination not dependent on gastrointestinal, hepatic, or renal function, coupled with the physician's ability to monitor drug levels easily by end-tidal gas analysis. The inhalational drugs have until recently included nitrous oxide (an inorganic gas) and isoflurane, enflurane, and halothane (volatile halogenated agents). Two newer halogenated agents, desflurane and sevoflurane, will probably make a significant impact on anesthesiology in the years to come. This chapter gives a brief introduction of each agent followed by a discussion of effects on important organ systems.

INHALATIONAL ANESTHETIC AGENTS

Isoflurane

Isoflurane was synthesized in 1965 by Terrell. Its introduction into clinical practice was delayed because of a later refuted claim of carcinogenicity.[1] It is a liquid at room temperature with a pungent vapor. The blood/gas partition coefficient of isoflurane is 1.4, and the oil/gas partition coeffi-

cient is 91.[2] Isoflurane has a minimum alveolar concentration (MAC) of 1.15 percent and undergoes little biotransformation (~1 percent).[3]

Enflurane

Enflurane was synthesized in 1963 by Terrell. Enflurane is a liquid at room temperature with a pungent vapor. The blood/gas and oil/gas partition coefficients of enflurane are 1.9 and 98, respectively.[2] Enflurane has a MAC of 1.7 percent and undergoes little biotransformation (~3 percent).[4] The clinical use of enflurane is limited primarily by its potential to cause seizures and nephrotoxicity (discussed subsequently).

Halothane

Halothane was first synthesized in 1951 and introduced into clinical practice in 1956.[5,6] It is a liquid at room temperature. Halothane vapor is not pungent; thus, the drug can be used for inhalational induction of anesthesia with or without the addition of nitrous oxide. The blood/gas and oil/gas partition coefficients of halothane are 2.3 and 224, respectively.[2] Halothane has a MAC of 0.77 percent and undergoes a moderate amount of biotransformation (~18 percent).[7] The drug is commonly employed in pediatric practice.

Sevoflurane

Sevoflurane was first synthesized by Wallin et al. in the early 1970s. Used clinically in Japan since the late 1980s, it is currently being evaluated for introduction into clinical practice in the United States. Sevoflurane is a liquid at room temperature. The vapor is not pungent. The blood/gas partition coefficient of sevoflurane is 0.6, and the oil/gas partition coefficient is 53.[2] Sevoflurane has a MAC of 2.05 percent and undergoes little biotransformation (~3.5 percent).[8] In the future, sevoflurane may supplant halothane as the anesthetic of choice for inhalation induction.

Desflurane

Desflurane is an analog of isoflurane, with an additional fluorine replacing the chlorine atom on the ether alpha carbon. It was introduced into clinical practice in 1992. Desflurane causes airway irritation.[9] The blood/gas and oil/gas partition coefficients of desflurane are 0.42 and 19, respectively.[10] The MAC of desflurane is 7.25 percent for 18- to 30-year-old patients and 6.0 percent for patients 31 to 65 years of age.[11] Desflurane undergoes little metabolism (less than 1 percent). The combination of a favorable solubility profile and a lack of metabolic transformation makes desflurane a promising anesthetic agent.

Nitrous Oxide

Nitrous oxide was first used clinically in the 1840s. It is an odorless inorganic gas. The blood/gas and oil/gas partition coefficients of nitrous oxide are 0.46 and 1.4, respectively. The MAC of nitrous oxide (administered under hyperbaric conditions) is 104 percent.[12] Nitrous oxide undergoes essentially no metabolism. Future clinical use of nitrous oxide may be limited by its propensity to accumulate in and expand closed air spaces, such as bowel and pneumothoraces, and its deleterious effects on hematopoiesis.

CENTRAL NERVOUS SYSTEM

Consciousness

Loss of consciousness occurs at roughly the same depth of anesthesia as does amnesia (MAC aware). In the past, it was held that the concentration of a

Table 25-1 Specific MAC-Aware Values

Agent	MAC-Aware
Isoflurane	0.25 MAC (0.29%)
Enflurane	0.27 MAC (0.46%)
Halothane	0.59 MAC (0.45%)

Abbreviations: MAC, minimum alveolar concentration. (From Gaumann et al.,[15] with permission.)

volatile agent required to achieve loss of consciousness was a common fraction of the MAC of each agent. This ratio was reported to be 0.25 MAC[13] or 0.4 MAC.[14] A recent report challenged the hypothesis of a uniform ratio between MAC and MAC aware[15] (see Table 25-1 for specific MAC-aware values).

Electroencephalographic Effects

Volatile anesthetics cause characteristic changes in the electroencephalogram (EEG). At low doses (less than 0.4 MAC), frequency and voltage increase.[16,17] At about 0.4 MAC, amplitude dominance shifts from posterior to anterior portions of the brain.[18]

Isoflurane

At light levels of isoflurane-induced anesthesia, low voltage fast activity (20 to 60 μV and 15 to 20 Hz) predominates. During surgical anesthesia, moderate voltage, low frequency (40 to 80 μV and 4 to 6 Hz) activity is seen. Deep surgical levels of anesthesia are associated with burst suppression. There is no evidence of epileptiform activity in the EEGs of subjects anesthetized with isoflurane.[16] Electrical silence occurs at isoflurane concentrations of 2.5 percent.[19]

Enflurane

As the depth of enflurane-induced anesthesia increases, voltage spikes of greater than 100 μV appear. With further increases of enflurane concentration, spike waves (voltage spikes followed by slow waves lasting as long as 1 second) occur with periods of burst suppression. Maximum depth is associated with a predominance of spike waves and burst suppression. Hypocarbia ($PaCO_2$ less than or equal to 34 mmHg) leads to increased EEG evidence of cerebral irritability.[20]

Halothane

At light levels of halothane-induced anesthesia, EEG activity in the 10- to 20-Hz range predominates. At 1.0 MAC, the dominant frequencies are 10 to 15 Hz. Deep surgical levels are associated with slowing to 1 to 3 Hz. Burst suppression is seen at concentrations well above MAC.[17]

Sevoflurane

Sevoflurane, at low concentrations, causes an increase in frequency and amplitude compared with awake values. Frequency and amplitude decrease at deeper concentrations. Deep anesthesia produces 10- to 14-Hz activity mixed with 5- to 8-Hz slow waves.[21] No EEG evidence of epileptiform activity is seen with sevoflurane.[22,23]

Desflurane

Desflurane-induced anesthesia produces EEG changes comparable to those observed with equipotent levels of isoflurane. No epileptiform activity is seen. Prominent burst suppression is seen at concentrations of 1.24 MAC and higher.[24]

Seizure Activity

At high doses (2.5 percent), enflurane administration can result in EEG activity that is indistinguishable from seizure activity. This is amplified in the presence of hypocapnia.[20] Clinically, tonic-clonic motor activity of the face and extremities can occur under these circumstances. Enflurane does not, however, activate pre-existing epileptic foci in animals.[25] Under normal clinical circumstances, enflurane decreases cerebral metabolic oxygen utilization ($CMRO_2$), but during enflurane-induced seizures there is a large increase in $CMRO_2$.[26] Cases of seizure-like motor activity have been reported during isoflurane anesthesia;[27] the exact causes of these events are unclear. Isoflurane has been used as a successful treatment for status epilepticus resistant to intravenous therapy.[28,29]

Cerebral Blood Flow and Autoregulation

Volatile anesthetics generally cause dose-dependent reductions of cerebral vascular resistance and increases in cerebral blood flow (CBF) at doses of 0.6 MAC and higher,[30] despite concurrent decreases in the cerebral metabolic rate for oxygen (see Cerebral Metabolic Oxygen Utilization and Cerebral Protection). Each of the anesthetics listed may perturb normal cerebral vascular autoregulation.

Isoflurane

Isoflurane administration causes a decrease in cerebral vascular resistance and an increase in CBF. This effect is not as great as with halothane or enflurane and occurs despite a decrease in the mean arterial pressure. Increases in CBF occur at doses of 1.0 MAC and higher.[31–34] In one study, however, isoflurane doses as high as 2.15 MAC were associated with only minimal increases in CBF.[23] This increased CBF is counteracted by hyperventilation, particularly in the cerebral cortex.[35,36] In the absence of inhaled anesthetics, autoregulation normally maintains CBF over a wide range of mean arterial pressures. Isoflurane administration appears to decrease the range of mean arterial pressures over which CBF is maintained in a dose-dependent fashion.[37] The effects of isoflurane on cerebral vascular resistance and CBF becomes less pronounced over time.[31]

Enflurane

Enflurane causes a decrease in cerebral vascular resistance and an increase in CBF. At 2.0 MAC, CBF is increased by roughly one-third.[26] This effect is not as great as with halothane but is more pronounced than with isoflurane and occurs despite a decrease in the mean arterial pressure.[26,38,39] Cerebral blood flow appears to increase linearly with $PaCO_2$ over a clinically relevant range in the presence of enflurane anesthesia.[26] Autoregulation of CBF appeared to be completely abolished at 1.0 MAC enflurane but was maintained over a narrow range of mean arterial pressures at 0.5 MAC.[40] Seizures induced in dogs anesthetized with enflurane at doses of 1.5 MAC were accompanied by a 50 percent additional increase in CBF.[26]

Halothane

Halothane causes dose-dependent decreases in cerebral vascular resistance and increases in CBF,[26,32,34,38,41] despite decreased mean arterial pressure. Halothane is a more potent cerebral vasodilator than either isoflurane or enflurane. The effect of halothane on CBF is attenuated by hyperventilation if instituted prior to halothane exposure.[22,42] CBF appears to increase linearly with $PaCO_2$ over a clinically relevant range during halothane anesthesia.[43] Halothane administration reduced the range of mean arterial pressures over which CBF was maintained in a dose-dependent fashion,[37] leading to ablation of autoregulation at doses greater than 1.0 MAC.[40] Cerebrovascular adaptation occurs during halothane administration such that CBF returned to near baseline levels after about 150 minutes.[44] This adaptation is caused by an increase in cerebral vascular tone and is unrelated to cerebrospinal fluid pH.[45]

Sevoflurane

Sevoflurane causes similar[22] or less profound[46] increases in CBF when compared with isoflurane. At doses of 0.5 and 1.0 MAC, neither agent caused an increase in global or cortical blood flow compared with baseline. At doses as high as 2.15 MAC, sevoflurane caused only minimal increases in CBF.[23]

Desflurane

Desflurane produces a dose-dependent decrease in cerebral vascular resistance.[47] When the desflurane concentration is increased from 0.5 to 1.0 MAC, CBF is increased; at higher doses (2.0 MAC), CBF is decreased, presumably on the basis of a marked decrease in mean arterial pressure. When phenylephrine was administered to support the arterial pressure under these circumstances, CBF increased. Cerebral vascular responsiveness to hypocarbia was maintained in the presence of high dose desflurane.[48]

Nitrous Oxide

The effects of nitrous oxide on CBF are controversial. Nitrous oxide did not appear to increase CBF in rats,[49] but in other models, it caused large increases in CBF.[50–52] An anesthetic consisting of nitrous oxide and morphine had no effect on cerebral vascular autoregulation.[53]

Cerebral Metabolic Oxygen Utilization and Cerebral Protection

Volatile anesthetics generally cause decreases in $CMRO_2$. As the concentration of the volatile anesthetic increases, there is a large initial decrease in the $CMRO_2$ followed by further dose-dependent decreases.[14] In the past, it was held that volatile anesthetics cause an "uncoupling" of CBF and $CMRO_2$. It appears that, although volatile anesthetics do not truly uncouple CBF and $CMRO_2$,[54] they do cause a dose-dependent increase in the ratio of CBF to $CMRO_2$.[32,55,56]

Isoflurane

Isoflurane causes dose-dependent decreases in $CMRO_2$, reaching a 30 to 50 percent reduction at isoflurane doses that result in an isoelectric EEG.[22,32,33,57] Higher isoflurane concentrations do not result in further decreases in $CMRO_2$.[57] Theoretically, this reduction in $CMRO_2$ could result in cerebral protection during temporary cerebral ischemia, such as occurs during carotid artery endarterectomies or cerebral aneurysm resections. Studies show both a protective effect[58] and no protective effect[59] of isoflurane under conditions of temporary or incomplete cerebral ischemia. A large retrospective study of patients undergoing carotid endarterectomies showed the CBF at which ischemic EEG changes occurred was lower with isoflurane than with either enflurane or halothane (10 ml/100 g/min versus 15 ml/100 g/min or 20 ml/100 g/min, respectively).[60] In this study, the incidence of ischemic EEG changes was less during isoflurane-induced anesthesia than that seen with enflurane or halothane, but there was no difference among the groups in neurologic outcome. A recent well-controlled animal study showed a lower cerebral ischemic flow threshold during isoflurane-nitrous oxide anesthesia than during halothane-nitrous oxide anesthesia.[61]

Enflurane

Enflurane causes a dose-dependent decrease in the $CMRO_2$.[39] The decrease in $CMRO_2$ seen with enflurane is not as dramatic as with isoflurane. Although frank seizure activity causes an increase in $CMRO_2$, enflurane concentrations associated with frequent voltage spikes result in a decreased

$CMRO_2$. When seizures were induced in dogs by enflurane anesthesia, there was a large increase in $CMRO_2$.[26] There is no evidence of cerebral protection during enflurane anesthesia.

Halothane

Halothane administration results in a dose-dependent decrease in the $CMRO_2$.[14,41] The decrease in $CMRO_2$ is not as significant as with isoflurane.[32] There is no evidence of cerebral protection during halothane anesthesia.

Sevoflurane

Sevoflurane appears to be similar to isoflurane in its effects on $CMRO_2$. It produced a dose-dependent decrease in $CMRO_2$, reaching a 50 percent reduction at 1.0 MAC.[13] Studies of cerebral protection in humans have not been performed, but preliminary data suggested that sevoflurane anesthesia decreased the neurologic deficit seen in rats after incomplete cerebral ischemia.[62]

Desflurane

Desflurane anesthesia causes a reduction in $CMRO_2$. A 20 percent reduction in $CMRO_2$ was seen in dogs anesthetized with 2.4 MAC (17.1 percent) desflurane.[63] High doses of desflurane (2.2 to 2.4 MAC) caused large (up to 60 percent) decreases in CBF and cerebral perfusion pressure and a decreased $CMRO_2$. These conditions were associated with moderately increased cerebral lactate levels and normal concentrations of high-energy phosphates, probably indicating that oxygen supply was adequate to meet metabolic utilization.

Nitrous Oxide

Data concerning the effects of nitrous oxide on $CMRO_2$ are frequently conflicting. Some authors found no effect of nitrous oxide on $CMRO_2$ in animals[49,64] or humans.[65] Others found small to significant increases in $CMRO_2$ during nitrous oxide administration.[50,51,52,66] There is no evidence of cerebral protection from nitrous oxide.

Cerebral Spinal Fluid Dynamics

Cerebrospinal fluid (CSF) volume is one determinant of intracranial pressure. The balance of CSF production and reabsorption determine the CSF

Table 25-2 Effects of Inhalational Anesthetics on Cerebrospinal Fluid Dynamics

Drug	CSF Production	CSF Reabsorption
Isoflurane[67,68]	↔	↑
Enflurane[68,69]	↑	↓
Halothane[70,71]	↓	↓
Nitrous oxide[72]	↔	

Abbreviations: ↑, increased; ↓, decreased; ↔, no change; CSF, cerebrospinal fluid.

volume. Inhaled anesthetics frequently affect dynamics of CSF production and reabsorption and are thus of concern to the anesthesiologist. The effects of specific anesthetics on CSF dynamics are given in Table 25-2.

Effects on Intracranial Pressure

Inhaled anesthetics affect intracranial pressure (ICP) by effects on CBF, cerebral blood volume, and CSF volume.

Isoflurane

Isoflurane caused an increase in cerebral blood volume in dogs but only a transient increase in ICP.[73] Intracranial hypertension has been seen in patients with intracranial lesions under isoflurane anesthesia.[74] Hyperventilation prevented or reversed an increase in ICP caused by isoflurane administration.[35,75]

Enflurane

Enflurane caused increased cerebral blood volume in dogs accompanied by prolonged increases in ICP.[76] Hyperventilation to prevent an enflurane-induced increase in ICP may not be wise given the drug's propensity to cause seizures in the presence of hypocarbia.

Halothane

Halothane causes increased cerebral blood volume in dogs accompanied by a prolonged increase in ICP.[76] In one study, hyperventilation prevented a halothane-induced increase in ICP reliably only if instituted prior to halothane administration.[42]

Sevoflurane

Sevoflurane caused small increases in ICP in rabbits at doses of 0.5 and 1.0 MAC.[22]

Desflurane

The ICP decreased in dogs anesthetized with high concentrations of desflurane (2.2 and 2.4 MAC), presumably on the basis of a decrease in CBF.[63] The effect on ICP of lower desflurane concentrations that may not be associated with a large decrease in mean arterial pressure and a decreased CBF has not been compared with awake values.

Nitrous Oxide

Nitrous oxide administration can cause intracranial hypertension.[77] It appears that the increase in ICP associated with nitrous oxide administration can be reversed or prevented by the administration of barbiturates or benzodiazepines or by hyperventilation.

Effects on Evoked Potentials

Evoked potentials used for neurosurgical procedures include visual, somatosensory, and brain stem auditory evoked potentials. Inhaled anesthetics may affect each type of evoked potential by increasing latency and decreasing amplitude. Long exposure to anesthetics may enhance the effects on evoked potentials.[78] The specific effects of inhalational anesthetics on evoked potentials are shown in Table 25-3.

VENTILATION

Ventilatory Pattern

Isoflurane caused a dose-dependent reduction of minute ventilation,[84] as a result of a decreased tidal volume. The ventilatory rate is increased during isoflurane anesthesia, but it is not dose dependent. Prolonged exposure to isoflurane results in partial reversal of these effects because tidal volume and minute ventilation increase over time.

Enflurane, halothane, and sevoflurane also caused a dose-dependent reduction of minute ventilation as a result of decreased tidal volume;[84–87] the ventilatory rate increases with increasing doses of anesthetic. In the case of enflurane, prolonged exposure results in partial reversal of these effects; the ventilatory rate remains unchanged. The tidal volume and minute ventilation increase over time.

Desflurane caused dose-dependent reduction of tidal volume and increases of ventilatory rate.[88] The minute ventilation was not changed at doses ranging from 0.83 to 1.66 MAC.

The substitution of nitrous oxide for an equipotent dose of a volatile anesthetic resulted in an increase in tidal volume and minute ventilation but typically no change in ventilatory rate.[89–91]

Control of Ventilation

Inhaled anesthetics alter the effects of both carbon dioxide and oxygen on ventilation. In general, resting $PaCO_2$ is elevated. The CO_2 response curve (increase in minute ventilation as a function of in-

Table 25-3 Effects of Inhalational Anesthetics on Evoked Potentials

Drugs	Effect on Amplitude	Effect on Latency	Maximum Concentration (in 60% N_2O) at Which Useful SEP Information Is Obtainable
Isoflurane[79,80,81]	↓	↑	0.5–1.0 MAC
Enflurane[79,81]	↓	↑	0.5–1.0 MAC
Halothane[79,81]	↓	↑	0.75–1.0 MAC
Nitrous oxide[82,83]	↓↓	↑	

Abbreviations: ↑, increase; ↓, decrease; ↓↓, larger decrease; MAC, minimal alveolar concentration; SEP, sensory evoked potentials.

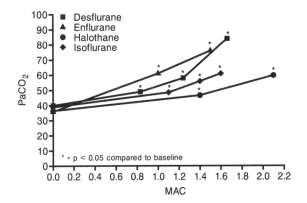

Fig. 25-1 Inhaled anesthetics administered to spontaneously breathing volunteers produced dose-dependent increases in $PaCO_2$. (Modified from Eger[30] and Lockhart et al.,[88] with permission.)

creasing arterial $PaCO_2$) is shifted to the right, and its slope is depressed. The hypoxic ventilatory drive is generally depressed. The following information was obtained from studies of healthy human volunteers unless otherwise noted (Fig. 25-1).

Isoflurane

Arterial $PaCO_2$ increased with increasing depth of isoflurane anesthesia;[84] the arterial $PaCO_2$ values during 1.0 and 1.5 MAC isoflurane were 50 and 65 mmHg, respectively. Surgical stimulation reduced the resting arterial $PaCO_2$ during isoflurane anesthesia by 5 to 13 mmHg.[92] The ventilatory response to CO_2 challenge is depressed in a dose-dependent fashion. During 1.0 MAC isoflurane, the slope of the CO_2 response curve is depressed by 70 percent. The hypoxic ventilatory drive is depressed in dogs by isoflurane but to a lesser extent than that seen with halothane or enflurane.[93] Isoflurane reduces (0.1 MAC) or abolishes (1.1 MAC) hypoxic ventilatory drive in humans.[94]

Enflurane

Enflurane produces dose-dependent increases of resting arterial $PaCO_2$;[85] the arterial $PaCO_2$ values during 1.0 and 1.5 MAC enflurane anesthesia were 61 and 76 mmHg, respectively. Prolonged anesthesia results in partial reversal of enflurane-induced

ventilatory depression. After 7 hours of enflurane-induced anesthesia, the arterial $PaCO_2$ values during 1.0 and 1.5 MAC were 46 and 56 mmHg, respectively. This adaptation of ventilatory effects is more dramatic with enflurane than with isoflurane or halothane. The ventilatory response to CO_2 challenge is depressed in a dose-dependent fashion. During 1.1 MAC enflurane, the slope of the CO_2 response curve is depressed by 77 percent.[89] The hypoxic ventilatory drive is depressed in dogs by enflurane, more so than with isoflurane.[93]

Halothane

Halothane administration results in dose-dependent increases of resting arterial $PaCO_2$;[86] the arterial $PaCO_2$ values during 1.0 and 1.5 MAC halothane anesthesia were 48 and 59 mmHg, respectively. Surgical stimulation reduces the resting arterial $PaCO_2$ during halothane anesthesia by about 5 mmHg.[86] The ventilatory response to CO_2 challenge is depressed in a dose-dependent fashion. During 1.5 MAC halothane, the slope of the CO_2 response curve is depressed by 55 percent.[84] The hypoxic ventilatory drive is depressed in dogs by halothane more than isoflurane.[93] Depression of hypoxic ventilatory response during halothane anesthesia has also been demonstrated in humans.[95] Halothane also causes a dose-dependent attenuation of the ventilatory stimulation normally produced by acute metabolic acidemia.[96]

Sevoflurane

Arterial $PaCO_2$ increased with increasing depth of sevoflurane anesthesia in surgical patients.[87] The arterial $PaCO_2$ values during 0.9 and 1.2 MAC sevoflurane were 49 and 55 mmHg, respectively. (These MAC values were adjusted from values given in the study cited. At the time this study was published, the MAC of sevoflurane was thought to be 1.7 percent. It is now thought to be 2.05 percent.[8]) The ventilatory response to CO_2 challenge was depressed by sevoflurane in a dose-dependent fashion. During 0.9 MAC sevoflurane, the slope of the CO_2 response curve was depressed by 66 percent.

Desflurane

Desflurane administration resulted in dose-dependent increases of resting arterial $PaCO_2$.[88] The arterial $PaCO_2$ values during 0.83 and 1.66 MAC desflurane anesthesia were 49 and 84 mmHg, respectively. The ventilatory response to CO_2 challenge was depressed in a dose-dependent fashion. During 0.83 and 1.66 MAC desflurane, the slope of the CO_2 response curve was depressed by 55 percent and 89 percent, respectively.[88]

Nitrous Oxide

Under hyperbaric conditions, 1.0 to 1.5 MAC nitrous oxide did not change $PaCO_2$ during spontaneous ventilation.[97] The substitution of nitrous oxide for an equipotent amount of volatile anesthetic resulted in a lower carbon dioxide tension during spontaneous breathing.[84,89,98] The ventilatory response to CO_2 challenge is depressed by nitrous oxide in a dose-dependent fashion. During 1.5 MAC nitrous oxide, the slope of the CO_2 response curve was depressed by 80 percent. This concentration of nitrous oxide is not used under normal circumstances, of course. Nitrous oxide in low concentrations depressed the ventilatory response to hypoxemia.[99]

Effects on Muscles of Breathing

Isoflurane

A recent study in humans showed that 1.0 MAC isoflurane does not selectively depress rib cage motion. During awake measurements, the rib cage contributed 33 percent of the total ventilation; during isoflurane-induced anesthesia, this contribution was 39 percent. Patients breathing spontaneously during isoflurane anesthesia did not recruit rib cage ventilation normally in response to a CO_2 challenge.[100]

Halothane

Patients breathing spontaneously during halothane anesthesia did not recruit rib cage ventilation normally in response to a CO_2 challenge.[101] This effect is much more significant than effects on the diaphragm. In dogs, it appeared that depression of diaphragmatic function was the result of effects of halothane on either the neuromuscular junction or the contractile processes of the muscle, or both.[102]

Sevoflurane

Sevoflurane appeared to impair diaphragmatic contractility in dogs through inhibitory effects on neuromuscular transmission.[103]

Bronchomotor Tone

Isoflurane

Isoflurane anesthesia results in reduced pulmonary compliance,[104] as a result of a decrease in pulmonary volumes. Bronchomotor tone is decreased.[105] Isoflurane has protective effects against antigen-induced bronchospasm. In a dog model, aerosolized Ascaris antigen caused both direct and reflex-mediated airway constriction. Isoflurane-induced anesthesia attenuated this constriction, as demonstrated by decreased pulmonary resistance and increased dynamic compliance compared with a control group after Ascaris challenge.[106] The change in pulmonary resistance was similar and the improvement of dynamic compliance was somewhat less than that seen with halothane in this model.

Enflurane

Enflurane blocked hypocapnic bronchoconstriction in isolated canine lungs.[107] Enflurane reduced Ascaris-induced bronchoconstriction in dogs as effectively as did halothane.[108]

Halothane

Halothane-induced anesthesia results in decreased bronchomotor tone.[105,109,110] Halothane was shown to block hypocapnic bronchoconstriction in isolated canine lungs.[107] Similar to isoflurane and enflurane, halothane protects against antigen-induced bronchospasm. Halothane anesthesia attenuated Ascaris-induced bronchoconstriction in dogs as demonstrated by decreased pulmonary resistance and increased dynamic compliance compared with a control group.[106] Halothane also attenuated histamine-induced bronchoconstriction.[111] Albuterol (intravenously) further reduced histamine, induced bronchoconstriction in dogs anesthetized with halothane, but atropine did not.[112] Halothane was no more effective than parenteral bronchodilators or steroids for the treatment of status asthmaticus in humans.[113]

Mucociliary Function

Enflurane

Enflurane caused a dose-dependent reduction of mucociliary flow velocity in dogs.[114] Flow rates quickly returned toward normal as end-tidal enflurane was reduced. Enflurane caused a dose-dependent reduction of ciliary beat frequency in rabbit trachea segments.[115]

Halothane

Halothane caused a dose-dependent reduction in mucociliary flow rates in dogs.[116] At 2.4 MAC, flow velocity was 27 percent of control. Flow rates quickly returned toward normal as end-tidal halothane was reduced. The reduction in mucociliary flow was at least partially caused by direct suppression of ciliary activity.[115] In humans, halothane-induced anesthesia has been associated with cessation of mucociliary flow after 90 minutes.[117] However, patients in this study received antisialagogue treatment and were intubated with cuffed endotracheal tubes, factors that probably affected mucociliary flow independent of halothane administration.

Nitrous Oxide

Nitrous oxide and morphine anesthesia caused dose-dependent reduction in mucociliary flow rates in dogs equal to that seen with halothane.[114] However, nitrous oxide did not appear to affect ciliary beat frequency in rabbit trachea segments.[115]

Pulmonary Vascular Resistance

Nitrous Oxide

Nitrous oxide and morphine anesthesia caused increased pulmonary vascular resistance and pulmonary artery pressure.[118] In patients with pre-existing pulmonary hypertension, administration of 50 percent nitrous oxide increased pulmonary vascular resistance but did not change pulmonary artery pressures.[119]

Hypoxic Pulmonary Vasoconstriction

Hypoxic pulmonary vasoconstriction is the ability of the pulmonary vasculature to constrict in response to regional hypoxemia, thereby helping to maintain ventilation-perfusion matching.

Isoflurane

The effect of isoflurane on hypoxic pulmonary vasoconstriction has been tested in animal models (in vitro and in vivo) and in humans. Isoflurane caused dose-dependent attenuation of the increase in pulmonary artery pressure in rat lungs that occurs in response to an hypoxic gas mixture.[120] Halothane and enflurane had similar effects on this model. In the intact dog model, isoflurane attenuated hypoxic pulmonary vasoconstriction.[121,122] However, addition of isoflurane to total intravenous anesthesia did not affect PaO_2 in patients undergoing thoracotomy with one-lung ventilation.[123]

Enflurane

Enflurane caused dose-dependent attenuation of the increase in pulmonary artery pressure that occurs in response to hypoxic ventilation in a rat lung model.[120] However, when an intact dog model was used, enflurane did not attenuate hypoxic pulmonary vasoconstriction.[122] Patients undergoing thoracotomy under total intravenous anesthesia (with ketamine) did not have increased intrapulmonary shunting when enflurane was added to the anesthetic during one-lung ventilation.[124]

Halothane

Halothane caused dose-dependent attenuation of the increase in pulmonary artery pressure that occurs in response to ventilation with an hypoxic gas mixture in a rat lung model.[120] When an intact dog model was used, however, halothane did not attenuate hypoxic pulmonary vasoconstriction.[122] Patients undergoing thoracotomy under intravenous anesthesia did not have further decreases in PaO_2 if halothane was added to the anesthetic during one-lung ventilation.[123]

Nitrous Oxide

Nitrous oxide had effects on hypoxic pulmonary vasoconstriction similar to isoflurane in intact dogs.[122] One-third MAC nitrous oxide caused attenuation of hypoxic pulmonary vasoconstriction in this model.

CARDIOVASCULAR SYSTEM

Myocardial Contractility

Volatile anesthetics cause a reduction in myocardial contractility and, usually, in cardiac output. The effects on myocardial contractility are dose dependent.[125] Changes in myocardial contractility are often independent of changes in cardiac output, because the latter is dependent on several variables, such as preload, afterload, and heart rate.

Isoflurane

Isoflurane has negative inotropic effects on isolated cat papillary muscles.[126] Maximal velocity of shortening was decreased by 36 percent, and peak developed force was decreased by 40 percent in the presence of 1.0 MAC isoflurane. These reductions were larger if muscle from failing hearts was used. The isoflurane-induced reduction in contractility in this model was somewhat less than that seen with halothane administration. In intact dogs, the administration of isoflurane decreased the maximum rate of left ventricular pressure rise (dP/dT) to a lesser extent than equipotent doses of enflurane or halothane.[127]

Enflurane

Isolated cat papillary muscle exposed to 1.0, 2.0 or 3.0 MAC enflurane had a lower peak developed tension and maximal velocity of contraction compared with control or muscle exposed to halothane.[125]

Halothane

Halothane has negative inotropic effects on isolated cat papillary muscles.[125,126] The decrease in contractility was less than with enflurane but greater than with isoflurane. No difference was noted when cat papillary muscle from normal hearts was compared with samples obtained from failing hearts.[126]

Sevoflurane

Sevoflurane and isoflurane produced similar reductions in left ventricular dP/dT in dogs at doses of 1.2 and 2.0 MAC.[128]

Desflurane

The effects of desflurane on myocardial contractility were compared with those of isoflurane in intact dogs.[129] Contractility was evaluated using the preload recruitable stroke work versus end-diastolic length relationship. This index was reduced by an equivalent amount by each agent, about 30 percent at 1.0 MAC and 50 percent at 1.5 MAC.

Nitrous Oxide

When 60 percent nitrous oxide was added to enflurane or halothane in dogs, there was no additional depression of myocardial contractility compared with the volatile agents alone.[130]

Systemic Vascular Resistance

Unless otherwise noted, each of the studies cited below involved measurement of cardiovascular indices in healthy volunteers, mechanically ventilated to maintain normocarbia. Anesthetic effects on systemic vascular resistance were different during spontaneous ventilation as a result of hypercarbia. (Fig. 25-2).[131]

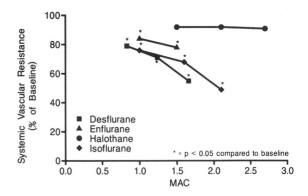

Fig. 25-2 Systemic vascular resistance in normocarbic volunteers was decreased in a dose-related manner by desflurane, enflurane, and isoflurane, but not by halothane. (Modified with permission from Eger[30] and Weiskopf et al.,[135] with permission.)

Isoflurane

Isoflurane, 1.5 MAC, decreased systemic vascular resistance 32 percent compared with awake values.[132] This is a greater decrease than caused by equivalent doses of halothane or enflurane.

Enflurane

Enflurane 1.5 MAC decreased systemic vascular resistance 22 percent compared with awake values,[133] a greater decrease than caused by an equivalent dose of halothane, but not as great as with isoflurane.

Halothane

Halothane 1.5 MAC decreased systemic vascular resistance 8 percent compared with awake values,[134] a smaller decrease than with equipotent doses of isoflurane or enflurane.

Sevoflurane

Invasive human volunteer cardiac studies had not been performed with sevoflurane at the time of writing this chapter. Sevoflurane caused decreases in systemic vascular resistance similar to isoflurane in intact dogs at doses of 1.2 and 2.0 MAC.[128] Sevoflurane reduced systemic vascular resistance by 22 percent of awake values at 1.2 MAC.

Desflurane

The effect of desflurane on systemic vascular resistance was measured at 1.24 MAC and 1.66 MAC.[135] During the first 90 minutes of anesthesia, systemic vascular resistance decreased 28 percent at 1.24 MAC and 45 percent at 1.66 MAC.

Nitrous Oxide

The administration of 40 percent nitrous oxide to healthy volunteers caused mild peripheral vasoconstriction.[136] This was also the case when nitrous oxide was added to isoflurane.[137] Systemic vascular resistance was unchanged when nitrous oxide was added to halothane or enflurane.[91,138]

Central Venous Pressure

The studies cited subsequently were performed in healthy volunteers, mechanically ventilated to maintain normocarbia unless otherwise noted (Fig. 25-3).

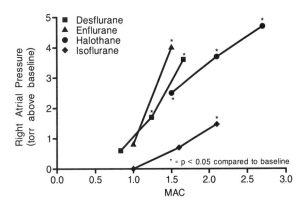

Fig. 25-3 In normocapnic volunteers, volatile anesthetics increased right atrial pressures as shown. (Modified from Eger[30] and Weiskopf et al.,[135] with permission.)

Isoflurane

Isoflurane anesthesia caused a small increase in central venous pressure.[97] This was manifest as a higher right atrial pressure at 2.0 MAC isoflurane compared with awake values.

Enflurane

Enflurane caused increased central venous pressure.[133] An enflurane dose of 1.5 MAC caused an increase in right atrial pressure compared with awake control values.

Halothane

Halothane anesthesia caused dose-dependent increases in central venous pressure.[134] Right atrial pressures were higher than awake control values at halothane doses of 1.2 MAC and higher.

Sevoflurane

Central venous pressure did not change in dogs when sevoflurane dose was increased from 1.0 to 3.0 MAC.[139] Baseline measurements were not made in this study.

Desflurane

Desflurane at 1.24 MAC and higher caused an increase in central venous pressure compared with awake controls.[135]

Nitrous Oxide

Nitrous oxide caused an increase in right atrial pressure at doses of 1.5 MAC but not at 1.0 MAC.[97] Given that the MAC of nitrous oxide is greater than 1 atm, this effect is of little clinical importance.

Baroreceptor Function

Anesthetics may alter baroreceptor function. This is commonly tested in humans by measuring changes in the R-R interval after a vasopressor or vasodilator is administered.

Isoflurane

Baroreceptor function was attenuated by isoflurane.[140] This effect was less dramatic than with either enflurane or halothane. In a more recent study, isoflurane and enflurane were found to have similar depressive effects on baroreceptor function, but the depression by enflurane persisted longer postoperatively.[141]

Enflurane

Enflurane depressed baroreceptor function to a greater degree than did isoflurane at equipotent concentrations.[140,142] Depression of baroreceptor function by enflurane persisted longer into the postoperative period than that caused by isoflurane.[141]

Halothane

Halothane depressed baroreceptor function in a dose-related fashion; at 1.5 MAC, halothane completely abolished heart rate changes resulting from pressor infusion.[143]

Nitrous Oxide

The addition of 67 percent nitrous oxide to halothane anesthesia in dogs attenuated baroreceptor function.

Cardiac Output

The cardiac output of anesthetized patients is affected by numerous factors, including myocardial contractility, systemic vascular resistance, preload, baroreceptor function, and heart rate. The information presented subsequently, unless otherwise

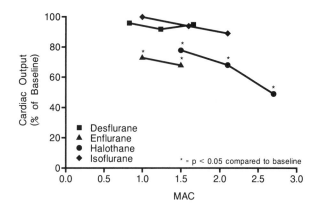

Fig. 25-4 Cardiac output decreased in a dose-dependent fashion in normocapnic volunteers given enflurane or halothane. Desflurane and isoflurane did not change cardiac output at the doses tested. (Modified from Eger[30] and Weiskopf et al.,[135] with permission.)

noted, was obtained from human volunteers (Fig. 25-4).

Isoflurane

Isoflurane anesthesia did not affect cardiac output at concentrations of 1.0, 1.5, or 2.0 MAC during normocarbia.[132] Stroke volume decreased in a dose-dependent fashion but was compensated for by an increased heart rate. Isoflurane administered to spontaneously breathing volunteers resulted in a 30 percent increase in cardiac output at 1.0 MAC.[98] Increasing the isoflurane concentration to 1.5 MAC did not further alter cardiac output. The effects of isoflurane on cardiac output were not influenced by duration of anesthesia during the first 5 hours of isoflurane administration.[132]

Enflurane

Enflurane administered to mechanically ventilated normocarbic volunteers resulted in a 20 percent reduction in cardiac output at 1.0 MAC and about a 30 percent reduction in cardiac output at 1.5 MAC.[133] Duration of anesthesia altered the effect of enflurane on cardiac output. After 6 hours of enflurane administration, cardiac output returned to baseline.

Halothane

Halothane administration to mechanically ventilated normocarbic volunteers resulted in a 22 percent reduction in cardiac output at 1.0 percent, a 32 percent reduction at 1.6 percent, and a 50 percent reduction at a concentration of 2.0 percent.[134] In spontaneously breathing volunteers, cardiac output was maintained at near normal levels at halothane doses below 2.0 MAC.[144] The duration of anesthesia appeared to influence the degree to which halothane altered cardiac output and other cardiac indices. After 5 hours of anesthesia, cardiac output returned to baseline.

Sevoflurane

Invasive human volunteer cardiac studies have not been performed with sevoflurane at the time of writing this chapter. In spontaneously breathing rats, sevoflurane did not alter cardiac output in doses as high as 1.5 MAC.[145] Sevoflurane produced a dose-dependent reduction in cardiac output similar to isoflurane in mechanically ventilated normocarbic dogs.[128] The effect of duration of anesthesia on sevoflurane-induced alterations in cardiac function was not examined.

Desflurane

Desflurane administered to mechanically ventilated normocarbic volunteers did not change the cardiac index in doses up to 1.66 MAC.[135] In spontaneously breathing volunteers, the cardiac index was increased;[146] this was not dose dependent. The duration of anesthesia appeared to influence the degree to which desflurane altered the cardiac output and other cardiac indices.[135] After 7 hours of desflurane anesthesia, the cardiac index of normocarbic volunteers was slightly higher than that seen after 90 minutes of anesthesia.

Nitrous Oxide

In normocapnic volunteers, 1.0 and 1.5 MAC (hyperbaric) nitrous oxide did not change cardiac output.[97] The addition of nitrous oxide to halothane, isoflurane, or desflurane did not change cardiac output.[137,146,147] The addition of nitrous oxide to enflurane increased cardiac output to near baseline levels.[138]

Heart Rate

Heart rates of patients anesthetized with inhalational anesthetics are affected by numerous factors, including baroreceptor function and direct effects

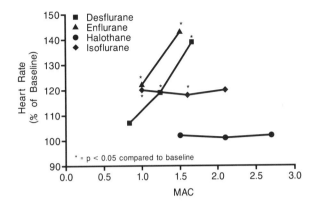

Fig. 25-5 Effect of volatile anesthetics on the heart rate of normocarbic volunteers. (Modified from Weiskopf et al.,[135] with permission, with data from Stevens et al.,[132] Calverly et al.,[133] and Eger et al.[134])

on the sinoatrial node. The information presented subsequently, unless otherwise noted, was obtained from human volunteers (Fig. 25-5).

Isoflurane

Isoflurane caused an increase in heart rate in normocarbic subjects that did not appear to be dose dependent.[132] Spontaneously breathing volunteers had a greater increase in heart rate compared with normocarbic subjects.[98] Young patients were more likely to have increased heart rates than were older patients.[148] Isoflurane had negative chronotropic effects on the sinoatrial node of guinea pigs.[149]

Enflurane

In normocarbic volunteers enflurane caused a dose-dependent increase in heart rate, 22 percent at 1.0 MAC and 40 percent at 1.5 MAC.[133] This increase in heart rate was not as dramatic as with isoflurane.[150] Enflurane had negative chronotropic effects on the sinoatrial node of guinea pigs.[149]

Halothane

Halothane administration did not change heart rate in doses up to 2.0 percent in normocarbic volunteers.[134] Halothane anesthesia caused an increase in heart rate during spontaneous ventilation.[144] Halothane had negative chronotropic effects on the sinoatrial node of guinea pigs.[149]

Sevoflurane

Sevoflurane administration to surgical patients was associated with a smaller increase in heart rate both before and after incision compared with isoflurane.[151]

Desflurane

In normocarbic volunteers, desflurane produced dose-dependent increases in heart rate at doses greater than 0.83 MAC.[135]

Nitrous Oxide

Nitrous oxide administered alone caused a small increase in heart rate.[97] The heart rate of volunteers increased when nitrous oxide was added to enflurane,[138] but not halothane, isoflurane, or desflurane.[137,146,147]

Arterial Blood Pressure

The information presented subsequently, unless otherwise noted, was obtained from human volunteers (Fig. 25-6).

Isoflurane

Isoflurane caused a dose-dependent reduction of mean arterial pressure in normocarbic volunteers.[132] The mean arterial pressure was reduced 27 percent at 1.0 MAC, 37 percent at 1.5 MAC, and 54 percent at 2.0 MAC. Spontaneous ventilation during isoflurane anesthesia resulted in a

slightly higher mean arterial pressure compared with normocarbic mechanical ventilation.[98]

Enflurane

Enflurane caused a reduction of mean arterial pressure in normocarbic volunteers.[133] The mean arterial pressure was reduced 35 percent at 1.0 MAC and 40 percent at 1.5 MAC.

Halothane

Halothane caused a dose-dependent reduction of mean arterial pressure in normocarbic volunteers.[134] The mean arterial pressure was reduced 24 percent at 1.0 percent halothane, 33 percent at 1.6 percent, and 51 percent at 2.0 percent. Spontaneous ventilation during halothane-induced anesthesia resulted in a slightly higher mean arterial pressure compared with normocarbic mechanical ventilation.[144]

Sevoflurane

The effects of sevoflurane on arterial blood pressure were similar to those of isoflurane in surgical patients.[151]

Desflurane

Desflurane caused a dose-dependent reduction of mean arterial pressure.[135] The mean arterial pressure was reduced about 40 percent by 1.24 MAC desflurane and 50 percent by 1.66 MAC desflurane. Spontaneous ventilation during desflurane administration resulted in a slightly higher mean arterial pressure compared to normocarbic mechanical ventilation, but only at the highest dose tested (1.66 MAC).[146]

Nitrous Oxide

Nitrous oxide administered alone caused either a small increase in mean arterial pressure or no change.[12,30] The blood pressure of volunteers increased when nitrous oxide was added to halothane, isoflurane, and desflurane[137,146,147] but not enflurane.[138]

Cardiac Rhythm/Response to Catecholamines

Volatile anesthetics frequently alter myocardial sensitivity to catecholamines. The magnitude of this effect varies from one agent to another and

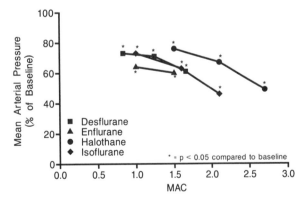

Fig. 25-6 The mean arterial pressure of normocapnic volunteers given volatile anesthetics decreased in a dose-related fashion. (Modified with permission from Eger[30] and Weiskopf et al.,[135] with permission.)

may not be dose dependent.[152] Volatile anesthetics may also cause changes in cardiac conduction pathways.

Isoflurane

Isoflurane did not lower the epinephrine dose that provokes ventricular dysrhythmias compared with the awake state.[153] The epinephrine dose required to cause dysrhythmias in 50 percent of patients during 1.25 MAC isoflurane anesthesia was 6.7 μg/kg.[154] Isoflurane had little effect on atrioventricular conduction times in dogs.[155] Isoflurane did not affect thresholds for pacemaker capture.[156]

Enflurane

The epinephrine dose required to cause dysrhythmias in 50 percent of patients during 1.25 MAC enflurane anesthesia was 10.9 μg/kg.[154] Enflurane administration prolonged atrioventricular conduction times in dogs.[155] Thresholds for pacemaker capture were not affected by enflurane anesthesia.[156]

Halothane

The epinephrine dose required to cause dysrhythmias in 50 percent of patients during 1.25 MAC halothane administration was 2.1 μg/kg.[154] The tendency for halothane to cause myocardial sensitization to catecholamines was less pronounced in children than in adults.[157] Addition of lidocaine antagonized the effect of epinephrine in patients anesthetized with halothane.[154] Atrioventricular conduction times in dogs were prolonged by halothane anesthesia.[155] Halothane administration did not affect thresholds for pacemaker capture.[156]

Sevoflurane

The effect of sevoflurane on the response to epinephrine administration was similar to that of isoflurane in dogs (less than halothane) at equal MAC doses.[158]

Desflurane

The effect of desflurane on the response to epinephrine administration was similar to that of isoflurane in pigs (less than that halothane) at equal MAC doses.[159]

Coronary Circulation and Ischemia

Inhaled anesthetics can affect the coronary circulation. Volatile anesthetics generally decrease myocardial oxygen consumption[140] and may alter coronary vascular resistance. Coronary steal may be induced by inhaled anesthetics, thereby affecting the myocardial oxygen supply. Coronary steal is the redistribution of coronary flow from collateral dependent zones of myocardium to noncollateral dependent zones in the presence of a coronary vasodilator. Potent coronary vasodilators, such as adenosine, can cause such regional redistribution of myocardial blood flow.[160] Volatile anesthetics cause coronary artery dilatation and could theoretically cause coronary steal in patients with susceptible coronary anatomy. In one study, 23 percent of patients undergoing coronary arteriography for coronary artery disease had steal prone anatomy.[161] Whether volatile anesthetics, isoflurane in particular, produce myocardial ischemia as a result of coronary steal in the clinical setting, remains controversial.

Isoflurane

Isoflurane causes dose-dependent coronary vasodilation, primarily at the arteriolar level.[162–165] Depending on the model used, isoflurane is a more[165] or less[162] potent coronary vasodilator than halothane. Several investigators studied the possibility that isoflurane causes regional redistribution of myocardial blood flow in chronically instrumented animals with steal prone coronary anatomy. Some of these showed isoflurane caused regional redistribution of myocardial blood flow with or without evidence of subsequent ischemia in the collateral-dependent zone.[166,167] Other animal studies did not find evidence of coronary steal over a wide range of coronary perfusion pressures.[168–170] Human studies are also contradictory. Some detected indirect evidence of regional redistribution of myocardial blood flow in patients with steal prone coronary anatomy anesthetized with isoflurane.[163,171,172] This evidence includes increased myocardial lactate production and ischemic electrocardiographic (ECG) changes despite increased global coronary blood flow and reduced metabolic demand. On the other hand, two recent studies do not support the hypothesis that isoflurane causes coronary steal. A large retrospective study compared the effects of isoflurane, enflurane, halothane, and sufentanil during coronary artery bypass surgery in patients with steal prone coronary anatomy.[173] The incidence of myocardial ischemia detected by ECG changes was not different among patients anesthetized with any of the four agents. Finally, one study compared the regional and global myocardial circulatory effects of isoflurane and halothane in patients with steal prone coronary anatomy undergoing coronary artery bypass surgery.[174] There was no difference in the incidence of myocardial ischemia between the groups, and no evidence of redistribution of regional myocardial blood flow in either group. Therefore, it appears that isoflurane does not cause clinically significant coronary steal in humans.

Isoflurane had a protective effect against ischemia induced by pacing in humans with coronary artery disease.[175] However, isoflurane did not mitigate ischemia induced by pacing in dogs.[176]

Enflurane

Enflurane is a coronary vasodilator.[177] It appears that coronary vasodilatation caused by enflurane is equivalent to or slightly less marked than that caused by isoflurane.[165,177] There is some evidence that enflurane causes regional redistribution of myocardial blood flow[177] but no large definitive studies. Enflurane has been compared with isoflurane in a large study of patients undergoing coronary artery bypass surgery.[178] The rates of postoperative myocardial infarction and perioperative death were lower in the enflurane group than in the isoflurane group.

Halothane

Halothane causes coronary vasodilatation that is either more or less profound than that seen with isoflurane, depending on the model tested.[162,165] There is no evidence that halothane causes regional redistribution of myocardial blood flow.[174] Halothane does not protect against ischemia induced by pacing in dogs.[176] The incidence of myocardial ischemia during coronary artery bypass surgery did not appear to be different during halo-

thane anesthesia compared with isoflurane or enflurane anesthesia.[173]

Sevoflurane

Sevoflurane caused a decrease in coronary vascular resistance and an increase in coronary blood flow similar to isoflurane.[125]

Desflurane

Desflurane caused a decrease in coronary vascular resistance and increase in coronary blood flow similar to isoflurane.[179] Desflurane did not appear to cause coronary steal in dogs.[180] In a relatively small study, the incidence of myocardial ischemia, myocardial infarction, and perioperative death with the use of desflurane as the primary anesthetic for coronary artery bypass surgery was similar to isoflurane.[181]

Nitrous Oxide

The addition of nitrous oxide to a volatile anesthetic appeared to result in further reduction of coronary vascular resistance.[177] Nitrous oxide did not appear to cause coronary steal in dogs.[166]

HEPATIC EFFECTS

Hepatic Blood Flow

The liver derives its blood flow from two sources, the hepatic artery and the portal vein. The portal vein normally supplies 65 to 75 percent of total liver blood flow and 50 to 60 percent of the oxygen utilized by the liver, and the hepatic artery supplies the balance. Hepatic blood supply is notable for the reciprocity of blood flow. When portal vein blood flow is reduced, hepatic artery resistance decreases resulting in increased hepatic artery blood flow. Likewise, when portal vein flow increases, hepatic artery resistance increases resulting in decreased hepatic artery flow. Inhaled anesthetics can affect both the reciprocity of hepatic blood flow and the total blood flow to the liver.

Isoflurane

Isoflurane in concentrations up to 2.0 MAC resulted in increased hepatic artery and decreased portal vein blood flow in dogs.[182] It appeared that hepatic oxygen supply was better preserved with isoflurane than with halothane at equipotent concentrations.[183] Isoflurane and halothane in doses resulting in 50 percent reduction of mean arterial pressure decreased hepatic oxygen delivery and total hepatic blood flow in guinea pigs, but the decrease was less dramatic with isoflurane (34 percent) than with halothane (65 percent).[184] Reciprocal hepatic circulation was better maintained with isoflurane than with halothane.[182,185]

Enflurane

Enflurane caused dose-dependent reductions of hepatic artery and portal venous blood flow in dogs.[186] Enflurane produced a drop in portal venous blood flow proportional to the drop in systemic blood pressure, but there was no change in portal venous resistance.[187,188] Reciprocity of hepatic blood flow was better maintained with enflurane than with halothane.[186]

Halothane

In dogs, 1.0 MAC halothane decreased portal vein blood flow but did not change hepatic artery flow.[182] An increase in halothane concentration to 2.0 MAC decreased both hepatic artery and portal vein blood flow. In one series of studies, halothane produced a drop in portal venous blood flow proportional to the drop in systemic blood pressure. There was no change in portal venous resistance, but hepatic artery resistance was increased resulting in a greater reduction of hepatic artery flow than of portal venous flow.[187,188] Isoflurane and halothane in doses resulting in 50 percent reduction of mean arterial pressure decreased hepatic oxygen delivery and total hepatic blood flow in guinea pigs, but the decrease was less dramatic with isoflurane (34 percent) than with halothane (65 percent).[184] Because halothane caused selective constriction of the hepatic artery, reciprocity of hepatic blood flow was not maintained.[186,189]

Sevoflurane

Hepatic blood flow and oxygen delivery during sevoflurane-induced anesthesia in dogs has been compared with that of isoflurane and halothane in doses up to 2.0 MAC.[190] Hepatic arterial blood flow was maintained with sevoflurane and isoflurane but not with halothane. Portal venous flow was re-

duced with sevoflurane and isoflurane, but halothane caused even greater reductions. Total hepatic blood flow was not changed by sevoflurane. Hepatic oxygen delivery was greater with sevoflurane and isoflurane than with halothane.

Desflurane

The effects of desflurane on canine hepatic blood flow were comparable to those of isoflurane in concentrations up to 2.0 MAC.[179] Hepatic arterial flows were maintained by desflurane and slightly increased by isoflurane. Portal blood flow was slightly decreased by both drugs. Total hepatic blood flow was reduced by desflurane but not changed by isoflurane in this model.

Nitrous Oxide

Nitrous oxide had no effect on hepatic blood flow in swine when added to isoflurane.[191]

Drug Clearance

The presence of clinically relevant concentrations of potent inhalational anesthetics may reduce hepatic drug clearance. This may be caused by the previously mentioned effects on hepatic blood supply, inhibition of biotransformation, or a combination of both. Volatile anesthetics inhibit hepatic metabolism of certain drugs,[192] and there is evidence in dogs that prolongation of the hepatic clearance rate for propranolol is primarily the result of inhibition of biotransformation.[193]

Isoflurane

Isoflurane prolonged the elimination half-life of the model drug, aminopyrine, in the rat.[194] This effect was apparent when tested 2 hours after anesthesia but not when tested 24 hours after anesthesia.

Enflurane

Enflurane, unlike isoflurane or halothane, did not prolong the elimination half-life of aminopyrine in the rat.[194]

Halothane

Halothane prolonged the elimination half-life of aminopyrine in the rat.[194] This effect was apparent when tested both 2 and 24 hours after anesthesia.

Other drugs whose elimination half-life was increased included fentanyl, ketamine, lidocaine, pancuronium, and propranolol. In the case of propranolol, the inhibition of metabolism was stereoselective.[195]

Protein Synthesis

Volatile anesthetics can affect hepatic protein synthesis, but the clinical significance of this is unclear.

Isoflurane

Isoflurane reduced protein synthesis in guinea pig liver slices but not as profoundly as halothane.[196]

Enflurane

Enflurane caused a dose-dependent reduction of protein synthesis in isolated rat liver preparations.[197] In guinea pig liver slices, the inhibition of protein synthesis by enflurane was less dramatic than with halothane or isoflurane.[198]

Halothane

Halothane caused a dose-dependent reduction of protein synthesis in isolated rat liver preparations.[197]

Sevoflurane

Sevoflurane reduced protein synthesis in guinea pig liver slices but not as profoundly as halothane, isoflurane, or enflurane.[198]

Desflurane

Desflurane inhibited protein synthesis in guinea pig liver slices but not as markedly as isoflurane.[199]

Hepatotoxicity

Potent inhalational anesthetics, primarily halothane, are associated with two forms of hepatotoxicity: a mild self-limited form with nonspecific increases of hepatic transaminases and a more severe hepatitis with significant associated morbidity and mortality rates. This discussion will focus on the more severe form of hepatic toxicity. The overwhelming majority of inhalational anesthetic related hepatic dysfunction has occurred after halothane administration.

Isoflurane

During the years 1981 to 1984, the Food and Drug Administration received reports of 45 cases of hepatic dysfunction, possibly related to isoflurane administration.[200] It was concluded that all but 16 were more likely explained by causes other than isoflurane administration. Each of the remaining 16 had possible causes other than isoflurane. The Food and Drug Administration concluded there is not a reasonable likelihood of an association between the use of isoflurane and hepatic dysfunction.

Enflurane

Halothane related hepatitis appears to be caused by an immune reaction with a neoantigen formed by a halothane metabolite bound to hepatic proteins (discussed later). There is evidence that an enflurane metabolite is also capable of binding hepatic proteins to form potential immunogens.[201] However, there is no strong clinical evidence of a syndrome of enflurane-induced hepatitis.[202]

Halothane

The incidence of hepatic injury related to halothane is between 1 in 7,000 and 1 in 30,000 halothane anesthetics.[203] Fatal hepatic necrosis had an apparent incidence of 1 in 35,000 halothane exposures when cases with other likely causes were excluded.[204] Halothane hepatotoxicity is thought to be mediated by one or more halothane metabolites. Halothane undergoes both reductive and oxidative biotransformation. In the past, it was thought that halothane related hepatitis was mediated by reductive metabolites, but this hypothesis has been largely abandoned for numerous reasons.[203] Currently, it is thought that a trifluoroacetyl halide compound derived from oxidative halothane biotransformation can covalently bind to hepatic microsomal proteins, thereby forming a hapten. Antibodies that react to such antigens have been found in the sera of patients with halothane related hepatitis.[205–207] Patients thus sensitized to halothane are susceptible to hepatic injury with repeat halothane exposure. There is evidence for a genetic predisposition to such injury.[208,209] Risk factors associated with halothane-induced hepatic injury include repeated halothane exposures, obesity, middle age, female gender, and Mexican-American ethnic origin.[203] The authors of a review of halothane related hepatic injury concluded that children are at low risk for such hepatitis, that there is no contraindication to halothane use in patients with pre-existing compensated hepatic dysfunction, that single exposure to halothane carries a very low risk of halothane related hepatitis, and that an immune response is most likely involved in the syndrome.[210]

Sevoflurane

There is no evidence of hepatic dysfunction in surgical patients anesthetized with sevoflurane.[211] More extensive clinical use will help determine whether sevoflurane can cause hepatotoxicity.

Desflurane

There is no evidence of hepatic dysfunction in human volunteers anesthetized with desflurane.[212,213] More extensive clinical use will help determine whether desflurane can cause hepatotoxicity; because desflurane undergoes little biotransformation, this is unlikely.

Nitrous Oxide

There is no clinical evidence that nitrous oxide administration causes hepatic dysfunction.[214]

RENAL EFFECTS

Renal Blood Flow and Glomerular Filtration Rate

Data concerning the effects of volatile anesthetics on renal blood flow and glomerular filtration rate seem to be conflicting, depending on whether animal models or surgical patients are examined. Information from both animal and human studies (when available) is presented below (Fig. 25-7).

Isoflurane

Renal blood flow was maintained in dogs given isoflurane in doses up to 2.0 MAC[215] and in doses necessary to reduce mean arterial pressure to 45

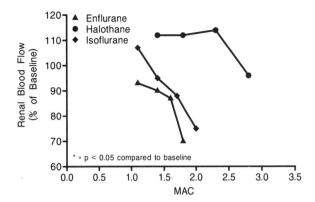

Fig. 25-7 The effect of halothane, enflurane, and isoflurane on renal blood flow in chronically instrumented dogs. None of the changes are statistically significant. (Data from Hysing et al.[216])

mmHg.[216] In surgical patients given 0.6 to 1.0 MAC isoflurane, reductions of renal blood flow (para-amino hippurate, or PAH clearance technique) to 50 percent of control and of glomerular filtration rate (inulin clearance technique) to 63 percent of control have been reported.[217]

Enflurane

Renal blood flow was maintained in dogs given enflurane in doses necessary to reduce mean arterial pressure to 45 mmHg.[216] In surgical patients given enflurane 0.6 MAC, reductions of renal blood flow (PAH clearance technique) to 77 percent of control and of glomerular filtration rate (inulin clearance technique) to 79 percent of control were reported.[218]

Halothane

Renal blood flow was maintained in dogs given halothane in concentrations up to 2.0 MAC[215] and in concentrations necessary to reduce mean arterial pressure to 45 mmHg.[216] In surgical patients given halothane 0.7 to 1.4 MAC, reductions of renal blood flow (PAH clearance technique) to 60 percent of control and of glomerular filtration rate (inulin clearance technique) to 72 percent of control have been reported.[219] Renal blood flow normally remains relatively constant over a wide range of renal artery perfusion pressures because of autoregulation. Autoregulation of renal blood flow in the isolated dog kidney was maintained in the presence of halothane 0.9 percent.[220]

Sevoflurane

Sevoflurane had effects similar to isoflurane on renal blood flow in rats.[46] Both maintained renal blood flow when administered at doses necessary to reduce mean arterial pressure to 70 mmHg and reduced renal blood flow when administered at doses necessary to reduce mean arterial pressure to 50 mmHg.

Desflurane

Desflurane had effects similar to isoflurane on renal blood flow in dogs.[179] Both maintained renal blood flow and reduced renal vascular resistance in concentrations up to 2.0 MAC.

Nephrotoxicity

Halogenated anesthetics that undergo biotransformation to inorganic fluoride are implicated in renal toxicity. The link between biotransformation of a halogenated anesthetic (methoxyflurane) to fluoride and renal damage was first made in 1970.[221] The cause and effect relationship between the free fluoride ion and methoxyflurane nephrotoxicity was established in 1971.[222] Methoxyflurane can cause high output renal failure characterized by a urine concentrating defect, azotemia, hypernatremia, and hyperosmolality that usually resolves within 10 to 20 days.[223] Nephrotoxic effects begin to occur when peak plasma fluoride concentrations reach 50 μM/L.[224] It appears that the occurrence of renal failure cannot be predicted on the basis of peak plasma fluoride levels alone and that the length of time the kidneys are exposed to fluoride must also be taken into account.[225]

Isoflurane

Prolonged isoflurane administration in critically ill patients was reported to cause a mean peak plasma fluoride level of 25 μM/L.[226] Serum and urine electrolytes, urine osmolality, and creatinine clearance were not altered in these patients, compared with those in a control group.

Enflurane

Urine concentrating ability was assessed after short (2.7 MAC-hours) exposures to enflurane or halothane in healthy surgical patients.[218] Urine concentrating ability was measured using urine osmolality in response to a vasopressin challenge. Neither agent caused a urine concentrating defect. The mean peak plasma fluoride in the enflurane group was 22 μM/L. However, after prolonged (9.6 MAC-hour for the enflurane group) exposures,[225] the mean peak plasma fluoride level in the enflurane group was 34 μM/L, and this was associated with a urine concentrating defect. Preoperative exposure to certain liver enzyme inducers resulted in higher plasma fluoride levels after enflurane exposure as a result of enhanced enflurane biotransformation.[227]

Halothane

The mean peak plasma fluoride level, in volunteers exposed to halothane for 13.7 MAC-hours, was 15 μM/L.[225] This was not associated with a urine concentrating defect.

Sevoflurane

Inorganic fluoride is a major metabolic product of sevoflurane.[228] In a study of healthy volunteers, sevoflurane 1.5 MAC administered for 1 hour resulted in peak plasma fluoride levels of 22 μM/L.[229] Prolonged sevoflurane exposure in surgical patients was reported to result in a mean peak plasma fluoride level of 42.5 μM/L.[230] No evidence of nephrotoxicity was found in these patients. Healthy volunteers had no urine concentrating defect after 9.6 MAC-hour exposure to sevoflurane as measured by desmopressin challenge (Frink EJ, Jr: Personal communication).

Desflurane

Desflurane undergoes little biotransformation. In humans, both volunteers and surgical patients, postoperative plasma fluoride levels did not differ from baseline levels.[231]

ENDOCRINE EFFECTS
Glucose/Insulin Balance
Isoflurane

Isoflurane anesthesia causes glucose intolerance.[232] This is partly the result of decreased insulin secretion, although growth hormone and norepinephrine levels are increased under anesthesia and probably contribute to the glucose intolerance. When surgical stimulation is superimposed on isoflurane anesthesia, growth hormone, cortisol, epinephrine, and norepinephrine levels all increase, resulting in increased glucose levels.

Enflurane

Enflurane produced a dose related inhibitory effect on glucose stimulated insulin release when tested in rat pancreatic islet cells in vitro.[233]

Halothane

Halothane anesthesia between 1.0 and 2.0 MAC in humans appeared to reduce insulin levels in the absence of surgical stimulation.[234] The reduction of insulin was dose related.[235]

Thyroid Function
Halothane

Thyroxine levels increased under halothane anesthesia.[236] However, halothane did not appear to affect thyroid stimulating hormone release.

Antidiuretic Hormone/Renin/Angiotensin
Halothane

Light halothane anesthesia did not cause antidiuretic hormone release.[237] The use of 1.0 to 2.0 percent halothane with 50 percent nitrous oxide increased plasma antidiuretic hormone levels.[238] Surgical stimulation during halothane anesthesia resulted in further increases in antidiuretic hormone levels. Plasma renin activity was unchanged during halothane-nitrous oxide anesthesia in the absence of surgery.[239]

Effects on Hormonal Stress Response

Normal responses to surgical stress include increased serum levels of β-endorphins, adrenocorticotrophic hormone, growth hormone, antidiuretic hormone, epinephrine, and norepinephrine. Inhalational anesthetic agents may alter some of these responses.

Isoflurane

Isoflurane caused an increase in serum norepinephrine levels in the absence of surgical stimulation.[240] Despite increased norepinephrine levels, isoflurane in adequate doses abolished the pressor response to intubation. Isoflurane and halothane had similar effects on intraoperative hormonal stress markers.[241]

Enflurane

Enflurane in a dose of 2.2 percent caused a reduction of both spontaneous and stress related release of epinephrine and norepinephrine in cats.[242] The dose of enflurane required to prevent a stress response to skin incision in 50 percent of patients was 1.6 MAC;[243] stress response in this study was defined as an increase in plasma norepinephrine, increased heart rate and/or blood pressure, or changes in pupil diameter.

Halothane

Halothane-nitrous oxide anesthesia in clinically relevant concentrations did not prevent stress related increases in plasma antidiuretic hormone levels and renin activity.[238,239] Moderate and deep halothane anesthesia (1.2 and 2.1 MAC) were not different with respect to blood glucose, cortisol, insulin, or catecholamine responses during abdominal hysterectomy.[244] The dose of halothane required to prevent a stress response to skin incision in 50 percent of patients was 1.45 MAC;[243] stress response in this study was defined as an increase in plasma norepinephrine, increased heart rate and/or blood pressure, or changes in pupil diameter.

HEMATOLOGIC/IMMUNE SYSTEM

Hematopoiesis

Nitrous Oxide

Nitrous oxide has been implicated in reversible bone marrow depression for many years.[245,246] Megaloblastic bone marrow changes have been seen after prolonged[247] or even relatively brief exposures[248] to nitrous oxide. It appears these effects are a result of the oxidation of the cobalt moiety in vitamin B_{12}.[249] Vitamin B_{12} is a coenzyme of methionine synthetase. Thus, nitrous oxide inhibits the activity of methionine synthetase, an enzyme necessary for folate metabolism and normal hematopoiesis. Pretreatment with folinic acid may prevent nitrous oxide-induced bone marrow changes.[250]

Red Blood Cells

Enflurane, halothane, or nitrous oxide exposure was shown to cause a small rightward shift of the normal oxyhemoglobin dissociation curve.[251] However, more recent data suggested a leftward shift[252] or no change[253] in the oxyhemoglobin dissociation curve in patients exposed to 50 percent nitrous oxide.

Leukocytes

Isoflurane

The ability of polymorphonuclear leukocytes to kill gram-negative bacteria when exposed to clinically relevant isoflurane concentrations was not different than when exposed to air.[254]

Enflurane

Enflurane anesthesia in volunteers caused a slight leukocytosis.[255] The ability of polymorphonuclear leukocytes to kill gram-negative bacteria when exposed to clinically relevant enflurane concentrations was not different than when exposed to air.[254]

Halothane

Halothane anesthesia in volunteers caused a slight leukocytosis.[255] Both nonspecific mobility and chemotaxis of leukocytes appeared to be inhibited by halothane anesthesia, but phagocytosis appeared to be normal.[255–257] Polymorphonuclear leukocytes exposed to clinically relevant halothane concentrations are less able to kill gram-negative bacteria than those exposed to air.[258] This effect was rapidly reversed when halothane exposure ceased. Halothane caused a dose-dependent inhibition of lymphocyte transformation after exposure to an antigen.[255]

Nitrous Oxide

Nitrous oxide-morphine anesthesia in volunteers caused a slight leukocytosis.[255] Phagocytosis by leukocytes did not appear to be affected.[255] The ability of polymorphonuclear leukocytes to kill gram-negative bacteria when exposed to clinically relevant nitrous oxide concentrations was not different than when exposed to air.[254]

Platelets

Isoflurane, enflurane, and nitrous oxide did not increase the standardized bleeding time, but there was a 33 percent increase with halothane.[259,260]

REPRODUCTIVE SYSTEM

Uterine Tone

Volatile anesthetics generally decrease muscle tone in the pregnant uterus. This may affect surgical blood loss during procedures such as cesarean section or termination of pregnancy.

Isoflurane

Isoflurane caused a dose-dependent decrease in uterine muscle contractility in vitro and in vivo.[261,262] This reduction in uterine muscle tone was the same with isoflurane as with equipotent concentrations of enflurane or halothane. The use of isoflurane in a general anesthetic for elective cesarean section was associated with a greater perioperative fall of hematocrit than regional anesthesia, indicating greater blood loss.[263]

Enflurane

Enflurane caused a dose-dependent decrease in uterine muscle contractility in vitro and in vivo.[261,262] This reduction in uterine muscle tone was the same with enflurane as with equipotent concentrations of isoflurane or halothane.

Halothane

Halothane caused a dose-dependent decrease in uterine muscle contractility in vitro and in vivo.[261,262] This reduction in uterine muscle tone was the same with halothane as with equipotent concentrations of enflurane or isoflurane. During therapeutic termination of pregnancy, 1 percent halothane anesthesia was associated with greater blood loss than 0.5 percent halothane plus 75 percent nitrous oxide or 80 percent nitrous oxide plus meperidine and thiopental.[264]

Nitrous Oxide

During therapeutic termination of pregnancy, 75 percent nitrous oxide with halothane 0.5 percent was associated with less blood loss than is 1.0 percent halothane.[264]

Fetal Effects

The potent inhalational anesthetics readily cross the placenta and are taken up by the fetus.

Isoflurane

When pregnant ewes were given isoflurane, 1.0 or 1.5 MAC, maternal blood pressure was decreased, but uterine vasodilatation occurred and uteroplacental blood flow was maintained.[262] Isoflurane, 2.0 MAC, caused greater depression of maternal blood pressure that was not completely compensated by uterine vasodilatation, resulting in fetal hypoxia and acidemia. In pregnant ewes, isoflurane 2.0 percent did not cause a reduction of fetal blood pressure, but there was a decrease in fetal pH.[265]

Halothane

When pregnant ewes were given halothane, 1.0 or 1.5 MAC, maternal blood pressure was decreased but uterine vasodilatation occurred and uteroplacental blood flow was maintained.[262] Halothane 2.0 MAC caused greater depression of maternal blood pressure that was not completely compensated by uterine vasodilatation, resulting in fetal hypoxia and acidemia. In pregnant ewes, halothane 1.5 percent caused a reduction of fetal blood pressure,

but regional fetal blood flow was maintained and no change in fetal acid base status or oxygenation occurred.[266] Asphyxiated fetal lambs, like normal fetal lambs, showed no ill effects from maternal halothane administration.[267]

REFERENCES

1. Corbett TH: Cancer and congenital anomalies associated with anesthetics. Ann N Y Acad Sci 271:58, 1976
2. Yasuda N, Targ AG, Eger EI II: Solubility of I-653, sevoflurane, isoflurane, and halothane in human tissues. Anesthesiology 69:A615, 1988
3. Stevens WC, Dolan WM, Gibbons RT et al: Minimum alveolar concentrations (MAC) of isoflurane with and without nitrous oxide in patients of various ages. Anesthesiology 42:197, 1975
4. Gion H, Saidman LJ: The minimum alveolar concentration of enflurane in man. Anesthesiology 35:361, 1971
5. Suckling CW: Some chemical and physical factors in development of Fluothane. Br J Anaesth 29:466, 1957
6. Johnstone M: Human cardiovascular response to Fluothane anaesthesia. Br J Anaesth 28:392, 1954
7. Saidman LJ, Eger EI II, Munson ES et al: Minimum alveolar concentrations of methoxyflurane, halothane, ether and cyclopropane in man: correlation with theories of anesthesia. Anesthesiology 28:994, 1967
8. Scheller MS, Saidman LJ, Partridge BL: MAC of sevoflurane in humans and the New Zealand white rabbit. Can J Anaesth 35:153, 1988
9. Van Hemelrigck J, Smith I, White PF: Use of desflurane for outpatient anesthesia: a comparison with propofol and nitrous oxide. Anesthesiology 75:197, 1991
10. Eger EI II: Partition coefficients of I-653 in human blood, saline, and olive oil. Anesth Analg 66:971, 1987
11. Rampil IJ, Lockhart SH, Zwass MS et al: Clinical characteristics of desflurane in surgical patients: minimum alveolar concentration. Anesthesiology 74:429, 1991
12. Hornbein TF, Eger EI II, Winter PM et al: The minimum alveolar concentration of nitrous oxide in man. Anesth Analg 61:553, 1982
13. Adams N: Effects of general anesthetics on memory functions in man. J Comp Physiol 83:294, 1973

14. Stulken EH, Jr, Milde JH, Michenfelder JD et al: The non-linear responses of cerebral metabolism to low concentrations of halothane, enflurane, isoflurane and thiopental. Anesthesiology 46:28, 1977

15. Gaumann DM, Mustaki JP, Tassonyi E: MAC-awake of isoflurane, enflurane and halothane evaluated by slow and fast alveolar washout. Br J Anaesth 68:81, 1992

16. Homi J, Konchigeri HN, Eckenhoff JE et al: A new anesthetic agent—Forane: preliminary observations in man. Anesth Analg 51:439, 1972

17. Clark DL, Rosner BS: Neurophysiologic effects of general anesthetics. Anesthesiology 38:564, 1973

18. Tinker JH, Sharbrough FW, Michenfelder JD: Anterior shift of the dominant EEG rhythm during anesthesia in the Java monkey. Anesthesiology 46:252, 1977

19. Eger EI II, Stevens WC, Cromwell TH: The electroencephalogram in man anesthetized with Forane. Anesthesiology 35:504, 1971

20. Neigh JL, Garman JK, Harp JR: The electroencephalographic pattern during anesthesia with Ethrane. Anesthesiology 35:482, 1971

21. Avramov MN, Shingu K, Omatsu Y, et al: Effects of different speeds of induction with sevoflurane on the EEG in man. J Anesth 1:1, 1987

22. Scheller MS, Tateishi A, Drummond FC et al: The effects of sevoflurane on cerebral blood flow, cerebral metabolic rate for oxygen, intracranial pressure, and the electroencephalogram are similar to those of isoflurane in the rabbit. Anesthesiology 68:548, 1988

23. Scheller MS, Nakakimura K, Fleischer JE et al: Cerebral effects of sevoflurane in the dog: comparison with isoflurane and enflurane. Br J Anaesth 65:388, 1990

24. Rampil IJ, Lockhart SH, Eger EI II et al: The electroencephalographic effects of desflurane in humans. Anesthesiology 74:434, 1991

25. Oshima A, Urabe N, Shingu K et al: Anticonvulsant actions of enflurane on epilepsy models in cats. Anesthesiology 63:29, 1985

26. Michenfelder JD, Cucchiara RF: Canine cerebral oxygen consumption during enflurane anesthesia and its modification during induced seizures. Anesthesiology 40:575, 1974

27. Poulton TJ, Ellingson RJ: Seizure associated with induction of anesthesia with isoflurane. Anesthesiology 61:471, 1984

28. Kofke WA, Snider MT, Young RS et al: Prolonged low flow isoflurane anesthesia for status epilepticus. Anesthesiology 62:653, 1985

29. Hilz MJ, Bauer J, Claus D et al: Isoflurane anaesthesia in the treatment of convulsive status epilepticus. J Neurol 239:135, 1992

30. Eger EI II: Isoflurane (Forane): A Compendium and Reference. 2nd Ed. Ohio Medical Products, Madison, WI, 1985

31. Boarini DJ, Kassell NF, Coester HC et al: Comparison of systemic and cerebrovascular effects of isoflurane and halothane. Neurosurgery 15:400, 1984

32. Todd MM, Drummond JC: A comparison of the cerebrovascular and metabolic effects of halothane and isoflurane in the cat. Anesthesiology 60:276, 1984

33. Cucchiara RF, Theye RA, Michenfelder JD: The effects of isoflurane on canine cerebral metabolism and blood flow. Anesthesiology 40:571, 1974

34. Drummond JC, Todd MM, Scheller MS et al: A comparison of the direct cerebral vasodilating potencies of halothane and isoflurane in the New Zealand white rabbit. Anesthesiology 65:462, 1986

35. Adams RW, Cucchiara RF, Gronert GA et al: Isoflurane and cerebrospinal fluid pressure in neurosurgical patients. Anesthesiology 54:97, 1981

36. Young WL, Bardai AI, Prohovnik I et al: Effect of PaCO$_2$ on cerebral blood flow distribution during halothane compared with isoflurane anaesthesia in the rat. Br J Anaesth 67:440, 1991

37. Hoffman WE, Edelman G, Kochs E et al: Cerebral autoregulation in awake versus isoflurane-anesthetized rats. Anesth Analg 73:753, 1991

38. Eintrei C, Leszniewski W, Carlsson C: Local application of [133]xenon for measurement of regional cerebral blood flow during halothane, enflurane, and isoflurane anesthesia in humans. Anesthesiology 63:391, 1985

39. Sakabe T, Fujii S, Ishikawa T: Cerebral circulation and metabolism during enflurane anesthesia in humans. Anesthesiology 59:532, 1983

40. Miletich DJ, Ivankovich AD, Albrecht RF: Absence of autoregulation of cerebral blood flow during halothane and enflurane anesthesia. Anesth Analg 55:100, 1976

41. Theye RA, Michenfelder JD: The effect of halothane on canine cerebral metabolism. Anesthesiology 26:1113, 1968

42. Adams RW, Gronert GA, Sundt TM et al: Halothane, hypocapnia, and cerebrospinal fluid pressure in neurosurgery. Anesthesiology 37:510, 1972

43. Alexander SC, Wollman G, Cohen PJ et al: Cerebro-

vascular response to $PaCO_2$ during halothane anesthesia in man. J Appl Physiol 19:561, 1964

44. Albrecht RF, Miletich DJ, Madala LR: Normalization of cerebral blood flow during prolonged halothane anesthesia. Anesthesiology 58:26, 1983

45. Warner DS, Boarini DJ, Kassell NF: Cerebrovascular adaptation to prolonged halothane anesthesia is not related to cerebrospinal fluid pH. Anesthesiology 63:243, 1985

46. Conzen PF, Vollmar B, Habazettl H et al: Systemic and regional hemodynamics of isoflurane and sevoflurane in rats. Anesth Analg 74:79, 1992

47. Lutz LJ, Milde JH, Milde LN: The cerebral functional, metabolic, and hemodynamic effects of desflurane in dogs. Anesthesiology 73:125, 1990

48. Lutz LJ, Milde JH, Milde LN: The response of the canine cerebral circulation to hyperventilation during anesthesia with desflurane. Anesthesiology 74:504, 1991

49. Carlsson C, Hagerdal M, Siesjo BK: The effect of nitrous oxide on oxygen consumption and blood flow in the cerebral cortex of the rat. Acta Anaesthiol Scand 20:91, 1976

50. Pelligrino DA, Miletich DJ, Hoffman WE: Nitrous oxide markedly increases cerebral cortical metabolic rate and blood flow in the goat. Anesthesiology 60:405, 1984

51. Sakabe T, Kuramoto T, Inove S et al: Cerebral effects of nitrous oxide in the dog. Anesthesiology 48:195, 1978

52. Oshito S, Ishikawa T, Tokutsu Y et al: Cerebral circulatory and metabolic stimulation with nitrous oxide in the dog. Acta Anaesthesiol Scand 23:177, 1979

53. Jobes DR, Kennell EK, Bitner R et al: Effects of morphine-nitrous oxide anesthesia on cerebral autoregulation. Anesthesiology 42:30, 1975

54. Kuramoto T, Oshita S, Takeshita H et al: Modification of the relationship between cerebral metabolism, blood flow, and electroencephalogram by stimulation during anesthesia in the dog. Anesthesiology 51:211, 1979

55. Smith AL, Wollman H: Cerebral blood flow and metabolism: effects of anesthetic drugs and techniques. Anesthesiology 36:378, 1972

56. Sakabe T, Kuramoto T, Kumagae S et al: Cerebral responses to the addition of nitrous oxide to halothane in man. Br J Anaesth 48:957, 1976

57. Newberg LA, Milde JH, Michenfelder JD: The cerebral metabolic effects of isoflurane at and above concentrations that suppress cortical electrical activity. Anesthesiology 59:23, 1983

58. Newberg LA, Michenfelder JD: Cerebral protection by isoflurane during hypoxemia or ischemia. Anesthesiology 59:29, 1983

59. Nehls DG, Todd MM, Spetzlet RF et al: A comparison of the cerebral protective effects of isoflurane and barbiturates during temporary focal ischemia in primates. Anesthesiology 66:453, 1987

60. Michenfelder JD, Sundt TM, Fode N et al: Isoflurane when compared to enflurane and halothane decreases the frequency of cerebral ischemia during carotid endarterectomy. Anesthesiology 67:336, 1987

61. Verhaegen MJ, Todd MM, Warner DS: A comparison of cerebral ischemic flow thresholds during halothane/N_2O and isoflurane/N_2O anesthesia in rats. Anesthesiology 76:743, 1992

62. Werner C, Kochs E, Hoffman WE et al: Sevoflurane reduces neurologic deficit following incomplete ischemia in rats. Anesthesiology 75:A603, 1991

63. Milde LN, Milde JH: The cerebral and systemic hemodynamic and metabolic effects of desflurane-induced hypotension in dogs. Anesthesiology 74:513, 1991

64. Dahlgren N, Ingvar M, Yokoyama H et al: Influence of nitrous oxide on local cerebral flow in awake, minimally restrained rats. J Cereb Blood Flow Metab 1:211, 1981

65. Algotsson L, Messeter K, Rosen I et al: Effects of nitrous oxide on cerebral haemodynamics and metabolism during isoflurane anaesthesia in man. Acta Anaesthesiol Scand 36:46, 1992

66. Theye RA, Michenfelder JD: The effects of nitrous oxide on canine cerebral metabolism. Anesthesiology 20:1119, 1964

67. Artru AA: Isoflurane does not increase the rate of CSF production in the dog. Anesthesiology 60:193, 1984

68. Artru AA: Effects of enflurane and isoflurane on resistance to reabsorption of cerebrospinal fluid in dogs. Anesthesiology 61:529, 1984

69. Artru AA, Nugent M, Michenfelder JD: Enflurane causes a prolonged and reversible increase in the rate of CSF production in the dog. Anesthesiology 57:255, 1982

70. Artru AA: Effects of halothane and fentanyl on the rate of CSF production in dogs. Anesth Analg 62:581, 1983

71. Artru AA: Effects of halothane and fentanyl anesthesia on resistance to reabsorption of CSF. J Neurosurg 60:252, 1984

72. Artru AA: Anesthetics produce prolonged altera-

tions of CSF dynamics. Anesthesiology 57:A356, 1982

73. Artru AA: Relationship between cerebral blood volume and CSF pressure during anesthesia with isoflurane or fentanyl in dogs. Anesthesiology 60:575, 1984

74. Grosslight K, Foster R, Colohan AR et al: Isoflurane for neuroanesthesia: risk factors for increases in intracranial pressure. Anesthesiology 63:533, 1985

75. Campkin TV: Isoflurane and cranial extradural pressure. A study in neurosurgical patients. Br J Anaesth 56:1083, 1984

76. Artru AA: Relationship between cerebral blood volume and CSF pressure during anesthesia with halothane or enflurane in dogs. Anesthesiology 58:533, 1983

77. Phirman JR, Shapiro HM: Modification of nitrous oxide-induced intracranial hypertension by prior induction of anesthesia. Anesthesiology 46:150, 1977

78. Rappaport M, Leonard J, Ruiz Portillo S: Effects of anesthesia and stimulus intensity on posterior tibial nerve somatosensory evoked potentials. Clin Electroencephalogr 23:24, 1992

79. Pathak KS, Ammadio M, Kalamchi A et al: Effects of halothane, enflurane, and isoflurane on somatosensory evoked potentials during nitrous oxide anesthesia. Anesthesiology 66:753, 1987

80. Samra SK, Vanderzant CW, Domer PA et al: Differential effects of isoflurane on human median nerve somatosensory evoked potentials. Anesthesiology 66:29, 1987

81. Peterson DO, Drummond JC, Todd MM: Effects of halothane, enflurane, isoflurane, and nitrous oxide on somatosensory evoked potentials in humans. Anesthesiology 65:35, 1986

82. McPherson RW, Mahla M, Johnson R et al: Effects of enflurane, isoflurane, and nitrous oxide on somatosensory evoked potentials during fentanyl anesthesia. Anesthesiology 62:626, 1985

83. Sebel PS, Flynn PJ, Ingram DA: Effect of nitrous oxide on visual, auditory and somatosensory evoked potentials. Br J Anaesth 56:1403, 1984

84. Fourcade HE, Stevens WC, Larson CP, Jr, et al: The ventilatory effects of Forane, a new inhaled anesthetic. Anesthesiology 35:26, 1971

85. Calverley RK, Smith NT, Jones CW et al: Ventilatory and cardiovascular effects of enflurane anesthesia during spontaneous ventilation in man. Anesth Analg 57:610, 1978

86. Munson ES, Larson CP Jr, Babad AA et al: The effects of halothane, fluroxene and cyclopropane on

ventilation: a comparative study in man. Anesthesiology 27:716, 1966

87. Doi M, Ikeda K: Respiratory effects of sevoflurane. Anesth Analg 66:241, 1987

88. Lockhart SH, Rampil IJ, Yasuda N et al: Depression of ventilation by desflurane in humans. Anesthesiology 74:484, 1991

89. Lam AM, Clement JL, Chung DC et al: Respiratory effects of nitrous oxide during enflurane anesthesia in humans. Anesthesiology 56:298, 1982

90. Murat I, Saint-Maurice JP, Beydon L et al: Respiratory effects of nitrous oxide during isoflurane anaesthesia in children. Br J Anaesth 58:1122, 1986

91. Hornbein TF, Martin WE, Bonica JJ et al: Nitrous oxide effects on the circulatory and ventilatory responses to halothane. Anesthesiology 31:250, 1969

92. Eger EI II, Dolan WM, Stevens WC et al: Surgical stimulation antagonizes the respiratory depression produced by Forane. Anesthesiology 36:544, 1972

93. Hirshman CA, McCullough RE, Cohen PJ et al: Depression of hypoxic ventilatory response by halothane, enflurane and isoflurane in dogs. Br J Anaesth 49:957, 1977

94. Knill LR, Kieraszewicz HT, Dodgson BG et al: Chemical regulation of ventilation during isoflurane sedation and anaesthesia in humans. Can J Anaesth 30:607, 1983

95. Duffin J, Triscott A, Whitwam JG: The effect of halothane and thiopentone on ventilatory responses mediated by the peripheral chemoreceptors in man. Br J Anaesth 48:975, 1976

96. Knill RL, Clement JL: Ventilatory responses to acute metabolic acidemia in humans awake, sedated, and anesthetized with halothane. Anesthesiology 62:745, 1985

97. Eger EI II: Isoflurane: a review. Anesthesiology 55:559, 1981

98. Cromwell TH, Stevens WC, Eger EI II et al: The cardiovascular effects of compound 469 (Forane) during spontaneous ventilation and CO_2 challenge in man. Anesthesiology 35:17, 1971

99. Knill RL, Clement JL: Variable effects of anaesthetics on the ventilatory response to hypoxaemia in man. Can J Anaesth 29:93, 1982

100. Lumb AB, Petros AJ, Nunn JF: Rib cage contribution to resting and carbon dioxide stimulated ventilation during 1 MAC isoflurane anaesthesia. Br J Anaesth 67:712, 1991

101. Tusiewicz K, Bryan AC, Froese AB: Contributions of changing rib cage-diaphragm interactions to the ventilatory depression of halothane anesthesia. Anesthesiology 47:327, 1977

102. Clergue F, Viires N, Lemesle P et al: Effect of halothane on diaphragmatic muscle function in pentobarbital-anesthetized dogs. Anesthesiology 64:181, 1986

103. Ide T, Kochi T, Isono S et al: Effect of sevoflurane on diaphragmatic contractility in dogs. Anesth Analg 74:739, 1992

104. Rehder K, Mallow JE, Fibuch EE et al: Effects of isoflurane anesthesia and muscle paralysis on respiratory mechanics in normal man. Anesthesiology 41:477, 1974

105. Heneghan CP, Bergman NA, Jordan C et al: Effect of isoflurane on bronchomotor tone in man. Br J Anaesth 58:24, 1986

106. Hirshman CA, Edelstein G, Peetz S et al: Mechanism of action of inhalational anesthesia on airways. Anesthesiology 56:107, 1982

107. Coon RL, Kampine JP: Hypocapnic bronchoconstriction and inhalation anesthetics. Anesthesiology 43:635, 1975

108. Hirshman CA, Bergman NA: Halothane and enflurane protect against bronchospasm in an asthma dog model. Anesth Analg 57:629, 1978

109. Colgan FJ: Performance of lungs and bronchi during inhalation anesthesia. Anesthesiology 26:778, 1965

110. Hickey RF, Graf PD, Nadel JA et al: The effects of halothane and cyclopropane on total pulmonary resistance in the dog. Anesthesiology 31:334, 1969

111. Shah MV, Hirshman CA: Mode of action of halothane on histamine-induced airway constriction in dogs. Anesthesiology 65:170, 1986

112. Tobias JD, Hirshman CA: Attenuation of histamine-induced airway constriction by albuterol during halothane anesthesia. Anesthesiology 72:105, 1990

113. Gold MI, Helrich M: Pulmonary mechanics during general anesthesia: status asthmaticus. Anesthesiology 32:422, 1970

114. Forbes AR, Horrigan RW: Mucociliary flow in the trachea during anesthesia with enflurane, ether, nitrous oxide, and morphine. Anesthesiology 46:319, 1977

115. Lee KS, Park SS: Effect of halothane, enflurane, and nitrous oxide on tracheal ciliary activity in vitro. Anesth Analg 59:426, 1980

116. Forbes AR: Halothane depresses mucociliary flow in the trachea. Anesthesiology 45:59, 1976

117. Lichtiger M, Landa JF, Hirsch JA: Velocity of tracheal mucus in anesthetized women undergoing gynecologic surgery. Anesthesiology 42:753, 1975

118. Lappas DG, Buckley MJ, Laver MB et al: Left ventricular performance and pulmonary circulation following addition of nitrous oxide to morphine during coronary-artery surgery. Anesthesiology 43:61, 1975

119. Hilgenberg JC, McCammon RL, Stoelting RK: Pulmonary and systemic vascular responses to nitrous oxide in patients with mitral stenosis and pulmonary hypertension. Anesth Analg 59:323, 1980

120. Marshall C, Lindgren L, Marshall BE: Effects of halothane, enflurane, and isoflurane on hypoxic pulmonary vasoconstriction in rat lungs in vitro. Anesthesiology 60:304, 1984

121. Domino KB, Borowec L, Alexander CM et al: Influence of isoflurane on hypoxic pulmonary vasoconstriction in dogs. Anesthesiology 64:423, 1986

122. Mathers J, Benumof JL, Wahrenbrock EA: General anesthetics and regional hypoxic pulmonary vasoconstriction. Anesthesiology 46:111, 1977

123. Rogers SN, Benumof JL: Halothane and isoflurane do not decrease PaCO$_2$ during one-lung ventilation in intravenously anesthetized patients. Anesth Analg 64:946, 1985

124. Rees DI, Gaines GY III: One-lung anesthesia—a comparison of pulmonary gas exchange during anesthesia with ketamine or enflurane. Anesth Analg 63:521, 1984

125. Brown BR Jr, Crout JR: A comparative study of the effects of five general anesthetics on myocardial contractility: isometric conditions. Anesthesiology 34:236, 1971

126. Kemmotsu O, Hashimoto Y, Shimosato S: Inotropic effects of isoflurane on mechanics of contraction in isolated cat papillary muscles from normal and failing hearts. Anesthesiology 39:470, 1973

127. Merin RG: Are the myocardial functional and metabolic effects of isoflurane really different from those of halothane and enflurane? Anesthesiology 55:398,1981

128. Bernard JM, Wouters PF, Doursout MF et al: Effects of sevoflurane and isoflurane on cardiac and coronary dynamics in chronically instrumented dogs. Anesthesiology 72:659, 1990

129. Pagel PS, Kampine JP, Schmeling WT et al: Influence of volatile anesthetics on myocardial contractility in vivo: desflurane versus isoflurane. Anesthesiology 74:900, 1991

130. Van Trigt P, Christian CC, Fagraeus L et al: Myocardial depression by anesthetic agents (halothane, enflurane, and nitrous oxide): quantitation based on end-systolic pressure-dimension relations. Am J Cardiol 53:243, 1984

131. Cullen DJ, Eger EI II: Cardiovascular effects of carbon dioxide in man. Anesthesiology 41:345, 1974

132. Stevens WC, Cromwell TH, Halsey MJ et al: The cardiovascular effects of a new inhalation anesthetic, Forane, in human volunteers at constant arterial carbon dioxide tension. Anesthesiology 35:8, 1971

133. Calverley RK, Smith NT, Prys-Roberts C et al: Cardiovascular effects of enflurane anesthesia during controlled ventilation in man. Anesth Analg 57:619, 1978

134. Eger EI II, Smith NT, Stoelting RK et al: Cardiovascular effects of halothane in man. Anesthesiology 32:396, 1970

135. Weiskopf RB, Cahalan MK, Eger EI II et al: Cardiovascular actions of desflurane in normocarbic volunteers. Anesth Analg 73:143, 1991

136. Eisele JH, Smith NT: Cardiovascular effects of 40 percent nitrous oxide in man. Anesth Analg 51:956, 1972

137. Dolan WM, Stevens WC, Eger EI II et al: The cardiovascular and respiratory effects of isoflurane-nitrous oxide anaesthesia. Can J Anaesth 21:557, 1974

138. Smith NT, Calverley RK, Prys-Roberts C et al: Impact of nitrous oxide on the circulation during enflurane anesthesia in man. Anesthesiology 48:345, 1978

139. Kazama T, Ikeda K: The comparative cardiovascular effects of sevoflurane with halothane and isoflurane. J Anesth 2:63, 1988

140. Kotrly KJ, Ebert TJ, Vucins E et al: Baroreceptor reflex control of heart rate during isoflurane anesthesia in humans. Anesthesiology 60:173, 1984

141. Takeshima R, Dohi S: Comparison of arterial baroreflex function in humans anesthetized with enflurane or isoflurane. Anesth Analg 69:284, 1989

142. Morton M, Duke PC, Ong B: Baroreflex control of heart rate in man awake and during enflurane and enflurane-nitrous oxide anesthesia. Anesthesiology 52:221, 1980

143. Duke PC, Fownes D, Wade JG: Halothane depresses baroreflex control of heart rate in man. Anesthesiology 46:184, 1977

144. Bahlman SH, Eger EI II, Halsey MJ et al: The cardiovascular effects of halothane in man during spontaneous ventilation. Anesthesiology 36:494, 1972

145. Crawford MW, Lerman J, Pilato M: Haemodynamic and organ blood flow responses to sevoflurane during spontaneous ventilation in the rat: a dose-response study. Can J Anaesth 39:270, 1992

146. Weiskopf RB, Cahalan MK, Ionescu P et al: Cardiovascular actions of desflurane with and without nitrous oxide during spontaneous ventilation in humans. Anesth Analg 73:165, 1991

147. Smith NT, Eger EI II, Stoelting RK et al: The cardiovascular and sympathomimetic responses to the addition of nitrous oxide to halothane in man. Anesthesiology 32:410, 1970

148. Forrest JB: Clinical evaluation of isoflurane—pulse and blood pressure. Can J Anaesth 29:S15, 1982

149. Bosnjak ZJ, Kampine JP: Effects of halothane, enflurane, and isoflurane on the SA node. Anesthesiology 58:314, 1983

150. Eger EI II: The pharmacology of isoflurane. Br J Anaesth 56:71S, 1984

151. Frink EJ, Jr, Malan TP, Atlas M et al: Clinical comparison of sevoflurane and isoflurane in healthy patients. Anesth Analg 74:241, 1992

152. Metz S, Maze M: Halothane concentration does not alter the threshold for epinephrine-induced arrhythmias in dogs. Anesthesiology 62:470, 1985

153. Joas TA, Stevens WC: Comparison of the arrhythmic doses of epinephrine during Forane, halothane, and fluroxene anesthesia in dogs. Anesthesiology 35:48, 1971

154. Johnston RR, Eger EI II, Wilson C: A comparative interaction of epinephrine with enflurane, isoflurane, and halothane in man. Anesth Analg 55:709, 1976

155. Atlee JL, Brownlee SW, Burstrom RE: Conscious-state comparisons of the effects of inhalation anesthetics on specialized atrioventricular conduction times in dogs. Anesthesiology 64:703, 1986

156. Zaidan JR, Curling PE, Craver JM, Jr: Effect of enflurane, isoflurane, and halothane on pacing stimulation thresholds in man. PACE Pacing Clin Electrophysiol 8:32, 1985

157. Karl HW, Swedlow DB, Lee KW et al: Epinephrine-halothane interactions in children. Anesthesiology 58:142, 1983

158. Imamura S, Ikeda K: Comparison of the epinephrine-induced arrhythmogenic effect of sevoflurane with isoflurane and halothane. J Anesth 1:62, 1987

159. Weiskopf RB, Eger EI II, Holmes MA et al: Epinephrine-induced premature ventricular contractions and changes in arterial blood pressure and heart rate during I-653, isoflurane, and halothane anesthesia in swine. Anesthesiology 70:293, 1989

160. Cheng DC, Moyers JR, Knutson RM et al: Dose-response relationship of isoflurane and halothane versus coronary perfusion pressures. Effects on flow

redistribution in a collateralized chronic swine model. Anesthesiology 76:113, 1992

161. Buffington CW, Davis KB, Gillispie S et al: The prevalence of steal-prone coronary anatomy in patients with coronary artery disease: an analysis of the coronary artery surgery study registry. Anesthesiology 69:721, 1988

162. Bollen BA, Tinker JH, Hermsmeyer K: Halothane relaxes previously constricted isolated porcine coronary artery segments more than isoflurane. Anesthesiology 66:748, 1987

163. Reiz S, Balfors E, Sorensen MB et al: Isoflurane—a powerful coronary vasodilator in patients with coronary artery disease. Anesthesiology 59:91, 1983

164. Priebe HJ: Differential effects of isoflurane on regional right and left ventricular performances, and on coronary, systemic, and pulmonary hemodynamics in the dog. Anesthesiology 66:262, 1987

165. Conzen PF, Habazettl H, Vollmar B et al: Coronary microcirculation during halothane, enflurane, isoflurane, and adenosine in dogs. Anesthesiology 76:261, 1992

166. Buffington CW, Romson JL, Levine A et al: Isoflurane induces coronary steal in a canine model of chronic coronary occlusion. Anesthesiology 66:280, 1987

167. Tatekawa S, Traber KB, Hantler CB et al: Effects of isoflurane on myocardial blood flow, function, and oxygen consumption in the presence of critical coronary stenosis in dogs. Anesth Analg 66:1073, 1987

168. Cason BA, Verrier ED, London MJ et al: Effects of isoflurane and halothane on coronary vascular resistance and collateral myocardial blood flow: their capacity to induce coronary steal. Anesthesiology 67:665, 1987

169. Hartman JC, Kampine JP, Schmeling WT et al: Volatile anesthetics and regional myocardial perfusion in chronically instrumented dogs: halothane versus isoflurane in a single-vessel disease model with enhanced collateral development. J Cardiothorac Vasc Anesh 4:588, 1990

170. Moore PG, Kien ND, Reitan JA et al: No evidence for blood flow redistribution with isoflurane or halothane during acute coronary artery occlusion in fentanyl-anesthetized dogs. Anesthesiology 75:854, 1991

171. Moffitt EA, Barker RA, Glenn JJ et al: Myocardial metabolism and hemodynamic responses with isoflurane anesthesia for coronary arterial surgery. Anesth Analg 65:53, 1986

172. Khambatta HJ, Sonntag H, Larsen R et al: Global and regional myocardial blood flow and metabolism during equipotent halothane and isoflurane anesthesia in patients with coronary artery disease. Anesth Analg 67:936, 1988

173. Slogoff S, Keats AS, Dear WE et al: Steal-prone coronary anatomy and myocardial ischemia associated with four primary anesthetic agents in humans. Anesth Analg 72:22, 1991

174. Pulley DD, Kervassilis GV, Kelermenos N et al: Regional and global myocardial circulatory and metabolic effects of isoflurane and halothane in patients with steal-prone coronary anatomy. Anesthesiology 75:756, 1991

175. Tarnow J, Markschies-Hornung A, Schulte-Sasse U: Isoflurane improves the tolerance to pacing-induced myocardial ischemia. Anesthesiology 64:147, 1986

176. Spahn DR, Smith LR, Veronee CD et al: Influence of anesthesia on the threshold of pacing-induced ischemia. Anesth Analg 74:14, 1992

177. Rydvall A, Haggmark S, Nyhman H et al: Effects of enflurane on coronary haemodynamics in patients with ischaemic heart disease. Acta Anaesthesiol Scand 28:690, 1984

178. Inoue K, Reichelt W, El-Banayosy A et al: Does isoflurane lead to a higher incidence of myocardial infarction and perioperative death than enflurane in coronary artery surgery? Anesth Analg 71:469, 1990

179. Merin RG, Bernard JM, Doursout MF et al: Comparison of the effects of isoflurane and desflurane on cardiovascular dynamics and regional blood flow in the chronically instrumented dog. Anesthesiology 74:568, 1991

180. Hartman JC, Pagel PS, Kampine JP et al: Influence of desflurane on regional distribution of coronary blood flow in a chronically instrumented canine model of multivessel coronary artery obstruction. Anesth Analg 72:289, 1991

181. Thomson IR, Bowering JB, Hudson RJ et al: A comparison of desflurane and isoflurane in patients undergoing coronary artery surgery. Anesthesiology 75:776, 1991

182. Gelman S, Fowler KC, Smith LR: Liver circulation and function during isoflurane and halothane anesthesia. Anesthesiology 61:726, 1984

183. Gelman S, Rimerman V, Fowler KC et al: The effect of halothane, isoflurane, and blood loss on hepatotoxicity and hepatic oxygen availability in phenobarbital-pretreated hypoxic rats. Anesth Anlg 63:965, 1984

184. Hursh D, Gelman S, Bradley EL, Jr: Hepatic oxy-

gen supply during halothane or isoflurane anesthesia in guinea pigs. Anesthesiology 67:701, 1987

185. Gelman S: General anesthesia and hepatic circulation. Can J Physiol Pharmacol 65:1762, 1987

186. Hughes RL, Campbell D, Fitch W: Effects of enflurane and halothane on liver blood flow and oxygen consumption in the greyhound. Br J Anaesth 52:1079, 1980

187. Andreen M, Irestedt L, Zetterstrom B: The different responses of the hepatic arterial bed to hypovolemia and to halothane anaesthesia. Acta Anaesthesiol Scand 21:475, 1977

188. Irestedt L, Andreen M: Effects of enflurane on haemodynamic and oxygen consumption in dogs, with reference to the liver and preportal tissue. Acta Anaesthesiol Scand 23:119, 1979

189. Benumof JL, Bookstein JJ, Saidman LJ et al: Diminished hepatic arterial flow during halothane administration. Anesthesiology 45:545, 1976

190. Frink EJ, Jr, Morgan SE, Coetzee A et al: The effects of sevoflurane, halothane, enflurane, and isoflurane on hepatic blood flow and oxygenation in chronically instrumented greyhound dogs. Anesthesiology 76:85, 1992

191. Lundeen G, Manohar M, Parks C: Systemic distribution of blood flow in swine while awake and during 1.0 and 1.5 MAC isoflurane anesthesia with and without 50% nitrous oxide. Anesth Analg 62:499, 1983

192. Brown BR, Jr: The diphasic action of halothane on the oxidative metabolism of drugs by the liver. Anesthesiology 35:241, 1971

193. Reilly CS, Wood AJ, Koshakji RP et al: The effect of halothane on drug disposition: contribution of changes in intrinsic drug metabolizing capacity and hepatic blood flow. Anesthesiology 63:70, 1985

194. Wood M, Wood AJ: Contrasting effects of halothane, isoflurane, and enflurane on in vivo drug metabolism in the rat. Anesth Analg 63:709, 1984

195. Whelan E, Wood AJ, Koshakji R et al: Halothane inhibition of propranolol metabolism is stereoselective. Anesthesiology 71:561, 1989

196. Ghantous HN, Fernando JL, Keith RL et al: Effects of halothane and other volatile anaesthetics on protein synthesis and secretion in guinea pig liver slices. Br J Anaesth 68:172, 1992

197. Bessesen A, Morlan DJ: Anaesthetic and protein synthesis in isolated rat hepatocytes. Naunyn Schmiedebergs Arch Pharmacol, suppl. R18:313, 1980

198. Ghantous HN, Fernando JL, Gandolfi AJ et al: Inhibition of protein synthesis and secretion by volatile anesthetics in guinea pig liver slices. Adv Exp Med Biol 283:725, 1991

199. Ghantous HN, Fernando JL, Gandolfi AJ et al: Minimal biotransformation and toxicity of desflurane in guinea pig liver slices. Anesth Analg 72:796, 1991

200. Stoelting RK, Blitt CD, Cohen PJ et al: Hepatic dysfunction after isoflurane anesthesia. Anesth Analg 66:147, 1987

201. Christ DD, Kenna JG, Kammerer W et al: Enflurane metabolism produces covalently bound liver adducts recognized by antibodies from patients with halothane hepatitis. Anesthesiology 69:833, 1988

202. Eger EI II, Smuckler EA, Ferrell LD et al: Is enflurane hepatotoxic? Anesth Analg 65:21, 1986

203. Brown BR, Jr, Gandolfi AJ: Adverse effects of volatile anesthetics. Br J Anaesth 59:14, 1987

204. Bunker JP, Forrest WH, Jr, Mosteller F et al (eds): National Halothane Study: A Study of the Possible Association Between Halothane Anesthesia and Post-Operative Hepatic Necrosis. United States Government Printing Office, Washington, D.C., 1969

205. Hubbard AK, Roth TP, Gandolfi AJ et al: Halothane hepatitis patients generate an antibody response toward a covalently bound metabolite of halothane. Anesthesiology 68:791, 1988

206. Neuberger J, Vergani D, Mieli-Vergani G et al: Hepatic damage after exposure to halothane in medical personnel. Br J Anaesth 53:1172, 1981

207. Lewis RB, Blair M: Halothane hepatitis in a young child. Br J Anaesth 54:349, 1982

208. Farrell G, Prendergast D, Murray M: Halothane hepatitis. Detection of a constitutional susceptibility factor. N Engl J Med 313:1310, 1985

209. Otsuka S, Yamamtot M, Kasuya S et al: HLA antigens in patients with unexplained hepatitis following halothane anesthesia. Acta Anaesthesiol Scand 29:497, 1985

210. Stock JG, Strunin L: Unexplained hepatitis following halothane. Anesthesiology 63:424, 1985

211. Frink EJ, Jr, Ghantous H, Malan TP et al: Plasma inorganic fluoride with sevoflurane anesthesia: correlation with indices of hepatic and renal function. Anesth Analg 74:231, 1992

212. Weiskopf RB, Eger EI II, Ionescu P et al: Desflurane does not produce hepatic or renal injury in human volunteers. Anesth Analg 74:570, 1992

213. Jones RM, Koblin DD, Cashman JN et al: Biotransformation and hepato-renal function in volunteers after exposure to desflurane (I 653). Br J Anaesth 64:482, 1990

214. Brodsky JB: Toxicity of nitrous oxide. p. 265. In Eger EI II (ed): Nitrous Oxide/N_2O. Elsevier, New York, 1985

215. Gelman S, Fowler KC, Smith LR: Regional blood flow during isoflurane and halothane anesthesia. Anesth Analg 63:557, 1984

216. Hysing ES, Chelly JE, Doursout MF et al: Comparative effects of halothane, enflurane, and isoflurane at equihypotensive doses on cardiac performance and coronary and renal blood flows in chronically instrumented dogs. Anesthesiology 76:979, 1992

217. Mazze RI, Cousins MJ, Barr GA: Renal effects and metabolism of isoflurane in man. Anesthesiology 40:536, 1974

218. Cousins MF, Greenstein LR, Hitt BA et al: Metabolism and renal effects of enflurane in man. Anesthesiology 44:44, 1976

219. Mazze RI, Schwartz FD, Slocum HC et al: Renal function during anesthesia and surgery. The effects of halothane anesthesia. Anesthesiology 24:279, 1963

220. Bastron RD, Perkins FM, Pyne JL: Autoregulation of renal blood flow during halothane anesthesia. Anesthesiology 46:142, 1977

221. Taves DR, Fry BW, Freeman RB et al: Toxicity following methoxyflurane anaesthesia. JAMA 214:91, 1970

222. Mazze RI, Shue GL, Jackson SH: Renal dysfunction associated with methoxyflurane anesthesia. JAMA 216:278, 1971

223. Crandell WB, Pappas SG, MacDonald A: Nephrotoxicity associated with methoxyflurane anesthesia. Anesthesiology 27:591, 1966

224. Cousins MJ, Mazze RI: Methoxyflurane nephrotoxicity. A study of dose response in man. JAMA 225:1611, 1973

225. Mazze RI, Calverley RK, Smith NT: Inorganic fluoride nephrotoxicity: prolonged enflurane and halothane anesthesia in volunteers. Anesthesiology 46:265, 1977

226. Spencer EM, Willatts SM, Prys-Roberts C: Plasma inorganic fluoride concentrations during and after prolonged (greater than 24 h) isoflurane sedation: effect on renal function. Anesth Analg 73:731, 1991

227. Mazze RI, Woodruff RE, Heerdt ME: Isoniazid-induced enflurane defluorination in humans. Anesthesiology 57:5, 1982

228. Hossain D, Fujii K, Yuge O et al: Dose-related sevoflurane metabolism to inorganic fluoride in rabbits. Hiroshima J Med Sci 40:1, 1991

229. Holaday DA, Smith FR: Sevoflurane anesthesia and biotransformation in man. Anesthesiology 51:S27, 1979

230. Kobayashi Y, Ochiai R, Takeda J et al: Serum and urinary fluoride concentrations after prolonged inhalation of sevoflurane in humans. Anesth Analg 74:753, 1992

231. Sutton TS, Koblin DD, Gruenke LD et al: Fluoride metabolites after prolonged exposure of volunteers and patients to desflurane. Anesth Analg 73:180, 1991

232. Diltoer M, Camu F: Glucose homeostasis and insulin secretion during isoflurane anesthesia in humans. Anesthesiology 68:880, 1988

233. Ewart RBL, Rusy BF, Bradford MW: Effects of enflurane on release of insulin by pancreatic islets in vitro. Anesth Analg 60:878, 1981

234. Merin RG, Samuelson PN, Schalch DS: Major inhalation anesthetics and carbohydrate metabolism. Anesth Analg 50:625, 1971

235. Gingerich R, Wright PH, Paradise PR: Effects of halothane on glucose-stimulated insulin secretion and glucose oxidation in isolated rat pancreatic islets. Anesthesiology 53:219, 1980

236. Oyama T, Matsuki A, Kudo T: Effect of halothane, methoxyflurane anaesthesia and surgery on plasma thyroid-stimulating hormone levels in man. Anaesthesia 27:2, 1972

237. Philbin DM, Coggins CH: Plasma antidiuretic hormone levels in cardiac surgical patients during morphine and halothane anesthesia. Anesthesiology 49:95, 1978

238. Oyama T, Sato K, Kimura K: Plasma levels of antidiuretic hormone in man during halothane anaesthesia and surgery. Can J Anaesth 18:614, 1971

239. Robertson D, Michelakis AM: Effect of anesthesia and surgery on plasma renin activity in man. J Clin Endocrinol Metab 34:831, 1971

240. Randell T, Seppala T, Lindgren L: Isoflurane in nitrous oxide and oxygen increases plasma concentrations of noradrenaline but attenuates pressore response to intubation. Acta Anaesthesiol Scand 35:600, 1991

241. Crozier TA, Morawietz A, Drobnik L et al: The influence of isoflurane on peri-operative endocrine and metabolic stress responses. Eur J Anaesthesiol 9:55, 1992

242. Göthert M, Wendt J: Inhibition of adrenal medullary catecholamine secretion by enflurane. Anesthesiology 46:400, 1977

243. Roizen MF, Horrigan RW, Frazer BM: Anesthetic doses blocking adrenergic (stress) and cardiovascu-

lar responses to incision—MACBAR. Anesthesiology 54:390, 1981

244. Lacoumenta S, Paterson JL, Burrin J: Effects of two differing halothane concentrations on the metabolic and endocrine responses to surgery. Br J Anaesth 58:844, 1986

245. Lassen HCA, Henriksen E, Neukirch F et al: Treatment of tetanus: severe bone marrow depression after prolonged nitrous oxide anaesthesia. Lancet 1:527, 1956

246. Lassen HCA, Kristensen HS: Remission in chronic myeloid leukaemia following prolonged nitrous oxide inhalation. Dan Med Bull 6:252, 1959

247. Amess JAR, Burman JF, Rees GM et al: Megaloblastic haemopoieisis in patients receiving nitrous oxide. Lancet 2:339, 1978

248. Nunn JF, Chanarin I, Tanner AG et al: Megaloblastic bone marrow changes after repeated nitrous oxide anaesthesia. Br J Anaesth 58:1469, 1986

249. Nunn JF: Clinical aspects of the interaction between nitrous oxide and vitamin B_{12}. Br J Anaesth 59:3, 1987

250. O'Sullivan H, Jennings F, Ward K et al: Human bone marrow biochemical function and megaloblastic hematopoiesis after nitrous oxide anesthesia. Anesthesia 55:645, 1981

251. Smith TC, Colton ET, Behar MG: Does anesthesia alter hemoglobin dissociation? Anesthesiology 32:5, 1970

252. Fournier L, Major D: The effect of nitrous oxide on the oxyhaemoglobin dissociation curve. Can J Anaesth 31:173, 1984

253. Shah MV, Anderson LK, Bergman NA: The influence of nitrous oxide on oxyhaemoglobin dissociation and measurement of oxygen tension. Anaesthesia 41:586, 1986

254. Welch WD: Effect of enflurane, isoflurane, and nitrous oxide on the microbicidal activity of human polymorphonuclear leukocytes. Anesthesiology 61:188, 1984

255. Duncan PG, Cullen BF: Anesthesia and immunology. Anesthesiology 45:522, 1976

256. Nunn JF, Sturrock JE, Jones AJ et al: Halothane does not inhibit human neutrophil function in vitro. Br J Anaesth 51:1101, 1979

257. Moudgill GC, Allan RB, Russell RJ et al: Inhibition by anaesthetic agents of human leukocyte locomotion towards chemical attractants. Br J Anaesth 49:97, 1977

258. Welch WD: Halothane reversibly inhibits human neutrophil bacterial killing. Anesthesiology 55:650, 1981

259. Dalsgaard-Nielsen J, Rsbo A, Simmelkjaer P et al: Impaired platelet aggregation and increased bleeding time during general anesthesia with halothane. Br J Anaesth 53:1039, 1981

260. Fyman PN, Triner L, Schranz H et al: Effect of volatile anaesthetics and nitrous oxide-fentanyl anaesthesia on bleeding time. Br J Anaesth 56:1197, 1984

261. Munson ES, Embro WJ: Enflurane, isoflurane, and halothane and isolated human uterine muscle. Anesthesiology 46:11, 1977

262. Palahniuk RJ, Shnider SM: Maternal and fetal cardiovascular and acid-base changes during halothane and isoflurane anesthesia in the pregnant ewe. Anesthesiology 41:462, 1974

263. Andrews WW, Ramin SM, Maberry MC et al: Effect of type of anesthesia on blood loss at elective repeat cesarean section. Am J Perinatol 9:197, 1992

264. Cullen BF, Margolis AJ, Eger EI II: The effects of anesthesia and pulmonary ventilation on blood loss during elective therapeutic abortion. Anesthesiology 32:108, 1970

265. Biehl DR, Yarnell R, Wade JG et al: The uptake of isoflurane by the foetal lamb in utero: effect on regional blood flow. Can J Anaesth 30:581, 1983

266. Biehl DR, Tweed WA, Cote J et al: Effect of halothane on cardiac output and regional flow in the fetal lamb in utero. Anesth Analg 62:489, 1983

267. Yarnell R, Biehl DR, Tweed WA et al: The effect of halothane anaesthesia on the asphyxiated foetal lamb in utero. Can J Anaesth 30:474, 1983

Chapter 26

Basic Pharmacology of α and β Adrenoceptors

Dan E. Berkowitz and Debra A. Schwinn

The sympathetic nervous system, one of two important components of the autonomic nervous system, mediates many diverse physiologic functions including states of consciousness, cardiovascular homeostasis, and cellular metabolism. The sympathetic nervous system relays information to cells by catecholamines—norepinephrine (NE) at the nerve terminal and circulating epinephrine (EPI) released from the adrenal gland. Adrenoceptors (adrenergic receptors; ARs) bind catecholamines and hence are the ultimate mediators of sympathetic function. Ahlquist,[1] in his classic article, proposed that adrenotropic responses be divided into two distinct classes called α and β. The development of selective agonists and antagonists confirmed this classification and enabled a further subdivision of these responses. In 1967, Lands et al.[2] subdivided β AR responses into β_1 and β_2 based on differences in affinity for the agonists isoproterenol (ISO), EPI, and NE. αAR responses were subdivided into the α_1 and α_2 based on the relative potencies of selective agonists and antagonists, with α_1 ARs stimulated by phenylephrine and blocked by prazosin and α_2 ARs stimulated by clonidine and blocked by yohimbine. Further pharmacologic subdivision has continued, but the greatest recent advances in adrenergic receptor biology occurred with molecular biologic approaches that resulted in the cloning (isolation of DNA sequence encoding

receptor protein), characterization, and expression of nine ARs (α_{1A}, α_{1B}, α_{1C}, α_{2C2}, α_{2C4}, α_{2C10}, in which C represents the human chromosome on which the receptor gene is located], β_1, β_2, and β_3).

Because EPI and NE are charged molecules, they are unable to traverse cellular lipid membranes. Thus, a system has evolved that notifies the cell of the presence of catecholamine ligand. This entire process is termed "signal transduction." The first component of this system is a membrane receptor that binds catecholamine agonists at the extracellular surface (Fig. 26-1). The second component of the signal transduction system is an intermediate molecule called a guanine nucleotide binding (G) protein, which couples the receptor on the intracellular surface to an effector system. Activation of the effector system results in a cascade of intracellular reactions, ultimately leading to the cellular and physiologic response. ARs bind to specific G protein subtypes and second messengers. Binding of agonists to β ARs results in activation of G_s, which then stimulates the enzyme adenylyl cyclase. α_2 ARs inhibit adenylate cyclase by the inhibitory G protein, G_i. α_1 ARs are thought to activate phospholipase C through a newly characterized G protein, G_q, resulting in the formation of two important cellular second messengers—inositol trisphosphate and diacylglycerol; the overall result of

581

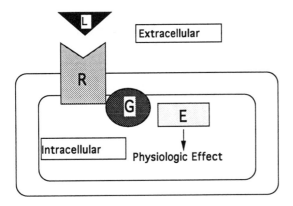

Fig. 26-1 Receptors (*R*) are transmembrane proteins that bind ligands (*L*) (either endogenous hormones or exogenous drugs). Many membrane receptors interact with a guanine nucleotide (*G*) protein that transduces the signal from the receptor to the effector (*E*). Energy derived from the hydrolysis of guanosine triphosphate to guanosine diphosphate enables the G protein to interact with the effector molecule, resulting in a change in intracellular chemistry and thereby a physiologic effect.

α_1 AR activation is an increase in intracellular Ca^{++}.

Receptors coupled to G proteins define a large and rapidly expanding superfamily of receptors, the genes for which have been cloned and expressed in cells; the resulting receptor proteins have been characterized pharmacologically. ARs (and other G protein-coupled receptors) are characterized structurally by the presence of seven transmembrane spanning domains, forming three extracellular and three intracellular loops (Fig. 26-2). A number of G protein-coupled receptors are or may become increasingly important in anesthesia and clinical medicine. These include adrenergic, opioid, muscarinic cholinergic, serotonergic, endothelin, dopamine, cannabinoid, substance P, and cholecystokinin receptors (for review, see ref. 3). ARs are one of the most intensively studied membrane receptors and, hence, make a good model for understanding the function of G protein-coupled receptors in general. Because the majority of studies regarding structure of ARs were performed using the β_2 AR, we will begin with this receptor as a model to discuss the structure and function of the ARs. Therefore, the pharmacology of β ARs and their general structure, G protein coupling, and regulation will be discussed in depth. This will be followed by a discussion highlighting similarities and differences between β ARs, α_2 ARs, and α_1 ARs. Because this chapter covers a large body of literature, reviews will be cited whenever possible to simplify the presentation and yet provide in-depth sources for those who wish to delve further into a given topic.

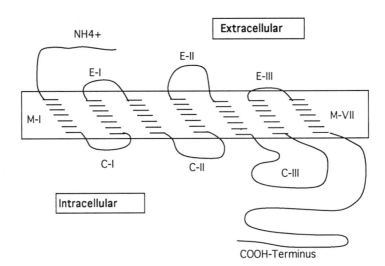

Fig. 26-2 Schematic diagram of the transmembrane structure of a G protein-coupled receptor. The amino terminus (*NH4+*) *is located on the extracellular surface of the cell; the carboxyl (COOH)* terminus is intracellular. There are seven putative transmembrane regions (*M-1 to M-VII*), three intracellular loops (*C-I to C-III*), and three extracellular loops (*E-I to E-III*).

β ADRENOCEPTORS

General Introduction

Receptors are distinguished by pharmacologists in terms of the potency of a series of agonists and selective antagonists. β AR subtypes are classically discriminated by agonist potency with the compounds ISO, EPI, and NE. Specifically, EPI and NE have similar potencies for the β_1 AR, but EPI has far greater potency for the β_2 AR compared with NE. The resulting agonist potency series are as follows: β_1-Ars, ISO > EPI $\geq$ NE and β_2 ARs, ISO > EPI >> NE. There are no selective agonists for the β_1 AR at present, but albuterol is a selective agonist at β_2 ARs. Selective antagonists include metoprolol (selective for the β_1 AR) and pindolol (selective for the β_2 AR). During the last two decades, selective β AR antagonists and agonists have been developed, which have enabled us, not only to confirm this receptor classification, but they have also become the mainstay of therapeutic intervention in human disease (β_1 AR antagonists in the treatment of hypertension and ischemic heart disease and β_2 AR agonists in the treatment of obstructive airways diseases, such as asthma).

During the last few years, increasing evidence has accumulated for the existence of a third β AR. This receptor was initially thought to be an atypical β_1 AR (for review, see ref. 4). This atypical β AR was suggested to mediate sympathetic control of various metabolic processes in adipose tissue, skeletal muscle, and gastrointestinal tract. The development of β AR agonists that are potent stimulators of metabolic rate, adipose tissue thermogenesis, and soleus muscle glycogen synthesis (but with minimal effects on β_1 and β_2 AR sites) confirmed the existence of a unique β AR. The existence of a third β AR was confirmed following the discovery of a gene encoding a novel β AR, now called the β_3 AR.[5] The β_3 AR demonstrates a different rank order of agonist potency compared with either the β_1 or β_2 AR, and the search for selective agonists and antagonists for this receptor continues.

Receptor subtypes can also be described by their mediated physiologic response. For example, β_1 ARs are predominantly found in the heart and are important in mediating increases in heart rate, contractility, conduction velocity, and arrhythmogenicity. β_2 ARs are also found in the heart where they mediate many of the same functions of β_1 ARs, and they are also thought to be involved in conduction. In addition, β_2 ARs are important in mediating bronchial, vascular, and uterine smooth muscle relaxation. The β_3 AR appears to be predominantly involved in mediating metabolic functions related to sympathetic stimulation.

Receptor Purification

One method of understanding receptor function is to purify the receptor protein to homogeneity and study its function in reconstituted lipid vesicles. This process has been used successfully over the last two decades to study many receptor systems. The initial purification of ARs was accomplished using a technique called affinity chromatography.[6–8] Briefly, affinity chromatography utilizes a long tube filled with a solid support to which side chain molecules are attached ending with a ligand that binds the receptor of interest. After freeing membrane-bound receptors from the membrane using a detergent, these receptors (in the form of a crude cell preparation) are poured into the top of the affinity chromatography column. As the membrane preparation passes down through the column under the influence of gravity, the receptor of interest binds to the column ligand. The column is washed to remove other receptors, and the purified receptor is then eluted off the column with higher salt or higher ligand concentrations. The result is a highly purified receptor. After repeating the process several times, membrane receptors can be purified to homogeneity and studied. Because this process can take weeks to months, studies of receptor function were completed slowly. However, this has radically changed with the recent development of molecular biologic techniques.

Molecular Biology

Every protein in the body, including enzymes and receptors, is encoded by DNA. By discovering the portion of DNA that encodes a given receptor (defined as a gene), the sequence of receptor protein can be deduced. Because it is easier to manipulate and mass-produce DNA, compared with receptor protein, molecular techniques are invaluable in the study of membrane receptor function. After the gene is isolated, it can be placed in circular DNA (plasmids) and introduced into cells; the cells then make the receptor protein (a process called receptor expression) from this genetic information—enabling a receptor to be individually expressed and studied with classic pharmacologic tools. After a receptor is purified to homogeneity as described, it can be cleaved into smaller polypeptide fragments that can be sequenced using an amino acid analyzer. From polypeptide sequence information, a DNA probe can be designed that is used to search for the entire receptor gene using standard molecular biologic methods (a process called cloning). Following this strategy, three ARs were initially cloned, a β_2,[9] an α_2,[10] and an α_1 AR.[11] This was soon followed by the cloning of homologous receptors. Currently, the genes for nine AR subtypes have been discovered and expressed in cells, and the resultant receptor protein have been characterized pharmacologically. These nine AR subtypes include the α_{1A}, α_{1B}, α_{1C}, α_{2C2}, α_{2C4}, α_{2C10}, β_1, β_2, and β_3.[5,9–20]

Receptor Structure

Seven Transmembrane Domains

G protein-coupled receptors have a common structural motif (Fig. 26-2). Hydropathic analysis (an algorithm devised by Kyte and Doolittle[21] that assigns a numeric value to each amino acid in a polypeptide sequence according to its hydrophobicity) reveals seven stretches of hydrophobic amino acids that most likely span the membrane. These membrane spanning regions are connected by three intracellular and three extracellular hydrophilic domains. In this model, the receptor protein amino terminus is extacellular, and the carboxyl terminus is intracellular. Extensive confirmation of this model has occurred using biochemical, immunohistochemical, and molecular techniques.

Transmembrane regions of the ARs appear to be conserved, with significant homology (amino acid identity) between individual receptors. When comparing transmembrane domains between AR subtypes, there is a 42 to 45 percent amino acid identity between ARs of different receptor subfamilies (i.e., and α_2 AR compared with an α_1 AR or β AR). However, transmembrane identity approaches 72 to 75 percent when comparing receptors within an

AR subfamily (i.e., an α_{1A} versus an α_{1B} AR). This was the first evidence that suggested that transmembrane domains might be important in ligand binding. We now know that specific transmembrane segments are important in agonist and antagonist binding, a concept that will be explored in detail later in this chapter. Other general receptor regions of physiologic significance include cytoplasmic loops and the carboxyl terminal, which are associated with G protein coupling and receptor regulation, respectively. The potential functional importance of each of these domains will be discussed in detail later.

Biophysical Structure

One of the best methods to determine the biophysical structure of a protein is to use x-ray crystallographic (diffraction) techniques. To apply these techniques to membrane receptors, the receptor must be purified to homogeneity and crystallized, a rather daunting task because of their relatively low abundance. However, in the retina, rhodopsin receptors occur in relatively high abundance, and they represent one of the few G protein-coupled receptors that have been crystallized and analyzed by x-ray crystallography. In general, there is significant homology between the photoreceptor rhodopsin and the β_2 AR at the molecular level, and their hydrophobicity profiles are similar.[22] Hence, information regarding the overall structure for rhodopsin is useful for studies with β_2 ARs. Using x-ray crystallography, Henderson and Unwin[23] determined the structure of bacteriorhodopsin and confirmed that the overall topology is consistent with seven α-helical rods (a spiral orientation of amino acids) spanning the membrane. This information strongly suggests that transmembrane domains of the β_2 AR (and potentially other ARs and G protein-coupled receptors) consists of α helices.

Post-Translational Modifications

The process of receptor protein synthesis from DNA occurs in a similar fashion for all proteins. First, the gene encoding the receptor is transcribed to messenger RNA (mRNA); this process moves the message from the nucleus to the cytoplasm. In the cytoplasm, the message is translated from mRNA to individual amino acids, according to the genetic code (in which three nucleotides encode a single amino acid). There, the receptor protein is built amino acid by amino acid. After the entire protein is completely synthesized, it is mobilized as required. For membrane receptors, this means moving the protein to the cell surface membrane and inserting it into the membrane in the proper orientation. The signals required for this mobilization are not yet known. In addition, after the receptor protein is synthesized, it can be modified further (a process called post-translational modification). In the case of G protein-coupled receptors, this includes the addition of sugar (oligosaccharide) moieties and covalent bonds that hold the receptor in its proper and final configuration. Each of these processes will be discussed subsequently (Fig. 26-3A).

ARs are glycoproteins with oligosaccharides covalently linked to specific asparagine residues close to the amino terminus. The function of receptor glycosylation is unclear. Glycosylation sites, however, do not appear to be involved in receptor ligand binding, signal transduction, or receptor regulation.[24] Glycosylation was postulated to prevent receptor degradation by extracellular proteases.[25] In addition, glycosylation sites may be signal sequences that direct receptor proteins to cell membranes.[26] One of the advantages of identifying the gene encoding a receptor protein is that DNA can be manipulated more easily than proteins. Hence, artificial changes in amino acids (mutations) can be induced in DNA sequences to make receptors that are not normally found in nature. The function of these changed, or mutated, receptors can be compared with the naturally occurring (or wild-type) receptor. One study showed that mutating the two asparagine glycosylation residues resulted in a decrease of receptor number at the cell surface without altering binding or coupling.[27] Thus, such studies reinforce the concept that glycosylation sites appear to be important in intracellular trafficking of receptors to the cell membrane.

In addition to glycosylation sites, other post-translational modifications occur in ARs. There are numerous cysteine residues in the extracellular region that are involved in the formation of disulfide bonds, which are important in maintaining the tertiary structure and ligand binding integrity of the AR.[28] The β_2 AR is palmitoylated (addition of a long chain fatty acid, palmitate) at cysteine[341] (a cysteine residue located 341 amino acids from the amino terminus). This, and homologous cysteines in the α_1 AR and α_2 AR, serve to anchor the proximal portion of the carboxyl terminal of the receptor to the internal surface of the plasma membrane, making in essence, a fourth intracellular loop. This region of the carboxyl terminal is structurally adjacent to the third intracellular loop, and these two regions appear to be important in G protein coupling. Mutagenesis experiments replacing the cysteine with a glycine that is not palmitoylated results in significantly impaired G protein coupling and signal transduction.[29]

Ligand Binding

As described earlier, the high degree of receptor transmembrane amino acid identifies within an AR subfamily (i.e., α_{1A}, α_{1B}, and α_{1C}) strongly suggested that transmembrane domains might be important in the binding of ligands to ARs. Several types of experiments have been performed to test this hypothesis, many of which take advantage of molecular biologic techniques to create new "designer" synthetic receptors (by altering the DNA sequence of the gene) and comparing the result with native receptor function. The first of such experiments involved the synthesis of chimeric receptors. Chimera refers to a Greek mythologic creature described as a "fire breathing female monster with the head of a lion, the body of a goat, and the tail of a serpent." This is a fitting description for a receptor created by combining different regions of two distinct receptor genes and then expressing these genes in cells to define their pharmacology and ability to couple to second messengers. By combining regions of receptors, we are able to assess whether a specific region will confer ligand binding characteristics or alter G protein-coupling specificity from one receptor to another receptor.[30] Using these types of experiments, the third and fourth transmembrane domains were shown to be important in agonist binding; the sixth and seventh transmembrane regions were shown to be important in antagonist binding.

To localize further where ligands bind to the β_2 AR, classic biochemical approaches were combined

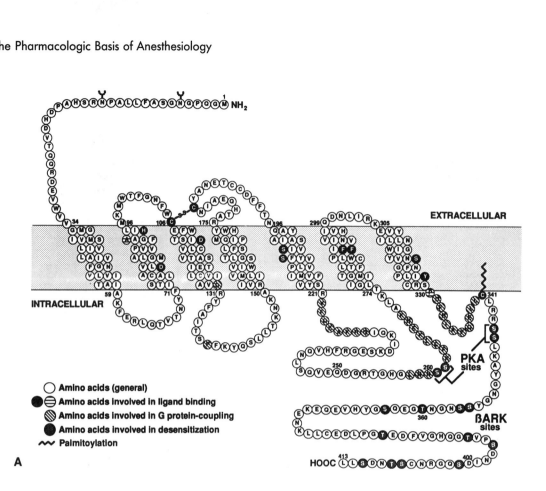

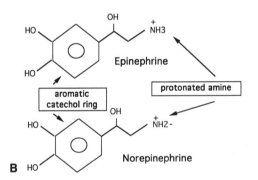

Fig. 26-3(A) Diagram demonstrating the regions of the β_2 adrenoceptor that are important in ligand binding, G protein coupling, and desensitization (see text for details) (From Schwinn et al.,[38] with permission.) **(B)** The chemical structure of the two endogenous catecholamines that bind adrenoceptors. It is important to understand ligand structure-activity relationships to understand specific requirements for binding of AR ligand in the receptor binding "pocket." (See text for a more detailed discussion.) (*Figure continues.*)

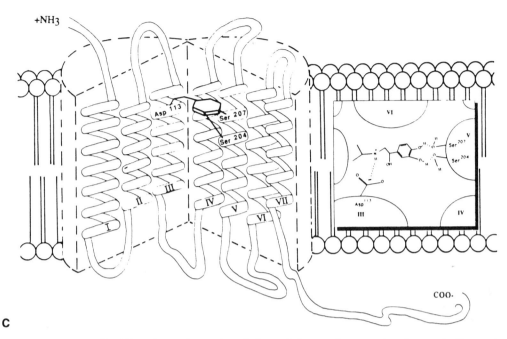

C

Fig. 26-3 (Continued) **(C)** A three-dimensional view of the β adrenoceptor demonstrating epinephrine binding in the ligand binding pocket of the transmembrane region of the receptor. The critical residues for ligand binding, aspartate[133] and serine[204] and serine[207]. (From Jasper and Insel,[34] with permission.)

with molecular biologic characterizations. Photoaffinity labeling of a receptor is a classic biochemical tool to study receptors. In photoaffinity labeling, a specially designed ligand binds specifically (and when exposed to light irreversibly [or covalently]) to the receptor. The receptor is then cleaved with proteases known to cleave at specific amino acid residues. For example, receptors can be cleaved with the protease trypsin into smaller fragments, and the fragments can be separated and purified chromatographically. The peptide that contains bound ligand is then sequenced using an amino acid analyzer to determine to which residue the ligand is bound. Because the putative amino acid sequence of all nine amino acids is known from the gene, the resulting fragments after protease digestion can be predicted. This process was used to identify ligand binding regions of a number of ARs.[31,32]

Up to this point, we have considered only general receptor areas involved in ligand binding or regions important in the covalent binding of photoaffinity labels. Indeed, we could ask at this point

how water soluble catecholamines (which are charged and therefore cannot cross the cell membrane) can interact with receptor transmembrane regions, which by definition, are lipophilic. It is important to remember in this context that an amino acid can be lipophilic and still have charged side groups. Hence, specific charged side groups may be important as counterions for charged groups in the ligand. Therefore, to determine if specific amino acid residues are critical in receptor-ligand interactions, we must first consider the structure of catecholamine ligands themselves. Endogenous catecholamines are defined structurally by an aromatic catechol ring and a protonated amine group connected by a β-OH-ethyl chain (Fig. 26-3B).[33] It is the catechol ring that distinguishes catecholamines from other G protein-coupled receptor ligands (e.g., acetylcholine). Structure-activity relationships have defined regions of the catecholamine structure that are functionally important. The β-OH and amine groups were shown to be important for both agonist and antagonist binding, whereas the catechol ring is characteristic of agonists only.[27] An in-depth analysis of catecholamine structure suggests that three counterions must be present in the receptor ligand binding pocket to provide (1) interactions with the protonated amine, (2) hydrogen bonding with the β-OH and catechol OH group, and (3) aromatic interactions with the catechol ring.[34] Figure 26-3C depicts this interaction in a three dimensional fashion.

Intricate mutagenesis experiments were performed to dissect out the exact amino acids involved in catecholamine binding to the β_2 AR. Aspartate[133] was shown to be important as a counterion for the cationic amine group of adrenergic ligands.[35] Because the amine group is present in many G protein-coupled receptor ligands, this aspartate[113] appears to be conserved in other receptors that bind amine ligands (e.g., histamine receptors). Serine(ser)[204], ser[207], and ser[319] (located in transmembrane regions 5 and 7) appear to be important in hydrogen ion bond formation[36] between (1) the -OH group of ser[204] and the meta-OH group of the ligand and (2) the -OH side chain of the ser[207] and the para-OH group of the ligand. Phenylalanine[289] and phe[290] are involved in interactions with the aromatic catechol ring, and specifically, they define agonist function.[37] Concepts that relate the structure and function of agonists, partial agonists, and antagonists to specific receptor binding sites and their interaction with G proteins remain complex and are beyond the scope of this chapter. However, the subject has been reviewed well.[34,38]

G Protein Coupling

As discussed previously, G proteins are a large family of proteins that act as transducers of signals generated by the interaction of agonists with membrane receptors. For a specific signal to be transduced without confusion and with the appropriate temporal relationship to the stimulus, G proteins must be specific for individual receptors. G proteins must also be able to be turned off rapidly so that the responses are proportional to the stimulus. G proteins are heterotrimeric proteins consisting of α, β, and γ subunits. It was initially believed that the α subunit defined the specificity of the interaction of a given G protein with the receptor. Many subtypes of G protein α subunits exist, effectively

dividing G proteins into many classes (e.g., G_i, G_s, G_q, and G_t). These will be discussed later in relation to distinct AR subtypes. In addition to specificity, the α subunit classically was thought to be important in interacting with the effector systems. The α subunit has a single high affinity site for guanine nucleotides and intrinsic guanosine triphosphatase (GTPase) activity. The hydrolysis of guanosine triphosphate (GTP) determines the ability of the G protein rapidly to switch on and off (G protein cycling) in response to receptor activation. In contrast, the βγ subunit has been viewed as the regulatory component for the α subunit; βγ subunits stabilize the guanosine diphosphate (GDP)-bound form of the α subunit, allow interaction of the α subunit with the receptor, and anchor the complex to the membrane. The βγ subunits are found in close association with one another and are difficult to separate. There is, however, a growing body of evidence to suggest that the βγ complex itself can interact with effector proteins. This complex was shown to interact with adenylyl cyclase and couple to certain ion channels. Recent findings also suggest that βγ may play an essential role in agonist-induced receptor phosphorylation and desensitization. G proteins are a subject of intense research and a detailed discussion of their biology is beyond the scope of this chapter (for review, see refs. 39 and 40).

The G Protein Cycle

To understand G protein interactions with membrane receptors, it is important to grasp each step in the G protein cycle. This cycle is summarized schematically in Figure 26-4. At the beginning of the G protein cycle, the receptor is in the inactive state. The agonist is not bound to the receptor, and the G protein is not coupled to the effector (e.g., adenylyl cyclase in the case of the β AR). On binding of the agonist to the receptor, a conformational change in the structure of the receptor takes place. This conformational change probably involves the rotation and movement of a transmembrane α helix, opening a binding site on the receptor for the G protein and, thereby, enabling receptor interaction with the G protein. The affinity of GDP for the α subunit of the G protein is decreased, and in the presence of Mg^{++}, GDP is replaced by GTP. The GTP-bound α subunit of G protein dissociates and

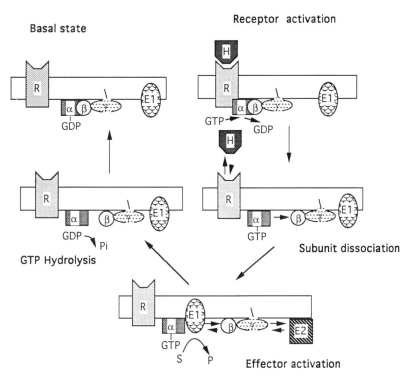

Fig. 26-4 G protein cycling and G protein-mediated transmembrane signaling. In the basal state, G proteins exist as heterotrimers with *GDP* bound tightly to the α subunit. The receptor (*R*) is unoccupied and the effector (*E*) is inactive. After binding of the hormone (*H*), the receptor undergoes a conformational change and interacts with the heterotrimer G protein. This results in the dissociation of GDP from the guanine nucleotide binding site. Binding of *GTP* to the G protein α subunit has two consequences. The first is that the G protein dissociates from the H-R complex, reducing the affinity of the hormone for the receptor. Second, a reduced affinity for the G protein α subunit for the $\beta\gamma$ subunits occurs, resulting in $\beta\gamma$ subunit dissociation from the α subunit. The α-GTP bound subunits binds effector (*E1*), which in turn, induces a change in intracellular chemistry. The $\beta\gamma$ subunit may interact directly with a different effector (*E2*) or may modulate the activity of the α-E1 complex. The α subunit possesses intrinsic GTPase activity. The α subunit catalyzed hydrolysis of GTP results in GDP being left in the α subunit nucleotide binding site, a process that results in deactivation of the activated complex. The GDP bound form of G protein α subunit has high affinity for $\beta\gamma$ subunits with subsequent reassociation of these three subunits and a return of the system to the basal state. GDP, guanosine diphosphate; GTP, guanosine triphosphate. (Adapted from Helper and Gilman,[39] with permission.)

couples with the effector molecule. The affinity of the receptor for the agonist then decreases, and the agonist dissociates from the receptor binding site. The intrinsic GTPase in the dissociated α subunit hydrolyzes GTP to GDP, and the receptor returns to its inactive state.[39]

Receptors and G Proteins

G proteins are located on the cytoplasmic surface of cell membranes. Because portions of G protein-coupled receptors are located on the intracellular surface of the cell (three intracellular loops and the entire carboxyl terminus), these regions were initially postulated to be important in receptor-G protein interactions. Initial studies with rhodopsin localized receptor-G protein interactions predominantly to the third intracellular loop of the receptor.[41] Subsequently, chimeric ARs, such as β_2/α_2 AR[30] and β_2/α_1,[42] and muscarinic receptor chimeras, such as M1/M2[43] and M1/β AR,[44] have defined the importance of the second and third intracellular loops and the initial carboxyl terminus in interactions with G proteins. To define further individual key amino acid residues important in receptor-G protein coupling, deletion mutations and conservative amino acid substitutions in regions of the third intracellular loop of the receptor have been tested.[45] It appears that the carboxyl terminus of the third loop is particularly important for G protein binding, specifically two distinct amino acids, histidine[269] and lysine[270] in the β_2 AR. Although specific interactions have been identified, it is important to remember that receptor interactions with G proteins and the interaction of activated G proteins with effector systems is a dynamic process and may be modified in various disease states.

Mechanisms of Regulation

The response to a particular hormone or drug stimulus may decrease over time. This process was initially referred to as tachyphylaxis. With the development of the science of receptor biology, it was discovered that receptors undergo dynamic regulation, giving rise to the observed pharmacologic dampening phenomenon. The most extensively investigated mechanism of regulation is that of desensitization, which is the reduction in a physiologic response to a stimulus that is constant over time.

Desensitization is the result of three interrelated processes: (1) receptor uncoupling, (2) sequestration, and (3) downregulation (Fig. 26-5A). Receptor uncoupling refers to a rapid process (seconds to minutes) that results in the inability of the receptor to bind G protein, causing uncoupling of the receptor from the signal transduction system. Uncoupling is caused by phosphorylation of the receptor and perhaps the G protein. Receptor sequestration is a process that occurs more slowly (minutes to hours) and results in the movement of receptors from the cell surface to intracellular compartments that are not accessible to hydrophilic ligands. However, with termination of agonist stimulation, sequestered receptors are available for recycling to the cell surface. Downregulation is a more prolonged process (hours to days) that also results in the movement of receptors from the cell surface to intracellular compartments, but then the receptors are destroyed. On termination of agonist

stimulation, downregulated receptors are not available for recycling to the cell surface; in fact, new receptor protein must be made from RNA to replace lost receptors at the cell surface (for review, see ref. 46).

Receptor Uncoupling

The most rapid form of desensitization, receptor uncoupling, is associated with phosphorylation of the carboxyl terminus of the β AR.[47] Phosphorylation is dependent on enzymes called protein kinases that catalyze the transfer of a phosphate group from adenosine triphosphate to a distinct amino acid in a specific receptor (consensus) sequence that binds the kinase. Two distinct protein kinases, protein kinase A (PKA, also called cyclic adenosine monophosphate [cAMP]-dependent kinase) and β AR kinase (β ARK), are thought to be involved in the regulation of the β AR. The involvement of each of these kinases in receptor uncoupling will now be explored.

Many biologic systems are regulated by negative feedback of a downstream product. Therefore, it is logical that cAMP-dependent protein kinase (a target protein for cAMP) would regulate β ARs, the downstream second messenger of which is cAMP. β ARs were shown to be phosphorylated by purified PKA,[48] and the β_2 AR has a number of PKA consensus sequences (R-R-X-S), one in the carboxyl terminal and one in the third intracellular loop. Substitution mutations of these consensus sequences result in the impairment of desensitization, confirming the importance of phosphorylation in this regulatory process.[49]

In 1981, Green et al.[50] demonstrated that G proteins were not essential for agonist specific desensitization of a line of cells devoid of G_s. This raised the question of whether another protein kinase is important in the process of desensitization. This in turn led to the discovery of β ARK[51] which phosphorylates the agonist occupied form of the β_2 AR with high efficiency. β ARK phosphorylation results in uncoupling of the receptor from G_s. Initially, β ARK was thought to phosphorylate only β ARs. However, more recently, it also was shown to phosphorylate both α_2 ARs (as described in the section on regulation of the α_2 AR[52]) and the light bleached form of rhodopsin.[53] The use of deletion

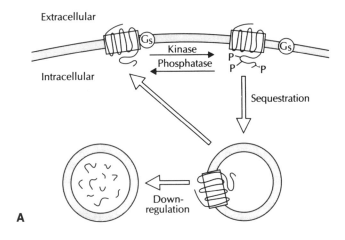

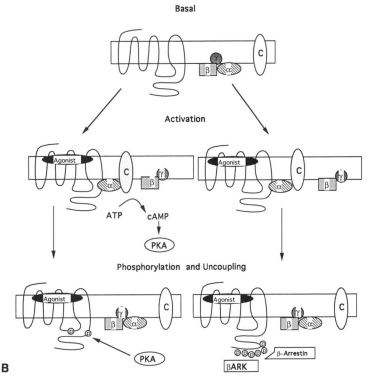

Fig. 26-5(A) Summary of the mechanisms of desensitization of the β adrenoceptor. (From Berkowitz and Schwinn,[3] with permission.) **(B)** Mechanisms of β uncoupling from G proteins, resulting in dampening of the physiologic response. The agonist binds to the β AR, resulting in activation of adenylate cyclase (C). This in turn results in the activation of cAMP-dependent protein kinase (or *PKA*). PKA phosphorylates sites in the third intracellular loop and carboxyl terminus of the β AR, resulting in uncoupling of the α subunit of the G protein from the receptor. β ARK has a high affinity for the agonist occupied form of the receptor and phosphorylates sites on the carboxyl terminus. β-arrestin binds to the phosphorylated form of the receptor, disrupting G protein coupling (see text for details). β-AR, β-adrenoceptor; β-ARK, β-adrenoceptor kinase; PKA, protein kinase A.

mutants clarified the site of phosphorylation by β ARK. In a mutant β_2 AR in which the seven serine and three threonines of the carboxyl terminal were deleted, agonist-promoted desensitization was significantly depressed.[54] This was associated with significant decreases in agonist-induced receptor phosphorylation. These results demonstrate that β ARK phosphorylation of serine and threonine residues in the carboxyl terminal of the receptor is important in receptor desensitization. Another protein was shown to be important in enhancing the desensitization process induced by β ARK phosphorylation. This protein was found serendipitously during the purification of β AR kinase. Whereas the β ARs that had been phosphorylated by crude preparations of β ARK were impaired in their ability to couple to Gs, β ARs phosphorylated by purer preparations of β ARK coupled relatively normally to the G protein.[55] The addition of arrestin, a protein in the visual system that enhances uncoupling, restored this process of uncoupling in the β AR system in the presence of pure preparations of β ARK. This discovery led to the cloning of a new protein similar to arrestin, called β arrestin. It appears that β arrestin binds to the phosphorylated receptor and covers the G protein binding site, effectively inhibiting receptor-G protein interactions.[56] Figure 26-5B summarizes the importance of PKA and β ARK in desensitization.

Sequestration

Sequestration involves internalization of surface receptors during the desensitization process.[57] The development of hydrophilic and hydrophobic β AR analogs allows differentiation of surface β ARs from total β ARs. Cell surface β ARs bind hydrophilic ligands; a cell surface and internalized (total) β ARs bind hydrophobic ligands. By subtracting surface receptors from total receptors, a determination of sequestered receptors can be made.[58,59] Although many laboratories have investigated the process of sequestration during the last decade, the mechanism(s) of sequestration remain unclear. Studies using inhibitors of PKA and β ARK,[60] and chimeric and mutant receptors with key serine and threonine residues mutated, demonstrate that phosphorylation is not required and does not regulate sequestration of receptors.[61] It was also shown

that G protein uncoupling is not part of the signal for receptor sequestration. Thus, receptor sequestration, although recognized as a mechanism of signal regulation, has not been fully characterized. However, physical removal of receptors from the cell membrane (sequestration) is an important process in desensitization in general.

Downregulation

Short-term regulation of receptors (including receptor uncoupling and sequestration) does not seem to be associated with long-term decreases in receptor number. This long-term process of regulation reflects steady state changes in the number of receptors,[62] which in turn, reflects changes in levels of mRNA and receptor protein.[63,64] This can be measured in vitro by solution hybridization and ribonuclease protection assays and by northern blotting. There are two major mechanisms responsible for altering steady state mRNA levels of receptors and G proteins, that is, gene expression and mRNA stability (post-transcriptional). Gene transcription is measured by experiments called nuclear run-off transcription assays, and mRNA stability is determined by measuring the half-life of a species of mRNA specific for ARs. These two mechanisms are responsible for the regulation of β AR mRNA levels in response to agonists. Studies highlighted the importance of adenylyl cyclase and cAMP in this process (e.g., agonist-promoted increases in transcription can be mimicked by cAMP analogs and variant SF49 mouse lymphoma cells with mutations in the cAMP pathway). In addition, studies of cells expressing β ARs with mutations in PKA binding sites demonstrated the importance of PKA in agonist-promoted down regulation of receptor and receptor mRNA.

The DNA sequence, or gene, encoding an individual receptor protein has regulatory regions on both ends. DNA sequences that are present just prior to the nucleotide triplet encoding the starting amino acid of the protein are called the 5' untranslated sequences; DNA sequences present after the nucleotides encoding the last amino acid in the protein's carboxyl terminus are called 3' untranslated sequences. Various DNA sequences (or domains) in each of these regions appear to be important in regulating the transcription rate of encoded receptor protein mRNA. Domains involved in the regulation of gene expression include glucocorticoid responsive elements in the 5′ noncoding region, which have been shown to increase β_2-AR transcription. In addition, a cAMP responsive element was also demonstrated to be present in the β_2 AR gene. In some receptor systems, cAMP responsive elements are associated with an increase in receptor expression. However, evidence for long-term increases in β AR expression was not observed. The reason for this was postulated to be associated with an agonist-induced mRNA destabilization. Although the sequences necessary for RNA destabilization remain to be identified, β AR mRNA contains possible consensus sequences in the 3′ noncoding region. In summary, the decline in mRNA on long-term exposure to β-agonists appears to involve a decrease in the stability of mRNA rather than a lowering in the rate of transcription. This is in part dependent on cAMP and PKA but may depend on many other regulatory factors (for review, see ref. 65)

α_1-ADRENOCEPTORS
General Introduction

α ARs are widely distributed in tissues and are responsible for many functions, ranging from modulation of the state of consciousness and nociception to cardiovascular regulation and energy metabolism.[66] The α ARs are subdivided into α_1 AR and α_2 AR families. Each of these receptor families is coupled to distinct signal transduction mechanisms and is divided into several subtypes.[67] To understand the subdivision of α ARs, we present a review of the evolution of the anatomic, functional, and pharmacologic classification of α ARs in general.

The demonstration that the release was inhibited by stimulation of prejunctional α ARs was an important step in the recognition of a class of α ARs distinct from classic postjunctional α ARs that mediate vasoconstriction.[68] Further studies demonstrated that compounds, such as clonidine (a relatively α_2 AR selective agonist) and phenoxybenzamine (an α_1 AR selective antagonist) could discriminate between pre- and postjunctional α ARs. This led Langer[69,70] to propose an anatomic classi-

cation of α ARs, with α_1 ARs described as postsynaptic and α_2 ARs described as presynaptic. The classification of α AR subtypes on the basis of anatomic distribution alone was shown to be inadequate following the demonstration by Schimmel[71] that the inhibition of isoproterenol-induced glycolysis and lipolysis in adipocytes (events mediated by postjunctional β AR stimulation) occurred only with highly selective α_2 AR agonists. These experiments demonstrated the presence of postjunctional α_2 ARs in addition to those previously described as prejunctional. This led to a functional classification of α ARs in which α_1 ARs were described as stimulatory and α_2 ARs inhibitory.[72] This classification was also shown to be inadequate with the demonstration by Drew and Whiting[73] that vasoconstrictive responses to NE were inhibited, not only by prazosin, but also by yohimbine, effectively defining stimulatory postjunctional α AR in the vasculature.

Pharmacologic classifications are based on agonist potency series and selective antagonists. The agonist potency series for α_1 and α_2 ARs are identical. It was not until selective antagonists were developed for each α AR subtype in the 1970s that these two families of receptors could be distinguished pharmacologically. Today, a series of agonists and antagonists that are relatively selective for α_1 versus α_2 ARs defines each α AR family. α_1 ARs are activated by phenylephrine, methoxamine, and cirazoline and are blocked in a competitive manner by low concentrations of prazosin and WB4101. α_2 ARs are stimulated by clonidine, dexmedetomidine, azepexole (also known as BHT933), and brimonidine tartrate (UK14,304) and competitively inhibited by yohimbine, rauwoscoline, and idazoxan.[67] The use of these ligands, and more recently developed selective compounds, led to the demonstration of α AR heterogeneity. Table 26-1 summarizes some adrenergic agonists and antagonists used in the classification of α_1 and α_2 ARs. Molecular cloning and characterization of encoded α AR subtypes, however, yielded the greatest information regarding α AR heterogeneity. There are now known to be at least six α AR subtypes—at least three α_1 ARs and three α_2 ARs. Differentiation of each of these subtypes will be discussed in the following sections.

Table 26-1 Adrenergic Agonists and Antagonists Used in the Classification of α_1 and α_2 Adrenoceptors

α_1 AR Selective	Nonselective	α_2 AR Selective
Agonists 　Phenylephrine 　Methoxamine 　Cirazoline	Agonists 　Norepinephrine 　Epinephrine	Agonists 　Clonidine 　α-Methylnorepinephrine 　Azepexole 　BHT920 　Brimonidine tartrate
Antagonists 　Prazosin 　WB4101	Antagonists 　Phentolamine 　Tolazoline	Antagonists 　Rauwolscine 　Yohimbine 　Idazoxan

Abbreviations: AR, adrenoceptor.
(Adapted from Ruffolo et al.,[67] with permission.)

Pharmacology

α_1 ARs are widely distributed and are responsible for mediating many physiologic functions. Stimulation of α_1 ARs results primarily in vasoconstriction (systemic arteries) and venoconstriction (veins). Examples of α_1 AR effects in other tissues include gluconeogenesis (liver) and positive inotropy (heart, approximately 10 percent of that seen with β ARs). In addition, selective α_1 AR antagonists protect against myocardial arrhythmias. When describing α_1 ARs in terms of pharmacology rather than physiology (end-organ response), agonist potency series and selective antagonists become important. The agonist potency series for α_1 ARs is EPI > NE > phenylephrine > ISO; the selective α_1 AR antagonist is prazosin. For many years, α_1 ARs were thought to represent one receptor subtype; however, recent pharmacologic and molecular cloning evidence suggests the existence of more than one α_1 AR.

During the last five years, both functional in vitro and pharmacologic radioligand binding data demonstrate the existence of α_1 AR heterogeneity. Prazosin was found to have a 100-fold range in antagonist affinity against a variety of α_1 AR responses in functional assays.[74] This led to the suggestion of two distinct populations of α_1 ARs. This was confirmed in vitro by Flavahan and Vanhoutte.[75] Radioligand binding studies showed the heterogeneity of α_1 ARs by the presence of biphasic competition curves of α_1 ARs with the an-

tagonists WB4101 and phentolamine in membranes isolated from the rat cerebral cortex. Each component represented approximately 50 percent of total binding. The α_1 AR subtype with a high affinity for WB4101 was designated α_{1A} and the subtype with a low affinity for WB4101, α_{1B}. More recent studies showed that another compound, 5-methyurapidil, is selective (40 to 80-fold higher affinity) for the α_{1A} subtype compared with WB4101 (10 to 40-fold higher affinity for the α_{1A}). Other compounds were described that discriminate between α_1 AR subtypes, including oxymetazoline, niguldipine, and benoxathian. In addition, the alkylating agent chloroethylclonidine irreversibly inactivates the α_{1B} subtype (the α_{1A} is resistant to inactivation by chloroethylclonidine); thus, chloroethylclonidine has become important in discriminating α_1 AR subtypes.[76] Wilson and Minneman[77] demonstrated the existence of two distinct α_1 AR subtypes based on coupling to distinct signal transduction pathways. This will be discussed in a later section.

Molecular Biology

During the years that α_1 AR heterogeneity was first suggested pharmacologically, molecular biologic techniques were rapidly being applied to ARs. The gene encoding the α_1 AR was isolated in 1988.[11] After the gene was isolated, it was placed in plasmids that enabled it to be expressed in cell lines. These cells then generated receptor protein from the cloned gene. Pharmacologic testing on the resultant α_1 AR protein showed low affinity for WB4101 and phentolamine and sensitivity to inactivation by the alkylating agent chloroethylclonidine. Thus, the cloned receptor had pharmacologic characteristics of the α_{1B} AR subtype. Soon after this receptor was identified, Schwinn et al.[19] isolated a gene encoding another α_1 subtype. Initial pharmacologic testing of this receptor that was expressed in cells demonstrated high affinity binding for the compounds WB4101 and phentolamine, suggesting that this gene encoded the α_{1A} AR subtype, but further testing demonstrated only partial sensitivity to inactivation by chloroethylclonidine, and a lack of expression of this receptor in rat tissues that should have contained α_{1A} ARs. Hence this receptor was named the α_{1C} AR. During ensuing years, the gene was cloned that encoded an α_1 AR with high affinity for WB4101 and phentolamine, resistance to inactivation by chloroethylclonidine, and an expected distribution in rat tissues, suggesting that this gene encoded that α_{1A} AR.[16] The receptor was initially named the α_{1A} AR on this basis. However, newer selective compounds that have high affinity for the cloned α_{1A} AR subtype have low affinity for the cloned α_{1A} AR.[78] Thus, for the time being, this receptor has been renamed the $\alpha_{1A/D}$ until this controversy can be successfully resolved. This leaves open the possibility that the α_{1A} AR has not yet been cloned; hence, there may be four α_1 ARs. Molecular techniques,

such as gene cloning, have added a tremendous amount to our understanding of α_1 AR heterogeneity and the pharmacology of individual α_1 ARs.

Tissue Localization and Species Heterogeneity

α_1 ARs are widely distributed throughout the human body. Because the rat is commonly used as an animal model, the expression of individual α_1 AR subtypes was first tested in rat tissues using ligand binding techniques. After genes encoding various α_1 ARs became available, molecular techniques were used to localize α_1 AR mRNA in various rat tissues. Northern blot analysis is a technique in which RNA is harvested from various tissues, separated according to size on an agarose gel through which an electric field is applied (smaller fragments migrate faster than larger fragments), transferred to a membrane, and then hybridized with radiolabeled DNA probes from cloned α_1 AR subtype genes. Using these approaches, each cloned α_1 AR subtype mRNA was localized to various rat tissues. It is important to note here that the presence of mRNA in a tissue does not guarantee high levels of receptor protein. However, the opposite is true (i.e., the absence of mRNA suggests that encoded receptor protein is not present). Fortunately, with only a few exceptions so far, mRNA concentrations tend to follow receptor protein concentrations in tissues. A summary of α_1 AR mRNA distribution in rat tissues is presented in Table 26-2.[76] It is impor-

Table 26-2 Distribution of α_1 Adrenoceptor Subtypes in the Rat

	α_{1B}	α_{1A}	α_{1C}
Hippocampus	+	+++	0
Brain stem	+++	++	0
Cerebellum	++	+	0
Cortex	+++	+++	0
Kidney	++	+	0
Liver	++++	0	0
Lung	++	+	0
Aorta	0	+++	0
Heart	++++	++	0
Skeletal muscle	0	+	0
Spleen	+	++	0
Vas deferens	0	++++	0

tant to note that the $\alpha_{1A/D}$ AR and the α_{1B} AR are present in many rat tissues, both in some tissues and only one subtype in other tissues. However, initial studies in peripheral tissues of the rat demonstrated the lack of expression of the α_{1C} AR subtype. More recently, this α_1 AR subtype was found in localized regions of rat brain,[79] but this receptor has a limited overall distribution in rat tissues.

Because some functional experiments on individual α_1 AR subtypes were performed using a rabbit model, the distribution of α_1 AR subtype mRNA was determined in rabbit tissues. In these experiments, striking species heterogeneity in the distribution of α_1 ARs was observed.[80] For example, rabbit liver contains only the α_{1C} AR subtype mRNA (whereas the rat liver contains only α_{1B} AR mRNA). Rabbit aorta contained only α_{1B} AR mRNA, whereas rat aorta contained the $\alpha_{1A/D}$ AR. Interestingly, $\alpha_{1A/D}$ mRNA was not demonstrated in any rabbit tissue studied, but it was present in many rat tissues. These findings make it imperative to define the location of each AR subtype in human tissue. These experiments are being performed currently. Because many of the drugs used in modulating cardiovascular responses are AR agonists and antagonists, defining the location of various AR subtypes in human tissue will enhance the development of more selective pharmacologic agents designed for specific human physiologic responses.

Coupling to Second Messengers

In this section, the latest knowledge of α_1 AR signal transduction will be reviewed briefly. In many cells, binding of agonist to α_1 ARs causes hydrolysis of membrane phospholipids (predominantly phosphoinositide bisphosphate), resulting in the formation of inositol triphosphate and diacylglycerol through a G protein coupled to phospholipase C.[81,82] Inositoltrisphosphate promotes the release of calcium (Ca^{++}) from nonmitochondrial intracellular stores. α_1 AR signal transduction, however, may be more complicated. Han et al.[83,84] reported on two subtypes of α_1 ARs that cause contractile responses through molecular mechanisms different from hydrolysis of membrane phospholipids. One α_1 AR subtype located in rat vas deferens and hippocampus demonstrated an absolute requirement for extracellular Ca^{++} and appears to control

the opening of dihydropyridine sensitive Ca^{++} channels. This subtype was given the name α_{1A} AR. In contrast, the α_{1B} AR subtype located in rat liver and spleen regulates phospholipid hydrolysis to give rise to contraction independent of extracellular Ca^{++}. Thus, the activation of α_{1A} and α_{1B} AR subtypes may result in the formation of different inositol phosphate second messengers, and the response to α_{1A} activation may require the influx of extracellular Ca^{++}.

Cotecchia et al.[11] initially demonstrated the coupling of the cloned hamster α_{1B} AR to phospholipase C by a pertussis toxin-insensitive G protein. They further demonstrated the importance of the third cytoplasmic loop at the α_1 AR in coupling to the specific G protein by constructing a chimeric receptor consisting of the β_2 AR gene in which the putative third cytoplasmic loop was replaced with the corresponding region of the α_{1B} gene.[85] When this synthetic gene was expressed in cells, the chimeric receptor activated phosphoinositide metabolism as effectively as the native α_{1B} AR. Later, it was determined that 27 amino acids of the α_{1B} AR derived from the amino terminal portion of the third intracellular loop (residues 233 to 259) represented the structural determinants conferring G protein coupling specificity and phosphoinositide hydrolysis.[86] Schwinn et al.,[80] following the cloning of the α_{1C} AR from bovine brain, characterized the transduction mechanisms for the α_{1C} AR and highlighted differences with the α_{1B} AR. Even though the α_{1B} and α_{1C} AR activate phosphoinositide hydrolysis, the α_{1C} AR couples to phospholipase C more efficiently than does the α_{1B} AR. At about the same time, Kjelsberg et al.[87] demonstrated that a single amino acid substitution at residue 293 of the third intracellular loop of the α_{1B} AR resulted in constitutive activation of the receptor. Thus, the receptor couples to G protein in the absence of agonist. Studies such as these clearly have contributed toward our understanding of cell regulation and growth and, potentially, of the cancer process. They also give important information regarding mechanisms of receptor-G protein coupling.

It is only within the last year that the G protein that couples to α_1 ARs was defined. The G_q class of G proteins, a family of pertussis toxin insensitive G proteins, was shown to couple to phospholipase C

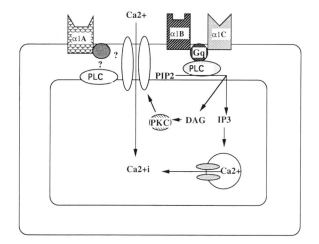

Fig. 26-6 This figure summarizes signal transduction mechanisms for the α_1 ARs. α_1 AR agonists bind receptor (*R*) and activate the G protein, G_q. G_q then activates *PLC*, which results in the hydrolysis of membrane phospholipids. The most common membrane phospholipid to be hydrolyzed is *PIP$_2$*, resulting in two predominant products—*IP$_3$* and *DAG*. IP$_3$ is responsible for mobilizing calcium from intracellular nonmitochondrial stores. The resultant increase in intracellular calcium is thought to be important in physiologic end points, such as vascular constriction. α_1 AR, α_1 adrenoceptor; DAG, diacylglycerol; IP$_3$, inositol trisphosphate; PIP$_2$, phosphoinositol-4,5-biphosphate; PLC, phospholipase C.

β_1.[88] Wu et al.,[89] in an elegant experiment in COS-7 cells cotransfecting genes encoding different members of the α_1 AR receptor family with genes encoding different members of the G_q family, showed that G_q and G_{11} couple to the α_{1A} AR; G_q, G_{11}, G_{14}, and G_{16} couple to the α_{1B} AR; and G_q, G_{11}, and G_{14} couple to the α_{1C} AR. The importance of this experiment is that it demonstrates that the response to a stimulus is not only dependent on the distribution of a subtype of receptor but also on the distribution and coupling to G protein subtypes. Figure 26-6 summarizes our current knowledge of signal transduction mechansims for α_1 AR subtypes.

Mechanisms of Regulation

Desensitization refers to the dampening of a biologic response during continuous exposure to a stimulus. The biology of β AR desensitization and

down regulation has been well characterized and was discussed in the previous section. In contrast to β ARs, mechanisms of α_1 AR desensitization are much less well defined. In cultured smooth muscle cells, Leeb-Lundberg et al.[90,91] demonstrated that phorbol esters (compounds that activate the enzyme protein kinase C directly), result in uncoupling of α_1 AR-mediated stimulation of phosphoinositide turnover. They also demonstrated a decrease in the affinity of α_1 ARs for agonist binding in the presence of phorbol esters. These findings suggest that protein kinase C phosphorylation of α_1 ARs may be involved (as was seen with phosphorylation of β ARs) with desensitization of α_1 ARs. Diacylglycerol, one of the products of α_1 AR stimulation, is known to activate protein kinase C. Hence, agonist-promoted activation of protein kinase C may serve as a negative feedback loop regulating the function of α_1 ARs. Subsequently, it was demonstrated that both the α_1 AR agonist NE and the naturally occurring vasoactive peptide bradykinin (that activates protein kinase C through the inositol trisphosphate-diacylglycerol pathway) phosphorylates and desensitizes the α_1 AR purified from hamster smooth muscle.[92] Protein kinase C is a multifunctional serine-threonine protein kinase that plays an important role in signal transduction and phosphorylates numerous receptors and proteins.[93] Although protein kinase C is less well understood than PKA or β ARK, it appears that the presence of a single basic amino acid residue (preferably arginine, but also lysine) one to two amino acids on either side of a serine or threonine is an important determinant of protein kinase C-mediated serine-threonine phosphorylation. Further studies are currently in progress to determine the mechanism of regulation of the α_1 ARs. Figure 26-7 summarizes the postulated mechanism of regulation of the α_1 ARs.

α_2 ADRENOCEPTORS

General Introduction

α_2 ARs, which couple with G_i to inhibit adenylyl cyclase activity, are important in the physiologic functions of platelet aggregation, smooth muscle contraction, neurotransmitter release, and modu-

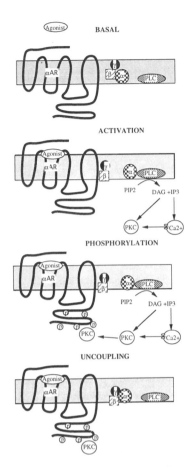

Fig. 26-7 Mechanisms of desensitization of α_1 ARs. Agonist binding to α_1 ARs results in coupling to *PLC* through a G protein, G_q resulting in the hydrolysis of membrane phospholipids (specifically *PIP$_2$* to produce *IP$_3$* and *DAG*. DAG binds and activates *PKC*, which in turn, phosphorylates consensus sequences in the receptor carboxyl terminus. It is postulated that this phosphorylation results in the uncoupling of α_1 ARs from G_q. α_1 AR, α_1 adrenoceptor; DAG, diacylglycerol; IP$_3$, inositol trisphosphate; PIP$_2$, phosphoinositol-4,5-biphosphate; PKC, protein kinase C; PLC, phospholiphase C.

lation of sympathetic outflow from the central nervous system. α_2 ARs are also known to play important roles in peripheral tissues, such as the liver (glycogenolysis and gluconeogenesis), pancreas (decreased secretion of insulin from islet β cells), spleen (contraction of capsule), and kidney (yet undetermined role in water reabsorption in both proximal and distal tubules).[66] The importance of the α_2 ARs in clinical anesthesia was highlighted after the demonstration of the potent hypnotic and analgesic effects of α_2 AR agonists. Clonidine, a centrally acting α_2 AR agonist was first introduced into clinical medicine for the treatment of hypertension. It was noted at that time that one of the side effects of clonidine was sedation. Although α_2 AR agonists have been used for years as anesthetics in veterinary medicine, the idea that α_2 AR agonists could be used as adjunctive anesthetic agents in human medicine has only recently been embraced. Kaukinen et al.[94] demonstrated that patients treated preoperatively with clonidine exhibited a "smoother" hemodynamic profile compared with those who did not receive the drug. A modest reduction in the minimum aveolar concentration for halothane was also demonstrated with clonidine administration. Bloor and Flacke[95] defined the dose-response curve for acutely administered clonidine during halothane anesthesia. They also demonstrated that the minimum alveolar concentration reducing effect of clonidine was reversed by tolazoline, a specific α_2 AR antagonist. Subsequently, numerous studies documented the effects of α_2 AR agonists, including the more potent and specific α_2 AR agonist dexmedetomidine, in reducing anesthetic requirements in many clinical scenarios (for review, see Ref. 96).

The locus ceruleus (a region of the brain adjacent to the fourth ventricle known to be a central noradrenergic cell body "traffic networking station") has become the focus of attention as the possible site of action of α_2 AR agonists. Maze and his colleagues have demonstrated that dexmedetomidine causes a dose-dependent hypnotic response when injected locally into the locus ceruleus of stereotactically cannulated awake rats.[97,98] They also demonstrated that the hypnotic effect of α_2 AR agonists is mediated through coupling to a pertussis sensitive inhibitory G protein with involvement of K^+ (hyperpolarization) and Ca^{++} channels.[99]

In addition to their hypnotic effect, the α_2 AR agonists are important in clinical anesthesia as analgesic agents. They have emerged as potentially important agents that may serve as alternatives to the opioid analgesics. At the turn of the century, Weber[100] demonstrated that EPI applied to the spinal cord could attenuate a thermally evoked withdrawal response. Recently, there have been numerous reports of the use of both epidural and intrathecal α_2 AR agonists as potent analgesics for labor, postoperative pain, and cancer pain. The mechanism of action of α_2 AR analgesia presumably includes modulation of opioid and substance P neurotransmission at spinal and supraspinal levels (for review, see ref. 96. These concepts are presented in detail in Chapter 27.

Classification and Subtypes

The pharmacologic classification of α_2 AR subtypes is extremely complex. However, the cloning of genes encoding three α_2 AR subtypes has enabled extensive crossreferencing between the cloned receptor profiles and previously described pharmacologic subtypes. Therefore, all the α_2 ARs that were previously described pharmacologically can now be fit into three receptor subtypes. A brief summary of these α_2 AR subtypes will be presented, then a review of the cloned subtypes, followed by the cross-referenced final classification.

Initial descriptions of α_2 AR subtypes were postulated by Bylund.[101] Based on ligand binding studies, three α_2 AR subtypes were postulated. Human and rat brain contain two α_2 AR subtypes, which differ in their affinities for prazosin. The α_{2A} subtype demonstrates a low affinity for prazosin but a high affinity for oxymetazoline, and it is typically found in platelets. The α_{2B} AR has a 30 to 40-fold higher affinity for prazosin, a low affinity for oxymetazoline, and is expressed in neonatal rat lung and renal cortex. There is evidence for a third pharmacologic subtype, the α_{2C} AR described in a specific cell line, the opossum kidney cells (for review, see ref. 102).

In addition to pharmacologic evidence for three subtypes of α_2 ARs, genes encoding three distinct α_2 ARs were cloned and characterized.[10,17,18] The first α_2 AR gene was cloned from human platelets. Isolation of this gene required purification of protein to homogeneity (using hundreds of batches of expired human platelets), followed by cleavage of receptor protein and poypeptide sequencing.[18] The gene encoding the platelet α_2 AR was located on human chromosome 10 and was thus called

α_{2C10}. The second gene to be cloned was the α_2 AR from human kidney using classic molecular cloning techniques. This gene resides on human chromosome 4 and was thus designated α_{2C4}.[10] Utilizing polymerase chain reaction technology (a technique that amplifies DNA sequences), a third α_2 AR was cloned and assigned to human chromosome 2; this receptor was therefore named the α_{2C2}.[17] Bylund et al.[103] investigated the relationship between pharmacologically defined α_2 ARs and α_2 ARs described by molecular cloning and expression in mammalian cells. They compared pharmacologic characteristics of each cloned α_2 AR subtype expressed in COS cells with the characteristics of pharmacologically defined α_2 ARs in their respective prototypic tissue or cell line. Using 12 subtype-selective ligands, they demonstrated convincingly that the pharmacologic α_{2A} subtype (as defined in the HT29 cell line), α_{2B} subtype (from neonatal rat lung), and the α_{2C} subtype (as defined by the opossum kidney cell line), corresponded to the cloned α_{2C10}, α_{2C2}, and α_{2C4} receptor subtypes, respectively.

Receptor Structure

α_2 ARs are G protein-coupled receptors with significant sequence homology to other ARs (42 to 45 percent amino acid identity in transmembrane regions with ARs from α_1 AR and β AR subfamilies). Within the α_2 AR subfamily, there is 72 to 75 percent amino acid identity in transmembrane domains. Despite these similarities, α_2 ARs have distinguishing features at the structural level. α_2 ARs differ from other ARs in that they have a large third intracellular loop and a short carboxyl tail that terminates just after the palmitoylated cysteine residue. The third intracellular loop of α_2 ARs contains potential phosphorylation sites (similar to those found in the carboxyl terminus of β ARs), which may be important in receptor regulation. In addition, the α_{2C2} AR is unique in comparison with the other α_2 ARs in having a short amino terminus that lacks sites for the N-linked glycosylation.[17] The role of glycosylation in receptor folding and G protein coupling remains unclear. The impact of α_2 AR structure on receptor regulation will be discussed in detail later.

Tissue Distribution

The distribution of the α_2 ARs in human tissues is poorly understood. Using northern blot analysis (a method described earlier), Lorenz et al.[104] demonstrated the presence of α_{2C10} ARs (corresponding to the α_{2A} subtype) in rat brain stem, cerebral cortex, hippocampus, pituitary, cerebellum, kidney, aorta, skeletal muscle, spleen, and lung. The α_{2C4} AR (corresponding to the α_{2C} AR) is present only in brain regions, not in peripheral tissues. The α_{2C2} AR (corresponding to the α_{2B} AR) is present in rat liver and kidney. Recent studies in our laboratories using ribonuclease protection assay techniques, suggest that the distribution of α_2 ARs, like α_1 ARs, is completely different in human and rat tissues. The distribution of α_2 ARs in human tissues will be more fully defined in the next few years. Using ligand binding studies, Lawhead et al.[105] demonstrated that rat and human spinal cord α_2 ARs are predominantly of the α_{2A} (or α_{2C10} AR) subtype. Defining the distribution of specific α_2 AR subtypes in human tissues becomes important for the design of subtype selective therapeutic agents (agonists and antagonists).

Coupling to Second Messengers

α_2 ARs are classically described as coupling to the G protein G_i,[106] with agonist stimulation resulting in decreases in intracellular cAMP. To understand the regions of the α_2 AR protein involved in coupling to G_i, chimeric receptor experiments have been performed using the α_{2C10} AR.[30] As described earlier, the third intracellular loop of α_2 ARs is considerably larger than the analogous region in β_2 or α_1 ARs (regions important in coupling to G_s and G_q, respectively). Easen et al.[107] demonstrated that α_2 ARs not only couple to G_i, but also to G_s. They found no difference in the efficiency of coupling of α_2 AR subtypes to G_i, but a significant difference was detected in the efficiency of α_2 AR subtype coupling to G_s with a rank order of $\alpha_{2C10} > \alpha_{2C4} > \alpha_{2C2}$. This is the first functional difference shown to exist between α_2 AR subtypes.

The decrease in cAMP associated with binding of α_2 AR agonists attenuates the activity of the cAMP-dependent PKA. PKA is a serine-threonine protein kinase that phosphorylates numerous intracellular

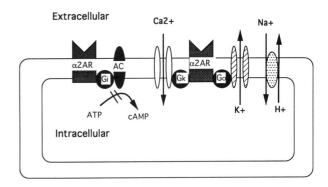

Fig. 26-8 Mechanisms of signal transduction for α_2 AR receptors. α_2 ARs classically inhibit *AC* through the inhibitory G protein, G_i. α_2 ARs also couple, through a poorly characterized G protein, to Ca^{++} channels. In addition, α_2 ARs couple to a K^+ channel through the G protein, G_k, resulting in hyperpolarization of the cell. Finally, α_2 ARs are also coupled to a H^+/Na^+ exchanger. AC, adenylate cyclose; α_2 AR, α_2 adrenoceptor. (Adapted from Maze and Tranquilli,[96] with permission.)

regulatory proteins with resultant alterations of the biologic response of a cell. cAMP was also shown to be an important regulator of specific ligand gated ion channels. Decreases in intracellular cAMP however, do not explain all the responses induced by α_2 AR agonists. In addition, α_2 ARs couple to a potassium (K^+) channel, resulting in hyperpolarization of the membrane. This process is dependent on a G protein and probably represents cAMP gating of the K^+ channel. α_2 AR agonists were also demonstrated to inhibit Ca^{++} channels and may play an important role in the suppression of Ca^{++} entry into nerve terminals, with subsequent prevention of neurotransmitter release. Coupling of α_2 ARs to Ca^{++} channels also appears to be through a G protein.[108] Figure 26-8 summarizes possible mechanisms of signal transduction of α_2 ARs.

Mechanisms of Regulation

As discussed previously, desensitization represents a dampening of a biologic response during continuous receptor exposure to an agonist. Among G protein-coupled receptors, desensitization has been studied most extensively in β ARs. Despite abundant knowledge regarding regulation of β ARs, little is known of mechanisms of regulation for α_2 ARs. Liggett et al.[109] investigated mechanisms of α_2 AR regulation using cloned native (wild-type) and mutant receptors. As previously discussed, the third intracellular loop of α_2 ARs is large and contains consensus sequences for the enzyme β ARK. To test desensitization of α_2 ARs, it is important to measure their ability to inhibit colforsin (also known as forskolin) stimulated adenylyl cyclase. Colforsin is a compound that directly stimulates adenylyl cyclase, which results in the increased production of cAMP. Because α_2 ARs inhibit the production of cAMP by stimulating G_i, which inhibits the function of adenylyl cyclase, this inhibition can be measured only if the cyclase is previously stimulated (as with colforsin). Desensitization, then, may be defined as an impaired ability of α_2 AR stimulation to inhibit colforsin-stimulated adenylyl cyclase. Liggett et al.[109] demonstrated that, in cells expressing wild-type α_2 AR, the EPI mediated inhibition of colforsin stimulated cAMP formation was decreased by 70 percent, demonstrating α_2 AR desensitization. This desensitization promoted by agonist was accompanied by α_2 AR phosphorylation. Mutated α_2 ARs, in which the β ARK consensus sequence was deleted, did not undergo desensitization or phosphorylation. Thus, β ARK is likely to be important in the regulation of α_2 ARs and β ARs.

ARs are important in many aspects of human physiology, in both health and disease. In addition to classic pharmacology, we reviewed in this chapter the molecular pharmacology of the nine currently known AR subtypes. Discrimination of AR subtypes using pharmacologic agents, mechanisms of coupling to intermediary G proteins and effector systems, and mechanisms of regulation for each AR subfamily (α_1, α_2, and β) was explored. A most interesting recent finding is the fact that the distribution of AR subtypes appears to be completely different in human tissues compared with that in rats and rabbits. This strongly suggests that the AR selective compounds developed in the future must be tested in humans to establish their efficacy in treating various human disease. An understanding of signal transduction mechanisms and G protein coupling is also important because drugs on the future may be aimed, not only at surface receptors, but also at the G proteins to which they couple downstream in the transduction pathway.[110] Although not exhaustive, this review should enable the reader to have a solid basis of understanding for the next two chapters on specific AR drugs used in anesthesiology.

REFERENCES

1. Ahlquist RP: A study of the adrenotropic receptors. Am J Physiol 153:586, 1948
2. Lands AM, Arnold A, Mcauliff JP et al: Differentiation of receptor systems activated by sympathomimetic amines. Nature 214:597, 1967
3. Berkowitz DE, Schwinn DA: New advances in receptor pharmacology. Curr Opin Anesthesiol 4:486, 1991
4. Zaagsma J, Hollenga C: Distribution and function of atypical β_3-adrenoreceptors. p. 47. In Adrenoreceptors: Structure, Mechanisms, Function. Verlag, Basel, 1991
5. Emorine LJ, Marullo S, Briend-Sutren MM et al: Molecular characterization of the human beta 3-adrenergic receptor. Science 245:1118, 1989
6. Lomasney JW, Leeb-Lundberg LMF, Cotecchia S et al: Mammalian α_1-adrenergic receptor: purification and characterization of the native receptor ligand binding subunit. J Biol Chem 261:7710, 1986
7. Benovic JL, Shorr RG, Caron MG, Lefkowitz RJ: The mammalian β_2-adrenergic receptor: purification and characterization. Biochemistry 23:4510, 1984
8. Regan JW, Nakata H, Demarinis RM et al: Purification and characterization of the human platelet α_2-adrenergic receptor. J Biol Chem 261:3894, 1986
9. Kobilka BK, Dixon RAF, Frielle T et al: cDNA for the human β_2-adrenergic receptor: a protein with multiple membrane spanning domains and a chromosomal location shared with the PDGF receptor gene. Proc Natl Acad Sci U S A 84:46, 1987
10. Kobilka BK, Matsui H, Kobilka TS et al: Cloning, sequencing, and expression of the gene coding for human platelet α_2-adrenergic receptor. Science 238:650, 1987
11. Cotecchia S, Schwinn DA, Randall RR et al: Molecular cloning and expression of the cDNA for the hamster α_1-adrenergic receptor. Proc Natl Acad Sci U S A 85:7159, 1988
12. Cowan AC, Zuker CS, Rubin GM: A rhodopsin gene expressed in photoreceptor cell R of the drosophila eye: homologies with other signal-transducing molecules. Cell 44:705, 1986

13. Emorine LJ, Marullo S, Delavier-Klutcho C et al: Structure of the gene for human β_2 adrenergic receptor: expression and promoter characterization. Proc Natl Acad Sci U S A 84:6995, 1987

14. Frielle T, Collins S, Daniel KW et al: Cloning of the cDNA for the human β_1-adrenergic receptor. Proc Natl Acad Sci U S A 84:7920, 1987

15. Kobilka BK, Frielle T, Dohlman HG et al: Delineation of the intronless nature of the genes for the human and hamster β_2-adrenergic receptor and their putative promoter regions. J Biol Chem 262:7321, 1987

16. Lomasney JW, Cotecchia S, Lorenz W et al: Molecular cloning and expression of the cDNA for the α_{1A}-adrenergic receptor. J Biol Chem 266:6365, 1991

17. Lomasney JW, Lorenze W, Allen LF et al: Expansion of the α_2-adrenergic receptor family: cloning and characterization of a human α_2-adrenergic receptor subtype, the gene for which is located on chromosome 2. Proc Natl Acad Sci U S A 87:5094, 1990

18. Regan JW, Kobilka TS, Yang-Feng TL et al: Cloning and expression of a human kidney cDNA for an α_2-adrenergic receptor subtype. Proc Natl Acad Sci U S A 85:6301, 1988

19. Schwinn DA, Lomasney JL, Szklut PJ et al: Molecular cloning and expression of the cDNA for a novel α_1-adrenergic receptor subtype. J Biol Chem 265:8183, 1990

20. Zeng D, Harrison JK, D'Angelo DD et al: Molecular characterization of a rat α_{2B}-adrenergic receptor. Proc Natl Acad Sci U S A 87:3102, 1990

21. Kyte J, Doolittle RF: A simple method for displaying the hydropathic character of protein. J Mol Biol 157:105, 1982

22. Dohlman HG, Caron MG, Lefkowitz RJ: Structure and function of the β_2-adrenergic receptor—homology with rhodopsin. Kidney Int, suppl. 23:S-2, 1987

23. Henderson R, Unwin PN: Three-dimensional model of purple membrane obtained by electron microscopy. Nature 257:28, 1975

24. George ST, Ruoho AE, Malbon CC: N-glycosylation in expression and function of β-adrenergic receptors. J Biol Chem 261:16559, 1986

25. O'Dowd BF, Lefkowitz RJ, Caron MG: Structure of the adrenergic and related receptors. Annu Rev Neurosci 12:67, 1989

26. Singer SJ, Maher PA, Yaffe MP: On the transfer of integral proteins into membranes. Proc Natl Acad Sci U S A 84:1960, 1987

27. Strader CD, Sigal IS, Dixon RAF: Mapping the functional domains of the β-adrenergic receptor. Am J Respir Cell Mol Biol 1:81, 1989

28. Dohlman HG, Caron MG, DeBlasi A et al: Role of extracellular disulfide-bonded cysteines in the ligand binding function of the β_2-adrenergic receptor. Biochemistry 29:2336, 1990

29. O'Dowd BF, Hnatowich M, Caron MG et al: Palmitoylation of the human β_2-adrenergic receptor. Mutation of CYS in the carboxyl tail leads to an uncoupled nonpalmitoylated form of the receptor. J Biol Chem 264:7564, 1989

30. Kobilka BK, Kobilka TS, Daniel K et al: Chimeric α_2-β_2-adrenergic receptors: delineation of domains involved in effector coupling and ligand binding specificity. Science 240:1310, 1988

31. Dohlman HG, Caron MG, Strader CD et al: Identification and sequence of a binding site peptide of the β_2-adrenergic receptor. Biochemistry 27:1813, 1988

32. Regan JW, Demarinis RM, Caron MG, Lefkowitz RJ: Identification of the subunit site of α_2-adrenergic receptors using [^{3}H]phenoxybenzamine. J Biol Chem 259:7864, 1984

33. Strader CD, Sigal IS, Dixon RAF: Structural basis of β-adrenergic receptor function. FASEB J 3:1826, 1989

34. Jasper JR, Insel PA: Evolving concepts of partial agonism. The β-adrenergic receptor as a paradigm. Biochem Pharmacol 43:119, 1992

35. Strader CD, Sigal IS, Candelore MR et al: Conserved aspartic acid residues 79 and 113 of the β-adrenergic receptor have different roles in receptor function. J Biol Chem 263:10267, 1989

36. Strader CR, Candelore MR, Hill WS et al: Identification of two serine residues involved in agonist activation of the β-adrenergic receptor. J Biol Chem 264:13572, 1989

37. Dixon RAF, Sigal IS, Strader CD: Structure-function analysis of the β-adrenergic receptor. Cold Spring Harb Symp Quant Biol 53:487, 1988

38. Schwinn DA, Caron MG, Lefkowitz RJ: The beta-adrenergic receptor as a model for molecular structure-function relationships in G-protein coupled receptors. p. 1657. In Fozzard HA et al. (eds): The Heart and Cardiovascular System: Scientific Foundation. 2nd Ed. Vol. 1. Raven Press, New York, 1992

39. Helper JR, Gilman AG: G proteins. Trends Biochem Sci 17:383, 1992

40. Olate J, Allende JE: Structure and function of G proteins. Pharmacol Ther 51:403, 1991

41. Findlay JGC, Pappin DJC: The ospin family of proteins. Biochem J 238:625, 1986

42. Cotecchia S, Exum S, Caron MG, Lefkowitz RJ: Regions of the α-adrenergic receptor involved in coupling to phosphoinositol hydrolysis and enhanced sensitivity of biological function. Proc Natl Acad Sci U S A 87:2896, 1990

43. Kubo T, Bujo H, Akiba I et al: Location of a region of the muscarinic acetylcholine receptor involved in selective effector coupling. FEBS Lett 241:119, 1988

44. Wong SK-F, Parker EM, Ross EM: Chimeric muscarinic cholinergic: β-adrenergic receptors that activate Gs in response to muscarinic agonists. J Biol Chem 265:6219, 1990

45. O'Dowd BF, Hnatowich M, Regan JW et al: Site-directed mutagenesis of the cytoplasmic domains of the human β_2-adrenergic receptor. J Biol Chem 263:15985, 1988

46. Hausdorff WP, Caron MG, Lefkowitz RJ: Turning off the signal: desensitization of β-adrenergic receptor function. FASEB J 4:2881, 1990

47. Sibley DR, Strasser RH, Benovic JL et al: Phosphorylation/dephosphorylation of the beta-adrenergic receptor regulates its functional coupling to adenylate cyclase and subcellular distribution. Proc Natl Acad Sci U S A 83:9408, 1986

48. Benovic JL, Pike LJ, Cerione RA et al: Phosphorylation of the mammalian beta-adrenergic receptor by cyclic AMP-dependent protein kinase: regulation of the rate of receptor phosphorylation and dephosphorylation by agonist occupancy and effects on coupling of the receptor to the stimulatory guanine nucleotide regulatory protein. J Biol Chem 260:7094, 1985

49. Liggett SB, Bouvier M, Hausdorff WP et al: Altered patterns of agonist-stimulated cAMP accumulation in cells expressing mutant β_2-adrendegic receptors lacking phosphorylation sites. Mol Pharmacol 36:641, 1989

50. Green DA, Clark RB: Adenylate cyclase coupling proteins are not essential for agonist-specific desensitization of lymphoma cells. J Biol Chem 256:2105, 1981

51. Benovic JL, Strasser RH, Caron MG, Lefkowitz RJ: β-Adrenergic receptor kinase: identification of a novel protein kinase that phosphorylates the agonist-occupied form of the receptor. Proc Natl Acad Sci U S A 83:2797, 1986

52. Benovic JL, Regan JW, Matsui H et al: Agonist-dependent phosphorylation of the α_2-adrenergic receptor by the β-adrenergic receptor kinase. J Biol Chem 262:17251, 1987

53. Benovic JL, Mayor F, Jr, Somers RL et al: Light-dependent phosphorylation of rhodopsin by β-adrenergic receptor kinase. Nature 322:869, 1986

54. Bouvier M, Hausdorff WP, De Blasi A et al: Removal of phosphorylation sites from the β_2-adrenergic receptor delays onset of agonist-promoted desensitisation. Nature 333:370, 1988

55. Benovic JL, Kuhn H, Weyland I et al: Functional desensitization of the isolated β-adrenergic receptor by the β-adrenergic receptor kinase: potential role of an analog of the retinal protein arrestin (48-kDa protein). Proc Natl Acad Sci U S A 84:8879, 1987

56. Lohse MJ, Benovic JL, Codina J et al: β-Arrestin—a protein that regulates β-adrenergic receptor function. Science 248:1547, 1990

57. Chuang D-M, Costa E: Evidence for internalization of the recognition site of beta-adrenergic receptors during receptor subsensiivity induced by ($-$)-isoproterenol. Proc Natl Acad Sci U S A 76:3024, 1979

58. Hertel C, Muller P, Portenier M, Staehelin M: Determination of the desensitization of beta-adrenergic receptors by [^{3}H]CGP-12177. Biochem J 216:669, 1983

59. Staechelin M, Hertel CJ: [^{3}H]CGP-12177, a beta-adrenergic ligand suitable for measuring cell surface receptors. J Recept Res 3:35, 1983

60. Lohse MJ, Benovic JL, Caron MG, Lefkowitz RJ: Multiple pathways of rapid β_2-adrenergic receptor desensitization: delineation with specific inhibitors. J Biol Chem 265:3202, 1990

61. Strader CD, Sigal IS, Blake AD et al: The carboxyl terminus of the hamster β-adrenergic receptor expressed in mouse L cells is not required for receptor sequestration. Cell 49:855, 1987

62. Su Y-F, Harden TK, Perkins JP: Isoproterenol-induced desensitization of adenylate cyclase in human astrocytoma cells: relation of loss of hormonal responsiveness and decrement in beta-adrenergic receptors. J Biol Chem 254:38, 1979

63. Doss RC, Perkins JP, Harden TK: Recovery of beta-adrenergic receptors following long term exposure of astrocytoma cells to catecholamine: role of protein synthesis. J Biol Chem 256:12281, 1981

64. Morishima I, Thompson WJ, Robison GA, Strada SJ: Loss and restoration of sensitivity to epinephrine in cultured BHK cells: effect of inhibitors of RNA and protein synthesis. J Mol Pharmacol 18:370, 1980

65. Hadock JR, Malbon CC: Agonist regulation of gene expression of adrenergic receptors and G proteins. J Neurochem 60:1, 1993

66. Nichols AJ, Ruffolo RR: Functions mediated by α-adrenoreceptors. p. 115. In Ruffolo RR (ed): Pro-

gress in Basic and Clinical Pharmacology. Vol. 8. Karger, Basel, 1991

67. Ruffolo RR, Nichols AJ, Stadel JM, Hieble JP: Structure and function of α-adrenoreceptors. Pharmacol Rev 43:475, 1991

68. Starke K, Montel H, Wagner J: Effect of phentolamine on noradrenaline uptake and release. Naunyn Schmiedesbergs Arch Pharmacol 271:181, 1971

69. Langer SZ: Presynaptic regulation of catecholamine release. Biochem Pharmacol 23:1793, 1974

70. Langer SZ, Shepperson NB: Recent developments in vascular smooth muscle pharmacology: the postsynaptic α2-adrenoreceptor. Trends Pharmacol Sci 3:440, 1982

71. Schimmel RJ: Role of α- and β-adrenoreceptors in the control of glucose oxidation in hamster epididymal adipocytes. Biochim Biophys Acta 428:379, 1976

72. Berthelsen S, Pettinger WA: A functional basis for classification of α-adrenergic receptors. Life Sci 21:595, 1977

73. Drew GM, Whiting SB: Evidence for two distinct types of postsynaptic α-adrenoreceptors in vascular smooth muscle in vivo. Br J Pharmacol 67:207, 1979

74. Agrawal DK, Triggle GR, Daniel EE: Pharmacological characterization of the postsynaptic α-adrenoreceptors in vascular smooth muscle from canine and rat mesenteric arterial beds. J Pharmacol Exp Ther 229:364, 1984

75. Flavahn NA, Vanhoutte PM: α1-Adrenoreceptor subclassification in vascular smooth muscle. Trends Pharmacol Sci 7:347, 1986

76. Lomasney JW, Cotechia S, Lefkowitz RJ, Caron MC: Molecular biology of a-adrenergic receptors: implications for receptor classification and for structure-function relationships. Biochim Biophys Acta 1095:127, 1991

77. Wilson KM, Minneman KP: Different pathways of [^{3}H]inositol phosphate formation mediated by α1A- and α1B-adrenergic receptors. J Biol Chem 265:17601, 1990

78. Schwinn DA, Lomasney JW: Pharmacologic characterization of cloned a1-adrenoreceptor subtypes: selective antagonists suggest the existence of a fourth subtype. Eur J Pharmacol 227:433, 1992

79. McCune SK, Voigt MM, Hill JM: Developmental expression of the alpha-1A, alpha-1B and alpha-1C adrenergic receptor subtype mRNA in the rat brain. J Neurosci 18:457, 1992

80. Schwinn DA, Page SO, Middleton JP et al: The alpha 1C-adrenergic receptor: characterization of signal transduction pathways and mammalian tissue heterogeneity. Mol Pharmacol 40:619, 1991

81. Berridge MJ, Dawson RMC, Downes CP et al: Changes in the levels of inositol phosphates after agonist-dependent hydrolysis of membrane phosphoinositides. Biochem J 212:473, 1983

82. Berridge MJ, Irvine R: Inositol trisphosphate, a novel second messenger in cellular signal transduction. Nature 312:315, 1984

83. Han C, Abel PW, Minneman KP: α1-Adrenoreceptor subtypes linked to different mechanisms for increasing intracellular Ca^{2+} in smooth muscle. Nature 329:333, 1987

84. Han C, Wilson KM, Minneman KP: α1-Adrenergic receptor subtypes and formation of inositol phosphates in dispersed hepatocytes and renal cells. Mol Pharmacol 37:903, 1990

85. Cotecchia S, Exum S, Caron MG, Lefkowitz RJ: Regions of the alpha 1-adrenergic receptor involved in coupling to phosphatidylinositol hydrolysis and enhanced sensitivity of biological function. Proc Natl Acad Sci U S A 87:2896, 1990

86. Cotecchia S, Ostrowski J, Kjelsberg MA et al: Discrete amino acid sequences of the alpha 1-adrenergic receptor determine the selectivity of coupling to phosphatidylinositol hydrolysis. J Biol Chem 267:1633, 1992

87. Kjelsberg MA, Cotecchia S, Ostrowski J et al: Constitutive activation of the alpha 1B-adrenergic receptor by all amino acid substitutions at a single site. Evidence for a region which constrains receptor activation. J Biol Chem 267:1430, 1992

88. Sternweis PC, Smrcka AV: Regulation of phospholipase C by G proteins. Trends Biochem Sci 17:502, 1992

89. Wu D, Katz A, Lee C, Simon MI: Activation of phospholipase C by α1-adrenergic receptors is mediated by the subunits of Gq family. J Biol Chem 267:25798, 1992

90. Leeb-Lundberg LM, Cotecchia S, Lomasney JW et al: Phorbol esters promote alpha 1-adrenergic receptor phosphorylation and receptor uncoupling from inositol phospholipid metabolism. Proc Natl Acad Sci U S A 82:5651, 1985

91. Cotecchia S, Leeb-Lundberg LM, Hagen PO et al: Phorbol ester effects on alpha 1-adrenoceptor binding and phosphatidylinositol metabolism in cultured vascular smooth muscle cells. Life Sci 37:2389, 1985

92. Leeb-Lundberg LMF, Cotecchia S, Caron MG, Lefkowitz RJ: Regulation of adrenergic receptor function by phosphorylation. Agonist-promoted desensitization and phosphorylation of α1-adrenergic

receptors coupled to inositol phospholipid metabolism in DDT1 MF2 smooth muscle cells. J Biol Sci 262:3098, 1986

93. Farago A, Nishizuka Y: Protein kinase C in transmembrane signalling. FEBS Lett 268:350, 1990

94. Kaukinen S, Kaukinen L, Eerola R: Postoperative use of clonidine with neuroleptanesthesia. Acta Anaesthesiol Scand 23:113, 1979

95. Bloor BC, Flacke WE: Reduction of halothane anesthetic requirement by clonidine, an alpha adrenergic agonist. Anesth Analg 61:741, 1982

96. Maze M, Tranquilli W: Alpha-2 adrenoceptor agonists: defining the role in clinical anesthesia. Anesthesiology 74:581, 1991

97. Correa-Sales C, Rabin BC, Maze M: A hypnotic response to dexmedetomidine, and $\alpha2$ agonist, is mediated in the locus coeruleus in rats. Anesthesiology 76:948, 1992

98. Scheinin M, Schwinn DA: The locus coeruleus. Site of hypnotic action of $\alpha2$-adrenergic agonists. Anesthesiology 76:873, 1992

99. Maze M, Regan JW: Role of signal transduction in anesthetic action of $\alpha2$-adrenergic agonists. Ann N Y Acad Sci 625:409, 1991

100. Weber H: Uber Anesthesie durch adrenalin. Verh Dtsch Ges Inn Med 21:616, 1904

101. Bylund DB: Heterogeneity of alpha-2 adrenergic receptors. Pharmacol Biochem Rev 22:835, 1985

102. Bylund DB: Subtypes of $\alpha1$ and $\alpha2$-adrenergic receptors. FASEB J 6:832, 1992

103. Bylund DB, Blaxall HS, Iversen LJ et al: Pharmacological characteristics of alpha-2 adrenergic receptors: comparison of pharmacologically defined subtypes with subtypes identified by molecular cloning. Mol Pharmacol 42:1, 1992

104. Lorenz W, Lomasney JW, Collins S et al: Expression of three $\alpha2$-adrenergic receptor subtypes in rat tissues: implications for $\alpha2$ receptor classification. Mol Pharmacol 38:599, 1990

105. Lawhead RG, Blaxall HS, Bylund DB: α-2A is the predominant α-2 adrenergic receptor subtype in human spinal cord. Anesthesiology 77:983, 1992

106. Limbird LE: Receptors linked to inhibition of adenylate cyclase: additional signaling mechanisms. FASEB J 2:2686, 1988

107. Eason MG, Kurose H, Holt BD et al: Simultaneous coupling of alpha 2-adrenergic receptors to two G-proteins with opposing effects. Subtype-selective coupling of alpha 2C10, alpha 2C4, and alpha 2C2 adrenergic receptors to Gi and Gs. J Biol Chem 267:15795, 1992

108. Dunlap K, Holz GG, Rane SG: G proteins are regulators of ion channel function. Trends Neurosci 14:103, 1987

109. Liggett SB, Ostrowski J, Chestnut LC et al: Sites in the third intracellular loop of the $\alpha2A$-adrenergic receptor confer short term agonist promoted desensitization. J Biol Chem 267:4740, 1992

110. Luttrell LM, Ostrowski J, Cotecchia S et al: Antagonism of catecholamine receptor signalling by expression of cytoplasmic domains of the receptors. Science 259:1453, 1993

Chapter 27

Drugs Affecting Adrenoceptors: α_2 Agonists

Yukio Hayashi and Mervyn Maze

MOLECULAR PHARMACOLOGY

Ahlquist[1] differentiated adrenoceptors into α and β based on the rank order of potency of various natural and synthetic catecholamines in different physiologic preparations. The next substantial advance in α adrenoceptor pharmacology was based on the identification of a receptor that regulated the release of neurotransmitters.[2] From this, it was inferred that the receptor was located presynaptically.[3] This led to a subdivision of α adrenoceptors based on their synaptic location into postsynaptic, α_1, and presynaptic, α_2.[4] A classification strictly based on anatomic location was proved to be untenable in the light of the finding of postsynaptically and even extrasynaptically located α_2 adrenoceptors not linked to neurotransmitter release.[5] As more selective α adrenoceptor antagonists became available, it was possible to separate definitively the α adrenoceptors into two subtypes on a pharmacologic basis based on the antagonists yohimbine and prazosin (Fig. 27-1).[6] At α_1 adrenoceptors, prazosin is more potent than yohimbine, whereas at the α_2 adrenoceptors, yohimbine is more potent than prazosin.

Subtypes of α_2 Adrenoceptors

Pharmacologic Subtypes of α_2 Adrenoceptors

Soon after the discovery of α_2 adrenoceptors on postsynaptic and extrasynaptic sites, it became apparent that all α_2 adrenoceptors do not have the same pharmacologic characteristics.[7] They were all activated by the classic adrenergic agonists epinephrine and norepinephrine and were sensitive to blockade by yohimbine (thus fulfilling the basic criteria for α_2 adrenoceptors), but variability was observed in the rank order of potency of other α adrenergic ligands at the receptors in different tissues.[8–10] The α_1 adrenergic ligands prazosin and oxymetazoline were found to discriminate between two classes of α_2-adrenoceptors, termed α_{2A} and α_{2B}; in binding studies, oxymetazoline was bound with 50-fold higher affinity to the α_{2A} subtype compared with α_{2B}, whereas prazosin bound to α_{2B} receptors with relatively high affinity (K_i, 5 nM) compared with α_{2A} receptors (K_i, 300 nM).

Some cells and tissues were found to express a single receptor subtype; examples include α_{2A}

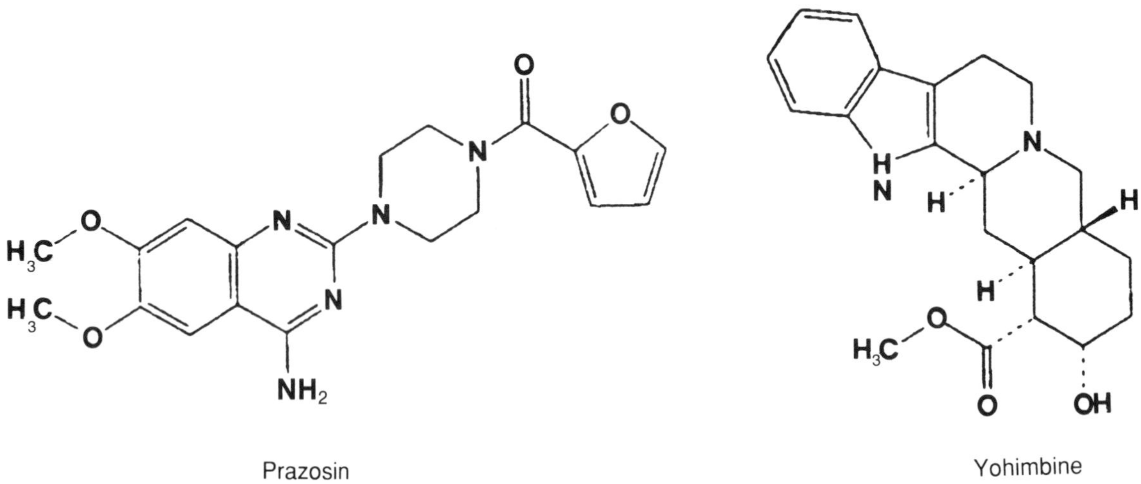

Fig. 27-1 Structures of the α adrenoceptor antagonists, prazosin and yohimbine. Prazosin is relatively more selective for α_1 adrenoceptors, whereas yohimbine is more selective for α_2 adrenoceptors.

adrenoceptors on blood platelets and α_{2B} adrenoceptors in neonatal rat lung.[9] Mixed receptor subtype populations were detected in rat brain and human caudate nucleus, whereas the human cerebral cortex was found to contain predominantly α_{2A} adrenoceptors.[8,11,12] More detailed pharmacologic studies suggested the existence of a third (α_{2C}) subtype.[13]

None of these pharmacologic subtypes has been conclusively identified as the presynaptic α_2-adrenoceptor regulating neuronal release of norepinephrine; in fact, recent results with 10 different α_2 adrenoceptor antagonists indicate that heterogeneity may exist in drug affinities also among presynaptic α_2 adrenoceptors.[14]

A definitive subtyping of α_2 adrenoceptor gene expression at the cellular level (e.g., by in situ hybridization) will be important for the understanding of noradrenergic mechanisms in the central nervous system and in peripheral tissues. This pertains especially to α_2 adrenoceptor gene expression in the locus ceruleus, where these receptors are important regulators of noradrenergic input to other brain centers and play a role in sleep, arousal, and anesthesia.[15–17] Likewise, the identification of α_2 adrenoceptor subtypes mediating the central antinociceptive and cardiovascular effects of α_2 adrenoceptor agonists, and their peripheral effects on vascular tone, endocrine, and renal functions, may have important practical consequences for drug development.

Imidazoline Binding Sites

Functional and radioligand binding studies indicate the existence of another class of receptors or binding sites that resemble the α_2 adrenoceptors. These sites selectively bind α_2 ligands that are either imidazolines (e.g., clonidine and idazoxan) or oxazolines (e.g., rilmenidine) but have very low affinity for agonists or antagonists without the imidazoline or oxazoline structure (e.g., epinephrine and yohimbine).[18] No imidazoline-preferring receptor has yet been cloned, and their structural and functional relationships to the α_2 adrenoceptors have not been clarified. In an attempt to find an endogenous ligand for the imidazoline-preferring receptor, a substance called "clonidine displacing substance" was derived from brain extracts.[19] The structure of this substance is not known, but it is not a catecholamine. It displaces [^{3}H]clonidine from brain membranes and has both clonidine-like and clonidine-antagonizing actions in the central nervous system and in isolated smooth muscle.

CLINICAL PHARMACOLOGY

α_2-Adrenergic agonists can be grouped, into three main classes; the imidazolines (e.g., clonidine), phenylethylamines (e.g., α-methylnorepinephrine), and oxaloazepines (e.g., rilmenidine and azepexole; Fig. 27-2). The ligands with an imidazole ring bind to nonadrenergic imidazole-preferring receptors and to the α_2-adrenoceptor.[18] The cardiovascular properties of α_2 ligands will vary considerably, depending on whether the imidazole-preferring receptor is also bound.[20]

Clonidine, an imidazole compound, is a selective agonist for α_2 adrenoceptors with a ratio of 200 : 1 (α_2/α_1). In many models of α_2 action, clonidine has been identified as a partial agonist. Clonidine is rapidly and almost completely absorbed after oral administration and reaches a peak plasma level within 60 to 90 minutes by this route. Clonidine can also be delivered using a time release transdermal patch, although a minimum of 2 days must elapse before therapeutic levels are achieved (see Ch. 31).[21] The elimination half-life of clonidine is 9 to 12 hours with about one-half of the drug being metabolized in the liver to inactive metabolites, while the rest is excreted unchanged in the kidney.

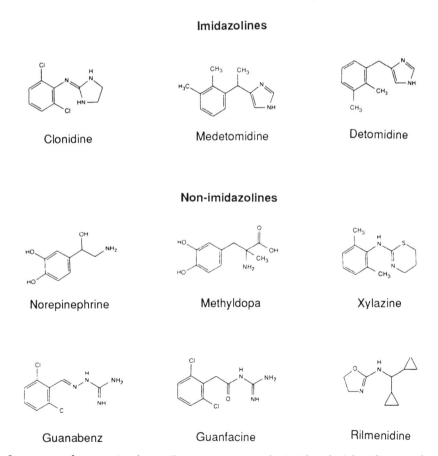

Imidazolines

Clonidine   Medetomidine   Detomidine

Non-imidazolines

Norepinephrine   Methyldopa   Xylazine

Guanabenz   Guanfacine   Rilmenidine

Fig. 27-2 Structures of α agonist drugs. Drugs containing the imidazole (clonidine, medetomidine, or detomidine) or oxazolamine (rilmenidine) rings also bind to nonadrenergic imidazole-preferring receptors.

Medetomidine, 4(5)-[1-2,3-dimethylphenyl)-ethyl]imidazole, is the prototype of the novel superselective α_2 agonists. It is an order of magnitude more selective than clonidine and is a full agonist at this class of receptor.[22] Medetomidine is extremely potent and is active at low nanomolar concentrations. It has been widely used in veterinary practice in Europe. Medetomidine is a chiral molecule, the D-enantiomer being more active. Thus, dexmedetomidine (D-medetomidine) has been developed for clinical use. At the time of writing this chapter, Phase II (preclinical) studies with this compound had been launched in the United States; in Europe, the drug was in clinical trials.

Methyldopa is metabolized to α-methylnorepinephrine, which is a full agonist at the α_2 receptor and has a 10-fold selectivity for the α_2 over the α_1 adrenoceptor. Because transformation into the active compound is necessary, effects are slow to develop (4 to 6 hours) and somewhat unpredictable. It is the only α_2 agonist available for parenteral use in the United States.

Azepexole (BHT 933) is an oxaloazepine that decreases anesthetic requirements by nearly 90 percent in dogs.[23] BHT 920 is a thiazolazepine that is chemically related to azepexole. Although BHT 920 is more potent than azepexole at the α_2-adrenoceptor,[24] it is relatively nonspecific because it also exerts considerable activity at dopamine receptors.

Guanabenz is similar to clonidine in its effects; however, it is less potent and shorter acting with a terminal elimination half-life of 6 hours. Doses for the antihypertensive effect range from 8 to 32 mg/day. Guanfacine has the longest half-life (14 to 18 hours) of all the clinically available α_2 agonists. Like guanabenz, guanfacine is a guanidine compound and is eliminated by renal excretion. This drug is administered once daily in a dose ranging from 1 to 3 mg.

Xylazine is a phenylamine that has been used in veterinary medicine to anesthetize dogs and cats. Detomidine, an imidazole compound related to dexmedetomidine, is a sedative and analgesic useful in horses and cattle. The sedative potency is approximately equal to that of clonidine and much higher than that of xylazine.[25]

Central Nervous System

Sedation is the most consistent central effect of α_2 adrenergic agonists.[26] Although this property is an undesirable side effect when α_2 agonists are used to treat hypertension, it is an advantage in anesthesia. This effect of α_2 agonists is significantly potentiated when administered together with a benzodiazepine (Fig. 27-3).[27] Recently, the locus ceruleus was shown to be a principal brain region responsible for the sedative effect in rats (Fig. 27-4).[17]

The α_2 agonists also produce anxiolysis, comparable to that produced by benzodiazepines.[28] Clonidine can also suppress panic disorder in humans.[29] However, higher doses of nonselective α_2 agonists may actually increase anxiety through activation of α_1 adrenoceptors.[30]

The α_2-adrenergic receptor activation produces potent analgesia, involving both supraspinal and spinal sites of action.[31,32] Clonidine exerts a more potent analgesic effect than does morphine in animals.[33] Furthermore, the analgesic potency of α_2

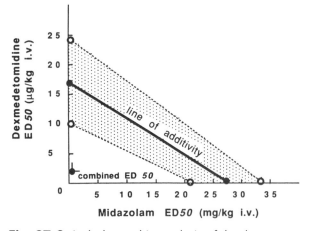

Fig. 27-3 Isobolographic analysis of the dose-response curves of midazolam and dexmedetomidine alone and in combination for the loss of the righting reflex. The ED$_{50}$ values for dexmedetomidine and midazolam alone were obtained by probit analysis of the individual drugs' dose-response curves and are plotted on the ordinate and abscissa, respectively. A line of additivity (solid line) connects these points and is banded by 95 percent confidence limits. The ED$_{50}$ value of the combination (●, lower left) is also plotted. The departure of the combined ED$_{50}$ from the line of additivity indicates synergistic activity. (From Salonen et al.,[27] with permission.)

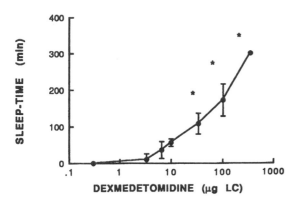

Fig. 27-4 Log dose-response curve for the hypnotic action of dexmedetomidine delivered into the left locus ceruleus of rats. The duration of loss of righting reflex was measured (sleep time). (From Correa-Sales et al.,[17] with permission.)

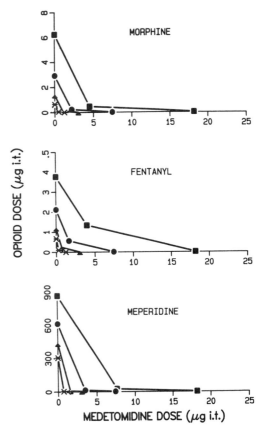

Fig. 27-5 Isobolograms for the 25 (*), 50 (▲), 75 (●), and 100 percent (■) effective intrathecal doses of medetomidine plotted against morphine (top), fentanyl (middle), and meperidine (bottom) in the rat tail flick test. The isobol points are shown for ratios of medetomidine to morphine (10:1), fentanyl (3:1), and meperidine (1:3). These results are characteristic of a synergistic interaction. (From Ossipov et al.,[35] with permission.)

agonists is synergistically enhanced by concomitant treatment with opioids (Fig. 27-5).[34,35] Both α_2 agonists and opioids mediate their analgesic actions through independent receptors, although these two classes of agents have a similar transduction pathway in their effector mechanism.[36] The transduction pathway may be the site of development of cross-tolerance between these two agents.[37] The α_2 agonists suppress the abstinance syndrome following withdrawal of opioids.[38] The α_2 agonists have also been used to treat abstinence syndromes related to alcohol and benzodiazepines.[39] Dexmedetomidine was reported to suppress ischemic pain[40] and to attenuate the affective component of ischemic pain.[41]

The α_2 agonists reduce anesthetic requirements. Kaukinen and Pyykko[42] demonstrated a modest reduction (15 percent) of halothane minimum alveolar concentration (MAC) following administration of clonidine in rabbits. Bloor and Flacke[43] observed that clonidine reduced halothane MAC by up to 50 percent, in a dose dependent fashion. This MAC reducing effect was antagonized by tolazoline, an α_2 antagonist. The ceiling to MAC reduction by clonidine is caused by stimulation of α_1 adrenoceptors. More selective α_2 agonists are able to reduce the MAC of volatile anaesthetics to a greater extent. Azepexole was shown to reduce isoflurane MAC by 85 percent in dogs.[23] Dexmedetomidine, a highly selective α_2 agonist, decreased halothane MAC by more than 95 percent in rats (Fig. 27-6),[44] suggesting that dexmedetomidine alone may produce an anesthetic state. The reduction in anesthetic requirement can also be demonstrated in humans and is not limited to volatile anesthetics (discussed subsequently).

The α_2 agonists can reduce intraocular pressure and also attenuate the rise in intraocular pressure associated with laryngoscopy and endotracheal in-

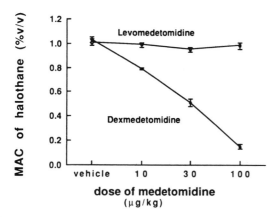

Fig. 27-6 The MAC for halothane was determined in rats before and after either the d or the l enantiomer of medetomidine. D-medetomidine (dexmedetomidine) produced a dose-related reduction in halothane MAC; l-medetomidine dod not. MAC, minimum alveolar concentration. (From Segal et al.,[44] with permission.)

tubation.[45] An early report showed that this action might be caused by a reduction in production and augmentation in outflow of aqueous humor; however, this has not been definitely established. The imidazole-preferring receptor has also been implicated in this action.[46]

The α_2 agonists and antagonists have been used experimentally for protection from cerebral ischemia. Hoffman et al.[47,48] reported that the α_2 agonists, clonidine and dexmedetomidine, could improve the outcome from incomplete global ischemia (Fig. 27-7). However, Gustafson et al.[49,50] demonstrated that idazoxan, an α_2 antagonist, could also protect against global ischemia. This paradox may have been reconciled by a study by Maiese et al.[51] They have shown that both an α_2 antagonist, idazoxan, and agonist, rilmenidine, with affinity for the imidazole-preferring receptor, are able to protect against cerebral ischemia. They

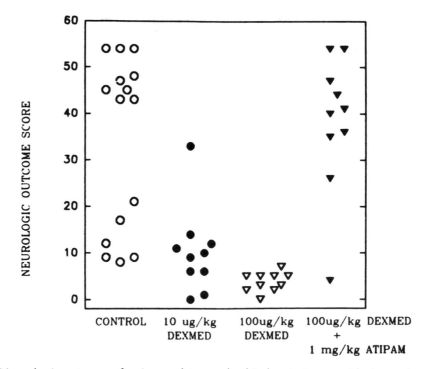

Fig. 27-7 Neurologic outcome after incomplete cerebral ischemia in rats with dexmedetomidine and atipamezole (α_2-adrenoceptor antagonist) treatment. A high score indicates a poor outcome. Neurologic outcome was improved with 10 and 100 μg/kg of dexmedetomidine compared with the control group ($P < 0.05$). (From Hoffman et al.,[48] with permission.)

hypothesized that the imidazole-preferring receptor, and not α_2 receptors, is involved in the neuroprotective mechanism.

Cardiovascular System

The cardiovascular actions of α_2 agonists may be classified as peripheral or central. The α_2 agonists inhibit norepinephrine release from peripheral prejunctional nerve endings; this property contributes to the heart rate lowering effect of α_2 agonists.[52] There is no evidence to support the existence of postsynaptic α_2 receptors in the myocardium.[53,54] Therefore direct effects of α_2 agonists on the heart are doubtful. Postjunctional α_2 receptors are present in both arteries and veins, in which they produce vasoconstriction.[55] A vasoconstrictive action of α_2 agonists on the coronary vasculature would be not favorable in the ischemic heart.[56,57] However, α_2 agonists can reduce sympathetic outflow, possibly ameliorating any direct vasoconstriction.[58] Furthermore, α_2 agonists released endothelial-derived relaxant factor in coronary arteries[59] and enhanced coronary blood flow induced by endogenous and exogenous adenosine in dogs.[60] Thus, the effect of α_2 agonists on coronary arteries may be very complicated.[61]

Clonidine is capable of producing hypotension and bradycardia. The mechanism of these actions may involve decreased sympathetic and increased parasympathetic activity. However, the precise mechanisms involved in these actions are not well understood. The nucleus tractus solitarius (a site known to modulate autonomic control, including vagal activity) is an important central site for the action of α_2 agonists.[62] However other nuclei, including the locus ceruleus,[63] the dorsal motor nucleus of the vagus,[64] and the nucleus reticularis lateralis,[65] may also mediate hypotension and/or bradycardia. Bousquet et al.[66] documented that imidazole-preferring receptors play an important role in the hypotensive effect of α_2 agonists. They also suggested that the α_2 agonists exert their hypotensive and sedative effects by different mechanisms.

The α_2 agonists have cardiac antiarrhythmic effects. Dexmedetomidine prevented epinephrine induced arrhythmias during halothane anesthesia in dogs (Fig. 27-8).[67] Central α_2 receptors and imidazole-preferring receptors are involved. The antiarrhythmic effects were totally abolished by vagotomy.[68]

The effect of α_2 agonists on the cerebral circulation has been studied during anesthesia. Zornow et al.[69] and Karlsson et al.[70] demonstrated that dexmedetomidine decreased cerebral blood flow in dogs anesthetized with isoflurane or halothane. McPherson and Traystman[71] reported that dexmedetomidine reduced the increase in cerebral blood flow that occurred in response to hypoxemia during isoflurane anesthesia.

Respiratory System

The respiratory depressant effects of clonidine are mild[72] unless massive doses are given.[73] The respiratory depressant effect of clonidine was less than that of opioids in rodents.[74] Clonidine blunts the ventilatory response to hypercarbia in humans.[75,76] However, clonidine did not potentiate opioid induced respiratory depression (Fig. 27-9).[76] Nebulized clonidine attenuated bronchoconstriction in asthmatic patients.[77] Eisenach[79] reported that intravenous clonidine produced hypoxemia in sheep as a result of the aggregation of platelets in the pulmonary circulation.[78]

Endocrine System

The α_2 agonists stimulate the secretion of growth hormone.[79] Devesa et al.[80] suggested that α_2-adrenoceptor activation is coupled to growth hormone releasing factor. The α_2 agonists that possess an imidazole ring may inhibit steroidogenesis. However with clinically relevant doses of α_2 agonists, this effect is not likely to have serious consequences.[81] The α_2 agonists decrease sympathoadrenal outflow, and they can suppress the stress response following surgical stimulation.[82] The α_2 agonists may regulate catecholamine secretion in the adrenal medulla,[83] but this effect has been questioned.[84] The α_2 agonists also directly inhibit the release of insulin from the pancreatic β cells.[85] However, this effect did not appear to be clinically significant.[86]

Gastrointestinal System

The α_2 agonists reduce salivary flow.[87] The α_2 agonists can modulate the release of gastric acid by a presynaptic mechanism.[88] However, no significant

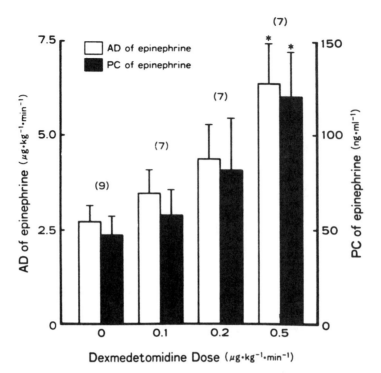

Fig. 27-8 Arrhythmogenic doses (*AD*) and plasma concentrations (*PC*) of epinephrine in the presence of dexmedetomidine during halothane anesthesia in dogs. *$P < 0.05$ compared with the 0 dose. (From Hayashi et al.,[67] with permission.)

change in gastric pH was observed in humans.[89] The α_2 agonists may prevent water and electrolyte secretion in the large bowel, suggesting possible utility in the treatment of watery diarrhea.[90]

Renal System

The α_2 agonists induce diuresis. Inhibition of the release of antidiuretic hormone,[91] antagonism of the renal tubular action of antidiuretic hormone,[92] and an increase in the glomerular filtration rate[93] have each been implicated in the mechanism. The α_2 agonist induced release of atrial natriuretic factor has also been suggested to contribute to the diuretic action.[94]

Hematologic System

The α_2 agonists induce aggregation of platelets.[95] In the clinical setting, this is probably offset by the decrease in circulating catecholamines.

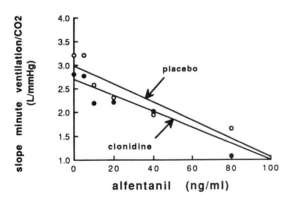

Fig. 27-9 Effect of alfentanil on the ventilatory response to hypercarbia with and without clonidine. (From Jarvis et al.,[76] with permission.)

PRACTICAL APPLICATIONS

Preanesthetic Administration

The sedative and anxiolytic effects of α_2 agonists make them suitable for use as anesthetic premedication.[96] Premedication with α_2 agonists potentiates the anesthetic actions of other agents and reduces anesthetic requirements during surgery. This effect has been observed with intravenous or volatile general anesthesia, or with regional anesthesia. Ghignone et al.[97] reported that premedication with oral clonidine, 5 μg/kg, reduced fentanyl requirements for induction and intubation by 45 percent in patients undergoing aortocoronary bypass surgery. Flacke et al.[98] demonstrated that clonidine reduced sufentanil requirements by 40 percent in a similar patient population. Engelman et al.[99] showed that preoperative clonidine (5 μg/kg) decreased the dose of droperidol required to prevent hypertension during aortic surgery. The dose of thiopental or propofol required for induction of anesthesia were reduced by preanesthetic administration of clonidine or dexmedetomidine.[89,100–102] Oral clonidine (150 μg) prolonged tetracaine spinal anesthesia.[103]

Minimizing the hemodynamic effects of endotracheal intubation and surgical stimulation is an important goal of anesthetic care. The α_2 agonists attenuate sympathoadrenal responses to stress. Carabine et al.[104] suggested that 200 μg of clonidine was an optimal dose and higher doses of clonidine did not offer any further advantage. Others recommended a higher dose.[45,105,106] The efficacy of dexmedetomidine has been extensively studied in Finland. Dexmedetomidine, 0.3 to 0.6 μg/kg intravenously, provided optimal premedication.[107–109] Aantaa et al.[110] also studied intramuscular dexmedetomidine and found that 1.0 μg/kg was adequate. However, the sedative effects may outlast the surgery at these doses. Flacke et al.[98] reported that the hemodynamic parameters were more favorable during aortocoronary bypass surgery and that lower doses of opioids were required when clonidine was administered. Ghignone et al.[97] corroborated the findings of Flacke et al.[98] in a similar patient population. Although these features also applied to patients undergoing aortic surgery,[111] this favorable property was absent in patients undergoing carotid artery surgery.[112] Oral clonidine was used successfully in geriatric patients undergoing eye surgery.[105] The use of α_2 agonist premedication in a pediatric population has not been reported.

Oral clonidine (300 μg) did not affect tidal volume, respiratory rate, or end-tidal carbon dioxide tension, but it did attenuate the ventilatory response to carbon dioxide, suggesting that clonidine has a respiratory depressant effect.[113] However, Bailey et al.[114] reported that oral clonidine (4 to 5 μg/kg) did not depress the CO_2 response. Jarvis et al.[77] also reported that CO_2 response was not affected. Oral clonidine did not potentiate the respiratory depression exerted by opioids.

Premedication with α_2 agonists may cause bradycardia and/or hypotension.[104] Atropine is the treatment of choice for bradycardia, but it should be noted that high doses of oral clonidine, 5 μg/kg, will slightly attenuate the effect of atropine (Fig. 27-10).[115] By contrast, clonidine potentiates the pressor effect exerted by ephedrine.[116]

Intraoperative Administration

Although α_2 agonists possess potent analgesic and sedative effects, these agents have not been widely used intraoperatively in place of other anesthetic agents. Segal et al.[119] reported that a combination of oral and transdermal clonidine (which maintained the plasma concentration of clonidine at therapeutic levels) provided lower anesthetic requirements, greater hemodynamic stability, more rapid recovery from anesthesia, and lower requirement for morphine for postoperative pain in patients undergoing lower abdominal surgeries. Quintin et al.[120] reported that an infusion of clonidine (7 μg/kg over 120 minutes) after removal of the aortic cross clamp reduced norepinephrine, epinephrine, and vasopressin concentrations during the postoperative recovery period. However, higher fluid volumes were required during the postoperative period. Intraoperative clonidine infusion (a loading dose of 4 μg/kg followed by 2 μg/kg/h until closure of the abdomen) enhanced the quality of postoperative morphine analgesia.[119]

The α_2 agonists have been administered into the intrathecal or epidural space. Racle et al.[120] showed that intrathecal clonidine (150 μg) prolonged bu-

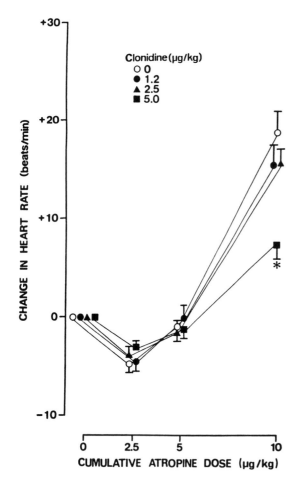

Fig. 27-10 Heart rate responses to atropine in patients receiving oral clonidine. Clonidine, 5.0 μg/kg, significantly attenuated the effect of atropine on heart rate (*$P < 0.05$). (From Nishikawa et al.,[115] with permission.)

pivacaine spinal anesthesia in elderly patients undergoing hip surgery, compared with the addition of epinephrine (200 μg). Bonnet et al.[121] demonstrated that clonidine prolonged tetracaine spinal anesthesia in a dose dependent fashion (Fig 27-11). The addition of clonidine to epidural lidocaine was reported to augment its anesthetic potency and provide sedation and relative hemodynamic stability compared with plain lidocaine or lidocaine with epinephrine.

Postoperative Administration

Epidural administration of α_2 agonists for postoperative pain control has been well investigated. The efficacy of postoperative clonidine depends on the

dose of the agonist and the severity of postoperative pain. In an early clinical study, Gordh[122] did not demonstrate any significant analgesic effect of epidural clonidine, 3 μg/kg, in patients after thoracotomy. Bonnet et al.[121] observed that epidural clonidine (2 μg/kg) produced brief but significant pain relief after peripheral orthopaedic surgery. Essen et al.[123] reported that 150 μg of epidural clonidine produce slight postoperative analgesia after abdominal hysterectomy. Eisenach et al.[124] examined the analgesic effect of epidural clonidine, ranging from 100 to 900 μg, in patients following total knee arthroplasty or abdominal surgery. Analgesia was estimated by verbal pain score and the need for supplemental morphine. Clonidine produced analgesia in a dose dependent manner, achieving complete pain relief for up to 5 hours without any sensory or motor blockade at the highest dose (700 to 900 μg) (Fig. 27-12). However, higher doses were associated with some disadvantages, including hypotension, bradycardia, and transient sedation, and they concluded that further studies would be required to evaluate these risks. Penon et al.[75] reported that 300 μg of epidural clonidine decreased the slope of the ventilatory response to CO_2 without changing unstimulated end-tidal CO_2, respiratory rate, or minute ventilation. Continuous epidural infusion following bolus injection of clonidine (800 μg bolus followed by 20 μg/h) has been suggested as an alternative method.[125] This regimen provided more than 6 hours of analgesia following cesarean section. Epidural clonidine has been combined with local anesthetics or opioids. The addition of 150 μg of clonidine to epidural fentanyl, morphine, and bupivacaine resulted in a longer duration of postoperative analgesia.[126–128] Furthermore, these combinations may reduce the effective dose of clonidine, resulting in less side effects. Intrathecal clonidine (150 μg) was used effectively as a sole analgesic agent after cesarean section without remarkable side effects.[129]

Systemic administration of clonidine for postoperative analgesia has also been reported. Bonnet et al.[130] compared the analgesic effect (visual analog scale) of intramuscular clonidine (2 μg/kg) with the same dose of epidural clonidine after minor orthopaedic or perineal surgery. The onset and duration of analgesia after intramuscular clonidine were

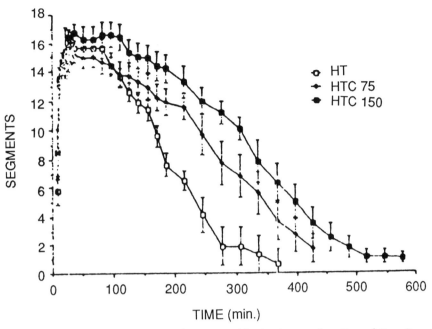

Fig. 27-11 Number of spinal segments with sensory blockade as a function of time (in minutes) with hyperbaric tetracaine (lower line), hyperbaric tetracaine plus clonidine, 75 μg (middle line), or hyperbaric tetracaine plus clonidine, 150 μg (upper line). (From Bonnet et al.,[121] with permission.)

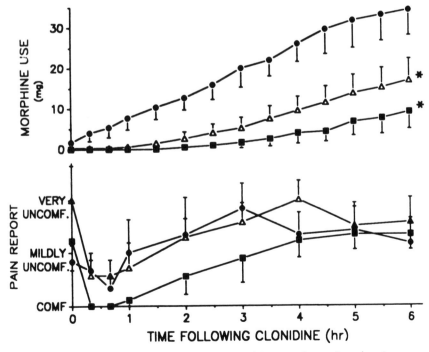

Fig. 27-12 Cumulative supplemental intravenous morphine use (upper) and pain scores (lower panel) following epidural injection of clonidine, 100 to 300 (●), 400 to 600 (▲), and 700 to 900 μg (■). *$P < 0.05$ versus 100 to 300-μg group. (From Eisenach et al.,[124] with permission.)

comparable to those of epidural clonidine. Although the peak plasma concentration of clonidine was higher in the intramuscular group, the side effects were similar, including hypotension, bradycardia, and drowsiness. Tryba et al.[131] reported that clonidine, 150 μg intravenously, produced analgesia similar to morphine, 5 mg, after orthopaedic surgeries. However, Striebel et al.[132] could not demonstrate an analgesic effect of intravenous clonidine after cholecystectomy. Aho et al.[133] compared the analgesic effect of intravenous dexmedetomidine (0.2 and 0.4 μg/kg) with that of an opioid, oxycodone (60 μg/kg), or a nonsteroidal anti-inflammatory drug, diclofenac (250 μg/kg), in women undergoing laparoscopic tubal ligation. They showed that dexmedetomidine, 0.4 μg/kg, could produce a comparable effect to that of oxycodone, but drowsiness and bradycardia were problematic in the dexmedetomidine group. Bernard et al.[134] documented the efficacy of intravenous clonidine after major spine surgery, 5 μg/kg, infused in the first 1 hour, followed by 0.3 μg/kg/h. They cautioned that adequate fluid administration must be maintained to prevent hypotension during this regimen.

Clonidine can decrease shivering and oxygen consumption during recovery from anesthesia.[135]

Other Uses

The α_2 agonists may be useful in the relief of pain other than acute postoperative pain. Epidural clonidine produced effective dose dependent (100 to 900 μg) analgesia in patients with neuropathic pain with few side effects.[136] Epidural clonidine was also a useful adjunct in the management of patients with refractory reflex sympathetic dystrophy.[137] Anecdotal reports suggest that intrathecal clonidine in combination with opioids is a suitable treatment for cancer pain.[138,139] A case report suggested that intrathecal clonidine was effective after tolerance to intrathecal morphine has developed.[140]

REFERENCES

1. Ahlquist RP: A study of the adrenotropic receptors. Am J Physiol 153:586, 1948
2. Paton WD, Vizi ES: The inhibitory action of nor-adrenaline and adrenaline on acetylcholine output by guinea-pig ileum longitudinal muscle strip. Br J Pharmacol 35:10, 1969
3. Langer SZ: Presynaptic regulation of catecholamine release. Biochem Pharmacol 23:1793, 1974
4. Berthelsen S, Pettinger WA: A functional basis for classification of a adrenergic receptors. Life Sci 21:595, 1977
5. Drew GM, Whiting SB: Evidence for two distinct types of postsynaptic α-adrenoceptors in vascular smooth muscle in vivo. Br J Pharmacol 67:207, 1979
6. Bylund DB, U'Pritchard DC: Characterization of α-1 and α-2 adrenergic receptors. Int Rev Neurobiol 24:343, 1983
7. Cheung Y-D, Barnett DB, Nahorski SR: [^{3}H]Rauwolscine and [^{3}H]yohimbine binding to rat cerebral and human platelet membranes: possible heterogeneity of α_2-adrenoceptors. Eur J Pharmacol 84:79, 1982
8. Bylund DB: Heterogeneity of α-2 adrenergic receptors. Pharmacol Biochem Behav 22:835, 1985
9. Bylund DB: Subtypes of α_2-adrenoceptors: pharmacological and molecular biological evidence converge. Trends Pharmacol Sci 9:356, 1988
10. Docherty JR: The pharmacology of α_1- and α_2-adrenoceptors: evidence for and against a further subdivision. Pharmacol Ther 44:241, 1989
11. Petrash AC, Bylund DB: α-2 adrenergic receptor subtypes indicated by [^{3}H]yohimbine binding in human brain. Life Sci 38:2129, 1986
12. De Vos H, Vauquelin G, De Keyser J et al: Regional distribution of α_{2A}- and α_{2B}-adrenoceptor subtypes in postmortem human brain. J Neurochem 58:1555, 1992
13. Bylund DB, Blaxall HS, Murphy TJ, Simonneaux V: Pharmacological evidence for α-2C and α-2D adrenergic receptor subtypes. p. 27. In Szabady E (ed): Adrenoceptors: Structure, Mechanisms, Function. Birkhauser, Berlin, 1991
14. Connaughton S, Docherty JR: Functional evidence for heterogeneity of peripheral prejunctional α_2-adrenoceptors. Br J Pharmacol 101:285, 1990b
15. Unnerstall J, Kopajtic TA, Kuhar MJ: Distribution of α_2 agonists bindind sites in the rat and human central nervous system. Analysis of some functional, autonomic correlates of the pharmacology effects of clonidine and related adrenergic agents. Brain Res Rev 7:69, 1984
16. DeSarro GB, Ascioti C, Froio F, et al: Evidence that locus coeruleus is the site where clonidine and drugs acting at α_1 and α_2 adrenoceptors affect sleep and arousal mechanisms. Br J Pharmacol 90:675, 1987

17. Correa-Sales C, Rabin BC, Maze M: A hypnotic response to dexmedetomidine, an α_2 agonist is mediated in the locus coeruleus in rats. Anesthesiology 76:948, 1992

18. Ernsberger P, Meeley MP, Mann JJ, Reis DJ: Clonidine binds to imidazole binding sites as well as α_2-adrenoceptors in the ventrolateral medulla. Eur J Pharmacol 134:1, 1987

19. Atlas D, Diamant S, Zonnenschein R: Is imidazoline site a unique receptor? A correlation with clonidine-displacing substance activity. Am J Hypertens 5:83S, 1992

20. Tibirica E, Feldman J, Mermet C et al: An imidazoline-specific mechanism for the hypotensive effect of clonidine. A study with yohimbine and idazoxan. J Pharmacol Exp Ther 256:606, 1991

21. Toon S, Hopkins KJ, Aarons L, Rowland M: Rate and extent of absorption of clonidine from a transdermal therapeutic system. J Pharm Pharmacol 41:17, 1989

22. Scheinin H, Virtanen R, MacDonald E et al: Medetomidine—a novel α_2-adrenoceptor agonist: a review of its pharmacodynamic effects. Prog Neuropsychopharmacol Biol Psychiatry 13:635, 1989

23. Maze M, Vickery RG, Merlone SC, Gaba DM: Anesthetic and hemodynamic effects of the α_2 adrenergic agonists, azepexole, in isoflurane-anesthetized dogs. Anesthesiology 69:689, 1988

24. Pichler L, Kobinger W: Centrally mediated cardiovascular effects of BHT 920. J Cardiovasc Pharmacol 3:269, 1981

25. Virtanen R, MacDonald E: Comparison of the effects of detomidine and xylazine on some α_2 adrenoceptor mediated responses in the central and peripheral nervous system. Eur J Pharmacol 115:277, 1985

26. Doze VA, Chen BX, Maze M: Dexmedetomidine produces a hypnotic-anesthetic action in rats via activation of central α_2 adrenoceptors. Anesthesiology 71:75, 1989

27. Salonen M, Reid K, Maze M: Synergistic interaction between α_2-adrenergic agonists and benzodiazepines in rats. Anesthesiology 76:1004, 1992

28. Ferrari F, Tartoni PL, Margiafico V: B-HT 920 antagonizes rat neophobia in the x-maze test. Arch Int Pharmacodyn Ther 298:71, 1989

29. Uhde TW, Stein MB, Vittone BJ et al: Behavioral and physiologic effects of short-term and long-term administration of clonidine in panic disorder. Arch Gen Psychiatry 46:170, 1989

30. Soderpalm B, Engel JA: Biphasic effects of clonidine on conflict behavior: involvement of different α-adrenoceptors. Pharmacol Biochem Behav 30:471, 1988

31. Pertovaara A, Kauppila T, Jyasjarvi E, Kalso E: Involvement of supraspinal and spinal segmental α-2-adrenergic mechanisms in the medetomidine-induced antinociception. Neuroscience 44:705, 1991

32. Yaksh TL, Reddy SVR: Studies in primate on the analgesic effects associated with intrathecal actions of opiates, α_2 adrenergic agonists, and baclofen. Anesthesiology 54:451, 1981

33. Fielding S, Wilker J, Hynes M et al: A comparison of clonidine with morphine for antinociceptive and anti-withdrawal actions. J Pharmacol Exp Ther 207:899, 1978

34. Omote K, Kitahata L, Collins JG et al: Interaction between opiate subtype and α_2 adrenergic agonists in suppression of noxiously evoked activity of WDR neurons in the spinal dorsal horn. Anesthesiology 74:737, 1991

35. Ossipov MH, Harris S, Lloyd P et al: Antinoceptive interaction between opioids and medetomidine: system additivity and spiral synergy. Anesthesiology 73:1227, 1990

36. Brown DA: G-proteins and potassium currents in neurons. Annu Rev Physiol 52:215, 1990

37. Paalzow G: Development of tolerance to the analgesic effect of clonidine in rats cross-tolerance to morphine. Naunyn Schmiedebergs Arch Pharmacol 304:1, 1978

38. Gold MS, Redmond DE, Jr, Kleber HD: Clonidine blocks acute opiate withdrawal symptoms. Lancet 2:599, 1978

39. Cushman P, Jr, Sowers JR: Alcohol withdrawal syndrome: clinical and hormonal responses to α_2 adrendergic treatment. Alcoholism 13:361, 1989

40. Jaakola ML, Salonen M, Lehinen R, Scheinin H: The analgesic action of dexmedetomidine a novel α_2-adrenoceptor agonist in healthy volunteers. Pain 46:281, 1991

41. Kauppila T, Kemppainen P, Tanila H, Pertovaara A: Effect of systemic medetomidine, an α_2 adrenoceptor agonist, on experimental pain in humans. Anesthesiology 74:3, 1991

42. Kaukinen S, Pyykko K: The potentiation of halothane anesthesia by clonidine. Acta Anaesthsiol Scand 23:107, 1979

43. Bloor BC, Flack WE: Reduction in halothane anesthetic requirement by clonidine, an α_2 adrenergic agonist. Anesth Analg 61:741, 1982

44. Segal IS, Vickery RG, Walton JK et al: Dexmedetomidine diminishes halothane anesthetic require-

ments in rats through a postsynaptic α_2 adrenergic receptors. Anesthesiology 69:818, 1988

45. Ghingnone MC, Calvillo O, Quintin L: Anesthesia for ophthalmic surgery in the elderly: the effects of clonidine on intraocular pressure, perioperative hemodynamics, and anesthesia requirement. Anesthesiology 68:707, 1988

46. Potter D, Ogidigben MJ: Medetomidine-induced alterations of intraocular pressure and contraction of the nictitating membrane. Invest Ophthalmol Vis Sci 32:2799, 1991

47. Hoffman WE, Cheng MA, Thomas C et al: Clonidine decreases plasma catecholamines and improves outcome from incomplete ischemia in the rat. Anesth Analg 73:460, 1991

48. Hoffman WE, Kochs E, Werner C et al: Dexmedetomidine improves neurologic outcome from incomplete ischemia in the rat. Anesthesiology 75:328, 1991

49. Gustafson I, Yoshimoto M, Wieloch TW: Postischemic administration of idazoxan, an α_2 adrenergic receptor antagonist, decreased neuronal damage in the rat brain. J Cereb Blood Flow Metab 9:171, 1989

50. Gustafson I, Westerberg E, Wielock T: Protection against ischemia-induced neural damage by the α_2-adrenoceptor antagonist idazoxan: influence of time of administration and possible mechanism of action. J Cereb Blood Flow Metab 10:885, 1990

51. Maiese K, Pek L, Berger SB, Resi DJ: Reduction in focal cerebral ischemia by agents acting at imadazole receptors. J Cereb Blood Flow Metab 12:53, 1992

52. De Jonge A, Timmermans PBMWM, Van Zweiten PA: Participation of cardiac presynaptic α_2 adrenoceptors in the bradycardic effects of clonidine and analogues. Naunyn Schmiedebergs Arch Pharmacol 317:8, 1981

53. Dukes ID, Williams EMV: Effects of selective α_1-, α_2-, β_1- and β_2-adrenoceptor stimulation on potentials and contractions in the rabbit heart. J Physiol 355:523, 1984

54. Houssmans PR: Effects of dexmedetomidine on contractility, relaxation and intracellular calcium transients of isolated ventricular myocardium. Anesthesiology 73:919, 1990

55. Ruffolo RR, Jr: Distribution and function of peripheral α-adrenoceptors on the cardiovascular system. Pharmacol, Biochem Behav 22:827, 1985

56. Chillian WN: Functional distribution of α_1 and α_2 adrenergic receptors in coronary microcirculation. Circulation 84:2108, 1991

57. Miyamoto MI, Rockman HA, Guth BD et al: Effect of α-adrenergic stimulation on regional contractile

function and myocardial blood flow with and without ischemia. Circulation 84:1715, 1991

58. Heusch G, Schipke J, Thamer V: Clonidine prevents sympathetic initiation and aggravation of poststenotic myocardial ischemia. J Cardiovasc Pharmacol 7:1176, 1985

59. Cocks TM, Angus JA: Endothelium-dependent relaxation of coronary arteries by noradrenaline and serotonin. Nature 305:627, 1983

60. Hori M, Kitakaze M, Tamai J et al: α_2-adrenoceptor stimulation can augment coronary vasodilation maximally induced by adenosine in dogs. Am J Physiol 57:H142, 1989

61. Schmeling WT, Kampine JP, Roerig DL, Warltier DC: The effects of the stereoisomers of the α_2 adrenergic agonist medetomidine on systemic and coronary hemodynamics in conscious dogs. Anesthesiology 75:499, 1991

62. Kubo T, Misu Y: Pharmacological characterization on the α-adrenoceptor responsible for a decrease of blood pressure in the nucleus tractus solitarii of the rat. Naunyn Schmiedebergs Arch Pharmacol 317:120, 1981

63. Svensson TH, Bunney BS, Aghajanian GK: Inhibition of both noradrenergic and serotonergic neurons in brain by the α-adrenergic agonsist clonidine. Brain Res 92:291, 1975

64. Ross CA, Ruggiero DA, Reis DJ: Projections from the nucleus tractus solitarii to the rostal ventrolateral medulla. J Comp Neurol 242:511, 1985

65. Ernsberger P, Guiliano R, Willette N, Reis D: Role of imidazole receptors in the vasodepressor response to clonidine analogs in the rostal ventrolateral medulla. J Pharmacol Exp Ther 253:408, 1990

66. Bousquet P, Feldman J, Tibirica E et al: New concepts on the central regulation of blood pressure. Am J Med 87:10s, 1989

67. Hayashi Y, Sumikawa K, Maze M et al: Dexmedetomidine prevents epinephrine-induced arrhythmias through stimulation of central α_2 adrenoceptors in halothane-anesthetized dogs. Anesthesiology 75:113, 1991

68. Kamibayashi T, Hayashi Y, Sumikawa K et al: A role of vagus nerve in antiarrhythmic effects of doxazosin and dexmedetomidine on halothane-epinephrine arrhythmias. Anesthesiology 77:A642, 1992

69. Zornow NH, Fleischer JE, Scheller MS et al: Dexmedetomidine, and α_2-adrenergic agonist, decreases cerebral blood flow in the isoflurane-anesthetized dog. Anesth Analg 70:624, 1990

70. Karlsson BR, Forsman M, Roald OK et al: Effect of

dexmedetomidine, a selective and potent α_2-agonist, on cerebral blood flow and oxygen consumption during halothane anesthesia in dogs. Anesth Analg 71:25, 1990

71. McPherson RW, Traystman RJ: Effect of dexmedetomidine on cerebrovascular response to hypoxia during isoflurane anesthesia. Anesthesiology 75:A174, 1991

72. Nguyen D, Abdul-Rasool I, Ward D et al: Ventilatory effects of dexmedetomidine, atipamezole, and isoflurane in dogs. Anesthesiology 76:573, 1992

73. Anderson RJ, Hart GR, Crumpler CP, Lerman MJ: Clonidine overdoses: report of six cases and review of the literature. Ann Emerg Med 10:107, 1989

74. Garty M, Ben-Zvi Z, Harwity A: Interaction of clonidine and morphine with lidocaine in mice and rats. Toxicol Appl Pharmacol 101:255, 1989

75. Penon C, Ecoffey C, Cohen SE: Ventilatory response to carbon dioxide after epidural clonidine injection. Anesth Analg 72:761, 1991

76. Jarvis DA, Duncan SR, Segal IS, Maze M: Ventilatory effects of clonidine alone and in the presence of alfentanil, in human volunteers. Anesthesiology 76:899, 1992

77. Lindgren BR, Ekstrom T, Anderson RG: The effect of inhaled clonidine in patients with asthma. Am Rev Respir Dis 134:266, 1986

78. Eisenach JC: Intravenous clonidine produces hypoxia by a peripheral α_2 adrenergic mechanism. J Pharmacol Exp Ther 244:247, 1988

79. Grossman A, Weerasuriya K, Al-Damluji S et al: α_2 adrenoceptor agonists stimulate growth hormone secretion but have no acute effects on plasma cortisol under basal conditions. Horm Res 25:65, 1987

80. Deveasa J, Diaz MJ, Tresquerres AI et al: Evidence that α_2 adrenergic pathways play a major role in growth hormone (GH) neuroregulation: α_2 adrenergic agonism counteracts the inhibitory effects of muscarinic cholinergic receptor blockade on the GH response to GH-releasing hormone, while α_2 adrenergic blockade diminishes the potentiating effect of increased cholinergic tone on such stimulation in normal men. J Clin Endocrinol Metab 73:251, 1991

81. Maze M, Virtanen R, Daunt D et al: Effects of dexmedetomidine, a novel imidazole sedative-anesthetic agent, on adenal steroidogenesis: in vivo and in vitro studies. Anesth Analg 73:204, 1991

82. Langer SZ: Presynaptic regulation of catecholamine release. Biochem Pharmacol 23:1793, 1974

83. Gutman Y, Boonyaviroj P: Suppression by noradrenaline of catecholamine secretion from adrenal medulla. Eur J Pharmacol 28:384, 1974

84. Powis DA, Baker PF: α_2-adrecoceptors do not regulate catecholamine secretion by bovine adrenal medullary cells: a study with clonidine. Mol Pharmacol 29:134, 1986

85. Angel I, Langer SZ: Adrenergic-induced hyperglycemia in anaesthetized rats. Involvement of peripheral α_2 adrenoceptors. Eur J Pharmacol 154:191, 1988

86. Massara F, Limone P, Cagliero E et al: Effects of naloxone on the insulin and growth hormone responses to α-adrenergic stimulation with clonidine. Acta Endocrinol (Copenh) 103:371, 1983

87. Karhuvaara S, Kallio AM, Salonen M et al: Rapid reversal of α_2-adrenoceptor agonist effects by atipamezole in human volunteers. Br J Clin Pharmacol 31:160, 1991

88. Blandiaai C, Bernardini MC, Vizi ES, Del Tacca M: Modulation of gastric acid secretion by peripheral presynaptic α_2 adrenoceptors at both sympathetic and parasympathetic pathways. J Auton Pharmacol 10:305, 1990

89. Orko R, Pouttu J, Ghignone M et al: Effect of clonidine on hemodynamic responses to endotracheal intubation and gastric acidity. Acta Anaesthesiol Scand 31:325, 1987

90. McArthur KE, Anderson DS, Durbin TE et al: Clonidine and lidamidine to inhibit watery diarrhea in a patient with lung cancer. Ann Intern Med 96:323, 1982

91. Peskind ER, Raskind MA, Leake RD et al: Clonidine decreases plasma and cerebrospinal fluid arginine vasopressin but not oxytocin in humans. Neuroendocrinology 46:395, 1987

92. Stanton B, Puglisi E, Gellai M: Localization of α_2-adrenoceptor-mediated increase in renal Na^+, K^+, and water excretion. Am J Physiol 252:F1016, 1987

93. Strandhoy JW: Role of α_2 receptors in the regulation of renal function. J Cardiovasc Pharmacol, suppl 8:S28, 1985

94. Chen M, Lee J, Huang BS et al: Clonidine and morphine increase atrial natriuretic peptide secretion in anesthetized rats. Proc Soc Exp Biol Med 191:299, 1989

95. Ruffolo RR, Nichols AJ, Hieble JP: Functions mediated by α_2 adrenergic receptors. p. 187. In Limbird LE (ed): The α_2 Adrenergic Receptors. Humana Press, Clifton, NJ, 1988

96. Aantaa RE, Jaakola ML, Kallio A et al: A comparison of dexmedetomidine, an α_2 adrenoceptor agonist, and midazolam as i. m. premedication for minor gynaecological surgery. Br J Anaesth 67:402, 1991

97. Ghignone M, Quintin L, Duke PC et al: Effects of clonidine on narcotic requirements and hemodynamic response during induction of fentanyl anesthesia and endotracheal induction. Anesthesiology 64:36, 1986

98. Flacke JW, Bloor BC, Flack WE et al: Reduced narcotic requirement by clonidine with improved hemodynamic and adrenergic stability in patients undergoing coronary surgery. Anesthesiology 67:11, 1987

99. Engelman E, Lipszyc M, Gilbart E et al: Effects of clonidine on anesthetic requirements and hemodynamic response during aortic surgery. Anesthesiology 71:178, 1989

100. Aantaa RE, Kanto JH, Scheinen M et al: Dexmedetomidine premedication for minor gynecological surgery. Anesth Analg 70:407, 1990

101. Aantaa RE, Kanto JH, Scheinen M et al: Dexmedetomidine, an α_2 adrenergic agonist, reduces anesthetic requirements for patients undergoing minor gynecological surgery. Anesthesiology 73:230, 1990

102. Richard MJ, Skues MA, Jarvis AP, Prys-Roberts C: Total i.v. anaesthesia with propofol and alfentanin: dose requirements for propranolol and the effect of premedication with clonidine. Br J Anaesth 65:157, 1990

103. Ota K, Namiki A, Ujike Y, Takahashi I: Prolongation of tetracaine spinal anesthesia by oral clonidine. Anesth Analg 75:262, 1992

104. Carabine UA, Wright PMC, Moore J: Preanaesthetic medication with clonidine: a dose-response study. Br J Anaesth 67:79, 1991

105. Kumar A, Bose S, Phattacharya A et al: Oral clonidine premedication for elderly patients undergoing intraocular surgery. Acta Anaesthesiol Scand 36:159, 1992

106. Wright RMC, Carabine UA, Orr DA et al: Preanesthetic medication with clonidine. Br J Anaesth 65:628, 1990

107. Aho M, Lehtinen AM, Erkola O et al: The effects of intravenous administered dexmedetomidine on perioperative hemodynamics and isoflurane requirements in patients undergoing abdominal hysterectomy. Anesthesiology 74:112, 1991

108. Jaakola ML, Ali-Melkkila T, Kanto J et al: Dexmedetomidine reduces intraocular pressure, intubation responses and anaesthetic requirements in patients undergoing ophthalmic surgery. Br J Anaesth 68:570, 1992

109. Scheinin B, Lindgren L, Randel T et al: Dexmedetomidine attenuates sympathoadrenal responses to tracheal intubation and reduces the need for thiopentone and preoperative fentanyl. Br J Anaesth 68:126, 1992

110. Aantaa RE, Kanto J, Scheinen H: Intramuscular dexmedetomidine, a novel α_2 adrenoceptor agonist, as premedication for minor gynaecological surgery. Acta Anesthesiol Scand 35:283, 1991

111. Quintin L, Bonnet F, Macquin I et al: Aortic surgery: effect of clonidine on intraoperative catecholaminergic and circulatory stability. Acta Anaesthesiol Scand 34:132, 1990

112. Pluskwa F, Bonnet F, Saada M et al: Effects of clonidine on variation of arterial blood pressure and heart rate during carotid artery surgery. Cardiothorac Vasc Anesth 5:431, 1991

113. Benhamou D, Veillette Y, Narchi P, Ecoffey C: Ventilatory effects of premedication with clonidine. Anesth Analg 73:799, 1991

114. Bailey PL, Sperry RJ, Johnson GK et al: Respiratory effects of clonidine alone and combined with morphine in humans. Anesthesiology 74:43, 1991

115. Nishikawa T, Dohi S: Oral clonidine blunts the heart rate response to intravenous atropine in humans. Anesthesiology 75:217, 1991

116. Nishikawa T, Kimura T, Taguchi N, Dohi S: Oral clonidine preanesthetic medication augments the pressor responses to intravenous ephedrine in awake or anesthetized patients. Anesthesiology 74:705, 1991

117. Segal IS, Javis DJ, Duncan SR et al: Clinical efficacy of oral-transdermal clonidine combinations during the perioperative period. Anesthesiology 74:220, 1991

118. Quintin L, Roudot F, Roux C et al: Effect of clonidine on the circulation and vasoactive hormones after aortic surgery. Br J Anaesth 66:108, 1991

119. Dekock M, Pichon G, Scholtes JL: Intraoperative clonidine enhances postoperative morphine patient controlled analgesia. Anesthesiology 75:A654, 1991

120. Racle JP, Benkhadra A, Poy JY, Gleizal B: Prolongation of isobaric bupivacaine spinal anesthesia with epinephrine and clonidine for hip surgery in the elderly. Anesth Analg 66:442, 1987

121. Bonnet F, Brun-Buisson V, Saada M et al: Dose-related prolongation of hyperbaric tetracaine spinal anesthesia by clonidine in humans. Anesth Analg 68:619, 1989

122. Gordh T, Jr: Epidural clonidine for treatment of postoperative pain after thoracotomy. A double-blind placebo-controlled study. Acta Anaesthesiol Scand 32:702, 1988

123. van Essen EJ, Bovill JG, Ploeger EJ, Houben JJG: Pharmacokinetics of clonidine after epidural admin-

istration in surgical patients. Lack of correlation between plasma concentration and analgesia and blood pressure changes. Acta Anaesthesiol Scand 36:300, 1992

124. Eisenach J, Lysak SZ, Viscomi CM: Epidural clonidine analgesia following surgery: phase 1. Anesthesiology 71:640, 1989

125. Mendez R, Eisenach JC, Kashtan K: Epidural clonidine analgesia after cesarean section. Anesthesiology 73:848, 1990

126. Carabine UA, Milligan KR, Moore J: Extradural clonidine and bupivacaine for postoperative analgesia. Br J Anaesth 68:132, 1992

127. Carabine UA, Milligan KR, Mulholland D, Moore J: Extradural clonidine infusions for analgesia after total hip replacement. Br J Anaesth 68:338, 1992

128. Rostaing S, Bonnet F, Levron JC et al: Effects of epidural clonidine on analgesia and pharmacokinetics of epidural fentanyl in postoperative patients. Anesthesiology 75:420, 1991

129. Filos KS, Goudas LC, Patroni O, Polyzou V: Intrathecal clonidine as a sole analgesic for pain relief after cesarean section. Anesthesiology 77:174, 1992

130. Bonnet F, Boico O, Rostaining S et al: Clonidine-induced analgesia in postoperative patients: epidural versus intramuscular administration. Anesthesiology 72:423, 1990

131. Tryba M, Zenz M, Strumpf M: Clonidine i.v. is equally effective as morphine i.v. for postoperative analgesia—a double blind study. Anesthesiology 75:A1085, 1991

132. Striebel HW, Gottschalk B, Kramer J: Clonidine does not reduce postoperative meperidine requirements. Anesthesiology 75:A659, 1991

133. Aho M, Erkola OA, Scheinen H et al: Effect of intravenous administered dexmedetomidine on pain after laparoscopic tubal ligation. Anesth Analg 73:12, 1991b

134. Bernard JM, Hommeril JL, Passuti N, Pinaud M: Postoperative analgesia by intravenous clonidine. Anesthesiology 75:577, 1991

135. Delaunay L, Bonnet F, Duvaldestin P: Clonidine decreases postoperative oxygen consumption in patients recovering from general anaesthesia. Br J Anaesth 67:397, 1991

136. Eisenach JC, Rauck RL, Buzzanell C, Lysak S: Epidural clonidine analgesia for intractable cancer pain: phase 1. Anesthesiology 71:647, 1989

137. Rauck RL, Eisenach JC, Jackson KE et al: Epidural clonidine for refractory reflex sympathetic dystrophy. Anesthesiology 75:A657, 1991

138. Coombs D, Saunder RL, Fratkin JD et al: Continuous intrathecal hydromorphine and clonidine for intractable cancer pain. J Neurosurg 64:890, 1986

139. van Essen EJ, Bovill JG, Ploeger EJ, Beerman H: Intrathecal morphine and clonidine for control of intractable cancer pain. A case report. Acta Anaesthesiol Belg 39:109, 1988

140. Coombs D, Saunders RI, Lachance D et al: Intrathecal morphine tolerance: use of intrathecal clonidine, DADLE, and intraventricular morphine. Anesthesiology 62:358, 1985

Chapter 28

Drugs Affecting Adrenoceptors: β Adrenergic Antagonists

Martin J. London

Perioperative use of β adrenergic blockade has increased dramatically over the past 20 years. Before this time, the use of these agents perioperatively was considered extremely hazardous. Because a number of studies dispelled many of these concerns, clinicians have pursued numerous clinical applications. These clinical studies in many instances provided persuasive data for the continuation of these agents. However, the clinician must carefully interpret them to avoid potentially life threatening complications, which unfortunately, are most likely to occur in the sickest patients (i.e., those we would like to help the most). In addition, most of these studies were conducted in low risk patients, the majority of whom will do well not matter how they are treated. Indeed, we tend to underestimate the advantages of an intact cardiac reserve and the capability of vascular autoregulation to deal with major changes in hemodynamics encountered perioperatively. Perhaps the greatest limitation of many of these studies is the inadequate sample size, which prevents the possibility of a firm generalization of results, particularly those relating to postoperative outcome. Yet, there is no doubt that many patients can accrue substantial clinical benefits from the skillful use of these agents in what remains a "stressful" perioperative environment.

This chapter reviews many, but not all, perioperative applications of β adrenergic blockade. Emphasis is placed on adult cardiovascular anesthesia, with critical examination of clinical studies. Although pertinent basic physiology and pharmacology is covered, the reader is also referred to comprehensive basic reviews of β adrenergic blockers, particularly those of Frishman.[1–8]

PHARMACOLOGY OF β ADRENERGIC BLOCKING AGENTS

Currently, there are more than 10 β adrenergic blockers available in the United States (Table 28-1). There are at least 7 more in use elsewhere. Despite this large number, there are a limited number suited for perioperative use, and only a few of these have received considerable attention from clinical researchers. In the United States, propranolol, labetalol, esmolol, and metoprolol are by far the most commonly used agents perioperatively. As a result, this chapter focuses almost exclusively on them and the pertinent clinical research about them.

β adrenoceptor blockers are competitive inhibitors of catecholamine binding at the beta adrenoceptor (see Ch. 26). They are generally categorized by four different pharmacologic properties.[9,10] *Po-*

Table 28-1 Pharmacologic Properties of β Adrenergic Blockers

Drug	β_1 Potency Ratio[a]	Relative β_1 Selectivity	Intrinsic Sympathomimetic Activity	Membrane Stabilizing Activity	Lipid Solubility	Elimination Half-Life (h)	Total Body Clearance (ml/min)	Metabolism
Acebutolol	0.3	+	+	+	Moderate	3–4	6–15	Renal/hepatic
Atenolol	1.0	++	0	0	Low	6–9	130	Renal
Esmolol	0.02	++	0	0	Low	9 min	27,000	Erythrocyte esterase
Labetalol	0.3	0	+?	0	Low	3–4	2,700	Hepatic
Metoprolol	1.0	++	0	0	Moderate	3–4	1,100	Hepatic
Nadolol	1.0	0	0	0	Low	14–24	200	Renal
Penbutolol	1.0	0	+	0	High	27	350	Renal
Pindolol	6.0	0	++	+	Moderate	3–4	400	Renal/hepatic
Propranolol	1.0	0	0	++	High	3–4	1,000	Hepatic
Sotalol	0.3	0	0	0	Low	9–10	150	Renal
Timolol	6.0	0	0	0	Low	4–5	660	Renal/hepatic

[a] Relative to propranolol = 1.
(Adapted from Frishman,[2] with permission.)

tency is the amount of drug that must be administered to inhibit the effects of an adrenergic agonist (usually isoproterenol). Interestingly, esmolol is the least potent of any of the β adrenergic blockers and thus is administered in the highest dosages. *Receptor selectivity* can be equated to a major degree with a particular agent's clinical safety profile. Nonselective agents that block both β_1 and β_2 adrenoceptors are more likely to precipitate bronchospasm and can result in peripheral vasoconstriction. However, selectivity is dose dependent, and at high doses, all of the so-called β-selective agents lose their selectivity. *Membrane stabilizing activity* is a so-called local anesthetic effect on the cardiac action potential, and it is unrelated to the β adrenoceptor. This effect is generally considered to be of significance only with very high doses of drug. *Intrinsic sympathomimetic activity* is the capacity of certain agents to manifest partial agonist activity at the receptor. Agents with this property (i.e., pindolol, practolol, and oxprenolol) result in less slowing of the heart rate at rest, although during exercise, the heart rate response is significantly attenuated. Ventricular function may be better preserved by partial agonists, as suggested by Taylor et al.[11] who demonstrated less myocardial depression in patients with stable coronary artery dis-

ease from practolol or oxprenolol compared with agents lacking intrinsic sympathomimetic activity (metoprolol or propranolol, Fig. 28-1). An additional property of significance is concomitant α-*adrenergic blocking activity*. Labetalol is the first agent available that produces significant α-adrenoceptor blockade.

ELECTROPHYSIOLOGIC EFFECTS OF PERIOPERATIVE β ADRENERGIC BLOCKADE

β blockers decrease sinoatrial node activity and increase atrioventricular (AV) node and intramyocardial conduction times. Thus, β adrenergic blockade is relatively contraindicated in patients with congenital or acquired heart block (particularly those with greater than first degree AV block) who are not paced. Also patients with left bundle branch block are particularly at risk for severe bradycardia. There is only a limited amount of clinical data on these effects and little in the perioperative setting. Several of these studies are reviewed here.

Wiener et al.[12] reported on the regional effects of propranolol on intramyocardial conduction in seven patients 1 week after coronary artery bypass graft (CABG) surgery. Measurements were made from surface electrocardiographic (ECG) leads and epicardial bipolar electrodes on the right atrium and ventricle (normally placed for temporary pacing) and on the left ventricle in the distribution of the bypassed left anterior descending coronary artery. The conduction interval to each ventricle, the QRS duration, and the "stimulus to Q interval" (a measure of the effect on the AV node) were recorded following acute administration of a 3-mg intravenous dose of propranolol. The atria were paced at 110 beats/min to avoid any effects related to the reduction in sinus node rate. No other drugs were administered, although four patients were receiving digoxin at the time of study. The conduction interval in the left ventricle increased by 10 percent (a statistically significant increase); right ventricular conduction did not change. The QRS duration was unchanged; the stimulus to Q interval increased by 16 percent. These findings were similar to previous data from dogs in which conduction through ischemic myocardium was decreased by propranolol, although no effect was observed in normal myocardium. This has been attributed to the local anesthetic effect (membrane stabilizing effect) of propranolol.

These investigators also evaluated responses to a single oral dose of labetalol using the same method. Three patients received labetalol 100 mg, and four received a 200-mg dose. In contrast to propranolol, there were no significant effects on conduction to either ventricle and no effect on AV

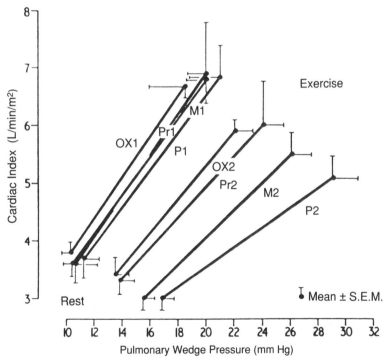

Fig. 28-1 Effects of four intravenous β adrenergic blockers on left ventricular function response to exercise in 24 patients with coronary artery disease (1 = control period, 2 = treatment period). The effects of cardioselectivity (metoprolol [M] and practolol [Pr]) and ISA (practolol and oxprenolol [Ox]) were compared with those of propranolol (P) (nonselective, no ISA). Agents with ISA induced significantly less depression of ventricular function. Cardioselectivity had no hemodynamic advantage. ISA, intrinsic sympathomimetic activity. (From Taylor et al.,[11] with permission.)

conduction. The authors postulated a lack of local anesthetic effect with labetalol. The lack of effect on AV conduction was postulated to be related to α adrenergic blocking properties, although the exact mechanism is unclear.

Henling et al.[14] investigated the risk of heart block following cardiopulmonary bypass in 140 patients undergoing CABG chronically treated with either β adrenergic blockers or calcium channel blockers alone or both types of drugs, compared with patients who received neither of the drugs. The anesthetic techniques consisted of halothane or enflurane, supplemented with fentanyl and pancuronium. Normothermic cardiopulmonary bypass with cold potassium crystalloid cardioplegia was used. The ECG data were collected intermittently. Patients receiving β adrenergic blockers, alone or in combination with calcium channel blockers, had lower heart rates at each measurement point, although only in those receiving diltiazem or verapamil was the difference statistically significant. Heart rates increased over time in all groups relative to preinduction. The PR intervals increased relative to control in all groups after induction; they were greatest in the combined therapy group. Ten minutes after cardiopulmonary bypass, the PR interval was increased relative to control, despite a 25 to 30 percent increase in heart rate, in patients receiving β adrenergic blockers or both. Despite these findings, the frequency of first degree heart block was not related to drug therapy. Higher degrees of block were not observed. Remarkably, no patient required pacing during or after weaning from bypass.

These data demonstrate that β adrenergic blockers, alone or in combination with calcium channel blockers, exert definite chronotropic and dromotropic effects, although the magnitude of these effects are generally not clinically significant. However, caution must be exercised in extrapolating these data to all anesthetic regimens. Clinically significant differences in heart rate and blood pressure exist between high dose opioid versus inhalational based techniques. The choice of neuromuscular blocker also results in significant differences in heart rate. In addition, patients with concurrent conduction abnormalities would be expected to behave differently.

PREOPERATIVE WITHDRAWAL VERSUS ADMINISTRATION OF β ADRENERGIC BLOCKERS

The controversies regarding β blocker withdrawal syndromes have been thoroughly reviewed by Frishman.[4] The risks of withdrawing therapy must be considered along with data on the safety and efficacy of their continuation perioperatively. It is well appreciated that the intravenous administration of propranolol to dogs anesthetized with depressant volatile anesthetics (particularly halothane) can result in significant depression of cardiac output (caused by depressed contractility and/or decreased heart rate or conduction). However, the significance of preoperative oral β blocker therapy on intraoperative hemodynamic management was controversial in the early 1970s.[15] Many believed that therapy should be withdrawn 2 weeks prior to surgery because the patient would need maximal sympathetic function to deal with the depressant anesthetic drugs and the major physiologic stresses, such as hemorrhage; others thought that continuing the primary therapy necessary to treat the patient's underlying cardiac disease was of greater importance. The finding that patients treated with propranolol for symptomatic angina pectoris were prone to develop unstable angina and even myocardial infarction when therapy was abruptly withdrawn (e.g., as was done at the termination of several drug trials) was recognized as a clinical problem in the early 1970s. Patients with the most severe angina prior to treatment and those who were ambulatory were found to be at greatest risk. Surprisingly, despite many other uses for β adrenergic blockers, patients with angina are the only group in which a withdrawal syndrome has been well documented.[4]

Paradoxically, at least one major clinical study has shown that withdrawal from β-adrenergic blockers following acute myocardial infarction is not associated with an increased incidence of new ischemic symptoms.[16] Patients in the Multicenter Investigation of the Limitation of Infarct Size study were randomized to either a propranolol eligible or ineligible group, based on the presence or absence of standard clinical contraindications for β adrenergic blockade (e.g., bradycardia, hypotension, and congestive heart failure). Patients meeting eligibility criteria for randomization to aggressive propranolol therapy (i.e., absence of heart failure, hypotension, and conduction block) in whom therapy was withdrawn appeared to manifest a rebound increase in heart rate (Fig. 28-2). However, there were no significant differences in any of the indices of infarct size, ventricular function, or other ischemic clinical complications in these patients relative to any other group. The finding that

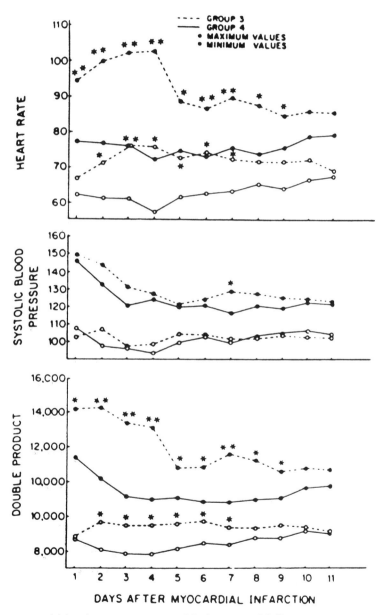

Fig. 28-2 Heart rate and blood pressure over an 11-day period following acute myocardial infarction in patients withdrawn from chronic β adrenergic blockade (group 3) compared with those maintained on therapy. The data suggest a rebound increase in heart rate in the first 4 days following withdrawal. Despite this, clinical outcomes were no different. (From Croft et al.,[16] with permission.)

withdrawal is not a problem during acute myocardial infarction, a condition associated with marked elevations of plasma catecholamines and renin, is puzzling. However, the often aggressive use of other anti-ischemic agents in this setting may offset any withdrawal phenomena.

Hypertensive patients (without known ischemic heart disease) have reported hyperadrenergic symptoms (palpitations, tremor, and sweating) following acute β adrenergic blocker withdrawal; however, there are no reported cases of rebound hypertension or hypertensive crisis in the literature. This is in distinct contrast to problems reported with the acute withdrawal of clonidine in these patients.

Various hypotheses have been advanced to explain β adrenergic blocker withdrawal.[4] The simplest is that it is not really a unique syndrome, rather an emergence of the underlying disease process. However, the pronounced severity of the symptoms and their higher incidence in patients treated with β adrenergic blockers in contrast to other classes of drugs makes this explanation implausible.

Several investigators demonstrated increased hemodynamic sensitivity to low dose isoproterenol infusion in patients withdrawn from propranolol and other pure "antagonist" β adrenergic blockers (i.e., those with no partial agonist properties). This is likely the result of receptor "up regulation" (increased density or sensitivity of β adrenoceptors in response to chronically decreased adrenergic tone). Following resumption of normal adrenergic tone, rebound occurs because an increased number of receptors are activated. A lack of clinical problems following withdrawal of agents with partial agonist activity (e.g., pindolol) fits this theory nicely.[4] Up regulation should not (or only minimally) occur with partial agonists because the basal level of adrenergic tone is maintained with their use. In fact, their major clinical advantage is that antagonist effects are manifest only during states of increased adrenergic tone (e.g., with exercise), a feature that makes their use in patients with impaired conduction or ventricular function attractive.

Increased platelet aggregation in response to epinephrine or adenosine diphosphate was re-

ported following withdrawal.[17] This could explain certain events, such as unstable angina or myocardial infarction that are mediated to a large extent by thrombosis. However, that correlation of in vitro platelet tests with in vivo phenomena remains controversial in this and in many other areas of coagulation research.

PERIOPERATIVE MYOCARDIAL ISCHEMIA

In adult cardiovascular anesthesia, prevention and/or therapy of myocardial ischemia is often cited as a major reason for perioperative β adrenergic blockade. Although some would argue that brief episodes of myocardial ischemia are well tolerated, clinicians have recently "tuned into" this problem, and many have adopted an aggressive posture with regard to treatment in light of recent studies relating perioperative ischemia to postoperative cardiac morbidity in both the cardiac and noncardiac surgical patient.[18–20] However, currently, no one has been able to prove convincingly that treatment of ischemia affects outcome.

The issue is somewhat complicated by differences between the two major clinical populations of interest. Patients with CABG undergo a primary therapeutic procedure; vascular surgery patients (a population with a high incidence of coronary artery disease) are subjected to significant perioperative "stress" without primary therapy for their disease. Most clinicians believe that minimizing the ischemic burden in both groups is an important clinical priority.

Interpreting results of clinical studies requires a consideration of several factors. The incidence of coronary artery disease in the clinical population is important, as is an adequate sample size (i.e., "statistical power"), to distinguish true differences between study groups. The type of monitor used to detect ischemia is also a major consideration. Most studies focus on ECG signs of ischemia. However, different types of monitors have varying frequency response, which may significantly alter the morphology of the QRS complex.[21,22]

An additional factor is adequate consideration of the patient's "ischemia pattern" or "ischemic burden."[23,24] More than 50 percent of patients with coronary artery disease develop ischemia in the absence of a clear-cut increase in myocardial oxygen demand.[25,26] In addition, many of these episodes are clinically "silent." Thus, some of the older clinical axioms that ischemia can be prevented solely by rigorously controlling myocardial oxygen demand (through heart rate and blood pressure) are no longer adequate.[20,27,28]

β Adrenergic Blockade During and Following Acute Myocardial Infarction

Prophylactic use of perioperative β adrenergic blockade is based in part on the strong evidence from a number of clinical trials in the early 1980s that suggest a significant reduction in morbidity and mortality rates with β adrenergic blockade in both the acute evolving phase of myocardial infarction and up to several years postinfarction. The topic was comprehensively reviewed by Hjalmarson and Olsson.[29] Based on an extensive review of the literature, they make the following generalizations and recommendations.

β Adrenergic blockers have a favorable effect on reducing ischemic chest pain during acute infarction. Their use is safe, and concerns that they may precipitate coronary vasospasm as a result of unopposed α adrenergic stimulation are generally unfounded. Their use in the early phase of infarction is associated with a 20 to 30 percent reduction in infarct size and decreased ventricular ectopy and ventricular fibrillation. The overall mortality rate is reduced by 15 percent, a larger reduction in the mortality rate is obtained in higher risk patients (30 to 45 percent), and the rates of morbidity and reinfarction are reduced when β adrenergic blockade is used together with thrombolytic therapy. Chronic β-adrenergic blockade postinfarction is associated with a 20 to 25 percent reduction in the long-term mortality rate. Interestingly, these beneficial effects were obtained with either selective (particularly, metoprolol) or nonselective (particularly, propranolol) agents, but not with agents with intrinsic sympathomimetic activity. Only about 15 percent of patients presenting with infarction have definite contraindications to the use of β-adrenergic blockers. Although this figure is probably higher in the

surgical population, particularly patients undergoing vascular surgery, these data provide a strong basis for their use in the perioperative setting.

Effects During Coronary Artery Bypass Graft Surgery

Prebypass Ischemia

Slogoff and Keats[30] studied the effects of preoperative calcium channel blockade or β adrenergic blockade either alone or in combination compared with a control group (n = 119, 71, 74, and 180, respectively) on the frequency of ECG ischemia on arrival to the operating room or during the prebypass period. The frequency of ischemia was lowest in the two groups receiving β adrenergic blockers (Table 28-2). These differences were attributed to a lower incidence of tachycardia (heart rate less than 89 beats/min) with β adrenergic blockade (3.4 versus 15.4 percent). An "ischemic threshold" heart rate of 110 was observed; at heart rates over 110, the incidence of ischemia was doubled (Fig. 28-3). Only 1 of the 145 patients receiving β adrenergic blockers exceeded this limit, in contrast to 29 of 299 patients who did not receive these drugs. With heart rates less than this limit, the incidence of ischemia was not different between the groups. However, roughly two-thirds of the ischemia occurred in the absence of any hemodynamic change. The limitations of this study include failure to randomize patients and the use of intermittent ECG sampling.[21]

Similar findings were presented by Chung et al.[31] in a study of 92 patients, although fewer time points were sampled. The heart rate and mean arterial pressure were higher at all times in patients receiving calcium channel blockers alone. In contrast to the results of Slogoff and Keats,[30] they found that the difference between groups was unrelated to changes in the heart rate. However, significant differences in experimental design preclude a close comparison of these studies.

These studies suggest that β adrenergic blockers are more effective than calcium channel blockers in preventing intraoperative ischemia in low risk patients undergoing CABG. However, the application of these findings to higher risk patients should

Table 28-2 Perioperative Ischemia and Its Relationship to Hemodynamic Abnormality in Patients Receiving Four Different Preoperative Antianginal Regimens

	None	β-Adrenergic Blocking Drugs	Calcium Entry Blocking Drugs	β-Adrenergic + Calcium Entry Blocking Drugs
Patients (n)	180	71	119	74
New perioperative ischemia (%)[a]	50.5	37[b]	56.3	32[b]
Arrival ischemia[c]				
Total (%)[a]	27.2	23	36.1	19
Hemodynamically unrelated (%)	13	14	26	16
Intraoperative ischemia[a]				
Total (%)	38.9	27	37.8	26
Hemodynamically unrelated (%)	21.7	18	26.1	18

[a] $P < 0.05$ for differences in incidences of ischemia among the four assignment groups.

[b] $P < 0.05$ compared with "none" or "calcium entry blocking drugs."

[c] Data for 67 patients with separate and distinct episodes of ischemia on arrival and during anesthesia are included in both groups.

(From Slogoff and Keats,[30] with permission.)

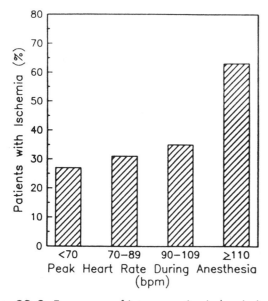

Fig. 28-3 Frequency of intraoperative ischemia in relation to peak heart rates observed in four groups of patients stratified by heart rate (n = 49, 229, 136, and 30, respectively). The incidence of ischemia increased dramatically with peak heart rate more than 110 beats/min. (From Slogoff and Keats,[30] with permission.)

be done with caution. The effects of calcium channel blockers on functional recovery of the "stunned myocardium" following cardiopulmonary bypass is an additional variable, not yet studied, that may be of clinical significance.[32]

Protective Effects During Global Ischemia

Several studies examined the role of β adrenergic blockade in minimizing ischemic injury during bypass. A quantitative assessment of creatine kinase (the MB fraction) is generally used as an index of injury, although the exact determination of myocardial injury in this setting is controversial and continues to evolve.[33] In addition, the complex biochemistry during reperfusion (i.e., following removal of the aortic cross clamp) requires that additional studies be performed to explain any beneficial effects that might be observed.[34]

Rao et al.[35] examined the effects of propranolol (0.05 mg/kg) administered just before aortic cross clamping in 46 patients undergoing CABG or valve replacement (with 34 patients serving as a control). Plasma levels ranged from 80 to 100 ng/ml in the treated group. Multiple creatine kinase MB isoenzyme determinations allowed an estimation of "infarct size" based on a complex calculation approximating the integrated area under the plasma concentration curve. With β adrenergic blockade, a 30 percent reduction in this score was observed. However, the data were complicated by the chronic use of β adrenergic blockers in both groups.

Berggren et al.[36] studied 30 patients in whom metoprolol was either withdrawn 3 days preoperatively or continued until surgery. An analysis of infarct size was performed. The mean area under the creatine kinase MB curve in the treated group was nearly one-half that of the withdrawn group. This study is complicated by the possibility that the greater degree of damage in the withdrawn patients may have been a result of withdrawing therapy rather than a direct protective effect of continued therapy.

Putting these studies in perspective, any effect that β adrenergic blockers may have during global ischemia is probably small in comparison to the effects of cardioplegia. Despite the controversies as to which technique of cardioplegia is best (i.e., retrograde coronary sinus, warm continuous, or blood cardioplegia), any standard form of cardioplegia is currently universally accepted as being more important than any pharmacologic adjuvants.

Ischemia in Patients Undergoing Noncardiac Surgery

Preoperative Administration in High Risk Patients

Stone et al.[37,38] presented data evaluating the effect of a single preoperative oral dose of a β adrenergic blocker on the incidence of intraoperative ischemia in 128 untreated hypertensive patients. Criteria for inclusion in the study were at least three preoperative blood pressures between 160/90 and 200/100 mmHg, with no antihypertensive therapy for at least 1 year. Curiously, patients with known coronary artery disease were excluded from the study, along with those having standard contraindications to β adrenergic blockade (congestive heart failure, bronchospastic lung disease, and conduction abnormalities). The majority of surgical procedures were abdominal or peripheral.

Two hours prior to induction, 89 patients received a single oral dose of labetalol, atenolol, or oxprenolol (an agent with intrinsic sympathomimetic activity). Thirty-nine untreated patients served as the control group. Anesthesia was not standardized, although clinicians were instructed to provide a smooth and atraumatic anesthetic. The V5 ECG lead was monitored, and plasma concentrations of β adrenergic blocker were measured prior to induction and on entry to the recovery room.

The incidence of ischemia was markedly lower in the treated group than in the untreated control group (2 versus 28 percent). The heart rate was lower at all time points in treated patients. Untreated patients with ischemia (all during either intubation or emergence) had a mean heart rate of 120 beats/min. However, all these episodes were self-limited, and no patient developed postoperative infarction.

Mean arterial pressures were similar preoperatively in all groups (115 to 119 mmHg). In the untreated patients, the mean arterial pressure increased significantly up to 127 mmHg. In patients with ischemic changes, the peak mean arterial pressure was 130 mmHg. These increases were transient and did not require specific therapy. The pressor responses during intubation and emergence seen in all groups were most effectively attenuated by labetalol and atenolol.

Bardycardia (heart rate less than 45 beats/min) did not occur in untreated patients. However, it occurred in 24 percent of those in the treated group, requiring treatment with atropine in one-half of these. Hypotension (systolic pressure less than 70 mmHg) occurred in 12 percent of treated patients versus 5 percent of untreated, although this difference did not attain statistical significance.

As noted in an accompanying editorial, the lack of true randomization or blinding and a distinctly higher incidence of nonspecific ST-T wave abnormalities on the preoperative ECG and prior myocardial infarction in the control group could have significantly influenced the results.[39]

Goldman and Caldera[40] found that untreated patients with mild to moderate hypertension (diastolic pressure less than 110 mmHg) had no greater incidence of postoperative infarction. From an outcome standpoint, the study by Stone et al.[37,38] seems to confirm this, although they clearly documented transient episodes of myocardial ischemia and, like Prys-Roberts et al.,[41–43] greater hemodynamic lability in untreated hypertensive patients.

Perioperative Use in Patients Undergoing Major Vascular Surgery

Pasternack et al.[44] reported on the efficacy of perioperative β adrenergic blockade with metoprolol in 32 patients undergoing abdominal aortic aneurysm repair, a patient population at high risk for postoperative cardiac morbidity. All patients received a 50-mg oral dose immediately prior to surgery and 10 to 15 mg IV (depending on blood pressure) every 12 hours for the first 5 days postoperatively. Roughly one-third of the group were receiving other β adrenergic blockers chronically and were switched to metoprolol 24 hours before surgery. A historic control group of 52 patients from a 5-year period before the study was analyzed. Although slightly more than one-third of these control patients were chronically receiving β adrenergic blockers, none of them received any β adrenergic blocker intra- or postoperatively. Frequent measurements of hemodynamics, including filling pressures and cardiac output, were performed. Postoperative myocardial infarction was diagnosed using elevations of the creatine kinase MB fraction alone, although specific details of sampling, the actual results, and any correlation with ECG findings were not presented.

Systolic pressures and heart rate, were significantly lower at all time periods in the treated group (only up to the first 48 hours postoperatively was reported, Figs. 28-4 and 28-5). Diastolic pressure was also significantly lower although only until 8 hours postoperatively. The cardiac index was significantly lower in treated patients intraoperatively and immediately postoperatively; at all later times, no differences were observed. Although pulmonary artery wedge pressure was not reported, there were no differences between groups in pulmonary systolic or diastolic pressures at any point. The incidence of postoperative infarction (all within 48 hours postoperatively) was significantly lower in the treated group (3.1 versus 17.6 percent). In addition, there were fewer atrial and ventricular arrhythmias in the treated group. The authors emphasize that β adrenergic blockade reduced myocardial oxygen demand (i.e., systolic arterial pressure and heart rate) while maintaining myocardial oxygen supply (stable systemic and pul-

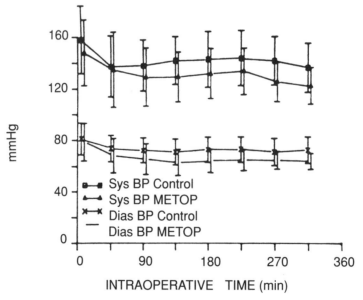

Fig. 28-4 Intraoperative systolic and diastolic blood pressures in metoprolol treated and control groups. Significant differences were present for all intervals after 45 minutes. (From Pasternack et al.,[44] with permission.)

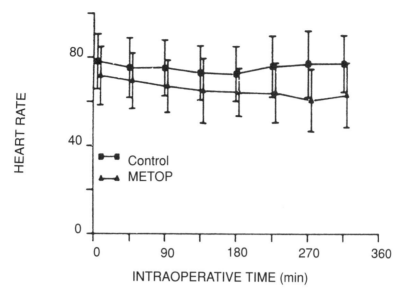

Fig. 28-5 Intraoperative heart rates in metoprolol treated and control groups. Significant differences were present for all intervals. (From Pasternack et al.,[44] with permission.)

monary artery pressure). There were no reported hemodynamic or other complications of therapy.

This study seems to indicate that β adrenergic blockade in this population is well tolerated and associated with substantial benefits. However, the use of historic controls and failure to randomize patients, and the controversial and incompletely reported criteria for the diagnosis of infarction, greatly weaken its results.

Effects on Silent Myocardial Ischemia in Vascular Patients

Pasternack et al.[45] extended their observations to include continuous Holter monitoring to detect myocardial ischemia in a cohort of 48 patients undergoing a variety of vascular procedures (aortic, carotid, and lower extremity) who had received metoprolol 50 mg orally immediately preoperatively. A concurrent control group (n = 152) was also monitored. Unfortunately, it is not stated whether the study group received any additional doses of metoprolol. As in their earlier study, nearly one-third of the control group was receiving chronic β adrenergic blocker therapy (although this would tend to minimize any potential differences).

As expected, intraoperative heart rates were sig-

nificantly different between groups, averaging 15 to 20 beats/min lower in those receiving metoprolol. The total number of ischemic episodes per patient, their duration, and the percent of time intraoperatively during which ischemia was present were significantly less in the treated group, although there was substantial variability in the data. Unfortunately, little raw data are presented (including the actual number of ischemic patients in each group, hemodynamics during the ischemic episodes, and outcome data). Thus, although this study suggests a significant difference in the incidence of silent ischemia with β adrenergic blockade, a firm generalization of the results to clinical practice is precluded. At this time, few clinicians in the United States utilize β adrenergic blockers prophylactically in patients undergoing vascular surgery.

USE DURING CORONARY ARTERY BYPASS GRAFT SURGERY

Studies of Clinical Safety

The anecdotal report of Viljoen et al.,[46] in which five patients receiving oral propranolol within 24 hours of CABG surgery died or had major complications, greatly influenced the clinical community with its recommendation that therapy be withdrawn 2 weeks preoperatively. Kaplan et al.[47] pointed out that these patients were at high risk because of other factors (complex surgery, poor ventricular function, and the use of the depressant anesthetic, methoxyflurane). However, the recommendation to withdraw therapy 2 weeks before surgery remained popular, despite the finding 1 year later that the negative inotropic effects of propranolol were no longer present 48 hours after discontinuation of oral therapy.[48]

Eventually, clinical practice started to shift toward the continuation of therapy. Kaplan et al.[47] reported a retrospective study of 143 patients undergoing cardiac surgery in whom therapy was discontinued less than 24 hours, 24 to 48 hours, or greater than 48 hours prior to induction. The average preoperative propranolol dose was 125 mg (range, 40 to 480 mg). Anesthesia consisted of morphine, diazepam, pancuronium, and nitrous oxide. The incidence of hypotension or bradycardia before or after cardiopulmonary bypass was no different between groups. However, 5 of the 46 patients in whom therapy was withdrawn 48 hours before surgery sustained preoperative infarction. The operative mortality rate was similar between groups (4 to 6 percent). The authors recommended that propranolol could be given safely within 24 to 48 hours of surgery and than be discontinued under close medical supervision. However, they *did not* recommend that it be administered the morning of surgery.

Slogoff et al.[49] were the first to present a prospective randomized trial of the safety of continuing propranolol in full dosage up to the time of operation. Thirty-eight patients scheduled for elective CABG (ejection fraction more than 0.3) were randomized to full dosage up to 12 hours before surgery, 40 patients were randomized to discontinuation of β adrenergic blockers between 24 and 72 hours, and 41 patients not taking propranolol served as controls. An anesthetic regimen similar to that of Kaplan et al.[47] was used, and the average doses of propranolol were similar. Lead II of the ECG was monitored for signs of ischemia (the more sensitive V5 lead was not yet popular). Fifteen patients in the withdrawal group developed worsened angina, prompting the authors to alter the study protocol such that patients were continued on one-half of their usual dose rather than being withdrawn completely. In the prebypass period, the incidence of ischemia (changes in lead II or the presence of ventricular arrhythmias) was much greater in this group (70 versus 26 percent). The incidence of ischemia in the control group (51 percent) was also greater than that in the treated group. Interestingly, despite these findings, there were no differences in emergence from bypass, postoperative infarction, or mortality rate (although the study groups were too small to detect such differences conclusively). They recommended that for "routine" CABG surgery, β adrenergic blockers should be continued until 6 to 12 hours before surgery.

Boudolas et al.[50] measured urinary catecholamine levels (epinephrine and norepinephrine), systolic time intervals (as an index of ventricular function) and 35-lead precordial ST segment mapping within 24 hours of surgery in 30 patients receiving chronic β adrenergic blocker therapy. Patients received their usual dose 4 to 10 hours before surgery (average dose, 155 mg), and plasma propranolol levels, drawn 1 hour before surgery, were in the therapeutic range. Urinary catecholamine concentrations were significantly elevated (three- to fourfold relative to a control group of hospitalized patients with no cardiac disease), indicating significant preoperative stress. Although details were not specifically reported, there were no hemodynamic complications. Four (13 percent) of the patients developed postoperative infarction. Interestingly, two of these had the highest preoperative urinary catecholamine excretion. Systolic time intervals suggested that the negative inotropic effects of propranolol lasted only 3 to 5 hours after oral dosing. They recommended dosing be continued up to 4 hours before surgery.

Plasma Concentrations and Hemodynamic Suppression

Sill et al.[51] investigated the relationship of plasma levels from chronic oral therapy continued until the day before or the morning of surgery to intraoperative hemodynamics (heart rate, mean arterial pressure, cardiac index, systemic vascular resistance, pulmonary capillary wedge pressure) in 26 patients undergoing CABG anesthetized with morphine-diazepam-pancuronium. In a subgroup of these patients, additional intravenous doses were administered to increase the range of plasma concentrations obtained intraoperatively. Plasma levels from 0 to 96 ng/ml were observed in the prebypass period. Postbypass, they declined significantly but, surprisingly, started to rise with no additional drug administered, suggesting release from a storage site. Hemodynamics obtained 5 minutes prior to skin incision served as control values from which the percent changes were calculated and compared with the logarithm of the plasma concentration.

In the resting state and with induction of anesthesia, no correlation of heart rate or mean arterial pressure with log plasma levels was evident (r = -0.05 and 0.25, respectively). With laryngoscopy and intubation, the heart rate and mean arterial pressure were significantly inversely correlated with the log concentration (r = -0.62 for both) (Figs. 28-6 and 28-7). With sternotomy and sternal

retraction, the heart rate and log concentration were correlated (r = -0.66 to -0.80). Correlation for the other hemodynamic variables was less significant. Following intubation, the mean arterial pressure was deliberately attenuated with halothane to prevent the deleterious effects of intraoperative hypertension. Likewise, postbypass correlations were poor as a result of low plasma concentrations and the use of other vasoactive agents and/or cardiac pacing required for clinical management. Although not conclusive, at higher log plasma concentrations, the cardiac index decreased, and systemic vascular resistance increased. Potential explanations for this include either direct negative inotropic effects and/or the unopposed α-adrenergic tone, leading to peripheral vasoconstriction. The data suggested that propranolol was most effective at blocking the hemodynamic response to intubation. Interestingly, counter to standard clinical teaching, the resting heart rate was a poor indicator of the degree of β adrenergic blockade.

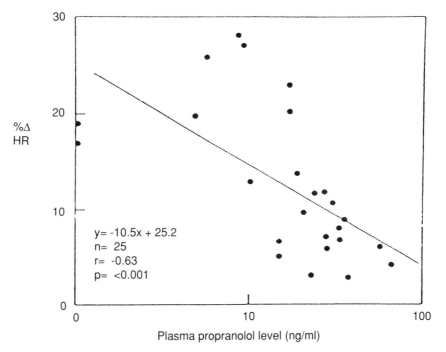

Fig. 28-6 A significant negative correlation between the percent change in heart rate from prelaryngoscopy to postintubation and the log plasma propranolol level was observed in contrast to a lack of correlation in the resting preoperative state. (From Sill et al.,[51] with permission.)

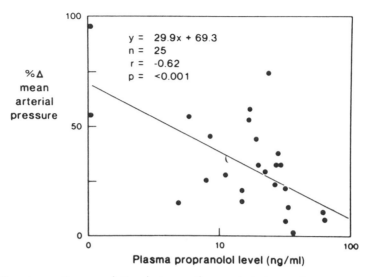

Fig. 28-7 A significant negative correlation between the percent change in mean arterial pressure from prelaryngoscopy to postintubation and the log plasma propranolol level was observed. (From Sill et al.,[51] with permission.)

These investigators subsequently presented additional pharmacokinetic data on 68 patients who were receiving propranolol or metoprolol to determine what intraoperative plasma levels occur with various preoperative doses.[52] Samples were obtained immediately prior to anesthetic induction, and the results were correlated with the time interval between preoperative dosing and intraoperative sampling. Patients receiving propranolol in doses less than 40 mg four times a day had plasma levels below 50 ng/ml, the lower limit for effective attenuation of hemodynamic responses to intubation (based on their earlier study), only 2 hours after dosing (Fig. 28-8). With doses of metoprolol of 50 mg two times a day, plasma levels were therapeutic for 4.5 hours. Interestingly, in 10 patients sampled repeatedly, the plasma levels declined sharply between induction and incision, suggesting a dilutional effect from intravenous fluid administration. They noted that propranolol levels as low as 8 ng/ml were shown to blunt tachycardia with exercise; levels of 30 ng/ml were associated with a significant reduction in the frequency of angina pectoris.[53] This study clearly demonstrates that, with commonly used preoperative doses of propranolol (and to a lesser extent metoprolol), therapeutic levels are not maintained for long. Thus, if β

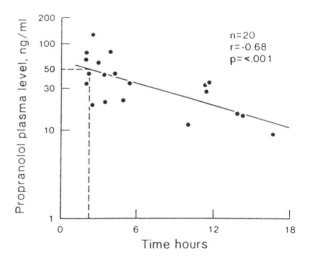

Fig. 28-8 Propranolol plasma levels at the time of induction of anesthesia in patients taking 40 mg four times a day chronically were determined. The time interval from the final preoperative dose to induction of anesthesia is shown. The lower limit of the therapeutic range for propranolol is 50 ng/ml. Thus, propranolol plasma levels are subtherapeutic approximately 2 hours after the last preoperative dose. (From Sill et al.,[52] with permission.)

adrenergic blockade is desired for intubation, therapy should be administered right up until the time of surgery.

Effects on Minimum Alveolar Concentration

Stanley et al.[54] were among the first to assess carefully the effect of β-adrenergic blockers on opioid requirements and intraoperative hemodynamics. Using sufentanil-pancuronium anesthesia, they noted a modest but statistically significant reduction in anesthetic doses required for loss of consciousness (3.8 versus 4.9 μg/kg without β adrenergic blockers) and maintenance of anesthesia (11.1 versus 15 μg/kg). The use of phentolamine and/or sodium nitroprusside was also significantly lower in the β-blocked patients. Interestingly, the time to awakening was similar in both groups.

Effects on Hemodynamics

Hammon et al.[55] studied the hemodynamic effects of perioperative β adrenergic blockade with propranolol on patients undergoing CABG. Fifty patients were randomized using a double blind design to receive propranolol (60 mg every 6 hours) or placebo, starting 24 to 48 hours preoperatively. Dosing was continued (by nasogastric tube) on arrival in the intensive care unit. The rate-pressure product was significantly lower in β-blocked patients during induction and sternotomy. Postoperative nitroprusside use was lower in these patients (3/24 versus 10/26 patients), as was the incidence of arrhythmias (7/24 versus 15/26 patients). Two patients, both in the placebo group, developed postoperative myocardial infarctions. Based on plasma concentrations, the authors postulate that a postoperative level of 75 ng/ml is necessary to reduce hypertension, ischemia, and/or arrhythmias.

Similar but less dramatic findings were reported by Heikkila et al.[56] in 20 patients who were receiving metoprolol (average daily dose, 1.9 mg/kg) and were randomized to either discontinuation 12 hours before surgery or continuation with the last dose administered 1.5 hours preoperatively. Plasma concentrations varied by three- to fourfold between the two groups. Hemodynamic changes were not significantly different between groups. The use of inotropes was no different between

groups. Despite the small sample size and the lack of outcome data, the authors concluded that continuation of metoprolol was safe and associated with a more favorable myocardial oxygen-supply demand balance intraoperatively.

Effects on Indices of Coronary Perfusion

The beneficial clinical effects of β adrenergic blockers on myocardial ischemia result from a complex interplay of a number of variables modulating myocardial oxygen demand and supply.[57] A reduction of myocardial oxygen consumption, primarily through a decrease in heart rate and negative inotropic effects, which decrease contractility, is the most important effect. A reduction in heart rate not only decreases demand but also increases myocardial oxygen supply because, in the left ventricle, coronary blood flow occurs almost exclusively during diastole. This effect is particularly important distal to a significant coronary stenosis.

Boudoulas et al.[58] extensively studied the effects of β adrenergic blockade on diastolic time at varying heart rates using systolic time intervals. This noninvasive approach uses high speed ECG recordings, carotid pulse tracings, and phonocardiography to measure precisely the left ventricular ejection time, pre-ejection period, and total electromechanical systole (QS_2).[59] The diastolic time was obtained by subtracting QS_2 from the total cardiac cycle length (R-R interval). It is related to the heart rate in a nonlinear fashion, increasing steeply with heart rates below 75 beats/min (Fig. 28-9).

Boudoulas et al.[58] studied 159 β-blocked or control patients with coronary artery disease. In selected patients, 2.5 mg of propranolol was given intravenously; others received chronic oral therapy. In all groups, the diastolic time significantly increased with β adrenergic blockade (as a result of a decrease in the heart rate); only modest increases in QS_2 were noted (Fig. 28-10). The blood pressure was unchanged.

Other experiments show that the ratio of subendocardial to subepicardial blood flow improves as diastolic time increases.[60] As long as left ventricular end-diastolic pressure stays constant (as it does at low and moderate doses of β adrenergic blockers), myocardial oxygen supply will improve. At higher

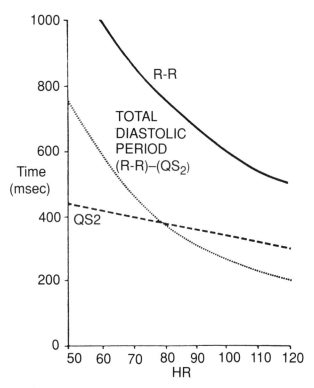

Fig. 28-9 Relationship between cardiac cycle length (R-R), total electromechanical systole (QS_2), total diastolic period (R-R) − (QS_2), and heart rate. Small changes in heart rate produce significant changes in diastolic time, most marked at lower heart rates. See text for details. (From Boudoulas et al.,[58] with permission.)

doses, which decrease contractility, left ventricular end-diastolic pressure may increase and mean arterial pressure decrease, leading to a decrease in coronary perfusion pressure. In this setting, an increase in diastolic time is especially critical to preserve the myocardial oxygen supply demand balance. However, given the complex interplay of multiple physiologic variables involved in the causes of ischemia, the precise scenario is difficult to predict clinically (Fig. 28-11).[57]

Propranolol and Postoperative Hypertension

Bolling et al.[61] found a significant relation between residual propranolol serum levels and postoperative hypertension in 15 patients undergoing CABG. Sodium nitroprusside was used as indicated to maintain the postoperative mean arterial pressure between 80 and 90 mmHg. The dosage requirements of this drug were significantly and positively correlated with residual plasma propranolol levels (r = 0.76) at 6 hours postcardiopulmonary bypass. No correlation was found with sex, age, ejection fraction, number of grafts, cross clamp or total bypass time, or preoperative propranolol dose. The authors postulate that unopposed α-adrenergic stimulation in the face of a nonselective β adrenergic blockade was the most likely etiologic factor. However, failure to measure catecholamine levels or to study patients taking cardioselective agents (which should have less effect on the systemic vascular resistances) weakens their study. Given that other studies have reported a lower frequency of postoperative hypertension with perioperative propranolol administration, their results are controversial.

Selective Agents and Those With Intrinsic Sympathomimetic Activity

The theoretic advantages of agents having β_1 adrenoceptor selectivity or intrinsic sympathomimetic action have been advanced. The former might be advantageous as a result of preservation of β_2 adrenoceptor mediated peripheral vasodilation; the latter might better preserve myocardial contractility. Agents with intrinsic sympathomimetic activity (e.g. pindolol, practolol, and oxprenolol) produce minimal slowing of the heart rate at rest, but during exercise, the heart rate response is significantly attenuated. Ventricular function may be better preserved following intravenous administration of practolol or oxprenolol compared with agents lacking intrinsic sympathomimetic activity (e.g., metoprolol or propranolol).[11] There is also evidence in a canine model that agents with such activity may better preserve contractility in the presence of depressant volatile anesthetics, such as halothane.[62]

Salmenpera et al.[63] evaluated agents with and without intrinsic sympathomimetic activity in a randomized study of 20 low risk patients 2 to 3 hours after CABG surgery. Ten patients received metoprolol (0.03 mg/kg), and 10 received pindolol (0.003 mg/kg) intravenously. The heart rate decreased an average of 5 beats/min in each group at 5 minutes postinjection. In the metoprolol group, there were no other significant changes in any of the hemodynamic variables. In contrast, pindolol caused a small but significant decline in cardiac index (approximately, 0.4 L/min/m²) and an increase in systemic vascular resistance (approximately, 100 dynes/sec/cm^{-5}). Changes in pulmonary artery wedge pressure were minimal, but a consistent small increase (less than 2 mmHg) was noted with pindolol, although small decreases occurred with metoprolol. Thus, the effects of pindolol appear to reflect its nonselective blocking properties over its intrinsic sympathomimetic activity. Post-CABG, given the high levels of sympathetic tone, the effects of such activity are not as evident.

Response to Inotropes in Patients With β Adrenergic Blockade

Although many studies have shown perioperative β adrenergic blockade to be beneficial, most only considered low risk patients, the majority of whom

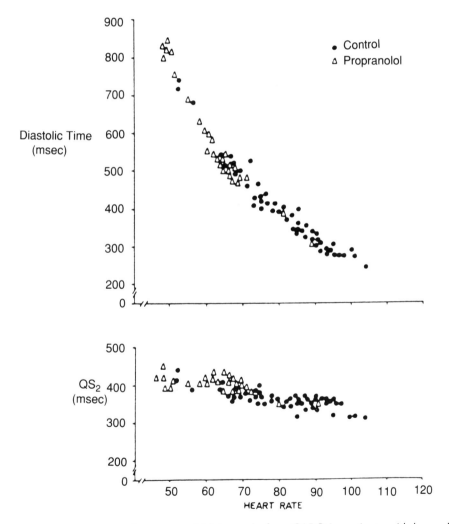

Fig. 28-10 Systolic time intervals measured 15 hours before CABG in patients withdrawn from chronic propranolol therapy (24 hours prior to study) compared surgery with those maintained on therapy. The latter patients had significantly longer diastolic times. (From Boudoulas et al.,[58] with permission.)

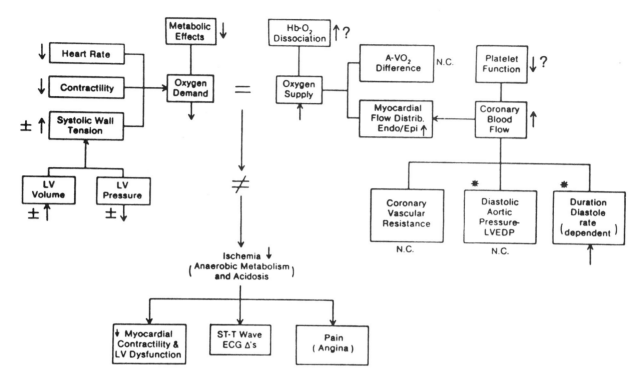

✱ *Limiting only in presence of coronary obstruction*

Fig. 28-11 Effect of β adrenergic blockade on the many factors influencing myocardial oxygen balance during ischemia. (From Frishman,[57] with permission.)

do not require inotropic support postoperatively. In fact, most of these patients will do well no matter how they are managed as they have a significant margin of "cardiac reserve." The effects of preoperative blockade on patients who subsequently require inotropes is controversial and until recently, was poorly studied. Given the increasing number of high risk patients coming to surgery, many of whom have significant impairment of ventricular function, this topic assumes greater clinical importance. Significant impairment of myocardial compliance and function occurs postbypass, particularly with a long ischemic time (often necessitated by multiple grafts or inadequate native vessels), dramatically increasing the need for postoperative inotropic support.

The effects of β adrenergic blockade on hemodynamic responsiveness to dobutamine and epinephrine were investigated by Tarnow et al.[64,65] in two studies. The first study consisted of 20 low risk patients treated chronically with either selective (n = 14) or nonselective β adrenergic blockers (n = 6) undergoing CABG. Eleven patients not receiving β adrenergic blockers served as controls. The study was performed after induction but prior to skin incision. Fentanyl-pancuronium-isoflurane anesthesia was used. The degree of β adrenergic blockade was assessed using the isoproterenol sensitivity test in which the heart rate response to small graded doses of intravenous isoproterenol is measured. The dose required to increase the heart rate by 25 beats/min (CD$_{25}$), was used as an index of β adrenergic blockade. After return to a steady state, dobutamine was infused in doses of 1.0, 2.0, and 4.0 μg/kg/min for 10-minute periods. Hemodynamic measurements were made at the end of each period. As expected, the isoproterenol dose-response curves showed a rightward shift in the β blocked patients (Fig. 28-12). The dose ratio between blocked and control patients was 6.5 (based on the geometric mean CD_{25} dose). A significant inverse correlation between log CD_{25} and the change in cardiac index was observed at each level of dobutamine infusion (r = −0.78 to −0.82, Fig. 28-13). Thus, with increasing levels of β adrenergic blockade, dobutamine did not increase the cardiac index. A positive correlation was noted between log CD_{25} and the systemic vascular resistance index (r = 0.75). Thus, a vasoconstrictive effect of dobutamine was observed despite the predominance of patients receiving selective agents. The authors concluded that higher degrees of β adrenergic blockade significantly reduced the inotropic response to dobutamine and allowed the systemic vascular resistance index to increase as a result of blockade of β_2 adrenoceptor mediated vasodilatation.

An identical experimental design was used to study the effects of epinephrine.[65] Following a determination of the CD_{25}, epinephrine was infused at doses of 0.01, 0.02, and 0.04 μg/kg/min. The augmentation of the cardiac index was antagonized by β adrenergic blockade, although the systemic vascular resistance index was increased, as with dobutamine. In addition, a significant positive correlation with the mean arterial pressure was observed (r = 0.59 to 0.76, Fig. 28-14). The heart rate showed a significant negative correlation (r = −0.65 to −0.74), presumably caused by baroreceptor reflexes.

These studies illustrate the complexity of the interactions between inotropes and β adrenergic blockers. Further investigation of this complex issue is necessary, especially during more critical and unstable conditions.

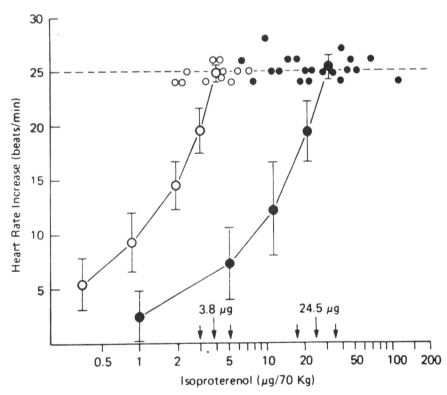

Fig. 28-12 Isoproterenol log dose-response curves for patients receiving β adrenergic blockers (●) and a control group (○). The mean isoproterenol doses producing an increase in heart rate of 25 beats/min (termed the CD_{25}) are shown. See text for details. (From Tarnow,[64] with permission.)

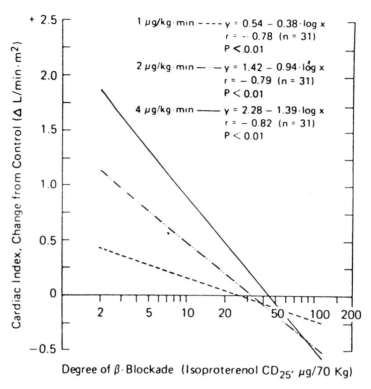

Fig. 28-13 Relationship between degree of β adrenergic blockade (based on the CD₂₅ dose) and the effects of three different doses of dobutamine on cardiac index. The effects of dobutamine were attenuated with increasing degree of β adrenergic blockade regardless of the dobutamine dosage studied. (From Tarnow,[64] with permission.)

USES DURING NONCARDIAC SURGERY

Kaplan et al.[66] reported a retrospective study of 73 patients undergoing a variety of noncardiac surgical procedures who were receiving propranolol for treatment of angina, arrhythmias, or hypertension (mean dose, 77 mg/day). A variety of anesthetic techniques were used, although enflurane was the most common. Seventy-two percent had their last dose within 24 hours of surgery, one-half of these within 12 hours. The incidence rates of hypotension, bradycardia, or arrhythmias were insignificant. Only one patient developed postoperative infarction, and there were no deaths. They concluded that propranolol need not be withdrawn preoperatively.

Goldman[67] presented two case reports of high

risk patients undergoing aortic vascular surgery in whom propranolol was continued immediately up to or within 24 hours of surgery. In the latter patient, the dose was tapered, starting 48 hours preoperatively. This patient did well intraoperatively but developed sinus tachycardia (120 beats/min) in the early postoperative period accompanied by frequent unifocal premature ventricular contractions. On the second postoperative day, he developed ischemic ECG changes with a slight rise in creatine kinase enzymes along with episodes of chest pain. On the fourth postoperative day, propranolol was restarted, and the sinus tachycardia resolved along with the chest pain and ECG changes. The second patient had a far more complicated course (bleeding, acute cholecystitis, pneumonia, and renal failure) but had labile hypertension and tachycardia that appeared to resolve once propranolol was re-

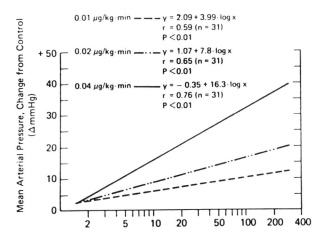

Fig. 28-14 Relationship between degree of β adrenergic blockade (based on the CD$_{25}$ dose) and the effects of three different doses of epinephrine on the mean arterial pressure. Higher degrees of β adrenergic blockade, particularly in patients receiving nonselective blockers, unmasked α adrenergic effects, increasing systemic vascular resistance and mean arterial pressure. (From Tarnow and Muller,[65] with permission.)

started 7 days postoperatively. Goldman hypothesized that these cases, particularly the first, illustrated propranolol withdrawal rebound. He recommended that oral, nasogastric, or intravenous administration of propranolol be started postoperatively when the patient is stable or whenever signs of increased adrenergic activity (unrelated to other acute postoperative complications) occur. He also noted that this withdrawal syndrome is relatively rare.

Ponten et al.[68] reported on 48 patients with ischemic heart disease and/or hypertension who were receiving chronic β adrenergic blocker therapy and undergoing either carotid or gallbladder surgery. Therapy included both selective and nonselective agents. Patients were randomly assigned to either withdrawal of therapy over 4 days preoperatively or continuation up to surgery. Nitrous-fentanyl-pancuronium anesthesia was used. This study is notable for its comprehensive physiologic data collection (including preoperative stress testing, intraoperative pulmonary artery catheterization in a subset of patients, perioperative Holter recording of arrhythmias, and postoperative ECG/cardiac enzyme levels). Three patients withdrawn from therapy developed severe arrhythmias, hypertension, tachycardia, or angina requiring reinstitution of therapy. As expected, the heart rates in the withdrawn patients (both surgical groups) were significantly higher preinduction (approximately 15 to 20 beats/min) and during intubation and extubation (approximately 25 to 40 beats/min). However, by the first postoperative morning, no significant differences were apparent. Changes in blood pressure were more variable between the four subgroups, although in general, a decline in blood pressure during induction was most evident in the β blocked patients. Interestingly, rebound increase in blood pressure with surgical stimulation was also most evident in these patients. In the subgroup of patients with pulmonary artery catheters, the cardiac index was lower, and the pulmonary artery wedge pressure and systemic vascular resistance index were higher in β blocked patients. There was no difference in the incidence of ventricular arrhythmias. Supraventricular arrhythmias were more common in the withdrawn patients, but transient bradycardia was more common in β blocked patients, particularly during reversal and extubation. Ischemic ST segment changes on the early postoperative 12-lead ECG were more common in patients withdrawn from β adrenergic blockers. The incidence of postoperative infarction was similar. There were no differences in hemodynamics between patients continued on selective versus nonselective β adrenergic blockers.

These findings, among the first to include detailed central hemodynamics, are consistent with all of the expected hemodynamic effects of β adrenergic blockade and illustrate the potential trade-offs that must be weighed when using these drugs. β Adrenergic blockers can be associated with both increased vasoconstriction and decreased contractility. The increase in pulmonary artery wedge pressure can reduce coronary perfusion pressure. However, the lower heart rates observed will tend to increase the diastolic coronary perfusion time. The lower incidence of myocardial ischemia with β adrenergic blockade observed in this and other studies suggests the latter effect is more significant.

AIRWAY REACTIVITY AND PERIOPERATIVE β ADRENERGIC BLOCKADE

The possibility that β adrenergic blockers may induce clinically significant bronchospasm is one of the major reasons these agents are used cautiously. Many patients with coronary artery disease or hypertension have smoked heavily and have clinically significant chronic obstructive pulmonary disease. Asthma in younger individuals is also relatively common. Acute bronchospasm during anesthesia or the postoperative period can be exceedingly dangerous. There are few clinicians that have not induced some degree of bronchospasm in a patient at least once following administration of a β adrenergic blocker. With the increasing popularity of the β_1-selective agents (e.g., metoprolol and esmolol), acute bronchospasm is less likely. However, nonselective agents (e.g., labetalol) are also widely used. Several recent studies provide useful clinical information on the effects of the selective agents on airway resistance, although none have been performed in the perioperative setting.

Sheppard et al.[69] studied the effects of esmolol compared with placebo in a double blind randomized crossover study of 10 mild asthmatic patients (defined by an increase in specific airway resistance of 100 percent in response to dry air inhalation) whose medications had been withdrawn for 24 hours. In addition, 6 of these patients were also studied following intravenous administration of 1 to 5 mg of propranolol. The response to each agent or placebo was evaluated during dry air provocation and following isoproterenol inhalation. Following loading doses of 500 μg/kg, esmolol was infused starting at 100 μg/kg/min and increased up to 300 μg/kg/min, with each infusion dose maintained for 30 minutes.

No significant differences were seen between esmolol and placebo in specific airway resistance at the maximal dose of esmolol. However, symptomatic bronchoconstriction developed in two of six subjects after only 1 mg of propranolol. One of the remaining patients had a 100 percent increase in specific airway resistance to dry air testing at the 5-mg dose of propranolol. Small but significant increases in sensitivity to dry air and decreases in sensitivity to isoproterenol were observed with esmolol. However, the latter effect was only evident following the first inhalation (Fig. 28-15). The authors concluded that esmolol is considerably safer than propranolol. However, it is not completely selective in that it causes some inhibition of airway muscle β_2 adrenoceptors. They caution that further testing in sicker asthmatic patients may reveal more significant effects.

Gold et al.[70] evaluated ventilatory function in 50 patients with chronic obstructive pulmonary disease (smoking history, chronic bronchitis, or emphysema, and obstructive pattern on pulmonary function testing) and active cardiac disease (angina, recent myocardial infarction, arrhythmias, or hypertension) in response to infusion of esmolol at 8, 16, and 24 mg/min. The forced expiratory volume in 1 second (FEV_1), forced vital capacity, and peak expiratory flow were measured at each dose. Twenty percent of the group was studied at the 16-mg/min dose but not at the 24-mg/min dose because they attained a hemodynamic end point precluding a further increase in dose. Remarkably, no patient developed clinical bronchospasm or dyspnea, and only three had a reduction in FEV_1 (by more than 20 percent). This study is particularly significant in that it is the first (and only) study to document safety in a chronically ill population commonly seen in the surgical setting. It also demonstrates that the drug can be used to exert its hemodynamic effects without significant risk to pulmonary function.

PROPHYLAXIS OF POSTOPERATIVE SUPRAVENTRICULAR TACHYCARDIA

The prophylactic use of agents with antiarrhythmic properties (e.g., β adrenergic blockers, digoxin, or verapamil) to prevent supraventricular arrhythmias following CABG surgery is controversial. During the past 10 to 15 years, several dozen articles have appeared on this subject. The number of articles lends itself well to meta-analysis, a statistical technique allowing pooling of data to detect treatment effects with greater statistical power than any of the individual studies allow.

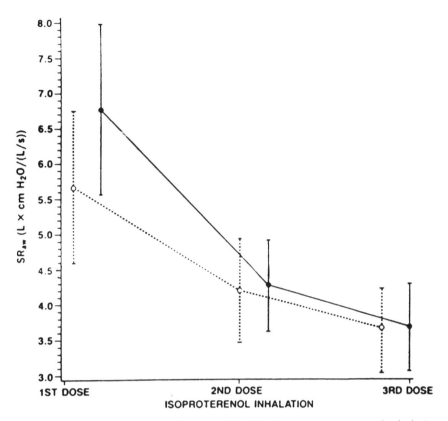

Fig. 28-15 Changes in specific airway resistance (SR_{aw}) following isoproterenol inhalation during esmolol (—) or placebo (---) infusion. A small but statistically significant decrease in bronchomotor sensitivity to isoproterenol is evident during the first inhalation. (From Sheppard et al.,[69] with permission.)

Andrews et al.[71] performed such an analysis, calculating proportions of patients developing supraventricular arrhythmia, odds ratios (an estimate of the likelihood of developing an arrhythmia between treatment and control groups), and the mean ventricular rate during the arrhythmia (if it occurred) in each treatment group. They identified 24 randomized controlled trials evaluating the use of digoxin, verapamil, or several β adrenergic blockers (propranolol, metoprolol, atenolol, timolol, nadolol, sotalol, or acebutolol) in which therapy was administered orally (pre- or postoperatively) and some type of ECG data was collected for at least 3 days postoperatively. They further anaylzed four β adrenergic blocker subgroups (therapy before versus after CABG, high versus low dose propranolol, propranolol versus other β adrenergic

blockers, and trials in which continuous Holter monitoring was used) to evaluate treatment effects further.

Supraventricular arrhythmias were present in 27 percent of patients in the control groups. They detected a striking difference in odds ratios between the drugs (Fig. 28-16). No significant treatment effect was detected for digoxin or verapamil; β adrenergic blockers imparted a significant beneficial effect (odds ratio = 0.28). This effect was present in each of the β blocker subgroups analyzed. Patients receiving treatment who developed supraventricular arrhythmias had a statistically significant (although not clinically significant) reduction in ventricular response (20 to 30 beats/min lower than in control patients).

The authors note that most of the subjects were

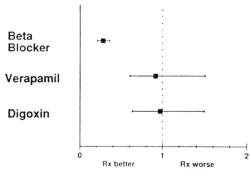

Fig. 28-16 Odds ratios for the development of postoperative supraventricular arrhythmias following CABG surgery in patients receiving prophylaxis with digoxin, verapamil, or β adrenergic blockers based on a meta-analysis of 24 published studies. The horizontal error bars indicate the 95 percent confidence intervals for the estimates. A significant protective effect of β adrenergic blockers was demonstrated. (From Andrews et al.,[71] with permission.)

relatively young, with normal or only mildly depressed ventricular function, and that many were already receiving β adrenergic blockers chronically, suggesting a potential confounding effect of drug withdrawal. However, given the strength of the protective effect, they recommended routine β adrenergic blocker use perioperatively in all appropriate candidates.

INHIBITION OF RENIN RELEASE: EFFECTS ON PERIOPERATIVE HYPERTENSION

The ability of β adrenergic blockers to inhibit renin release has been studied as a means to prevent "rebound hypertension" following termination of vasodilator therapy, particularly with sodium nitroprusside. Although not directly affecting the intraoperative portion of deliberate hypotensive anesthesia, rebound hypertension can jeopardize postoperative hemostasis. Given the popularity of nitroprusside for hypotensive anesthesia, this issue continues to be clinically significant.

Fahmy et al.[72] studied 20 American Society of Anesthesiologists class I to II patients undergoing deliberate hypotensive anesthesia for hip arthroplasty. Nitroprusside was used in addition to halothane, nitrous oxide, and curare to maintain mean arterial pressure at 50 to 55 mmHg. Ten patients were pretreated (just prior to induction) with propranolol 0.1 mg/kg. Plasma renin activity and catecholamine levels were measured.

With nitroprusside induced hypotension, the heart rate increased (by 16 percent) in untreated controls, leading to an increase in cardiac output. Patients given propranolol had no increase in heart rate or cardiac output. The plasma renin activity rose fivefold in the controls along with plasma epinephrine, norepinephrine, and dopamine levels (Fig. 28-17). These values remained elevated for 30 to 60 minutes following discontinuation of nitroprusside. In propranolol treated patients, the plasma renin activity did not increase, and catecholamine levels increased to a lesser degree. Following termination of the nitroprusside infusion, the mean arterial pressure rose significantly over preinfusion levels as a result of a doubling of systemic vascular resistance (Fig. 28-18) and heart rate and cardiac output remained elevated for 30 to 60 minutes in the control group. Overshoot was not observed in the treated group. Of note was the fact that the control group required twice as much nitroprusside.

Aortic cross clamping during vascular surgery can also significantly increase the plasma renin activity, although conflicting data have been reported.[73] Grant and Jenkins[74] reported an observational study of plasma renin activity in 13 patients undergoing infrarenal cross clamping, 5 of whom were receiving oral propranolol therapy. The plasma renin activity doubled with cross clamping and remained elevated at 30 minutes postoperatively in patients not receiving propranolol therapy. Patients who were receiving propranolol had lower basal plasma renin activities to start and did not show any significant increase perioperatively. However, there was no correlation between plasma renin activity and postoperative hypertension (which occurred in approximately the same percentage of patients in each group).

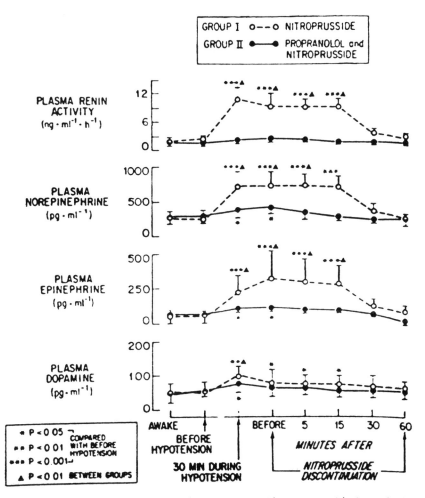

Fig. 28-17 Hormonal responses to deliberate hypotension with nitroprusside in patients pretreated with 0.1 mg/kg of propranolol prior to induction of anesthesia versus those not treated. Propranolol significantly attenuated the hormonal response. (From Fahmy et al.,[72] with permission.)

PERIOPERATIVE USE IN OBSTETRICS

β Adrenergic blockers can be useful for treating cardiovascular disorders during pregnancy, including hypertension, supraventricular arrhythmias (such as those caused by mitral valve prolapse or stenosis), idiopathic hypertrophic subaortic stenosis, and hyperthyroidism. Acutely, β adrenergic blockers can be used for treating severe hypertension during eclamptic states. However, they must be used with a considerable degree of caution.

Ethical considerations limit investigation of the physiologic effects of β adrenergic blockers to pregnant animal models, particularly pregnant sheep.[5] Obviously, adverse effects on the fetus are the major concern. Early in pregnancy, organogenesis is a concern. Intrauterine growth retardation has been associated with β adrenergic blockers; however, in most instances, the high risk nature of the pregnancy is a more likely cause. In later pregnancy, adverse effects on the regulation of maternal-fetal physiology are of major concern, including the regulation of umbilical blood flow, uterine

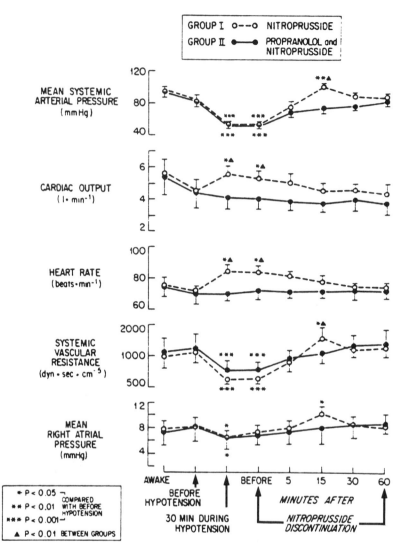

GROUP I o--o NITROPRUSSIDE
GROUP II •--• PROPRANOLOL and NITROPRUSSIDE

Fig. 28-18 Hemodynamic responses in the same group of patients described in Figure 28-17. Elevation of heart rate and cardiac output were attenuated by propranolol. A rebound increase in mean arterial pressure following discontinuation of nitroprusside was also attenuated. (From Fahmy et al.,[72] with permission.)

tone and contractility, and fetal heart rate. These physiologic effects are complex and have been reviewed elsewhere in detail.[5]

The body of evidence suggests that the effects of β adrenergic blockade in the unstressed fetus are minimal. However, in the compromised fetus, β adrenergic blockade may significantly impair the fetal response to stress, particularly in response to a decline in uterine blood flow and may lead to life

threatening bradycardia. Recent interest has focused on the use of cardioselective agents (e.g., metoprolol and esmolol) and on the use of labetalol. The vasodilating properties of labetalol could be helpful in treating the vasoconstriction associated with eclamptic states.

There is substantial clinical interet in esmolol for acute perioperative management of eclampsia because of the ultrashort half-life and lack of dependence on renal or hepatic function for metabolism (i.e., intravascular ester hydrolysis). The first published data on transplacental transfer of esmolol were obtained in pregnant ewes near term.[75] Despite low lipid solubility and intravascular hydrolysis, esmolol crossed the placenta rapidly, exerting fetal hemodynamic effects. An infusion of 500 μg/kg/min for 4 minutes followed by 300 μg/kg/min for 6 minutes resulted in a detectable serum concentration at 10 minutes following the termination of the infusion but not thereafter. The mean fetal to maternal ratio of concentrations varied from 0.13 to 0.20. Maximal changes in maternal heart rate and mean arterial pressure were −14 and −7 percent, respectively. In the fetus, the maximal heart rate change was −12 percent. The mean arterial pressure declined by 7 percent. No other physiologic changes were noted (i.e., fetal arterial blood gases or intra-amniotic pressure).

Eisenach and Castro[76] extended these observations, studying the dose-response characteristics and the degree of fetal β adrenergic blockade, using selective maternal and fetal isoproterenol sensitivity testing in a similar model. A wide range of doses was evaluated (15-minute infusions of 4 to 200 μg/kg/min). Esmolol decreased maternal, but not fetal, mean arterial pressure. In contrast, fetal, but not maternal, heart rate declined significantly, persisting for 30 minutes following termination of the infusion. Fetal PO_2 and pH declined significantly but rose to control levels at 30 minutes postinfusion. Based on the isoproterenol sensitivity plots, they suggested that esmolol is more potent in sheep than in dogs or humans. Residual β adrenergic blockade persisted 30 minutes following termination of the infusion. The authors suggested that esmolol should be used cautiously in pregnancy.

The first report of the effects of esmolol on human fetal heart rate were reported by Losasso et al.[77] during monitoring of a pregnant patient at 22 weeks undergoing resection of a cerebellar arteriovenous malformation. The fetal weight was estimated at 350 g, and its resting heart rate was 139 to 144 beats/min. Bolus doses up to 2 mg/kg and infusion up to 200 μg/kg/min prior to induction produced small reductions in the fetal heart rate (131 to 137 beats/min). Coadministration of esmolol with thiopental during intubation had greater ef-

fects (120 beats/min). During surgery, with isoflurane and fentanyl, a further decline to 112 to 120 beats/min was noted. Following termination of surgery and discontinuation of esmolol, the fetal heart rate returned to baseline.

Ducey and Knape[78] reported fetal bradycardia, which resulted in emergency cesarean section, with the use of esmolol to treat supraventricular tachycardia in a women at term. The patient, suspected to be thyrotoxic, was given a bolus of 500 μg/kg followed by an infusion of 50 μg/kg/min for 20 minutes, at which time severe fetal bradycardia (70 to 80 beats/min) occurred. The mother's blood pressure was normal. The fetus was born with Apgar scores of only 1 and 5 but subsequently did well. The mother's supraventricular tachycardia was treated successfully with verapamil, and her placenta, and the workup for thyroid or cardiac disease, proved completely normal. Perhaps, the supraventricular tachycardia induced a reduction in uterine blood flow, compromising the fetus, and the addition of β adrenergic blockade further reduced uterine perfusion. This case illustrates the potential risks of β adrenergic blockade. Verapamil has been used safely in this setting and probably should be the first line therapy.

OTHER PERIOPERATIVE APPLICATIONS OF β ADRENERGIC BLOCKADE

Pheochromocytoma

Intraoperative management of pheochromocytoma is often complicated by acute elevation of blood pressure and/or heart rate, especially during manipulation of the tumor, the majority of which secrete norepinephrine and epinephrine.[79] Given the predominance of α adrenergic mediated vasoconstriction, α adrenergic blockade and/or primary vasodilatation is required. With the routine use of preoperative α adrenergic blockade with phenoxybenzamine, severe systemic vasoconstriction and hypovolemia are relatively uncommon. Following removal of the tumor, profound hypotension can occur as elevated catecholamine levels rapidly decline. Intravenous phentolamine or nitroprusside are commonly used for perioperatively blood pressure control, allowing precise titration of hemodynamic effect, with rapid termination of action.

Several case reports document the use of intraoperative esmolol infusion for the control of tachycardia (as a result of unblocked epinephrine activity or as a reflex response to primary vasodilators).[80,81] It is also helpful for blood pressure control, although it should not be used without concurrent α adrenergic blockade because it might result in unopposed α adrenergic mediated vasoconstriction. Although other β adrenergic blockers, particularly labetalol, have also been used, the ultrashort half-life of esmolol probably makes it a safer choice.

Treatment of Tetralogy of Fallot

Esmolol has been found to be effective in the treatment of the hypercyanotic spells of tetralogy of Fallot. Nussbaum et al.[82] presented the cases of two pediatric patients (14 weeks premature and 6 months old) who responded intraoperatively with dramatic improvement in oxygen saturation to standard bolus and infusion doses of esmolol (on a per kilogram basis).

Treatment of Drug Overdosage

Esmolol and other β adrenergic blockers have been used successfully for the treatment of hyperadrenergic states resulting from overdosage of catecholamines or drugs with significant sympathomimetic effects, such as cocaine or theophylline.[83,84]

Use During Electroconvulsive Therapy

With a resurgence in popularity of electroconvulsive therapy for the treatment of depression, anesthesiologists have investigated strategies to minimize the hyperadrenergic response this therapy elicits. The anesthesiologist must balance the need for an adequate seizure against the antiseizure effects of most anesthetics. Despite adequate blockade of recall, severe hypertension and tachycardia are common and may be a problem in patients with cardiovascular disease. β Adrenergic blockers are an obvious adjuvant to block these hemodynamic responses.

The effects of labetolol (0.3 mg/kg) and esmolol (1 mg/kg) administered just prior to induction of anesthesia, were evaluated by Weinger et al.[85,86] in

Table 28-3 Effect of Pretreatment on Seizure Duration

Treatment	Seizure Duration (s)	Number Requiring Second Stimulus	Number of Inadequate Seizures
Labetalol	36.9 ± 4.5^a	2	1
Fentanyl	43.6 ± 4.1^a	2	0
Esmolol	45.8 ± 5.9	1	0
Lidocaine	26.5 ± 7.2^a	6	3
Saline	56.5 ± 12.5	0	0

^{a} Significantly different from saline control value ($P < 0.05$).
(From Weinger et al.,[86] with permission.)

a placebo controlled trial. Lidocaine (1.0 mg/kg) and fentanyl (1.5 μg/kg) were also evaluated, and each patient received each of the five therapies during their electroconvulsive treatment schedule.

Either β adrenergic blocker significantly attenuated the hemodynamic responses, although blood pressure was better controlled with esmolol. All drugs except esmolol significantly reduced seizure duration (Table 28-3). Only esmolol attenuated both norepinephrine and epinephrine release in response to electroconvulsive therapy.

Howie et al.[87] extended these observations by performing a dose-response placebo controlled study of esmolol. Following a bolus dose of 500 μg/kg, an infusion of either 100, 200, or 300 μg/kg/min for 3 minutes was administered. Although control of hemodynamic response was superior with the higher doses, only the 100 μg/kg/min dose did not alter the seizure duration. Similar results were reported by Ramsay et al.[88]

Thus, it appears that esmolol is effective in controlling adverse hemodynamic responses to electroconvulsive therapy. However, the total dose should be limited to 1 mg/kg to avoid reducing the seizure duration.

ESMOLOL

Esmolol is an ultrashort acting β adrenergic blocker ideally suited for perioperative use. There are more clinical reports on the use of this agent than on most of the older agents combined. A symposium on esmolol published in the American Journal of Cardiology is highly recommended,[89–96] as is a more recent review by Frishman.[7]

Its rapid onset, ultrashort elimination half-life (9 minutes), the rapid offset of its sympathetic blockade, and its high degree of β_1 adrenergic selectivity are advantageous intraoperatively when a variety of physiologic conditions change rapidly. Jacobs et al.,[97] using an extensively instrumented canine model, demonstrated that depressed ventricular function induced by a massive esmolol dose of 3,000 μg/kg/min returned to baseline by 30 minutes after termination of infusion (Fig. 28-19). The depression of the heart rate will normalize to baseline much sooner (usually by 15 minutes or less) as a result of the distinctly lower dose at which the

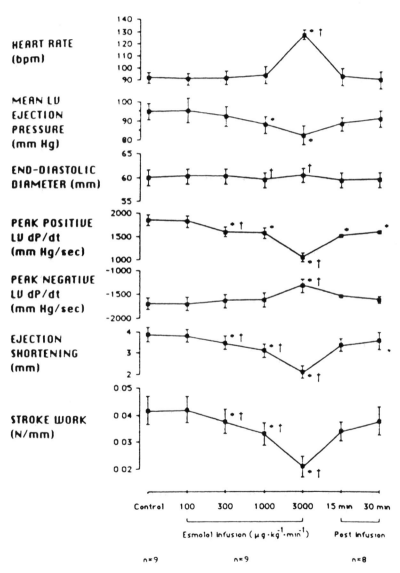

Fig. 28-19 Effects of increasing doses of esmolol on indices of ventricular contractility in an instrumented canine preparation. Reversal of adverse effects following termination of infusion is evident by 30 minutes. (From Jacobs et al.,[97] with permission.)

sinoatrial node is depressed (less than 100 μg/kg/min) relative to the dose required for negative inotropic effects (more than 300 μg/kg/min) (Fig. 28-20).[98] This difference confers distinct advantages in treating perioperative atrial and sinus tachycardia. It has also led some clinicians to use it to control severe tachycardia in patients requiring high doses of inotropes (albeit with great caution).[99]

However, these short acting properties makes long-term use impractical and in some instances hazardous (discussed later). Thus, if β adrenergic blockade is to be continued, a longer acting agent must be instituted. In most instances, metoprolol can be instituted because it has similar properties, aside from a longer elimination half-life. If a nonselective agent can be tolerated, propranolol or labetalol can be used.

Intraoperative Pharmacokinetics

de Bruijn et al.[100] were the first to report the pharmacokinetics of esmolol in anesthetized subjects. All 19 subjects were receiving chronic propranolol therapy. Esmolol was infused at doses varying from 100 to 500 μg/kg/min starting 7 minutes before induction up until 5 minutes after sternotomy (mean duration, 55 minutes). Venous sampling continued for 40 minutes after discontinuation of the infusion, and the data were fitted to a two-compartment model. The half-lives for the distribution and elimination phases were 1.34 $\pm$ 0.77 and 9.9 $\pm$ 1.2 minutes, respectively. Intersubject variation in the volume of distribution, clearance, and half-lives was substantial, up to 300 percent (similar to data in nonanesthetized subjects). However, given the short half-lives involved, this variation is not clinically significant.

Prophylactic Infusion During Coronary Artery Bypass Graft Surgery

Menkhaus et al.[101] were the first to evaluate the cardiovascular effects of esmolol during induction and intubation in 40 low risk patients undergoing CABG. Four equal groups were studied: placebo and 100, 200, and 300 μg/kg/min administered for 3 minutes prior to laryngoscopy. Loading doses of 500 μg/kg preceded the infusion. The heart rate and rate-pressure product responses were significantly attenuated by esmolol during intubation and for 5 minutes following cessation of infusion. Plasma levels were undetectable in most treated patients by 15 minutes after termination.

Girard et al.[102] reported on the safety and efficacy of esmolol in 37 patients undergoing CABG during high dose fentanyl anesthesia. In 9 patients, esmolol was administered at rates between 100 and 300 μg/kg/min after intubation but before sternotomy. The only significant effect was a small increase in pulmonary artery wedge pressure in the esmolol group from 8 to 13 mmHg. The heart rate decreased from the preinfusion baseline in both the placebo and the esmolol group. In 11 other patients, esmolol was infused from preintubation until cardiopulmonary bypass. The increase in heart rate with intubation was attenuated, although the difference was clinically insignificant (mean difference of only 5 beats/min between groups).

Harrison et al.[103] studied the effects of esmolol on myocardial ischemia in 30 patients randomized to receive either esmolol or placebo using continuous Holter monitoring in the prebypass period. An

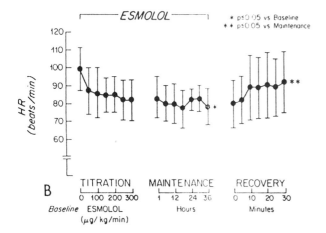

Fig. 28-20 Mean heart rates ($\pm$ standard deviation) in 16 patients with acute myocardial ischemia or infarction in response to esmolol titration and maintenance (up to 300 μg/kg/min or until hemodynamic end points or adverse effects reached). Note the rapid return of heart rate to baseline levels following termination of infusion. (From Kirshenbaum et al.,[98] with permission.)

unusual lead set (modified V6 and a lateral V9) was used to detect ischemia and arrhythmias. Esmolol was infused at 300 μg/kg/min (after a 500-μg/kg bolus) until institution of bypass. Fentanyl-pancuronium anesthesia was used with isoflurane supplementation for control of blood pressure. Three patients in the control group and one in the esmolol group developed prebypass ischemia, although this difference was not statistically significant. During aortic dissection and cannulation, complex ventricular arrhythmias were greater in the control group (73 versus 27 percent). Although an identical number of patients in each group required supplemental isoflurane, the total number of minutes of isoflurane (1 percent inspired concentration) administered was significantly lower in the esmolol group (16 versus 32 minutes). There were no apparent differences in outcome between the groups. The incidence of ischemia detected was low relative to the findings in other published clinical studies. However, the use of an atypical lead set may have contributed to this difference.

These studies, which evaluated small numbers of low risk patients, show minor differences in hemodynamics with the prophylactic use of esmolol but do not prove any substantial differences that justify its routine use.

Bolus Dosing During Coronary Artery Bypass Graft Surgery

The use of bolus dosing of esmolol, followed by infusion, for the treatment of intraoperative tachycardia and/or hypertension was studied by Reves et al.[104] in 45 patients undergoing CABG surgery. The study was randomized, double blind, and placebo controlled, and it included an initial dose ranging phase. All patients were receiving chronic β adrenergic blocker therapy (although not administered the morning of surgery), and many were also receiving calcium channel blockers. Anesthesia included midazolam, vecuronium, and enflurane.

In the initial dose ranging phase (performed randomly during surgery), a bolus of 80 mg followed by an infusion of 12 mg/min, was found to reduce the heart rate or systolic blood pressure by 15 percent within 3 minutes. Interestingly, one patient experienced a 50 percent decrease in cardiac output with only one-half this dose; this patient had been taking clonidine preoperatively. This dose was then used in the treatment phase of the study. The criteria for treatment included systolic blood pressure more than 140 mmHg and heart rate more than 70 beats/min. A significant reduction in the heart rate (average, 9 percent) was observed at 1 minute, with a peak effect of 14 percent by 1.6 minutes. The systolic blood pressure was reduced by 11 percent at 1.6 minutes. No differences in central pressures or cardiac output or in the incidence of hypotension, bradycardia, or ischemia were observed between treatment and placebo groups.

Dose-response and clinical safety data for the use of 100- or 200-mg boluses of esmolol during induction in patients undergoing general surgery were reported in a Canadian multicenter study of 548 patients at 12 institutions.[105] Anesthesia was induced with thiopental, 3 to 5 mg/kg, and succinylcholine. Some patients also received fentanyl, 2 to 3 μg/kg, or sufentanil, 0.3 μg/kg. The subjects were evenly distributed between the two doses of esmolol or placebo. American Society of Anesthesiologists class I to III patients (predominantly, class II) were studied. Standard exclusion criteria for the use of β adrenergic blockade were used. Only 8 percent of subjects were receiving chronic oral therapy.

The heart rate and systolic blood pressure values were significantly higher after intubation in the placebo group (Fig. 28-21). The proportion of patients with heart rates greater than 110 beats/min and/or peak systolic blood pressure more than 180 mmHg in the placebo group was twice that in the esmolol treatment groups. Opioid supplementation improved the control of systolic blood pressure. The incidence of hypotension (systolic blood pressure less than 90 mmHg) was significantly greater with esmolol, 200 mg (33 percent), intermediate with 100 mg (25 percent), and lowest with placebo (16 percent). The incidence of bradycardia or bronchospasm did not differ between groups. The authors concluded that the 100-mg dose along with low dose narcotic supplementation (fentanyl, 2 to 3 μg/kg), allows adequate control of hemodynamics during intubation with a low incidence of side effects.

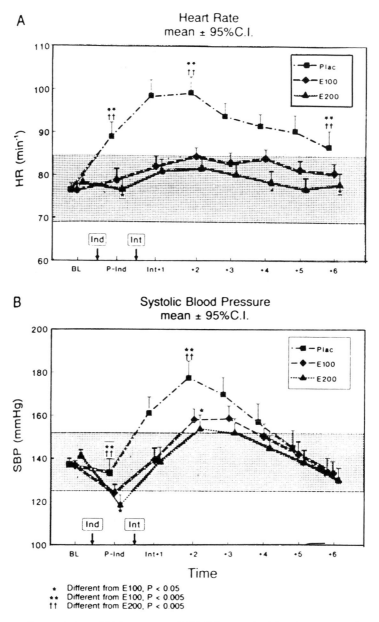

A

Heart Rate
mean ± 95%C.I.

B

Systolic Blood Pressure
mean ± 95%C.I.

* Different from E100, P < 0 05
** Different from E100, P < 0.005
†† Different from E200, P < 0.005

Fig. 28-21 Effects of esmolol on **(A)** heart rate (HR) **(B)** systolic blood pressure (SBP) during induction (Ind), intubation (Int), and the first 6 minutes thereafter. Placebo or 100- or 200-mg doses of esmolol were administered (Plac, E100, and E200, respectively). Stippled areas represent the mean ± 10 percent of baseline values. (From Miller et al.,[105] with permission.)

Treatment of Postoperative Hypertension

Gray et al.[106] evaluated the efficacy of esmolol compared with nitroprusside for treatment of hypertension in 20 patients postcardiac surgery (primarily, CABG), using a randomized crossover study design. The study was performed following extubation in patients who were hypertensive after surgery and had been receiving nitroprusside. Therapy was titrated to decrease systolic blood pressure by 15 percent or go between 90 to 120 mmHg. Esmolol was titrated up to a maximum infusion rate of 300 μg/kg/min with 500 μg/kg boluses between incremental increases in the infusion. Nitroprusside was titrated up to a maximum of 10 μg/kg/min. After 20 minutes of infusion and a 20-minute washout period, the patient was crossed over to the other agent.

Both drugs were effective in reducing the systolic blood pressure to target levels (from 170 to 140 mmHg). Diastolic blood pressure was reduced to a significantly greater degree with nitroprusside (27 versus 10 percent). The heart rate decreased by 14 percent with esmolol; it increased 8 percent with nitroprusside. The mean dose of esmolol was 147 μg/kg/min, and the mean dose of nitroprusside was 1.8 μg/kg/min. Pulmonary capillary wedge pressure did not change with esmolol but fell significantly with nitroprusside. The cardiac index decreased with esmolol and increased with nitroprusside. PaO$_2$ was unchanged with esmolol but fell significantly with nitroprusside, as did oxygen saturation (Fig. 28-22). The incidence of adverse reactions was equal in each group, although the administration of esmolol to a patient with a preoperative ejection fraction of 15 percent resulted in the elevation of the pulmonary capillary wedge pressure to 29 mmHg. The authors concluded that esmolol is as safe and effective as nitroprusside, with better effects on arterial oxygenation. However, they cautioned against its use in patients with severe left ventricular dysfunction.

Use During Hypotensive Anesthesia

Although nitroprusside is commonly used for deliberate intraoperative hypotension, there are a number of risks associated with its use. Reflex activation of the renin-angiotensin and sympathetic

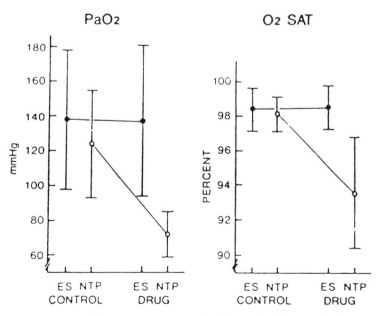

Fig. 28-22 Effects of esmolol (ES) and nitroprusside (NTP) on **(A)** PaO$_2$ and **(B)** oxygen saturation used for treatment of hypertension following coronary artery bypass graft surgery. See text for details. (From Gray et al.,[106] with permission.)

nervous system may lead to rebound hypertension and tachycardia. Inhibition of hypoxic pulmonary vasoconstriction commonly increases shunt fraction, leading to a decrease in arterial oxygen tension. Cyanide toxicity, although uncommon, can cause major morbidity and mortality rates.[107] Based on earlier observations demonstrating that propranolol pretreatment prevented increased plasma renin activity during nitroprusside infusion, there has been considerable interest in the use of esmolol along with nitroprusside, or esmolol alone, for use during deliberate hypotension.

Shah et al.[108] evaluated the effects of esmolol on 11 American Society of Anesthesiologists class I to II patients undergoing lymph node dissection during nitroprusside induced hypotension. Fentanyl, vecuronium, and 60 percent nitrous oxide were used for anesthesia. Esmolol at doses of 200, 300 and 400 μg/kg/min was administered after nitroprusside to lower the mean arterial pressure to 55 to 60 mmHg. The nitroprusside was then adjusted downward as needed to maintain the pressure stable while the esmolol was infused for 20 minutes. In six patients, transesophageal echocardiography

allowed a detailed assessment of left ventricular contractility (end-systolic wall stress [ESWS] to rate-corrected velocity of circumferential shortening relationship [VCFC]).

Esmolol decreased the nitroprusside dose requirements by 50 percent and decreased the heart rate by approximately 25 percent. The cardiac index decreased by nearly 50 percent at 400 μg/kg/min. The stroke volume declined by approximately 20 percent, and systemic vascular resistance increased by approximately 40 percent. Pulmonary capillary wedge pressure increased significantly with esmolol but never exceeded the baseline level. A dose dependent downward and leftward shift of the ESWS versus VCFC relationship was observed, suggesting a primary decrease in myocardial contractility (Fig. 28-23). The plasma renin activity declined significantly. The hemodynamic changes associated with esmolol persisted for 20 minutes after the termination of nitroprusside and esmolol. The shunt fraction decreased significantly, and the PaO_2 increased with esmolol, although the differences were clinically insignificant.

Blau et al.[109] evaluated the efficacy of esmolol

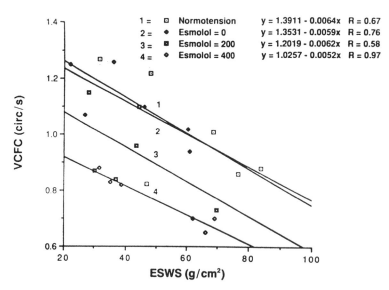

Fig. 28-23 Effects of esmolol on myocardial contractility during nitroprusside induced hypotension assessed by the end-systolic wall stress (ESWS) to rate-corrected velocity of circumferential shortening relationship (VCFC) obtained by transesophageal echocardiography (see text for details). Nitroprusside induced hypotension had no effect on contractility (relative to normotensive measurements). Increasing doses of esmolol caused a significant downward shift of the relationship indicative of diminished contractility. (From Shah et al.,[108] with permission.)

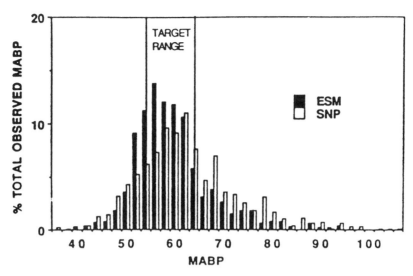

Fig. 28-24 Average frequency distributions for mean arterial pressure (MABP) (2-minute epochs) in patients receiving esmolol (ESM) or nitroprusside (SNP) during controlled hypotension. The data suggest somewhat better control of blood pressure with esmolol given the shift of the frequency distribution toward the lower limits of the target range relative to SNP. (From Blau et al.,[109] with permission.)

compared with nitroprusside for controlled hypotension in 30 American Society of Anesthesiologists class I to II patients undergoing orthognathic surgery. The patients received esmolol (500-μg/kg boluses until the target mean arterial pressure range of 55 to 65 mmHg was reached, followed by infusion of 100 to 300 μg/kg/min) or nitroprusside. A substantial amount of isoflurane was used (2 percent) to reach the target pressure and was continued at 1 percent (along with 65 percent nitrous oxide) during the hypotensive period. Blood loss and the surgeon's assessment of bleeding in the surgical field were recorded.

A frequency distribution of mean arterial pressure values (2-minute epochs) revealed lower average values with esmolol than nitroprusside (Fig. 28-24). The surgical field was rated drier with esmolol, and blood loss was significantly reduced by 49 percent compared with nitroprusside. The plasma renin activity was significantly lower with esmolol. Interestingly, despite a trend toward a greater decline in postoperative hematocrit (−10 versus −6.6 percent) with nitroprusside, the difference was not statistically significant. This study demonstrated that esmolol is effective for controlled hypotension without nitroprusside. Curi-

ously, the authors take the middle road in their summary, recommending the use of both agents rather than esmolol alone, to limit their respective doses.

Use for Treatment of Unstable Angina

The efficacy of routine esmolol infusion in patients hospitalized for unstable angina was reported by Hohnloser et al.[110] in a multicenter placebo controlled European study. Fifty-nine patients received esmolol (in addition to nitrates, thrombolytic agents, oral β adrenergic blockers, or calcium channel blockers), that was titrated to decrease rate pressure product by 25 percent; 54 received placebo. This dose was then infused for 24 to 72 hours. It is not clearly stated how the dose for the placebo group was derived. Two-lead Holter monitoring (V5 and a V_F) was used to detect ischemia.

The mean dose infused was 12 mg/min for a mean duration of 34 hours. The groups were well matched with regard to demographic and clinical characteristics (although no information on coronary anatomy was provided). Progression of unstable angina to myocardial infarction, urgent surgery, or angioplasty was higher in the placebo group (17 versus 5 percent), although the difference did not reach statistical significance. The incidence of symptomatic ischemia was similar in both groups. Although there was a trend toward a lower number of episodes of silent ischemia, and a lower average duration, with esmolol, the difference was not statistically significant. The incidence of adverse effects was higher in the esmolol group (39 versus 22 percent). A greater percentage of patients in the esmolol group were withdrawn from the study than in the placebo group.

This interesting study suggests some trends but does not prove any statistically significant differences between esmolol and placebo, despite maintenance of a lower rate-pressure product. The authors claimed that esmolol is safe and effective and can be considered a first line drug for unstable angina, but these conclusions appear not to be well supported by the data.

Barth et al.[111] reported on the use of esmolol in 21 patients with acute unstable angina unresponsive to "conventional medical therapy" (although this is not well defined). Esmolol was titrated to similar criteria as the European multicenter study (more than 20 percent reduction in rate-pressure product). A complete two dimensional Doppler and M-mode echocardiographic examination was performed at baseline and at 30 minutes into the maintenance infusion. Cardiac output, ejection fraction, regional wall motion, and other indices of systolic function were derived from the echo examination. Diastolic function was assessed based on the mitral inflow velocity Doppler profile.

At the target response, the mean dose of esmolol was 17 mg/min, although the range was great, 8 to 24 mg/min. Chest pain resolved during titration in 86 percent of patients, although 66 percent eventually went on to either CABG or percutaneous transluminal coronary angioplasty. The cardiac output decreased significantly (−14 percent), as a result of a decrease in stroke volume, not heart rate. The mean change in ejection fraction was not significant, increasing or decreasing in nearly equal number of patients. Segmental wall motion was unchanged in the majority of patients. Diastolic relaxation appeared to improve in the majority of patients, based on the Doppler indices.

Thirty-eight percent of patients developed hypotension, the majority of which was transient. One patient developed transient congestive failure treated with diuresis. The other patients with a history of congestive failure were asymptomatic, although all developed impairment of echo indices of systolic or diastolic function.

This study provides insights into the effects of esmolol in the setting of acute myocardial ischemia, suggesting a beneficial effect in the majority of patients. However, the absence of a randomized placebo controlled design limits the conclusions. That the majority of patients went on to require definitive therapy suggests that the effect of esmolol on outcome was probably small. The adverse effects on ventricular function suggest caution with its use in patients with a history of congestive failure.

Use in Patients With Left Ventricular Dysfunction

Iskandrian et al.[112] described the effects of graded infusions of esmolol in 10 patients with coronary artery disease and left ventricular dysfunction (mean ejection fraction, 27 percent; range, 20 to 36 percent). All subjects were clinically stable without overt signs of heart failure, and all cardiac medications were withheld for 2 half-lives prior to the study. Pulmonary artery catheterization and radionuclide angiography were performed, including repeated measurement of ejection fraction. Esmolol was infused incrementally up to approximately 200 μg/kg/min. At each titration step, measurements were performed after 5 minutes of infusion.

Surprisingly, esmolol was well tolerated with no clinical side effects. The heart rate declined starting at the lowest dose, 2 mg/min; the systolic pressure started to decline at 4 mg/min. Pulmonary capillary wedge pressure increased while cardiac output and ejection fraction decreased; the fall in cardiac output was primarily the result of the decrease in heart rate (Fig. 28-25). The changes were variable among patients. As expected, the changes in ejection fraction were dose dependent. An increase in systemic vascular resistance appeared to be secondary to the decline in cardiac output and not a primary effect.

The authors hypothesized that the deleterious effects of a reduction in ejection fraction and an increase in ventricular volumes, which increase wall stress (and thus, myocardial oxygen demand),

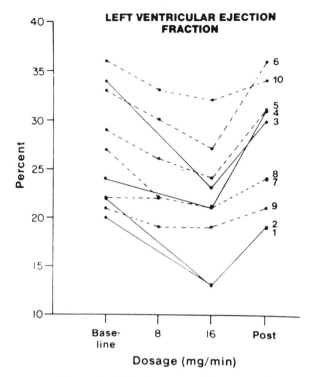

Fig. 28-25 Individual changes in left ventricular ejection fraction in response to increasing doses of esmolol in 10 patients with moderate to severe resting impairment of left ventricular function (mean ejection fraction 27 percent). However, all patients were clinically stable with no signs of congestive heart failure. (From Iskandrian et al.,[112] with permission.)

was offset by a reduction in systolic pressure (also a determinant of wall stress). These data suggest that esmolol can be used safely in patients with moderate degrees of left ventricular dysfunction (and no other contraindications to β adrenergic blockade) as long as the dose is carefully titrated and evaluated.

Adverse Effects of Esmolol

With proper attention to dosing, esmolol is well tolerated for a variety of perioperative applications. The most common adverse reaction is hypotension. This is most likely to occur in the patient with hypovolemia and/or pre-existent left ventricular dysfunction. Being an effect of β adrenergic blockade, it is not unique to esmolol. However, given esmolol's rapid elimination half-life, many clinicians are more willing to use it in situations in which they would otherwise probably avoid β adrenergic blockers with longer half-lives.

In a multicenter trial of efficacy for treatment of supraventricular tachycardia, cardiovascular and central nervous system side effects were the most common,[94] including somnolence (7 percent); agitation, headache, and dizziness (4 percent each); and confusion (3 percent). However, this trial involved prolonged infusion of the drug (up to 24 hours). Nausea was noted in 13 percent of patients; bronchospasm or dyspnea was noted in only 3 percent.

The author of this chapter has anecdotally observed profound obtundation in two geriatric patients treated with prolonged infusions. Fortunately, this was reversed rapidly by termination of therapy.

LABETALOL

Labetalol is a nonselective β adrenergic blocker, with significant α adrenergic blocking properties.[6,113] The ratio of β to α blockade varies from 4 to 16 in the literature, with a ratio of 7 commonly stated. It is not a potent α adrenergic blocker, being 6 to 10 times less potent at the α_1 adrenoceptor than phentolamine. It has no blocking effect on the α_2 adrenoceptor (see Ch. 26).

In the supine chronic hypertensive patient, acute intravenous administration of doses from 50 to 200 mg lower blood pressure approximately 20 percent. The primary physiologic change is a reduction in systemic vascular resistance (10 to 15 percent); heart rate and cardiac output are altered minimally.[114] Stroke volume actually increases slightly. These changes have been shown to persist with chronic (up to 6 years) therapy.[115] Indeed, the markedly elevated systemic vascular resistance, characteristic of the long standing severe hypertensive patient, may be completely normalized as a result of structural remodeling of the left ventricle and peripheral vasculature. Preventing the increase in systemic vascular resistance by the use of β adrenergic blockers appears to facilitate the treatment of hypertension.[116] In addition to chronic therapy, it has been shown to be useful when administered orally (doses from 100 to 1,200 mg) for the treatment of "hypertensive urgency" (diastolic pressure from 110 to 140 mmHg in a patient with no end-organ damage) and has compared favorably with multiple doses of oral clonidine.[117,118]

In the perioperative setting, the α adrenergic blocking properties of labetalol may obviate the need for a primary vasodilator. Theoretically, β_1 selective agents should help prevent major increases in systemic vascular resistance as a result of preservation of β_2 adrenoceptor mediated peripheral vasodilation in skeletal muscle. However, β_1 adrenergic selectivity is dose dependent, and at the higher doses required to treat hypertension, this selectivity is usually of little benefit.[6] Obviously, an agent similar to labetalol that is also β_1 adrenoceptor selectivity would be ideal, although such a drug is not currently available. Dilevalol, a stereoisomer of labetalol, is also a nonselective β adrenergic blocker.[114] Although it lacks α adrenergic blocking properties, dilevalol has partial β_2 adrenergic agonist activity, which imparts some vasodilating properties. Its perioperative use has not been reported.

Use During Coronary Artery Bypass Graft Surgery

Meretoja et al.[119] were the first to report the use of labetalol to treat hypertension following CABG and valve surgery. They administered a mean dose of 15 mg (range, 3 to 50 mg) to 11 patients 6 hours postoperatively. The mean arterial pressure declined 15 to 20 percent. However, the mean cardiac index fell from 2.2 to 1.65 L/min/m². Glucagon, 3 mg, was given to four patients, improving the cardiac index by 16 percent. It was unclear what caused a decline in cardiac index, given that filling pressures appeared adequate and systemic vascular resistance remained constant.

Cruise et al.[120] reported the first randomized study comparing labetalol to nitroprusside for control of hypertension following CABG surgery. Forty patients with preoperative ejection fractions more than 40 percent, not requiring inotropes, were randomized to receive either nitroprusside (starting at 0.5 μg/kg/min and titrated up in 0.5 μg/kg/min increments) or labetalol (three intravenous boluses of 25 mg initially if needed plus an infusion starting at 2 mg/min up to a maximum total dose of 300 mg) when systolic blood pressure exceeded 140 mmHg or mean arterial pressure exceeded 90 mmHg. The end pionts for therapy were systolic blood pressure less than 120 or mean arterial pressure less than 80 mmHg, at which point hemodynamic variables were followed for 30 minutes.

Mean arterial pressure decreased to a greater degree with nitroprusside as a result of a significant decline in diastolic blood pressure (approximately a 15-mmHg difference). The heart rate increased significantly with nitroprusside (+9 beats/min); it decreased significantly with labetalol (−6 beats/min). Central venous pressure and pulmonary capillary wedge pressure increased slightly with labetalol (approximately +3 and +2 mmHg). The same parameters decreased slightly with nitroprusside. The cardiac index declined to a small but significant degree with labetalol (approximately 0.3 L/min/m²); it rose with nitroprusside. Systemic vascular resistance did not change with labetalol, but it fell with nitroprusside (approximately 500 dyne-sec/cm⁻⁵). An average labetalol dose of 150 mg was required. No side effects occurred in either group. The authors concluded that labetalol appeared safe and speculated that, despite its negative inotropic effects (decrease in cardiac index and increase in filling pressure), it better maintained myocardial oxygen supply demand balance because it reduced heart rate and maintained diastolic pressure.

Use During Noncardiac Surgery

Amar et al.[121] evaluated anesthetic requirements and hemodynamic and hormonal responses when labetalol was administered immediately prior to induction in a placebo controlled study of 16 American Society of Anesthesiologists class I female patients undergoing major gynecologic surgery. The drug was administered incrementally, up to a total dose of 1 mg/kg, to reduce mean arterial pressure by 15 percent. Isoflurane, nitrous oxide, and vecuronium were used for anesthesia.

During tracheal intubation, the heart rates were significantly lower in the treated group; blood pressures were similar. Two patients receiving 0.75 mg/kg or greater developed transient hypotension.

Before induction, plasma norepinephrine levels actually increased significantly (63 percent) with labetalol. With surgical stimulation, plasma norepinephrine, epinephrine, cortisol, and aldosterone concentrations increased significantly in both groups. A small, but statistically significant, reduction in serum potassium concentration occurred in the control group. This was attributed to β_2 adrenoceptor mediated potassium uptake that was blocked in the labetalol group. Anesthetic requirements were similar in both groups. The authors concluded that labetalol is effective in reducing the heart rate response to induction and that hypotension may occur with doses greater than 0.5 mg/kg.

Use for Controlled Hypotension

Goldberg et al.[122] compared labetalol with nitroprusside for deliberate hypotension in a randomized double blind study of 20 American Society of Anesthesiologists class I to II patients undergoing major spinal surgery. Anesthesia included fentanyl, isoflurane, nitrous oxide, and vecuronium. Both boluses and infusion of either drug or a placebo were administered. Up to a total dose of 10 μg/kg/min of nitroprusside or 300 mg of labetalol (in increments of 10 mg) were used to reduce mean arterial pressure to 55 to 60 mmHg. The mean dose per hour was 15 to 30 mg for labetalol and 1.3 to 5.0 mg for nitroprusside.

With nitroprusside, the heart rate and cardiac output increased significantly and systemic vascular resistance decreased. With labetalol, systemic vascular resistance decreased significantly; there was no significant change in the heart rate or cardiac output. The time required to return the blood pressure to baseline levels was twice as long with labetalol. No differences in blood loss were observed. Intrapulmonary shunt increased with nitroprusside.

This study appears to demonstrate a significant α_1 adrenergic blocking effect of labetalol. The authors concluded that labetalol had a more desirable hemodynamic effect than did nitroprusside. However, they caution that the significantly longer time required to return pressure to baseline (required to ensure that surgical hemostasis will be adequate) could be detrimental, although it could be aug-

mented by the use of pressors. The differences in pulmonary shunting in the prone position (one that favorably affects ventilation perfusion matching) were of no clinical significance.

Postoperative Use

Chauvin et al.[123] reported on the hemodynamics and pharmacokinetics of labetalol in six patients with normal ventricular function after aortic surgery. The patients were studied 15 hours postoperatively (after extubation). A mean arterial pressure greater than 120 mmHg and a cardiac index more than 2.0 L/min/m² were the criteria for administration of a 1.5-mg/kg bolus followed by a maintenance infusion of 0.2 mg/kg/h for 5.5 hours. Hemodynamics and plasma levels were measured frequently. Within 5 minutes of the loading dose, the mean arterial pressure decreased by 32 percent, heart rate by 20 percent, and cardiac index (which had been elevated) by 26 percent. Initial changes in systemic vascular resistance were variable, but by 3 hours, it had declined in all patients (22 percent). Filling pressures were not affected. The plasma concentrations were stable (less than 15 percent variation) during hours 2 to 6 of the infusion. Therapy was well tolerated.

Orlowski et al.[124] compared labetalol to nitroprusside following neurosurgery (arteriovenous malformation or aneurysm surgery) in 15 patients. All patients were initially treated with nitroprusside but required high doses (mean, 10 μg/kg/min). Labetalol was administered as a bolus or infusion, although the dosing was not standardized. Eleven patients were weaned from nitroprusside, and the remaining required between 1 and 2 μg/kg/min of nitroprusside. The total labetalol doses were not reported. Cerebral perfusion pressure was well maintained, and intracranial pressure remained stable or declined. The authors recommended the use of labetalol, particularly in patients requiring high doses of nitroprusside, which place the patient at risk for cyanide toxicity.

Muzzi et al.[125] compared labetalol and esmolol for control of hypertension after neurosurgery in a randomized trial of 50 patients. Anesthesia included low doses fentanyl (6 to 8 μg/kg), isoflurane, and nitrous oxide. Hypertension, hypotension, and bradycardia were all defined as a 20 percent change from the preoperative values. Labetalol was administered in incremental doses of 0.25 mg/kg, up to a total of 2.5 mg/kg cumulative dose, during emergence from anesthesia (but not after). Esmolol was administered with a 500 μg/kg loading dose followed by infusion of 50 to 300 μg/kg/min until 10 minutes after extubation.

Either drug controlled hypertension initially in about 90 percent of the patients (mean labetalol dose, 0.97 mg/kg; mean esmolol dose, 160 μg/kg/min). In the recovery room, hypertension recurred in about 35 percent of patients in each group within 18 to 27 minutes. The incidence of hypotension was not statistically different. The incidence of bradycardia was significantly greater in the labetalol group (60 versus 10 percent); however, the mean low heart rate was 56 beats/min (range, 40 to 62), a level of no clinical significance.

Hepatotoxicity of Labetalol

Although labetalol is considered a safe drug, probably safer than nitroprusside, there is recent evidence for idiosyncratic hepatotoxicity. Clark et al.[126] analyzed the Food and Drug Administration's adverse drug reaction data base and found 11 cases of unexplained serious hepatotoxicity in which labetalol was considered the most likely etiologic agent. An additional 6 to 7 cases were not analyzed prior to publication of the report. All patients were receiving labetalol orally for chronic hypertension, and 82 percent were female. The median duration of therapy was 60 days. Severe hepatocellular necrosis was observed in 5 patients in whom liver biopsy was performed. Nine of the 11 patients improved with discontinuation of labetalol, but 3 died (one shortly after a liver transplant).

The authors noted that the findings were similar to isoniazid or hydralazine induced hepatoxicity and that the most likely cause is metabolic idiosyncrasy. They recommended periodic screening of all patients undergoing prolonged therapy. There are no reported cases in patients exposed for short periods of time or with intravenous dosing. These findings are of concern, but probably should not have an immediate impact on the use of labetalol perioperatively (except perhaps in patients with known liver disease). However, after such an association is detected, caution and vigilance are required.

REFERENCES

1. Frishman WH: β-Adrenoceptor antagonists: new drugs and new indications. N Engl J Med 305:500, 1981
2. Frishman WH: Clinical Pharmacology of the β-Adrenoceptor Blocking Drugs. 2nd Ed. Appleton-Century-Crofts, Norwalk, CT, 1984
3. Frishman W, Furberg C, Friedewald W: β-Adrenergic blockade for survivors of acute myocardial infarction. N Engl J Med 310:830, 1984
4. Frishman WH: β-Adrenergic blocker withdrawal. Am J Cardiol 59:26, 1987
5. Frishman WH, Chesner M: β-Adrenergic blockers in pregnancy. Am Heart J 115:147, 1988
6. Frishman WH: β-Adrenergic blockers. Med Clin North Am 72:37, 1988
7. Frishman WH, Murthy VS, Strom JA: Ultra-short-acting β-adrenergic blockers. Med Clin North Am 72:359, 1988
8. Frishman WH: β-Adrenergic blockers as cardioprotective agents. Am J Cardiol 70:2, 1992
9. Harrison DC: Beneficial effects of β blockers: class action or individual pharmacologic spectrum? Circulation, suppl. 1:I-77, 1983
10. Shand DG: Clinical pharmacology of β-blocking drugs: implications for the postinfarction patient. Circulation, suppl. 1:I2, 1983
11. Taylor SH, Silke B, Lee PS: Intravenous β-blockade in coronary artery disease: is cardioselectivity or intrinsic sympathomimetic activity hemodynamically useful? N Engl J Med 306:631, 1982
12. Wiener I, Mindich B, DiStefano D, Kupersmith J: Regional effects of propranolol on intraventricular conduction in coronary artery disease. Clin Pharmacol Ther 26:696, 1979
13. Reder RF, Mindich R, Halperin J et al: Acute effects of oral labetalol on myocardial conduction after coronary artery bypass grafting. Clin Pharmacol Ther 35:454, 1984
14. Henling CE, Slogoff S, Kodali SV, Arlund C: Heart block after coronary artery bypass—effect of chronic administration of calcium-entry blockers and β-blockers. Anesth Analg 63:515, 1984
15. Slogoff S, Keats AS, Hibbs CW et al: Failure of general anesthesia to potentiate propranolol activity. Anesthesiology 47:504, 1977
16. Croft CH, Rude RE, Gustafson N et al: Abrupt withdrawal of β-blockade therapy in patients with

myocardial infarction: effects on infarct size, left ventricular function, and hospital course. Circulation 73:1281, 1986

17. Frishman WH, Weksler BB: Effects of β-adrenoceptor blocking agents on platelet function. p. 273. In Frishman WH (ed): Clinical Pharmacology of the β-Adrenoceptor Blocking Drugs. 2nd Ed. Appleton-Century-Crofts, Norwalk, CT, 1984

18. Slogoff S, Keats AS: Does perioperative myocardial ischemia lead to postoperative myocardial infarction? Anesthesiology 62:107, 1985

19. Raby KE, Goldman L, Creager MA et al: Correlation between preoperative ischemia and major cardiac events after peripheral vascular surgery. N Engl J Med 321:1296, 1989

20. Mangano DT, Browner WS, Hollenberg M et al: Association of perioperative myocardial ischemia with cardiac morbidity and mortality in men undergoing noncardiac surgery. N Engl J Med 323:1781, 1990

21. London MJ: Monitoring for myocardial ischemia. p. 249. In: Kaplan JA (ed): Vascular Anesthesia. 1st Ed. Churchill Livingstone, New York, 1991

22. London MJ, Kaplan JA: Advances in electrocardiographic monitoring. In Kaplan JA (ed): Cardiac Anesthesia. 3rd Ed. WB Saunders, Philadelphia, 1992 (in press)

23. London MJ: Preoperative assessment: the role of ambulatory electrocardiography, imaging techniques, and cardiac catherization. J Cardiothorac Vasc Anesth, suppl. 1:2, 1990

24. London MJ: Silent ischemia and postoperative infarction. J Cardiothorac Vasc Anesth, suppl. 1:58, 1990

25. Cohn PF: Silent myocardial ischemia: an update. Adv Intern Med 34:377, 1989

26. Gottlieb SO: Asymptomatic or silent myocardial ischemia in angina pectoris: pathophysiology and clinical implications. Cardiol Clin 9:49, 1991

27. Knight AA, Hollenberg M, London MJ et al: Perioperative myocardial ischemia: importance of the preoperative ischemic pattern. Anesthesiology 68:681, 1988

28. London MJ, Hollenberg M, Wong MG et al: Intraoperative myocardial ischemia: localization by continuous 12 lead electrocardiography. Anesthesiology 69:232, 1988

29. Hjalmarson A, Olsson G: Myocardial infarction. Effects of β-blockade. Circulation 84:VI-101, 1991

30. Slogoff S, Keats AS: Does chronic treatment with calcium entry blocking drugs reduce perioperative myocardial ischemia? Anesthesiology 68:676, 1988

31. Chung F, Houston PL, Cheng DC et al: Calcium channel blockade does not offer adequate protection from perioperative myocardial ischemia. Anesthesiology 69:343, 1988

32. Przyklenk K, Ghafari GB, Eitzman DT, Kloner RA: Nifedipine administered after reperfusion ablates systolic contractile dysfunction of postischemic "stunned" myocardium. J Am Coll Cardiol 13:1176, 1989

33. Jain UJ: Myocardial infarction during coronary artery bypass surgery. J Cardiothorac Vasc Anesth 6:612, 1992

34. Bolling SF, Groh MA, Mattson AM et al: Acadesine (AICA-riboside) improves postischemic cardiac recovery. Ann Thorac Surg 54:93, 1992

35. Rao PS, Brock FE, Cleary K et al: Effect of intraoperative propranolol on serum creatine kinase MB release in patients having elective cardiac operations. J Thorac Cardiovasc Surg 88:562, 1984

36. Berggren H, Ekroth R, Herlitz J et al: Myocardial protective effect of maintained β-blockade in aortocoronary bypass surgery. Scand J Thorac Cardiovasc Surg 17:29, 1983

37. Stone JG, Foex P, Sear JW et al: Myocardial ischemia in untreated hypertensive patients: effect of a single small dose of a β-adrenergic blocking agent. Anesthesiology 68:495, 1988

38. Stone JG, Foex P, SEar JW et al: Risk of myocardial ischaemia during anaesthesia in treated and untreated hypertensive patients. Br J Anaesth 61:675, 1988

39. Roizen MF: Should we all have a sympathectomy at birth? Or at least preoperatively? Anesthesiology 68:482, 1988

40. Goldman L, Caldera DL: Risks of general anesthesia and elective operation in the hypertensive patient. Anesthesiology 50:285, 1979

41. Prys-Roberts C, Meloch R, Foëx P: Studies of anaesthesia in relation to hypertension. I: Cardiovascular responses of treated and untreated patients. Br J Anaesth 43:122, 1971

42. Prys-Roberts C, Greene LT, Meloche R, Foëx P: Studies of anaesthesia in relation to hypertension. II: Haemodynamic consequences of induction and endotracheal intubation. Br J Anesth 43:531, 1971

43. Prys-Roberts C, Foëx P, Biro GP, Roberts JG: Studies of anaesthesia in relation to hypertension. V: Adrenergic β-receptor blockade. Br J Anaesth 45:671, 1973

44. Pasternack PF, Imparato AM, Baumann GF et al: The hemodynamics of β-blockade in patients un-

dergoing abdominal aortic aneurysm repair. Circulation, supp. 3:1, 1987

45. Pasternack PF, Grossi EA, Baumann G et al: β Blockade to decrease silent myocardial ischemia during peripheral vascular surgery. Am J Surg 158:113, 1989

46. Filjoen J, Estafanous F, Kellner G: Propranolol and cardiac surgery. J Thorac Cardiovasc Surg 64:826, 1972

47. Kaplan JA, Dunbar RW, Bland JW et al: Propranolol and cardiac surgery: a problem for the anesthesiologist? Anesth Analg 54:571, 1975

48. Falkner S, Hopkins J, Boerth R et al: Time required for complete recovery from chronic propranolol therapy. N Engl J Med 289:607, 1973

49. Slogoff S, Keats AS, Ott E: Preoperative propranolol therapy and aortocoronary bypass operation. JAMA 240:1487, 1978

50. Boudoulas H, Snyder GL, Lewis RP et al: Safety and rationale for continuation of propranolol therapy during coronary bypass operation. Ann Thorac Surg 26:222, 1978

51. Sill JC, Nugent M, Moyer TP et al: Influence of propranolol plasma levels on hemodynamics during coronary artery bypass surgery. Anesthesiology 60:455, 1984

52. Sill JC, Nugent M, Moyer TP et al: Plasma levels of β-blocking drugs prior to coronary artery bypass surgery. Anesthesiology 62:67, 1985

53. Pine M, Favrot L, Smith S et al: Correlation of plasma propranolol concentration with therapeutic response in patients with angina pectoris. Circulation 52:886, 1975

54. Stanley TH, de LS, Boscoe MJ, de BN: The influence of chronic preoperative propranolol therapy on cardiovascular dynamics and narcotic requirements during operation in patients with coronary artery disease. Can J Anaesth 29:319, 1982

55. Hammon JJ, Wood AJ, Prager RL et al: Perioperative β blockade with propranolol: reduction in myocardial oxygen demands and incidence of atrial and ventricular arrhythmias. Ann Thorac Surg 38:363, 1984

56. Heikkila H, Jalonen J, Laaksonen V et al: Metoprolol medication and coronary artery bypass grafting operation. Acta Anaesthesiol Scand 28:677, 1984

57. Frishman WH: Multifactorial actions of β-adrenergic blocking drugs in ischemic heart disease: current concepts. Circulation, suppl. 1:I-11, 1983

58. Boudoulas H, Lewis RP, Rittgers SE et al: Increased diastolic time: a possible important factor in the beneficial effect of propranolol in patients with cor-

onary artery disease. J Cardiovasc Pharmacol 1:503, 1979

59. Lewis RP, Rittgers SE, Forester WF, Boudoulas H: A critical review of the systolic time intervals. Circulation 56:146, 1977

60. Buckberg GD, Fixler DE, Archie JP, Hoffman JIE: Experimental subendocardial ischemia in dogs with normal coronary arteries. Circ Res 30:67, 1972

61. Bolling SF, Flaherty JT, Potter AM, Gardner TJ: Propranolol-induced postoperative hypertension following coronary artery bypass grafting. J Thorac Cardiovasc Surg 87:112, 1984

62. Foëx P, Roberts JG, Saner CA, Bennett MJ: Oxprenolol and the circulation during anaesthesia in the dog: influence of intrinsic sympathomimetic activity. Br J Anesth 53:463, 1981

63. Salmenpera M, Yrjola H, Heikkila J: Hemodynamic responses to β-adrenergic blockade with metoprolol and pindolol after coronary artery bypass surgery. Chest 83:739, 1983

64. Tarnow J: Altered hemodynamic response to dobutamine in relation to the degree of preoperative β-adrenoceptor blockade. Anesthesiology 68:912, 1988

65. Tarnow J, Muller RK: Cardiovascular effect of low-dose epinephrine infusions in relation to the extent of preoperative β-adrenoceptor blockade. Anesthesiology 74:1035, 1991

66. Kaplan JA, Dunbar RW: Propranolol and surgical anesthesia. Anesth Analg 55:1, 1976

67. Goldman L: Noncardiac surgery in patients receiving propranolol. Case reports and recommended approach. Arch Intern Med 141:193, 1981

68. Ponten J, Biber B, Henriksson BA et al: β-receptor blockade and neurolept anaesthesia. Withdrawal vs continuation of long-term therapy in gall-bladder and carotid artery surgery. Acta Anaesthesiol Scand 26:576, 1982

69. Sheppard D, DiStefano S, Byrd RC et al: Effects of esmolol on airway function in patients with asthma. J Clin Pharmacol 26:169, 1986

70. Gold MR, Dec GW, Cocca-Spofford D, Thompson BT: Esmolol and ventilatory function in cardiac patients with COPD. Chest 100:1215, 1991

71. Andrews TC, Reimold SC, Berlin JA, Antman EM: Prevention of supraventricular arrhythmias after coronary artery bypass surgery. A meta-analysis of randomized control trials. Circulation 3:236, 1991

72. Fahmy NR, Mihelakos PT, Battit GE, Lappas DG: Propranolol prevents hemodynamic and humoral events after abrupt withdrawal of nitroprusside. Clin Pharmacol Ther 36:470, 1984

73. Gridlinger GA, Vegas AM, Williams GH et al: Independence of renin production and hypertension in abdominal aortic aneurysmectomy. Am J Surg 141:472, 1981

74. Grant RP, Jenkins LC: Modification by preoperative β-blockade of the renin response to infrarenal aortic cross-clamping. Can J Anaesth 30:480, 1983

75. Ostman PL, Chestnut DH, Robillard JE et al: Transplacental passage and hemodynamic effects of esmolol in the gravid ewe. Anesthesiology 69:738, 1988

76. Eisenach JC, Castro MI: Maternally administered esmolol produces fetal β-adrenergic blockade and hypoxemia in sheep. Anesthesiology 71:718, 1989

77. Losasso TJ, Muzzi DA, Cucchiara RF: Response of fetal heart rate to maternal administration of esmolol. Anesthesiology 74:782, 1991

78. Ducey JP, Knape KG: Maternal esmolol administration resulting in fetal distress and cesarean section in a term pregnancy. Anesthesiology 77:829, 1992

79. Sheps SG, Jiang NS, Klee GG, van HJ: Recent developments in the diagnosis and treatment of pheochromocytoma. Mayo Clin Proc 65:88, 1990

80. Gabrielson GV, Guffin AV, Kaplan JA et al: Continuous intravenous infusions of phentolamine and esmolol for preoperative and intraoperative adrenergic blockade in patients with pheochromocytoma. J Cardiothorac Vasc Anesth 1:554, 1987

81. Zakowski M, Kaufman B, Berguson P et al: Esmolol use during resection of pheochromocytoma: report of three cases. Anesthesiology 70:875, 1989

82. Nussbaum J, Zane EA, Thys DM: Esmolol for the treatment of hypercyanotic spells in infants with tetralogy of Fallot. J Cardiothorac Vasc Anesth 3:200, 1989

83. Boldt J, Kling D, Zickmann B et al: The effects of esmolol on the hemodynamics of acute theophylline toxicity. Ann Emerg Med 16:1334, 1987

84. Price KR, Fligner DJ: Acute theophylline toxicity and the use of esmolol to reverse cardiovascular instability. Ann Emerg Med 19:671, 1990

85. Weinger MB, Partridge BL, Hauger R, Mirow A: Prevention of the cardiovascular and neuroendocrine response to electroconvulsive therapy: I. Effectiveness of pretreatment regimens on hemodynamics. Anesth Analg 73:556, 1991

86. Weinger MB, Partridge BL, Hauger R et al: Prevention of the cardiovascular and neuroendocrine response to electroconvulsive therapy: II. Effects of pretreatment regimens on catecholamines, ACTH, vasopressin, and cortisol. Anesth Analg 73:563, 1991

87. Howie MB, Hiestand DC, Zvara DA et al: Defining the dose range for esmolol used in electroconvulsive therapy hemodynamic attenuation. Anesth Analg 75:805, 1992

88. Ramsay JG: Comparison of two esmolol bolus doses on the haemodynamic response and seizure duration during electroconvulsive therapy. Can J Anaesth 38:204, 1991

89. Gorczynski RJ: Basic pharmacology of esmolol. Am J Cardiol 56:3, 1985

90. Lowenthal DT, Porter RS, Saris SD et al: Clinical pharmacology, pharmacodynamics and interactions with esmolol. Am J Cardiol 56:14, 1985

91. Greenspan AM, Spielman SR, Horowitz LN et al: Electrophysiology of esmolol. Am J Cardiol 56:19, 1985

92. Iskandrian AS, Hakki AH, Laddu A: Effects of esmolol on cardiac function: evaluation by noninvasive techniques. Am J Cardiol 56:27, 1985

93. Morganroth J, Horowitz LN, Anderson J, Turlapaty P: Comparative efficacy and tolerance of esmolol to propranolol for control of supraventricular tachyarrhythmia. Am J Cardiol 56:33, 1985

94. Kloner RA, Kirshenbaum J, Lange R et al: Experimental and clinical observations on the efficacy of esmolol in myocardial ischemia. Am J Cardiol 56:40, 1985

95. Gray RJ, Bateman TM, Czer LS et al: Use of esmolol in hypertension after cardiac surgery. Am J Cardiol 56:49, 1985

96. Reves JG, Flezzani P: Perioperative use of esmolol. Am J Cardiol 56:57, 1985

97. Jacobs JR, Maier GW, Rankin JS, Reves JG: Esmolol and left ventricular function in the awake dog. Anesthesiology 68:373, 1988

98. Kirshenbaum JM, Kloner RF, McGowan N, Antman EM: Use of an ultrashort-acting β-receptor blocker (esmolol) in patients with acute myocardial ischemia and relative contraindications to β-blockade therapy. J Am Coll Cardiol 12:773, 1988

99. Jacobs JR: Use of esmolol during anesthesia to treat tachycardia and hypertension. Anesth Analg 68:101, 1989

100. de Bruijn NP, Reves JG, Croughwell N et al: Pharmacokinetics of esmolol in anesthetized patients receiving chronic β blocker therapy. Anesthesiology 66:323, 1987

101. Menkhaus PG, Reves JG, Kissin I et al: Cardiovascular effects of esmolol in anesthetized humans. Anesth Analg 64:327, 1985

102. Girard D, Shulman BJ, Thys DM et al: The safety

and efficacy of esmolol during myocardial revascularization. Anesthesiology 65:157, 1986

103. Harrison L, Ralley FE, Wynands JE et al: The role of an ultra short-acting adrenergic blocker (esmolol) in patients undergoing coronary artery bypass surgery. Anesthesiology 66:413, 1987

104. Reves JG, Croughwell ND, Hawkins E et al: Esmolol for treatment of intraoperative tachycardia and/or hypertension in patients having cardiac operations. J Thorac Cardiovasc Surg 100:221, 1990

105. Miller DR, Martineau RJ, Wynands JE, Hill J: Bolus administration of esmolol for controlling the haemodynamic response to tracheal intubation; the Canadian multicentre trial. Can J Anesth 38:849, 1991

106. Gray RJ, Bateman TM, Czer LS et al: Comparison of esmolol and nitroprusside for acute post-cardiac surgical hypertension. Am J Cardiol 59:887, 1987

107. Robin ED, McCauley R: Nitroprusside-related cyanide poisoning. Time (long past due) for urgent, effective interventions. Chest 102:1842, 1992

108. Shah N, Del VO, Edmondson R et al: Esmolol infusion during nitroprusside-induced hypotension: impact on hemodynamics, ventricular performance, and venous admixture. J Cardiothorac Vasc Anesth 6:196, 1992

109. Blau WS, Kafer ER, Anderson JA: Esmolol is more effective than sodium nitroprusside in reducing blood loss during orthognathic surgery. Anesth Analg 75:172, 1992

110. Hohnloser SH, Meinertz T, Klingenheben T et al: Usefulness of esmolol in unstable angina pectoris. European Esmolol Study Group. Am J Cardiol 67:1319, 1991

111. Barth C, Ojile M, Pearson AC, Labovitz AJ: Ultra short-acting intravenous β-adrenergic blockade as add-on therapy in acute unstable angina. Am Heart J 121:782, 1991

112. Iskandrian AS, Bemis CE, Hakki H et al: Effects of esmolol on patients with left ventricular dysfunction. J Am Coll Cardiol 8:225, 1986

113. Frishman WH, MacCarthy EP, Kimmel B et al: Labetalol: a new β-adrenergic blocker-vasodilator. In Frishman WH (ed): Clinical Pharmacology of the β-Adrenoceptor Blocking Drugs. 2nd Ed. Appleton-Century-Crofts, Norwalk, CT, 1984

114. Lund-Johansen P: Hemodynamic effects of β-blocking compounds possessing vasodilating activity: a review of labetalol, prizidilol, and dilevalol. J Cardiovasc Pharmacol 11:S12, 1988

115. Lund-Johansen P, Bakke OM: Haemodynamic effects and plasma concentrations of labetalol during long-term treatment of essential hypertension. Br J Clin Pharmacol 7:169, 1979

116. Blakey B, Williams LL, Lopez LM, Stein GH: Labetalol HCl: α- and β-blocking properties may offer advantages over pure β-blockers. Hosp Formulary 22:864, 1987

117. Gonzalez EF, Peterson MA, Racht EM et al: Dose-response evaluation of oral labetalol in patients presenting to the emergency department with accelerated hypertension. Ann Emerg Med 20:333, 1991

118. Atkin SH, Jaker MA, Beaty P et al: Oral labetalol versus oral clonidine in the emergency treatment of severe hypertension. Am J Med Sci 303:9, 1992

119. Meretoja OA, Allonen H, Arola M, Laaksonen VO: Combined α- and β-blockade with labetalol in post-open heart surgery hypertension. Reversal of hemodynamic deterioration with glucagon. Chest 78:810, 1980

120. Cruise CJ, Skrobik Y, Webster RE et al: Intravenous labetalol versus sodium nitroprusside for treatment of hypertension postcoronary bypass surgery. Anesthesiology 71:835, 1989

121. Amar D, Shamoon H, Frishman WH et al: Effects of labetalol on perioperative stress markers and isoflurane requirements. Br J Anaesth 67:296, 1991

122. Goldberg ME, McNulty SE, Azad SS et al: A comparison of labetalol and nitroprusside for inducing hypotension during major surgery. Anesth Analg 70:537, 1990

123. Chauvin M, Deriaz H, Viars P: Continuous i.v. infusion of labetalol for postoperative hypertension. Haemodynamic effects and plasma kinetics. Br J Anaesth 59:1250, 1987

124. Orlowski JP, Shiesley D, Vidt DG et al: Labetalol to control blood pressure after cerebrovascular surgery. Crit Care Med 16:765, 1988

125. Muzzi DA, Black S, Losasso TJ, Cucchiara RF: Labetalol and esmolol in the control of hypertension after intracranial surgery. Anesth Analg 70:68, 1990

126. Clark JA, Zimmerman HJ, Tanner LA: Labetalol hepatotoxicity. Ann Intern Med 113:210, 1990

Chapter 29

Nonsteroidal Anti-Inflammatory Drugs

Peter M. Brooks

Nonsteroidal anti-inflammatory drugs (NSAIDs) are widely used throughout the world for the treatment of pain and inflammation associated with musculoskeletal disease. This class of drugs constitutes one of the most commonly taken by humans. It has been estimated that each year more than one in seven Americans is treated with a NSAID,[1] and in Australia, up to 20 percent of patients are receiving an NSAID at the time of hospital admission.[2] To a certain extent, their wide usage reflects the high prevalence of rheumatic disease, although many people still receive NSAIDs for soft tissue conditions, such as sports injuries. Over the last decade, increasing emphasis has been placed on NSAID use for the relief of a wide variety of pain, such as peri- and postoperative pain, renal and biliary colic, cancer pain, and periodontal disease. A number of NSAIDs have been introduced for intramuscular or intravenous administration, and rectal and transcutaneous formulations may also have a place in the management of pain. This chapter reviews the mechanisms of action, the role that NSAIDs may play in the relief of pain, particularly in the peri- and postoperative period, and adverse drug reactions.

There are more than 100 NSAIDs under trial or marketed around the world, of which the salicylates are probably the best known.[3] In general, the therapeutic effects of the newer NSAIDs are not significantly different from those of the older drugs, such as aspirin, phenylbutazone, and indomethacin, although there is some evidence to suggest that the newer agents are tolerated better. What is clear, however, is that there is marked interpersonal variability in response to these drugs, although the exact mechanism(s) for this variability are unknown.[4] Subtle differences seem to exist between these agents in their mechanism of action. More pronounced pharmacokinetic differences between agents will influence the duration of analgesia and the length of time required for platelet function to return to normal after the drug has been discontinued.

MECHANISM OF ACTION

Inhibition of Prostaglandin Biosynthesis

The major mechanism by which NSAIDs exert their anti-inflammatory, analgesic, and adverse effects is inhibition of prostaglandin biosynthesis (Fig. 29-1).[5] Prostaglandin inflammatory mediators promote vasodilation, erythema, and hyperalgesia when released in response to injury (Table 29-1). Cyclooxygenase inhibition explains many of the

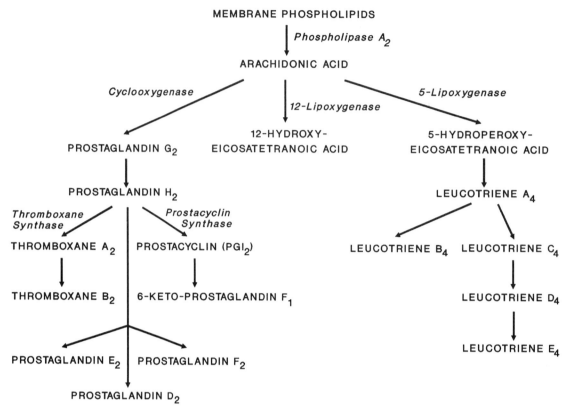

Fig. 29-1 Pathways of arachidonic acid metabolism.

anti-inflammatory effects of NSAIDs and some of the analgesic properties.[6] NSAID anti-inflammatory potency in vivo tends to reflect the rank order of potency for inhibition of prostaglandin synthesis in vitro.[4] The effect on prostaglandins primarily affects those of the E series by inhibition of the enzyme prostaglandin H synthase (cyclooxygenase), which converts arachidonic acid to prostaglandin G_2 and then acts as a peroxidase, converting prostaglandin G_2 to prostaglandin H_2. Aspirin irreversibly acetylates and inactivates cyclooxygenase; the other NSAIDs are reversible competitive antagonists of cyclooxygenase. Wu et al.[7] recently showed that aspirin not only inhibits prostaglandin H synthase directly, but it also reduces interleukin-1-induced prostaglandin H synthase gene expression in cultured endothelial cells. This activity was also seen with sodium salicylate but not indomethacin, suggesting that the effect is independent of a direct functional inhibition of the prostaglandin H synthase enzymes. These data suggest that aspirin might limit the biosynthesis of eicosanoids at inflammatory sites while exerting a lesser effect on basal prostaglandin production in other tissues. The effect of NSAIDs on prostaglandin production is also the principal cause of toxicity, as reflected in the platelet dysfunction, bronchospasm, decreased renal function, hypertension, and peptic ulceration commonly associated with their use.

Nonprostaglandin Processes

During the last decade, it has been increasingly appreciated that NSAIDs have multiple effects on inflammatory processes in addition to inhibition of prostaglandin biosynthesis (Table 29-2). Early studies showed that the NSAID doses necessary to supress inflammation were greater than those required to inhibit prostaglandin synthesis.[4] The capacity of an NSAID to inhibit prostaglandin syn-

Table 29-1 Some Functions of Eicosanoids Related to Inflammatory Reactions

PGE_2 and PGI_2	Vasodilation
	Act synergistically with other mediators, including bradykinin, histamine, C5a, and LTB_4 to increase vascular permeability
	Bronchodilation
	Inhibition of platelet aggregation
	Stimulation of osteoclastic bone resorption
PGD_2	Vasodilation
	Increased vascular permeability
	Bronchoconstriction
	Stimulation of random migration of neutrophils and eosinophils
LTC_4, LTD_4, and LTE_4	Vasoconstriction and bronchoconstriction
	Production of wheal and flare reaction in skin
	Augment bronchial mucus secretion
LTB_4	Chemotaxis and chemokinesis of neutrophils, eosinophils, and monocytes
	Promotion of leukocyte adhesiveness and adherence to endothelium
	Promotion of secretion of reactive oxygen species and hydrolytic enzymes by neutrophils

Abbreviations: LT, leukotriene; PG, prostaglandin.

Table 29-2 Multiple Effects of Nonsteroidal Anti-Inflammatory Drugs on Inflammatory Processes

Prostaglandin production
Leukotriene synthesis
Superoxide anion generation
Lysosomal enzyme release
Neutrophil aggregation and adhesion
Cell membrane functions
    Enzyme activity (NADPH oxidase and phospholipase C)
    Transmembrane anion transport
    Oxidative phosphorylation
    Uptake of arachidonate
Lymphocyte function

Abbreviations: NADPH, nicotinamide adenine dinucleotide phosphate.

thesis does not correlate well with the anti-inflammatory activity.[6] Similarly, the anti-inflammatory efficacy of salicylate, a weak cyclooxygenase inhibitor, equals that of aspirin, a potent cyclooxygenase inhibitor.[4]

Significant NSAID effects probably occur as a consequence of neutrophil function inhibition, interference with lymphocyte function, and inhibition of lipoxygenase, all of which are independent of cyclooxygenase inhibition. All NSAIDs inhibit some neutrophil functions, although assorted agents variably affect different neutrophil functions, such as cell aggregation and peroxide generation. Many effects on neutrophil function result from inhibition of membrane processes, such as G protein activation, which interrupts chemoattractant signals and inhibits cell activation.[8] This leads to a modulation of cell function, reducing cell adhesion and the subsequent release of inflammatory mediators, such as activated oxygen radicals. NSAIDs also interfere with lymphocyte function, specifically both T-helper and T-suppressor cells. NSAIDs will influence the release of a variety of cytokines by inhibiting various lipoxygenase enzymes (Fig. 29-1).[4,7,9]

NSAIDs may have a central and peripheral effect. For example, salicylates may act within the central nervous system to inhibit inflammation at the periphery, but this effect is not shared by indomethacin.[10] NSAIDs administered spinally produce significant analgesia, at doses several hundredfold less than those required after systemic administration.[11] These data are important, considering that both the central and peripheral nervous systems play an important role in modifying the inflammatory process.[12] A variety of observations now demonstrate a link between the nervous system and inflammation. Inflammatory mediators, such as bradykinin, prostaglandins, and leukotrienes, cause hyperalgesia. Conversely, interference with neural connections attenuates the characteristic signs of inflammation (swelling and hyperalgesia) in the contralateral paw of rats with chronic hind paw inflammation.[12] Neuropeptides such as substance P and somatostatin may induce the release of histamine and leukotriene B_4 from mast cells and modulate lymphocyte function. Treatment of neonatal rats with capsaicin reduces the severity of joint injury in arthritic rats; intra-articular infusion of substance P worsens arthritis. Studies of patients with rheumatoid arthritis clearly show sparing of inflammatory joint damage in limbs that have been paralyzed as a result of a stroke. The pain and swelling of a reflex sympathetic dystrophy will respond to sympathetic blockade. These studies have opened up a fascinating area of research that clearly links inflammatory mediators and the nervous system, both of which may be influenced by NSAIDs.

PHARMACOKINETICS

Physicochemical Differences

There are several different chemical classes of NSAIDs (Table 29-3). The physicochemical properties of NSAIDs govern their tissue distribution, and therefore, differences in these characteristics may influence therapeutic efficacy.[4] The most important factors are lipid solubility and pKa. More lipid soluble NSAIDs will penetrate the central nervous system more effectively and produce greater central nervous system effects. The antipyretic, and to some extent analgesic, activity of NSAIDs is dependent on penetration into the central nervous system. Similarly, NSAID side effects, such as mild changes in mood, perception, and cognition, are centrally mediated and, therefore, more common with lipid soluble agents.[13,14]

Most NSAIDs are weak acids with ionization constants (pKa) ranging from 3 to 5. The proportion of drug existing in the un-ionized lipid soluble state at physiologic pH will influence tissue distribution. Acidic NSAIDs will be preferentially taken up and sequestered by inflamed synovial tissue because of ion trapping (Fig. 29-2).[15] These agents will also tend to concentrate in gastric mucosa and the kidney, major sites of adverse NSAID effects. Some NSAIDs, such as sulindac, are delivered as prodrugs from which the active component is produced by metabolism in vivo. This may also produce differential exposure of various tissues to the active metabolite and, therefore, a potential reduction in side effects. For example, sulindac does not seem to affect the renal synthesis of prostaglandins as much as other NSAIDs and, therefore, has been

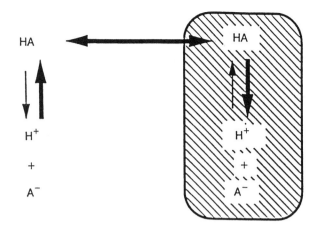

Fig. 29-2 Ion trapping of weak acids in an acidic milieu. The proportion of the nonionized form of a weak acid (HA) is higher in an acidic environment (left) than in a more neutral environment, such as that within cells (right). Because the nonionized form of the drug must be in equilibrium across the cell membrane ($\longleftrightarrow$), the total intracellular drug concentration ($HA + A^-$) must be higher than that outside the cell. (From Brooks and Day,[4] with permission.)

suggested as preferable in patients with renal disease or those with compromised renal function.[16] Other workers, however, have not found that sulindac is advantageous in these situations.[17]

Absorption, Metabolism, Distribution, and Excretion

NSAIDs have varying pharmacokinetic properties but, in general, are absorbed rapidly and extensively if administered orally, have low hepatic clearances (which are not blood flow dependent), undergo little first pass metabolism, are highly bound to plasma proteins (particularly albumin), possess small volumes of distribution (approaching the plasma volume owing to extensive protein binding), and demonstrate minimal urinary excretion of the parent drug. The pharmacokinetic characteristics of various NSAIDs are provided in Table 29-3. Fenbufen, sulindac, and nabumetone are prodrugs, which are transformed in vivo to active metabolites.

NSAIDs can be conveniently divided into those with a short (less than 6 hours) half-life (aspirin, diclofenac, etodolac, fenoprofen, flufenamic acid,

Table 29-3 Nonsteroidal Anti-Inflammatory Drug Classification and Pharmacokinetic Parameters

Drug Class and Members	Volume of Distribution (L/kg)	Clearance (ml/kg/min)	Half-Life[a] (h)	Plasma Protein Binding (%)	Urinary Excretion (%)
Salicylic acid derivatives					
Aspirin[b]	0.15	9.3	0.25 ± 0.03	85–90	<2
Salicylate[c]	0.17	0.14–0.86	2–19[d]	80–95[e]	2–30[f]
Diflunisal	0.10	0.11	13 ± 2	99.9	3–9
Arylacetic acids					
Alclofenac	0.10	1.5–2.5	1.5–2.5	>99	10–50
Diclofenac	0.12	3.7	1.1 ± 0.2	>99.5	<1
Arylpropionic acids					
Benoxaprofen		0.03–0.14	25–32	>98	<5
Carprofen		0.29–0.57	9–16	>99	3–5
Fenbufen	2–4	2.1–3.6	8–17	>98	<2
(active metabolites)					
γ-Hydroxy-4-biphenyl			7–17		<3
Biphenyl-4-acetic acid			7–12		1–15
Fenprofen	0.10	0.6–1.3	2.5 ± 0.5	>99	30
Flurbiprofen	0.10	0.3	3.8 ± 1.2	>99	<1
Ibuprofen	0.1–0.15	0.6–1.4	2.0 ± 0.5	>99	<1
Ketoprofen	0.11	1.2	1.8 ± 0.3	>99	<1
Naproxen	0.10–0.12	0.07–0.14	14 ± 2	>99	<1
Oxaprozin	0.16	0.04	58 ± 10	>99	1–4
Pirprofen			$3.8; 7.1 \pm 1.2$[g]	>99	<5
Suprofen	0.17	1.4–1.8	1–3	>99	<1
Tiaprofenic acid	0.1–0.25	0.6–1.4	3 ± 0.2	98	<5
Heterocyclic acetic acids					
Etodolac	0.4	0.68	$3.0; 6.5 \pm 0.3$[g]	>99	<1
Indomethacin	0.3–1.6	1–2	4.6 ± 0.7	>99	16
Ketorolac	0.1–0.25	0.36–0.57	4–10	>99	58
Sulindac			8	>99	7
(active metabolite)					
sulindac sulfide	2	1.5	15.8 ± 11.6	93.1	<1
Tolmetin	0.04	1.8	1.0 ± 0.3	>99	7
Zomepirac	1.8	2.6	4–8	98.5	0–5
Pyrazolones					
Apazone	0.14		15 ± 4	>99	62
Oxyphenbutazone	0.17	0.02	27–64	>98	>2
Phenylbutazone	0.17		68 ± 25	>99	1–3
Oxicams					
Isoxicam	0.17	0.001	29–34	96	1–2
Piroxicam	0.12–0.15	0.04	57–22	>99	4–10
Tenoxicam	0.12–0.15	0.0014	60–75	>98	<1
Fenamic acids					
Flufenamic acid			$1.4; 9$[g]	>90	<1
Mefenamic acid	1.3		3–4	>99	<6
Meclofenamic acid		2.6–2.9	3	99	2–4
Nonacidic Drugs					
Nabumetone					
(active metabolite)					
6-Methoxy-2-naphthylacetic acid	7.5		26 ± 5	99	1

[a] Mean ± standard deviation, or range.

[b] Acetylated; rapidly hydrolyzed to salicylate.

[c] Includes choline, magnesium, and sodium salts.

[d] Dose dependent; half-life increases with increasing plasma concentration.

[e] Dose dependent; binding decreases with increasing plasma concentration.

[f] Increases as urinary pH increases.

[g] Two-phase elimination (indicated by semicolon). First phase is generally more important.

Data from Day et al.[18] and Murray and Brater.[24]

ibuprofen, indomethacin, ketoprofen, ketorolac, pirprofen, tiaprofenic acid, and tolmetin) and those with a long (more than 10 hours) half-life (apazone, diflunisal, fenbufen, nabumetone, naproxen, oxaprozin, phenylbutazone, piroxicam, salicylate, sulindac, and tenoxicam). It must be remembered that these figures relate to plasma half-life rather than length of time that the drug remains in either the synovial fluid or other sites of action. NSAIDs diffuse slowly into synovial fluid and then maintain relatively stable concentrations of approximately 60 percent of the mean concentration in plasma.[18] Interestingly, the effect of an NSAID on prostaglandin production within the synovial fluid persists long after the synovial drug concentration has become undetectable.[19] Dose-response effects have been demonstrated for the anti-inflammatory effects of naproxen,[20] carprofen,[21] and ibuprofen,[22] and dose-effect relationships have also been shown for adverse events, such as gastrointestinal bleeding.[23]

Hepatic excretion is important for the elimination of most NSAIDs. Most NSAIDs are extensively metabolized in the liver by oxidation or conjugation (to several compounds, including glucuronides and acetyl coenzyme A), with little parent drug excreted intact in the urine.

Renal excretion is important for the elimination of some NSAIDS. Alclofenac, oxaprozin, indomethacin, ketorolac, and apazone undergo clinically important renal elimination and may accumulate in patients with impaired renal function.[24] Another important aspect of NSAID elimination and renal insufficiency concerns the arylpropionic acids. These NSAIDs, and other such as ketorolac, form acyl-glucuronide conjugates, which are easily cleaved back to the parent drug, forming a "futile cycle" of metabolism. Normally excreted renally, the acyl-glucuronide conjugate accumulates in patients with renal insufficiency and hydrolyzes to release the parent NSAID. Thus, the parent drug, which normally undergoes minimal renal excretion, nonetheless accumulates in renal failure.

A number of NSAIDs are available for intravenous or intramuscular use. These include asprin (available as glycine acetyl salicylate, 0.9 and 1.8 g, corresponding to 0.5 and 1 g of aspirin, respectively, and dissolved in 5 ml of sterile water immediately before use), ketoprofen (100 mg of freeze-dried drug reconstituted in normal saline or 5 percent dextrose in water), diclofenac sodium (approved for intramuscular use but sometimes given intravenously),[25] indomethacin (as a water soluble trihydrate salt for neonates or as 50 mg of indomethacin, freeze-dried, for reconstitution in sterile water or normal saline), and ketorolac tromethamine (10 mg in 1 ml of 10 percent alcohol).[26] The pharmacokinetics of these intravenous preparations are shown in Table 29-4. These NSAIDs, together with tenoxicam, tiaprofenic acid, and proxicam, may also be used by the intramuscular route.[27]

Table 29-4 Pharmacokinetic Parameters Following Intravenous Administration of Nonsteroidal Anti-Inflammatory Drugs

Drug	Dose (mg)	$T_{1/2\beta}$ (h)	CL (mL/min/kg)	V_d (l/kg)	V_{ss} (l/kg)	Reference
Aspirin	898	0.25	12.2		0.219	43
Salicylic acid		[1.65]	1.2	1.25	0.19	44
Diclofenac sodium	50	1.1	[4.2]	(0.12–0.17)[a]		45
Indomethacin	50	7.0	1.8	1.0		46
Ketoprofen	100	1.9	0.87		0.1	47
Ketorolac tromethamine	10	5.09	0.35	0.17	0.11	28

Abbreviations: CL, plasma clearance; $T_{1/2\beta}$, plasma elimination half-life; V_d, apparent volume of distribution; V_{ss}, volume of distribution at steady state.

[a] Data given in parentheses correspond to ranges.

The pharmacokinetics of intravenous, intramuscular, and oral administration have been compared for a few NSAIDs. Compared with oral administration, intramuscular injection results in a shorter time to peak plasma concentration. However, peak plasma concentrations after oral administration are achieved only slightly later than those after intramuscular injection (less than 1 hour), reducing the theoretic advantage of intramuscular administration. Maximum plasma concentrations achieved with intramuscular injection may be higher with some but not all NSAIDs than those achieved with oral forms[25,27–29] and might provide more rapid pain relief. The absorption concepts are illustrated for ketorolac (Fig. 29-3). After intramuscular administration, peak concentrations were achieved after 46 minutes.[28] Peak analgesia occurs at approximately 2 hours,[30] suggesting a lag time for the onset of effect. Compared with young patients (20 to 39 years old), the pharmacokinetics of oral and intramuscular ketorolac in elderly patients (65 to 78 years old) were characterized by slightly diminished clearance and increased half-life, prolonged oral absorption, and unchanged plasma protein binding and intramuscular absorption, with similar peak plasma concentrations achieved in all patient groups.[29]

In general, the total bioavailability is similar between intramuscular and oral NSAIDs, except for diclofenac. This NSAID is metabolized rapidly by the liver; thus, parenteral administration decreases first pass metabolism and significantly improves the bioavailability.[25]

Stereochemistry

Many NSAIDs have an asymmetric carbon atom and exist as two optical isomers, or (R) and (S) enantiomers, which are mirror images of each other. For the majority of the NSAIDs, the (S) enantiomer is the inhibitor of prostaglandin synthesis; the (R) enantiomer has minimal inhibitory activity toward cyclooxygenase. The majority of enantiomeric NSAIDs exist as racemates, or equal mixtures of (R) and (S) enantiomers,[4] although naproxen is marketed exclusively as the active (S) enantiomer.

The pharmacokinetic disposition of some NSAIDs is complicated by stereochemistry, both by enantioselective disposition and by chiral metabolic interconversion. Enantioselective disposition of oral ibuprofen in plasma, synovial fluid, and fat has been shown by Day et al.,[31,32] who demonstrated a markedly different pharmacokinetic profile for (R)- and (S)-ibuprofen enantiomers (Fig. 29-4). Similarly, following intravenous ketorolac administration plasma concentrations of (S)-ketorolac were

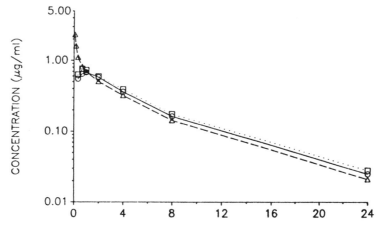

Fig. 29-3 Mean plasma concentration-time profiles of ketorolac after intravenous (△), intramuscular (□), and oral (○) administration of 10 mg of ketorolac tromethamine to 15 healthy subjects. After intravenous, intramuscular, and oral administration, the mean peak concentrations were 2.39, 0.77, and 0.81 μg/ml, achieved after 5, 46, and 53 minutes, respectively. The systemic bioavailability of intramuscular and oral ketorolac was 100 percent. (From Jung et al.,[28] with permission.)

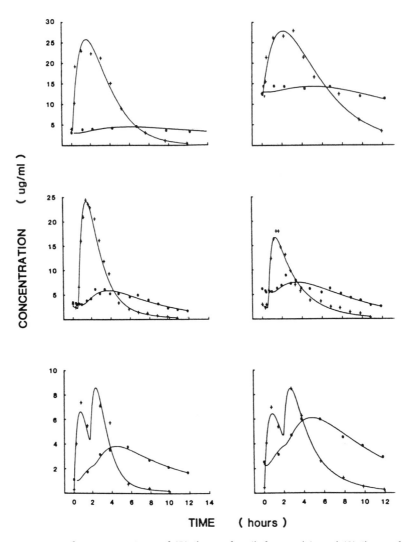

Fig. 29-4 Time course of concentrations of (R)-ibuprofen (left panels) and (S)-ibuprofen (right panels) enantiomers in synovial fluid (○) and plasma (+) in three patients. Concentrations of the active (S)-enantiomer in synovial fluid exceeded those of the (R)-enantiomer at all times. Variable ibuprofen absorption in one patient (lower panels) resulted in two concentration peaks. (From Day et al.,[31] with permission.)

significantly less than those of (R)-ketorolac, and the elimination half-life of (S)-ketorolac was less than that of (R)-ketorolac.[33] Chiral metabolic interconversion refers to the unique in vivo metabolism of inactive (R) to active (S) NSAID enantiomers. Such interconversion is unidirectional, occurring exclusively from (R) to (S), and it happens to varying extents with different chiral NSAIDs. Chiral conversion explains the higher plasma concentration of (S)-compared with (R)-ibuprofen after oral administration of the racemate. Some of the variability in response to NSAIDs may be the result of variable in vivo interconversion from (R) to (S) enantiomers,[31] which enhances anti-inflammatory activity, depending on the drug and the individual subject.[34]

Drug Interactions

The potential for drug interactions with NSAIDs is great because many patients who receive NSAIDs for musculoskeletal conditions are relatively elderly and have significant comorbidites or because the perioperative period includes polypharmaceutical therapy. NSAID interactions, both pharmacokinetic and pharmacodynamic, have been reviewed extensively recently and are summarized in Table 29-5.[35] The majority of these interactions have been described with a relatively long-term use of NSAIDs, but there is no reason to suspect that short-term administration, either orally or parenterally, will not produce the same potential interactions, particularly those involving the antihypertensive agents and diuretics. The administration of an NSAID should be preceded by a careful evaluation of any coexisting pathologic conditions, such as cardiovascular or renal dysfunction or concurrent drug therapy, which may predispose the patient to the development of a drug interaction with potentially serious consequences.

EFFICACY

Musculoskeletal Diseases

NSAIDs have been shown to be efficacious in the treatment of inflammatory forms of arthritis, such as rheumatoid arthritis and the seronegative arthropathies, and in the "less inflammatory" rheumatic diseases, such as osteoarthritis.[4] Although NSAIDs are used widely in sports injuries, controlled clinical trials do not show major differences between NSAIDs and placebo.[36] Where differences do exist, they are relatively small, and patients in both groups respond rapidly.

Comparative trials of NSAIDs have rarely identified clinically important differences between agents, with similar responses to average doses of NSAIDs among patients with rheumatoid arthritis or osteoarthritis.[4] There is, however, marked variation in individual responses and patient preferences for NSAIDs,[37,38] although the exact reasons for these differences are unclear. From a practical perspective, if appropriate for a particular musculoskeletal problem, a suitable NSAID should be se-

lected after considering the diagnosis and any previous experiences of the physician and the patient.[3] The dose is increased over 1 to 2 weeks until a satisfactory response is achieved or the maximum recommended dose is reached. If the patient does not respond, then that NSAID should be discontinued and another started. The use of analgesic agents without anti-inflammatory activity, such as acetaminophen, has been shown to allow a significant reduction in the dose of concurrently prescribed NSAIDs.[39] In less inflammatory musculoskeletal syndromes, such as back pain and osteoarthritis, physical therapy and analgesic agents should be prescribed initially, and NSAIDs should be prescribed only if there is a significant inflammatory component or the patient has not responded to simpler measures.

Analgesia

NSAIDs have been used extensively in the treatment of cancer pain.[40] World Health Organization guidelines stress NSAID use alone or in conjunction with opioids to diminish opioid requirements and enhance effects.[41] Although some studies have indicated that NSAIDs can be effective as an opioid analgesic,[42] this is usually seen in the short term. Little synergism is observed when NSAIDs and opioids are used together, although the effects of the two are additive. NSAIDs are used commonly for the treatment of disabling dysmenorrhea; they have been shown to decrease uterine prostaglandin production, intrauterine pressure, and uterine contractility.[48]

NSAID use in the management of mild to moderate acute pain (such as tension headaches; musculoskeletal pain; dental pain; and postoperative, postpartum, and postepisiotomy pain) was reviewed recently.[48] Sunshine et al.[49] were the first to demonstrate the analgesic properties of indomethacin for postoperative pain, and since then, a large number of studies have suggested that aspirin, acetaminophen, and other NSAIDs are equal or superior to weak opioids (such as codeine, proproxyphene, or combinations of these drugs with aspirin or acetaminophen) in the management of postepisiotomy pain,[50] dental procedures,[51] and postpartum uterine pain.[52]

Table 29-5 Interactions of Nonsteroidal Anti-Inflammatory Drugs With Other Drugs

Drug Affected	NSAID Implicated	Effect	Approach to Management
Pharmacokinetic Interactions			
NSAID affecting other drug			
Oral anticoagulants	Phenylbutazone Oxyphenbutazone Apazone	Inhibition of metabolism of S-warfarin, increasing anticoagulant effect.	Avoid NSAID if possible or use careful monitoring.
Lithium	Probably all (except possibly sulindac and aspirin)	Inhibition of renal excretion of lithium, increasing plasma lithium concentrations and risk of toxicity.	Use sulindac or aspirin if NSAID must be used. Monitor lithium concentration carefully and make appropriate dose reduction.
Oral hypoglycemic agents	Phenylbutazone Oxyphenbutazone Apazone	Inhibition of metabolism of sulfonylurea drugs, prolonging their half-life and increasing the risk of hypoglycemia.	Avoid these NSAIDs if possible; if not, monitor blood glucose level closely.
Phenytoin	Phenylbutazone Oxyphenbutazone	Inhibition of metabolism of phenytoin, increasing plasma phenytoin concentration and risk of toxicity.	Avoid these NSAIDs if possible; if not, intensify therapeutic drug monitoring.
	Others	Displacement of phenytoin from plasma protein, reducing total concentration for the same unbound (active) concentration.	Interpret total plasma concentration of phenytoin carefully; measuring the unbound concentration may be helpful.
Methotrexate (high nonrheumatologic dose)	Probably all	Reduced clearance of methotrexate (by unknown mechanism), increasing plasma methotrexate concentration and risk of toxicity.	Simultaneous dosing is contraindicated. Use of NSAIDs between cycles of chemotherapy is probably safe. Interaction not seen with rheumatologic doses of methotrexate.

Sodium valproate	Aspirin	Inhibition of valproate metabolism, increasing plasma valproate concentration.	Avoid aspirin; monitor plasma valproate concentration closely if another NSAID is used.
Digoxin	All	Potential reduction in renal function (particularly in very young and very old patients), reducing digoxin clearance and increasing plasma digoxin concentration and risk of toxicity (no interaction if renal function normal).	Avoid NSAIDs if possible; if not, measure plasma digoxin and creatinine concentrations frequently.
Aminoglycosides	All	Reduction in renal function in susceptible persons, lowering aminoglycoside clearance and increasing plasma aminoglycoside concentration.	Monitor plasma aminoglycoside concentration closely and adjust the dose accordingly.
Other drug affecting NSAID			
Antacids	Indomethacin	Variable effects of different preparations: rate and extent of absorption of indomethacin reduced by aluminum-containing antacids, but increased by sodium bicarbonate.	No action required unless markedly reduced absorption results in a poor response to the NSAID; dose may need to be increased. Rate of absorption of other NSAIDs can be slowed by antacids.
Probenecid	Probably all	Reduction in metabolism and renal clearance of NSAIDs and acyl-glucuronide metabolites, which are hydrolyzed back to parent drug.	
Barbiturates	Phenylbutazone, possibly others	Increased metabolic clearance of NSAID.	May require higher doses of phenylbutazone.
Caffeine	Aspirin	Increased rate of absorption of aspirin.	No action required.
Cholestyramine	Naproxen and probably others	Anion-exchange resin binding of NSAIDs in gut, reducing rate (and possibly extent) of absorption.	Separate dosing times by 4 h; may need larger than expected doses of NSAID.
Metoclopramide	Aspirin and others	Increased rate and extent of absorption of aspirin in patients with migraine.	

(Continues)

679

Table 29-5 (Continued)

Drug Affected	NSAID Implicated	Effect	Approach to Management
Pharmacodynamic Interactions			
NSAID affecting other drug			
Antihypertensive agents			
β-Blockers	Indomethacin	Reduction in hypotensive effect, probably related to inhibition of prostaglandin synthesis in kidneys (producing retention of salt and water) and blood vessels (producing increased vasoconstriction).	Avoid all NSAID use in patients receiving treatment for hypertension if possible; if not, use sulindac preferentially. Check blood pressure measurements repeatedly after starting NSAID. Additional antihypertensive therapy may be needed.
Diuretics	Others (possibly except sulindac)		
Angiotensin-converting enzyme inhibitors			
Diuretics	Indomethacin	Reduction in natriuretic and diuretic effects; may exacerbate congestive cardiac failure.	Avoid NSAID use in patients with cardiac failure, if possible; use sulindac and monitor clinical signs of fluid retention.
	Others (possibly except sulindac)		
Anticoagulants	All	Damage to mucosa of gastrointestinal tract and inhibition of platelet aggregation, both increasing risk of gastrointestinal bleeding in patients taking anticoagulants.	Avoid all NSAIDs, if possible.
Hypoglycemic agents	Salicylate (high dose)	Potentiation of hypoglycemic effects (by unknown mechanism).	Monitor blood glucose level.
Combination with increased risk of toxicity			
Diuretics			
General	All	Combination associated with increased risk of hemodynamic renal failure.	Avoid combination if possible.
Triamterene	Indomethacin	Potentiation of nephrotoxicity, even in subjects with normal renal function.	Combination contraindicated.
Potassium-sparing	All	Potassium retention and hyperkalemia.	Avoid combination; monitor plasma potassium level.

Abbreviations: NSAID, nonsteroidal anti-inflammatory drugs.
(Adapted from Brooks and Day,[4] with permission.)

Visceral Pain

Intravenous or intramuscular doses of diclofenac (50 to 75 mg), indomethacin (50 to 100 mg), ketoprofen (100 to 200 mg), and piroxicam (20 to 40 mg) have all been shown to be rapidly effective in the management of ureteral and biliary colic. In most studies, more than two-thirds of patients responded within 30 minutes. Rectal administration of these drugs may also be useful. In this regard, indomethacin solution, 100 mg per rectum, has been shown to be almost as effective in the treatment of renal colic pain as 50 mg administered intravenously.[53] If given intravenously, NSAIDs are generally administered as a bolus or as an infusion over 5 to 30 minutes. In the treatment of ureteral colic, ketoprofen has been used with a loading dose of 35 mg and a maintenance infusion rate of 25 mg/h over 24 hours.[54]

Postoperative Pain

The use of NSAIDs either as a sole postoperative analgesic or as an adjunct to opioid analgesics is not new,[55-57] but it has been the subject of increasing interest. This interest is the result primarily of the recent North American introduction of an NSAID for use by parenteral injection, that is, ketorolac. The postoperative use of NSAIDs has been the subject of two recent reviews.[26,58] Although it is clear that NSAIDs can be extremely useful in this situation, there are relatively few well conducted clinical trials with significant numbers of patients. Available studies have compared NSAIDs with placebo and compared NSAIDs with conventional opioid therapy, either alone or in combination.

The majority of studies demonstrate that NSAIDs are more effective than placebo in decreasing postoperative pain and/or postoperative opioid requirements following major abdominal surgery.[58] Similarly, intravenous, intramuscular, or oral NSAIDs decreased postoperative pain intensity and/or opioid requirement following orthopaedic surgery, although the magnitude of the effect was less than that following more painful procedures. Compared with placebo, NSAIDs are able to reduce, but not eliminate, postoperative opioid analgesic requirements. Therefore, NSAIDs are said to have an "opioid-sparing effect."[59,60] The magnitude of this opioid-sparing effect has been estimated to be between 20 and 35 percent.[58]

Numerous investigations have compared the efficacy of perioperative NSAIDs with that of opioids. The effect of intravenous or intramuscular postoperative NSAID administration on subsequent opioid analgesic demand has been well characterized. Lysine acetyl salicylate (14.67 mg/kg IV) was as effective as meperidine (1 mg/kg IM) after cholecystectomy,[61] as effective as oxycodone (6 mg IV) after upper abdominal surgery,[62] and as effective as pentazocine (60 mg IV) after thoracotomy.[63] Similar findings have been reported in some, but not all, studies of lysine acetyl salicylate after gynecologic and orthopaedic surgery.[58] The majority of these studies found that perioperative lysine acetyl salicylate is not a complete analgesic, having moderate efficacy in the treatment of mild to moderate postoperative pain, but primarily, it has an opioid-sparing effect.[58] Intravenous infusions of indomethacin, ketoprofen (200 to 600 mg/day), or diclofenac (150 mg/day) similarly reduced the postoperative requirements for oxycodone following lower extremity surgery or cesarean section.[64-66]

The clinical effects of ketorolac have been carefully summarized.[67] In one set of studies, the time to peak analgesia was slower following ketorolac (2 hours) than following morphine (1 hour) or fentanyl.[68,69] Another study found that ketorolac and morphine had similar analgesic onset times.[70] It is apparent that major surgery is a more sensitive indicator of ketorolac analgesic efficacy compared with minor surgery.[30,58,67] In patients undergoing major abdominal or orthopaedic surgery, a single dose of ketorolac (30 or 90 mg IM) was equieffective with morphine (12 mg IM) up to 3 hours.[68] Ketorolac (10 or 30 mg IM) was as effective as morphine (12 mg IM) for 6 hours, and ketorolac (90 mg IM) was more effective than morphine (12 mg IM) for the 6 hour observation period.[30] Ketorolac given by postoperative intramuscular infusion (1.5 to 3 mg/h) significantly reduced morphine requirements in patients who had undergone upper abdominal surgery.[60] In a further study, in patients following abdominal surgery, continuous postoperative intramuscular infusion of ketorolac (6.25 mg loading dose over 30 minutes followed by 2.5 mg/h) was superior to intermittent intramuscular injections of ketorolac (10 mg every 4 hours) in terms of reducing morphine requirements.[71] In patients who had undergone ambulatory surgery, ketorolac (60 to 120 mg IV followed by 10 mg orally) provided delayed but equieffective analgesia compared with fentanyl (50 μg) followed by oral acetaminophen plus codeine.[69] In contrast, following cholecystectomy, ketorolac (30 mg IM) administered on demand as often as every 2 hours was less effective than morphine (10 mg IM) on demand as often as every 2 hours in providing analgesia on the first day postoperatively, and patients receiving ketorolac required earlier and more frequent opioid rescue medication.[72] These studies reinforce the concept that NSAIDs do not provide complete analgesia following severe postoperative pain but rather possess an opioid-sparing effect.

NSAIDs have also been given preoperatively or perioperatively in an attempt to reduce postoperative pain. Premedication with ketorolac (10 mg or 30 mg IM) was shown to be as effective as morphine (10 mg, IM) for minor surgery, as assessed by drowsiness, anxiolysis, and reduction in postoperative pain.[73] Intravenous lysine acetyl salicylate (14 mg/kg) administered during anesthesia reduced postoperative pain after minor maxillofacial surgery.[74] Intravenous diclofenac (75 mg) significantly reduced pain after dental surgery.[75] Diclofenac (50 mg per rectum) administered 1 hour before anesthesia reduced 24-hour postoperative pain scores and the number of patients needing additional postoperative analgesics.[76]

More recent studies with postoperative NSAIDs have explored the concept of "balanced analgesia," using NSAIDs in combination with other analgesic modalities.[58] The rationale for combination therapy is that drugs acting by different receptors or mechanisms will have additive or synergistic effects. Thus, rather than simply exerting an opioid-sparing effect, NSAIDs might produce additive or synergistic effects to reduce pain more effectively. Although opioid-sparing effects and additive analgesic effects have been well documented, other beneficial effects are not yet as apparent.[58,77,78] More data are needed before specific therapeutic NSAID balanced analgesia regimens can be recommended.[58]

The theoretic advantage of NSAIDs over opioids is that NSAIDs do not suppress respiration and have no effect on cardiovascular function.[79–81] Because NSAIDs are incomplete analgesics and are customarily used in combination with opioids, the theoretic advantage of the opioid-sparing effect of NSAIDs is a reduction in the opioid dose and, therefore, a reduction in opioid-induced ventilatory depression or other side effects. Early studies showed that, compared with placebo, patients receiving postoperative NSAIDs required less morphine, and this was accompanied by a slightly diminished rise in postoperative PCO_2.[59,60] In contrast, Liu et al.[82] showed more recently in a double-blind protocol that the opioid-sparing effect of ketorolac following laparoscopic cholecystectomy was not accompanied by any decrease in postoperative nausea, vomiting, or ventilatory impairment as measured by formal respirometry.

Pediatric Use

Compared with adults, relatively less is known about perioperative NSAID use in pediatric patients. The elimination half-life of ketorolac in children is similar to that in adults, although the plasma clearance and volume of distribution are twice that in adults.[83] In children undergoing either myringotomy or adenoidectomy with or without myringotomy, oral preinduction ketorolac or diclofenac was compared with acetaminophen (paracetamol) and placebo, respectively.[84,85] Children receiving ketorolac or diclofenac required less postoperative analgesic therapy than did those receiving acetaminophen, or placebo, although discharge times and side effect profiles were similar in all groups. In children undergoing more painful operations, intravenous indomethacin reduced postoperative morphine requirements compared with placebo.[86] Intravenous ketorolac and morphine were equieffective as judged by pain scores and analgesic requirements.[87,88]

ADVERSE EFFECTS

Adverse reactions to NSAIDs constitute the most commonly reported adverse drug effect. The spectrum of side effects is broad, with gastrointestinal problems reported most commonly.[89,90] Rare adverse reactions include blood dyscrasias, skin reactions, hepatic syndromes, pneumonitis, and neurologic problems, such as headache, aseptic meningitis, and nausea.[89] Central nervous system reactions, such as dizziness, and skin reactions are relatively frequent but usually not severe. Gastrointestinal effects and renal adverse reactions are of greatest interest for the anesthesiologist and will be emphasized here because these may occur soon after the institution of NSAID therapy. Gastrointestinal and renal side effects are often precipitated in situations of compromised regional blood flow, such as diminished renal perfusion in the perioperative or postoperative period.

Gastrointestinal Effects

It is now clear that both acute and chronic NSAID use are associated with an increased risk of gastrointestinal mucosal erosive damage, which can take place throughout the gastrointestinal tract.[91,92] For NSAID-induced serious upper gastrointestinal adverse effects, an increased risk of between 2 cases per 10,000 person months of prescriptions[93] and a 7-fold increase in the risk of hospitalization in patients with rheumatoid arthritis[94] have been reported. Peptic ulceration is most frequent within the first 3 to 4 months of therapy,[95] but the risk continues throughout the period of treatment.[96] Of particular recent interest is the study from Piper et al.,[97] which demonstrated that glucocorticoid therapy per se does not increase the risk of peptic ulceration in patients older than age 65 years but that patients taking both glucocorticoids and NSAIDs have a 15-fold increase in risk over individuals using neither of these drugs. Significant risk factors for serious NSAID-associated upper gastrointestinal events in patients with rheumatoid arthritis include age (older than age 65 years), a history of previous NSAID-associated gastrointestinal side effects, significant disability, the dose of the NSAID, and current prednisolone use.[98] The incidence of peptic ulceration can be significantly reduced by H_2 antagonists, omeprazole, and a prostaglandin analog, such as misoprostol.[92,99] Whether these agents reduce the complications of peptic ulceration has not yet been proved. Parenteral NSAID administration does not reduce the risk of peptic ulceration, caused by breakdown of the gastric mucosal barrier, compared with oral ad-

ministration. There is increasing evidence that small and large bowel mucosal abnormalities occur in patients receiving NSAIDs.[100] This may be a particular problem in elderly patients with compromised vascular supply to the gut, potentially complicated by the diminished splanchnic blood flow that accompanies abdominal surgery.

Renal Effects

NSAIDs may cause adverse renal events, particularly in patients with compromised renal function. Because prostaglandins are responsible for autoregulation of renal blood flow and glomerular filtration, NSAID inhibition of renal cyclooxygenase activity may diminish renal blood flow and glomerular filtration rate.[101] NSAIDs can cause reversible or permanent impairment of glomerular filtration, acute renal failure, peripheral edema, interstitial nephritis, papillary necrosis, chronic renal failure, and hyperkalemia.[4,24,32] The most common form of NSAID-induced nephrotoxicity is acute renal insufficiency caused by diminished renal blood flow and glomerular filtration rate, which can occur within hours after a single NSAID dose.[24] NSAID-induced renal ischemia is usually reversible after discontinuation of the NSAID. Acute interstitial nephritis and analgesic-associated nephropathy caused by papillary necrosis are far less common and typically occur after chronic NSAID use. Because prostaglandins also modulate vascular tone, NSAIDs may cause hypertension and also interfere with the action of antihypertensive medications.[102] Healthy individuals receiving therapeutic NSAID doses are minimally at risk of renal toxicity. Risk factors for NSAID nephrotoxicity include hypovolemia as a result of dehydration, hemorrhage, cirrhosis with ascites, or concurrent diuretic therapy; pre-existing chronic renal insufficiency caused by atherosclerosis, hypertension, intrinsic renal disease, or increasing age; and congestive heart failure.[24,32]

Hemostasis

Another important issue in regard to the use of NSAIDs in the perioperative period is their effect on bleeding. NSAIDs interfere with platelet cyclooxygenase (aspirin, irreversibly, and the other NSAIDs, reversibly).[103] This has important implications if NSAIDs are to be used in the perioperative period. Because the platelet is derived from a megakaryocyte, it does not have the ability to produce more cyclooxygenase after this enzyme has been inactivated. Thus, the effect of aspirin is to reduce platelet adhesion during the lifetime of the platelet (7 to 10 days). Because new platelets are being released all the time, functional bleeding tests will return to normal 3 or 4 days after aspirin is discontinued. NSAIDs will only interfere with platelet function while they remain in sufficient concentration in the blood (determined by the plasma half-life). As a rough rule of thumb, NSAIDs will maintain their pharmacologic activity for about three to four half-lives and will inhibit platelet function during this time.

Prolonged bleeding times have been reported compared to placebo in patients on indomethacin,[64] diclofenac,[104] and ketorolac.[105] However, even patients receiving indomethacin as a perioperative analgesic did not show a dramatic increase in peri- or postoperative blood loss,[106] and patients receiving diclofenac during total hip replacements did not show an increased blood loss.[78] From a practical point of view, the issue of increased bleeding does not seem to be a major problem, although great care needs to be taken in any patient with an underlying disorder of coagulation.[107]

SUMMARY

The use of NSAIDs as adjunctive analgesic therapy in the perioperative period seems to provide a means of reducing opioid requirements and providing effective pain relief. Given either intramuscularly or intravenously, these drugs have a rapid effect, and their analgesia lasts for a varying length of time, depending on the plasma half-life. Great variability in individual response to NSAIDs has been noted in other situations in which these drugs were used and may also occur in relation to perioperative analgesia.

Potential adverse reactions to NSAIDs in the perioperative period may be important, particularly because prostaglandins may be involved in maintaining regional blood flow to the kidney and gut in situations of hypoperfusion. Great care should be taken in patients with evidence of atherosclerosis or underlying renal disease. There are already reports associating parenteral NSAIDs with acute renal failure[108] or gastrointestinal bleeding.[109] Further studies are required to assess these issues, but parenteral NSAIDs should be used with caution, particularly in elderly patients.

REFERENCES

1. Clive DM, Stoff JS: Renal syndromes associated with non-steroidal anti-inflammatory drugs. N Engl J Med 310:563, 1984
2. Henry DA: Side effects of non-steroidal anti-inflammatory drugs. Baillieres Clin Rheumatol 2:425, 1988
3. Champion GD: Therapeutic usage of the non-steroidal anti-inflammatory drugs. Med J Aust 149:203, 1988
4. Brooks PM, Day RO: Non-steroidal anti-inflammatory drugs—differences and similarities. N Engl J Med 324:1716, 1991
5. Vane JR: Inhibition of prostaglandin synthesis as a mechanism of action of the aspirin-like drugs. Nature 231:232, 1971
6. Jeremy JY, Mikhailidis JP: NSAID efficacy and side effects: are they wholly prostaglandin mediated? J Drug Rev 3:3, 1990
7. Wu KK, Sanduja R, Tsai AL et al: Aspirin inhibits interleukin-1-induced prostaglandin H synthase expression in cultured endothelial cells. Proc Natl Acad Sci USA 88:2384, 1991
8. Abramson SB, Lescczynska-Piziak J, Haines H, Reibman J: Non-steroidal anti-inflammatory drugs: effects on a GTP binding protein within the neutrophil membrane. Biochem Pharmacol 41:1567, 1991
9. Abramson S: Therapy and mechanisms of non-steroidal anti-inflammatory drugs. Curr Sci 3:336, 1991
10. Catania A, Arnold J, MacAluso A et al: Inhibition of acute inflammation in the periphery by central action of salicylates. Proc Natl Acad Sci USA 88:8544, 1991
11. Malmberg AB, Yaksh TL: Antinociceptive actions of spinal nonsteroidal anti-inflammatory agents on the formalin test in the rat. J Pharmacol Exp Ther 263:136, 1992
12. Levine JD, Goetzl EJ, Basbaum AL: Contribution of the nervous system to the pathophysiology of rheu-

matoid arthritis and other polyarthritides. Rheum Clin North Am 13:369, 1987

13. Netter P, Lapicque F, Bannwarth B et al: Diffusion of intramuscular ketoprofen into the cerebrospinal fluid. Eur Clin Pharmacol 29:319, 1985

14. Goodwin JS, Regan M: Cognitive dysfunction associated with naproxen and ibuprofen in the elderly. Arthritis Rheum 25:1013, 1982

15. Brune K, Graft P: Non-steroidal anti-inflammatory drugs: influence of extracellular pH on biodistribution and pharmacological effects. Biochem Pharmacol 27:525, 1978

16. Ciabattoni G, Gnotti GA, Pierucci A et al: Effects of sulindac and ibuprofen in patients with chronic glomerular disease: evidence for the dependence of renal function on prostacyclin. New Engl J Med 310:279, 1984

17. Quintero E, Gines P, Arroyo V et al: Sulindac reduces the urinary excretion of prostaglandins and impairs renal function in cirrhosis with ascites. Nephron 42:298, 1986

18. Day RO, Graham GG, Williams KM: Pharmacokinetics of non-steroidal anti-inflammatory drugs. Baillieres Clin Rheumatol 2:363, 1988

19. Dromgoole SH, Furst DE, Desiraja RK et al: Tolmetin kinetics and synovial fluid prostaglandin E levels in rheumatoid arthritis. Clin Pharmacol Ther 32:371, 1982

20. Day RO, Furst DE, Dromgoole SH et al: Relationship of serum naproxen concentration to efficacy in rheumatoid arthritis. Clin Pharmacol Ther 31:733, 1982

21. Furst DE, Caldwell JR, Klugman MP et al: Serum concentration and dose-response relationships for carprofen in rheumatoid arthritis. Clin Pharmacol Ther 44:186, 1988

22. Grennan DM, Aarons L, Siddiqui M et al: Dose-response study with ibuprofen in rheumatoid arthritis: clinical and pharmacokinetic findings. Br J Clin Pharmacol 18:311, 1983

23. Carson JL, Strom BL, Morse ML et al: The relative gastrointestinal toxicity of the nonsteroidal anti-inflammatory drugs. Arch Intern Med 147:1054, 1987

24. Murray MD, Brater DC: Renal toxicity of the nonsteroidal anti-inflammatory drugs. Annu Rev Pharmacol Toxicol 33:434, 1993

25. Campbell WI, Waters CH: Venous sequelae following IV administration of diclofenac. Br J Anaesth 62:545, 1989

26. Bannwarth B, Netter P, Giroud J-P: Intravenous use of NSAIDs. p. 413. In Famaey JP, Paulus HE (eds): Therapeutic Applications of NSAIDs—Subpopulations and New Foundations. Marcel Dekker, New York, 1992

27. Avoual B: Intramuscular use of NSAIDs. p. 400. In Famaey JP, Paulus HE (eds): Therapeutic Applications of NSAIDs. Marcel Dekker, New York, 1992

28. Jung D, Mroszczak E, Bynum L: Pharmacokinetics of ketorolac tromethamine in humans after intravenous, intramuscular and oral administration. Eur J Clin Pharmacol 35:423, 1988

29. Jallad NS, Garg DC, Martinez JJ et al: Pharmacokinetics of single-dose oral and intramuscular ketorolac tromethamine in the young and elderly. J Clin Pharmacol 30:76, 1990

30. Yee JP, Koshiver JE, Allbon C, Brown CR: Comparison of intramuscular ketorolac tromethamine and morphine sulfate for analgesia of pain after major surgery. Pharmacol Ther 6:253, 1986

31. Day RO, Williams KM, Graham GG et al: Stereoselective disposition of ibuprofen enantiomers in synovial fluid. Clin Pharmacol Ther 43:480, 1988

32. Day RO, Graham GG, Williams KM et al: Clinical pharmacology of non-steroidal anti-inflammatory drugs. Pharmacol Ther 33:383, 1987

33. Hayball PJ, Tamblyn JG, Holden Y, Wrobel J: Stereoselective analysis of ketorolac in human plasma by high-performance liquid chromatography. Chirality 5:31, 1993

34. Williams KM, Day RO, Knihinicki RD, Duffield A: The stereoselective uptake of ibuprofen enantiomers into adipose tissue. Biochem Pharmacol 35:3403, 1986

35. Tonkin AL, Wing LMH: Interactions of non-steroidal anti-inflammatory drugs. Baillieres Clin Rheum 2:455, 1988

36. Weiler JM, Albright JP, Buckwater JA: Non-steroidal anti-inflammatory drugs in sports medicine. p. 71. In Lewis AT, Furst DE (eds): Non-Steroidal Anti-Inflammatory Drugs—Mechanisms and Clinical Use. Marcel Dekker, New York, 1987

37. Huskisson EC, Woolf DL, Balme WH et al: Four new anti-inflammatory drugs: responses and variations. BMJ 1:1048, 1976

38. Gall EP, Caperton JF, McComb JE et al: Clinical comparison of ibuprofen, fenoprofen calcium, naproxen and tolmetin sodium in rheumatoid arthritis. J Rheumatol 9:402, 1982

39. Seideman P, Melander A: Equianalgesic effects of paracetamol and indomethacin in rheumatoid arthritis. Br J Rheumatol 27:117, 1988

40. Gilman SC, Chang J: Non-steroidal anti-inflammatory drugs in cancer therapy. p. 157. In Lewis AJ, Furst DE (eds): Non-Steroidal Anti-Inflammatory Drugs—Mechanisms and Clinical Use. Marcel Dekker, New York, 1987

41. World Health Organization: Cancer Pain Relief. Geneva, World Health Organization, 1986

42. Ventafridda V, Fochi C, DeConno D, Sganzerla E: Use of non-steroidal anti-inflammatory drugs in the treatment of pain in cancer. Br J Clin Pharmacol 10:343, 1980

43. Aarons L, Hopkins K, Rowland M et al: Route of administration and sex differences in the pharmacokinetics of aspirin, administered as its lysine salt. Pharmacol Res 6:660, 1989

44. Bochner F, Williams DB, Morris PMA et al: Pharmacokinetics of low-dose oral modified release, soluble and intravenous aspirin in man, and on platelet function. Eur J Clin Pharmacol 35:287, 1988

45. Willis JV, Kendall MJ, Flinn RM et al: The pharmacokinetics of diclofenac sodium following intravenous and oral administration. Eur J Clin Pharmacol 16:405, 1979

46. Jensen KM, Grenabo L: Bioavailability of indomethacin after intramuscular injection and rectal administration of solution and suppositories. Acta Pharmacol Toxicol 57:322, 1985

47. Monmay G, Le Liboux A, Chashard D et al: Pharmacokinetics and bioavailability of ketoprofen after intravenous, intramuscular and oral administration. Eur J Clin Pharmacol, Suppl.:A317, 1989

48. Deck CC, Bloomfield SS, Radacke KL: Occasional use of NSAIDs for dysmenorrhea, pain or injuries. p. 299. In Famaey JP, Paulus HE (eds): Therapeutic Applications of NSAIDs—Subpopulations and New Formulations. Marcel Dekker, New York, 1992

49. Sunshine A, Laske E, Meisner M: Analgesic studies of indomethacin as analyzed by computer techniques. Clin Pharmacol Ther 5:699, 1964

50. Hopkinson JH: Ibuprofen versus propoxyphene hydrochloride and placebo in the relief of post episiotomy pain. Curr Ther Res 27:55, 1980

51. Cooper SA, Beever W: A model to evaluate mild analgesics in oral surgery outpatients. Clin Pharmacol Ther 20:241, 1976

52. Bloomfield SS, Barden TP, Mitchell J: Naproxen, aspirin and codeine in post partum uterine pain. Clin Pharmacol Ther 21:414, 1977

53. Nelson CE, Mulander C, Olsson AM et al: Rectal v. intravenous administration of indomethacin in the treatment of renal colic. Acta Chir Scand 154:253, 1988

54. De Bruyne O, Hurault DE, Ligny B et al: Clinical pharmacokinetics of ketoprofen after a single dose bolus or infusion. Clin Pharmacokinet 12:214, 1987

55. Stetson JB, Robinson K, Wardell WM, Lasagna L: Analgesic activity of oral naproxen in patients with postoperative pain. Scand J Rheumatology, suppl. 2:50, 1973

56. Reasbeck PG, Rice ML, Reasbeck JC: Double-blind controlled trial of indomethacin as an adjunct to narcotic analgesia after major abdominal surgery. Lancet 2:115, 1982

57. Dionne RA, Campbell RA, Cooper SA et al: Suppression of postoperative pain by preoperative administration of ibuprofen in comparison to placebo, acetaminophen, and acetaminophen plus codeine. J Clin Pharmacol 23:37, 1983

58. Dahl JB, Kehlet H: Non-steroidal anti-inflammatory drugs: rationale for use in severe postoperative pain. Br J Anaesth 66:703, 1991

59. Hodsman NBA, Burns J, Blyth A et al: The morphine sparing effects of diclofenac sodium following abdominal surgery. Anaesthesia 42:1005, 1987

60. Gillies GWA, Kenny GNC, Bullingham RES, McArdle CS: The morphine sparing effect of ketorolac tromethamine. Anaesthesia 42:727, 1987

61. Cattaneo AD, Rivara A, Launo C: Valutazione clinica dell' acetilsalicilato di lisinanel contròllo del dolóre postoperatòrio. Minerva Anestesiol 41:599, 1975

62. Tammisto T, Tigerstedt I: Mild analgesics in postoperative pain. Br J Clin Pharmacol 10:3475, 1980

63. Henriques F, De Martins G: L'asl nélla terapía antalgiga dell' operatòrio toracico: confronto tra acl e pentazolina. Minerva Anestesiol 47:247, 1981

64. Taivanen T, Hiller A, Rosenberg PH, Neuvonen P: The effect of continuous intravenous indomethacin in fusion on bleeding time and postoperative pain in patients undergoing emergency surgery of the lower extremities. Acta Anesthesiol Scand 33:58, 1989

65. Schillinge D, Gipeauz M, Dollet JM: Intérêt du kétoprofène en chirurgie obstétricale. Presse Med 17:1651, 1988

66. Rorarius MGF, Suominen P, Baer GA et al: Diclofenac and ketoprofen for pain treatment after elective caesarean section. Br J Anaesth 70:293, 1993

67. Buckley MM-T, Brogden RN: Ketorolac: a review of its pharmacodynamic and pharmacokinetic properties, and therapeutic potential. Drugs 39:86, 1990

68. O'Hara DA, Fragen RJ, Kinzer M, Pemberton D: Ketorolac tromethamine as compared with mor-

phine sulfate for treatment of postoperative pain. Clin Pharmacol Ther 41:556, 1987

69. Wong HY, Carpenter RL, Kopacz DJ et al: A randomized, double-blind evaluation of ketorolac tromethamine for postoperative analgesia in ambulatory surgery patients. Anesthesiology 78:6, 1993

70. Rice ASC, Lloyd J, Miller CG et al: A double-blind study of the speed of onset of analgesia following intramuscular administration of ketorolac tromethamine in comparison to intramuscular morphine and placebo. Anaesthesia 46:541, 1991

71. Burns JW, Aitken HA, Bullingham RES et al: Double blind comparison of the morphine sparing effect of continuous and intermittent IM administration of ketorolac. Br J Anaesth 67:235, 1991

72. Power I, Noble DW, Douglas E, Spence AA: Comparison of i.m. ketorolac trometamol and morphine sulphate for pain relief after cholecystectomy. Br J Anaesth 65:448, 1990

73. Alexander JI, Harris C, Johnson RW, Thomas TA: A double-blind randomized comparison of the analgesic and side effects of ketorolac and morphine when used as premedicants for surgery. Curr Ther Res 49:1, 1991

74. Velzeboer SJ: An evaluation of lysine acetyl salicylate as an analgesic in maxillofacial surgery. S Afr Med J 62:135, 1982

75. Valanne J, Kortilla K, Ylkiorwala O: Intravenous diclofenac sodium decreases prostaglandin synthesis and postoperative symptoms after general anaesthesia in outpatients undergoing dental surgery. Acta Anaesthesiol Scand 31:722, 1987

76. Gillberg LE, Harsten AS, Stahl LB: Preoperative diclofenac sodium reduces post-laparoscopy pain. Can J Anaesth 40:406, 1993

77. Grass JA, Sakima NT, Valley M et al: Assessment of ketorolac as an adjuvant to fentanyl patient-controlled epidural analgesia after radical retropubic prostatectomy. Anesthesiology 78:642, 1993

78. Laitinen J, Nuutinen LS: Intravenous diclofenac coupled with P.C.A. fentanyl for pain relief after total hip replacement. Anesthesiology 76:194, 1992

79. Murray AW, Brockway MS, Kenny GNC: Comparison of the cardiorespiratory effects of ketorolac and alfentanil during propofol anaesthesia. Br J Anaesth 63:601, 1989

80. Camu F, Overberge LV, Bullingham R, Lloyd J: Hemodynamic effects of two intravenous doses of ketorolac tromethamine compared to morphine. Pharmacol Ther 10:1225, 1990

81. Brandon Bravo LJC, Mattie H, Spierdijk J et al: The effects on ventilation of ketorolac in comparison with morphine. Eur J Clin Pharmacol 35:491, 1988

82. Liu J, Ding YF, White PF et al: Effects of ketorolac on postoperative analgesia and ventilatory function after laparoscopic cholecystectomy. Anesth Analg 76:1061, 1993

83. Olkkola KT, Maunuksela E-L: The pharmacokinetics of postoperative intravenous ketorolac tromethamine in children. Br J Clin Pharmacol 31:182, 1991

84. Watcha MF, Ramirez-Ruiz M, White PF et al: Perioperative effects of oral ketorolac and acetaminophen in children undergoing bilateral myringotomy. Can J Anaesth 39:649, 1992

85. Baer GA, Rorarius MGF, Kolehmainen S, Selin S: The effect of paracetamol or diclofenac administered before operation on postoperative pain and behaviour after adenoidectomy in small children. Anaesthesia 47:1078, 1992

86. Maunuksela E-L, Olkkola KT, Korpela R: Does prophylactic intravenous infusion of indomethacin improve the management of postoperative pain in children? Can J Anaesth 35:123, 1988

87. Maunuksela E-L, Kokki H, Bullingham RES: Comparison of intravenous ketorolac with morphine for postoperative pain in children. Clin Pharmacol Ther 52:436, 1992

88. Watcha MF, Jones B, Lagueruela RG et al: Comparison of ketorolac and morphine as adjuvants during pediatric surgery. Anesthesiology 76:368, 1992

89. O'Brien WM, Bagby GF: Rare adverse reactions to nonsteroidal anti-inflammatory drugs. J Rheumatol 12:13, 1985

90. Brooks PM: Side effects of non-steroidal anti-inflammatory drugs. Med J Aust 148:248, 1988

91. Langman MJS, Brooks P, Hawkey CJ et al: Nonsteroidal anti-inflammatory drug associated ulcer: epidemiology, causation and treatment. J Gastroenterol Hepatol 6:442, 1991

92. Simons LS: Toxicities of the nonsteroidal anti-inflammatory drugs. Curr Sci 4:301, 1992

93. Langman MJS: Epidemiologic evidence on the association between peptic ulceration and anti-inflammatory drug use. Gastroenterology suppl. 2:640, 1989

94. Fries JF, Miller SR, Spitz PW et al: Towards an epidemiology of gastropathy associated with nonsteroidal anti-inflammatory drug use. Gastroenterology suppl. 2:647, 1989

95. Larson JC, Strom BC, Soper KA et al: The association of non-steroidal anti-inflammatory drugs with

upper g.i. tract bleeding. Arch Intern Med 147:85, 1987

96. Kurata JH, Abbey DE: The effect of chronic aspirin use on duodenal and gastric ulcer hospitalizations. J Clin Gastroenterol 12:260, 1990

97. Piper JM, Ray WA, Daugherty JR, Griffin MR: Corticosteroid use and peptic ulcer disease: role of nonsteroidal anti-inflammatory drugs. Ann Intern Med 114:735, 1991

98. Fries JF, Williams CA, Bloch DA, Michel BA: Nonsteroidal anti-inflammatory drug associated gastropathy: incidence and risk factor models. Am J Med 91:213, 1991

99. Howard JM, Le Riche NGH: The management of NSAID gastropathy. Baillieres Clin Rheumatol 4:269, 1990

100. Bjarnason I, Zanelli G, Smith T et al: Nonsteroidal anti-inflammatory drug induced intestinal inflammation in humans. Gastroenterol 93:480, 1987

101. Garella S, Matarese RA: Renal effects of prostaglandins and clinical adverse effects of nonsteroidal anti-inflammatory agents. Medicine (Baltimore) 64:165, 1984

102. Houston MC: Nonsteroidal anti-inflammatory drugs and antihypertensives. Am J Med suppl. 5A:42S, 1991

103. Kantor T: NSAIDs, salicylates and blood coagulation. p. 265. In Famaey JP, Paulus HE (eds): Therapeutic Applications of NSAIDs. Marcel Dekker, New York, 1992

104. Power I, Chambers WA, Greer IA et al: Platelets function after intramuscular diclofenac. Anaesthesia 45:916, 1990

105. Greer IA: Effects of ketorolac tromethamine on hemostasis. Pharmacol Ther 10:715, 1990

106. Rorarus MGF, Baer GA, Metsaketela T et al: Effects of peri-operatively administered diclofenac and indomethacin on blood loss bleeding time and plasma prostanoids in man. Europ J Anaesth 6:335, 1989

107. Nuutinen LS, Laitinen JO, Salomaki TE: A risk benefit assessment of moderate to severe pain: the impact of injectable NSAIDs. Drug Safety. In press 1993

108. Boras-Uber LA, Bracket NC: Ketorolac-induced acute renal failure. Am J Med 92:450, 1992

109. Canadian pharmacists briefed on risk of GI bleeding with toradol. Reactions 4, 1993

Chapter 30

Antiemetics

Mark Dershwitz

Postoperative nausea and vomiting remain the most common manifestations of anesthesia-related morbidity and the most common indication for the unanticipated overnight admission of a patient scheduled for ambulatory surgery. Postoperative nausea and vomiting has been described as "the big 'little problem'" in anesthesia today in spite of a number of antiemetic agents available to the anesthesiologist.[1]

This chapter presents the anatomy and physiology of vomiting as it occurs in the perioperative period, followed by a presentation of the five classes of agents used as antiemetics. The use of antiemetics in the perioperative period is then discussed.

Further information on the physiology of nausea and vomiting may be found in the review by Borison and Wang.[2] An exhaustive review of postoperative nausea and vomiting was recently published.[3]

ANATOMY AND PHYSIOLOGY OF VOMITING

Vomiting is a complex and well orchestrated series of actions, and it may be defined as the forceful expulsion of gastric contents through the mouth.[4] It is often, although not always, accompanied by nausea. Nausea is both a physiologic and psychological phenomenon that is difficult to define or describe. It is usually manifested by such symptoms and signs as aversion to food, a desire to vomit, hypersalivation, perspiration, pallor, dizziness, or bradycardia.

A large number of disparate stimuli may lead to vomiting as shown in Figure 30-1. These stimuli cause a stereotypical series of events:[4]

1. The diaphragm descends, and the abdominal muscles contract, causing a rise in intragastric pressure.
2. The gastric pylorus contracts, preventing gastric emptying into the duodenum.
3. The gastric fundus and cardia and the lower esophageal sphincter relax and the gastric contents are forced upward into the esophagus.
4. The hyoid bone and larynx move superiorly and anteriorly, accelerating the upward movement of the vomitus.
5. The soft palate is elevated, thereby preventing the vomitus from entering the nasopharynx.
6. The glottis closes, preventing aspiration of the vomitus into the trachea.
7. After the glottis closes, intrathoracic pressure increases, exerting pressure on the esophagus.
8. The esophagus contracts, or waves of reverse peristalsis rise upward in the esophagus. The esophagus empties, and the vomitus is propelled through the mouth.

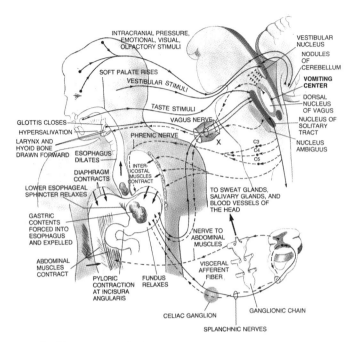

Fig. 30-1 Vomiting is a highly integrated, chiefly somatic, motor act. Visceral motor activity prepares the gastrointestinal tract for the efficient expulsion of vomitus. However, the expulsive force is supplied by skeletal muscles. The diaphragm contracts sharply (descends) accompanied by contraction of the abdominal musculature. The cranial nerves that bring afferent stimuli to act on the vomiting center are also illustrated, as are the efferent neural pathways concerned with the somatic aspects of the vomiting act. (From Clearfield and Roth,[4] with permission.)

The vomiting center is located in the medullary reticular formation and may receive stimuli from the cerebral cortex (e.g., olfactory, visual, or emotional stimuli), the gastrointestinal tract (through the autonomic afferent fibers), the vestibular system, and the chemoreceptor trigger zone (CTZ). These stimuli are integrated by the vomiting center, and when a certain threshold is exceeded, the events listed earlier, which comprise the act of vomiting, begin. There are no compounds that are known to act directly at the vomiting center to cause vomiting or to function as antiemetics.[3]

The CTZ exists outside of the functional blood-brain barrier and is located in the area postrema in the floor of the fourth ventricle. This area is therefore exposed to whatever chemicals are circulating in the blood. The CTZ contains a multitude of receptor types, including those for dopamine, histamine, acetylcholine (muscarinic), serotonin (5-hy-droxytryptamine or 5-HT), and opioids. The presence of these receptors may explain the mechanism of the antiemetic actions of antagonists at the dopamine, histamine, muscarinic, and 5-HT receptors and the emetic effects of opioid analgesics.[3]

Postoperative nausea and vomiting are more common in certain subsets of the population, in persons undergoing certain types of operative procedures, and in persons anesthetized with certain agents or techniques.[3] Postoperative nausea and vomiting occur more frequently in children compared with adults; in women compared with men; in obese patients compared with the lean; in persons who have a history of motion sickness or prior history of postoperative nausea or vomiting; in persons experiencing anxiety in the preoperative period; and in persons with various abnormalities of the gastrointestinal tract, such as hiatus hernia, diabetic gastroparesis, intestinal obstruction, or peritonitis. Some operative procedures are associated with higher incidence rates of postoperative nausea and vomiting, including laparoscopy; strabismus repair; and surgery on the biliary tract, intestines, and inner ear.

With the abandonment of ether and cyclopropane as anesthetic agents, postoperative nausea and vomiting have become less common. There are no convincing data that any of the available inhalational anesthetic gases (i.e., halothane, enflurane, isoflurane, desflurane, and nitrous oxide) has a greater or lesser propensity for causing nausea. The intravenous induction agents etomidate and ketamine are associated with higher incidence rates of postoperative nausea and vomiting; propofol has an unusually low incidence. The inclusion of opioids in the anesthetic regimen also contributes to an increased incidence.

Insufflation of the stomach, as might occur during positive pressure ventilation with a face mask, predisposes patients to postoperative emesis. Paradoxically, emptying the stomach with a nasogastric or orogastric tube intraoperatively does not seem to lower the incidence of postoperative nausea or vomiting. Other factors that may influence the likelihood of postoperative nausea or vomiting include excessive movement (e.g., too early ambulation or less than gentle transport to or from the recovery room) or premature administration of food or drink in the postoperative period.[3]

Postoperative emetic symptoms are more common after general compared with regional anesthesia. However, nausea or vomiting may occur during regional anesthesia, and they may be a result of anesthetic or surgical factors. The hypotension that commonly occurs after the induction of spinal or epidural anesthesia is often accompanied by nausea or vomiting. The mechanism of this effect may be hypoxemia in the medulla because it is less likely to occur in patients breathing supplemental oxygen.[5] Restoration of normotension by the administration of intravenous fluids and/or vasopressors, such as ephedrine or phenylephrine, effectively treats the emetic symptoms. Nausea or vomiting may occur during spinal or epidural anesthesia in the absence of hypotension, probably as a

result of withdrawal of sympathetic tone from the gut; this usually responds to atropine. Nausea or vomiting may also be among the symptoms of local anesthetic toxicity that might occur as a result of overdosage or inadvertent intravenous injection. Intraoperative emetic symptoms are also more common during intra-abdominal surgery and herniorrhaphy compared with surgery on the extremities. Even when the patient is experiencing no pain, certain surgical manipulations (e.g., traction on the spermatic cord, peritoneum, or intestines or exteriorization of the uterus during cesarean section) may result in nausea or vomiting. Such symptoms may be treated effectively with atropine or glycopyrrolate, indicating that these surgical maneuvers may be affecting vagal tone.

In controlled studies comparing propofol by infusion with an inhaled volatile agent for anesthesia maintenance in women undergoing breast biopsy or egg harvest, the patients given propofol experienced less nausea and vomiting, requested less antiemetic therapy, and were less likely to require unscheduled admission to the hospital.[6,7] Maintenance with propofol compared with halothane in children undergoing strabismus repair was also shown to result in a lower incidence of postoperative nausea and vomiting. However, children in the propofol group were more likely to experience episodes of bradycardia as a result of the oculocardiac reflex.[8,9]

Propofol was even shown to be effective as a postoperative antiemetic when administered in subhypnotic doses (10 mg).[10] The lipid emulsion vehicle was postulated to contribute to the antiemetic effect of propofol; however, this was refuted by clinical trials.[10,11]

ANTIEMETIC AGENTS
Dopaminergic Antagonists

Agonists at the dopamine receptor, such as levodopa and bromocriptine, frequently cause nausea, and dopaminergic antagonists are antiemetic. Agents in this group are classified as antipsychotics, and they are also known as neuroleptics or major tranquilizers. There are two chemical subtypes of dopaminergic antagonists that are clinically relevant, that is, phenothiazines and butyrophenones.

Chlorpromazine and prochlorperazine are phenothiazines. They are also antagonists at the α adrenoceptor. Chlorpromazine is also a potent antihistamine and has weak antagonistic activity at the muscarinic receptor. Both of these agents may cause hypotension as a result of α adrenergic blockade, and they should be diluted and administered slowly when given intravenously. Phenothiazines cause profound sedation that may be useful in the management of the agitated or psychotic patient. When administered to normal individuals, phenothiazines may produce dysphoria. The phenothiazines have a high incidence of dose-related extrapyramidal effects, for example, acute dystonia (usually manifested as spasm of the muscles of the head and neck), akathisia (extreme restlessness which is not the result of anxiety), and Parkinson-like rigidity.

Droperidol is a butyrophenone. It is the dopaminergic antagonist with which anesthesiologists have the most experience. It may also be used in combination with opioids in the technique of neuroleptanesthesia (see Ch. 4). Droperidol has weak α adrenoceptor blocking activity and may cause hypotension. Droperidol causes sedation that may be accompanied by dysphoria and may cause extrapyramidal effects.

The dose-response effects and pharmacokinetics of droperidol as an antiemetic are complex. Antiemetic effects may be achieved by doses that cause minimal sedation (i.e., 0.5 to 1.25 mg IM or IV). However, delayed awakening or increased sedation in the recovery room may occur. Despite this, there is no overall prolongation of recovery time when droperidol is used prophylactically because postoperative nausea and vomiting is a frequent cause of delayed discharge from the recovery room.[12–15]

The terminal elimination half-life of droperidol was reported to be 1.7 to 2.1 hours.[16,17] However, droperidol has a prolonged antiemetic effect, perhaps as long as 24 hours.[18] Droperidol is more effective when given before the onset of nausea, and the initial dose that controls or prevents the nausea is followed by a long "tail".

When droperidol is given intraoperatively during certain procedures (e.g., strabismus repair), it is more effective if given at the beginning of the anesthesia compared with just prior to emergence. Its antiemetic effect may be more effective if the drug is given prior to the surgical manipulation that contributes to postoperative nausea and vomiting.[19,20]

Droperidol does not depress ventilation. In a study in normal volunteers in which a large dose of droperidol was given (0.3 mg/kg), there was no change in two measures of ventilatory drive.[21] Droperidol does appear to potentiate the analgesic activity of opioids; patients given droperidol intraoperatively had less postoperative pain and requirements for analgesics.[22,23]

Metoclopramide

Metoclopramide is considered in a class by itself because of its unique pharmacologic properties. Metoclopramide is an antagonist of the dopamine receptor like the neuroleptic drugs. In addition, it has important actions in the gastrointestinal system, which decrease nausea and vomiting. Metoclopramide was described as a gastrointestinal prokinetic drug because it increases the tone of the lower esophageal sphincter, increases gastric emptying, and increases the frequency and amplitude of longitudinal propulsive contractions of gastrointestinal smooth muscle.[24] The mechanism of action in the periphery appears to be blockade of dopaminergic neurons that modulate acetylcholine release; the prokinetic effects of metoclopramide may be antagonized by levodopa or by atropine. Metoclopramide, in contrast to cholinergic agonists, does not increase gastric acid secretion. Metoclopramide produced reproducible hypertensive crises in patients with pheochromocytoma.[25]

The usual doses of metoclopramide used in conjunction with anesthesia (10 to 20 mg) cause mild sedation. However, in contrast to droperidol, there is no increase in the time to awakening or recovery room sedation.[12,15] The large doses of metoclopramide (e.g., 1 mg/kg) used in the antiemetic regimens for patients receiving cancer chemotherapy are associated with a high incidence of extrapyramidal reactions. These do not usually occur with the doses used in anesthesia. Restlessness and hunger were reported after preoperative administration of metoclopramide.[26]

Metoclopramide is commonly used as part of a premedication regimen, either alone or in combination with a histamine H_2 antagonist. In a study of day surgery patients who received cimetidine, metoclopramide, or both prior to coming to the hospital, it was found that cimetidine reliably raised the gastric juice pH but did not decrease its volume; metoclopramide had a complementary effect, decreasing gastric juice volume but having no effect on its pH.[27] Thus, the combination of metoclopramide and a H_2 antagonist is suitable when attempting to minimize the risks of aspiration of gastric contents.

The reported terminal elimination half-life of metoclopramide is about 4 hours.[24] However, its antiemetic effect appears short in comparison with that of droperidol. Thus, in operations longer than 1 to 2 hours, the effectiveness of metoclopramide as an antiemetic may be increased if a second dose is given at the end of the procedure or in the recovery room.

Metoclopramide was shown to be an effective antiemetic in women undergoing dilatation and curettage,[22,28] elective cesarean section under epidural anesthesia,[29] and laparotomy,[30] in men (but not in women) undergoing orthopedic surgery,[31] and in children undergoing strabismus repair.[32] However, there are studies that found metoclopramide to be much less effective than droperidol[22,23,33,34] or indistinguishable from placebo.[12] These conflicting results must be interpreted in terms of the timing of metoclopramide administration. Because the effective duration of the antiemetic effect of metoclopramide is short and antiemetics may be more effective if given prior to certain surgical maneuvers, metoclopramide may need to be given prior to induction of anesthesia and at the end of the anesthetic for optimum efficacy.

Anticholinergics

Scopolamine crosses the blood-brain barrier more readily than does atropine or glycopyrrolate. Despite the fact that the CTZ is considered to be outside the blood-brain barrier, scopolamine is also the more effective antiemetic.

Scopolamine has long been used as a premedication before anesthesia; however, antiemesis was not primary among its desirable effects. Scopolamine causes profound sedation, often accompanied by anterograde amnesia and sometimes delirium. Its antisialagogue activity is superior to that of atropine or glycopyrrolate. In addition, scopolamine causes less tachycardia and ileus and greater mydriatic and cycloplegic effects compared with atropine or glycopyrrolate.[35] The duration of action is short, with an elimination half-life of about 1 hour.[36]

A transdermal preparation of scopolamine is available. The scopolamine patch is formulated to deliver a loading dose of 140 μg followed by 5 μg/h over 72 hours. The patch is indicated for the prophylaxis of motion sickness. It must be applied to the postauricular area at least 4 to 6 hours *prior* to the emetogenic stimulus.[35]

Transdermal scopolamine was found to be effective for preventing postoperative nausea and vomiting in female patients undergoing major[37,38] and minor[39] gynecologic surgery, laparoscopy,[36] and elective cesarean section under epidural anesthesia.[40] Dry mouth is a common side effect.[36,39] In a study of children undergoing ocular surgery, transdermal scopolamine produced a trend toward less vomiting (lacking statistical significance), and 21 percent of the children had to have the patches removed prematurely because of hallucinations or agitation compared to 0 percent in the placebo group.[41]

Care is required when placing the patch to avoid getting any of the medication on the fingers because inadvertent topical application of scopolamine to the eye results in mydriasis and cycloplegia lasting 1 week or more. Transdermal scopolamine is contraindicated in patients with narrow angle glaucoma or urinary obstruction.[35]

Antihistamines

Antagonists of the histamine H_1 receptor have antiemetic properties, especially against motion sickness. The contribution of H_1 receptor antagonism to antiemetic efficacy is difficult to assess because all the histamine H_1 antagonists evaluated for antiemesis also possess significant antagonistic activity at central nervous system cholinergic receptors.

Promethazine, hydroxyzine, and diphenhydramine are the antihistamines most commonly used by anesthesiologists. Promethazine is chemically related to the phenothiazines but is thought to have little antipsychotic or neuroleptic activity. These drugs have their major utility as part of a preoperative medication regimen when both significant sedation and antiemesis are the desired effects. Patients do not perceive the sedative effects of these drugs as unpleasant, in contrast to the sedative effects produced by the neuroleptics. In addition, diphenhydramine is particularly useful in treating the acute extrapyramidal effects caused by neuroleptic drugs, by virtue of its potent anticholinergic activity.

Serotonin Antagonists

Specific antagonists at the $5-HT_3$ receptor have recently been introduced. There are many such agents under development; however, ondansetron is the only $5-HT_3$ antagonist approved for use in postoperative nausea and vomiting in the United States. It was approved for nausea and vomiting related to cancer chemotherapy in 1991 and for postoperative nausea and vomiting in 1993.

Cisplatin chemotherapy is highly emetogenic, and one of its actions appears to be the release of 5-HT from the enterochromaffin cells of the gut.[42] Circulating 5-HT presumably stimulates the CTZ. The efficacy of high dose metoclopramide therapy (1 mg/kg) may be caused in part by its ability to act as a competitive antagonist of the $5-HT_3$ receptor.

At present, the antiemetic mechanism of $5-HT_3$ antagonists is unknown. Anesthetic agents may cause the release of 5-HT from central or peripheral sites, or surgical manipulation of the gastrointestinal tract may cause 5-HT release. However, ondansetron does not appear to be more effective in treating the nausea and vomiting following intra-abdominal procedures; in one study, just the opposite was found, although this observation must be confirmed before any generalizations can be made.[43]

Ondansetron is well absorbed after oral administration, with a bioavailability of approximately 60 percent. The optimum time for ondansetron administration has not yet been determined; oral administration 1 hour prior to surgery[44,45] or intravenous administration at the time of anesthesia induction[43,46,47] were effective prophylactic regimens. In the treatment of postoperative vomiting, its efficacy after intravenous administration was apparent in 10 minutes or less.[48] The elimination half-life of ondansetron in normal volunteers aged 19 to 40 years was 3.5 hours; this value increased to 5.5 hours in subjects 75 years old.[49] When ondansetron was given prophylactically at the time of anesthesia induction, a second dose given 8 hours later provided antiemetic effects for 24 hours.[43,46]

Ondansetron does not cause extrapyramidal effects, sedation, or ventilatory depression, nor does it potentiate opioid-induced ventilatory depression.[50] Its adverse event profile when it is used for the prophylaxis of postoperative nausea and vomiting was indistinguishable from that of placebo.[46,47]

Ondansetron was shown to be effective in the prophylaxis of nausea and vomiting in women undergoing intra-abdominal pelvic surgery,[44–46] extra-abdominal surgery,[43,45] dilatation and curettage,[51] and lithotripsy.[52] It was also effective treatment for nausea and vomiting after arrival in the recovery room following laparoscopy,[53] orthopaedic surgery, or gynecologic surgery.[48] Many questions remain regarding ondansetron's efficacy; in single studies, it was more effective in patients who had undergone extra-abdominal compared with intra-abdominal surgery[43] and was effective against vomiting but not nausea.[51] It has not been adequately studied in men (one study evaluating treatment efficacy enrolled 68 male patients; however, only 5 required antiemetic therapy[48]) or in children. In two studies, ondansetron was shown to be more effective than droperidol[51] or metoclopramide.[51,52] Ondansetron has no efficacy against experimental motion sickness.[54]

The optimal effective dose of ondansetron also remains to be determined. Doses of 8 or 16 mg have similar efficacy when used for prophylaxis or treatment.[45] Three preliminary reports found equivalent efficacy with doses of 4 and 8 mg, but conflicting results using a 1-mg dose were reported.[55–57] A determination of the minimum effective dose of ondansetron will be important because ondansetron is expensive. Presently, a 4-mg dose of ondansetron, the minimum dose recommended by the manufacturer for the management of postoperative nausea and vomiting, is about 30 times the cost of a 1.25-mg dose of droperidol.

ANTIEMETIC THERAPY

The appraisal of clinical studies of antiemetic drugs is complicated by the lack of uniformity of the experimental conditions; a comparison of the efficacies of different agents evaluated in different trials is almost impossible. For example, in some studies of metoclopramide, the drug was given as a single dose prior to anesthesia induction, even though the operations lasted many hours. Most trials compare a treatment with placebo; few compare different treatments with each other. Finally, the efficacy of combinations of agents that act by different mechanisms is uncharted experimental territory.

For certain surgical procedures, such as strabis-

mus repair (and possibly intra-abdominal surgery), antiemetics are more effective if given prior to surgery. For a short-acting drug like metoclopramide, an additional dose at the end of the anesthetic may increase its efficacy.

The routine prophylactic use of antiemetics prior to all general anesthetics is probably not necessary. The overall incidence of postoperative nausea and vomiting requiring pharmacologic intervention is low enough that the potential toxicity of the drug (e.g., droperidol-induced delayed awakening) or the cost of the drug (e.g., ondansetron) preclude indiscriminate prophylactic administration. However, in subsets of patients in whom the incidence of postoperative nausea and vomiting is high (e.g., women undergoing pelvic surgery or children undergoing strabismus repair), there is little argument against prophylactic administration.

Table 30-1 lists the most commonly used antiemetic agents for postoperative nausea and vomiting along with recommended doses and routes of administration. It is difficult to recommend one drug or one regimen over another for the majority of patients.

Table 30-1 Comparison of Commonly Available Antiemetics for Postoperative Nausea and Vomiting

Receptor Antagonist	Drug	Usual Adult Dose	Usual Pediatric Dose
Dopamine	Chlorpromazine	10–25 mg PO, IM, *slow* IV[a]	0.5 mg/kg PO, IM, *slow* IV[a]
		100 mg PR	1 mg/kg PR
	Prochlorperazine	5–10 mg PO, IM, *slow* IV[a]	0.15 mg/kg IM, *slow* IV[a]
		25 mg PR	2.5–5 mg PR
	Droperidol	0.5–1.25 mg IM, IV	25–75 μg/kg IM, IV
	Metoclopramide	10–20 mg PO, IM, IV	0.1–0.2 mg/kg IM, IV
Muscarinic cholinergic	Scopolamine	1 patch for 72 h	*Not recommended*
Histamine H_1	Diphenhydramine	25–50 mg PO, IM, IV	0.5–1.0 mg/kg PO, IM, IV
	Hydroxyzine	25–50 mg PO, IM	0.75–1.5 mg/kg PO, IM
	Promethazine	25–50 mg PO, IM, *slow* IV, PR	0.75–1.5 mg/kg PO, IM, *slow* IV, PR
$5\text{-}HT_3$	Ondansetron	4 mg IV; 8 mg PO	*Unknown*[b]

[a] May cause severe hypotension when injected intravenously.

[b] Has not been studied in children for postoperative nausea and vomiting.

If a patient has severe nausea and vomiting unrelieved by a particular agent, it is reasonable to administer another antiemetic drug that acts through a different receptor mechanism. As stated previously, data are lacking on the efficacy of combinations of antiemetic drugs; however, there is little risk (other than perhaps additional sedation) because there is no substantial overlap in their adverse effects.

REFERENCES

1. Kapur PA: Editorial: the big "little problem." Anesth Analg 73:243, 1991
2. Borison HL, Wang SC: Physiology and pharmacology of vomiting. Pharmacol Rev 5:193, 1953
3. Watcha MF, White PF: Postoperative nausea and vomiting. Anesthesiology 77:162, 1992
4. Clearfield HR, Roth JLA: Anorexia, nausea, and vomiting. p. 48. In Berk JE (ed): Gastroenterology. 4th Ed. WB Saunders, Philadelphia, 1985
5. Ratra CK, Badola RP, Bhargava KP: A study of factors concerned in emesis during spinal anesthesia. Br J Anaesth 44:1208, 1972
6. Sung YF, Reiss N, Tillette T: The differential cost of anesthesia and recovery with propofol-nitrous oxide anesthesia versus thiopental sodium-isoflurane-nitrous oxide anesthesia. J Clin Anesth 3:391, 1991
7. Raftery S, Sherry E: Total intravenous anesthesia with propofol and alfentanil protect against postoperative nausea and vomiting. Can J Anaesth 39:37, 1992
8. Watcha MF, Simeon RM, White PF, Stevens JL: Effect of propofol on the incidence of postoperative vomiting after strabismus surgery in pediatric outpatients. Anesthesiology 75:204, 1991
9. Larsson S, Asgeirsson B, Magnusson J: Propofol-fentanyl anesthesia compared to thiopental-halothane with special reference to recovery and vomiting after pediatric strabismus surgery. Acta Anaesthesiol Scand 36:182, 1992
10. Borgeat A, Wilder-Smith OH, Saiah M, Rifat K: Subhypnotic doses of propofol possess direct antiemetic properties. Anesth Analg 74:539, 1992
11. Ostman PL, Faure E, Glosten B et al: Is the antiemetic effect of the emulsion formulation of propofol due to the lipid emulsion? Anesth Analg 71:536, 1990
12. Cohen SE, Woods WA, Wyner J: Antiemetic efficacy of droperidol and metoclopramide. Anesthesiology 60:67, 1984
13. Tigerstedt I, Salmela L, Aromaa U: Double-blind comparison of transdermal scopolamine, droperidol and placebo against postoperative nausea and vomiting. Acta Anaesthesiol Scand 32:454, 1988
14. O'Donovan N, Shaw J: Nausea and vomiting in day-case dental anaesthesia. The use of low-dose droperidol. Anaesthesia 39:1172, 1984
15. Korttila K, Kauste A, Auvinen J: Comparison of domperidone, droperidol, and metoclopramide in the prevention and treatment of nausea and vomiting after balanced general anesthesia. Anesth Analg 58:396, 1979
16. Fischler M, Bonnet F, Trang H et al: The pharmacokinetics of droperidol in anesthetized patients. Anesthesiology 64:486, 1986
17. Lehmann KA, Van Peer A, Ikonomakis M et al: Pharmacokinetics of droperidol in surgical patients under different conditions of anaesthesia. Br J Anaesth 61:297, 1988
18. Loeser EA, Bennett G, Stanley TH, Machin R: Comparison of droperidol, haloperidol and prochlorperazine as postoperative anti-emetics. Can J Anaesth 26:125, 1979
19. Nicolson SC, Kaya KM, Betts EK: The effect of preoperative oral droperidol on the incidence of postoperative emesis after paediatric strabismus surgery. Can J Anaesth 35:364, 1988
20. Lerman J, Eustis S, Smith DR: Effect of droperidol pretreatment on postanesthetic vomiting in children undergoing strabismus surgery. Anesthesiology 65:322, 1986
21. Prokocimer P, Delavault E, Rey F et al: Effects of droperidol on respiratory drive in humans. Anesthesiology 59:113, 1983
22. Madej TH, Simpson KH: Comparison of the use of domperidone, droperidol and metoclopramide in the prevention of nausea and vomiting following gynaecological surgery in day cases. Br J Anaesth 58:879, 1986
23. Madej TH, Simpson KH: Comparison of the use of domperidone, droperidol and metoclopramide in the prevention of nausea and vomiting following major gynaecological surgery. Br J Anaesth 58:884, 1986
24. Albibi R, McCallum RW: Metoclopramide: pharmacology and clinical application. Ann Intern Med 98:86, 1983
25. Agabiti-Rosie E, Alicandri CL, Corea L: Hypertensive crisis in patients with phaeochromocytoma given metoclopramide. Lancet 1:600, 1977

26. Dundee JW, Clarke RSJ, Howard PJ: Studies of drugs given before anaesthesia. XXIII: Metoclopramide. Br J Anaesth 46:509, 1974

27. Rao TLK, Suseela M, El-Etr AA: Metoclopramide and cimetidine to reduce gastric juice pH volume. Anesth Analg 63:264, 1984

28. Clark MM, Storrs JA: The prevention of postoperative vomiting after abortion: metoclopramide. Br J Anaesth 41:890, 1969

29. Chestnut DH, Vandewalker GE, Owen CL et al: Administration of metoclopramide for prevention of nausea and vomiting during epidural anesthesia for elective cesarean section. Anesthesiology 66:563, 1987

30. Lind B, Breivik H: Metoclopramide and perphenazine in the prevention of postoperative nausea and vomiting. Br J Anaesth 42:614, 1970

31. Diamond MJ, Keeri-Szanto M: Reduction of postoperative vomiting by preoperative administration of oral metoclopramide. Can J Anaesth 27:36, 1980

32. Broadman LM, Ceruzzi W, Patane PS et al: Metoclopramide reduces the incidence of vomiting following strabismus surgery in children. Anesthesiology 72:245, 1990

33. DeSilva PHDP, McDonald SM, Darvish AH et al: Evaluation of droperidol, perphenazine and metoclopramide for the prophylaxis of emetic symptoms after major gynecological surgery. Anesthesiology 75:A35, 1991

34. Kauste A, Tuominen M, Heikkinen H et al: Droperidol, alizapride and metoclopramide in the prevention and treatment of post-operative emetic sequelae. Eur J Anaesthesiol 3:1, 1986

35. Clissold SP, Heel RC: Transdermal hyoscine (scopolamine). A preliminary review of its pharmacodynamic properties and therapeutic efficacy. Drugs 29:189, 1985

36. Bailey PL, Streisand JB, Pace NL et al: Transdermal scopolamine reduces nausea and vomiting after outpatient laparoscopy. Anesthesiology 72:977, 1990

37. Loper KA, Ready LB, Dorman BH: Prophylactic transdermal scopolamine patches reduce nausea in postoperative patients receiving epidural morphine. Anesth Analg 68:144, 1989

38. Uppington J, Dunnet J, Blogg CE: Transdermal hyoscine and postoperative nausea and vomiting. Anaesthesia 41:16, 1986

39. Tolksdorf W, Meisel R, Müller P, Bender HJ: Transdermales scopolamin (TTS-scopolamin) zur prophylaxe postoperativer übelkeit und erbrechen. Anaesthesist 34:656, 1985

40. Kotelko DM, Rottman RL, Wright WC et al: Transdermal scopolamine decreases nausea and vomiting following cesarean section in patients receiving epidural morphine. Anesthesiology 71:675, 1989

41. Gibbons PA, Nicolson SC, Betts EK et al: Scopolamine does not prevent post-operative emesis after pediatric eye surgery. Anesthesiology 61:A435, 1984

42. Cubeddu LX, Hoffmann IS, Fuenmayor NT, Finn AL: Efficacy of ondansetron (GR38032F) and the role of serotonin in cisplatin-induced nausea and vomiting. N Engl J Med 322:810, 1990

43. Dershwitz M, Rosow CE, Di Biase PM et al: Ondansetron is effective in decreasing postoperative nausea and vomiting. Clin Pharmacol Ther 52:96, 1992

44. Leeser J, Lip H: Prevention of postoperative nausea and vomiting using ondansetron, a new, selective 5-HT$_3$ receptor antagonist. Anesth Analg 72:751, 1991

45. Kenny GNC, Oates JDL, Leeser J et al: Efficacy of orally administered ondansetron in the prevention of postoperative nausea and vomiting: a dose ranging study. Br J Anaesth 68:466, 1992

46. McKenzie R, Sharifi-Azad S, Dershwitz M et al: A randomized, double-blind pilot study examining the use of intravenous ondansetron in the prevention of postoperative nausea and vomiting in female inpatients. J Clin Anesth 5:30, 1993

47. Sung YF, Wetchler BV, Duncalf D, Joslyn AF: A double-blind, placebo controlled pilot study examining the effectiveness of intravenous ondansetron in the prevention of postoperative nausea and emesis. J Clin Anesth 5:22, 1993

48. Larijani GE, Gratz I, Afshar M, Minassian S: Treatment of postoperative nausea and vomiting with ondansetron: a randomized, double-blind comparison with placebo. Anesth Analg 73:246, 1991

49. Cerenex Pharmaceuticals: Zofran (ondansetron hydrochloride) injection product information. Cerenex Pharmaceuticals, Research Triangle Park, NC, 1994

50. Dershwitz M, Di Biase PM, Rosow CE et al: Ondansetron does not affect alfentanil-induced ventilatory depression or sedation. Anesthesiology 77:447, 1992

51. Alon E, Himmelseher S: Ondansetron in the treatment of postoperative vomiting: a randomized, double-blind comparison with droperidol and metoclopramide. Anesth Analg 75:561, 1992

52. Monk TG, White PF, Lemon D: Ondansetron reduces nausea following outpatient lithotripsy. Anesthesiology 77:A19, 1992

53. Bodner M, White PF: Antiemetic efficacy of ondansetron after outpatient laparoscopy. Anesth Analg 73:250, 1991

54. Stott JRR, Barnes GR, Wright RJ, Ruddock CJS: The

effect on motion sickness and oculomotor function of GR 38032F, a 5-HT$_3$-receptor antagonist with anti-emetic properties. Br J Clin Pharmacol 27:147, 1989

55. Hantler C, Baughman V, Shahvari M et al: Ondanse-tron treats nausea and vomiting following surgery. Anesthesiology 77:A16, 1992

56. Khalil S, Kallar S, Zahl K et al: Ondansetron prevents postoperative nausea and vomiting in outpatient fe-males. Anesthesiology 77:A18, 1992

57. Shahvari M, Epstein BS, Weintraub HD et al: Treat-ment of postoperative nausea and vomiting with I.V. ondansetron in outpatient surgery. Anesthesiology 77:A46, 1992

Chapter 31

Novel Drug Delivery

James B. Streisand and Jie Zhang

Optimal drug therapy includes the absorption and transport of drugs to specific receptor sites in the body, the maintenance of concentrations at these sites for as long as appropriate, and the rapid elimination of the drug when the effect is no longer desired. Time contingent oral or parenteral drug administration is often ineffective in achieving these goals. Oral administration of certain drugs is impossible if they are broken down in the acid milieu of the stomach, by gastrointestinal enzymes, or undergo significant first-pass hepatic metabolism. Bolus injections of drugs may be painful, require trained medical personnel, and create peaks and valleys in plasma drug concentrations that might be undesirable when a prolonged consistent effect is sought.

Recent advances in biopharmaceutical technology have produced sophisticated delivery systems that permit precise control of drug input into the body by unorthodox routes of administration. Greater knowledge of the physiology of the skin and mucous membranes has led to the development of new drug formulations that permit systemic drug delivery by these routes. This chapter examines some of these new systems and drug formulations as they relate to anesthetics and anesthetic adjuvants.

TRANSDERMAL DRUG ADMINISTRATION

The skin has been recognized as a site for drug administration for centuries. Early transdermal drug delivery involved creams and ointments applied primarily for their local effect. The dose absorbed was variable and not easy to reproduce. Thus, until recently, the skin had been overlooked as a site for systemic drug delivery. Rapid advances in biopharmaceutical technology have given rise to the development of several transdermal drug delivery systems. These systems are designed to deliver the active constituent into the systemic circulation through the skin at a sustained, predictable rate. The drugs in transdermal systems currently available in the United States include nitroglycerin, scopolamine, estrogen, clonidine, fentanyl, and nicotine.

Development of transdermal systems has escalated because transdermal drug delivery is convenient, noninvasive, and painless, therefore it has the potential to improve patient compliance. Adverse effects associated with fluctuations in serum concentration (typical of most time contingent, pulsed methods of drug administration) are minimized because transdermal delivery leads to sustained serum drug concentrations. Transdermal delivery circumvents gastrointestinal absorption and hepatic first pass metabolism and, therefore, provides greater bioavailability. It is an alternative route of drug administration for patients not able to swallow.

Physiology of Transdermal Drug Delivery

The skin is the largest organ of the body (by surface area), weighing approximately 2 kg in a 70-kg man. The stratum corneum, the thick, avascular, lipophilic, keratinized outermost layer of the skin serves as a barrier to the intrusion of most toxins, chemicals, and microorganisms.[1] Thus, most drugs do not penetrate the skin and are not suitable for transdermal drug delivery. Moving inward from the stratum corneum, the epidermis and dermis have a more aqueous structure that is the site of uptake into the systemic circulation for drugs that permeate the skin. Transdermal permeability requires that drug molecules have biphasic solubility; lipid solubility to pass through the stratum corneum and aqueous solubility to move through the dermis.[2] Other properties of a drug essential for transdermal delivery include high potency (a drug must be potent enough to allow a therapeutic dose to pass through a small convenient area of skin), a low molecular weight (favors increased permeability), and insignificant cutaneous metabolism. Finally, the skin itself must be able to tolerate long-term contact with the drug delivery system.

Under basal conditions, approximately 10 percent of the cardiac output passes through the skin.[3] Under thermal stress, skin blood flow can increase as much as 10-fold. Yet cutaneous vasoconstriction from cold stress can virtually abolish skin blood flow. In addition, the transdermal permeability of a drug may vary over different areas of the body. For example, the postauricular area is approximately 10 times more permeable to scopolamine than is the skin on the thigh.[4] Therefore, to maintain a constant rate of absorption, the design of transdermal drug delivery systems must allow for great variability in skin blood flow and the variability in permeability of different skin sites. This has been accomplished by the addition of a rate-controlling membrane to the transdermal delivery apparatus. The rate-controlling membrane limits the release rate of drug to a fraction of the maximum rate of absorption of the skin. Thus, the transdermal system, not the skin, dominates in controlling the rate of drug input to the skin surface and, therefore, to the systemic circulation.

Transdermal Fentanyl

The transdermal therapeutic system for fentanyl received regulatory approval in the United States in 1990. This system is a transparent rectangular unit composed of four layers.[5] The outermost layer, made of a polyester film, provides an impermeable backing that prevents the loss of drug from the system or the entry of foreign substances into the drug reservoir. The drug reservoir contains fentanyl, 2.5 mg/10 cm^2 in a patch, and alcohol, 0.1 ml/10 cm^2, gelled with hydroxyethyl cellulose. Alcohol is added to enhance the absorption of fentanyl. The microporous rate-controlling membrane is composed of an ethylene-vinyl acetate copolymer. The fourth layer, a silicone skin adhesive, also contains fentanyl. This allows the skin directly under the patch to absorb fentanyl rapidly just after the patch is placed. There are four sizes of fentanyl patches available. The rate of fentanyl delivered from each patch is directly proportional to the size of the patch (Table 31-1). The doses are additive. Indeed, some opioid tolerant patients may require more than one patch at a time (fentanyl dose greater than 100 μg/h).

Table 31-1 Transdermal Therapeutic System for Fentanyl: Size, Delivery Rate, and Plasma Concentrations Achieved

Fentanyl Size (cm^2)	Content (mg)	Dose		Plasma Concentration Range (ng/ml)
		(μg/h)	(mg/24 h)	
10	2.5	25	0.6	0.3–0.6
20	5	50	1.2	0.5–2
30	7.5	75	1.8	0.8–3
40	10	100	2.4	1–4

(Data from Lehmann and Zech.[137])

Pharmacokinetics

Because substantial variations exist in the pharmacokinetics of intravenous fentanyl,[6,7] it is not surprising that the same is true for the pharmacokinetics of transdermal fentanyl. Nevertheless, the goal of fentanyl transdermal delivery, to mimic a constant rate intravenous infusion and provide a constant plasma concentration of fentanyl over a 24- to 72-hour period, was confirmed by several investigators.[8–10]

Varvel et al.[10] determined the absorption characteristics of transdermal fentanyl (100 μg/h) by obtaining serum fentanyl concentrations after transdermal and intravenous administration in the same subject on different occasions and using deconvolution to extract the absorption profile (Fig. 31-1). When the system is first applied, fentanyl rapidly partitions from the drug-saturated adhesive layer of the patch into the skin. Nevertheless, absorption of fentanyl into the systemic circulation is slow during the first 4 hours after patch application (Fig. 31-1). Serum concentrations reach steady state by 12 to 14 hours. These concentrations are then maintained for the life of the patch. After the patch is removed, concentrations decrease slowly, and fentanyl is still detectable in the circulation after 36 hours. The terminal elimination half-life of transdermal fentanyl is approximately 17 hours, two to three times that reported for intravenous fentanyl.

Continuing absorption from a depot of fentanyl in the stratum corneum accounts for the prolonged half-life found after patch removal. The bioavailability of transdermally administered fentanyl is 92 percent (compared with intravenous administration).

These pharmacokinetic data for transdermal fentanyl delivery were derived primarily from healthy surgical patients. Patients with hepatic, renal, cardiac, or other systemic impairment of physiologic function have not been studied. The clearance of fentanyl is markedly reduced in patients with cancer.[11] Thus, in this patient population, the kinetic profile of transdermal fentanyl would be expected to show a longer terminal elimination half-life.

Because of the long terminal half-life, the system does not reliably reach a steady state by 24 hours. Also, peak serum concentrations of fentanyl are greater when the patch is replaced every 24 hours for 3 days compared with a patch that is worn for 72 hours. Therefore, the manufacturer recommends that the patch should not be changed more frequently than once every 3 days.[5]

Acute Postoperative Pain

The analgesic effectiveness of transdermal fentanyl for acute pain was first investigated in postoperative pain studies. Approximately 350 patients have

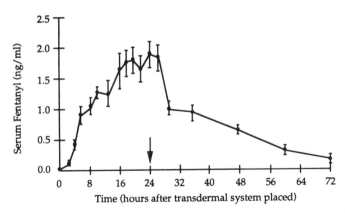

Fig. 31-1 Fentanyl plasma concentrations (mean ± standard error of the mean) following the placement of a 100-μg/h transdermal drug delivery system. The patch was removed at 24 hours shown by the arrow. (From Varvel et al.,[10] with permission.)

been studied in a variety of open label and double blind placebo controlled studies.[9,12–17] Transdermal fentanyl doses ranging from 25 to 100 μg/h were used. Pain control was usually assessed by a visual analog scale and by sparing of other parenteral opioids provided for "breakthrough pain" (available to subjects by intramuscular or intravenous intermittent dosing or by a patient-controlled analgesia pump).

Caplan et al.,[16] Rowbotham et al.,[12] McLesky[15] and others[18] found that patients receiving transdermal fentanyl had lower pain scores than did placebo groups. Patients who received transdermal fentanyl expressed a significantly higher overall satisfaction rating of their pain control.[16] Rowbotham et al.[12] noted an improvement in the peak expiratory flow rate in patients receiving transdermal fentanyl, presumably from their improved analgesia. The need for supplementary analgesics was greatest in the early postoperative period, reflecting the long lag time to attain effective plasma concentrations (12 to 24 hours).

The incidence of nausea and vomiting, the principal adverse effect observed with transdermal fentanyl, ranged from 30 to 70 percent, but this incidence was not different from patients wearing placebo patches.[12,15,16]

Hypoventilation, defined by a respiratory rate less than 8 breaths/min or a $PaCO_2$ more than 55 mmHg was the most serious adverse effect observed. Six of the 177 patients (3.4 percent) receiving 75 μg/h and 7 of the 105 patients (6.6 percent) receiving 100 μg/h experienced one or more episodes of hypoventilation.[17] Although there were no serious adverse outcomes in these patients, because they were closely monitored and treated rapidly with either naloxone or verbal prompting to breathe, the high incidence of respiratory side effects was worrisome to the manufacturer and the Food and Drug Administration (FDA) of the United States. As a result, transdermal fentanyl is not recommended or approved in the United States for use in acute postoperative pain.[5,17] Plasma concentrations rise and fall too slowly to meet the rapidly changing states of acute postoperative pain. The patches should only be changed every 72 hours, and thus, this system is not easily

titrated for acute pain. Finally, there is a significant risk of hypoventilation in unmonitored patients.

Cancer Pain Management

Most patients with long-standing pain from cancer ultimately receive potent opioid analgesics. Unlike acute postoperative pain, most cancer pain is constant, or nearly constant, and goes on for extended lengths of time. Therefore, an effective analgesic regimen for cancer pain aims at maintaining consistent concentrations of opioids in the blood. Continuous intravenous and subcutaneous infusions of opioids provide consistency, but their use requires equipment and experienced health care workers to supervise administration. Transdermal fentanyl, on the other hand, is simple to administer, is noninvasive, provides consistent serum concentrations, and therefore, is ideally suited for cancer pain management.

Miser et al.[11] were the first to report their findings from five patients with cancer pain treated with transdermal fentanyl. These patients were chosen because oral administration of opioids was either ineffective or not possible. The transdermal dose was selected by matching the microgram per hour dose of an intravenous infusion of fentanyl that had been titrated to obtain satisfactory pain control. All five patients reported good to excellent pain control, using doses of transdermal fentanyl that ranged from 75 to 300 μg/h for as long as 156 days. The delay in achieving steady state plasma concentrations led to minor overdosing in two patients. The prolonged effect of fentanyl after the system was removed became a significant clinical problem when new medical complications arose such that cessation of the opioid effect was desirable.

One hundred fifty-seven patients with cancer pain have received transdermal fentanyl in a variety of clinical studies.[11,13,17,19–21] The findings from these studies reinforce the concept that cancer pain is a dynamic process. Thus, the effects of a single intervention are difficult to analyze. Nevertheless, most of the patients who received transdermal fentanyl preferred this treatment to other choices because of satisfactory pain relief with a convenient, easy to use system.

Because of the problems that occur in opioid-naive patients (difficulty with titration or respiratory depression), transdermal fentanyl should not be used as a first line analgesic.[5,22] After the patient has achieved adequate pain relief from conventional oral or parenteral opioids, the initial dose selection of transdermal fentanyl can be determined using the morphine equivalence chart found in the package insert and in Table 31-2.[5] The conversion ratio is conservative; thus, 50 percent of patients are likely to require an increase in dose after the initial application. Upward titration of the dose of transdermal fentanyl should occur no more frequently than every 3 days after the initial dose or every 6 days thereafter because it may take that long to achieve equilibrium following a new dose. The majority of patients who use transdermal fentanyl will require "rescue" dosing of rapid acting, short duration oral or transmucosal opioids for the treatment of breakthrough pain, which may occur with routine daily activity. Although dermatologic reactions from transdermal fentanyl are mild and likely caused by skin occlusion rather than contact dermatitis, it is advisable to rotate the sites of patch applications to minimize

Table 31-2 Transdermal Fentanyl Dose Prescription Based on Daily Morphine Equivalence Dose

Oral 24-h Morphine (mg/day)	Intramuscular 24-h Morphine (mg/day)	Transdermal Fentanyl Dose (μg/h)
45–134	8–22	25
135–224	23–37	50
225–314	38–52	75
315–404	53–67	100
405–494	68–82	125
495–584	83–97	150
585–674	98–112	175
675–764	113–127	200
765–854	128–142	225
855–944	143–157	250
945–1,034	158–172	275
1,035–1,124	173–187	300

(From Janssen Pharmaceutica,[5] with permission.)

Table 31-3 Transdermal Fentanyl: Guidelines for Clinical Use

Apply standard guidelines for chronic opioid use
Stable pain baseline
Minimal incident pain
Provide rescue analgesic
Liberal use of rescue analgesics in first 48 h
Use average daily dose of rescue analgesics to calculate dose increment
Rotate skin sites
Clarify patient and family expectations
Allow several weeks for therapeutic trial

(From Payne,[23] with permission.)

local irritation. Table 31-3 summarizes the guidelines for the clinical use of transdermal fentanyl in cancer pain.[23]

Transdermal Scopolamine

Transdermal scopolamine was the first transdermal system to gain regulatory approval in the United States. Although originally developed for the prophylaxis of motion sickness, interest in the use of transdermal scopolamine for the prophylaxis of postoperative nausea and vomiting has emerged.

Transdermal scopolamine is a 2.5-cm^2 round, flat disc that is 0.2 mm thick and consists of four layers as follows: (1) an impermeable backing membrane (composed of an aluminized polyester film) to prevent the drug from escaping from the reservoir and water from entering the system; (2) a drug reservoir containing scopolamine (1.5 mg), mineral oil, and polyisobutylene; (3) a microporous polypropylene membrane that controls the rate of delivery of scopolamine to the skin; and (4) a skin adhesive that contains a priming dose of scopolamine, 0.2 mg.[24]

Pharmacokinetic Considerations

Oral and parenteral scopolamine often produce drowsiness, confusion, and blurred vision in association with peak blood levels. Yet the antiemetic effects are short-lived because drug levels fall to subtherapeutic levels within 6 hours. In contrast, transdermal scopolamine is designed to maintain a constant therapeutic serum concentration of scopolamine below the threshold for major side effects by delivering 0.5 mg of scopolamine over a 3-day period (140 μg initially then 5 μg/h).[24] However, it has never been demonstrated that this aim has been achieved. Furthermore, Schmitt et al.[25] found that scopolamine levels were significantly higher 12 to 24 hours after disc application compared with other times during a 72-hour study period. In addition, Graybiel et al.[4] and Pyykkö et al.[26] reported four- and sixfold variations in urinary scopolamine excretion rates 12 and 24 hours after the application of transdermal scopolamine.

Because effective drug concentrations are achieved slowly, 6 to 8 hours after administration, it is recommended that the disc be applied at least 4 hours before the desired antiemetic effect is desired (e.g., the night before surgery). Patients are instructed to place the disc behind the ear because the permeability of the postauricular skin to scopolamine is 10-fold higher than the skin of the thigh.[27] Like transdermal fentanyl, drug concentrations decline slowly after disc removal, reflecting the continued absorption from a scopolamine depot in the stratum corneum.

Clinical Experience

Price et al.[28] and others[29] demonstrated the prevention of motion-induced nausea at sea in the majority of patients wearing transdermal scopolamine patches. The efficacy of this drug for the prophylaxis of nausea and vomiting after general anesthesia is variable. Tigerstedt et al.[18] reported no antiemetic benefit from transdermal scopolamine in 96 female patients undergoing ambulatory surgery with the disc placed on the morning of surgery. However, earlier placement of the disc might have improved the effectiveness. Likewise, Koski et al.[30] did not detect any antiemetic value from transdermal scopolamine in a large placebo controlled trial. Many other investigators detected antiemetic efficacy with preoperative placement of transdermal scopolamine. Bailey et al.[31] studied 191 female patients undergoing outpatient laparoscopy surgery. Scopolamine treated patients had less severe nausea, required less rescue antiemetic, and were discharged from the hospital sooner than were the

patients wearing the placebo disc. Uppington et al.[32] also found that transdermal scopolamine reduced the incidence of postoperative nausea and vomiting in major gynecologic surgery.

The treatment of acute postoperative pain with epidural or parenteral opioids is often associated with nausea and vomiting. Prophylactic transdermal scopolamine decreased nausea and vomiting in patients receiving epidural[33] or patient-controlled intravenous morphine[34] following major gynecologic surgery and in patients receiving epidural morphine after cesarean section.[35]

Transdermal scopolamine commonly produces drowsiness, amblyopia, and dry mouth.[31,35] Infrequent adverse reactions include toxic psychosis, confusion, and hallucinations, especially in children and elderly patients.[36,37] Thus, the likelihood of the patient developing nausea and vomiting must be weighed against the potential side effects when considering prophylactic transdermal scopolamine administration.

IONTOPHORESIS

Because of the limitations in passive transdermal drug delivery, physical and chemical methods of enhancing transdermal drug delivery are being developed. Iontophoresis is the introduction of ions of soluble salts into the skin or mucosal surfaces by means of an electric current. Although interest in this technique for drug delivery has waxed and waned during the past 50 years, technologic advances have expanded the capabilities of this simple technique. Numerous applications of iontophoresis have been reported for disorders of the skin, muscles, joints, ears, nose, eyes and teeth.[38–44] Ashburn et al.[45] recently reported the systemic delivery of morphine by iontophoresis.

An iontophoresis system consists of a power source, a delivery electrode, and a current return electrode (Fig. 31-2). When used on the skin, the delivery electrode contains an enclosed receptacle for the drug. For iontophoresis in small or enclosed areas, such as the tympanic membrane[39] or tip of the nose,[46] the delivery electrode is brought in contact with a pledget or gauze saturated with the drug solution at the desired site. The current return electrode is placed on any convenient site, usually

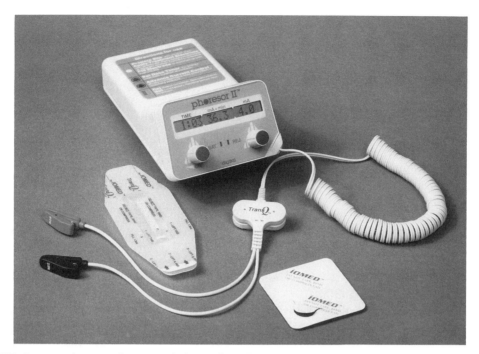

Fig. 31-2 Iontophoresis device and electrodes. There are variable controls for the milliamperage and time of therapy.

the skin near the delivery electrode. With activation of the current, electrons flow through the skin or mucosa beneath the electrode, through interstitial fluids, and back through the skin to the other electrode. An appropriately charged molecule will migrate along the same path. Positively charged drugs inserted into the reservoir at the anode are repelled toward the negative electrode. Conversely, negatively charged drugs placed at the cathode are repelled toward the positive electrode.

Dexamethasone

Iontophoresis of dexamethasone sodium phosphate for the treatment of acute and chronic musculoskeletal inflammatory conditions was reported in both experimental animals and humans. By using a current of 5 mA for 20 minutes, significant quantities of radiolabeled dexamethasone were delivered into all joint layers (skin, muscle, synovium, joint capsule, and cartilage) of rhesus monkeys.[47] Harris[41] reported improvement (89 percent of pa-

tients treated) in pain scores, swelling, and range of motion after iontophoresis of dexamethasone to a localized joint inflammation (lateral epicondylitis of the elbow, subacromial bursitis of the shoulder, or patellar tendonitis). Most patients required three treatments over a 1-week period with improvement of symptoms occurring 24 to 48 hours after a treatment. Hasson et al.[48] found that dexamethasone administered by iontophoretic treatment to an inflamed knee joint in a patient with rheumatoid arthritis improved muscle strength and joint range of motion and decreased joint swelling.

Although documentation of dexamethasone iontophoresis for the treatment of acute localized inflammatory disease is limited, this technique has several potential advantages over the injection of steroids into inflamed joints; the treatment is nontraumatic and painless and tissue damage as a result of needle penetration and subcutaneous injection of fluid is avoided. With the development of modern iontophoretic equipment, improved electrode systems, and commercially available ionized drugs, this technique may gain wider acceptance.[49]

Lidocaine

Injections of local anesthetics into the skin often cause distortion of surface anatomy, making superficial surgical procedures more difficult. Bezzant et al.[38] achieved painless cauterization of multiple spider veins after iontophoresis of the effected site with 4 percent lidocaine plus epinephrine 1:50,000. Epinephrine added to the iontophoretic solution increased the duration of anesthesia and enhanced the delineation of the abnormal vessels compared with iontophoresis of lidocaine alone. Local anesthesia by iontophoretically administered 4 percent lidocaine enabled pulsed dye laser treatment of port-wine stains with minimal discomfort.[50] Thus, this technique may allow children to undergo laser treatment without a general anesthetic. Sisler,[43] citing the difficulties in injecting local anesthetics into the blepharoconjunctiva, described successful lidocaine inotophoresis before conjunctival surgery. Finally, topical anesthesia of the oral mucosa with iontophoretically administered lidocaine decreased the pain and anxiety of dental procedures in children.[40]

Morphine

The two previous examples of iontophoretic drug delivery have shown how this technology may be used for local drug administration. Because new technologies in iontophoresis equipment and electrodes permit longer safe iontophoresis times, it is now possible to use iontophoresis for systemic drug administration. Morphine hydrochloride is a highly ionized molecule suitable for delivery through the skin by iontophoresis.

Initial trials in human volunteers established that analgesic morphine plasma concentrations were attained after only 20 minutes of iontophoretic treatment.[51] The plasma concentrations were proportional to the iontophoretic current. Subsequently, Ashburn et al.[45] reported the use of morphine iontophoresis for acute postoperative pain in 38 patients undergoing total hip or knee arthroplasty. Iontophoresis machines were attached on the morning of the first postoperative day, and the current was turned on for 6 hours. Patients received either morphine HCl or Ringer's lactate (placebo) in the chamber at the positive electrode. Meperidine by patient-controlled analgesia was available to all patients for pain not controlled by iontophoresis. Significant plasma concentrations of morphine were attained and patient-controlled analgesic meperidine requirements were decreased in the morphine group compared with placebo (Fig. 31-3). Other than a "wheal and flare" circular pattern under the positive electrode (only observed in patients receiving morphine), no significant adverse effects were reported.

Although these initial reports demonstrate that systemic administration of morphine by iontophoresis is feasible, many questions remain about the utility of this system for acute pain management. The main advantages of morphine iontophoresis over passive transdermal drug delivery (e.g., transdermal fentanyl) are the ability to change the dose of morphine rapidly that is delivered by adjusting the iontophoretic current and immediate discontinuation of drug delivery with removal of the delivery current (no "depot" effect as seen with transdermal fentanyl). Whether iontophoretic drug delivery can be adapted for patient-controlled analgesia remains to be seen. The safety of prolonged (greater than 6 hours) iontophoresis times is unknown. Finally, the iontophoresis of other more potent opioids needs to be investigated.

ORAL TRANSMUCOSAL DRUG ADMINISTRATION

For more than a century, nitroglycerin has been delivered by oral transmucosal absorption.[52] More recently, a number of drugs were found to penetrate the oral mucosa with sufficient speed to permit therapeutic plasma levels to be achieved. These drugs include β-adrenergic blockers,[53,54] β-adrenergic agonists,[55] and a variety of opioids.[56–71] Insulin, a peptide with a molecular weight of 6,000, was also systemically absorbed from the oral mucosa with the help of permeation enhancing agents (agents that increase the permeability of the oral mucosa).[72–75]

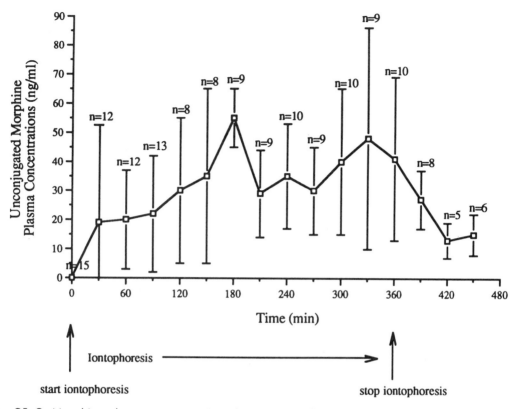

Fig. 31-3 Morphine plasma concentrations (mean ± standard deviation) detected in 17 postoperative patients during and after 6 hours of morphine iontophoresis. (From Ashburn et al.,[45] with permission.)

In oral transmucosal drug absorption, the drug in solid dosage form, such as a tablet or a lozenge, is allowed to dissolve into saliva under the tongue (sublingual) or in the cheek (buccal). Driven by the concentration gradient, the drug molecules in the saliva penetrate the oral mucosa to reach the submucosal interstitial fluid and capillary blood vessels. From this site, they are carried into the systemic circulation.

The advantages of an oral transmucosal drug delivery over traditional routes of delivery include

1. *Rapid absorption*. The oral mucosa's high vascularity aids in rapid absorption.
2. *No gastrointestinal or hepatic first-pass metabolism*. The systemic absorption of drugs may be greater (higher bioavailability) and less erratic than after oral administration. Some drugs that are broken down in the acid milieu of the stomach or by gastrointestinal enzymes can be absorbed through the oral mucosa.
3. *Simple and noninvasive means of administration*. Drugs are easily applied to the mucosa without special delivery devices or painful injections.
4. *Titratability*. Medications can be removed from the mouth when the desired effect is achieved.
5. *Permeability*. The oral mucosa is much more permeable than is the skin. Therefore, a greater variety of drugs can be administered through the oral mucosa than through the skin. Depots of drugs tend to form in the skin but not in the oral mucosa. Continuous absorption of drug from a depot is undesirable when rapid discontinuation of drug effect is required. Finally, because the oral mucosa maintains a relatively constant temperature and blood flow, there is less variation in drug absorption than there is in the skin, where the blood flow may be variable.

Physiology of Oral Transmucosal Drug Delivery

One of the important functions of the oral epithelium is to restrict the entry of microorgasms and toxic substances into the systemic circulation, but unlike the skin, there is no need for the oral mucosa to restrict the loss of salts and water because they can be recycled by swallowing. Hence, although the oral mucosa is a permeation barrier, it is far more permeable than is the skin.

The entire oral cavity is lined with stratified squamous epithelium. As a result of different functions, two kinds of epithelia exist, keratinized and nonkeratinized.[76] The parts that are subject to abrasion and mechanical insult, such as the gingiva and hard palate, are composed of keratin (about 24 percent of the total area) and resemble the epidermis of the skin. The outermost layer of keratinized epithelium consists of densely packed, flattened, hexagonal cells that have a low drug permeability. The parts of the oral mucosa that need to be flexible and extensible, such as the sublingual and buccal areas and the underside of the tongue, are nonkeratinized (about 60 percent of the total area). The outermost layer of the nonkeratinized epithelium consists of cells still containing organelles that allow greater drug permeability. For most drugs, the sublingual area and underside of the tongue have the highest permeability, followed by the buccal area of the oral mucosa. Beneath the epithelium, there are abundant capillary blood vessels in the submucosal tissues. Thus, after a drug permeates across the epithelium, it rapidly enters the systemic circulation.

Walton pioneered research in oral mucosal permeability in 1935. He found that the oil/water partition coefficient (lipid solubility) was one of the most important factors in determining whether a drug will pass through biological membranes.[77] In general, drugs that are lipophilic, un-ionized, and of small molecular weight have the highest oral transmucosal permeability. Applying permeation enhancing substances (e.g., bile salts) to the oral mucosa is one way of improving drug permeability.[78] Oral transmucosal absorption may also be improved by optimizing the formulation, for example, changing the pH to favor the un-ionized state.[79]

Buccal/Sublingual Morphine

Buccal and sublingual morphine administration has been extensively used in patients with cancer.[56–66] Buccal and sublingual morphine are useful when oral morphine is impractical (patients with nausea and vomiting, difficulty swallowing, or gastrointestinal problems) and parenteral injections are inconvenient. Special formulations for sublingual and buccal morphine have not been developed by pharmaceutical companies. Therefore, ordinary tablets or solutions have been used for oral mucosal morphine administration.

Pharmacokinetic Considerations

The bioavailability of buccal/sublingual morphine was reported to be as low as 9 percent.[57,61] Thus, morphine is not an ideal choice for transmucosal opioid administration because of low lipid solubility and poor transmucosal permeability (Fig. 31-4).

Clinical Experience

Buccal and sublingual morphine have been used for preoperative sedation and anxiolysis,[29] postoperative analgesia,[66] and pain relief in patients with chronic cancer pain.[60,61] Some authors reported that buccal or sublingual morphine was longer lasting, produced similar or better analgesia, and caused less adverse effects than similar doses of intramuscular morphine.[63,66] However, these findings have not been consistent. Also, many patients complain of the bitter taste. When buccal morphine was used for premedication before surgery, the reduction in anxiety and wakefulness was not as reliable as that of intramuscular morphine.[80]

A concentrated morphine solution (20 mg/ml) has been used sublingually with the hope that the onset of analgesia would be faster than with the oral route. However, there is no evidence of improved morphine absorption or faster onset of analgesia with this formulation.

Sublingual Buprenorphine

Buprenorphine is a long acting and potent agonist-antagonist opioid (see Ch. 5). Buprenorphine is lipophilic and well absorbed across mucosal membranes; thus, it is suitable for sublingual administration. The portion of the drug that is

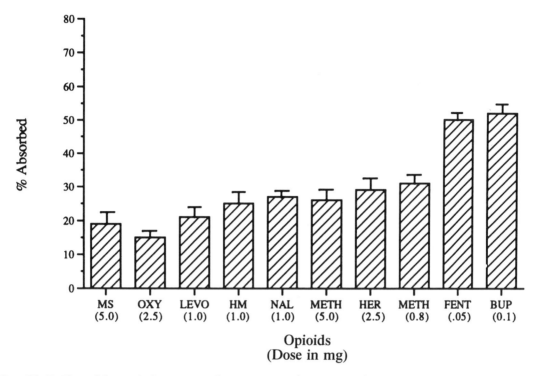

Fig. 31-4 The sublingual absorption of various opioid agonist and antagonist solutions in volunteers. BUP, buprenorphine; FENT, fentanyl; HER, heroin; HM, hydromorphone, LEVO, levorphanol; METH, methadone; MS, morphine sulfate; NAL, naloxone; OXY, oxycodone (From Weinberg et al.,[57] with permission.)

swallowed undergoes extensive first-pass hepatic metabolism. Sublingual buprenorphine has been used as an analgesic for the control of moderate to severe pain, for premedication before surgery, and for the detoxification of persons addicted to opioids. Parenteral buprenorphine is available for clinical use in the United States, but the sublingual formulation has not been approved by the FDA. Nevertheless, sublingual buprenorphine is used in 14 countries across Europe and Asia.

Pharmacokinetic Considerations

Clinical trials demonstrate that sublingual buprenorphine is 15 to 25 times more potent than is intramuscular morphine.[70,71] Buprenorphine is readily absorbed following sublingual administration, with an average bioavailability of 55 percent (range, 15 to 95 percent); 30 percent is absorbed in

the first 3 hours.[81] The oral bioavailability is only about 15 percent. Sublingual absorption is slow. Following the administration of 0.8 mg, measurable plasma concentrations do not occur until after 30 minutes (Fig. 31-5). Peak concentrations are reached 200 minutes after administration, significantly slower than after intramuscular[82] or intranasal administration.[83] The rapid disappearance of the tablet from the mouth (a few minutes) and the slow rise in plasma concentrations suggest the existence of a submucosal depot.

The analgesic effect that results following sublingual buprenorphine lasts 8 to 10 hours, much longer than the terminal elimination half-life.[84] This unusual finding may be the result of buprenorphine's slow dissociation from opioid receptors.[85] The receptor interaction may also explain the inability of naloxone to reverse buprenorphine-induced respiratory depression easily.[86]

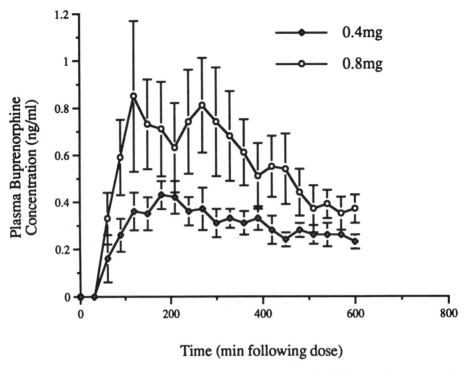

Fig. 31-5 Buprenorphine plasma concentrations (mean ± standard deviation) measured in healthy patients after a 0.4- or 0.8-mg sublingual tablet. (From Bullingham et al.,[81] with permission.)

Clinical Experience

Sublingual buprenorphine provides long-lasting postoperative analgesia with less drowsiness and sedation than comparable doses of intramuscular morphine,[87] meperidine,[88,89] or buprenorphine.[88] In addition, the sublingual route is more acceptable to children who dislike and sometimes refuse injections of analgesics despite significant pain.[70] Because buprenorphine is a partial agonist, it may not be as efficacious as a pure μ agonist, such as morphine, in treating severe pain. Long-lasting respiratory depression, even after a single dose, is the most alarming side effect reported with sublingual buprenorphine.[86,90]

Experience with sublingual buprenorphine for premedication has been mixed. Although avoidance of an injection is an advantage, preoperative anxiolysis and sedation are unreliable.[90,91] Furthermore, premedication with fentanyl or morphine is more likely to prevent hypertension and tachycardia following tracheal intubation than a comparable dose of sublingual buprenorphine.

Oral Transmucosal Fentanyl Citrate

Oral transmucosal fentanyl citrate is a new formulation of fentanyl being evaluated for transmucosal delivery at the time of writing this chapter. It consists of 100 to 800 μg of fentanyl in a sweetened lozenge on a stick (Fig. 31-6). When placed in the mouth, the fentanyl in the lozenge gradually dissolves into the saliva and is rapidly absorbed through the oral mucosa. The fast onset allows the patient or clinician to regulate delivery by removing the lozenge when the desired effect is reached. This drug is currently undergoing clinical trials in the United States for use in children for premedication before surgery and for painful procedures not requiring general anesthesia and in cancer patients for breakthrough pain.

Novel Drug Delivery 711

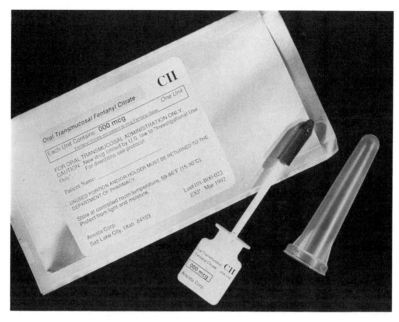

Fig. 31-6 Oral transmucosal fentanyl citrate.

Pharmacokinetics

Streisand et al.[92] determined the pharmacokinetics of transmucosal, oral, and intravenous fentanyl in the same volunteers on different occasions. Plasma concentrations peak at 3.0 ± 1.0 ng/ml (mean $\pm$ standard error of the mean), 23 minutes after oral transmucosal fentanyl citrate administration, then decline to less than 1 ng/ml 1 hour later (Fig. 31-7). Plasma concentrations exceed analgesic thresholds (0.6 to 1.0 ng/ml[93]) during drug consumption. This implies that oral transmucosal fentanyl citrate might be titratable for acute pain.

The elimination half-life of this drug is 7.7 hours, which is similar to the intravenous route. Unlike transdermal fentanyl, oral transmucosal fentanyl citrate leaves no significant depot in the mucosal tissues after it is removed.[67,79] However, some absorption of fentanyl continues after the drug is removed or completely consumed. This is caused by absorption of swallowed fentanyl from the gastrointestinal tract. The systemic bioavailability of oral transmucosal fentanyl citrate, 50 percent, reflects a combination of buccal and gastro-intestinal absorption. The bioavailability of swallowed fentanyl is low as a result of first-pass hepatic metabolism. The drug's bioavailability is similar to buprenorphine's (55 percent)[81] but much greater than that of buccal morphine and other opioids with low lipid solubility (Fig. 31-4).[57,61]

Clinical Experience

Initial clinical trials with oral transmucosal fentanyl citrate were performed in pediatric patients because of the need for less painful and less frightening methods of opioid administration in children. More than 800 doses have been administered to children for premedication in 13 clinical trials at 9 different hospitals in the United States (Moeller W: personal communication). Children receiving this drug before surgery were rapidly sedated and showed reduced anxiety within 30 minutes of administration.[68,94–97] Oral transmucosal fentanyl citrate produced only small clinically insignificant decreases in respiratory rate and oxygen saturation during these trials. However, close monitoring of respiration (pulse oximetry and respiratory rate)

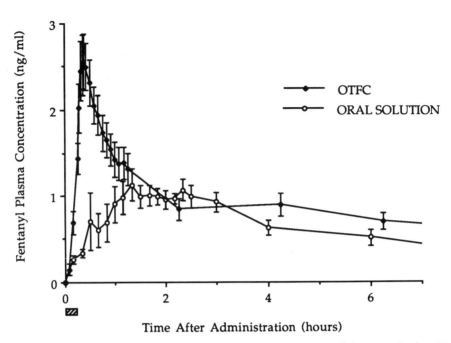

Fig. 31-7 Plasma concentrations of fentanyl (mean ± standard error of the mean) after 15-μg/kg of oral transmucosal fentanyl citrate (OTFC) or an oral fentanyl solution. The crosshatched bar represents the consumption time of oral transmucosal fentanyl citrate (15 minutes). (From Streisand,[68] with permission.)

and the availability of resuscitation equipment is recommended when this drug is used. In addition to being used as a premedication before surgery, it has been used in children with leukemia to provide analgesia for lumbar punctures and bone marrow biopsies (general anesthesia is usually not given for these procedures).[98]

Oral transmucosal fentanyl citrate is not an ideal premedication for children undergoing ambulatory surgery because of the high incidence of postoperative nausea and vomiting that may delay discharge in this setting.[99] Although the risk of aspiration is a possible concern with this type of premedication, Stanley et al.[97] demonstrated that the gastric volume and pH were not different whether children received the drug, a placebo lozenge, or no premedication.

Adults may also benefit from oral transmucosal fentanyl citrate. Ashburn et al.[69] reported on a patient who self-administered the drug, on an ambulatory basis, to provide analgesia for breakthrough cancer pain. For breakthrough cancer pain, it may fill a niche because it rapidly provides analgesic blood levels of a potent opioid without the use of expensive invasive equipment, such as pumps or catheters. Finally, it has the potential to be used for sedation and analgesia for procedures outside of the operating room environment, such as in the emergency room,[100] dermatology clinic, and surgeon's office.

INTRANASAL DRUG DELIVERY

Recently, a number of drugs have been delivered systemically through nasal absorption, including propranolol,[101] midazolam,[102] oxytocin,[103–106] calcitonin (with a permeation enhancer),[107] insulin (with permeation enhancer),[108–112] and human growth hormone.[113]

Intranasal drug delivery offers many of the same advantages as oral transmucosal drug delivery, including avoidance of the hepatic first-pass metabolism and a rapid onset of effect. It is a simple and noninvasive. Sustained delivery may also be achieved with techniques, such as bioadhesives and microcapsulation.[114]

Physiology of Intranasal Drug Delivery

The drug is administered into the nasal cavity in a suitable vehicle (solution or aerosol) by a nasal spray, nasal drop, saturated cotton pledget, or metered dose nebulizer. Ideally, the drug deposits on and dissolves in the mucus covering the mucosa. It then penetrates across the mucosa to reach the submucosal capillary blood vessels and is carried into the systemic circulation. In reality, the fate of intranasally administered drugs vary. Drugs delivered by nasal drops are deposited on the mucus covering the nasal mucosa; small inhaled particles pass into the lungs, and large inhaled particles are retained in the upper respiratory tract. Drugs that are soluble in the mucus are absorbed into the systemic circulation; insoluble drugs are carried posteriorly into the pharynx by a moving mucus blanket and then swallowed.[115–118]

The nasal mucosa lines the nasal cavity and is composed of olfactory and nonolfactory epithelium. The nonolfactory epithelium is a highly vascular tissue of the pseudostratified columnar ciliated type.[119] The olfactory epithelium is of the pseudostratified columnar type and consists of specialized olfactory cells, supporting cells and serous and mucous glands. Drug absorption from the nasal mucosa can be extremely rapid because it is highly vascular. However, blood flow to the nose is variable and can be affected by pathologic conditions (polyposis, rhinitis, allergy, and the common cold), emotions, environmental temperature, hyperventilation, and exercise. This, in turn, can lead to a wide variability in nasal drug absorption. Other factors that may influence intranasal drug absorption include the speed of mucus flow, atmospheric conditions, and loss out the anterior nares or into the esophagus.

The nasal mucosa is covered by a thin layer of "mucus" (90 to 95 percent water, 1 to 2 percent salt, and 2 to 3 percent mucin) secreted from the mucous and serous glands in the nasal mucosa and submucosa. The mucus layer behaves as an adhesive and acts as a retainer for the substances in the nasal ducts. In addition, the mucus has a two-layer composition, the watery layer located immediately adjacent to the mucosal surface and the superficial mucus (gel) layer. Thus, a drug must be both lipid and water soluble to pass through mucus and be absorbed by the nasal mucosa. Other physical properties of a drug that favor nasal absorption include low molecular weight and an un-ionized form.[120] However, the rules governing nasal absorption are complex because there are nonpassive permeation mechanisms in the nasal mucosa. These include a portal in the olfactory epithelium for substances to enter the central nervous system and the peripheral circulation and a port of entry for viruses responsible for some of the most common viral diseases.[121]

Certain factors in the drug formulation can affect absorption. For example, surfactants were found to increase the permeability of the nasal mucosa.[109,122–124] Because the nasal mucosa is highly sensitive, the formulation must be pH controlled and contain no caustic agents. Finally, the size of the droplets or aerosol can affect absorption.

Intranasal Sufentanil

Sufentanil is potent and lipid soluble. Thus, it should be easily absorbed through the nasal mucosa. Nasal sufentanil has been investigated in children and adults as a premedication before surgery. There is no special formulation for nasal administration; therefore, the commercially available parenteral solution is administered as nasal drops.

Pharmacokinetics

Helmers et al.[125] measured plasma concentrations of sufentanil after a 15-µg intranasal or intravenous dose. The maximum plasma concentration, 0.08 ± 0.03 ng/ml, occurs just 10 minutes after administration. The plasma concentration profiles of intranasal and intravenous sufentanil are virtually identical 30 minutes after administration. Nasal sufentanil provides the highest bioavailability, 78 percent, of any transmucosally administered opioid.

Clinical Experience

Although nasal sufentanil acts rapidly to sedate children within 10 minutes of administration, routine use as a premedication may be precluded by side effects (intravenous doses of 2 µg/kg are sufficient to produce unconsciousness and anesthesia in many patients). Nasal doses of 2 µg/kg and above produced an unacceptable incidence of low oxygen saturation and chest wall rigidity.[126,127] Nasal midazolam provided more reliable sedation than did nasal sufentanil without the respiratory side effects of sufentanil.[126] Most children were disturbed by this route of administration.[127]

Vercauteren et al. and Helmers et al.[125] reported excellent sedation with a low incidence of side effects with an intranasal sufentanil dose of 10 to 20 µg in adults. Many of the side effects reported in children were not observed in adults, probably because the dose used in adults was much lower than the dose used in children, normalized by weight.

The rapid absorption of nasally administered sufentanil suggests possible utility in acute pain management. However, there have been no reports of use for this indication.

Intranasal Fentanyl

Rapid absorption of fentanyl through the nasal mucosa suggests that this route might be useful for managing acute pain. Striebel et al.[129] recently reported on the intranasal administration of fentanyl (commercially available solution, 50 µg/ml) for acute postoperative pain using six metered nasal sprays (0.09 ml/spray) per dose, such that each dose equaled a total of 27 µg of fentanyl. The onset of analgesia occurred within 10 minutes and was nearly as effective as the same dose of intravenous fentanyl, suggesting a high bioavailability of fentanyl after nasal administration. The authors suggested intranasal fentanyl might be particularly useful during the late postoperative period after intravenous access has been remoted or for patients with breakthrough cancer pain. Further clinical investigation is necessary to examine the chronic effects of intranasal fentanyl on the nasal mucosa and to establish how upper respiratory viral infections affect the absorption and bioavailability before this technique can be recommended for long-term use.

Intranasal Midazolam

Although midazolam is intended for parenteral administration; oral administration is possible by mixing the injectable form with highly concentrated fruit juices or chocolate syrup to hide the bitter taste. As a result of hepatic first-pass metabolism, oral midazolam has a bioavailability less than 25 percent of the parenteral route.[130] Therefore, the oral dose, 0.5 to 0.75 mg/kg, is approximately five times greater than the parenteral dose. The clinical effect is variable and relatively slow (30 to 45 minutes after administration).

As an alternative to oral administration, intranasal midazolam has been used as a sedative agent in pediatric patients. Because there is no commercially available formulation for intranasal midazolam administration, the injectable solution is delivered by nose drops.

Pharmacokinetic Considerations

Plasma concentrations following 0.1 mg/kg of nasal midazolam are illustrated in Figure 31-8.[102] Peak midazolam concentrations of 50 to 100 ng/ml (mean 75 ng/ml) were reached 10 minutes following intranasal administration, much faster than peak concentrations found after oral (53 minutes)[130] or rectal (16 to 30 minutes)[130,131] routes. Walbergh et al.[102] found that the minimum effective plasma concentration to produce sedation in adults (40 ng/ml) was reached 3 minutes after administration of 0.1 mg/kg and exceeded this threshold for greater than 30 minutes.[132] The elimination half-life after nasal administration (2.2 hours) was similar to that after intravenous administration (2.4 hours). Therefore, there is no evidence for a depot of midazolam in the nasal mucosa. The bioavailability of intranasal midazolam is 55 to 57 percent,[102,132] which is significantly higher than that of the oral (19 percent)[130] and rectal (18 percent)[131] routes of administration.

Clinical Experience

Intranasal midazolam (0.1 to 0.3 mg/kg) is used for the sedation of children in a variety of clinical settings, including premedication before general anesthesia,[125,153] during diagnostic radiologic and echocardiographic procedures,[134,135] and for the insertion of central venous catheters.[136] Sedation occurs rapidly, generally within 5 to 10 minutes, and lasts for 30 to 60 minutes. A low incidence of side effects was reported. Unfortunately, most chil-

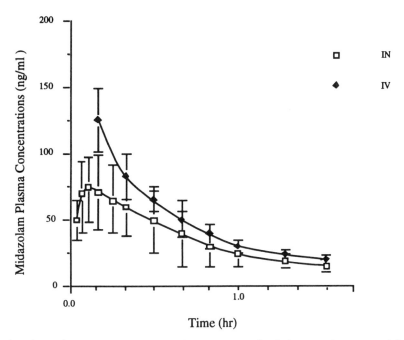

Fig. 31-8 Midazolam plasma concentrations (mean ± standard deviation) measured from children receiving intravenous or intranasal midazolam, 0.1 mg/kg. (From Walbergh et al.,[102] with permission.)

dren cry on administration and complain of the bitter taste. These factors may limit the popularity of this route of midazolam administration. As with some other drugs administered by the nasal route, no special formulation is available.

Intranasal Buprenorphine

Eriksen et al.[83] compared the pharmacokinetic profiles of buprenorphine (0.3 mg) following intranasal and intravenous administration to nine healthy volunteers. Unlike sublingual buprenorphine, the absorption of intranasal buprenorphine was rapid, with peak plasma concentrations ranging from 0.6 to 4.78 ng/ml (mean, 1.77 ng/ml), 10 to 60 minutes (mean, 30.6 minutes) after administration. Furthermore, the elimination half-life of intranasal buprenorphine was virtually the same as that of intravenous buprenorphine and much shorter than that of sublingual buprenorphine. The bioavailability, 48 percent, was comparable to that occurring after sublingual administration. Clinical experience with intranasal buprenorphine has not been reported.

REFERENCES

1. Elias PM: Protective role of the skin: the special role of the stratum corneum. p. 213. In Fitzpatrick TD (ed): Dermatology in Medicine. Vol. 3. McGraw-Hill, New York, 1987
2. Guy RH, Hadgraft J, Bucks DAW: Transdermal drug delivery and cutaneous metabolism. Xenobiotica 17:325, 1987
3. Hertzmann AB, Randall WC: Regional differences in the basal and maximal rates of blood flow in the skin. J Appl Physiol 1:234, 1948
4. Graybiel A, Knepton J, Shaw J: Prevention of experimental motion sickness by scopolamine absorbed through the skin. Aviat Space Environ Med 47:1096, 1976
5. Janssen Pharmaceutica: Duragesic package insert. Piscataway, NJ, 1991
6. McClain DA, Hug CC: Intravenous fentanyl kinetics. Clin Pharmacol Ther 28:106, 1980
7. Reilly CS, Wood AJJ, Wood M: Variability of fentanyl pharmacokinetics in man. Anaesthesia 40:837, 1984
8. Duthrie DJR, Rowbotham DJ, Wyld R et al: Plasma fentanyl concentrations during transdermal deliv-

ery of fentanyl to surgical patients. Br J Anaesth 60:614, 1988

9. Holley FO, Van Steenis C: Postoperative analgesia with fentanyl: pharmacokinetics and pharmacodynamics of constant-rate iv and transdermal delivery. Br J Anaesth 60:608, 1988

10. Varvel JR, Shafer SL, Hwang SS et al: Absorption characteristics of transdermally administered fentanyl. Anesthesiology 70:928, 1989

11. Miser AW, Narang PK, Dothage JA et al: Transdermal fentanyl for pain control in patients with cancer. Pain 37:15, 1989

12. Rowbotham DJ, Wyld R, Peacock JE et al: Transdermal fentanyl for the relief of pain after upper abdominal surgery. Br J Anaesth 63:56, 1989

13. Zech D, Daur HG, Stollenwerk B et al: PCA and TTS fentanyl in the treatment of cancer pain. Pain 5:S356, 1990

14. Gourlay GK, Kowalski SR, Plummer JL et al: The transdermal administration of fentanyl in the treatment of postoperative pain: pharmacokinetics and pharmacodynamic effects. Pain 37:193, 1989

15. McLesky CH: Fentanyl TTS for postoperative analgesia. Eur J Pain 11:92, 1990

16. Caplan RA, Ready LB, Oden RV et al: Transdermal fentanyl for postoperative pain management: a double blind placebo study. JAMA 261:1989

17. Wright C: Medical officer review, NDA #19813, Alza Corporation TTS fentanyl, pharmacokinetics and pharmacodynamics. 2:1990

18. Tigerstedt I, Salmela L, Aromaa U: Double-blind comparison of transdermal scopolamine, droperidol and placebo against postoperative nausea and vomiting. Acta Anaesthesiol Scand 32:454, 1988

19. Simmonds MA, Payne R, Richenbacher J et al: TTS (fentanyl) in the management of pain in patients and cancer. Proc Am Soc Clin Oncol 8:324, 1989

20. Levy MH, Rosen SM, Kedziera P: Transdermal fentanyl: seeding trial in patients with chronic cancer pain. J Pain Symptom Manage 7:48, 1992

21. Patt RB, Hogan LA: Transdermal fentanyl for chronic cancer pain: detailed case reports and the influence of confounding factors. J Pain Symptom Manage 7:51, 1992

22. Bailey PL, Stanley TH: Package inserts and other dosage guidelines are especially useful with new analgesics and new analgesic delivery systems. Anesth Analg 75:873, 1992

23. Payne R: Transdermal fentanyl: suggested recommendations for clinical use. J Pain Symptom Manage 7:40, 1992

24. Ciba-Geigy: Transderm Scop. Scopolamine transdermal therapeutic system package insert. Ciba-Geigy, Piscataway, NJ 1988

25. Schmitt LG, Shaw JE, Carpenter PF et al: Comparison of transdermal and intravenous administration of scopolamine. Clin Pharmacol Ther 29:282, 1981

26. Pyykkö I, Schalén L, Jäntti V: Transdermally administered scopolamine vs. dimenhydrinate: effect on nausea and vertigo. Acta Otolaryngol (Stockh) 99:588, 1985

27. Shaw JE: Development of transdermal therapeutic systems. Dev Ind Pharm 9:579, 1983

28. Price NM, Schmitt LG, McGuire J et al: Transdermal scopolamine in the prevention of motion sickness at sea. Clin Pharmacol Ther 29:414, 1981

29. van Marion WF, Bongaerts MCM, Christiaanse JC et al: Influence of transdermal scopolamine on motion sickness during 7 days exposure to heavy seas. Clin Pharmacol Ther 38:301, 1985

30. Koski EMJ, Mattila MAK, Knapik D et al: Double blind comparison of transdermal hyoscine and placebo for the prevention of postoperative nausea. Br J Anaesth 64:16, 1990

31. Bailey PL, Streisand JB, Pace NL et al: Transdermal scopolamine reduces nausea and vomiting after outpatient laparoscopy. Anesthesiology 72:977, 1990

32. Uppington J, Dunnet J, Blogg CE: Transdermal hyoscine and postoperative nausea and vomiting. Anaesthesia 41:16, 1986

33. Loper KA, Ready BL, Dorman BH: Prophylactic transdermal scopolamine patches reduce nausea in postoperative patients receiving epidural morphine. Anesth Analg 68:144, 1989

34. Harris SN, Sevarino FB, Sinatra RS et al: Nausea prophylaxis using transdermal scopolamine in the setting of patient-controlled analgesia. Obstet Gynecol 78:673, 1991

35. Kotelko DM, Rottman RL, Wright WC et al: Transdermal scopolamine decreases nausea and vomiting following cesarean section in patients receiving epidural morphine. Anesthesiology 71:675, 1989

36. Gibbons PA, Nicholson SC, Betts EK et al: Scopolamine does not prevent post-operative emesis after pediatric eye surgery. Anesthesiology 61:A435, 1984

37. Rodysill KJ, Warren JB: Transdermal scopolamine and toxic psychosis. Ann Intern Med 98:561, 1983

38. Bezzant JL, Pentelenz TJ, Jacobsen SC: Painless cauterization of spider veins using iontophoretic local anesthesia. J Am Acad Dermatol 19:869, 1988

39. Comeau M, Brummett R: Anesthesia of the human tympanic membrane by iontophoresis of a local anesthetic. Laryngoscope 88:277, 1978

40. Davis WT, Jr: Use of iontophoresis for oral mucosal anesthesia. SC Dent J 39:53, 1981

41. Harris PR: Iontophoresis: clinical research in musculoskeletal inflammatory conditions. Journal of Orthopaedic and Sports Physical Therapy 4:109, 1982

42. Kern DA, McQuade MJ, Scheidt MJ et al: Effectiveness of sodium fluoride on tooth hypersensitivity with and without iontophoresis. J Periodontol 60:386, 1989

43. Sisler HA: Iontophoretic local anesthesia for conjunctival surgery. Ann Ophthalmol 10:597, 1978

44. Sloan JB, Soltani K: Iontophoresis in dermatology. J Am Acad Dermatol 15:671, 1986

45. Ashburn MA, Stephen RL, Ackerman E et al: Iontophoretic delivery of morphine for postoperative analgesia. J Pain Symptom Manage 7:27, 1991

46. Maloney JM: Local anesthesia obtained via iontophoresis as an aid to shave biopsy. Arch Dermatol 128:331, 1992

47. Glass JM, Stephen RL, Jacobson SC: The quantity and distribution of radiolabeled dexamethasone delivered to tissue by iontophoresis. Int J Dermatol 19:519, 1980

48. Hasson SH, Henderson GH, Daniels JC et al: Exercise training and dexamethasone iontophoresis in rheumatoid arthritis: a case study. Physiother Can 43:11, 1991

49. Petelenz TJ, Buttke JA, Bonds C et al: Iontophoresis of dexamethasone: laboratory studies. J Controlled Release 20:55, 1992

50. Kennard CD, Whitaker DC: Iontophoresis of lidocaine for anesthesia during pulsed due laser treatment of port-wine stains. J Dermatol Surg Oncol 18:287, 1992

51. Petelenz TJ: Selected topics in iontophoresis. PhD thesis, University of Utah, 1989

52. Murrell W: Nitroglycerine as a remedy for angina pectoris. Lancet 1:234, 1879

53. Schürmann W, Turner P: A membrane model of the human oral mucosa as derived from buccal absorption performance and physiochemical properties of the β-blocking drugs atenolol and propranolol. J Pharm Pharmacol 30:137, 1978

54. Kates RE: Absorption kinetics of sublingually administered propranolol. J Med 8:393, 1977

55. Zhang J, Ebert CE, McJames S et al: Transbuccal permeability of isoproterenol—a dog model. Pharmacol Res 6:S135, 1989

56. Al-Sayed-Omar O, Johnston A, Turner P: Influence of pH on the buccal absorption of morphine sulphate and its major metabolite, morphine-3-glucuronide. J Pharm Pharmacol 39:934, 1987

57. Weinberg DS, Inturrisi CE, Reidenberg B et al: Sublingual absorption of selected opioid analgesics. Clin Pharmacol Ther 44:335, 1988

58. Manara AR, Shelly MP, Quinn KG et al: Pharmacokinetics of morphine following administration by the buccal route. Br J Anaesth 62:498, 1989

59. Bardgett D, Howard C, Murray GR et al: Plasma concentration and bioavailability of a buccal preparation of morphine sulphate. Proc Br Pharm Soc 198, 1983

60. Fisher AP, Fung C, Hanna M: Absorption of buccal morphine. Anaesthesia 43:552, 1988

61. Fisher AP, Fung C, Hanna M: Serum morphine concentrations after buccal and intramuscular morphine administration. Br J Clin Pharmacol 24:685, 1987

62. Hoskin PJ, Hanks GW, Aherne GW et al: The bioavailability and pharmacokinetics of morphine after intravenous, oral and buccal administration in healthy volunteers. Br J Clin Pharmacol 27:499, 1989

63. Pitorak EF: Pain control with sublingual or buccal morphine. Oncology Nursing Forum 18:941, 1991

64. Shepard KV, Bakst AW: Alternate delivery methods for morphine sulfate in cancer pain. Cleve Clin J Med 57:48, 1990

65. Pannuti F, Rossi AP, Iaefelice G et al: Control of chronic pain in very advanced cancer patients with morphine hydrochloride administered by oral, rectal and sublingual route. Clinical report and preliminary results on morphine pharmacokinetics. Pharmacol Res 14:369, 1982

66. Bell MDD, Mishra P, Weldon BD et al: Buccal morphine—a new route for analgesia? Lancet 1:71, 1985

67. Streisand J, Ashburn M, LeMaire L: Bioavailability and absorption of oral transmucosal fentanyl citrate. Anesthesiology 71:A230, 1989

68. Streisand JB, Stanley TH, Hague B et al: Oral transmucosal fentanyl citrate premedication in children. Anesth Analg 69:28, 1989

69. Ashburn MA, Fine PG, Stanley TH: Oral transmucosal fentanyl citrate for the treatment of breakthrough cancer pain: a case report. Anesthesiology 71:615, 1989

70. Maunnuksela E-L, Korpela R, Olkkola KT: Comparison of buprenorphine with morphine in the treatment of postoperative pain in children. Anesth Analg 67:233, 1988

71. Wallenstein S, Kaiko R, Rogers A: Crossover trials

in clinical analgesic assays: studies of buprenorphine and morphine. Pharmacotherapy 6:228, 1986

72. Aungst BJ, Rogers NJ: Site dependence of absorption-promoting action of laureth-9, Na-salicylate, Na₂EDTA, and aprotinin on rectal, nasal, and buccal insulin delivery. Pharmacol Res 5:305, 1988

73. Aungst BJ, Rogers NJ, Shefter E: Comparison of nasal, rectal, buccal, sublingual, and intramuscular insulin efficacy and the effects of a bile salt absorption promoter. J Pharmacol Exp ther 244:23, 1988

74. Ishida M, Machida Y, Nambu N et al: New mucosal dosage form of insulin. Chem Pharm Bull (Tokyo) 29:810, 1981

75. Zhang J, Niu S, McJames S et al: Buccal absorption of insulin in an in vivo dog model—evidence of mucosal storage. Pharmacol Res 8:S155, 1991

76. Wertz PW, Squier CA: Cellular and molecular basis of barrier function in oral epithelium. Crit Rev Ther Drug Carrier Syst 8:237, 1991

77. Gibaldi M, Kanig J: Absorption of drugs through the oral mucosa. J Oral Ther Pharmacol 1:440, 1965

78. Siegel I, Gordon H: Effects of surfactants on the permeability of canine oral mucosa. Toxicol Lett 26:153, 1985

79. Streisand J, Zhang J, Niu S et al: pH and oral transmucosal fentanyl absorption in dogs. Anesthesiology 77:A365, 1992

80. Fisher A, Vine P, Whitlock J et al: Buccal morphine premedication. Anaesthesia 41:1104, 1986

81. Bullingham RES, McQuay HJ, Porter EJB et al: Sublingual buprenorphine used postoperatively: ten hour plasma drug concentration analysis. Br J Clin Pharmacol 13:665, 1982

82. Bullingham RES, McQuay HJ, Moore RA et al: Buprenorphine kinetics. Clin Pharmacol Ther 28:667, 1980

83. Eriksen J, Jensen N-H, Kamp-Jensen M et al: The systemic availability of buprenorphine administered by nasal spray. J Pharm Pharmacol 41:803, 1989

84. Bullingham RES, McQuay HJ, Dwyer D et al: Sublingual buprenorphine used postoperatively: clinical observations and preliminary pharmacokinetic analysis. Br J Clin Pharmacol 12:117, 1981

85. Boas R, Villiger J: Clinical actions of fentanyl and buprenorphine: the significance of receptor binding. Br J Anaesth 57:192, 1985

86. Thörn S-E, Rawal N, Wennhager M: Prolonged respiratory depression caused by sublingual buprenorphine. Lancet 1:179, 1988

87. Cuschieri R, Morran C, McArdle C: Comparison of morphine and sublingual buprenorphine following abdominal surgery. Br J Anaesth 56:855, 1984

88. Carl P, Crawford ME, Madsen NBB et al: Pain relief after major abdominal surgery: a double-blind controlled comparison of sublingual buprenorphine intramuscular buprenorphine, and intramuscular meperidine. Anesth Analg 66:142, 1987

89. Shah MV, Jones DI, Rosen M: "Patient demand" postoperative analgesia with buprenorphine: comparison between sublingual and i.m. administration. Br J Anaesth 58:508, 1986

90. Korttila K, Hovorka J: Buprenorphine as premedication and as analgesic during and after light isoflurane-N₂O-N₂ anaesthesia: a comparison with oxycodone plus fentanyl. Acta Anaesthesiol Scand 31:673, 1987

91. O'Sullivan G, Bullingham R, McQuay H et al: A comparison of intramuscular and sublingual buprenorphine, intramuscular morphine, and placebo as premedication. Anaesthesia 38:977, 1983

92. Streisand JB, Stanley TH: Transmucosal narcotic delivery. p. 256. In Estafanous FG (ed): Opioids in Anesthesia. Vol. 2. Butterworth-Heinemann, Boston, 1991

93. Gourlay GK, Kowalski SR, Plummer JL et al: Fentanyl blood concentration-analgesic response relationship in treatment of postoperative pain. Anesth Analg 67:329, 1988

94. Feld LH, Champeau MW, van Steennis CA et al: Pre-anesthetic medication in children: a comparison of oral transmucosal fentanyl citrate versus placebo. Anesthesiology 71:374, 1989

95. Friesen RH, Lockhart CH: Oral transmucosal fentanyl citrate for preanesthetic medication of pediatric day surgery patients with and without droperidol as a prophylactic anti-emetic, Anesthesiology 76:46, 1992

96. Nelson PS, Streisand JB, Mulder SM et al: Comparison of oral transmucosal fentanyl citrate and an oral solution of meperidine, diazepam, and atropine for premedication in children. Anesthesiology 70:616, 1989

97. Stanley TH, Leiman BC, Rawal N et al: The effects of oral transmucosal fentanyl citrate premedication of preoperative behavioral responses and gastric volume and acidity in children. Anesth Analg 69:328, 1989

98. Schechter NL, Weisman SJ, Rosenblum M et al: Sedation for painful procedures in children with cancer using the fentanyl lollipop: a preliminary report.

p. 209. In Tyler D, Krane E (eds): Advances in Pain Research Therapy. Vol. 15. Raven Press, New York, 1990

99. Ashburn MA, Streisand JB, Tarver SD et al: Oral transmucosal fentanyl citrate for premedication in paediatric outpatients. Can J Anaesth 37:857, 1990

100. Lind GH, Marcus MA, Ashburn MA et al: Oral transmucosal fentanyl citrate for analgesia and anxiolysis in the emergency room. Anesth Analg 70:S241, 1990

101. Hussain AA, Foster T, Hirai S et al: Nasal absorption of propranolol in humans. J Pharm Sci 69:1240, 1980

102. Walbergh EJ, Wills RJ, Eckhert J: Plasma concentrations in midazolam in children following intranasal administration. Anesthesiology 74:233, 1991

103. Hendricks C, Gabel RA: Use of intranasal oxytocin in obstetrics. I. Laboratory evaluation. Am J Obstet Gynecol 79:780, 1960

104. Hendricks CH, Pose SV: Intranasal oxytocin in obstetrics. JAMA 175:384, 1961

105. Stander RW, Thompson JF, Gibbs CP: Evaluation of intranasal oxytocin in amniotic fluid pressure recordings. Am J Obstet Gynecol 85:193, 1963

106. Sandholm LE: The effect of intravenous and intranasal oxytocin on intramammary pressure during early lactation. Acta Obstet Gynecol Scand 47:145, 1968

107. Pontiroli A, Alberetto M, Pozza G: Intranasal calcitonin and plasma calcium concentrations in normal subjects. BMJ 290:1390, 1985

108. Pontiroli AE, Alberetto M, Secchi M et al: Insulin given intranasally induces hypoglycaemia in normal and diabetic subjects. BMJ 284:303, 1982

109. Moses AC, Gordon GS, Carey MC et al: Insulin administered intranasally as an insulin-bile salt aerosol: effectiveness and reproducibility in normal and diabetic subjects. Diabetes 32:1040, 1983

110. Flier JS, Moses AC, Gordon GA et al: Intranasal administration of insulin: efficacy and mechanism. p. 217. in Chien YW (ed): Transnasal Systemic Medications. Elsevier, Amsterdam, 1985

111. Gordon GS, Moses AC, Silver RD et al: Nasal absorption on insulin: enhancment by hydrophobic bile salts. Proc Natl Acad Sci U S A 82:7419, 1985

112. Salzman R, Manson JE, Griffling GT et al: Intranasal aerosolized insulin: mixed-meal studies and long-term use in type I diabetes. N Engl J Med 312:1078, 1985

113. Evans WS, Borges JLC, Kaiser DL et al: Intranasal administration of human pancreatic tumor GH-releasing factor-40 stimulates GH release in normal men. J Clin Endocrinol Metab 57:1081, 1983

114. Hussain A, Hirai S, Bawarshi R: Absorption of propranolol from different dosage forms by rats and dogs. J Pharm Sci 69:1411, 1980

115. Proctor DF, Anderson IB, Lundqvist G: Clearance of inhaled particles from the human nose. Arch Intern Med 131:132, 1973

116. Proctor DF: Nasal mucous transport and our ambient air. Laryngoscope 93:58, 1983

117. Proctor DF, Wagner HN: Clearance of particles from the human nose. Arch Environ Health 11:366, 1965

118. Sakakura Y, Ukai K, Majima Y et al: Nasal mucociliary clearance under various conditions. Acta Otolaryngol (Stockh) 96:167, 1983

119. Geurkink N: Nasal anatomy, physiology, and function. J Allergy Clin Immunol 72:123, 1983

120. Hussain AA, Bawarshi-Nassar R, Huang CH: Physiocochemical consideration in intranasal drug administrations. p. 121. In Chien YW (ed): Transnasal Systemic Medications. Elsevier, Amsterdam, 1985

121. Chien Y, Chang S: Intranasal drug delivery for systemic medications. Crit Rev Ther 4:67, 1987

122. Duchateau GSMJE, Zuidema J, Merkus FWHM: Bile salts and intranasal drug absorption. Int J Pharmacol 31:193, 1986

123. Longenecker JP, Moses AC, Flier JS et al: Effects of sodium taurodihydrofusidate on nasal absorption of insulin in sheep. J Pharm Sci 76:351, 1987

124. Hersey SJ, Jackson RT: Effect of bile salts on nasal permeability in vitro. J Pharm Sci 76:876, 1987

125. Helmers JH, Noorduin H, Van Peer A et al: Comparison of intravenous and intranasal sufentanil absorption and sedation. Can J Anaesth 36:494, 1989

126. Karl HW, Keifer AT, Rosenberger JL et al: Comparison of the safety and efficacy of intranasal midazolam or sufentanil for preinduction of anesthesia in pediatric patients. Anesthesiology 76:209, 1992

127. Henderson JM, Brodsky DA, Fisher DM et al: Preinduction of anesthesia in pediatric patients with nasally administered sufentanil. Anesthesiology 68:671, 1988

128. Vercauteren M, Boeckx E, Hanegreefs G et al: Intranasal sufentanil for pre-operative sedation. Anaesthesia 43:270, 1988

129. Striebel H, Koenigs D, Kramer J: Postoperative pain management by intranasal demand-adapted fentanyl titration. Anesthesiology 77:281, 1992

130. Payne K, Mattheyse FJ, Liebenberg D et al: The pharmacokinetics of midazolam in paediatric patients. Eur J Clin Pharmacol 37:267, 1989

131. Saint-Maurice C, Meistelman C, Rey E et al: The pharmacokinetics of rectal midazolam for premedication in children. Anesthesiology 65:536, 1986

132. Rey E, Delauney L, Pon G et al: Pharmacokinetics in midazolam in children: comparative study of intranasal and intravenous administration. Eur J Clin Pharmacol 41:355, 1991

133. Wilton NCT, Leigh J, Rosen DR et al: Preanesthetic sedation of preschool children using intranasal midazolam. Anesthesiology 69:972, 1988

134. Saint-Maurice C, Landais A, Delleur M et al: The use of midazolam in diagnostic and short surgical procedures in children. Acta Anaesthesiol Scand 34:39, 1990

135. Latson LA, Cheatham JP, Gumbiner CH et al: Midazolam nose drops for outpatient echocardiography sedation in infants. Am Heart J 121:209, 1991

136. Rice TL, Kyff JV: Intranasal administration of midazolam to a severely burned child. Burns 14:307, 1990

137. Lehmann KA, Zech D: Transdermal fentanyl: clinical pharmacology. J Pain Symptom Manage (suppl 3):58, 1992

Chapter 32

Nitric Oxide

Raymond M. Quock

An emerging concept with immediate impact on anesthesiology is the biologic role of nitric oxide (NO), the first of a novel class of neurochemical messengers. There has been such an exponential explosion of new knowledge about NO and its multifaceted role in biology (Table 32-1) that it is virtually impossible to keep abreast of all the developments in the NO field. This chapter reflects information available through mid-1993.

For many years, NO was of concern mainly to environmentalists and toxicologists because it is an atmospheric pollutant produced by internal combustion engines.[1] Only recently has the physiologic significance of NO been recognized. Initially, NO was found to be the active bactericidal and tumoricidal agent generated by macrophages.[2] Then endothelium-derived relaxing factor (EDRF), an endogenous regulator of physiologic and pharmacologic vasodilation, was identified as NO (or some other species either closely related to NO or able to generate NO). Further studies demonstrated NO to be a novel type of intracellular or secondary messenger involved in the relaxation of vascular smooth muscle and inhibition of platelet aggregation.[3,4] More recently, NO was implicated as an *inter*cellular messenger in both the peripheral[5] and central nervous systems.[6,7] The accumulated evidence demonstrates that NO fulfills all the classic requirements of a neurotransmitter (Table 32-2), yet it is not a typical one (Table 32-3). Within the past 5 years, the number of scientific reports dealing with NO has literally skyrocketed and continues to grow at an astounding rate.

Increasing recognition of the complex biologic implications of this simple inorganic gaseous molecule (Table 32-1) prompted *Science* magazine to declare NO as "The Molecule of the Year" for 1992.[8] This chapter will serve as a primer on NO, its biologic functions, and its possible importance in anesthesiology.

CHEMISTRY

NO is the NO form of nitrogen monoxide and is a manifestly simple inorganic molecule, which is composed of one nitrogen atom coupled to a single oxygen atom. Nitrogen contributes seven electrons to NO and oxygen eight. The single unpaired electron confers paramagnetism and free radical properties on the molecule and renders it highly reactive.[1] NO is related but not identical to two other forms of nitrogen monoxide, nitrosonium (NO^+) and nitroxyl anion (NO^-). NO should also not be mistaken for nitrous oxide (N_2O), a far more chemically stable oxide of nitrogen that is widely used in anesthesiology and dentistry.

Table 32-1 Suspected or Proven Functions of Nitric Oxide

Peripheral Functions
Nonspecific immunity
Inhibition of platelet aggregation
Endothelium-dependent vasodilation
Renal sodium excretion
NANC nerve-induced gastrointestinal relaxation
NANC nerve-induced penile erection
Sensory signal transduction
Regulation of norepinephrine release from sympathetic nerves
Central Nervous System Functions
Learning and memory
Pain, analgesia, and anesthesia
Behavior and psychotropic drug effects
Neuroendocrine regulation
Appetite regulation
Epileptogenesis
Neurotoxicity
Regulation of neurotransmitter release from central nervous system neurons

Abbreviations: NANC, nonadrenergic noncholinergic.

Table 32-2 Is NO a Neurochemical Transmitter?

Classic Criteria for Identifying a Neurochemical Transmitter	Evidence for NO Being a Neurochemical Transmitter
1. The substance and the enzymes involved in its synthesis must be present in nervous tissue.	1. Histochemical studies have localized NOS in nervous tissues where NO is suspected to be a neurochemical transmitter.
2. The substance must be released from nervous tissue during nerve stimulation.	2. A chemical substance identified as NO is released following nerve stimulation.
3. The exogenously administered substance must produce effects identical to those evoked by nerve stimulation.	3. Exogenously administered NO produces effects identical to those evoked by nerve stimulation.
4. The effects of exogenously administered substance and of nerve stimulation must be influenced in a consistent and predictable manner by other drugs.	4. Effects of nerve stimulation but not exogenous NO are blocked by NOS inhibitors; effects of both nerve stimulation and exogenous NO are blocked by hemoglobin and methylene blue.

Abbreviations: NO, nitric oxide; NOS, nitric oxide synthase.

Table 32-3 How Does NO Differ From Typical Neurochemical Transmitters?

General Characteristics of a Typical Neurochemical Transmitter	Atypical Characteristics of NO
1. Neurochemical transmitters are synthesized and then stored in synaptic vesicles for eventual neuronal release.	1. NO is synthesized and immediately diffuses out of the neuron to the target cell; there is no storage of NO in synaptic vesicles.
2. Neurochemical transmitters act on specific receptors on the surface of the target cell.	2. NO readily diffuses through the membrane of the target cell and binds to the metal component of an intracellular enzyme.
3. The actions of neurochemical transmitters are terminated by neuronal reuptake or by enzymatic degradation.	3. NO is nonenzymatically converted by oxygen and water to various nitrites and nitrates.

Abbreviations: NO, nitric oxide.

NO is extremely labile and has a life span measured in mere seconds. In the presence of abundant oxygen, NO is highly reactive and spontaneously oxidizes to nitrite (NO_2^-) and nitrate (NO_3^-). This is a nonenzymatic reaction, but it can be accelerated by superoxide anion and, conversely, inhibited by the enzyme superoxide dismutase or by low oxygen tension. The usually minute levels of NO found endogenously together with its brief half-life in the presence of oxygen have greatly complicated direct measurement of NO in biologic samples. Various assay techniques for quantifying NO were recently reviewed.[9]

NO also readily interacts with the metal ions in a variety of proteins and enzymes.[10] The binding of NO to the heme iron in soluble guanylate cyclase results in a stimulation of catalytic activity and increased production of cyclic guanosine monophosphate (GMP). In other cases, the binding of NO to other metalloproteins may result in a diminution or loss of enzymatic activity. Therefore, NO is capable of playing a regulatory function, either facilitating or inhibiting the activity of selected enzymes. Binding to heme also appears to be the primary mechanism of toxicity of NO. A constituent of polluted air, NO can be inhaled into the lungs where it can bind to the heme of hemoglobin, thus inhibiting its ability to carry oxygen.

SYNTHESIS OF NITRIC OXIDE

NO is the product of a multistep reaction catalyzed by what is now recognized as a family of NO synthase (NOS) isoenzymes.[4] These enzymes are flavoproteins that contain bound flavin mononucleotide and flavin adenine dinucleotide. Critical cofactors for enzymatic activity include reduced nicotinamide adenine dinucleotide phosphate (NADPH) and tetrahydrobiopterin. The nitrogen of NO is derived from the terminal guanidino moiety of L-arginine, and the oxygen in NO is incorporated from molecular oxygen. The byproduct of this reaction is L-citrulline (Fig. 32-1). The precise biosynthetic pathway is not clear, but hydroxyarginine seems to be a key intermediate.

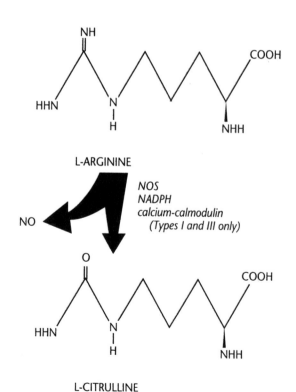

Fig. 32-1 A schematic diagram of the conversion of L-arginine to NO and L-citrulline, catalyzed by NOS. NO, nitric oxide; NOS, nitric oxide synthese.

Nitric Oxide Synthase

Originally, NOS was divided into two types, constitutive or inducible, based on the mode of enzyme activation.[4] The constitutive form of NOS (cNOS) is found in the vascular endothelium and central nervous system (CNS), among other places. cNOS is continuously active at a basal level and provides spontaneous production and release of NO. Its enzymatic activity is calcium- and calmodulin-dependent because increased intracellular calcium levels can increase cNOS activity, rapidly enhancing NO production; accordingly, cNOS activity is inhibited by calcium chelating agents or calmodulin antagonists.[11] Picomolar quantities of NO are released in bursts for short periods following stimulation of the vascular endothelium. The NO released in this way acts as a transduction mechanism underlying various physiologic processes, including endothelium-dependent vasodilation, and as a mechanism of neurotransmission in the CNS.

The inducible form of NOS (iNOS) is found in macrophages but is also known to occur in the vascular endothelium and various other cell types. This NOS activity is relatively quiescent until induced by cytokines and γ-interferon. Unlike cNOS, iNOS is so closely coupled to calmodulin that enzyme activity is not influenced by changes in intracellular concentrations of calcium ion.[12] Also unlike cNOS, protein synthesis is required for the expression of iNOS, which makes it susceptible to suppression by anti-inflammatory glucocorticoids. The induction of NOS may take 15 to 18 hours, and the activated macrophage will continue to release nanomolar amounts of NO for more prolonged periods (20 to 30 hours) after induction. Whereas cNOS is active as a monomer, the iNOS from macrophages appears to be active only as a dimer.

A more recent classification, however, lists three distinct types of NOS (Table 32-4). In this system, iNOS or macrophage NOS is labeled type II NOS. cNOS is further divided into two types, based on the cytosolic or particulate localization of the enzyme in the cell. Type I NOS (cytosolic) is exemplified by the enzyme found in brain neurons; type III NOS (particulate) is found primarily in the vascular endothelium.

The two types of cNOS appear to be otherwise

Table 32-4 Comparative Characteristics of the Three Types of NOS

Characteristic	Type I	Type II	Type III
Isoform of enzyme	Constitutive (cNOS)	Inducible (iNOS)	Constitutive (cNOS)
Trivial name	Brain NOS	Macrophage NOS	Endothelial NOS
Location in cell	Usually cytosolic	Usually cytosolic	Usually particulate
Cofactors	NADPH, FAD/FMN, BH_4	NADPH, FAD/FMN, BH_4	NADPH, FAD/FMN, BH_4
Mode of regulation	Ca^{++}/calmodulin	Transcription after cell is stimulated by endotoxins/cytokines; calcium independent	Ca^{++}/calmodulin
Production and release of NO	Picomolar quantities of NO for short periods after enzyme activation	Nanomolar quantities of NO for prolonged periods after enzyme induction	Picomolar quantities of NO for short periods after enzyme activation
Localization in body	Brain neurons Vascular endothelium Blood platelets Adrenal glands NANC nerves Macula densa of kidney Pulmonary tissue Gastrointestinal tract	Macrophages Neutrophils Fibroblasts Lymphocytes Chrondrocytes Megakaryocytes Hepatocytes Vascular endothelium	Vascular endothelium

Abbreviations: BH_4, tetrahydrobiopterin; FAD, flavin adenine dinucleotide; FMN, flavin mononucleotide; NADPH, reduced nicotinamide adenine dinucleotide phosphate; NANC, nonadrenergic noncholinergic; NO, nitric oxide; NOS, nitric oxide synthase.

closely related, if not identical. Rat cerebellar NOS was isolated and purified.[13] This permitted the raising of antisera against brain NOS for immunohistochemical localization studies. Brain and endothelial forms of NOS were both recognized by this brain cNOS-specific antiserum, and their distribution in the CNS and periphery was characterized. NOS protein which was purified to homogeneity from rat cerebellum, was cloned and expressed. The amino acid sequence of brain NOS was proved to be closely homologous to that of cytochrome P-450 reductase.[14]

Macrophage NOS was not labeled by the brain NOS antiserum, which is not surprising because this enzyme is inducible and its activity is not dependent on calcium. Macrophage NOS has also been cloned, expressed, and characterized.[15,16] Despite its differences from cNOS, macrophage NOS also shares a close homology with cNOS and cytochrome P-450 reductase.[17] Purified iNOS from neutrophils differs from macrophage, brain, and endothelial NOS in requiring calcium but not calmodulin.[18]

NADPH diaphorase has been identified as a

NOS enzyme.[19] Although the biologic function of NADPH diaphorase was unknown, it was long recognized that neurons containing this enzyme were darkly stained by the dye tetrazolium. Capitalizing on the ability of tetrazolium to stain NADPH diaphorase-containing neurons, the distributions of NOS immunoreactivity and NADPH diaphorase staining were localized to virtually identical sites in the CNS and periphery.[20] Further in situ hybridization studies reinforced the idea that these enzymes are closely associated.[14]

Recent evidence suggests that, consistent with other neurotransmitters, NO may be capable of self-regulating its own synthesis by modulating the activity of NOS. Both neuronal cNOS and macrophage-derived iNOS appear to be subject to a negative feedback inhibition by NO itself,[21] although cNOS appears to be more sensitive to such endproduct inhibition than is iNOS.[22] Inhibition of NOS by NO may be irreversible,[21] but whether NO binds directly to the heme of NOS (as it does other metalloenzymes) or by some other mechanism remains to be determined.

Most of the physiologic effects of NO are presently attributed to binding of NO to iron-containing proteins. By coupling to iron, NO can activate or inhibit the enzymatic activity of metalloenzymes. The most widely investigated example is the activation of soluble guanylate cyclase by NO, resulting in an increase in the intracellular second messenger cyclic GMP.

Nitric Oxide Synthase Inhibitors

Elucidation of the synthetic pathway for NO was greatly facilitated by studying the tumoricidal activity of macrophages. The presence of cytotoxic nitrates and nitrites produced by immunologically activated macrophages is determined by the amount of L-arginine in the medium, citrulline being a coproduct.[2] An analog of L-arginine, N^G-monomethyl-L-arginine (L-NMMA), but not its D-isomer, enhanced microbial growth and simultaneously reduced levels of nitrites, nitrates, and citrulline generated by activated macrophages.[23] L-NMMA competitively inhibits the conversion of L-arginine to NO and L-citrulline (Fig. 32-2).

The recognition of L-NMMA as a potent selective inhibitor of NOS has given rise to a host of related compounds that have become widely used in studying the biologic significance of NO (Fig. 32-3). The major criterion today for establishing an involvement of the L-arginine-NO pathway in a particular physiologic, pathophysiologic, or pharmacologic process is largely based on the response to the inhibition of NO production and the stereoselective reversal of inhibition by L-arginine. L-NMMA, N^G-nitro-L-arginine (L-NOARG), N^G-nitro-L-arginine methyl ester (L-NAME), and N-iminoethyl-L-ornithine (L-NIO) are qualitatively similar in inhibiting endothelial NOS in vivo and in vitro; their quantitative differences are attributed to differences in uptake, distribution, and breakdown.[4] L-NIO is reportedly the most potent of these inhibitors. In vitro assays comparing different arginine analogs show L-NOARG to be the most selective in inhibiting brain and endothelial forms of NOS.[25] A new agent, aminoguanidine, was introduced as a selective inhibitor of iNOS.[26]

Other Nitric Oxide Investigative Drugs

There are other useful investigative tools in the pharmacologic arsenal. The production or facilitation of a NO-mediated response is one tack, but this is dependent on whether the role of NO is critical in the mediation of the response or merely modulates its expression. L-arginine has been used to increase NO levels, but whether plasma levels of L-arginine are indeed rate limiting in regard to the synthesis of NO is questionable. Alternatively, NO-like or NO-generating drugs should mimic the effects of NO but not be sensitive to blockade by NOS inhibitors. One such drug is S-nitrosocysteine, which is considered by some investigators to be the actual EDRF rather than NO.[27] Time-honored vasodilators, now called nitrovasodilators, including such drugs as sodium nitroprusside and nitroglycerin, are now known to produce NO by simple dissociation. Newer NO donors include sydnonimine-1, the active metabolite of milsidomine;

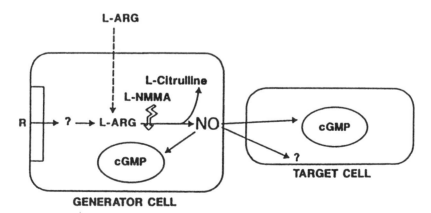

Fig. 32-2 A schematic diagram of the L-arginine-NO pathway. Question marks indicate areas requiring clarification. (From Moncada et al.,[24] with permission.)

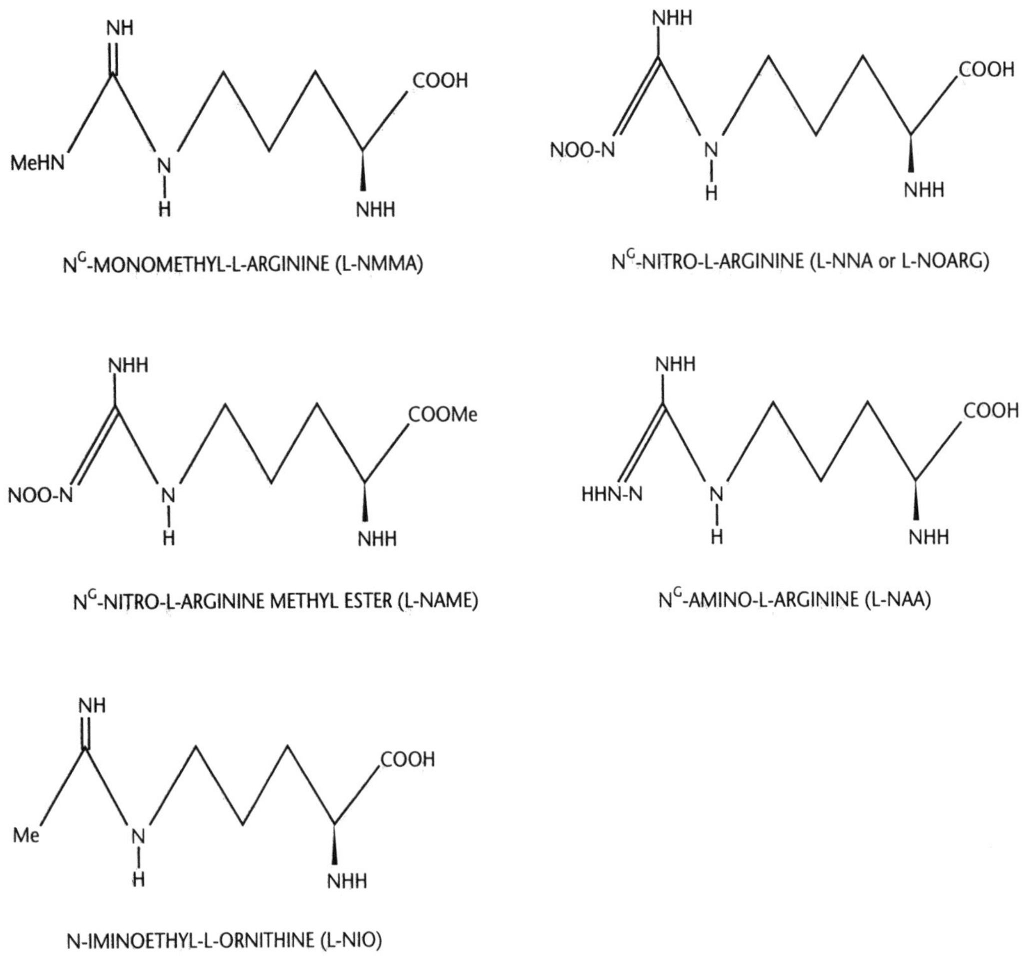

Fig. 32-3 Chemical structures of arginine analogs that can inhibit NOS. NOS, nitric oxide synthase.

S-nitroso-N-acetylpenicillamine, which releases NO in the presence of oxygen; and hydroxylamine, which is metabolized to NO by neuronal enzymes.[28]

Other experimental drugs can influence NO-mediated effects at other points in the L-arginine-NO-cyclic GMP system. Antagonism by hemoglobin, a natural protein scavenger of NO,[29] is generally accepted as evidence of extracellular transit by NO. If the result is mediated by cyclic GMP, antagonism and potentiation of the NO effect will be produced by inhibitors of soluble guanylate cyclase, such as methylene blue,[30] or inhibitors of cyclic GMP phosphodiesterase.[31]

FUNCTIONS IN THE PERIPHERY

Endothelium-Dependent Vasodilation

NO is required to produce acetylcholine-induced vasodilation.[32] In aortic strips in which the endothelium was inadvertently rubbed off, acetylcholine did not evoke its expected relaxant response. Other preparations that retained at least a portion of the original endothelium readily relaxed in response to acetylcholine. Such observations led to the conclusion that acetylcholine might not act directly on the vascular smooth muscle itself, but perhaps, it might act on the endothelium, causing it to release some substance actually responsible for the vasodilation.[33] Accordingly, this substance was termed EDRF.

In addition to acetylcholine, other vasodilators appear to share the same dependence on an intact endothelium; these include muscarinic receptor agonists, hydralazine, serotonin, adenosine triphosphate, and adenosine diphosphate, selected peptides (such as bradykinin and substance P), and the calcium ionophore A23187 (calcimycin).[33,34] However, the vascular endothelium is not a universal requirement for all vasodilators. An endothelium-*independent* relaxation is produced by other drugs and endogenous substances such as β_2-adrenergic agonists, calcium channel blockers, papaverine, selected eicosanoids (prostacyclin), and nitrovasodilators (sodium nitroprusside, nitroglycerin, and isosorbide dinitrate).

A close correlation between elevated cyclic GMP levels and the relaxation of vascular smooth muscle cells was previously recognized.[35] Research into the mechanism of vasodilatation evoked by nitrovasodilators showed that these drugs break down and yield nitrosothiol byproducts, which in turn, generate NO.[36] Nitrovasodilators were also shown to inhibit the aggregation of blood platelets, another cyclic GMP-mediated process.[37] When NO was also found to be capable of stimulating guanylate cyclase and elevating cellular cyclic GMP levels in vascular smooth muscle to cause vasodilatation[38] and in blood platelets to inhibit aggregation,[39] these previously separate lines of research converged. Endothelial cells produced NO, and the quantities released were sufficient to account for the relaxation of adjacent vascular smooth muscle cells.[39] Furchgott[40] and Ignarro et al.[41] independently proposed that EDRF was, in fact, NO. Although EDRF and NO were demonstrated to share virtually identical chemical characteristics and pharmacologic properties,[3,42] some investigators maintain that EDRF may not be NO itself but possibly an unstable nitroso derivative, such as S-nitrosocysteine.[43]

Vasodilatation is the typical physiologic response to acetylcholine (released from parasympathetic nerve terminals) and circulating bradykinin (Fig. 32-4). Acetylcholine and bradykinin act on specific receptors on the surface of endothelial cells to trigger synthesis of EDRF/NO from L-arginine. NO is released from the endothelial cell and diffuses into underlying smooth muscle cells. NO binds with high affinity to the heme of guanylate cyclase and activates the enzyme. The resulting increase in intracellular cyclic GMP stimulates a cyclic GMP-dependent protein kinase, which leads to protein phosphorylation and the relaxation of vascular smooth muscle. Although there are multiple forms of guanylate cyclase, only the soluble heme-containing enzyme is sensitive to activation by NO.[44] It is also critical to point out that soluble guanylate cyclase may not be the only "receptor" for NO; it is merely the most extensively studied of probably a wide range of metalloenzymes that interact with NO.

The question arises as to whether NO is important in the regulation of vascular tone and blood pressure. Systemic and oral treatment with various NOS inhibitors can cause an elevation in the blood pressure of experimental animals, suggesting that a basal release of NO may help to regulate vascular tone.[45] There is evidence of altered endothelium-dependent vasodilatation in hypertension, diabetes, atherosclerosis, and other disease states.[46] It appears that NO participates in homeostatic control of the cardiovascular system, but whether this is solely dependent on endothelium-derived NO is not clear. The resolution of this issue is likely to be complicated by the involvement of NO in the regulation of catecholamine release from the sympathetic nervous system[47] and by the participation of NO in central cardiovascular control.[48]

Nonspecific Immunity

NO is thought to be a critical component of the defense mechanism against invading microbes and other foreign organisms that are too large to be phagocytosed.[2] Macrophages in culture exposed to bacterial endotoxin and γ-interferon become immunologically activated and increase their production of nitrite and nitrate. The involvement of these reactive nitrogen intermediates in the cytotoxic effects of activated macrophages was deduced from the apparent inverse correlation between the output of nitrites and nitrates and susceptibility to infection. Subsequent study showed that macrophage production of nitrite and nitrate was depen-

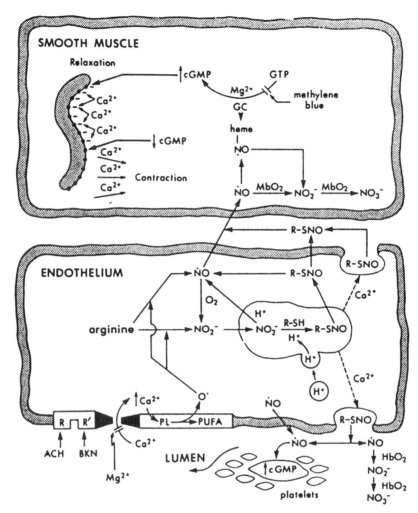

Fig. 32-4 Possible mechanisms for the formation, release, action, and inactivation of endothelium-derived NO (EDNO). NO formation from L-arginine is triggered by oxygen radicals or other products of calcium-dependent phospholipid metabolism, which in turn, is triggered by endothelium-dependent vasodilators interacting with selective receptors at the endothelial cell surface. Arginine may be converted to NO or to nitrate, which in turn, is stored in acidic vesicles and converted to a stabilized form of NO. The release of NO from endothelial cells may occur by diffusion or by secretion of a more stable form of NO that spontaneously liberates NO at neutral pH. NO is rapidly inactivated by oxidation to inorganic nitrite and nitrate in the presence of oxyhemoglobin or oxymyoglobin. NO causes vascular smooth muscle relaxation and inhibition of platelet adhesion by activating soluble guanylate cyclase by heme-dependent mechanisms, thereby elevating intracellular cyclic GMP levels. Cyclic GMP elicits its biologic effects by lowering the intracellular concentration of free calcium. ACH, acetylcholine; BKN, bradykinin; cGMP, cyclic GMP; EDNO, endothelium-derived NO; GC, soluble guanylate cyclase; HbO_2, oxyhemoglobin; MbO_2, oxymyoglobin; NO, nitric oxide radical; O˙, oxygen radical. PL, phospholipid; PUFA, polyunsaturated fatty acid; R, muscarinic receptor; R′, bradykinin receptor; R-SH, thiol; R-SNO, S-nitrosothiol. (From Ignarro,[3] with permission.)

dent on L-arginine and that L-citrulline was a co-product.

The elucidation of the L-arginine-NO pathway in the vascular endothelium resulted in the identification of NO as the most likely source of nitrite and nitrate from activated macrophages. Currently, it is thought that endotoxin induces NOS in macrophages and increases production of NO. The activated macrophages produce NO, which kills microbes by inhibiting iron-containing respiratory enzymes. Interference with NO production by the removal of arginine from the incubation medium or by the addition of substituted arginines that inhibit NOS interferes with the cytotoxic actions of macrophages against a variety of microorganisms.

Neutrophils were also identified as a source of NO, but how this contributes to the defensive function of the neutrophil remains to be determined. There is suspicion that NO of neutrophil origin may react with superoxide anion to form super-toxic peroxynitrite that decomposes to hydroxide free radical and NO_2 (nitrogen dioxide), both of which are cytotoxic.[49]

Nonadrenergic Noncholinergic Neurotransmission

Inhibitory nonadrenergic noncholinergic (NANC) nerves constitute a portion of the peripheral autonomic nerves that innervate the gastrointestinal tract. The transmitter released by these nerves has been sought for more than three decades. NO is now considered a likely candidate. NO fulfills many of the classic criteria for establishing a substance as a neurochemical transmitter,[5] that is, (1) NO production in gastrointestinal tract neurons, as shown by the immunohistochemical localization of NOS; (2) antagonism of the inhibitory effects of NANC nerve stimulation by arginine analogs that block NO synthesis; (3) restoration of the inhibitory effects by L-arginine but not D-arginine; (4) NO release by NANC nerve stimulation, as demonstrated by bioassay; and (5) exogenously applied NO mimicking the effects of NANC nerve stimulation. Moreover, oxyhemoglobin, which binds to NO, can block the effects of exogenously administered NO and NANC nerve stimulation.

Another structure innervated by NANC nerves is the corpus cavernosum, the relaxation of which produces penile erection. Electrical stimulation of strips of corpus cavernosum increases NO and cyclic GMP levels[50] and induces relaxation of the muscle, an effect that is abolished by NOS inhibitors.[51,52] Immunohistochemical studies found NOS in rat penile neurons that innervate the corpus cavernosum.[51]

FUNCTIONS IN THE CENTRAL NERVOUS SYSTEM

Glutamate Neurotransmission

Excitatory amino acid neurotransmitters have been studied extensively; foremost among these is glutamate. Glutamate receptors linked to ion channels have been divided into N-methyl-D-aspartate (NMDA) receptors (see Ch. 16) and non-NMDA receptors, which are further subdivided into kainate and α-amino-3-hydroxy-5-methyl-isoxazole-4-propionate receptors.[53] NMDA receptors appear to govern calcium influx; non-NMDA receptors control sodium and potassium influx. Activation of the NMDA receptor increased intracellular levels of cyclic GMP in the cerebellar cortex; however, the increase in intracellular cyclic GMP did not occur in the same neurons that were stimulated by glutamate.[54] Highly reminiscent of the mechanism by which acetylcholine elevated cyclic GMP in vascular smooth muscle cells, it was strongly implied that there was an intercellular messenger involved.

Earlier studies suggested the existence of an endogenous activator of soluble guanylate cyclase in rat brain that was inhibited by hemoglobin.[55] The endogenous activator was subsequently identified as L-arginine, but another soluble factor was also implicated.[56] NMDA-induced elevations in cyclic GMP in the cerebellum were potentiated by superoxide dismutase and inhibited by hemoglobin.[57] A factor produced by NMDA-stimulated cerebellar cells caused relaxation of vascular smooth muscle, which was reminiscent of EDRF[6] The cyclic GMP response to NMDA receptor activation was also enhanced by L-arginine but not by D-arginine. This response was inhibited by L-NMMA, and stereospecific reversal of this inhibition by L-arginine indicated that the mysterious factor was NO.

In a current view of NO involvement in glutamate neurotransmission (Fig. 32-5),[54,57] neuronally

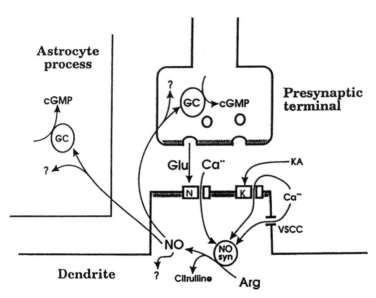

Fig. 32-5 A proposed mechanism for the synthesis and action of NO in the rat cerebellum. GC, guanylate cyclase; Glu, glutamate; KA, kainate; K, kainate receptor; N, NMDA receptor; NO syn, NO synthase; VSCC, voltage-sensitive Ca^{++} channel. (From Collier and Vallance,[58] with permission).

released glutamine can stimulate postsynaptic NMDA and non-NMDA receptors. As exemplified by mossy fiber-granule cell synapses in the cerebellum, low-frequency transmission activates non-NMDA receptors, and high-frequency transmission stimulates NMDA receptors. The latter receptors, after they are activated, mediate an influx of calcium ion, which in turn, activates cNOS. NO acts as a retrograde messenger to stimulate the production of cyclic GMP by soluble guanylate cyclase in the presynaptic nerve terminal and in adjacent astrocytes. The physiologic consequences of this NO-induced elevation in neuronal and glial cyclic GMP await further characterization; however, the presence of this L-arginine-NO-cyclic GMP system suggests some regulatory role.

Synaptic Plasticity

CNS neurons are capable of modifying their synaptic connections, a process called synaptic plasticity. Synaptic transmission and neuronal excitability can be either enhanced (long-term potentiation, LTP) or reduced (long-term depression, LTD) in response to a brief conditioning stimulus of high frequency; the alteration may persist long after the initial stimulus.

There has been great interest in LTP in particular. LTP in the CA1 region of the hippocampus is associated with learning and memory formation. This process is known to involve NMDA receptors and is also dependent on calcium and calmodulin. It was also suspected that synaptic plasticity must involve a retrograde messenger that mediates postsynaptic to presynaptic communication. NO is a prime candidate for retrograde diffusion across the synapse for the purpose of regulating presynaptic neuronal activity.[59]

Inhibition of NO production by L-NMMA resulted in the blockade of LTP in the hippocampus[60,61] and also of LTD in the cerebellum[62]; this inhibition was reversed by L-arginine but not D-arginine.[61] The NOS inhibitor, L-NAME, induced learning deficits in experimental animals.[63] NO donors enhance LTP.[61] Such findings strongly imply a role for endogenous NO in synaptic plasticity. However, the actual presynaptic action of NO remains to be determined.

Neurotoxicity

Excessive amounts of the excitatory neurotransmitter, glutamate, can produce neurotoxicity, which is mediated by NMDA receptors. Glutamate is thought to be involved in the neuronal degeneration associated with diseases such as Alzheimer's dementia, Parkinson's disease, Huntington's disease,[64] and acquired immunodeficiency syndrome.[65] NOS is central to glutamate neurotoxicity.[66] The potential for NO-induced toxicity was already seen in the role of NO in nonspecific immunity against various microorganisms and tumor cells.

A NMDA receptor-mediated calcium influx activates NOS and increases NO production (Fig. 32-6). NO is either itself directly toxic or reacts with superoxide anion to form toxic free radicals by way of an intermediate, peroxynitrite. Glutamate neurotoxicity is attenuated by NOS inhibitors, hemoglobin, and superoxide dismutase.[66]

Paradoxically, the neurons that produce NO appear to be resistant to the neurotoxic effects of NO.[67,68] One possibility is that the NADPH diaphorase portion of the NOS enzyme may play a protective role. Another possibility is that NOS-containing cells may contain high levels of manganese superoxide dismutase. Whatever the mechanism, NO is not toxic to the cells that elaborate it.

Pain

Chronic pain may represent a type of synaptic plasticity. There are parallels between LTP and hyperalgesia.[69] Both continue for sustained periods following high frequency afferent input. Both are thought to be mediated by NMDA receptor stimulation. NMDA facilitates LTP and thermal reflexes. Selective blockers of the NMDA receptor can reduce LTP without affecting normal synaptic activity and can similarly reverse hyperalgesia to a thermal stimulus without affecting normal thermal reflexes.

NO appears to be a mediator of hyperalgesia. High- but not low-frequency stimulation of the spinal cord activates NMDA receptors, resulting in increased intracellular calcium ion and increased production of NO, which mediates the hyperalgesia.[69] NMDA-induced hyperalgesia is blocked by L-NAME, methylene blue, and hemoglobin; these same pretreatments did not affect normal nociceptive responsiveness.[70,71] Treatment with L-arginine, but not D-arginine, caused a rapid transient dose-dependent thermal hyperalgesia reminiscent

of the NMDA-induced hyperalgesia.[71] These findings suggest that NO may play a similar role in the mechanisms of NMDA-induced hyperalgesia in the spinal cord and of NMDA-induced elevation in cerebellar cyclic GMP.

Consequently, drugs that interfere with the synthesis and actions of NO might be effective analgesic drugs. L-NAME applied topically onto the spinal cord reduced the response induced by acute electrical stimulation and prolonged chemical stimulation.[72] The expression of *fos* (a transcription factor regulating gene expression) by noxious stimulation was also effectively suppressed by intrathecal administration of L-NAME.[73]

The NOS inhibitors L-NOARG, L-NAME, and 7-nitro indazole (7-NI) are all effective in producing analgesia in experimental animals.[74–76] This analgesic effect is directly related to the inhibition of NO synthesis and involves adrenoceptors and serotonergic receptors[77] but is apparently independent of opioid mechanisms.[75,77] The 7-NI-induced analgesia occurred without an alteration of the blood pressure, suggesting that 7-NI might be selective for brain NOS.[76]

Analgesia

Although NO promotes hyperalgesia in the spinal cord, it mediates analgesia at sensory afferent nerve endings. Such paradoxic actions of NO reinforce the concept that NO is endowed with multiple and complex regulatory functions throughout the body. Inhibition of NOS production can antagonize either peripherally or centrally mediated analgesia. Drugs that enhance NO activity, such as NO donors or L-arginine, can produce or facilitate analgesic responses.

Activation of the L-arginine-NO-cyclic GMP system was demonstrated to produce analgesia in inflammatory states.[31] Prostaglandin E_2 (PGE$_2$) produces hyperalgesia by sensitization of nerve endings, accompanied by elevation in intracellular cyclic adenosine monophosphate (AMP) and calcium ions. Acetylcholine antagonizes PGE$_2$ by elevating cyclic GMP in the nerve endings. Hence, the sensitivity of sensory afferent nerve endings is determined by the balance between cyclic AMP and cyclic GMP. The hyperalgesic effect of PGE$_2$ is also blocked by sodium nitroprusside and methylene

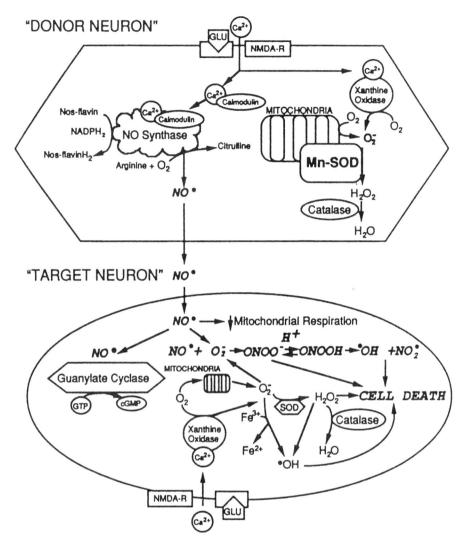

Fig. 32-6 NO as a neurotoxin. Excessive NO is formed during sustained glutamate stimulation of NMDA-R. NO freely diffuses to adjacent target neurons where it combines with O_2^- produced by mitochondria and xanthine oxidase to yield the $ONOO^-$, which is an extremely potent oxidant. $ONOO^-$ is protonated and decomposes to the OH free radical and the NO_2 free radical, both of which are potent activators of lipid peroxidation. Although NO can function as a toxin directly, by inhibiting mitochrondrial respiration by the inhibition of iron and sulfur-containing enzymes, the $ONOO^-$ pathway may be the major pathway of cell death because superoxide dismutase attenuates NMDA neurotoxicity. NOS (donor) neurons function as "killer neurons" and possess "factors" that allow them to survive in an environment rich in NO. The diaphorase portion of the NOS enzyme may play such a protective role. In addition, these neurons are enriched in Mn-SOD, which could prevent the formation of the peroxynitrite anion, allowing these cells to survive. Mn-SOD, manganese superoxide dismutase; NMDA, N-methyl-D-aspartate; NMDA-R, NMDA receptors; NO, nitric oxide; NO_2, nitrogen dioxide; NOS, NO synthase; O_2^-, superoxide anion; OH, hydroxyl; $ONOO^-$, peroxynitrite. (From Dawson,[66] with permission.)

blue and enhanced by the inhibition of cyclic GMP phosphodiesterase. The analgesic effect of cholinergic drugs, but not sodium nitroprusside, was blocked by L-NMMA. Peripherally acting analgesic drugs, such as cholinergic agents and selected nonnarcotic drugs (myrcene and dipyrone) are hypothesized to work through the NO-cyclic GMP system to down regulate hyperreactive nociceptors in inflammatory hyperalgesia. The effectiveness of sodium nitroprusside in the reversal of PGE_2-induced hyperalgesia led to the hypothesis that NO donors could be analgesic drugs. Topically applied nitroglycerin has analgesic effects in humans.[78]

The central analgesic effect of cholinergic agents is also mediated by the L-arginine-NO-cyclic GMP system. As is the case peripherally, central cholinergic analgesia is antagonized by NOS inhibition and methylene blue.[79,80] By comparison, the analgesic effect of morphine was blocked by methylene blue, but not by NOS inhibition, and was potentiated by inhibition of cyclic GMP phosphodiesterase. NO donors also induce an analgesic effect that is antagonized by methylene blue. However, the guanylate cyclase activity required for morphine analgesia may not be stimulated by NO derived from L-arginine.

In spite of such results, other evidence indicates that certain opioid receptor-mediated analgesic responses involve the L-arginine-NO-cyclic GMP system. L-arginine was reported to potentiate β-endorphin analgesia; this potentiation was reversed by inhibition of NOS.[81] Because it was shown that β-endorphin acting on ε-opioid receptors stimulated the release of methionine-enkephalin in the spinal cord[82] and because L-arginine did not potentiate the analgesic effects of other opioid drugs,[83] it was suggested that NO can selectively modulate a ε-opioid analgesic pathway.

The analgesic effect of N_2O was attributed to stimulated release of endogenous opioid peptides that stimulate central opioid receptors.[84] N_2O analgesia is sensitive to antagonism by the NOS inhibitors L-NOARG, L-NAME, and L-NMMA; this antagonism of N_2O analgesia was stereoselectively reversed by L-arginine.[85,86] Because NOS inhibition does not antagonize the analgesic effects of morphine and other direct acting opioid agonists, NO may be involved in the mechanism of neuronal release of endogenous opioid peptides by analgesic drugs, such as N_2O and β-endorphin, the analgesic action of which depends on the release of central opioid peptides.

Anesthesia

The possible role of NMDA and NO in general anesthesia is being widely investigated. Inhibition of NMDA transmission was found to reduce the minimum alveolar concentration for halothane anesthesia in experimental animals.[87] The relationship between NMDA receptors and NO naturally led to suspicion that NO might underlie certain aspects of anesthesia. Inhibition of NO synthesis by L-NAME reportedly causes a dose-related reduction in the minimum alveolar concentration for halothane anesthesia; this effect was stereospecifically reversed by L-arginine.[88] A disruption of NO activity appears to decrease the level of consciousness and augment anesthesia.

This is supported by evidence that halothane and other inhalational anesthetic agents can interfere with NO production in brain tissue[89] and the vascular endothelium.[90] Intravenous anesthetics, such as pentobarbital and ketamine, lack this effect.[89] Halothane and enflurane also decrease cyclic GMP levels in a variety of brain regions.[91] In addition, halothane can influence synaptic transmission by L-glutamate-stimulated cortical neurons[92] and NMDA-stimulated hippocampal neurons.[93] Based on these observations, inhibition of the L-arginine-NO-cyclic GMP pathway in the CNS may be a contributory factor to anesthesia.

Anxiolysis

Benzodiazepines are important in anesthesiology for the suppression of preoperative anxiety, among other applications. Inhibition of NO production with L-NOARG antagonized the anxiolytic effects of chlordiazepoxide; this antagonistic effect was reversed by L-arginine, but not D-arginine, thus implicating NO in the mechanism of anxiolysis.[94] N_2O, which is widely used in dentistry for inducing conscious sedation, evokes behavioral effects identical to those produced by benzodiazepines in various animal models of anxiety.[95] These effects of N_2O are apparently mediated by benzodiazepine receptors because they are reduced in the presence of a benzodiazepine antagonist or benzodiazepine tolerance. These benzodiazepine-like effects of N_2O are likewise sensitive to antagonism by L-NOARG, that is reversible by L-arginine.[96]

CLINICAL APPLICATIONS

There are important clinical ramifications of NO in the study of physiology, pathophysiology, and pharmacology. Some of these are applicable to anesthesiology.[97,98] Currently, there are several realized or expected clinical applications of drugs that can influence the L-arginine-NO pathway.

Nitric Oxide

The first clinical application of NO was as a pulmonary vasodilator. When inhaled, NO has the same pharmacologic activity as EDRF. It rapidly diffuses into the pulmonary vasculature, activates guanylate cyclase, and stimulates synthesis of cyclic GMP, resulting in smooth muscle relaxation. The high affinity of NO for hemoglobin results in virtually complete binding of NO in the pulmonary circulation, thus preventing systemic vasodilation. Consequently, inhalation of NO produces a selective reversible dose-dependent vasodilation of the pulmonary vasculature. This has been demonstrated in experimental animals[99] and human subjects.[100,101] A brief (10-minute) inhalation of NO was reported to reduce pulmonary vascular resistance in patients with primary pulmonary hypertension.[101,102] Inhalation of NO for up to 24 hours rapidly and significantly improved oxygenation in babies with severe hypoxemia from persistent pulmonary hypertension of the newborn.[103–105] The therapeutic efficacy of NO in other pulmonary disorders, such as adult respiratory distress syndrome, remains to be seen.[98]

NO inhalation is not without risk because high levels of NO react with oxygen to form toxic oxides of nitrogen that can damage tissues and cause methemoglobinemia, asphyxia, and death.[106] Low concentrations of NO react more slowly, reducing the production of toxic products. Studies of long-term administration of NO inhalation remain to be done.

Nitric Oxide Synthase Inhibitors

Overproduction of NO may be a contributing factor to various pathologic conditions. There is strong evidence that excessive NO may play a key role in septic shock, which is characterized by hypotension and by reduced responsiveness to vasoconstrictor drugs.[107] When administered in an experimental model of endotoxic shock, low doses of L-NMMA prevented the hypotension and lowered plasma levels of nitrate and nitrite. Higher doses of L-NMMA transiently improved the blood pressure and then caused a sustained hypotension, accompanied by signs of tissue damage and increased mortality rates.[108] Hence, excessive NO is suspected of mediating dual effects, prolonged and detrimental vasodilatation and the salubrious effect of counteracting sepsis-related vasoconstrictor mediators and preventing thrombogenesis.

Treatment with L-NMMA was reported to reduce the hypotension induced in experimental animals by tumor necrosis factor[109] and bacterial endotoxin.[110] Treatment with L-NAME significantly reduced the mortality rate associated with anaphylaxis induced in mice by an antigen or by a mast cell degranulator.[111] In a clinical study, L-NMMA, a nonselective inhibitor of NOS, increased the blood pressure and reduced the need for vasoconstrictor therapy in one patient with severe sepsis.[112] In the same study, a second septic patient was treated with L-NAME, which is more selective for cNOS than iNOS; the patient initially improved then deteriorated and died. It would appear that iNOS is readily inducible in sepsis and that NO is intimately involved in the pathogenesis of septic shock. A practical application of NOS inhibitors in sepsis, anaphylaxis, and related states may depend on the development of drugs with greater selectivity for iNOS.

Glucocorticoids

The glucocorticoids are drugs long used in medicine for their ability to suppress inflammation and maintain the integrity of the cardiovascular system; yet, their mechanism of action remained unclear. The clinical efficacy of glucocorticoids in the treatment of endotoxic shock, for instance, may be directly related to NO.[4,113] Macrophage NOS activity is dramatically increased following activation of macrophages by *Escherichia coli* lipopolysaccharide and γ-interferon, and it is evident that the increased production and release of NO underlies many of the signs of endotoxic shock. Unlike cNOS, macrophage NOS requires protein synthesis for its expression; this process is blocked by glucocorticoids, such as hydrocortisone and dexamethasone, while sparing cNOS. A direct correlation was demonstrated between the anti-inflammatory potency of steroid drugs and their potency in inhibiting NOS induction. The mechanisms of other drugs may also be shown to involve the L-arginine-NO system, similar to those of the glucocorticoids and nitrovasodilators.

REFERENCES

1. Lancaster JR, Jr: Nitric oxide in cells. Am Scientist 80:248, 1992
2. Nathan CF, Hibbs JB, Jr: Role of nitric oxide synthesis in macrophage antimicrobial activity. Curr Opin Immunol 3:65, 1991
3. Ignarro LJ: Endothelium-derived nitric oxide: actions and properties. FASEB J 3:31, 1989
4. Moncada S, Palmer RMJ, Higgs EA: Nitric oxide: physiology, pathophysiology, and pharmacology. Pharmacol Rev 43:109, 1991
5. Sanders KM, Ward SM: Nitric oxide as a mediator of nonadrenergic noncholinergic neurotransmission. Am J Physiol 262:G379, 1992
6. Garthwaite J, Charles SL, Chess-Williams R: Endothelium-derived relaxing factor release on activation of NMDA receptors suggests role as intercellular messenger in the brain. Nature 336:385, 1988
7. Bredt DS, Snyder SH: Nitric oxide, a novel neuronal messenger. Neuron 8:3, 1992
8. Culotta E, Koshland DE, Jr: NO news is good news. Science 258:1862, 1992
9. Archer S: Measurement of nitric oxide in biological models. FASEB J 7:349, 1993
10. Stamler JS, Singel DJ, Loscalzo J: Biochemistry of nitric oxide and its redox-activated forms. Science 258:1898, 1992
11. Bredt DS, Snyder SH: Isolation of nitrix oxide synthetase, a calmodulin-requiring enzyme. Proc Natl Acad Sci U S A 87:682, 1990
12. Cho HJ, Xie QW, Calaycay J et al: Calmodulin is a subunit of nitric oxide synthase from macrophages. J Exp Med 176:599, 1992
13. Bredt DS, Hwang PM, Snyder SH: Localization of nitric oxide synthase indicating a neural role for nitric oxide. Nature 347:768, 1990
14. Bredt DS, Hwang PM, Glatt CE et al: Cloned and expressed nitric oxide synthase structurally resembles cytochrome P-450 reductase. Nature 351:714, 1991
15. Xie Q, Cho HJ, Calaycay J et al: Cloning and characterization of inducible nitric oxide synthase from mouse macrophages. Science 256:225, 1992
16. Lowenstein CJ, Glatt CS, Bredt DS, Snyder SH: Cloned and expressed macrophage nitric oxide synthase contrasts with brain enzyme. Proc Natl Acad Sci U S A 89:6711, 1992
17. Lowenstein CJ, Snyder SH: Nitric oxide, a novel biologic messenger. Cell 70:705, 1992
18. Yui Y, Hattori R, Kosuga K et al: Calmodulin-independent nitric oxide synthase from rat polymorphonuclear neutrophils. J Biol Chem 266:12544, 1991
19. Hope BT, Michael GJ, Knigge KM, Vincent SR: Neuronal NADPH diaphorase is a nitric oxide synthase. Proc Natl Acad Sci U S A 88:2881, 1991
20. Dawson TM, Bredt DS, Fotuhi M et al: Nitric oxide synthase and neuronal NADPH diaphorase are identical in brain and peripheral tissues. Proc Natl Acad Sci U S A 88:7797, 1991
21. Assreuy J, Cunha FQ, Liew FY, Moncada S: Feedback inhibition of nitric oxide synthase activity by nitric oxide. Br J Pharmacol 108:833, 1993
22. Griscavage JM, Rogers NE, Sherman MP, Ignarro LJ: Negative feedback modulation of constitutive and inducible nitric oxide synthase by NO. FASEB J 7:A243, 1993
23. Hibbs JB, Jr, Vavrin Z, Taintor RR: L-Arginine is required for expression of the activated macrophage effector mechanism causing selective metabolic inhibition in target cells. J Immunol 138:550, 1987
24. Moncada S, Palmer RMJ, Higgs EA: Biosynthesis of nitric oxide from L-arginine. A pathway for the regulation of cell function and communication. Biochem Pharmacol 38:1709, 1989
25. Lambert LE, Whitten JP, Baron BM et al: Nitric oxide synthesis in the CNS, endothelium and macrophages differs in its sensitivity to inhibition by arginine analogues. Life Sci 48:69, 1991
26. Misko TP, Moore WM, Kasten TP et al: Selective inhibition of the inducible nitric oxide synthase by aminoguanidine. Eur J Pharmacol 233:119, 1993
27. Myers PR, Geurra R, Jr, Bates JN, Harrison DJ: Vasorelaxant properties of the endothelium-derived

relaxing factor more closely resemble S-nitrosocysteine than nitric oxide. Nature 345:161, 1990

28. Southam E, Garthwaite J: Comparable effects of some nitric oxide donors of cyclic GMP levels in rat cerebellar slices. Neurosci Lett 130:107, 1991

29. Martin W, Smith JA, White DG: The mechanisms by which haemoglobin inhibits the relaxation of rabbit aorta induced by nitrovasodilators, nitric oxide or bovine retractor penis inhibitory factor. Br J Pharmacol 89:562, 1986.

30. Gruetter CA, Gruetter DY, Lyon JE et al: Relationship between cyclic guanosine 3',5'-monophosphate formation and the relaxation of coronary arterial smooth muscle by glyceryl trinitrate, nitroprusside, nitrite and nitric oxide: effects of methylene blue and methemoglobin. J Pharmacol Exp Ther 219:181, 1981

31. Duarte IDG, Lorenzetti BB, Ferreira SH: Peripheral analgesia and activation of the nitric oxide-cyclic GMP pathway. Eur J Pharmacol 186:289, 1990

32. Furchgott RF, Zawadzki JV: The obligatory role of endothelial cells in the relaxation of arterial smooth muscle by acetylcholine. Nature 288:373, 1980

33. Furchgott RF: Role of endothelium in responses of vascular smooth muscle. Circ Res 53:557, 1983

34. Marin J, Sanchez-Ferrer CF: Role of endothelium-formed nitric oxide on vascular responses. Gen Pharmacol 21:575, 1990

35. Katsuki S, Murad F: Regulation of adenosine cyclic 3',5'-monophosphate levels and contractility in bovine tracheal smooth muscle. Mol Pharmacol 13:330, 1977

36. Ignarro LJ, Lippton H, Edwards JC et al: Mechanism of vascular smooth muscle relaxation by organic nitrates, nitrites, nitroprusside and nitric oxide: evidence for the involvement of S-nitrosothiols as active intermediates. J Pharmacol Exp Ther 218:739, 1981

37. Mellion BT, Ignarro LJ, Ohlstein EH et al: Evidence for the inhibitory role of cyclic GMP in ADP-induced human platelet aggregation in the presence of nitric oxide and related vasodilators. Blood 57:946, 1981

38. Gruetter CA, Barry BK, McNamara DB et al: Relaxation of bovine coronary artery and activation of coronary arterial guanylate cyclase by nitric oxide, nitroprusside and a carcinogenic nitrosoamine. J Cyclic Nucleotide Res 5:211, 1979

39. Palmer RMJ, Ferrige AG, Moncada S: Nitric oxide release accounts for the biological activity of endothelium-derived relaxing factor. Nature 327:524, 1987

40. Furchgott RF: Studies on relaxation of rabbit aorta by sodium nitrite: the basis for the proposal that the acid-activatable inhibitory factor from retractor penis is inorganic nitrite and the endothelium-derived relaxing factor is nitric oxide. p. 401. In Vanhoutte PM (ed): Vasodilatation: Vascular Smooth Muscle, Peptides, Autonomic Nerves and Endothelium. Raven Press, New York, 1988

41. Ignarro LJ, Byrns RE, Wood KS: Biochemical and pharmacological properties of endothelium-derived relaxing factor and its similarity to nitric oxide radicals. p. 427. In Vanhoutte PM (ed): Vasodilatation: Vascular Smooth Muscle, Peptides, Autonomic Nerves and Endothelium. Raven Press, New York, 1988

42. Moncada S, Radomski MW, Palmer RMJ: Endothelium-derived relaxing factor: identification as nitric oxide and role in the control of vascular tone and platelet function. Biochem Pharmacol 37:2495, 1988

43. Myers RR, Minor RL, Guerra R et al: Vasorelaxant properties of the endothelium-derived relaxing factor more closely resemble S-nitrocysteine than nitric oxide. Nature 365:161, 1990

44. Chinkers M, Garbers DL: Signal transduction by guanylyl cyclases. Annu Rev Biochem 60:553, 1991

45. Rees DD, Palmer RMJ, Moncada S: Role of endothelium-derived nitric oxide in the regulation of blood pressure. Proc Natl Acad Sci U S A 86:3375, 1989

46. Bassenge E: Clinical relevance of endothelium-derived relaxing factor (EDRF). Br J Clin Pharmacol 34:37S, 1992

47. Halbrugge T, Lutsch K, Thyen A, Graefe K-H: Role of nitric oxide formation in the regulation of haemodynamics and the release of noradrenaline and adrenaline. Naunyn Schmiedebergs Arch Pharmacol 344:720, 1991

48. Togashi H, Sakuma I, Yoshioka M et al: A central nervous system action of nitric oxide in blood pressure regulation. J Pharmacol Exp Ther 262:343, 1992

49. McCall TB, Boughton-Smith NK, Palmer RMJ, Moncada S: Synthesis of nitric oxide from L-arginine by neutrophils. Release and interaction with superoxide anion. Biochem J 261:293, 1989

50. Ignarro LJ, Bush PA, Buga GM et al: Nitric oxide and cyclic GMP formation upon electrical field stimulation can cause relaxation of corpus cavernosum smooth muscle. Biochem Biophys Res Commun 170:843, 1990

51. Burnett AL, Lowenstein CJ, Bredt DS et al: Nitric

oxide: a physiologic mediator of penile erection. Science 257:401, 1992

52. Rajfer J, Aronson WJ, Bush PA et al: Nitric oxide as a mediator of relaxation of the corpus cavernosum in response to nonadrenergic, noncholinergic neurotransmission. N Engl J Med 326:90, 1992

53. Monaghan DT, Bridges RJ, Cotman CW: The excitatory amino acid receptors: their classes, pharmacology, and distinct properties in the functions of the central nervous system. Annu Rev Pharmacol Toxicol 29:365, 1989

54. Garthwaite J: Glutamate, nitric oxide and cell-cell signalling in the nervous system. Trends Neurosci 14:60, 1991

55. Deguchi T: Endogenous activating factor for guanylate cyclase in synaptosomal-soluble fraction of rat brain. J Biol Chem 252:7617, 1977

56. Deguchi T, Yoshioka M: L-Arginine identified as an endogenous activator for soluble guanylate cyclase from neuroblastoma cells. J Biol Chem 257:10147, 1982

57. Garthwaite J: Nitric oxide synthesis linked to activation of excitatory neurotransmitter receptors in the brain. p. 115. In Moncada S, Higgs EA (eds): Nitrix Oxide From L-Arginine: A bioregulatory System. Elsevier Science Publishing, Amsterdam, 1990

58. Collier J, Vallance P: Second messenger role for NO widens to nervous and immune systems. Trends Pharmacol Sci 10:427, 1989

59. Gally JA, Montague PR, Reeke GN, Jr, Edelman GM: The NO hypothesis: possible effects of a short-lived, rapidly diffusable signal in the development and function of the nervous system. Proc Natl Acad Sci U S A 87:3547, 1990

60. Schuman EM, Madison DV: A requirement for the intercellular messenger nitric oxide in long-term potentiation. Science 254:1503, 1991

61. Bohme GA, Bon C, Stutzman JM et al: Possible involvement of nitric oxide in long-term potentiation. Eur J Pharmacol 199:379, 1991

62. Shibuki K, Okada D: Endogenous nitric oxide release required for long term synaptic depression in the cerebellum. Nature 349:326, 1991

63. Chapman PF, Atkins CM, Allen MT et al: Inhibition of nitric oxide synthesis impairs two different forms of learning. Neuroreport 3:567, 1992

64. Meldrum B, Garthwaite J: Excitatory amino acid neurotoxicity and neurodegenerative disease. Trends Pharmacol Sci 11:379, 1990

65. Lipton SA, Sucher NJ, Kaiser PK, Dreyer EB: Synergistic effects of HIV coat protein and NMDA receptor-mediated neurotoxicity. Neuron 7:111, 1991

66. Dawson TM, Dawson VL, Snyder SH: A novel neuronal messenger molecule in brain: the free radical, nitric oxide. Ann Neurol 32:297, 1992

67. Dawson VL, Dawson TM, London ED et al: Nitric oxide mediates glutamate neurotoxicity in primary cortical cultures. Proc Natl Acad Sci U S A 88:6368, 1991

68. Hyman BT, Marzloff K, Wenniger JJ et al: Relative sparing of nitric oxide synthase-containing neurons in the hippocampal formation in Alzheimer's disease. Ann Neurol 32:818, 1992

69. Meller ST, Gebhart GF: Nitric oxide and nociceptive processing in the spinal cord. Pain 52:127, 1993

70. Kitto KF, Haley JE, Wilcox GL: Involvement of nitric oxide in spinally mediated hyperalgesia in the mouse. Neurosci Lett 148:1, 1992

71. Meller ST, Dykstra C, Gebhart GF: Production of endogenous nitric oxide and activation of soluble guanylate cyclase are required for N-methyl-D-aspartate-produced facilitation of the nociceptive tail flick reflex. Eur J Pharmacol 214:93, 1992

72. Haley JE, Dickenson AH, Schacher M: Electrophysiological evidence for a role of nitric oxide in prolonged chemical nociception in the rat. Neuropharmacology 31:251, 1992

73. Lee J-H, Wilcox GL, Beitz AJ: Nitric oxide mediates *fos* expression in the spinal cord induced by mechanical noxious stimulation. Neuroreport 3:841, 1992

74. Hart SL, Oluyomi AO, Wallace P et al: L-N-^{G}-nitroarginine (L-NOARG), a selective inhibitor of nitric oxide biosynthesis exhibits anti-nociceptive activity in the mouse. Eur J Pharmacol 183:1440, 1990

75. Moore PK, Oluyomi AO, Babbedge RC et al: L-N^G-nitro arginine methyl ester exhibits antinociceptive activity in the mouse. Br J Pharmacol 102:198, 1991

76. Moore PK, Babbedge RC, Wallace P et al: 7-Nitroindazole, an inhibitor of nitric oxide synthase, exhibits anti-nociceptive activity in the mouse without increasing blood pressure. Br J Pharmacol 108:296, 1993

77. Mustafa AA: Mechanisms of L-N^G-nitroarginine methyl ester-induced antinociception in mice: a role for serotonergic and adrenergic neurons. Gen Pharmacol 23:1177, 1992

78. Ferreira SH, Lorenzetti BB, Facciolio LH: Blockade of hyperalgesia and neurogenic oedema by topical application of nitroglycerin. Eur J Pharmacol 217:207, 1992

79. Duarte IDG, Ferrira SH: The molecular mechanism of central analgesia induced by morphine or carbachol and the L-arginine-nitric oxide-cGMP pathway. Eur J Pharmacol 221:171, 1992

80. Iwamoto ET, Marion L: Nitric oxide mediates cholinergic antinociception in rats. FASEB J 7:A260, 1993

81. Tseng LF, Xu JY, Pieper GM: Increase of nitric oxide production by L-arginine potentiates i.c.v. administered β-endorphin-induced antinociception in the mouse. Eur J Pharmacol 212:301, 1992

82. Tseng LF, Higgins MJ, Hong JS et al: Release of immunoreactive met-enkephalin from the spinal cord by intraventricular β-endorphin but not by morphine in anesthetized rats. Brain Res 343:60, 1985

83. Xu Y, Pieper GM, Tseng LF: Supraspinal activation of a NO-cGMP system selectively potentiates β-endorphin- but no morphine-, DAMGO-, DPDPE-, or U50,488H-induced antinociception. Pharmacologist 34:171, 1992

84. Berkowitz BA, Finck AD, Hynes MD, Ngai SH: Tolerance to nitrous oxide analgesia in rats and mice. Anesthesiology 51:309, 1979

85. McDonald CE, Ellenberger EA, Tousman SA, Quock RM: Antagonism of nitrous oxide antinociception in mice by inhibitors of nitric oxide synthesis. FASEB J 7:A488, 1993

86. Gagnon MJ, Hodges BL, Quock RM: Inhibition of nitric oxide production antagonizes antinociception in the rat hot plate test. p. 50. In Wayner MJ (ed): Abstracts of the Second International Behavioral Neuroscience Conference. Vol. 2. International Behavioral Neuroscience Society, Tampa, 1993

87. Perkins WJ, Morrow DR: A dose dependent reduction in halothane M.A.C. in rats with a competitive N-methyl-D-asparate (NMDA) receptor antagonist. Anesth Analg 74:S233, 1992

88. Johns RA, Moscicki JC, DiFazio CA: Nitric oxide synthase inhibitor dose-dependently and reversibly reduces the threshold for halothane anesthesia. Anesthesiology 77:779, 1992

89. Tobin JR, Martin LD, Breslow MJ, Traystman RJ: Anesthetic inhibition of brain nitric oxide synthase. FASEB J 7:A257, 1993

90. Uggeri MJ, Proctor GJ, Johns RA: Halothane, enflurane, and isoflurane attenuate both receptor- and non-receptor-mediated EDRF production in rat thoracic aorta. Anesthesiology 76:1012, 1992

91. Kant GJ, Muller TW, Lenox RH, Myerhoff JL: *In vivo* effects of pentobarbital and halothane anesthesia on levels of adenosine 3′,5′-monophosphate and guanosine 3′,5′-monophosphate in rat brain regions and pituitary. Biochem Pharmacol 29:1891, 1980

92. Richards CD, Smaje JC: Anaesthetics depress the sensitivity of cortical neurones to L-glutamate. Br J Pharmacol 58:347, 1976

93. Pearce RA, Stringer JL, Lothman EW: Effect of volatile anesthetics on synaptic transmission in the rat hippocampus. Anesthesiology 71:591, 1989

94. Quock RM, Nguyen E: Possible involvement of nitric oxide in chlordiazepoxide-induced anxiolysis in mice. Life Sci 51:PL255, 1992

95. Johnson C, Emmanouil DE, Quock RM: Nitrous oxide anxiolytic effect in mice in the elevated plus maze: antagonism by flumazenil and cross-tolerance with benzodiazepines. Pharmacologist 34:137, 1992

96. Caton PW, Tousman SA, Quock RM: Involvement of nitric oxide in nitrous oxide-induced anxiolysis in mice in the elevated plus maze. p. 50. In Wayner MJ (ed): Abstracts of the Second International Behavioral Neuroscience Conference. Vol. 2. International Behavioral Neuroscience Society, Tampa, 1993

97. Johns RA: EDRF/nitric oxide. The endogenous nitrovasodilator and a new cellular messenger. Anesthesiology 75:927, 1991

98. Pearl RG: Inhaled nitric oxide. The past, the present and the future. Anesthesiology 78:413, 1993

99. Kinsella JP, McQueston J, Rosenberg AA, Abman SH: Hemodynamic effects of exogenous nitric oxide in the ovine transitional pulmonary circulation. Am J Physiol 263:H875, 1992

100. Frostell C, Fratacci M-D, Wain JC et al: Inhaled nitric oxide: a selective pulmonary vasodilator reversing hypoxic pulmonary vasodilatation in pulmonary vasoconstriction. Circulation 83:2038, 1991

101. Pepke-Zaba J, Higenbottam TW, Tuan ADX et al: Inhaled nitric oxide as a cause of selective pulmonary vasodilatation in pulmonary hypertension. Lancet 338:1173, 1991

102. Frostell CG, Blomquist H, Hedenstierna G et al: Inhaled nitric oxide selectively reverses human hypoxic pulmonary vasoconstriction without causing systemic vasodilation. Anesthesiology 78:427, 1993

103. Roberts JD, Polaner DM, Lang P, Zapol WM: Inhaled nitric oxide in persistent pulmonary hypertension of the newborn. Lancet 340:818, 1992

104. Kinsella JP, Neish SR, Shaffer E, Abman SH: Low-dose inhalational nitric oxide in persistent pulmonary hypertension of the newborn. Lancet 340:819, 1992

105. Sellden H, Winberg P, Gustafsson LE et al: Inhalation of nitric oxide reduced pulmonary hypertension after cardiac surgery in a 3.2-kg infant. Anesthesiology 78:577, 1993

106. Nakajima T, Oda H, Kusomoto S, Nogami H: Biological effects of nitrogen dioxide and nitric oxide. p. 121. In Lee SD (ed): Nitric Oxides and Their Effects on Health. Ann Arbor, Ann Arbor Science, 1980

107. Palmer RMJ: The discovery of nitric oxide in the vessel wall. A unifying concept in the pathogenesis of shock. Arch Surg 128:396, 1993

108. Nava E, Palmer RMJ, Moncada S: Inhibition of nitric oxide synthesis in septic shock: how much is beneficial? Lancet 338:1555, 1991

109. Kilbourn RG, Gross SS, Jurdan A et al: N^G-methyl-L-arginine inhibits tumor necrosis factor-induced hypotension: implications for the involvement of nitric oxide. Proc Natl Acad Sci U S A 87:3629, 1990

110. Thiemermann C, Vane J: Inhibition of nitric oxide synthesis reduces the hypotension induced by bacterial lipopolysaccharides in the rat *in vivo*. Eur J Pharmacol 182:591, 1990

111. Amir S, English AM: An inhibitor of nitric oxide production, N^G-nitro-L-arginine-methyl ester, improves survival in anaphylactic shock. Eur J Pharmacol 203:125, 1991

112. Petros A, Bennett D, Vallance P: Effect of nitric oxide synthase inhibitors on hypotension in patients with septic shock. Lancet 338:1557, 1991

113. Moncada S, Palmer RMJ: Inhibition of the induction of nitric oxide synthase by glucocorticoids: yet another explanation for their anti-inflammatory effects? Trends Pharmacol Sci 12:130, 1991

Chapter 33

Emerging Concepts in Pharmacokinetics

Thomas K. Henthorn

Thiopental was introduced into clinical practice by Ralph Waters at the University of Wisconsin in 1934. Its early popularity was not as an induction agent but as a sole anesthetic or in combination with nitrous oxide.[1] Dosing regimens were totally empiric because pharmacokinetic applications were virtually unknown at the time. These unguided ventures often met with disastrous results, such as the tragic application of thiopental at the Battle of Pearl Harbor, reported in *Anesthesiology* in 1943.[2] Fortunately for the future of intravenous anesthesia, the editor of *Anesthesiology* saw fit to include another article in which a trauma patient was successfully given thiopental[3] and editorialized that perhaps thiopental was not inherently dangerous, rather that the danger resulted from the manner in which it was administered.

A rational approach to dosing was undertaken through the gathering of pharmacokinetic data. It was initially thought that the rapid recovery of a patient following a single intravenous dose of thiopental must be the result of rapid metabolism. However, Brodie et al.[4] developed an assay for thiopental and found that subjects emerged from the effects of thiopental while nearly the entire dose was still present in the body. They discovered that the drug distributes from the blood to pharmacologically inert tissues, thus lowering the

plasma and brain concentrations and terminating its effects, before a significant degree of biotransformation occurs. This critical observation led to an entirely different way of conceptualizing the processes of drug disposition. During the past 40 years, understanding of the pharmacokinetics of anesthetic drugs has been refined considerably. However, many questions remain unanswered. The purpose of this chapter is first to review fundamental pharmacokinetic principles briefly and to discuss significant emerging pharmacokinetic concepts, including context-sensitive offset, computer assisted infusion regimens, pharmacodynamic models, high resolution sampling, and first-pass pulmonary uptake.

PHYSIOLOGIC MODELS

Kety[5] developed mathematic constructs with which to describe the movement and distribution of inert gases within the body. Models were developed based on blood flow, tissue volume or mass, and partitioning between plasma and tissue. Eger[6] and Mapleson[7] gathered data for the anesthetic gases to explain and quantify the pharmacokinetics of inhalation anesthesia.

Price et al.[8] used the physiologic modeling technique for inert gases developed by Kety[5] to describe the disposition of thiopental. It was demonstrated that these techniques were readily transferable to lipid soluble chemicals, such as thiopental. Lipid-soluble drugs, like the inert gases, easily cross capillary membranes; thus, blood flow to the tissue is an important determinant of tissue distribution. Price et al. graphically quantified (Fig. 33-1) the original finding of Brodie et al.[4] that the fall in brain thiopental concentrations was a result of its continuing distribution to the tissue. They treated thiopental as if it were inert and did not even include its elimination in their model. A few years later, Saidman and Eger[9] included elimination clearance in a similar model and demonstrated its minimal impact; the overwhelming importance of the distribution process in the termination of effect was substantiated by their findings.

Physiologic modeling provides a useful predictive function. Price[10] provided a revealing simulation study shortly after publishing his original experimental work. By altering the tissue blood flow parameters of his model to reflect a hyperdynamic, anxious patient on the one hand and a hypoperfused, hemorrhaging patient on the other hand, he demonstrated a twofold decrease and increase, re-

spectively, in the predicted brain concentrations of thiopental during the first 10 minutes after an intravenous induction dose. This provided a pharmacokinetic rationale for what was originally observed at Pearl Harbor.

Bischoff and Dedrick[11] used the physiologic modeling approach to develop interspecies scaling (Fig. 33-2). Data obtained in animal experiments can be used to predict thiopental concentrations in humans, based on known differences in tissue volumes and perfusions (e.g., human brain capacity and the percentage of cardiac output it receives normally differs from that of a rat). This has appeal because the detailed anatomic and physiologic data needed to construct human physiologic drug disposition models is nearly impossible to obtain experimentally.

PHARMACOKINETIC MODELS
One Compartment Concepts

Quantities in biologic systems tend to increase or decrease at a rate that is directly proportional to the magnitude of the variable itself.[12] Hull[13] re-

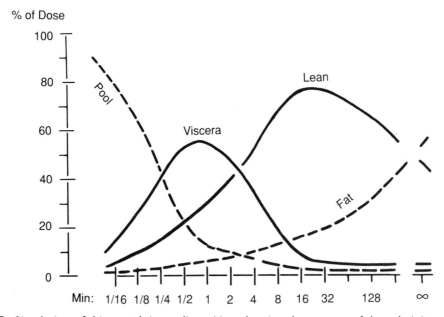

Fig. 33-1 Simulation of thiopental tissue disposition showing the amount of the administered dose in tissues. The tissues are grouped into the central pool (e.g., blood, lungs, and brain), viscera, lean, and fat. Note elimination was not included in this early model. (From Price et al.,[8] with permission.)

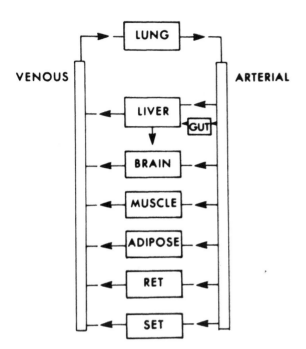

Fig. 33-2 Schematic of a typical physiologic model of a drug that has flow-limited tissue distribution. The *arrows* between compartments represent blood flow and the one leaving the liver is for elimination. Tissue volumes are calculated from the tissue mass and the blood/tissue partition ratio for the drug. (From Rowland,[39] with permission.)

ferred to this as "the universal rule of constant proportion." Stated mathematically, for decreasing concentration,

$$dx/dt = -kx_t \quad (1)$$

where x is the amount of drug, t is time, and k is the rate constant describing the proportional change. Solving for the integral of equation 1 so that we can determine what happens to x over a given period (from t = 0 to t), we obtain

$$x_t = x_0 e^{-kt} \quad (2)$$

with a negative exponent for decreasing amounts of x. Equation 2 can be rearranged to

$$x_t/x_0 = e^{-kt} \quad (3)$$

so that the left side is the fraction of the dose remaining in the body. When this fraction is $1/2$,

$$1/2 = e^{-kt_{1/2}} \quad \text{or} \quad \ln 1/2 = -kt_{1/2} = -kt_{1/2}$$
$$\text{or} \quad k = 0.693/t_{1/2} \quad (4)$$

Because $e^{-0.693} = 1/2$, then

$$x_t/x_0 = (1/2)^n \quad (5)$$

so that the amount of drug in the body falls by 50 percent in one half-life, 75 percent in two half-lives and so on.

Equation 1 is the mathematical expression of a one compartment pharmacokinetic model (Fig. 33-3), and equation 2 is its solution.

The plasma drug content is expressed as a concentration. Therefore, to convert from the amount of drug in the body to the concentration in plasma requires the introduction of a volume term, V.

$$\text{Amount} = V \cdot \text{Concentration} \quad (6)$$

Similarly, clearance (Cl) relates the rate of transfer (generally elimination) to concentration.

$$\text{Rate of transfer} = Cl \cdot \text{Concentration} \quad (7)$$

From equation 1, the rate of elimination = $k \cdot x_t$. Using equation 6, expressions for elimination clearance, Cl_E, can be constructed as follows:

$$\text{Rate of elimination} = k \cdot V \cdot \text{Concentration} \quad (8)$$

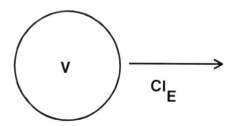

Fig. 33-3 Compartmental representation of a monoexponential pharmacokinetic model. Such a model is completely defined by the volume of distribution and the elimination clearance.

with equation 7

$$Cl_E = k \cdot V \qquad (9)$$

or with equation 4

$$Cl_E = 0.693 \cdot V/t_{1/2} \qquad (10)$$

During a constant rate infusion, the concentration will rise from zero to a plateau concentration, which will result in exactly equal rates of administration and elimination. Thus, a steady state is established at this concentration, C_{SS}. The infusion rate to maintain a target concentration (in this case, C_{SS}) is calculated as

$$\text{Infusion rate} = C_{SS} \cdot Cl_E \qquad (11)$$

C_{SS} may be similarly used to calculate a bolus dose to accompany the infusion (from equation 6)

as follows:

$$\text{Bolus Dose} = C_{SS} \cdot V \qquad (12)$$

One way of characterizing the time course of the approach of the drug concentration towards C_{SS} during an infusion is to consider a bolus (from equation 12) plus infusion regimen. The concentration at any time attributable only to the infusion, C_{INF}, will be the difference between the eventual C_{SS} (equation 11) and the residual concentration resulting from the bolus dose targeted for C_{SS} (equation 12) given at the time the infusion started or

$$C_{INF} = C_{SS} - C_{SS} \cdot e^{-kt} \qquad (13)$$

$$C_{INF} = C_{SS}(1 - e^{-kt}) \qquad (14)$$

To express the accumulation of drug during a constant infusion, or the plateau principle, in

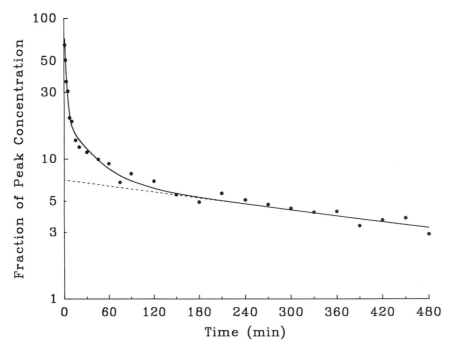

Fig. 33-4 The solid line is the three compartmental unit disposition function for thiopental from the pharmacokinetics in Table 14-2. The curve may be divided into a monoexponential terminal elimination phase defined as the log-linear regression through the data on the terminal slope and back extrapolated (- - -) to the ordinate. The function describing this line is the one compartmental model shown in Figure 33-3. Concentrations above this line represent the distribution phase.

terms of half-lives, n can be defined as the number of the infusion ($t/t_{1/2}$) so that equation 14 becomes

$$C_{INF} = C_{SS}(1 - (\tfrac{1}{2})^n) \qquad (15)$$

Therefore, in one half-life (n = 1), 50 percent of the eventual C_{SS} is reached; in two half-lives, it is 75 percent. Note that for each additional time increment equal to a half-life, the percentage of the steady state is increased by one-half of the previous increase. Therefore, in three half-lives, 12.5 percent is added to the previous total of 75 percent to yield 87.5 percent. For clinical purposes, reaching 90 percent of C_{SS} is usually sufficient for considering the concentration at its plateau. Solving for n yields the value of 3.3 half-lives. Thus, with shorter half-lives, the plateau is reached proportionately faster because this is the only factor of importance for this process.

Multicompartmental Concepts

The concepts and the equations in the preceding section require that the drug in question is instantaneously mixed and distributed throughout the body. Brodie et al.[4] and Price et al.[8] demonstrated the flaw in this assumption when applied to thiopental. Figure 33-4 shows graphically that the mixing of thiopental is not instantaneous. Not until approximately 150 minutes following a bolus dose does thiopental's kinetics conform to a one compartment model.

A more complex model is needed to characterize the concentration versus time relationship displayed in Figure 33-4. The fundamental principle is that the body is not pharmacokinetically homogeneous; concentrations rise and fall at different rates in different tissues. Because blood is generally the point of drug delivery, the sampled tissue, and also the means of drug delivery to various other tissues, the compartment that includes blood volume is called the central compartment or central volume, V_C, or V_1 (Fig. 33-5).

The so-called universal rule of constant proportion is also applied to drug transfer between compartments and is presumed to be driven by the law of mass action, with peripheral tissue transfer characterized by rate constants to and from V_1. Drug in

each tissue, then, is driven to reach an apparent concentration equal to that in the blood (V_1). The thermodynamics (or partitioning) may dictate that the actual tissue concentration is much different from that in the blood, but the mathematic model assumes them to be equal and adjusts volumes accordingly. Thus, the volumes are apparent.

We might imagine that each tissue would be represented by a distinct compartment (this is the underlying premise for the construction of "physiologic" models). However, pharmacokinetic models are typically models of plasma concentration data alone and cannot predict discrete tissue concentrations.

The mathematical function describing the concentration versus time curve is usually relatively simple because the myriad tissues have kinetic characteristics that result in them being lumped

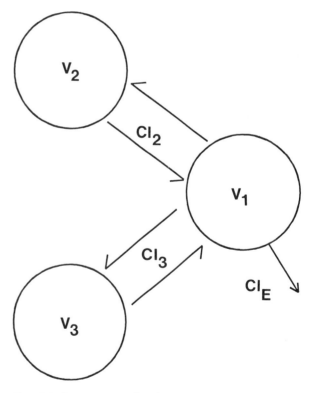

Fig. 33-5 Diagram of a three compartment open mammillary model. V_1, V_2, and V_3 are the central, rapid equilibrating, and slow equilibrating volumes, respectively. Cl_1 and Cl_2 are the intercompartmental clearances, and Cl_E is the elimination clearance.

into one of three groups. These groups are (1) tissues that equilibrate rapidly enough to be indistinguishable from the blood, V_1; (2) tissues that equilibrate rapidly (V_2) but not as rapidly as those in V_1; and (3) tissues that equilibrate slowly (V_3). The number of compartments that can be realized is partly a function of experimental design. For example, referring to Figure 33-4, we can see that, if blood sampling were restricted to between 150 and 600 minutes after the dose, only a one compartment model would be described. To expand pharmacokinetic models beyond the typical three groups mentioned above generally requires either additional "extraordinary" concentration data collected frequently, early, and/or for extended periods or other independent information, such as concentration data from a simultaneously administered drug or additional concentration data collected from another tissue or site.

The model in Figure 33-5 is a model that is typical for intravenous anesthetic agents and is called a three compartment open mammillary model. The term open refers to elimination of the drug from the model or body, and mammillary refers to the arrangement of the peripheral compartments relative to the central compartment. The change in each compartment with time is governed by the same laws of mass action operating in the one compartment model of equation 1. Therefore, the amounts in each compartment at time t, x_{it}, are modified by rate constants describing a proportional change with time as follows:

$$dx_1/dt = k_{21} \cdot x_{2t} + k_{31} \cdot x_{3t} - x_{1t}(k_{10} + k_{12} + k_{13}) \tag{16}$$

$$dx_2/dt = k_{12} \cdot x_{1t} - k_{21} \cdot x_{2t} \tag{17}$$

$$dx_3/dt = k_{12} \cdot x_{1t} - k_{31} \cdot x_3 \tag{18}$$

where k_{ij} is the rate constant describing the transfer from compartment i to compartment j.

Equations describing this three compartment model can be solved using numeric methods (e.g., Euler's approximation and a fourth order Runge-Kutta method) to yield estimates of the amount of drug in each compartment at any given time. Although these results must be considered estimates, most numeric techniques have accuracies several orders of magnitude better than the methods used to measure drug concentrations. Also, this series of linear differential equations can be integrated to yield an exponential equation. The triexponential equation for the central compartment is

$$x_{1t} = Ae^{-k_{1t}} + Be^{-k_{2t}} + Ce^{-k_{3t}} \tag{19}$$

in which A, B, and C are the t = 0 intercepts for the line describing each phase and k_1, k_2, and k_3 are the respective hybrid rate constants describing the slope of each exponential term. Although these hybrid rate constants describe proportional change, they are not to be confused with the rate constants for intercompartmental transfer of a multicompartmental model (equations 16 to 18).

Half-life is the time for the amount of drug in the body to fall by one-half. For a one compartment model, this is also the time required for the concentration to fall by one-half. For the multicompartment system, this rule applies only during the terminal pharmacokinetic phase (Fig. 33-4), which often occurs hours after a patient arrives in the recovery room. Prior to the terminal slope, the time required for the concentration to fall by one-half will be less than the elimination-phase half-life and the halving of the concentration will not mean that one-half of the drug has left the body; it merely signifies that one-half of the drug has left the central compartment because of distribution and/or elimination.

During a continuous infusion with multicompartmental kinetics, the rise toward the eventual steady-state concentration will be more rapid than by multiples of the elimination half-life as delineated in equation 15. Instead, the actual rise proceeds at a rate determined by a function of all the hybrid rate constants of the multiexponential equation (e.g., equation 19). Each hybrid rate constant contributes according to the overall "importance" of its portion of the pharmacokinetic curve. The "weight" of each exponential term is determined by the ratio of the area under the curve (AUC) for a particular term (AUC_i) where

$$f = AUC_i/AUC_{tot} \tag{20}$$

and the AUC for the entire concentration versus time curve (AUC_{tot}) for a triexponential function is

$$AUC_{tot} = A/k_1 + B/k_2 + C/k_3 \qquad (21)$$

Figure 33-6 shows that, as the fraction of the AUC corresponding to the elimination phase $[(C/k_3)/AUC_{tot}]$ decreases, the rate of rise to the eventual steady state increases. In more general terms, the more important the distribution phase is, as reflected by the portion of the AUC_{tot} attributable to these exponential terms, the less consideration should be given to a one compartment (elimination phase only) model described by a $t_{1/2}$, V_β, and Cl_E (where V_β is the total distribution volume) because the degree of error between the results predicted and actual events will become greater. This kinetic principle has important implications when anesthetic agents that undergo extensive distribution are given by infusion; it helps explain

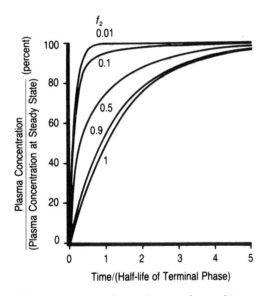

Fig. 33-6 Rise toward steady state for multicompartmental pharmacokinetic models where f is the fraction of the AUC of the unit disposition function that is accounted for by the terminal phase and its back-extrapolated line (- - -, Fig. 33-4). Note as the distribution phase becomes relatively more important to the unit disposition function (decreasing f), the time (number of half-lives) to reach any fraction of the steady-state concentration becomes less. AUC, area under the curve. (From Rowland and Tozer,[40] with permission.)

why the clinical effect is attained more rapidly than that predicted by the rule of 3.3 times the elimination-phase half-life that is calculated on the basis of a one compartment model. The rise to eventual steady state is closer to 3.3 times the "distribution" half-lives, but more accurately, it involves calculations that incorporate all of the pharmacokinetic parameters.

The greater the potential for a drug to distribute to the tissues is, the greater is the importance of the distribution phases and the less important is the elimination-phase half-life in determining the time course of drug effects. Unfortunately, this simple concept introduces some rather large complexities, at least in regard to computing the expected time course of drug concentrations. Nevertheless, this degree of computational complexity is necessary if intravenous anesthetics are to be used beyond the narrow scope of the peri-induction period. For many intravenous anesthetic agents, the importance of tissue distribution is evident in terms of large apparent peripheral distribution volumes and rapid rates of intercompartmental transfer.

Computer simulations indicate that the time required for concentrations to fall by a predetermined fraction is a complex function of the duration of the infusion that is not easily predictable from elimination-phase half-lives.[14] Therefore, a parameter designated the "context-sensitive half-time," was proposed.[15,16] This parameter is the time required for the steady-state plasma concentration to fall by 50 percent following the termination of a steady-state infusion of a specified duration. This term may have more utility than traditional pharmacokinetic half-lives in most clinical situations; however, it is descriptive of a narrowly defined situation and is not a pharmacokinetic parameter. For example, a fall in concentration to one-quarter of the starting concentration is not two context-sensitive half-times.

A computer is really necessary to make reasonable predictions of the behavior of drugs with multicompartmental kinetics. Alternatively, some pocket calculators can be programmed to perform real time estimates of current plasma concentrations as the clinician enters dosing information.[17]

One method for bringing computational power into the operating room is by using a computer controlled infusion pump. Two examples are computer assisted continuous infusion[18] and the Stanford pump.[14] These systems use a set of multicompartmental pharmacokinetic parameters to make calculations that adjust the current rate of infusion almost on a second-to-second basis to compensate for central compartment drug loss caused by tissue distribution and elimination clearance. The user has only to indicate the target concentration. Upward concentration changes are accomplished nearly instantaneously by a bolus dose and infusion change; downward adjustments proceed at the rate determined by the pharmacokinetic decay. Calculations to appraise the user of the expected rate of concentration decline are also made by the computer. Because the patient's individual pharmacokinetic parameters may differ from the "average" parameters used by the computer and drug concentrations are not actually measured, there is no certainty that the target concentration has actually been attained.

Computer controlled infusion pumps also have many research uses. An example is the so-called "concentration clamping" technique in which a plasma concentration is held steady long enough for the effect site to reach equilibrium, usually requiring only several minutes (Fig. 33-7).[19] The plasma concentration then reflects the concentra-

tion at the effect site, and a useful concentration-effect relationship can be established.

Minimum requirements for using a computerized infusion system are a full-feature computer, software, an appropriate pump connected to the computer, the wherewithal to assemble all these parts, and the knowledge and ability to judge the pharmacokinetic calculations being made.

Another way to bring computational power into the operating room is to determine a dosing scheme prior to entering the operating room. There are many software packages that can simulate infusion schemes. Dosing regimens are designed largely by trial and error until a suitable concentration profile is obtained. The choice of a dosing regimen generally represents a balance between tolerance for concentration fluctuation on the one hand and for the number of dosing interventions (bolus administration or infusion rate changes) on the other hand. Two possible extremes would be represented by a single "up front" bolus versus a small bolus plus a constantly adjusting infusion rate.

Another variation on the prior simulation strategy are the isoconcentration nomograms developed by Shafer.[20] These nomograms (Fig. 33-8) display the plasma concentration as a function of the duration of infusion for various infusion rates.

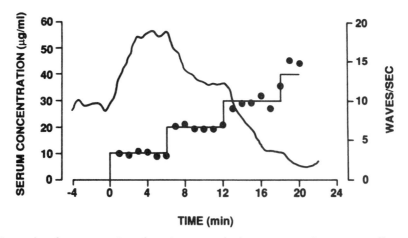

Fig. 33-7 Example of concentration clamping to study the concentration versus effect relationship. Serum thiopental concentrations were stepped up and held steady for 6 minutes by a computer controlled thiopental infusion. The EEG response (in waves per second) at each serum thiopental concentration is evaluated during the final 2 minutes of each 6-minute segment. EEG, electroencephalogram. (From Bührer et al.,[19] with permission.)

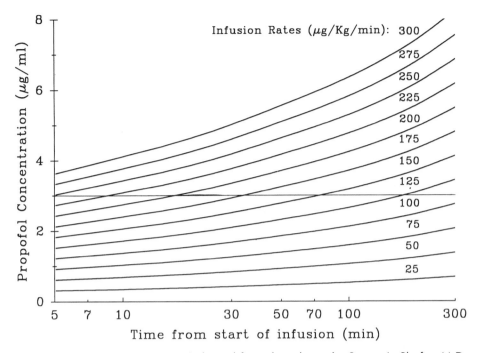

Fig. 33-8 Isoconcentration nomogram (adapted from the scheme by Steven L. Shafer, M.D., personal communication). For this example, to maintain a plasma propofol concentration of at least 3 µg/ml, start with an infusion rate of 275 µg/kg/min. Then from the horizontal line drawn at 3 µg/ml, change to the next infusion rate (250 µg/kg/min) at the time its concentration versus time curve intersects the horizontal (approximately 5 minutes). Continue changing infusion rates at the times specified by the nomogram until the target concentration is no longer desired. For this example, the new infusion rates in micrograms per kilogram per minute at time (in minutes) are 225 at 8.5, 200 at 17, 175 at 33, 150 at 72, and 125 at 170. (See Figure 14-7 for the propofol recovery curves.)

To maintain a given concentration, the physician "jumps" to the different infusion rates at the times their respective curves intersect the desired concentration.

PHARMACOKINETIC/ PHARMACODYNAMIC MODELS

The time courses of the drug concentrations in plasma and the resultant drug effects are frequently different. There is a counterclockwise hysteresis seen when drug effects are plotted as a function of the plasma concentrations obtained at the same time (Fig. 33-9A). Two practical features of this hysteresis are that the peak plasma concentration is reached before the peak effect is observed and that the same intensity of effect is observed first at a high concentration when plasma concen-

trations are rising during an infusion and then again at a lower plasma concentration when they are falling, following termination of the infusion.

Concentrations in the effect tissue, or biophase, are kinetically distinct from those of the plasma, just as those of any other peripheral tissue would be.[21,22] That is, the biophase is just another tissue compartment in which first order rate constants describe drug transfer. If the drug effect is plotted as a function of biophase drug concentration, there is no hysteresis (Fig. 33-9B). The description of the kinetics of the biophase compartment is made by a rate constant that has been termed, k_{e0}, which is the rate of transfer from the effect compartment out of the system (Fig. 33-10). The mathematical models are stated such that biophase kinetics do not influence the plasma pharmacokinetics; k_{e0} is often reported as a half-life, $t_{1/2}k_{e0}(0.693/k_{e0}$; equa-

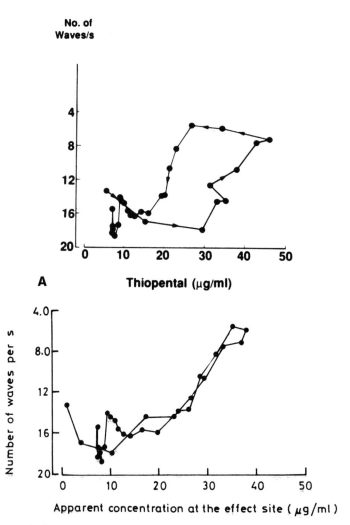

Fig. 33-9 **(A)** Thiopental plasma concentration versus EEG effect (in waves per second). The arrows demonstrate the counterclockwise hysteresis, reflecting that changes in plasma concentration occur before changes in drug effect. **(B)** Thiopental effect site concentration versus EEG effect. Note that there is no hysteresis, reflecting the changes in effect site concentration occur at the same time as changes in drug effect. EEG, electroencephalogram. (From Stanski,[41] with permission.)

tion 4). $t_{1/2}k_{e0}$ can be used in the manner of the $t_{1/2}$ in equation 14 to estimate the rate of equilibration between the plasma and biophase during a constant infusion (i.e., 3.3 $t_{1/2}k_{e0}$ to reach 90 percent of the steady-state biophase concentration).

In general, the greater the k_{e0} is, the more rapid the equilibration is between plasma and the biophase and the sooner the peak effect is reached (t_{max}) following a bolus dose. It should be pointed out that k_{e0} is not model independent. That is, this

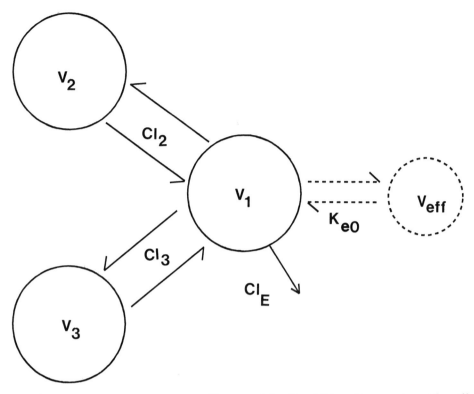

Fig. 33-10 Three compartment open mammillary model with additional compartment for effect site (biophase, V_{eff}). Note that the biophase and the transfer into and from it are designated by --- to indicate that its kinetics are to collapse the hysteresis only (see Fig. 9); therefore, no net drug transfer takes place. The rate constant leaving V_{eff}, k_{e0}, defines the kinetics of the biophase.

parameter merely links observed effects to a given set of pharmacokinetics. If the pharmacokinetic model differs, so will the k_{e0}. For the intravenous induction agents, all reach their peak effect near 1.5 minutes after a bolus, and there are minimal differences between them. However, there are important differences in k_{e0} and t_{max} for the benzodiazepines, opioids, and muscle relaxants.

Figure 33-10 shows a pharmacokinetic/pharmacodynamic model. Note that the biophase or effect compartment communicates with the central compartment, like the peripheral tissue compartments. The biophase concentrations are in turn linked to the observed effect by an effect model. Effect models often use classic sigmoid concentration-response relationships. This relationship is described by the Hill equation as follows:

$$E = EC^s \cdot E_{max}/(EC_{50}{}^s + EC^s) \qquad (22)$$

where E is the fraction of maximal response (E_{max}), EC_{50} is effect compartment concentration (EC) at one-half the maximal response, and s is a dimensionless term that determines the steepness of the sigmoidicity.

The effect model is dependent on the nature of the data collected. For instance, if a study only managed to collect data between 20 and 80 percent of the maximal response, the concentration-response relationship would appear entirely linear, and a maximum response could not be predicted.[23] In this case, the effect model would be a simple proportionality (linear regression), and predictions beyond the limits of the data could not be made. For this reason, pharmacokinetic/pharmacodynamic studies should make a point to include a maximum response.

The biophase is kinetically distinct from the plasma; thus, V_C can usually be considered pharmacologically inert. The relevance of drug concentrations produced in V_C is that they drive the drug concentrations in the biophase. This principle can be put to use to calculate a loading dose. A bolus dose may be determined from the relationship in equation 6, as the product of the desired concentration and the volume of distribution. However, a problem arises with respect to choosing the appropriate volume of distribution because the volume of distribution changes during the course of drug disposition, beginning with V_C and increasing continuously until reaching V_β during the terminal phase.[24,25] For thiopental, if we multiply a target concentration (based on its EC_{50} for hypnosis) of 12 μg/ml by the V_{SS} (the volume of distribution at steady state) of 1.7 L/kg, we arrive at the excessive dose of 20.4 mg/kg. The problem is that the biophase concentrations will exceed the target concentration until all body tissues have equilibrated with V_C. Conversely, a dose derived by multiplying the same target concentration by V_C (approximately 0.1 L/kg) would be 1.2 mg/kg. This dose is too small; the predicted peak plasma concentration would be 12 μg/ml, but the peak effect compartment concentration would be much lower. By the time the effector tissue attains pseudoequilibration with the plasma and momentarily has the same concentration, the concentrations will have fallen well below those needed for hypnosis. It is clear that we need a more useful distribution volume. By definition, the peak drug effect occurs at the time of pseudoequilibration of V_C with the effect compartment (at t_{max}). We can designate the distribution volume at the time of pseudoequilibration of V_C and the biophase as V_{pe} (pe standing for pseudoequilibrium).[26] The pseudoequilibration volume of distribution has also been termed the peak effect volume of distribution.[27]

Returning to our thiopental example, multiplying the target concentration of 12 μg/ml by the V_{pe} (see Table 14-2) of 0.29 L/kg yields the customary induction dose of 3.5 mg/kg. Following such a bolus dose of thiopental, V_C concentrations will exceed our target concentration in plasma prior to pseudoequilibration. However, peak biophase concentrations will exactly equal our target at t_{max}. Larger doses will enable the biophase to attain the target concentration earlier, but there will be an ever increasing overshoot of the biophase concentration until t_{max} is reached.

Because intravenous induction agents have a t_{max} in the range of 1 to 2 minutes, increasing emphasis has been placed on describing plasma concentrations accurately during this time so that we can better understand the relationship of these observable concentrations and the onset of effect (i.e., more valid pharmacokinetic/pharmacodynamic models). Also, if we are ever to make sense of interindividual differences in sensitivity to these agents, we must focus our attention on the time of significant drug effect. For pharmacokinetic studies, investigators now generally obtain blood samples at 30-second intervals beginning at 1 minute and not slowing to less frequent intervals until at least 5 minutes after drug administration. In addition, arterial blood samples are preferred. This is because arterial drug concentrations drive the biophase in the brain tissue and because it is much easier to draw blood samples from an arterial catheter at the frequency demanded. This method of sampling has been termed "high resolution" arterial sampling.

Pulmonary Uptake and Recirculatory Models

Measurement and characterization of blood drug concentrations within the first minute after bolus administration have relevance because significant pharmacologic effects for hypnotic drugs are observed during this period. New experimental and data analysis techniques have been developed that enable characterization of the pharmacokinetics from the moment of intravenous injection.[28,29] The first circulatory pass of injected drug produces a concentration peak in arterial blood that is determined by central (or thoracic) blood volume, pulmonary tissue uptake, and cardiac output.[30] This peak and the subsequent smaller peak associated with recirculation have been termed the circulatory mixing transient.

Whether the arterial blood concentrations during the mixing transient have relevance is debatable because there have been no studies correlating these drug concentrations with drug effects. However, it seems likely that there is such a relationship because the onset of effect for thiopental is related to the arm-brain circulation time. In addition, current pharmacokinetic and pharmacodynamic studies do not completely explain interindividual dose-response differences for thiopental.

The best evidence to date linking interindividual differences with distribution pharmacokinetics appeared in two recent studies[31,32] that described a significant correlation between adult patient age and the "conventional" pharmacokinetic parameter, that is, intercompartmental clearance for the rapidly equilibrating peripheral compartment (Fig. 33-11). These studies ignored plasma thiopental concentrations during the first minute after administration and, therefore, do not include the mixing transient. The association of age with intercompartmental clearance may be the result of age-related changes in cardiac output.[33]

The role of the lung in drug distribution following intravenous administration has been recently recognized. Drugs that bind extensively to α_1-acid glycoprotein tend to have significant pulmonary tissue uptake and binding. Basic amines, such as fentanyl and its analogs, propranolol, and lidocaine, exhibit significant pulmonary uptake.[34–37] Factors that alter pulmonary uptake, such as disease or displacement by other drugs, may affect the dose-response relationships for these agents. In contrast, the lipid-soluble intravenous induction agents distribute into the lungs, but they apparently do not bind to any large extent with lung tissue. Unless there is significant tissue binding, little of the drug in the body actually remains in the

lung tissue. For example, thiopental was retained in the lung only 14 percent more than was indocyanine green, which is so extensively bound to plasma albumin that it remains only in the intravascular space.[38]

REFERENCES

1. Organe GSW, Broad RJB: Pentothal with nitrous oxide and oxygen. Lancet 2:1170, 1938
2. Halford FJ: A critique of intravenous anesthesia in war surgery. Anesthesiology 4:67, 1943
3. Adam RC, Gray HK: Intravenous anesthesia with Pentothal sodium in the case of gunshot wound associated with accompanying severe traumatic shock and loss of blood: report of a case. Anesthesiology 4:70, 1943
4. Brodie BB, Mark LC, Papper EM et al: The fate of thiopental in man and a method for its estimation in biological material. J Pharmacol Exp Ther 98:85, 1950
5. Kety SS: The theory and applications of the exchange of inert gas at the lung and tissues. Pharmacol Rev 3:1, 1951
6. Eger EI II: A mathematical model of uptake and distribution. p. 72. In Papper EM, Kitz RJ (eds): Uptake and Distribution of Anesthetic Agents. McGraw-Hill, New York, 1963
7. Mapleson WW: Circulation-time models of the uptake of inhaled anaesthetics and data for quantifying them. Br J Anaesth 45:319, 1973
8. Price HL, Kovnat PJ, Safer JH et al: The uptake of thiopental by body tissues and its relation to the duration of narcosis. Clin Pharmacol Ther 1:16, 1960
9. Saidman LJ, Eger EI: The effect of thiopental metabolism on duration of anesthesia. Anesthesiology 27:118, 1966
10. Price HL: A dynamic concept of the distribution of thiopental in the human body. Anesthesiology 21:40, 1960
11. Bischoff KB, Dedrick RL: Thiopental pharmacokinetics. J Pharm Sci 57:1346, 1968
12. Riggs DS: The Mathematical Approach to Physiological Problems: A Critical Primer. MIT Press, Cambridge, 1963
13. Hull CJ: Pharmacokinetics for Anaesthesia. Butterworth-Heinemann, Oxford, 1991
14. Shafer SL, Varvel JR: Pharmacokinetics, pharmacodynamics, and rational opioid selection. Anesthesiology 74:53, 1991
15. Shafer SL, Stanski DR: Improving the utility of

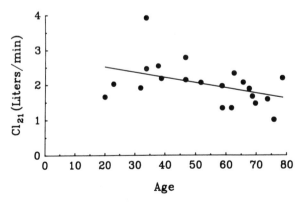

Fig. 33-11 The relationship of the intercompartmental clearance of thiopental from V_1 to V_2 versus age. (From Avram et al.,[31] with permission.)

anesthetic drug pharmacokinetics. Anesthesiology 76:327, 1992

16. Hughes MA, Glass PS, Jacobs JR: Context-sensitive half-time in multicompartment pharmacokinetic models for anesthetic drugs. Anesthesiology 76:334, 1992

17. Maitre PO, Shafer SL: A simple pocket calculator approach to predict anesthetic drug concentrations from pharmacokinetic data. Anesthesiology 73:332, 1990

18. Alvis JM, Reves JG, Govier AV et al: Computer-assisted continuous infusion of fentanyl during cardiac anesthesia: comparison with a manual method. Anesthesiology 63:41, 1985

19. Bührer M, Maitre PO, Hung OR et al: Thiopental pharmacodynamics: I. Defining the pseudo-steady-state serum concentration-EEG effect relationship. Anesthesiology 77:226, 1992

20. Shafer SL: Towards optimal intravenous dosing strategies. Semin Anesth 42:222, 1993

21. Segre G: Kinetics of interaction between drugs and biological systems. Farmaco 23:907, 1968

22. Sheiner LB, Stanski DR, Vozeh S et al: Simultaneous modeling of pharmacokinetics and pharmacodynamics: application to d-tubocurarine. Clin Pharmacol Ther 25:358, 1979

23. Eudeikis JR, Henthorn TK, Lertora JJL et al: Kinetic analysis of the vasculature and GABAergic blocking actions of n-acetylprocainamide. J Cardiovasc Pharmacol 4:203, 1982

24. Niazi S: Volume of distribution as a function of time. J Pharm Sci 65:452, 1976

25. Avram MJ, Henthorn TK, Shanks CA, Krejcie TC: The initial rate of change in distribution volume is the sum of intercompartmental clearances. J Pharm Sci 75:919, 1986

26. Henthorn TK, Krejcie TC, Shanks CA, Avram MJ: Time-dependent distribution volume and the kinetics of the pharmacodynamic effector site. J Pharm Sci 81:1136, 1992

27. Stanski DR, Shafer SL, Kern SE: The Scientific Basis of Infusion Techniques in Anesthesia. CR Bard, North Reading, MA, 1990

28. Henthorn TK, Avram MJ, Krejcie TC et al: A minimal compartmental model of circulatory mixing of indocyanine green. Am J Physiol 262:H903, 1992

29. Henthorn TK, Krejcie TC, Gupta DK et al: Recirculatory kinetics of ICG, inulin, and antipyrine. Clin Pharmacol Ther 53:217, 1993

30. Upton RN, Huang YF: Influence of cardiac output, injection time and injection volume on the initial mixing of drugs with venous blood after i.v. bolus administration to sheep. Br J Anaesth 70:333, 1993

31. Avram MJ, Krejcie TC, Henthorn TK: The relationship of age to the pharmacokinetics of early drug distribution: the concurrent disposition of thiopental and indocyanine green. Anesthesiology 72:403, 1990

32. Stanski DR, Maitre PO: Population pharmacokinetics and pharmacodynamics of thiopental: the effect of age revisited. Anesthesiology 72:412, 1990

33. Henthorn TK, Krejcie TC, Avram MJ: The relationship between alfentanil distribution kinetics and cardiac output. Clin Pharmacol Ther 52:190, 1992

34. Roerig DL, Kotrly KJ, Ahlf SB et al: Effect of propranolol on the first pass uptake of fentanyl in the human and rat lung. Anesthesiology 71:62, 1989

35. Taeger K, Weninger E, Schmelzer F et al: Pulmonary kinetics of fentanyl and alfentanil in surgical patients. Br J Anaesth 61:425, 1988

36. Howell RE, Lanken PN: Pulmonary accumulation of propranolol in vivo: sites and physiochemical mechanism. J Pharmacol Exp Ther 263:130, 1992

37. Post C: Studies on the pharmacokinetic function of the lung with special reference to lidocaine. Acta Pharmacol Toxicol (Copenh) 1:53, 1979

38. Roerig DL, Kotrly KJ, Dawson CA et al: First-pass uptake of verapamil, diazepam, and thiopental in the human lung. Anesth Analg 69:461, 1989

39. Rowland M: Physiologic pharmacokinetic models. p. 79. In Rowland M, Tucker G (eds): Pharmacokinetics: Theory and Methodology. Pergamon Press, New York, 1986

40. Rowland M, Tozer TN: Clinical Pharmacokinetics. Concepts and Applications. 2nd Ed. Lea & Febiger, Malvern, PA, 1989

41. Stanski DR: Pharmacodynamic measurement and modelling of anesthetic depth. p. 172. In van Boxtel CJ, Holford NHG, Danhof M (eds): The In Vivo Study of Drug Action. Elsevier, New York, 1992

Index

Page numbers followed by f *denote figures; those followed by* t *denote tables.*